Anesthesia and Uncommon Pediatric Diseases

Jordan Katz, M.D.
Professor, Department of Anesthesiology
School of Medicine
University of California, San Diego
    and
Staff Anesthesiologist
University Hospital and
Veterans Administration
    Medical Center
La Jolla, CA

David J. Steward, M.B., F.R.C.P. (C)
Anaesthetist-In-Chief
British Columbia's Children's Hospital
Vancouver, B.C.
Canada
    and
Professor of Anaesthesia
University of British Columbia
Canada

1987
W. B. SAUNDERS COMPANY
Philadelphia   London   Toronto   Mexico City
Rio de Janeiro   Sydney   Tokyo   Hong Kong

W. B. Saunders Company: West Washington Square
Philadelphia, PA 19105

Library of Congress Cataloging-in-Publication Data

Katz, Jordan
Anesthesia and uncommon pediatric diseases.

1. Pediatric anesthesia.   2. Children—Diseases.
I. Steward, David J., 1934–   II. Title. [DNLM: 1.
Anesthesia—in infancy & childhood. 2. Pediatrics. WO 440
K19a]

RD139.K38 1987   617'.96798   86–10178
ISBN 0–7216–1360–8

Editor: Dean Manke
Developmental Editor: David Kilmer
Designer: Terri Siegel
Production Manager: Frank Polizzano
Manuscript Editor: Mark Coyle
Illustration Coordinator: Walt Verbitski
Indexer: Dennis Dolan

Anesthesia and Uncommon Pediatric Diseases   ISBN   0–7216–1360–8

Last digit is the print number: 9   8   7   6   5   4   3   2

To Ruby
Eamus quo ducit fortuna
Jordan

This book is dedicated to all children unfortunate enough
to have an unusual disease. We hope that by reference to it
the anesthesiologist gains a better insight into the child's
disease and will thus be able to afford the most appropriate care.

JORDAN KATZ
DAVID STEWARD

CONTRIBUTORS

FREDERICK A. BURROWS, M.D., F.R.C.P.C.

Assistant Professor of Anaesthesia, University of Toronto, Faculty of Medicine; Staff Anaesthetist, The Hospital for Sick Children, Toronto, Ontario, Canada
Immune and Allergic Disorders

D. RYAN COOK, M.D.

Professor of Anesthesiology and Pharmacology, University of Pittsburgh School of Medicine; Director of Anesthesiology, Children's Hospital of Pittsburgh, Pittsburgh, Pennsylvania
Pharmacology of Pediatric Anesthesia

G. MARK CRAMOLINI, M.D., F.A.A.P.

Assistant Clinical Professor of Pediatrics and Anesthesiology, University of California, San Francisco, School of Medicine, San Francisco, California; Attending Anesthesiologist and Pediatric Intensivist, Director of Pediatric Intensive Care Education, Valley Children's Hospital, Fresno, California
Diseases of the Renal System

R. E. CREIGHTON, M.D.

Associate Professor, Department of Anaesthesia, University of Toronto; Anaesthetist-in-Chief, Department of Anaesthesia, The Hospital for Sick Children, Toronto, Ontario, Canada
Central Nervous System Diseases

PETER G. DUNCAN, M.D., F.R.C.P.(C.)

Professor and Chairman, Department of Anesthesia, University of Saskatchewan, Saskatoon, Saskatchewan, Canada
Neuromuscular Diseases

NANCY KNUTSEN FRANCE, M.D.

Associate Professor and Chief of Pediatric Anesthesia, Medical College of Wisconsin; Director of Pediatric Anesthesia, Children's Hospital of Wisconsin, Milwaukee, Wisconsin
Ophthalmological Diseases

NISHAN G. GOUDSOUZIAN, M.D., M.Sc.

Associate Professor of Anaesthesia, Harvard Medical School; Director, Pediatric Anesthesia, and Associate Anesthetist, Massachusetts General Hospital, Boston, Massachusetts
Anatomy and Physiology in Relation to Pediatric Anesthesia

WILLIAM R. HAIN, M.B., B.S., F.F.A.R.C.S.

Clinical Teacher, University of Nottingham; Consultant Paediatric Anaesthetist, City Hospital and University Hospital, Nottingham, England
Diseases of Blood

INGRID B. HOLLINGER, M.D.

Associate Professor of Anesthesiology, Assistant Professor of Pediatrics, Albert Einstein College of Medicine; Attending Anesthesiologist, Montefiore Medical Center, New York, New York
Diseases of the Cardiovascular System

HELEN M. K. HOLTBY, M.D., B.S. (London), F.R.C.P.(C.)

Clinical Teacher, Faculty of Medicine, University of Toronto; Staff Anaesthesiologist, The Hospital for Sick Children, Toronto, Ontario, Canada
Orthopedic Diseases

JORDAN KATZ, M.D.

Professor, Department of Anesthesiology, School of Medicine, University of California, San Diego; Staff Anesthesiologist, University Hospital and Veterans Administration Medical Center, La Jolla, California

THOMAS P. KEON, M.D.

Assistant Professor of Anesthesia, University of Pennsylvania School of Medicine; Senior Anesthesiologist, The Children's Hospital of Philadelphia, Philadelphia, Pennsylvania
Diseases of the Endocrine System

JERROLD LERMAN, M.D., F.R.C.P.(C.)

Assistant Professor of Anaesthesia, University of Toronto; Staff Anaesthetist, Department of Anaesthesia; Director of Anaesthesia Research, The Hospital for Sick Children, Toronto, Ontario, Canada
Immune and Allergic Disorders

M. E. McLEOD, M.D.

Assistant Professor, Department of Anaesthesia, University of Toronto; Staff Anaesthetist, The Hospital for Sick Children, Toronto, Ontario, Canada
Central Nervous System Diseases

JAMES D. MORRISON, B.Sc., M.D., F.F.A.R.C.S.

Assistant Professor of Anaesthesia, Dalhousie University; Active Staff, The Izaak Walton Killam Hospital for Children, Halifax, Nova Scotia, Canada

Otolaryngological Diseases

JOHN E. S. RELTON, M.B., F.F.A.R.C.S. (Eng.), F.R.C.P.(C.)

Associate Professor, Faculty of Medicine, University of Toronto; Staff Anaesthesiologist, The Hospital for Sick Children, Toronto, Ontario, Canada

Orthopedic Diseases

MICHAEL F. SMITH, M.D., F.R.C.P.(C.)

Clinical Instructor, University of British Columbia; Attending Anaesthesiologist, Children's Hospital of British Columbia, Vancouver, British Columbia, Canada

Skin and Connective Tissue Diseases

LINDA C. STEHLING, M.D.

Professor, Departments of Anesthesiology and Pediatrics, State University of New York Health Science Center at Syracuse, Syracuse, New York

Genetic Metabolic Diseases

DAVID J. STEWARD, M.B., F.R.C.P.(C.)

Professor of Anaesthesia, University of British Columbia;

Anaesthetist-in-Chief, British Columbia's Children's Hospital, Vancouver, British Columbia, Canada

Infectious Diseases; Diseases of the Gastrointestinal System

JOSEPHINE J. TEMPLETON, M.D.

Assistant Professor of Anesthesia, University of Pennsylvania School of Medicine; Senior Anesthesiologist, The Children's Hospital of Philadelphia, Philadelphia, Pennsylvania

Diseases of the Endocrine System

I. DAVID TODRES, M.D.

Associate Professor of Anaesthesia (Paediatrics), Harvard Medical School, Cambridge, Massachusetts; Anesthetist, Department of Anesthesia; Pediatrician, Children's Service; Director, Neonatal and Pediatric Intensive Care Units, Massachusetts General Hospital, Boston, Massachusetts

Diseases of the Respiratory System

C. F. WARD, M.D.

Associate Clinical Professor of Anesthesiology, University of California, San Diego, School of Medicine

Pediatric Head and Neck Syndromes

D. A. ZIDEMAN, B.Sc., M.B., B.S., F.F.A.R.C.S.

Senior Lecturer, Royal Postgraduate Medical School, University of London; Consultant in Anesthesia, Hammersmith Hospital, London, England

Infectious Diseases

PREFACE

There is a bewildering array of diseases of infancy and childhood, some relatively common but still challenging, some truly uncommon. Associated with many of these are surgically correctable malformations, either congenital or acquired, which will require repair under general anesthesia. In addition, unrelated surgical conditions may present in these children. The anesthesiologist, in the broader role as an acute care physician, may be asked to participate in the general management of some of these children. Hence, it is essential to understand the underlying pathophysiology of the disease process.

We, therefore, have attempted to assemble more than simply a book of anesthesia-related facts. We have designed this volume to provide a detailed summary of background knowledge related to each disease. We have added to this, where it is available, specific information that will be of additional direct importance to the anesthesiologist. Unfortunately, many diseases that are discussed in this book have not been the subjects of detailed anesthesia-oriented reviews, and there is little or no reported experience with these diseases in the anesthesia literature. In such instances it was necessary to extrapolate from the available knowledge of the disease process what might be the important anesthetic implications. This approach hopefully will enable the reader to meet the challenge of collaborating with specialists in other disciplines in providing optimal total care in and outside the operating room.

It is obvious that a book of this scope required the diligent effort of many dedicated physicians. We hope that the resultant text meets all of their expectations.

JORDAN KATZ
DAVID STEWARD

CONTENTS

ANATOMY AND PHYSIOLOGY IN RELATION TO PEDIATRIC ANESTHESIA

1

NISHAN G. GOUDSOUZIAN, M.D.

Of primary importance for the clinical anesthesiologist is the realization that the newborn infant is not simply a small adult. The infant is unique both in distinctive anatomical and physiological features and in the variable rate of different aspects of development. In the newborn, for instance, weight is one twentieth of that of the adult, surface area is one eighth, and length one third. With growth, weight increases markedly, doubling within the first 4 months, tripling in 1 year, and quadrupling in 2 years (Table 1–1). During these 2 years height increases 1.5 times and surface area 2.5 times.

The difference in growth between the infant and the adult is nowhere more dramatic than in the head. Whereas the head surface is only 9 percent of the total surface area in the adult, it is 20 percent in the infant and even more in the premature infant. The head of the infant is large because of his relatively large brain. Consequently the occiput rather than the face is the biggest area. Most of the postnatal growth of the skull occurs during the first 2 years of life, during which time the weight of the brain increases from 350 g to about 800 g. The brain reaches 90 percent of adult size (1400 g) at the fifth year and 95 percent at the tenth year.[1] As expected the circumference of the skull increases similarly, expanding from 33 to 35 cm in the newborn to 47 cm at the second year and 53 cm in the adult.

The large head of the infant necessitates special clinical consideration. Because the head, often with minimal hair, is a source of heat loss, it must be covered to protect against hypothermia.[2] This source of heat loss is especially important in the hydrocephalic infant, whose head is shaved and repeatedly cleaned with surgical preparation solutions. Conversely, the feverish infant can be cooled by bathing the head carefully. Since the head is often accessible to the anesthesiologist, these maneuvers can easily be done in the operating room.

CARDIOVASCULAR SYSTEM

One of the major transitions during delivery is the change from a fetal circulatory pattern (Figure 1–1) to an adult pattern. At birth, the newborn's lungs must assume the function of gas exchange, which in the fetal stages was performed by the placenta.

Fetal Circulation

In the fetus the placenta receives about 55 percent of the combined output of the two ventricles pumping in parallel. This unsaturated blood passes through the two umbilical arteries to the placenta, where it is oxygenated (80 percent saturation) and then returned to the fetus via a single umbilical vein. A small part of the blood present in the umbilical vein is mixed in the liver with the blood of the portal vessels, but most of it is directed by the ductus venosus to the inferior vena cava. The blood from the inferior vena cava as it reaches the heart is preferentially directed by the valve of the inferior vena cava to the left atrium through the foramen ovale. The left atrium pumps this blood to the left ventricle, from which it goes into the aorta and is distributed via the branches of the ascending

Table 1–1. APPROXIMATE VALUES FOR HEIGHT, WEIGHT, AND SURFACE AREA OF CHILDREN AND ADULTS

Age	Height (cm)	Weight (kg)	Surface Area (m²)
Newborn	50	3.2	0.2
3 mo	60	5.7	0.3
1 yr	70	10	0.45
3 yr	84	15	0.6
7 yr	120	25	0.8
10 yr	140	32	1
12 yr	150	40	1.2
15 yr	165	53	1.5
Adult	170	70	1.7

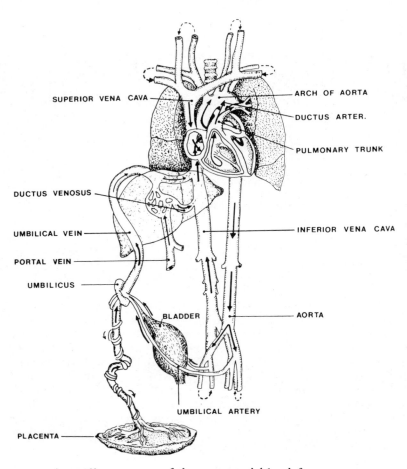

Figure 1–1. The fetal circulation. (*From* Goudsouzian N, Karamanian A: Physiology for the Anesthesiologist. 2nd ed. Norwalk, CT, Appleton-Century-Crofts, 1984, p. 110. Reproduced by permission of Appleton-Century-Crofts, Publishing Division of Prentice-Hall, Inc., Englewood Cliffs, NJ.)

aorta. A smaller amount of deoxygenated blood from the superior vena cava goes through the right ventricle to the pulmonary arteries. In the fetus, the pulmonary arterial pressure is higher than the aortic pressure because of the high pulmonary vascular resistance. Consequently, most of the blood leaving the right ventricle passes through the ductus arteriosus to the lower part of the aorta. The ductus joins the aorta distal to the innominate and left carotid arteries; therefore, much of the blood with the lowest saturation pumped by the right ventricle is directed peripherally to the umbilical arteries to be oxygenated in the placenta. Part of this poorly saturated blood perfuses the lower part of the fetus. In contrast, the relatively highly saturated blood of the left ventricles supplies the head of the fetus.

Circulatory Changes at Birth

With the delivery of the fetus, the sporadic ventilatory muscle activity present antenatally becomes continuous. These postnatal respiratory efforts create a markedly negative intrathoracic pressure (40 to 60 cm H_2O), which leads to expansion of the lung and a consequent drop in pulmonary vascular resistance. This causes a marked increase in pulmonary circulation; consequently, oxygenation improves. As a result, vasodilation occurs and pulmonary vascular pressure is further decreased.

Most of the drop in pulmonary vascular resistance (80 percent) occurs shortly after birth, with a gradual fall continuing for the next 8 weeks.[3] In general infants delivered by cesarean section have higher pulmonary vascular resistance at birth than infants delivered by the vaginal route. In such infants a decrease to the normal range usually occurs within 3 hours of birth.[4] The drop of pulmonary vascular resistance and the consequent increase in pulmonary blood flow lead to an increase in the blood returned to the left atrium. This increases left atrial pressure above the right atrial levels and the "flap valve" foramen ovale restricts left-to-right blood flow, thus causing the functional closure of the previously patent foramen ovale.

As placental circulation is interrupted, the systemic arterial resistance increases concurrent with a diminution in pulmonary arterial pressure. This leads to a reversal of the shunt at the ductus. Initially the flow in the ductus is bidirectional, but at 15 hours of age the shunt becomes entirely left-to-right.

Closure of the ductus arteriosus is dependent mainly on the arterial oxygenation. Functional closure, which is mainly due to contraction of smooth muscles of the wall of the ductus, usually occurs in the first 2 days. Permanent anatomical closure takes another 2 to 3 weeks and results primarily from destruction of endothelium, proliferation of subintimal layers, and eventual fibrosis. Vasoactive agents such as epinephrine and norepinephrine as well as prostaglandins (PGE_1 and PGE_2) are also involved. This has led to the use of prostaglandin E_1 in cyanotic congenital heart disease to keep the ductus open,[5] and the prostaglandin inhibitor indomethacin to help close the ductus.[6] The ductus venosus is usually the last structure to close, taking several more weeks.

Hypoxia, hypercarbia, and acidosis produce marked pulmonary vasoconstriction. Such an occurrence can lead to a marked rise in right atrial pressure over left atrial pressure, thus reopening the foramen ovale. Hypoxia will also lead to a reopening of the ductus arteriosus with a consequent right-to-left shunting and hence further hypoxia, a self-perpetuating vicious circle known as persistent fetal circulation.

Functional Behavior of the Myocardium

Throughout the fetal and early neonatal stages, the myocardial tissues contain a large number of nuclei and mitochondria and an extensive endoplasmic reticulum to support rapid cell growth and protein synthesis.[7] Since these tissues are not contractile, the neonatal myocardium is less compliant (stiffer) and probably less efficient than the adult myocardium.[8] With diminished ventricular compliance, small changes in end-diastolic volume cause marked changes in end-diastolic pressure. Diminished compliance thus makes the Frank-Starling mechanism less effective in infants in increasing the stroke volume in response to increases of the preload; hence, in infants the stroke volume is relatively fixed.[9] Consequently, the only effective way to increase their cardiac output is to increase heart rate.

In contrast to adult cardiac muscle, which is predominantly dependent on oxygen for its metabolism, the fetal myocardium is capable of anaerobic glycolytic metabolism,[10] probably because exogenous glucose can be metabolized during anaerobic conditions because of the presence of high concentrations of glycogen coupled with high hexokinase activity. This circumstance allows the fetal and newborn myocardia to be more resistant to the destructive effects of hypoxia, provided that oxygenation and perfusion are reestablished within a reasonable interval. It is interesting to note that glucose administration prolongs survival of anoxic newborn lambs, whereas insulin injection reduces survival time.[11]

With the infant's growth, the cardiac myofibers increase in number until all are formed, after which only their diameter and mass increase. The contractile elements become well organized and, during the first 3 months of extrauterine life, the left ventricle gradually becomes the dominant chamber owing to progressive ventricular remodeling.[12]

Innervation of the Heart

The sympathetic innervation of the fetal and neonatal myocardium is relatively sparse. In fact, in animals it has been demonstrated that the fetal myocardium has a diminished store of catecholamines and an increased sensitivity to exogenous norepinephrine.[8] In contrast, the parasympathetic supply to the myocardium is completely developed at birth and the heart is sensitive to vagal stimulation.[13] This relative imbalance between cholinergic tone and sympathetic innervation predisposes the fetal and neonatal heart to bradycardia, as evidenced by the bradycardic response of the infant to hypoxia. A similar response is seen in infants upon the administration of a single dose of succinylcholine.[14, 15] In adults such bradycardia is seen after a second dose but rarely after an initial dose.

These anatomical and autonomic characteristics of the neonatal myocardium put the neonate at a disadvantage relative to the adult. The infant's cardiac output can be increased by raising the heart rate, but little can be gained by changing the end-diastolic pressure. It has been demonstrated in fetal and newborn lambs that ventricular output is linearly related to heart rate over a wide range up to more than 200 beats per minute.[11, 16] In the newborn infant, this unbalanced cholinergic tone also predisposes to negative inotropy. Consequently, the neonate is more prone to develop congestive heart failure.[17] Further distinguishing the neonate is the fact that digoxin does not increase contractility as effectively as it does in older children and adults. The infant's myocardium performs in lower Frank-Starling curves and cannot increase contractility by shifting to another curve.[18]

Cardiovascular parameters are of course much different for the infant and the adult. The infant's heart rate is higher, decreasing to adult levels at about age 5 years (Table 1–2). Cardiac output is also higher in infants, especially when calculated according to body weight, and it parallels oxygen consumption. A more constant figure is obtained by relating cardiac output to surface area (cardiac index) because of the infant's high ratio of surface area to body weight. Blood pressure is lower in infants.[19] This, with a high cardiac output, implies that the child's systemic vascular resistance is lower, a factor that correlates well with the high oxygen consumption of the infant. This reflects the simple concept that cardiac output in normal situations is mostly governed by the requirement of tissues, whereas the control mechanisms and myocardial intrinsic properties help in adjusting it to perform at the most optimal conditions.[20]

Table 1–2. CIRCULATORY VARIABLES IN INFANTS AND CHILDREN

Age	Heart Rate (Beats/min)	Systolic Blood Pressure (mm Hg)	Diastolic Blood Pressure (mm Hg)	Cardiac Index (L/min/m²)	Oxygen Consumption (ml/kg/min)
Preterm	150 ± 20	50 ± 3	30 ± 3		8 ± 1.4
Term	133 ± 18	73 ± 8	50 ± 8	2.5 ± 0.6	6 ± 1.0
6 mo	120 ± 20	89 ± 29	60 ± 10	2.0 ± 0.5	5 ± 0.9
1 yr	120 ± 20	96 ± 30	66 ± 25	2.5 ± 0.6	5.2 ± 0.1
2 yr	105 ± 25	99 ± 25	64 ± 25	3.1 ± 0.7	6.4 ± 1.2
5 yr	90 ± 10	94 ± 14	55 ± 9	3.7 ± 0.9	6.0 ± 1.1
12 yr	70 ± 17	109 ± 16	58 ± 9	4.3 ± 1.1	3.3 ± 0.6
Young adult	75 ± 5	122 ± 30	75 ± 20	3.7 ± 0.3	3.4 ± 0.6

Adapted from Crone,[9] Kaplan and Graves.[19]

RESPIRATORY SYSTEM

Upper Airway

The upper airway of the newborn infant not only is smaller than that of adults but also is anatomically different. The tongue is relatively large and occupies fully the cavity of the mouth and oropharynx. Because the oral cavity is also compromised by the absence of teeth, the anesthesiologist must be aware of how easily airway obstruction can occur. The airway can usually be cleared by holding the mouth in an open position while lifting the jaw. It must also be remembered that infants in the first few weeks of life are *obligate nasal breathers* because the epiglottis, positioned high in the pharynx, almost meets the soft palate, making oral ventilation difficult. Consequently, clearing the nose of an infant during and after the administration of an anesthetic is extremely important. If a nasal obstruction does occur, it can usually be relieved by causing the infant to cry.

The larynx is located at a high position. In the baby the body of the hyoid bone is situated approximately at the level of the disc between the second and third cervical vertebrae, whereas in the adult it is about the level of the fourth cervical vertebra.[21] The high position of the epiglottis and larynx allows the infant to breathe and swallow simultaneously.[1]

The technique of endotracheal intubation in the newborn differs from that in the adult because of the newborn's anatomical features.[22] The relatively large head obviates the need for its support by a pillow or a blanket. The angle of the jaw is approximately 140°, whereas in a young adult it is about 120°. The epiglottis is more U-shaped, usually resembling the Greek letter omega (Ω), and protrudes over the larynx at a 45° angle. Because the larynx of the infant is high and has an anterior inclination, the straight laryngoscope blade is the more useful. The view can be markedly improved by external pressure on the larynx, pushing it backward.

With the growth of the child the larynx descends. Most of this descent occurs in the first year, but it is not until the fourth year that the adult position is reached. The change in position is essential for the development of speech and means that the child can no longer breathe and drink simultaneously.[1]

The narrowest area of the adult's airway is between the vocal cords, but that of the infant is in the cricoid region of the larynx.[22] Because the cricoid is a circular cartilaginous structure and consequently nonexpansile, an endotracheal tube may pass easily through an infant's vocal cords but be tight at the cricoid area. The limiting factor therefore becomes the cricoid ring. Additionally, the vocal cords of the neonate are slanted such that the anterior commissure is more caudal than the posterior commissure.

The tracheal direction in the infant is downward and posteriorly, whereas in the adult it is straight downward. Consequently, cricoid pressure is more effective in passing the endotracheal tube in an infant. This is especially important during nasotracheal intubation when the tube tends to get caught in the subglottic region. The tonsils and adenoids are very small in the neonate. They grow markedly during childhood and reach their largest size at 4 to 7 years of age but then recede gradually.

In the newborn infant the distance between the bifurcation of the trachea and the vocal cords is 4 to 5 cm. Thus an endotracheal tube must be very carefully positioned and fixed. Because of the large size of the infant's head, the tip of the tube can move about 2 cm during flexion or extension of the head. Consequently, it behooves the anesthesiologist to check the position of the endotracheal tube every time the head is moved.

The diameter of the trachea in the newborn is 4 to 5 mm. Airflow resistance is directly related to the length and inversely related to the fourth power of the diameter of a tube. Consequently, 1 mm of edema in the trachea of the newborn will reduce its cross sectional area by about 75 percent and will increase the resistance to air flow sixteenfold. The same degree of edema in an adult would decrease the cross sectional area by only 44 percent and increase the flow resistance only threefold.

In general the right main bronchus is less angled than the left. Hence the right main bronchus is the one most frequently intubated during endobronchial intubation and foreign bodies tend to lodge in the right side more frequently.

The configuration of the thoracic cage differs between infant and adult. The infant's ribs are more horizontal and therefore can rise less during inspiration. In addition, the chest has less anterioposterior movement during inspiration. The diaphragm is therefore more important in ventilation, and the consequences of abdominal distention are worse.

The Lung

The newborn lung is not a miniature of the adult lung. Each of its components has a different pattern of growth. At the fetal stage the pattern of the bronchial tree is fully developed by the 16th week of gestation. Alveoli develop later and increase in number until age 8 years[24] and in size until the full development of the chest wall. Of the blood vessels, the preacinar vessels (arteries and veins) develop concomitantly with the airways, whereas the intra-acinar vessels develop with the alveoli.

The lining of the respiratory saccules and the alveoli is derived from two types of cells: Type I pneumocytes produce the lining and supporting cells of the alveoli and contribute to the blood gas barrier. Type II pneumocytes are more glandular and contain osmiophilic cytoplasmic inclusion granules. Pulmonary surfactant is synthesized in these granular pneumocytes (Type II) and is stored in the lamellar bodies. It is released by fusion of the lamellar body membrane with the cell wall.

The lung surfactant is a complex, multicomponent system containing various surface-active molecules including phospholipids such as phosphatidylcholine and phosphatidylglycerol with broad fatty acid distribution. It is not identical with dipalmitoyl phosphatidylcholine.[25] Eighty-five percent of its lipid (mostly phospholipids) and 10 to 15 percent is protein unique to the lung.[26] The surfactant orients itself so that its hydrophilic choline group is in the aqueous phase and its hydrophobic palmitic side chains are above the air-liquid interface. This arrangement reduces the surface tension at the air-tissue interface in the alveoli, thus preventing the alveoli from collapsing during expiration.

Surfactant appears at approximately 20 weeks of gestational age. Its production increases slowly and then accelerates at about 30 to 34 weeks. This can be hastened by the administration of glucocorticoids during pregnancy and increases during such compromised situations as prolonged rupture of the membranes (probably also glucocorticoid-mediated). Whether glucocorticoids have a specific effect on normal surfactant development is speculative. In animals thyroxine accelerates its production. Beta-adrenergic and cholinergic stimulation can release surfactant, whereas pure oxygen accelerates its breakdown.

In the uterus, fetal lung fluid flows up in the trachea and can be detected in the amniotic fluid. It appears in the second trimester and then increases markedly in the last trimester.

Onset of Respiration

In the human embryo breathing movement can be detected as early as the 11th week of gestation. Such movement is irregular until the 20th week, after which it becomes more patterned; by 36 weeks it is entirely regular at a rate of 30 to 70 per minute. These intrauterine breathing movements show a circadian rhythm and are more accentuated in the evening than in the early morning. Fetal breathing may decrease or even stop with alterations of the fetal environment, such as those caused by bimanual examination, surgical procedures, hypoglycemia and even maternal cigarette smoking.

At birth, with the influence of physical stimuli such as gravity and lowering of skin temperature, the small fetal respiratory movements become strong and continuous. It seems, however, that they are finally maintained by clamping of the cord. It is also true that the chemoreceptors become sensitive at birth to small changes in arterial gas tension. All these factors combine to induce the newborn to gasp and aerate his lungs and generate inspiratory pressures of about 70 cm H_2O. These high inspiratory pressures act against the viscosity of the fluids in the airways and the elastic recoil of the lungs and chest wall to establish the resting lung volumes. As the alveoli expand, lower intrathoracic pressures are required to maintain air movement.

About one third of the fluid present in the airways at birth is drained through the mouth. The remainder is absorbed through the pulmonary lymphatics and capillaries.

Respiratory Function

When calculated according to body weight, respiratory parameters in the newborn, including tidal volume (V_T), dead spaces (V_D), V_D/V_T, vital capacity, functional residual capacity (FRC), and specific compliance are rather similar to those in the adult (Table 1–3). Because of the infant's higher metabolic rate, more marked differences are seen in respiratory frequency and hence in alveolar ventilation. The lungs of the infant therefore have less oxygen reserve than do the lungs of the adult; thus the infant can become hypoxic much more quickly than the adult. Furthermore, this high alveolar ventilation relative to the functional residual capacity makes it a less effective

Table 1–3. RESPIRATORY VARIABLES IN INFANTS AND CHILDREN

	Newborn	1 Yr	8 Yr	Adult
Weight (kg)	3	10	25	70
Height (cm)	48	75	130	170
Respiratory frequency (breaths/min)	40	25	18	12
Tidal volume (v_T)				
ml	21	78	180	500
ml/kg	7	8	7	7
Dead space V_D				
ml	7	21	70	150
ml/kg	2	2	2.8	2
V_D/V_T	0.3	0.3	0.3	0.3
Alveolar ventilation				
ml/min	400	1200	2200	4000
ml/min/kg	130	120	80	60
Vital capacity				
ml	120	450	1500	4000
ml/kg	40	45	60	60
Functional residual capacity				
ml	80	250	1000	2400
ml/kg	28	25	40	35
Specific compliance C_L/FRC				
ml/cm H_2O/ml	0.04		0.06	0.05
Resting alveolar ventilation				
ml/min	400	1200	2200	3000
ml/kg/min	130	120	90	45
Hematocrit g/100 ml	55	35	40	42
PaO_2 (mm Hg)	60–90	90	95	95

Data adapted from Crone,[9] Kaplan and Graves,[19] Motoyama and Cook,[51] and Goudsouzian and Karamanian.[20]

buffer between inspired gases and pulmonary circulation. Inspired anesthetic gases will therefore equilibrate much faster in an infant than in an adult.

Lung compliance depends on the amount of elastic tissue present in the lungs and varies with age. At birth the few elastic fibers present in the walls of terminal air sacs extend as far as the alveolar opening. With time, the elastic tissue increases as the alveoli grow in size. At the age of 18 years elastic tissue is fully developed, and from then on it gradually deteriorates. Consequently, lung compliance is relatively low in the very young and the very old, with a peak in late adolescence.[27]

Since the infant's chest wall is soft and the ribs are cartilaginous and horizontal, the chest wall is more compliant and does not contribute significantly to respiratory motion; hence, the negative intrapleural pressure is generated by diaphragmatic and abdominal muscles. This compliance of the chest wall and the lung lowers the resting lung volume, making the functional residual capacity more difficult to establish and maintain.

The closing volume is the lung volume at which terminal airways begin to close off, which creates a discontinuity between the trapped gases and the conducting airways. It is much higher in neonates and infants than in adults because of the decrease in elastic tissues. Consequently, in infants the terminal alveoli

at the base of the lungs would be close to atelectasis at the end of each breath.[27] Healthy infants overcome this tendency through constant activity and reach total lung volume through crying. By contrast, in a sedated infant with shallow breathing or in an infant with residual muscle paralysis airway closure can be exaggerated.

Respiratory Rate

In general the rate and the depth of respiration are controlled to result in the least expenditure of energy. At a rate of 35 to 40 breaths per minute in the newborn and 12 to 16 breaths per minute in an adult, the work of the respiratory muscles to overcome elastic and resistive work is at a minimum. At these rates, both the infant and the adult expend about 1 percent of their metabolic energy in ventilation.

In adults respiration is stimulated by hypoxia and depressed by hyperoxia. In the newborn, however, the initial hyperventilation of hypoxia can be followed rapidly by a sustained decrease in ventilation.[26] This response is more apparent in the premature infant than in the term infant, in whom it is aggravated by a cool environment and tends to disappear within a few weeks.

Periodic breathing can be observed in the newborn; a greater incidence has been noted in premature than in term infants. It is usually manifested as rapid ventilation followed by apnea of less than 10 seconds; arterial oxygen tension remains in the normal range. This pattern is not seen in healthy infants after 6 weeks of age. In premature neonates, however, apneic spells longer than 20 seconds can be observed and are usually associated with bradycardia and cyanosis.[28] This is also seen in infants who have survived an apneic episode related to sudden infant death syndrome. Such apneic episodes seem to be exaggerated during stressful situations such as respiratory infections or in the postanesthetic and postsurgical states.[29]

In both premature and term infants the arterial PCO_2 is lower than in the adult. This is because the metabolic acidosis induced by labor stimulates the chemoreceptors while the relative hypoxemia and exposure to the cold environment stimulate respiration. At term the chemoreceptors are functional; hence, an increase in the inspired CO_2 concentration will stimulate breathing. Interestingly, term infants will respond to CO_2 like adults and increase the tidal volume, whereas premature infants will increase mostly the respiratory rate with only a small increase in tidal volume.[26]

Oxygen Transport

The blood volume of the newborn is 70 to 90 ml/kg depending on whether the cord is clamped early or late. The hemoglobin content of the blood of the healthy newborn is high (19 g/100 ml) and consists mostly of fetal hemoglobin.

Fetal hemoglobin (HbF) has a greater affinity for oxygen than adult hemoglobin. In HbF, one histidine

Figure 1–2. The approximate amount of fetal hemoglobin (HbF) and adult hemoglobin (HbA) present in 100 ml of blood during infancy.

molecule of the beta chain is replaced by serine, thus preventing 2,3-DPG from sliding easily between the beta chains. Hence, O_2 is more strongly attracted to the hemoglobin molecule than is 2,3-DPG.[20, 30] Fetal hemoglobin has the teleological advantage of loading more oxygen at the placenta from the mother. However, because it does not give up the oxygen easily at the tissues, cyanosis occurs at a lower Po_2 than in the adult. The P_{50} (the partial pressure of oxygen when only 50 percent of the hemoglobin is saturated with oxygen) is about 27 mmHg in the normal adult, while in the newborn it is 20 mmHg. With the growth of the infant the fetal hemoglobin is replaced by adult hemoglobin and the P_{50} approximates the adult's, thus enhancing oxygen release. This partially compensates for the physiological anemia of infancy, the lowest level of which is reached at 3 months when the hemoglobin concentration can fall below 10 g/100 ml (Fig. 1–2).

In premature infants and in those with the respiratory distress syndrome, 2,3-DPG levels are lower than in term infants, and thus the P_{50} values are lower.[31] Such infants experience a greater fall in hemoglobin concentration than term infants, with hemoglobin levels reaching their lowest point at 2 or 3 months of age.

The regulation of erythropoiesis in the newborn is a complicated process. In the fetus anemia or hypoxia induces increased erythropoietin activity. After birth, however, erythropoiesis virtually ceases.[32] The reticulocyte count and the hemoglobin concentration fall after the first day of life and plasma-erythropoietin is not detectable thereafter for 2 to 3 months. In situations of decreased oxygen supply to the tissues (as in severe anemia or congenital heart disease) increased plasma erythropoietin is seen, indicating that tissue oxygen tensions or requirements are probably involved in modulating its production.

RENAL FUNCTION

In the fetus the placenta is the main excretory organ. Although anephric infants survive intrauterine life, fetal malformation may occur owing to oligohydramnios caused by the absence of fetal urine. The formation of the glomeruli is not complete until the 34th week of gestation, most of the growth occurring in the third trimester. Between 34 and 36 weeks of gestation, when the fetus weighs about 2000 grams, the glomeruli mature considerably. In prematurely born infants (less than 34 weeks) the glomerular function is markedly depressed and develops more slowly in the postnatal stage, whereas in infants born after this critical age glomerular and tubular function increases at the same rate as in a term infant.[34]

The healthy term infant has the same number of nephrons at birth but the glomeruli are smaller than their adult counterparts. However, their filtration surface related to body weight is similar. The tubules are not fully grown at birth and may not pass into the medulla.

The glomerular filtration rate at birth is about 30 percent of the adult value of 125 ml/min/1.73m². It increases rapidly during the first 2 weeks of age and then relatively slowly to approach the adult level by the end of the first year.[35] The rate of increase is practically the same in the premature infant born after the 34 weeks gestation and the full term infant, but it begins from a lower point in the premature one.[36]

Several factors contribute to the increase in glomerular function that is seen with development. These include an increase in cardiac output, changes of renovascular resistance, altered regional blood flow, and changes in the glomeruli. Maturation of glomerular function is complete at 5 to 6 months of age.

In general maturation of tubular function lags behind that of the glomeruli. Reasons for decreased tubular function in the premature infant include low blood flow to peritubular regions, immaturity of the energy-supplying process, the small number of the tubular working cells, and the size of the tubules themselves. Peak renal capacity is reached at 2 to 3 years of age, after which it decreases at a rate of 2.5 percent per year.[37]

Tubular function is not fully mature at birth and is even less so in the premature than in the term neonate. Although the kidney of the newborn can excrete dilute urine up 50 mOsm/L, it can rarely concentrate more than 700 mOsm/L (adults 1200 mOsm/L), owing in part to the lack of urea-forming solids in the diet. The kidney of the newborn does, however, respond to antidiuretic hormone. The inability to concentrate urine and maintain outflow may result in plasma hyperosmolarity, especially when the child is dehydrated from diarrhea or exposure to high environmental temperature. This may occur when small infants are kept under radiant heat sources for a prolonged period.

Because of the anabolic state of the newborn and the small muscle mass relative to body weight, the normal value for creatinine is lower in infants than in adults (0.4 mg/100 ml vs 1 mg/100 ml). The renal threshold for bicarbonate is also lower in the newborn (20 mmol/L vs adult 25 mmol/L). With a normal value of plasma bicarbonate 20 mmol/L, the infant has lower plasma pH of about 7.34.

THE LIVER AND METABOLISM

Glucose from the mother is the main metabolic energy source in the fetus. It is transferred through the placenta from the maternal circulation by the mechanism of facilitated diffusion and stored as fat and glycogen. The fetal plasma glucose level averages 70 to 80 percent of the maternal level throughout pregnancy, but storage mostly occurs in the last trimester. At a gestational age of 28 weeks, the fetus has practically no fat stored. At 34 weeks 7 to 8 percent of fetal body weight is fat and 9 g of glycogen is stored; at term 16 percent of the body is fat with 34 g of stored glycogen.

In the first few hours following delivery glucose is the infant's main energy source. During this period hepatic and muscle glycogen stores are rapidly depleted. Fat then becomes the principal energy source. As fat is metabolized, the respiratory quotient falls to 0.7. Ketone bodies and probably lactate are also utilized by the brain.

In the first 4 hours of extrauterine life, depletion of liver glycogen leads to a rapid drop in plasma glucose levels. The lower limit of normal is 30 mg/100 ml in the term infant but is as low as 20 mg/100 ml in the small infant. Although at this level infants usually do not show any neurological signs or symptoms, they may develop pallor, sweating, or tachycardia. A blood glucose level below 20 mg/100 ml usually produces neurological symptoms such as apnea or convulsions.

Since glucose stores are limited at birth, it is imperative that the newborn not be kept for a long period without enteral or parenteral nutrition. This is especially true for premature infants, in whom the tendency to hypoglycemia may persist for weeks. In fasting infants waiting for surgery an intravenous solution will prevent hypoglycemia. Small healthy infants may be given sugar water solution by mouth up to 2 hours before the surgery. If a change in schedule occurs the liquid contents of the stomach can be easily emptied by an orogastric tube.

The liver is of primary importance in neonatal metabolism and is relatively large compared with the adult's. In utero it performs several important functions essential for fetal survival.[38] Starting as early as 10 to 12 weeks of gestation, it maintains glucose regulation, protein and lipid synthesis, and drug metabolism. Its excretory products (such as lipid-soluble unconjugated substances like bilirubin) traverse the placenta and are detoxified and excreted by the maternal liver.

In the neonate the liver volume represents 4 percent of the total body weight, whereas in an adult it is 2 percent of body weight. However, the enzyme concentration and activity are lower in the neonatal liver.[37, 39, 40] Most of the metabolic biotransformation of drugs in the liver occurs through two major pathways. Phase I or degradative reactions include the oxidation, reduction, and hydrolysis reaction. Phase II or synthetic reactions occur mostly by conjugation. Most of the phase I reactions occur in the microsomal fraction of the liver and are known collectively as the cytochrome p450 enzyme system. It appears that the enzyme systems responsible for conjugation reactions (phase II) are more immature than enzymes responsible for phase I reactions. Consequently neonates, and especially the preterm, are less effective in conjugating bilirubin, chloramphenicol, sulfonamides, acetaminophen, and meprobamate.[41, 42] Glucuronide conjugation does not reach adult values until 3 years of age.[43] As the enzymes mature at this age and as the liver is relatively large, children demonstrate a high level of hepatic metabolic activity during childhood. Increased activity becomes manifest at 3 months of age, reaches its peak at 2 to 3 years, and then starts declining, reaching adult values after puberty.

Renin, angiotensin, aldosterone, cortisol, and thyroxine levels are high in the newborn and decrease in the first few weeks of life.

TEMPERATURE REGULATION

Although newborns have an active central temperature regulatory mechanism, it is limited by certain anatomical and physiological factors. As does the adult, the infant attempts to maintain a constant body temperature, but he succeeds only within a narrow range of environment conditions. While an adult can sustain body temperature in an environment as cold as 0°C, a full term infant starts developing hypothermia at an ambient temperature of about 22°C. Premature infants are even more vulnerable, requiring higher environmental temperatures to maintain normothermia.[44]

The important mechanisms for heat production are metabolic activity, shivering, and non-shivering thermogenesis. Newborn babies usually do not shiver. Heat is generated instead by non-shivering thermogenesis. Exposure to cold leads to increased production of norepinephrine, which in turn increases the metabolic activity of brown fat.[45] *Brown fat* is a highly specialized tissue with a high number of mitochondrial cytochromes; it is these that provide the tissue with its brown color. The cells have several small vacuoles of fat and are richly endowed with sympathetic nerve endings. They are mainly located in the nape of the neck and between the scapulae but are found as well in the mediastinal and perirenal regions.

Once released, norepinephrine acts on the alpha- and beta-adrenergic receptors on the brown adipocytes. This stimulates the release of lipase,[46] which in turn splits triglycerides into glycerol and fatty acids, thus increasing heat production. The increase in brown fat metabolism raises the proportion of cardiac output diverted through the brown fat, which in turn facilitates the direct warming of blood. The increased levels of norepinephrine have secondary effects, most notably pulmonary and peripheral vasoconstriction. Pulmonary vasoconstriction will increase pulmonary arterial pressure, which will predispose to increased right-to-left shunt through the foramen ovale and ductus arteriosus and lead to hypoxemia. Peripheral vasoconstriction also produces a mottled appearance of the skin.

Because the infant has a high ratio of surface area to body weight, heat loss through the skin is more marked than in the older child or adult. The infant's skin is also thinner and more permeable and therefore predisposes to heat loss by evaporation. One advantage of this is the ease with which the infant can be warmed by a warming blanket in the operating room.[47] The sweating mechanism is present in the term infant. It is not as efficient in the premature infant and is practically absent in infants less than 32 weeks of gestational age.[36]

In the infant, oxygen consumption is at its minimum when the environmental temperature is within 3 to 5 percent (1 to 2°C) of body temperature (an abdominal skin temperature of 36°C).[48] This is known as the neutral thermal state, and a deviation in either direction from this state increases oxygen consumption.

A major source of heat loss in an infant is the respiratory system. A 3-kg infant with a minute ventilation of 500 ml spends 3.5 cal/min to raise the temperature of the inspired gases. To saturate the gases with water vapor takes an additional 12 cal/min. The total—15 cal/min (900 cal/h) or approximately 1 kcal/h represents about 10 to 20 percent of the total oxygen consumption of an infant.[49]

In the spontaneously breathing child, the temperature of the inspired gases at the pharynx reaches 32°C with a relative humidity of 86 percent. Full saturation is achieved in the distal bronchi. In the anesthetized patient, an open breathing system delivers gases that are practically devoid of humidity. With a semiclosed system, relative humidity can be raised up to 80 percent at 20°C (water content 14 mg/L). The introduction of a heated humidifier into this system can ensure a water content of 30 mg/L at 30°C.[42, 50] Such humidification is similar to that occurring normally at the pharynx and minimizes the calories lost through the respiratory system.

DEVELOPMENT OF MYONEURAL JUNCTIONS

During development several organizational changes occur in the myoneural junctions. In the early stages polyneuronal innervation is a characteristic feature, and some axons innervate a very large number of muscle fibers. However, near full term these large motor units rapidly decrease in size as the superfluous nerve terminals are eliminated, probably by withdrawal. It is interesting that this elimination process is activity-dependent.[52, 53] Experimental tenotomy of the muscle or paralyzing the nerve with drugs delays the loss of the superfluous nerve terminals, whereas increasing the activity by chronic nerve stimulation accelerates the loss.[53]

After birth, as the motor activity increases, the activation of the muscles by acetylcholine increases and induces the release of enzymes into the synaptic clefts. These enzymes tend to digest the nerve terminal, and the ability of the terminal to survive will ultimately depend on the supply of reparative material that it received from the cell body. As the weaker terminals are withdrawn, the neuron is able to divert more reparative material to its surviving terminal, thus maintaining it. Ultimately the nerve terminal where the rate of repair balances the rate of digestion will survive.

Another maturational change that occurs in the muscle is in the distribution of receptors. In the normal situation the postsynaptic receptors for the cholinergic transmitter are primarily located at the crests of the junctional folds as part of the integral membrane protein. These receptors can be delineated at the binding sites at an approximate concentration of 20,000 per μm^2. The deeper region of the junctional cleft and the remainder of the muscle membrane are practically devoid of receptors.[54, 55]

Normally, almost all of the cholinergic receptors are localized around the nerve endings. These are known as junctional receptors. However there are also a very small number of extrajunctional receptors on the muscle membrane. These extrajunctional receptors are structurally similar to the junctional ones—they are glycoproteins and have a similar mode of action. In abnormal states the number of these extrajunctional receptors increases. For example denervation produces a fivefold to thirtyfold rise in the number of the acetylcholine receptors. The density of extrajunctional receptors is less than that of the junctional receptors, but they are large in number and widespread over the muscle. Extrajunctional receptors are more loosely attached to the cell membrane, and are characterized by having a rapid turnover rate. Their half-life is on the order of 17 to 22 hours, while that of the junctional receptors is 1 to 2 weeks.

Characteristically extrajunctional receptors are resistant to curare; up to three times the usual dose of curare is required to prevent acetylcholine from opening these channels.[54]

Clinically, resistance to nondepolarizing muscle relaxants can be found in the affected side of a hemiplegic patient, during prolonged immobilization, or after a severe burn.[56, 57, 58] Extrapolating animal studies, one can presume that resistance to muscle relaxants is due to the development of extrajunctional receptors.

The presence of extrajunctional receptors is not unique to denervation or immobilization . They are also found in embryonic muscle fiber; whether they are identical with the extrajunctional receptors of denervation is a matter of debate. Consequently the acetylcholine sensitivity is found all along the muscle of embryonal tissues. Also, the turnover rate of these receptors is rapid and rather similar to that of extrajunctional receptors (half-life of approximately 24 hours).[59, 60] However, within a few days of established innervation the turnover increases to the values characteristic of adult junctional receptors.[61] These developmental changes vary from one animal to another and even in the same animal from one group of muscles to another.[62]

For obvious reasons detailed studies on the myoneural junctions cannot be performed in human neonates. Indirect studies indicate immaturity of the junctions; for example, train-of-four values are lower in neonates than in older infants and children.[63, 64] Also, tetanus is poorly sustained,[65] as has also been seen in the frequency sweep electromyogram.[66]

Pharmacokinetic studies demonstrate that the same level of neuromuscular depression as is achieved in older children with a given plasma concentration of a relaxant can be achieved in infants with a similar or lesser concentration.[67, 68] However, a very interesting feature that appears in relaxant studies in infants is the marked variation in response; some infants are markedly sensitive to nondepolarizers, whereas others are resistant.[68, 69] Extrapolating from animal data one can presume that infants who are sensitive are the ones who have immature myoneural junctions, whereas the resistant ones are the ones with large numbers of extrajunctional receptors. Within a short interval, probably in less than a month, this variation diminishes and the myoneural junction behaves rather similarly to that of the adult.

REFERENCES

1. Crelin ES: Functional Anatomy of the Newborn. New Haven, Yale University Press, 1973, p 1–40.
2. Goudsouzian NG: Anatomical differences between the child and the adult and their clinical sequelae. In Ramez-Salem M (Ed.): Pediatric Anesthesia: Current Practice. New York, Academic Press, 1981, pp 1–3.
3. Rudolph AM: The changes in the circulation after birth: their importance in congenital heart disease. Circulation 41:343, 1970.
4. Jacobstein MD, Hirschfield SS, Flinn C, et al.: Neonatal circulatory changes following elective cesarean section. Pediatrics 69:374, 1982.
5. Heyman MA, Rudolph AM: Ductus arteriosus dilation by prostaglandin E$_1$ in infants with pulmonary atresia. Pediatrics 59:325, 1977.
6. Elliot RB, Starling MD, Neutra JM: Medical manipulation of the ductus arteriosus. Lancet 1:140, 1975.
7. Legato MJ: Ultrastructural changes during normal growth in the dog and rat ventricular myofiber. In Lieberman M, Sano T (Eds.): Developmental and Physiological Correlates of Cardiac Muscles. New York, Raven Press, 1976, pp 249–274.
8. Friedman WF: Intrinsic physiologic properties of the developing heart. Prog Cardiovasc Dis 15:87, 1972.
9. Crone RK: Pediatric critical care: supporting the developing organ systems. In Shoemaker WC, Thompson WL, Holbrook PR (Eds.): Society of Critical Care Medicine: Textbook of Critical Care. Philadelphia, W. B. Saunders Co., 1984.
10. Mott JC: The ability of young mammals to withstand total oxygen lack. Br Med Bull 17:145, 1961.
11. Enhoring G, Westin B: Experimental studies of the human fetus in prolonged asphyxia. Acta Physiol Scand 31:359, 1954.
12. Spotnitz WD, Spotnitz HM, Truccome NJ, et al.: Relation of ultrastructure and function. Sarcomere dimensions, pressure-volume curves and geometry of the intact left ventricle of the immature canine heart. Circ Res 44:679, 1979.
13. Gootman PM: Perinatal neural regulation of cardiovascular function. In Gootman N, Gootman PM (Eds.): Perinatal Cardiovascular Function. New York, Marcel Dekker, 1983, p 287.
14. Craythorne NW, Turndorf H, Dripps RD: Changes in pulse rate and rhythm associated with the use of succinylcholine in anesthetized children. Anesthesiology 21:465, 1960.
15. Goudsouzian NG: Turbe del ritmo cardiaco durante intubazione tracheale nei bambini. Acta Anesth Ital 32:293, 1981.
16. Rudolph AM, Heymann MA: Cardiac output in the fetal lamb: the effects of spontaneous and induced changes in heart rate and left ventricular output. Am J Obstet Gynecol 124:183, 1976.
17. Rudolph AM, Heymann MA: Fetal and neonatal circulation and respiration. Ann Rev Physiol 36:187, 1974.
18. Berman W Jr, Yabek SM, Dillon T, et al.: Effects of digoxin in infants with a congestive circulatory failure due to ventricular septal defect. N Engl J Med 308:363, 1983.
19. Kaplan RF, Graves SA: Anatomic and physiologic differences of neonates, infants and children. Semin Anesth 3:1, 1984.
20. Goudsouzian N, Karamanian A: Physiology for the Anesthesiologist. Norwalk, CT, Appleton-Century-Crofts, 1984, pp 242–254.
21. Ardran GM, Kemp FH: The mechanism of changes in form of the cervical airway in infancy. Med Radiolog Photog 44:26, 1968.
22. Eckenhoff JE: Some anatomic considerations of the infant larynx influencing endotracheal anesthesia. Anesthesiology 12:401, 1951.
23. Cote C, Eavey R, Todres ID: Providing for the needs of the pediatric larynx. Wellcome Trends in Anesthesiology, December 1983, p 2.
24. Reid L: The lung: its growth and remodeling in health and diseases. Am J Roentgenol 129:777, 1977.
25. Notter R, Shapiro DL: Lung surfactant in an era of replacement therapy. Pediatrics 68:781, 1981.
26. Roberton NRC: Perinatal physiology. In Godfrey S, Baum JD (Eds.): Clinical Paediatric Physiology. Oxford, Blackwell Scientific Publications, 1979, pp 134–192.
27. Mansell A, Bryan C, Levison H: Airway closure in children. J Appl Physiol 33:711, 1972.
28. Shannon DC, Kelly DH: SIDS and near SIDS. N Engl J Med 306:1022, 1982.
29. Liu LMP, Cote CJ, Goudsouzian NG, et al.: Life threatening apnea in infants recovering from anesthesia. Anesthesiology 59:506, 1983.
30. Perutz MF: Hemoglobin structure and respiratory function. Sci Am 239:92, 1978.
31. Stockman JA, Garcia JF, Oski FA: The anemia of prematurity. Factors governing the erythropoietin response. N Engl J Med 296:647, 1977.
32. Gairdner D, Marks J, Roscoe JD: Blood formation in infancy. I. The normal bone marrow. Arch Dis Child 27:128, 1952.

33. Arant B: Developmental patterns of renal functional maturation compared in the human neonate. J Pediatr 92:705, 1978.

34. Aperia A, Broberger O, Elinder G, et al.: Postnatal development of renal function in preterm and full term infants. Acta Pediatr Scand 70:183, 1981.

35. Fawer CL, Torrado A, Guignard JP: Maturation of renal function in full term and premature neonates. Helv Paediatr Acta 34:11, 1979.

36. Oh W: Renal function and clinical disorders in the neonate. Clin Perinatol 8:213, 1981.

37. Rane A, Wilson JT: Clinical pharmacokinetics in infants and children. Clin Pharmacokinet 1:2, 1976.

38. DeLaiglesia FA, Sturgess J, McGuire EJ, et al.: Quantitative microscopic evaluation of endoplasmic reticulum in developing human liver. Am J Pathol 82:61, 1976.

39. Morselli PL: Clinical pharmacokinetics in neonates. Clin Pharmacokinet 1:81, 1976.

40. Currin MR: Pharmacology of the neonate. S Afr Med J 56:101, 1979.

41. Weiss CF, Glazko AG, Weston JK: Chloramphenicol in the newborn infant: a physiological explanation of its toxicity when given in excessive doses. N Engl J Med 262:787, 1960.

42. Yu WL, Aldrich RA: The glucuronide transferase system in the newborn infant. Pediatr Clin N Am 7:381, 1960.

43. Dalton GJ: Developmental aspects of drug conjugation with special reference to glucuronidation. Ann Rev Pharmacol Toxicol 18:17, 1978.

44. Heiser MS, Downes JJ: Temperature regulation in the pediatric patient. Semin Anesth 2:37, 1980.

45. Schiff D, Stern L, Leduc J: Chemical thermogenesis in newborn infants. Catecholamine excretion and the plasma nonesterified fatty acid response to cold exposure. Pediatrics 37:577, 1966.

46. Himms-Hagen: Cellular thermogenesis. Ann Rev Physiol 38:315, 1966.

47. Goudsouzian NG, Morris RH, Ryan JF: The effects of a warming blanket in the maintenance of body temperature in anesthetized infants and children. Anesthesiology 39:351, 1973.

48. Adamsons K, Towell ME: Thermal hemostasis in the fetus and newborn. Anesthesiology 26:531, 1965.

49. Goudsouzian NG: Temperature regulation in the operating room. In Ramez-Salem M (Ed.): Pediatric Anesthesia: Current Practice. New York, Academic Press, 1981, pp 31–33.

50. Weeks DB, Bromank E: A method of quantitating humidity in the anesthesia circuit by temperature control semiclosed circle. Anesth Analg 49:292, 1970.

51. Motoyama EK, Cook CD: Respiratory physiology. In Smith RM (Ed.): Anesthesia for Infants and Children. St. Louis, CV Mosby Co., 1980, p 38.

52. Brown MG, Jansen JKS, van Essen D: Polyneuronal innervation of skeletal muscles in newborn rats and its elimination during maturation. J Physiol 261:387, 1976.

53. O'Brien RAD, Ostberg AJC, Vebova G: The reorganization of neuromuscular junctions during development in rats. In Hoffman JF, Giebisch GH (Eds.): Membranes in Growth and Development. New York, Alan R. Liss, 1982, pp 247–257.

54. Fambrough DM: Control of acetylcholine receptors in skeletal muscles. Physiol Rev 59:165, 1979.

55. Peper K, Bradley RJ, Dreyer F: The acetylcholine receptor at the neuromuscular junction. Physiol Rev 62:1271, 1982.

56. Graham DH: Monitoring neuromuscular block may be unreliable in patients with upper-motor-neuron lesions. Anesthesiology 52:74, 1980.

57. Moorthy SS, Hilgenberg JC: Resistance to nondepolarizing muscle relaxants in paretic upper extremities of patients with residual hemiplegia. Anesth Analg 59:624, 1980.

58. Martyn JAJ, Szyfelbein SK, Ali HH, et al.: Increased d-tubocurarine requirement following major thermal injury. Anesthesiology 52:352, 1980.

59. Bennett MR: Development of neuromuscular synapses. Physiol Rev 63:915, 1983.

60. Reiness CG, Weinberg CB: Metabolic stabilization of acetylcholine receptors at newly formed neuromuscular junctions in rats. Develop Biol 84:247, 1981.

61. Linden DC, Fambrough DM: Biosynthesis and degradation of acetylcholine receptors in rat skeletal muscles. Effects of electrical stimulation. Neuroscience 4:517, 1979.

62. Nag AC, Cheng M: Differentiation of fibre types in an extraocular muscle of the rat. J Embryol Exp Morph 71:171, 1982.

63. Goudsouzian NG: Maturation of neuromuscular transmission in the infant. Br Anaesth 52:205, 1980.

64. Goudsouzian NG, Crone RK, Todres ID: Recovery from pancuronium blockade in the neonatal intensive care unit. Br J Anaesth 53:1303, 1981.

65. Koenigsberger MR, Patten B, Lovelace RE: Studies of neuromuscular function in the newborn. I. A comparison of myoneural function in the full term and the premature infant. Neuropaediatrie 4:350, 1973.

66. Crumrine RS, Yodlowski EY: Assessment of neuromuscular function in infants. Anesthesiology 54:29, 1981.

67. Fisher DM, O'Keeffe C, Stanski DR, et al.: Pharmacokinetics and dynamics of d-tubocurarine in infants, children and adults. Anesthesiology 52:703, 1982.

68. Matteo RS, Lieberman IG, Salanitre E, et al.: D-Tubocurarine concentration and neuromuscular blockade in the neonate. Anesthesiology 53:S281, 1980.

69. Goudsouzian NG, Donlon JV, Savarese JJ, et al.: Reevaluation of D-tubocurarine dosage and duration in the pediatric age groups. Anesthesiology 43:416–525, 1975.

2 | PHARMACOLOGY OF PEDIATRIC ANESTHESIA

D. RYAN COOK, M.D.

The young infant, especially during the neonatal period, differs from the adult in his quantitative responses to many anesthetic drugs and adjuncts. During the first several months of life there is rapid physical growth and rapid change and maturation in the factors involved in the uptake, distribution, redistribution, metabolism, and excretion of drugs.[1-6] Important differences in these processes between the infant and adult have been identified to explain the young infant's different response to many drugs. In addition, variations in penetration of the blood-brain barrier and in receptor sensitivity have been observed in infants for some anesthetics and adjuncts. This chapter will discuss the factors that influence the infant's handling of drugs in general and give examples of pharmacological differences for certain anesthetic drugs and adjuncts, along with their probable explanations.

DRUG ABSORPTION

Most anesthetic drugs (other than inhalation anesthetics) are given parenterally. The intravenous route is the most direct, bypassing the absorption barriers. Drugs in aqueous solution injected intramuscularly are often absorbed fairly rapidly; subcutaneously injected drugs are usually more slowly absorbed. Absorption from intramuscular and subcutaneous sites depends mainly on tissue perfusion and if perfusion is adequate this absorption is similar in children and adults. The vasomotor instability in the newborn period theoretically might delay absorption from peripheral sites, although in practice the therapeutic effectiveness of drugs given via these routes suggests that this is not an important factor.[7]

On rare occasions anesthesiologists give either oral or rectal sedative-hypnotics to infants, usually for neurodiagnostic procedures. Such drugs are given in solution, not as tablets or capsules, so that disintegration and dissolution are irrelevant. They are absorbed across the gut by passive diffusion, which depends upon the physicochemical properties of the drug and the surface area of the gut available for diffusion.[8, 9] Since most drugs are weak acids or weak bases the nonionized fraction that is available for diffusion will vary with the pH of the fluid in the gut (for example, the pH of gastric fluid varies between 1.5 and 6.0, whereas the intestinal fluid is considerably more alkaline).

In adults, the total absorptional area of the small intestine is probably 200 m^2 compared with 1 m^2 for the stomach. Because of this larger surface area acidic drugs are absorbed more rapidly from the alkaline small intestine than from the acidic stomach in spite of their being highly nonionized in the intestine. In large part, therefore, the rate of gastric emptying is a controlling factor in drug absorption from the gut (that is, slower gastric emptying delays a drug's access to the small intestine and vice versa). Gastric emptying may be slowed by food, drugs, or surgical conditions. Once a drug is in the small intestine, up to 4 to 10 hours are available for absorption; however, most drugs reach peak concentrations by 30 to 40 minutes. Thus, changes in intestinal transit time have little effect on drug absorption. Likewise, very few drugs are absorbed rapidly enough for blood flow to be a rate-limiting factor, although ethanol may be an exception. Methyldopa, levodopa, and 5-fluorouracil are the few drugs actively transported across cell membranes against a concentration gradient. Ethanol is probably the only drug that, in part, crosses the gut by filtration through pores. There are no functional differences among the older infant, child, and adult that should affect gastrointestinal absorption. The rate, but not extent, of absorption of many drugs may be increased by using liquid preparations. In the newborn period and after the first day of life, gastric contents are less acidic, and the gastric emptying time and intestinal transit time are considerably slower than at any other age.[10] Consequently, drugs such as penicillin G and ampicillin, which are partially inactivated by a low pH, have greater overall absorption when swallowed. The slow gastric emptying time reduces the absorption of some drugs, whereas others may achieve greater absorption because of prolonged contact with the bowel wall during the longer transit period through the intestine.

DRUG DISTRIBUTION

The distribution process regulates the amount of drug reaching specific body compartments or tissues and hence the concentration of the drug at the receptor site. Distribution is influenced mainly by the degree of protein binding and red cell binding, tissue volumes, tissue solubility coefficients, and blood flow to various tissues. Extracellular inert binding to plasma proteins depends on the amount of binding protein available and the drug affinity constant for proteins; these factors are directly or indirectly modified by pathophysiological conditions and by other drugs and compounds.[11-18]

In blood, drugs may bind to albumin and several other serum proteins. The degree to which this occurs is usually measured as the percentage of total nondialyzable drug in the blood, that is, the percentage bound to large molecules. Binding to nonreceptor proteins also takes place outside the vascular compartment and may account for a significant fraction of the total drug in the body. The volume of distribution of a drug is directly proportional to the fraction of free drug in the plasma. Drug molecules bound to inert binding sites are not available for diffusion or interaction with receptors but are in equilibrium with free drug. Thus alterations in the concentration of free drug will result in changes in the amount (but not the percentage) bound. Nonreceptor protein binding sites are not very specific; many weak acids with different pharmacological effects bind to the same or closely related plasma protein sites. Therefore, different drugs may compete for the same binding sites. This can have important consequences when a high percentage of a potent drug (A) is bound; the binding sites must be loaded to achieve a therapeutic concentration of free drug in the plasma. Addition of a second drug (B) that competes for the same inert binding site (but not the receptor site) may result in a marked increase in the concentration of free drug A and thereby precipitate toxicity. A quantitative and qualitative reduction in plasma protein binding occurs in the newborn period.[19-21] At this stage infants, particularly preterm infants, have lower plasma albumin concentrations than at other ages (30 to 40 g/L), and the albumin is qualitatively different and has a lower affinity for drugs. Further modification of plasma protein binding is likely to occur at this age as a result of the higher free fatty acid and bilirubin concentrations and the lower blood pH. Concentrations of alpha-acid glycoproteins, which bind many basic drugs, are lower in the newborn than in the adult. Decreased protein binding may, therefore, contribute to the larger apparent volume of distribution for many drugs, for example, ketamine.[22]

In the neonate, differences in the size of the body fluid compartments, relatively smaller muscle mass and fat stores, and presumably greater blood flow per unit or organ weight influence the distribution of drugs to their active site and secondary redistribution. Metabolism and excretion may take place during redistribution. Total body water, extracellular fluid, and blood volume of the neonate are larger on a weight basis than those of an adult (Table 2–1).[23] The initial larger volume for distribution of a parenterally administered drug may explain, in part, why neonates appear to require larger amounts of some drugs on a weight basis to produce a given effect. Differences in fat stores and muscle mass at different ages are shown in Table 2–1.[24] Table 2–2 gives developmental estimates of tissue volumes and tissue blood flow derived from physiological studies and from autopsy of normal tissue at the Children's Hospital of Pittsburgh.[24-27] A high proportion of the cardiac output is distributed to the vessel-rich organs, particularly the brain. Smaller muscle mass and fat stores provide less uptake to inactive sites and tend to keep plasma concentration higher. The smaller amount of fat tissue in neonates provides a relatively small reservoir for fat-soluble drugs.

Blood-Brain Barrier

The blood-brain barrier, a lipid membrane interface between the endothelial cells of the brain vasculature

Table 2–1. BODY COMPOSITION DURING GROWTH

Body Compartment	Premature (1.5 kg)	Full Term (3.5 kg)	Adult (70 kg)
Total body water (% body weight)	83	73	60
Extracellular fluid (% body weight)	62	44	20
Blood volume (ml/kg)	60	85–105	70
Intracellular water (% body weight)	25	33	40
Muscle mass (% body weight)	15	20	50
Fat (% body weight)	3	12	18

Data from Friss-Hansen[23] and Widdowson.[24]

Table 2–2. AGE-RELATED ESTIMATES OF TISSUE VOLUME AND BLOOD FLOW

	Gas and Tissue Volumes (ml/kg)		Tissue Blood Flows (% CO)	
	Adult	*Infant*	*Adult*	*Infant*
Tidal volume	7	7		
Functional residual capacity	40	25		
Volume	70	90		
Brain	21	90	14.3	34
Heart	4	4.5	4.3	3
Splanchnic	57	70	28.6	25
Kidney	6	10	25.7	18
Muscle	425	180	11.4	10
Fat	150	100	5.7	5
Poorly perfused tissue	270	270	10.0	5

Data from Widdowson,[24] Smith and Nelson,[25] Guignard et al.,[26] and Altman and Dittmer.[27]

and the extracellular fluid of the brain, may be "immature" at birth.[28–35] The intercellular clefts of brain are closed; these are tight junctions. Transport of drugs into and out of brain depends on principles identical to those determining the movement of substances across other biological membranes. The rate of penetration of nonionized drugs into brain increases with the degree of lipid solubility. Active transport mechanisms or specific carrier systems allow rapid exchange of certain biologically active compounds and of certain inorganic and organic anions either into or from the brain. Some polar metabolites are cleared from the brain by diffusion into cerebrospinal fluid (sink action).

Oldendorf[36–39] has measured the blood-brain barrier permeability during a single capillary pass for a number of drugs relative to a highly diffusible tracer like water or butanol. The uptake of the drug is expressed as a percentage of the uptake of the highly diffusible tracer, the brain uptake index (BUI). Drugs with an oil-water partition coefficient below 0.01 hardly penetrate the cerebral capillaries during a single pass, whereas those with a partition coefficient above 0.1 are likely to have 50 percent or more penetration. Drugs having a partition coefficient greater than about 0.03 will undergo substantially complete clearance during a single brain passage (Fig. 2–1). For example, in adults morphine, with a limited lipid solubility, has rather limited brain uptake, whereas heroin, with a high lipid solubility, has high brain uptake. If the lipid solubility of a compound is very high, rapid diffusion across the barrier leads to rapid equilibration between blood and brain. The rate of entry is then determined by blood flow. Since in the infant the brain receives a large proportion of cardiac output, it is not surprising that the brain concentration of many drugs is higher in the infant than in the adult. Regional differences in brain perfusion will also affect the uptake of compounds into brain.

BIOTRANSFORMATION AND EXCRETION

Renal excretion plays a pivotal role in terminating the biological activity of a few drugs that have small molecular sizes or have polar characteristics at physiologic pH. Most drugs do not possess such physicochemical properties. Pharmacologically active organic molecules tend to be highly lipophilic and remain nonionized or only partially ionized at physiologic pH. They are often strongly bound to plasma proteins. Such substances are not readily filtered at the glomerulus. The lipophilic nature of renal tubular membranes also facilitates the reabsorption of hydrophobic compounds following their glomerular filtration. Consequently, most drugs would have a prolonged duration of action if termination of activity depended solely on renal excretion.

An alternative process that may lead to the termination or alteration of biological activity is metabolism. In general, lipophilic drugs are transformed to more polar and hence more readily excretable products. Most metabolic biotransformations occur at some point between absorption of the drug into the general circulation and its renal elimination. A few transformations occur in the intestinal lumen or intestinal wall. In general, all of these reactions can be assigned to two major categories called phase I and phase II reactions.

Phase I Reactions

Phase I reactions usually convert the parent drug to a more polar metabolite by introducing or unmasking a functional group (—OH, —NH₂, —SH). Often these metabolites are inactive, although in some instances activity is only modified. Metabolic products are often less active than the parent drug and may even be inactive. However, some biotransformation products have enhanced activity or toxic properties, including mutagenicity, teratogenicity, and carcinogenicity.

If phase I metabolites are sufficiently polar, they may be readily excreted. However, many phase I products are not eliminated rapidly and undergo a subsequent reaction in which an endogenous substrate such as glucuronic acid, sulfuric acid, acetic acid, or an amino acid combines with the newly established functional group to form a highly polar conjugate. Such conjugations or synthetic reactions are the hallmarks of phase II metabolism. A great variety of drugs undergo these sequential biotransformation reactions, although in some instances the parent drug may already have a functional group that may form a conjugate directly.

Although at all ages every tissue has some ability to metabolize drugs, the liver is the principal organ of drug metabolism. The overall rate of metabolism probably depends on both the size of the liver and the metabolizing ability of the appropriate microsomal enzyme system. Liver volume relative to body weight decreases from birth to adulthood, the relative volume in the first year of life being twice that at 14 years. Other sites of considerable metabolic acitivity include gastrointestinal tract, lungs, skin, and kidney. After oral administration, many drugs (for example, isoproterenol, meperidine, pentazocine, and morphine) are absorbed intact from the small intestine and transported first via the portal system to the liver, where they undergo extensive metabolism. This process has been called a first-pass effect. Some orally administered drugs (such as clonazepam and chlorpromazine) are more extensively metabolized in the intestine than in the liver. Thus, intestinal metabolism may contribute to the overall first-pass effect. First-pass effects may so greatly limit the bioavailability of orally administered drugs that alternative routes of administration must be used to achieve therapeutically effective blood levels. The lower gut harbors intestinal microorganisms that are capable of many biotransformation reactions. In addition, drugs may be metabolized by gastric acid (penicillin), digestive enzymes (polypeptides such as

insulin), or enzymes in the wall of the intestine (catecholamines).

Although drug biotransformation in vivo can occur by spontaneous, noncatalyzed chemical reactions, the majority are catalyzed by specific cellular enzymes. Many drug-metabolizing enzymes are located in the lipophilic membranes of the endoplasmic reticulum of the liver and other tissues. When these lamellar membranes are isolated by homogenization and fractionation of the cell, they re-form into vesicles called microsomes. Microsomes retain most of the morphological and functional characteristics of the intact membranes, including the rough and smooth surface features of the rough (ribosome-studded) and smooth (no ribosomes) endoplasmic reticulum. Whereas the rough microsomes tend to be dedicated to protein synthesis, the smooth microsomes are relatively rich in enzymes responsible for oxidative drug metabolism. In particular, they contain the important class of enzymes known as the mixed function oxidases.

Microsomal drug oxidations require cytochrome P-450, cytochrome P-450 reductase, NADPH, and molecular oxygen. The relative abundance of cytochrome P-450, as compared with that of the reductase

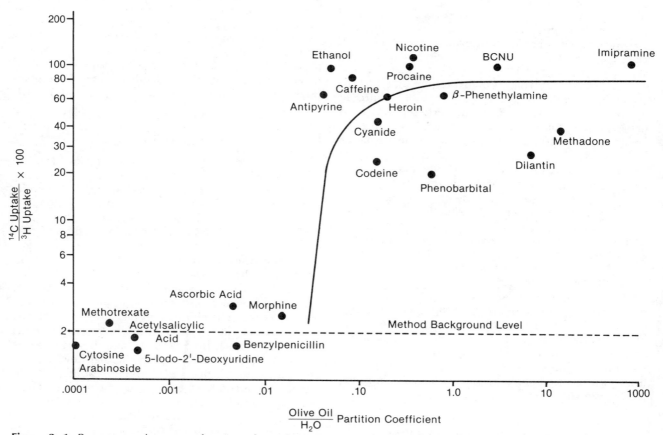

Figure 2–1. Percentage clearance of various drugs during a single brain circulatory passage vs. olive oil–water partition coefficients.

in the liver, contributes to making cytochrome P-450 heme reduction the rate-limiting step in hepatic drug oxidations. The potent oxidizing properties of this activated oxygen permit oxidation of a large number of substrates. Substrate specificity is very low for this enzyme complex. High solubility in lipids is the only common feature of the wide variety of structurally unrelated drugs and chemicals that serve as substrates in this system.

Phase II Reactions

Parent drugs or their phase I metabolites that contain suitable chemical groups often undergo coupling or conjugation reactions with an endogenous substance to yield drug conjugates. In general, conjugates are polar molecules that are readily excreted and often inactive. Certain conjugation reactions (sulfation of N-hydroxyacetylaminofluorine and N-acetylation of isoniazid) may lead to the formation of reactive species responsible for the hepatotoxicity of the drug. Conjugate formation involves high-energy intermediates and specific transfer enzymes. Such enzymes (transferases) may be located in microsomes or in the cytosol. They catalyze the coupling of an activated endogenous substance (such as the uridine 5'-diphosphate [UDP] derivative of glucuronic acid) with a drug or of an activated drug with an endogenous substrate. Because the endogenous substrates originate in the diet, nutrition plays a critical role in the regulation of drug conjugations.

The hepatic enzyme systems responsible for the metabolism of drugs are incompletely developed or absent in the neonate. Rats and ferrets develop the cytochrome P-450 system in liver microsomes to adult levels by 10 to 20 days. Of phase I biotransformation processes, the ability to oxidize drugs is most deficient in neonates, the ability to reduce substrates is much less so, and the ability to hydrolyze substrates is as effective as in adults. The activity of oxidative and reductive enzymes increases to adult levels within the first few days of life. Phase II processes—conjugation with sulfate, acetate, glucuronic acid, or amino acids—are severely limited at birth.[39-40] Neonatal hepatic tissues, for example, are unable to synthesize glucuronides because of low tissue levels of uridine diphosphate, glucuronic acid, and UDP-transferase, the last of which catalyzes transfer of glucuronic acid to foreign molecules.[41] Conjugation reactions with acetate occur by 1 month of age, with glucuronide by 2 months, and with amino acids by 3 months. Some of these metabolized drugs are recirculated and excreted in the urine; other metabolites or unmetabolized drugs are excreted in the bile.

Enzyme Induction and Inhibition

An interesting feature of some of these chemically dissimilar drug substrates is their ability, on repeated administration, to "induce" cytochrome P-450 by enhancing the rate of its synthesis or reducing its rate of degradation. Induction accelerates metabolism and usually results in a decrease in the pharmacological action of the inducer and also of coadministered drugs. However, in the case of drugs metabolically transformed to reactive intermediates, enzyme induction may exacerbate drug-mediated tissue toxicity. Various substrates appear to induce forms of cytochrome P-450 that have different molecular weights and exhibit different substrate specificities and immunochemical and spectral characteristics. In infants the enzyme activity of the cytochrome P-450 systems can be increased by known enzyme inducers such as benzopyrene or phenobarbital. Thus, the low enzyme activity for various substrates reflects lack of stimulation rather than inability of the enzyme system to be stimulated.[42] The age from birth determines the maturation of these enzyme systems, not the duration of gestation. Premature and full-term infants develop the ability to metabolize drugs to the same degree at the same time period after birth.

Other drug substrates may inhibit cytochrome P-450 enzyme activity. Proadifen (SK&F 525-A) and cimetidine bind avidly to the cytochrome molecule and thereby competitively inhibit the metabolism of potential substrates.[43-44] Some substrates irreversibly inhibit cytochrome P-450 via covalent interaction of a metabolically generated reactive intermediate that may react with either the apoprotein or the heme moiety of the cytochrome (for example, ethinyl estradiol, norethindrone, and spironolactone; fluroxene, secobarbital, and allobarbital; carbon disulfide; and propylthiouracil).[44]

Excretion

The ultimate route of elimination of most drugs or their metabolites is by way of the kidney. Since many drugs are simply filtered by the kidney, glomerular filtration rate (GFR) influences drug excretion and action. Inulin and thiosulfate clearances that reflect GFR are lower in newborns and young children than in adults. Volume clearance, when related to surface area, approaches adult values at about 3 months. If, on the other hand, clearance is related to weight, adult values are reached in about 10 days to 2 weeks. The time-clearance method resolves the question of which basis to select. The elimination half-life for thiosulfate is about three times slower in newborns than in older children or adults; by 3 weeks of age these differences disappear. The maturation of glomerular function may be related to changes in the permeability of the glomerular membrane or to conversion of nonfunctional glomeruli to functional participants in the process of filtration. Proximal tubular secretion assumes adult values in the first 4 to 5 months of age.[39] The glucuronide and sulfate metabolites of drugs may be secreted through the proximal tubules by an acid pump mechanism.

INHALATION ANESTHETICS

Age-Related Differences in Uptake and Distribution

The uptake of nitrous oxide, cyclopropane, and halothane is more rapid in infants and small children than in adults.[45-50] Salanitre and Rackow[46] compared the uptake of nitrous oxide among infants 0 to 6 months of age, 15-year-olds, and two groups of adults. An FE/FI (expiration/inspiration) ratio of 1.0 occurred in infants in about 25 minutes, in children in about 30 minutes, and in adults at about 60 minutes. Steward and Creighton[48] likewise noted more rapid wash-out of nitrous oxide in infants than in adults. These age-related differences in anesthetic uptake are more striking with halothane, which has a five-fold higher blood solubility than nitrous oxide. Salanitre and Rackow[46] showed that the uptake of halothane was more rapid in children 15 years of age than in adults. However, the uptake of halothane was determined concurrently with that of nitrous oxide. The rapid uptake of nitrous oxide may have influenced the early uptake of halothane because of the so-called second gas effect. More recently, Brandom and colleagues[50] measured the uptake of halothane in infants. FE/FI for halothane in these infants increased more rapidly than has been described in adults (Fig. 2–2).

Major differences between adults and infants in blood-gas solubility coefficients, body composition, alveolar ventilation, and the distribution of cardiac output explain the concomitant differences in their rates of uptake of anesthetic. Tidal volume on a weight basis (7 ml/kg) is relatively constant throughout life. However, the infant has a relatively high alveolar ventilation, particularly in relation to his functional residual capacity (FRC). The ratio of alveolar ventilation to FRC is about 5:1 in infants, contrasted with 1.4:1 in adults. The lung time constant is estimated to be 0.19 minute in infants and 0.73 minute in adults, for a gas with limited blood solubility (helium and nitrous oxide). Thus, lung wash-in or lung wash-out of inhalation anesthetics is relatively more rapid in infants than in adults. In infants controlled ventilation that increased alveolar ventilation would further increase this ratio; in adults it would appear difficult to utilize tidal breaths approaching FRC in magnitude.

The blood-gas solubility coefficients for halothane have been shown to vary with age.[51-52] Halothane is less soluble in blood taken from the fetal circulation of the placenta than it is in blood taken from adults. The influence of hematocrit, hemoglobin type, and plasma protein fractions on anesthetic solubility has not been well defined. The blood-gas solubility coefficient of nitrous oxide varies about 3 percent as hematocrit increases from 30 to 52 percent. If all other things were equal, the high cardiac output of the infant (on a weight basis about twice that of the adult) would retard the uptake of inhalation anesthetics. However, this effect is minimized by other factors. More important, a larger percentage of the infant's cardiac output is distributed to the vessel-rich tissue group. Compared with the adult the infant has increased brain mass and limited muscle mass and fat; significant differences in tissue blood flow correspond to these differences in tissue compartments.

We constructed an 11-compartment model incorporating age-dependent differences in respiratory variables, lung and tissue volumes, and (tissue regional) blood flow to illustrate these differences.[50] Such a model allows one to predict FE/FI ratios over time and, more important, tissue anesthetic concentrations

Figure 2–2. Predicted versus observed FE/FI for halothane in infants and adults.

Figure 2–3. Predicted concentration of halothane in the brain. The values in Figure 2–4 were derived from our computerized model of anesthetic uptake and distribution. The model infant weighed 4 kg; the model adult weighed 70 kg. In both cases normal ventilation and a constant inspired fraction of 0.5 percent halothane were employed. Tissue levels are given in mg/100 ml of tissue.

for any given anesthetic. Tissue solubility coefficients for adults were used in this model and may have introduced minor errors. For example, brain water content decreases with increasing age; this may influence the brain tissue solubility coefficient.[53] Our model predicts that the concentration of halothane in tissues (such as the brain and heart) will increase more rapidly in infants (Figs. 2–3 and 2–4) than in adults, given the same inspired concentration of halothane. The reduced muscle mass of the infant compared with the adult, and the concurrent reduction of the proportion of cardiac output perfusing muscle, tends to concentrate the cardiac output in infants toward the more highly perfused vessel-rich organs such as the brain and heart. Early in an anesthetic induction the infant has higher tissue concentration of anesthetic than the

adult; at some relatively distant time both will have the same tissue concentrations, if one assumes the partition coefficients to be the same in infants and adults. Another way to state this difference is in terms of tissue time constants, $\lambda V/Q$ (blood-tissue solubility coefficient times volume divided by tissue blood flow). Given the same concentration of anesthetic in arterial blood, the anesthetic concentration will increase more rapidly in a tissue with a shorter time constant. We derived tissue time constants for infants and adults using the anatomical and physiological assumptions of our model (Table 2–3). Time constants of infant tissues are less than the corresponding time constants in the adult. Although the volume of some vessel-rich tissues (such as brain) relative to total body weight is greater in the infant than in the adult, these tissues have so much more blood flow in the infant that their time constants are smaller than those in adults.

Influence of Intracardiac Shunts on Uptake

Intracardiac shunts can alter the uptake of inhalation anesthetics.[54-55] Their influence is more pronounced with relatively insoluble agents. A right-to-left shunt slows the uptake of anesthetic as the anesthetic tension or concentration in the arterial blood increases more slowly. Induction of anesthesia is prolonged. Using overpressure to achieve a more rapid induction in infants with significant right-to-left shunts from congenital heart disease can be hazardous. If significant cardiovascular depression occurs from a relative anesthetic overdose, it is equally difficult to decrease the anesthetic concentration. The influence of a left-to-right shunt on anesthetic uptake depends on the size of the shunt and on whether a right-to-left shunt exists. A large (> 80 percent) left-to-right shunt increases the rate of anesthetic transfer from the lungs to the arterial blood; smaller shunts (< 50 percent) have a negligible effect on uptake. A left-to-right shunt may speed induction when it coexists with a large right-to-left shunt. Increases in pulmonary vascular resistance or decreases in systemic vascular resistance occasionally can reverse left-to-right shunts.

Anesthetic Requirements

The anesthetic requirements for various inhalation anesthetics (cyclopropane, halothane, and enflurane)

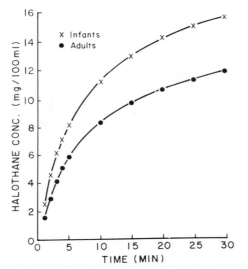

Figure 2–4. Predicted concentration of halothane in the heart. See Figure 2–3 for legend.

Table 2–3. TIME CONSTANTS (MINUTES)

	Adult	Infant
Brain	3.4	2.2
Heart	2.3	1.4
Splanchnic	5.0	2.5
Kidney	0.35	0.30
Muscle	49.0	8.4
Fat	2000.0	540.0

Tissue time constants = $\lambda V/Q$. (See text.)

generally are related inversely to age.[56-60] Anesthetic requirements are usually quantitated by the minimum alveolar concentration (MAC) of anesthetic at which 50 percent of the patients do not move in response to a surgical stimulus. Alternatively, one can estimate MAC for an individual patient as an intermediate concentration between a concentration associated with movement and a concentration associated with no movement. The MAC (also called the median effective dose, or ED50) for halothane in infants and children has been determined by several groups of investigators.

In the first month of life the relation between age and MAC is somewhat complex. During the first week of life the response of the newborn to pain is attenuated even in the awake state. During the first few months of life both the sensitivity to pain and the behavioral response to pain rapidly mature. Gregory and associates[60] noted that the MAC for halothane is lower in the fetal lamb than in the newborn lamb; in addition, the MAC for halothane increased over the first 12 hours of life in the newborn lambs. The increase in MAC in the newborn lambs was associated with a decrease in serum progesterone. At pharmacological doses progesterone is an anesthetic in the rat. No causal relationship exists.[61] Increased metabolic rate and oxygen consumption after birth may also contribute to the increase in anesthetic requirements. Increased plasma peptide concentrations have been documented in newborns during the immediate postnatal period; in the first month of life these concentrations decrease to adult concentrations.[62] In adults peptides do not cross the blood-brain barrier. In neonates one could postulate increased permeability of the blood-brain barrier to these peptides although CSF concentrations have not been documented. However, Gregory and associates[60] could not reverse the early "analgesia" in newborn lambs with naloxone.

As perplexing as the progressive increase in MAC through the first month or so of life is the gradual and progressive decrease after 6 months. Is this related to changes in oxygen consumption, is it related to differences in anesthetic solubilities, or is it a conundrum of definition?

MAC is an indirect measurement of the anesthetic partial pressure at the anesthetic sites of action. At equilibrium the partial pressure of anesthetic is equal in all tissue compartments of the body. However, the tissue concentration (mg/100 g tissue) of anesthetic will vary with the solubulity of the anesthetic in that tissue. Miller and colleagues[63] have suggested that a certain anesthetic molar concentration at the site of action is necessary to produce anesthesia. The molar concentration of anesthesia at the site of action is the product of the anesthetic partial pressure and the anesthetic solubility at the site. Measuring of anesthetic concentration in the brain allows one to estimate the molar concentration required in the brain to produce anesthesia. Cook and coworkers[53] noted that the ED50 for halothane was higher in 15-day-old rats than in 30- or 60-day-old rats. In contrast, the concentration of halothane in the brain under anesthesia was lower in the 15-day-old rats than in the older rats. This difference in brain concentration for halothane as a function of age is most likely due to the difference in water content in the younger rats. When corrected for differences in water content, the estimated halothane concentrations in brain dry weight appear comparable in the three age groups of rats. This suggests that nearly equal concentrations of halothane in the nonaqueous phase of the brain are achieved at the end point of anesthesia in different aged animals. A higher partial pressure of anesthetic (ED50 or MAC) may be necessary in the younger animal to compensate for the high water content of the developing brain.

Age-related differences in blood-gas solubility coefficients may also influence the brain anesthetic concentration and hence contribute to age-related differences in MAC. Brandom examined this issue using our model of anesthetic distribution (Brandom BW, unpublished data). She altered the blood gas solubility coefficient of halothane while holding all other physiological variables constant, to assess the effect of this change on brain anesthetic concentrations. With a blood-gas solubility coefficient of 2.3 the FE/FI ratio was 0.813 after 45 minutes of exposure to 0.5 percent halothane; the corresponding estimate of brain halothane concentration was 15.6 mg/100 ml. With a solubility coefficient of 1.9, that measured in neonatal cord blood, the FE/FI ratio was 0.843 after 45 minutes; the corresponding brain halothane concentration was 13.2 mg/100 ml. The decrease in the blood-gas solubility coefficient caused a more rapid increase in FE/FI and a slower increase in tissue anesthetic concentration. FE/FI was 3 percent higher with the less soluble anesthetic but the associated brain concentration was 17 percent lower. These data suggest that changes in blood-gas solubility may contribute to age-dependent differences in the movement of anesthetic through the body to the brain, and hence to age-dependent differences in anesthetic requirements.

Cardiovascular Effects of Inhalation Anesthetics

The incidence of bradycardia, hypotension, and cardiac arrest during induction of anesthesia is higher in infants and small children than in adults.[58, 64-66] This has been attributed to an increased sensitivity of the cardiovascular system to potent agents. Rao and associates[67] noted that halothane, isoflurane, and enflurane depress the force of contraction in isolated neonatal rat atria significantly more than in the adult atria. This may be related to the decreased contractile element in the neonatal myocardium. However, the greater incidence of untoward effects can be attributed partly to differences in uptake and to the use of higher-than-necessary inspired concentrations of potent agents. The myocardial and brain concentration of anesthetic at equal inspired concentrations may be higher early in anesthetic induction in the infant than in the adult. These higher tissue concentrations may produce what appears to be augmented cardiovascular effect. To define clearly the issue of age-related cardiovascular sensitivity it is necessary to measure simultaneously the determinants of cardiac output in anesthetized patients (or animals) at known end-tidal concentrations of anesthetic and at known MAC multiples. In addition, it is necessary to define the sensitivity of cardiovascular "protective" reflexes (baroreceptor reflex) at MAC multiples of the anesthetic. Direct measurement of cardiac output, contractility, preload, and afterload involves invasive techniques. Few patient studies have been done, but the results of several key animal studies are available.

The hemodynamic effects of halothane have been determined in the developing piglet.[68] MAC for halothane in piglets (1 to 11 days) was 0.87 percent (range 0.73 to 0.99 percent). Cardiac index (CI), mean arterial pressure (MAP), heart rate (HR), and all contractility indexes (LV peak dP/dT, left ventricular shortening fraction [SF], and mean rate of left ventricular circumferential fiber shortening [VCF]) decreased relative to concentration after 0.5 percent and 1 percent halothane (Table 2–4). When heart rate was kept constant with atrial pacing, dP/dT/DP40, CI, and MAP remained severely depressed at the two concentrations of halothane. Estimates of preload, stroke volume index (SVI), and total peripheral vascular index (TPVI) did not change significantly. Thus, the major adverse hemodynamic effect of halothane was its negative inotropic action, not negative chronotropic or

Table 2–4. HEMODYNAMIC VALUES FOR END-TIDAL HALOTHANE IN PIGLETS

Variable	Control	0.5%	1%	0.5%	0%
MAP (mmHg)	96.2 (21.2)	81.0 (17.4)	63.5 (20.3)	78.8 (18.0)	88.5 (15.5)
CI (L/min/kg)	0.288 (0.098)	0.237 (0.054)	0.205 (0.056)	0.264 (0.073)	0.293 (0.086)
dP/dT (mmHg/sec)	3640 (860)	2480 (800)	1560 (600)	2260 (720)	3500 (920)
SF	0.45 (0.11)	0.30 (0.15)	0.21 (0.10)	0.21 (0.11)	0.35 (0.09)
VCF (circ/sec)	3.40 (1.35)	2.32 (0.73)	1.51 (0.86)	1.76 (0.64)	2.93 (0.93)
LVEDP (mmHg)	4.1 (3.5)	4.9 (3.2)	6.6 (4.4)	5.0 (4.3)	4.4 (3.6)
LVIDd (cm)	1.49 (0.36)	1.46 (0.32)	1.63 (0.37)	1.63 (0.31)	1.45 (0.44)
HR (beats/min)	215 (41)	185 (40)	156 (33)	186 (51)	229 (54)
SVI (ml/beat/kg)	1.39 (0.54)	1.13 (0.61)	1.24 (0.51)	1.32 (0.78)	1.39 (0.64)
TPRI (mmHg/L/ min/kg)	0.364 (0.133)	0.357 (0.097)	0.323 (0.094)	0.317 (0.114)	0.328 (0.112)

Values are means ± 1 standard deviation.

MAP = mean aortic pressure; CI = cardiac index; dP/dT = Maximum first derivative of left ventricular (LV) pressure with respect to time; SF = LV shortening fraction; VCF = mean rate of LV circumferential fiber shortening; LVEDP = LV end-diastolic pressure; LVIDd = LV internal diastolic dimension; HR = heart rate; SVI = stroke volume index; TPRI = total peripheral resistance index.

Variables were obtained at end-tidal halothane values ascending to 1 percent and then returning to 0 percent.

loading activity. This effect occurred at a concentration less than MAC. These cardiovascular changes were not age-related. In piglets studied by Bailie and colleagues,[69] profound bradycardia and hypotension were associated with an unexplained increase in peripheral resistance. The change in cardiovascular response to halothane with age in the piglet is similar to that in newborn infants and children. In our study, the degree of change of each variable with the administration of 1 percent halothane did not correlate with age over the first 2.5 weeks of life. However, the pattern of cardiovascular response to halothane in pigs appears to change with increasing age beyond this period. At equal end-tidal halothane concentrations supplemented by 60 to 70 per cent nitrous oxide, 3-month-old pigs (21 to 28 kg) studied by Merin and associates[70] had a depression of CI comparable to that observed in our younger animals. However, MAP was considerably lower in the older animal study than in ours and was accompanied by peripheral vasodilation and marked reduction in dP/dT. Our newborn piglets had less profound reductions in CI, MAP, and dP/dT, and no important change in peripheral resistance. Of note, bradycardia occurred regularly only in the newborn piglets. These differences in HR among pigs of different ages under halothane anesthesia were probably due to the more highly developed baroreceptor responses of the older animals.[71] Recently, Lerman and coworkers,[59] found that at equipotent concentrations of halothane, the incidence of hypotension and bradycardia was equal in neonates and infants. These data agree with our findings that the maximal degrees of change in MAP and HR did not correlate significantly with age.

In a similar study by us, the MAC for isoflurane in piglets was determined to be 1.20 percent ± 0.4 percent (unpublished data). At 0.5 MAC, isoflurane caused a large, significant reduction in MAP, TPRI, and dP/dT/DP40 (Table 2–5). At 1 MAC, MAP and dP/dT/DP40 decreased further, and TPRI and SF remained depressed. At 1.3 MAC, these four variables remained low. Preload (left ventricular end-diastolic pressure, or LVEDP) and SVI did not change significantly during the study period. CI and HR were significantly less than baseline only at 1.3 MAC, although bradycardia did not occur in all animals. We used atrial pacing at baseline HR in five piglets that developed bradycardia at 1.3 MAC, to determine the influence of HR on the other variables. CI then remained within 2 percent of baseline, while MAP and TPRI each decreased 49 percent and dP/dT/DP40 decreased 45 percent from baseline values. The large decrease in MAP at 1 MAC isoflurane was offset by a similar decrease in afterload, leaving CI unchanged. During pacing dP/dT/DP40 is a particularly reliable indicator of LV contractility, since it is independent of changes in HR, preload, and afterload. The large reduction in afterload may have also partly offset the effect of reduced contractility on CI. However, the

Table 2–5. HEMODYNAMIC VALUES FOR ISOFLURANE

	Baseline	0.5 MAC	1 MAC	1.3 MAC
CI (L/min/kg)	0.263 (0.039)	0.293 (0.051) +11%	0.251 (0.039) −5%	0.225 (0.042) −14%
MAP (mmHg)	120 (23)	92 (20) −23%	76 (16) −37%	66 (15) −45%
HR (beats/min)	194 (43)	187 (41) −4%	164 (22) −15%	157 (24) −19%
dP/dT (mmHg/sec)	3457 (843)	2360 (577) −33%	1827 (328) −48%	1573 (433) −56%
dP/dT/DP40 (mmHg/sec)	2560 (519)	2040 (448) −20%	1733 (327) −32%	1480 (319) −42%
SF (%)	40 (10)	35 (8) −13%	32 (9) −20%	28 (7) −30%
TPRI (mmHg/L/min/kg)	.444 (.137)	.314 (.77) −29%	.303 (.79) −32%	.298 (.73) −33%
SVI (ml/beat/kg)	1.5 (0.5)	1.7 (0.4) −13%	1.7 (0.4) −13%	1.6 (0.3) −7%
LVEDP (mmHg)	4.0 (3.4)	2.9 (2.8)	4.7 (1.7)	4.5 (1.8)

Abbreviations as in Table 2–4.

reduced MAP should have caused tachycardia via the baroreceptor response. The lack of tachycardia signifies either an immature baroreflex or a drug-induced attenuation of baroreceptor responsiveness.

Isoflurane had fewer adverse cardiovascular effects than 1.3 MAC halothane in the same animal model. Although the drugs similarly reduced dP/dT and HR at 1.3 MAC, isoflurane reduced TPRI 3 times as much and MAP 1.5 times as much as did halothane; the resulting reduction in CI with isoflurane was thus only half that with halothane. At 0.5 MAC, isoflurane increased CI, whereas halothane reduced it. During anesthesia in the newborn isoflurane may permit greater hemodynamic stability than halothane. The alarming reduction in MAP caused by isoflurane may reflect only a decrease in peripheral resistance in the face of normal cardiac output.

Effects of Anesthetics on Baroreceptor Reflexes

Baroreceptor reflexes modulate changes in blood pressure by altering heart rate, myocardial contractility, and systemic vascular resistance. In the unanesthetized infant, particularly the premature infant, these protective reflexes may be limited. Anesthetic agents may further blunt these reflexes. To evaluate baroresponses, Gregory[72] examined the relationship among changes in heart rate and blood pressure in premature infants anesthetized with halothane in preparation for

ligation of a patent ductus arteriosus. After the ductus was ligated and systemic blood flow increased, the arterial pressure increased 38 percent (to about control values) without a change in heart rate. These data suggest that potent anesthetics abolish baroreceptor activity in premature infants.

In subsequent studies the effects of halothane and nitrous oxide on the baroresponse in adult and baby rabbits were evaluated.[73–74] In these studies, the baroreceptor response was tested by increasing the systolic pressure 20 to 30 percent with phenylephrine. When the baroreflexes are functioning, this increase in systolic pressure decreases heart rate (Fig. 2–5). The slope of the curve relating heart rate to systolic pressure, a reflection of baroreflex sensitivity, was decreased in adults and babies with halothane in a concentration-dependent manner (Table 2–6). More important, the sensitivity of the reflex was lower in the awake baby rabbits than in the awake adults, at equal MAC multiples of halothane. Halothane (1.0 MAC) effectively abolished the baroresponse in baby rabbits. In the newborn rabbit, nitrous oxide also diminishes

Figure 2–5. Relationship between heart rate and arterial pressure (FAP) in a baby rabbit. P ↑ indicates the point at which phenylephrine was injected. With the rabbit awake, the heart rate began to decrease within three beats after the initial rise in arterial pressure. During anesthesia the decrease in heart rate occurred later (after nine beats). The time from the onset of the rise in pressure to the onset of the decrease in heart rate is defined as the lag time.

Table 2–6. RELATIONSHIP BETWEEN HALOTHANE AND BARORECEPTOR RESPONSE

| | Slope of Heart Rate vs. Systolic Pressure (MS/mmHg) | | Log Time (S) | |
	Baby	Adult	Baby	Adult
Awake	1.94±0.27	2.90±0.41	0.67±0.25	0.75±0.67
0.5 MAC	0.40±0.21*	1.33±0.28*	1.11±0.26*†	1.19±0.61*
1.0 MAC	0.23±0.08*	1.05±0.35*	1.75±0.51*	1.50±0.63*†
1.5 MAC	0.07±0.08*†	0.60±0.20*†	2.44±0.44*†	1.87±0.30*†

Values are means ± 1 standard deviation.

*Significantly different from values obtained when animals were awake (p<0.001).

†Significantly different from values obtained at 0.5 MAC halothane (p<0.005).

baroreceptor activity in a concentration-dependent manner, to the same degree as does halothane (at equal MAC multiples).

The reasons why anesthesia depresses the baroreceptor reflexes more in baby rabbits are unknown. Most likely they are related to developmental differences in the autonomic nervous system. Baroresponses may be mediated in part by acute changes in plasma catecholamines. Young animals have significant amounts of norepinephrine in their adrenergic terminals, but the nerves fail to arborize, and incompletely penetrate the myocardium. In addition, the vascular response to vasopressors is also less in the neonate than in the adult. The baroresponse includes a reduction in sympathetic outflow. Since the neonate's sympathetic nervous system is inadequately developed, an increase in systolic pressure may not permit the heart rate to decrease as much. The parasympathetic nervous system is very active in the newborn.

The lack of responsiveness of the baroreflexes places the infant at considerable disadvantage during anesthesia with potent inhalation anesthetics. For reasons previously discussed, the incidence of hypotension and bradycardia is high in this age group.

Margin of Safety

The separation between MAC and the lethal concentration of a potent inhalation anesthetic defines the safety margin or therapeutic ratio. Wolfson and colleagues[75–76] determined the therapeutic ratio (TR) of the potent anesthetic in adult rats. This ratio is defined as the mean anesthetic heart concentration at cardiovascular failure divided by the mean anesthetic heart concentration at anesthesia. In their study, isoflurane had a higher therapeutic ratio than did halothane. Kissen and associates[77] confirmed this and in addition noted that the standard safety margin, the percentage by which the effective dose in 95 percent (ED95) has to be increased before the dose that is lethal in 5 percent (LD5) is reached, is also higher with isoflurane than with halothane.

Cook and colleagues[53] noted that the therapeutic

ratio for halothane was decreased about 50 percent in young rats compared with older rats. This study suggests that at higher anesthetic concentrations myocardial contractility and protective cardiovascular reflexes are not preserved in the infant. Recently, we determined that isoflurane and halothane have similar therapeutic ratios in the newborn piglet (2.5:1) (unpublished data).

Biotransformation of Inhalation Anesthetics

Significant biotransformation of inhalation anesthetics occurs in the liver. The metabolites may be toxic to tissue. Carbon tetrachloride and chloroform are hepatotoxic in adult animals; however, they are not hepatotoxins in animals less than 1 to 2 weeks of age. In the newborn rat the metabolism of halothane takes several weeks to reach adult levels.[78] The concentration of free fluoride, a nephrotoxic metabolite of methoxyflurane, is lower in infants and children.[79] Nephrotoxicity from free fluoride has, likewise, been reported after enflurane anesthesia in obese patients. This is unlikely in infants because of their limited fat deposits. Likewise, biotransformation of isoflurane is unlikely. Differences in the relative rates of metabolism of inhalation anesthetics in infants and adults have not been compared, nor has any determination been made of differences in intermediate metabolites.

INTRAVENOUS DRUGS

Sedative-Hypnotics

A variety of sedative-hypnotic drugs appear to have increased toxic effects in the neonate.[80] The mechanism of this increased sensitivity has been elucidated for some of the barbiturates and benzodiazepines.

Diazepam

Diazepam is a widely used sedative-hypnotic and anticonvulsant. Infants born of mothers who have had diazepam for sedation during labor have shown lethargy and impaired thermoregulation for several days. The probable reasons for this prolongation of effect are several. Brain levels of diazepam and N-demethyldiazepam, a demethylated metabolite, have been noted to be higher in newborn rats and guinea pigs for up to 180 minutes after subcutaneous administration. This higher brain concentration probably explains why diazepam also gives greater protection against Metrazol convulsions in newborn rats and guinea pigs than in adult animals.[81]

The plasma half-life of diazepam and the nature of the diazepam metabolites formed vary with maturity.[82] The premature infant and the mature infant at term eliminate diazepam at a slower rate than do older infants, children, and adults. Also, in premature infants N-demethyldiazepam could not be measured in plasma until 4 hours after injection; its plasma concentration was still rising at 48 hours. In contrast, N-demethyldiazepam was measured in the plasma of older infants and children by 1 hour and had peaked by 24 hours. In the premature infant hydroxylated metabolites of diazepam did not form; in term infants they formed in limited amounts. In adults 71 percent of diazepam or its metabolites was excreted in the urine and about 10 percent in the feces. No quantification of urinary excretion has been performed in infants or children.

Barbiturates

On a mg/kg basis barbiturates are more lethal to newborns than to more mature animals.[83-85] The sleeping times of newborn animals are markedly prolonged at sublethal doses given on an equal mg/kg basis.[85] Greater penetration of the blood-brain barrier by barbiturates has been found in neonates as opposed to older animals.[86] We have recently determined the brain uptake index (BUI) at 15 seconds for pentobarbital in developing rats (Table 2–7). BUI was higher in the younger rats and exceeded 100 percent. These data suggest that capillary transit time is less than 15 seconds in younger rats. High brain blood flow rather than differential permeability probably explains these observations for pentobarbital, which is highly lipid-soluble. In addition, the brain levels of hexobarbital on arousal or following death from respiratory failure are lower in neonates than in adults. This suggests that the barbiturates are more potent in the neonatal brain.

Neonates have a decreased ability to metabolize barbiturates.[87] The longer-acting barbiturates, which are in part excreted unmetabolized in the urine, would be expected to have prolonged or elevated blood levels.[88-89] Glucuronic acid conjugation of barbiturates develops rapidly and increases thirtyfold during the first 3 weeks of life.[40] For the ultrashort-acting barbiturates redistribution is as important as metabolism in the liver in lowering the brain concentration.[90] Blood concentrations of thiopentone decrease about as rapidly in newborns as in their mothers.[91] The use of these ultrashort-acting barbiturates for induction of anesthesia is, therefore, not a pharmacological problem, although the lack of a suitable intravenous route is often a practical deterrent.

Table 2–7. AGE-RELATED CHANGES IN BRAIN UPTAKE OF MORPHINE AND PENTOBARBITAL

Age (Days)	Brain Uptake Index (%)		Brain Water Content (%)
	Morphine	*Pentobarbital*	
7	36.2 ± 3.5	213.3 ± 20.6	87.9 ± 0.05
15	17.2 ± 3.2	78.0 ± 1.5	84.1 ± 0.1
30	7.4 ± 0.8	61.2 ± 5.0	79.6 ± 0.1
60	5.6 ± 1.3	44.0 ± 3.0	78.0 ± 0.1

Mean ± standard error.

Table 2–8. PHARMACOKINETICS OF KETAMINE AS A FUNCTION OF AGE

Age	β	AUC (μg/kg/min)	Cl (ml/min/kg)	Vd (L/kg)	t½β min
< 3 months	0.004	153.8	12.9	3.46	184.7
4–12 months	0.012	58.7	35.0	3.03	65.1
4 years	0.023	83.6	25.1	1.18	31.6
Adults	0.0315	99.0	20.0	.75	107.3

AUC = area under the curve; Cl = clearance; Vd = volume of distribution.

Ketamine

Ketamine is a nonbarbiturate cyclohexamine derivative that produces dissociation of the cortex from the limbic system; it may also act on the brain stem. There is frequently electroencephalographic seizure activity, particularly in the limbic system and cortex without clinical manifestations. This may be the mechanism of its action. On a μg/kg basis the amount of ketamine required to prevent gross movements is four times greater in infants under 6 months than in 6-year-olds.[92] Acute studies show little metabolism of ketamine by the newborn.[93]

Waterman and Livingstone[94] noted that after ketamine the sleeping times of rats decreased with increasing age; the onset time of sleep was significantly shorter in younger rats than in older ones. The demethylated metabolite of ketamine was present at recovery from anesthesia in 1-week-old rats; the oxidated metabolite was not present until 2 to 4 weeks of age. A dramatic decrease in sleeping time after ketamine was associated with the appearance of the oxidated metabolite.

Recently we have determined the pharmacokinetics of ketamine in patients of different ages (Table 2–8). In infants less than 3 months of age the volume of distribution was similar to that in older infants but the elimination half-life was prolonged. Hence, clearance was reduced in the younger infants. Reduced metabolism and renal excretion in the young infant are the likely causes.

In the "anesthetic" state associated with ketamine, respiration and blood pressure are usually well maintained. However, use of ketamine in infants, particularly at the high doses required for lack of movement, has been associated with respiratory depression and apnea.[95] Generalized extensor spasm with opisthotonus also has been seen in infants.[96] Intracranial pressure may increase in infants with hydrocephalus.[97] In addition, acute increases in pulmonary artery pressure occasionally have been seen in an infant with congenital heart disease when ketamine was used as an anesthetic for cardiac catheterization.[98] Recent studies suggest that pulmonary vascular resistance is not changed by ketamine in infants with either normal or elevated pulmonary vascular resistance as long as the airway and ventilation are maintained.[99-100]

Morphine and Meperidine

Meperidine (0.5 to 1 mg/kg) and morphine (0.05 to 0.1 mg/kg) are used to reinforce nitrous oxide–

oxygen anesthesia in the neonate. Such low doses attenuate the cardiovascular responses to surgical stress. In the past, high-dose meperidine and morphine anesthesia was given with oxygen-air to critically ill infants, particularly those requiring palliative heart surgery. The cardiovascular effects of these narcotics seemed minimal.

Narcotics are more toxic to newborn animals than to older animals.[80] In neonates, morphine depresses respiration more than meperidine does at a ratio of 1:10; in adults 10 mg of morphine produces respiratory depression equal to that from 100 mg meperidine.[101] The blood-brain barrier is more permeable to morphine and dihydromorphinone in newborn animals than in older animals. Brain concentration of morphine several hours after injection was two to four times greater in brains of younger rats despite equal blood concentration. This finding may be related to greater perfusion or to greater permeability, or both, in the newborn. We recently determined the brain uptake index, BUI, for morphine in developing rats (Table 2–7). The BUI was higher in younger rats than in the older rats. Such developmentally increased permeability is not seen with meperidine.[102] This is not surprising since the lipid solubility of meperidine is quite high.

Morphine is inactivated by N-demethylation and glucuronide conjugation; the inactive forms are largely excreted in the urine. In spite of the inefficient metabolism of morphine there is little difference in the plasma half-life of morphine between newborn and older animals.[103] Meperidine in inactive forms is also largely excreted. De-esterification and N-demethylation occur mainly in the liver. In adults the rate of transformation ranges from 10 to 20 percent per hour.[41] In newborn animals the plasma half-life of meperidine is about twice that of the adult. Neonates excrete 25 to 40 percent of a dose of meperidine in about 48 hours, almost exclusively in the demethylated form.[103]

Fentanyls

Fentanyl (3 to 5 μg/kg) is used to reinforce nitrous oxide–oxygen anesthesia in the neonate; high-dose fentanyl (25 to 50 μg/kg) is popular as the primary anesthetic in infants undergoing cardiac anesthesia. Bradycardia and chest wall rigidity are potential features of high-dose fentanyl anesthesia. For these reasons it is common to administer muscle relaxants with wanted cardiovascular side effects (pancuronium or gallamine) to ameliorate the effects of fentanyl. The cardiovascular effects of fentanyl at doses of 30 to 75 μg/kg fentanyl (with pancuronium) are minimal.[104] Modest decreases in mean arterial pressure and systemic vascular resistance index were noted by Hickey and colleagues.[105] Other indexes of cardiac function were unchanged. Schieber and coworkers[106] documented that the cardiovascular effects of fentanyl (without relaxant) are concentration-dependent; a similar relationship between decreases in systolic blood pressure and concentration was noted by Koren and associates.[107] Respiratory depression is probably concentration-related.

The dose of fentanyl needed to guarantee satisfactory anesthesia for infants is unknown. Age-related differences in the kinetics and sensitivity to fentanyl and changes in kinetics associated with profound pathophysiological conditions make generalizations difficult.[108–111] However, in the neonate fentanyl clearance seems comparable to that in the older child or adult; fentanyl clearance is markedly reduced in the premature infant. The elimination half-life is prolonged in neonates and in premature infants. These marked variations in kinetics reflect age differences and perhaps differences in anesthetic, dose, and duration of sampling. We noted that in infants having cardiac surgery fentanyl (50 μg/kg) was not uniformly effective in blunting cardiovascular responses nor hormonal responses to surgery despite rather uniform fentanyl plasma concentrations.

Several new analogues of fentanyl are undergoing clinical trials. Sufentanil is about seven times more potent than fentanyl and has minimal cardiovascular effects. Bradycardia is an uncommon feature. Alfentanil is equally potent to fentanyl but has a shorter duration of action. Because of its relatively short duration of action alfentanil may be particularly useful in neonatal anesthesia. Unfortunately, this has not been studied.

LOCAL ANESTHETICS

The rates of plasma decay for lidocaine and mepivacaine are similar in adults and newborns. However, the plasma levels of lidocaine and mepivacaine in the neonate that produce cardiovascular and respiratory depression are about one-half those in adults.[103] The convulsive dose for infants on a mg/kg basis of either ester-type (benzocaine) or amide-type (lidocaine) local anesthetics is not known. The rate of metabolism of the ester-type local anesthetics is decreased in the infant because pseudocholinesterase levels are low.[112] The newborn metabolizes lidocaine,[113] but the rates of metabolism of the amide-type local anesthetics in the neonate are not known.[114–115]

ATROPINE

Strong cholinergic stimulation, such as from cyclopropane, halothane, methoxyflurane, and succinylcholine, can produce profound bradycardia and reduce cardiac output in infants. The primary purpose of atropine in pediatric anesthesia is to protect against cholinergic challenge; its secondary purpose is to inhibit the production of secretions.

If atropine is given intravenously in incremental doses, more atropine is needed in children less than 2 years of age on a weight basis to accelerate the heart rate; however, acceleration uniformly occurs with 14.3 μg/kg.[116] A dose of 30 μg/kg appears to be vagolytic in infants, children, and adults. This dose provides adequate protection against a cholinergic challenge. In all age groups, 5 to 10 µg/kg atropine will minimally decrease salivation.[117]

MUSCLE RELAXANTS

Throughout infancy the neuromuscular junction matures physically and biochemically, the contractile properties of skeletal muscle change, the amount of muscle in proportion to body weight increases, and the neuromuscular junction is variably sensitive to relaxants. In addition, the apparent volume of distribution of relaxants, their redistribution and excretion (clearance), and possibly their rate of metabolism change. These factors influence the dose-response relationship of relaxants and the duration of neuromuscular blockade. It is not surprising, therefore, that the infant's or child's response to relaxants is different from that of the adult.[118]

Structural and Functional Development of the Neuromuscular System

The structural and functional development of the neuromuscular system is incomplete at birth.[119-123] The conduction velocity of motor nerves increases throughout gestation as nerve fibers myelinate. The myotubules connect to mature muscle fibers in the latter part of intrauterine life and in the first several weeks after birth. Some slow-contracting muscle (intrinsic muscles of the hand) is progressively converted to fast-contracting muscle, with a concomitant change in the force-velocity relationship. The percentage of slow muscle fibers in both the diaphragm and the intercostal muscles of infants increases during the first months of life. Synaptic transmission is relatively slow at birth, but more important, the rate at which acetylcholine is released during repetitive nerve stimulation is limited in the infant. Thus the margin of safety for neurotransmission is reduced in infants compared with adults.

Unanesthetized newborn infants appear to have less neuromuscular reserve during tetanic stimulation than do adults. In neonates there is no fade of twitch height with repetitive stimulation at rates of 1 to 2 Hz; at 20 Hz, however, there is significant fade. Premature infants may show post-tetanic exhaustion for 15 to 20 minutes.[124] Goudsouzian[125] noted slower contraction times of the thumb following slow and rapid rates of stimulation in term infants (1 to 10 days of age, anesthetized with halothane) than in older children. The percent of fading at 20, 50, or 100 Hz did not differ between the infants and the older children; however, the tetanic stimulus was applied for only 5 seconds. The train-of-four ratio (the ratio of the amplitude of the fourth evoked response to the amplitude of the first response in the same train), the degree of post-tetanic facilitation, and the tetanus twitch ratio increase with age. Crumrine and Yodlowski[126] noted a

decrease in the amplitude of the frequency sweep electromyogram (FS-EMG) at frequencies of 50 to 100 Hz in infants less than 12 weeks of age (Fig. 2–6). The FS-EMG is a recording of the action potential from an electrical stimulus rate that increases exponentially from 1 pulse per second to 100 Hz over a stimulation period of 10 seconds. The exponential increase in frequency allows assessment of neuromuscular transmission at tetanic rates without inducing fatigue. In older infants and children Crumrine and Yodlowski found that there was little or no decrement in the FS-EMG at the higher frequencies of stimulation. Similarly, the FS-EMG response of full-term infants less than 12 weeks old was depressed after administration of 70 percent nitrous oxide, whereas that of the older patients did not change.

Age-Related Differences in Sensitivity of the Cholinergic Receptor to Relaxants

The sensitivity of the postjunctional cholinergic receptor to acetylcholine may vary with age. When allowance is made for differences in the volume of distribution and for type and concentration of anesthesia, infants appear relatively resistant to succinylcholine and relatively sensitive to nondepolarizing relaxants.

Depolarizing Muscle Relaxants

On a weight basis, more succinylcholine is needed in infants than in older children or adults to produce apnea, to depress respiration, or to depress neuromuscular transmission. Cook and Fischer[127] noted that in

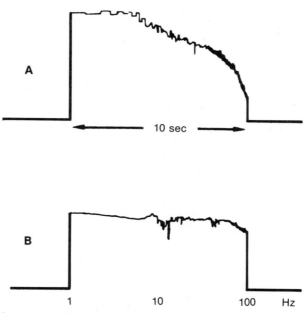

Figure 2–6. Tracings of the frequency sweep electromyogram (FS-EMG) responses from the tibialis anterior muscles of a 1-day-old infant (*A*) and a 4-month-old infant (*B*) premedicated with methohexital.

Figure 2–7. Mean dose-response curve (log-probit) for succinylcholine (mg/kg) for infants. Data calculated from Cook and Fischer.[127, 128]

infants succinylcholine (1 mg/kg) produced neuroblockade about equal to that produced by 0.5 mg/kg in children 6 to 8 years old. At these equipotent doses there is no statistically significant difference between the times to recover to 50 percent (T50) and 90 percent (T90) neuromuscular transmission in the two groups. Complete neuromuscular blockade develops in children given 1.0 mg/kg of succinylcholine. The ED95 of succinylcholine (the estimated dose of relaxant required to give 95 percent neuromuscular blockade) in infants is 2.2 mg/kg (Fig. 2–7).[127–128]

Goudsouzian and Liu[129] needed three-fold higher infusion rates of succinylcholine (mg/kg/hr) to maintain 90 percent twitch depression in young infants than in older infants or children. Phase II block occurred after a slightly larger dose of succinylcholine in infants than in the other age groups. Differences in cholinesterase activity, receptor sensitivity, or volume of distribution may explain these age-related differences in succinylcholine requirements.

The infant has about one-half the pseudocholinesterase activity of the older child or adult. Thus it is unlikely that augmented cholinesterase activity is responsible for the infant's resistance to succinylcholine. When succinylcholine was given in equal dose on a surface area basis (40 mg/m²), Walts and Dillon[130] found no difference between infants and adults in the times to recover to 10, 50, or 90 percent neuromuscular transmission; this dose of succinylcholine produced complete neuromuscular blockade in all patients. Cook and Fischer[127] noted a linear relationship between the log dose on a mg/m² basis and the maximum intensity of neuromuscular blockade for infants, children, and adults. They also saw a linear relationship between the logarithm of the dose on a mg/m² basis and either 50 to 90 percent recovery time for infants and children as a combined group. Because of its relatively small molecular size succinylcholine is rapidly distributed throughout the extracellular fluid. The blood volume and extracellular fluid (ECF) volume of the infant are significantly greater than the child's or adult's on a weight basis. Therefore, on a weight basis (mg/kg) twice as much succinylcholine is needed in the infant as in adults to produce 50 percent neuromuscular blockade. Since ECF and surface area bear a nearly constant relationship throughout life (6 to 8 L/m²), it is not surprising that there is a good correlation between succinylcholine dose (in mg/m²) and response throughout life. The data of Goudsouzian and Liu[129] suggest that relative resistance to succinylcholine persists in some infants even when the dose is transformed to mg/m²/min. These data suggest that the acetylcholine receptor matures with age.

Nondepolarizing Muscle Relaxants

Long-Acting Relaxants. On the basis of clinical criteria it has been suggested that the newborn is more sensitive than the adult to D-tubocurarine. However, EMG studies demonstrate no increased sensitivity of hand muscles to D-tubocurarine in infants compared with adults. In infants respiratory depression parallels the neuromuscular blockade noted in the hands; in adults neuromuscular blockade of the hand occurs before respiratory depression.[131] This important observation suggests that the respiratory muscles of the infant may be more sensitive to D-tubocurarine than those of the adult, or that the infant has less respiratory reserve than the adult. Both may be true.

In adults, Donlon and colleagues[132] have determined cumulative dose-response curves and noted recovery times for D-tubocurarine, gallamine, pancuronium, and metocurine during nitrous oxide–oxygen–narcotic anesthesia. At equipotent doses of these relaxants the recovery time from 95 percent block to 50 percent block averaged 45 minutes. Similar studies have been performed in children during halothane and balanced anesthesia by other investigators.[133–137] The ED95 for these relaxants during balanced anesthesia in children tended to be higher than that in adults and the recovery times tended to be shorter. The dose requirements (ED95) for pancuronium, metocurine, D-tubocurarine, and gallamine are reduced by halothane anesthesia in children as they are in adults. During halothane–nitrous oxide anesthesia there was little difference in the ED95 on a weight basis for the longer-acting muscle relaxants in infants and children (Table 2–9).

Recently we[138] estimated the dose of D-tubocurarine on a surface-area basis that would be needed to produce 95 percent twitch depression in infants, in children, and in adults during halothane anesthesia. In this estimate, adjustment is needed for the wide variation in extracellular fluid volume that exists in infants,

Table 2–9. COMPARISON OF AGE-RELATED DOSE REQUIREMENTS OF NONDEPOLARIZING RELAXANTS AND RECOVERY TIMES

Age	ED95 (mg/kg)*	Recovery Times T5–T25 (min)†
D-Tubocurarine		
1–7 yr	0.32	28.3
2–12 mo	0.29	17.8
11–60 d	0.34	22.4
1–10 d	0.34	32.7
Metocurine		
1–7 yr	0.18	49.7
10 d–1 yr	0.22	36.7
0–9 d	0.19	25.7
Pancuronium		
5 wk–7 yr	0.05	23.6
2–10 yr	0.06	—
Gallamine		
2–10 yr	1.90	—

*ED95 = estimated dose of relaxant required to produce 95 percent neuromuscular blockade.

†T5–T25 = time for neuromuscular transmission to recover from 5 percent to 25 percent.

children, and adults. The extracellular fluid volume mirrors the volume of distribution for the nondepolarizing muscle relaxants. Also, the comparison is between like anesthetics—halothane with halothane. The adult and child require about 7 to 8 mg/m² of D-tubocurarine; the 6- to 9-month-old infant, 5 to 6 mg/m²; but the neonate only about 4 mg/m². This suggests that the neonate, and to a lesser degree the infant, is quite sensitive to D-tubocurarine if compensation is made for the wide variation in volumes of distribution.

Fisher and associates[139] documented the sensitivity to D-tubocurarine of infants as compared with older patients during equipotent nitrous oxide–halothane anesthesia. Since the MAC of halothane is higher in infants than in adults, infants received higher end-tidal concentrations of halothane. The volume of distribution for D-tubocurarine is quite high in the newborn infant compared with the older child or adult, but plasma clearance of D-tubocurarine does not differ with age (Table 2–10). The volume of distribution for D-tubocurarine appears relatively constant on a L/m² basis (estimated by DRC). More important, the plasma

concentration associated with 50 percent neuromuscular block (CPss) was age-related; CPss in neonates was about one-third that noted for adults. The largest variability in elimination half-life and volumes of distribution was seen in the data for the neonates. Likewise, Goudsouzian and colleagues[136] noted wide variations in the ED95 for D-tubocurarine in neonates during halothane anesthesia. Some infants were paralyzed with 0.18 mg/kg and others required 0.6 mg/kg; the mean ED95 was similar to that in older children. This suggests that the neonate's response to nondepolarizing relaxants is quite unpredictable and that the clinician should titrate the dose of relaxant to produce the desired effect. The recovery times from all relaxants are dose-related: if the infant were overdosed by a factor of two, recovery time would be quite prolonged.

Intermediate-Acting Relaxants. Atracurium, a muscle relaxant of intermediate duration, is metabolized by nonspecific esters and spontaneously decomposes by Hofmann degradation. Both processes are sensitive to pH and temperature. Under physiologic conditions the breakdown of atracurium is mainly by ester hydrolysis; Hofmann elimination plays a minor role. Deficient or abnormal pseudocholinesterases have little or no effect on atracurium degradation.[140–141]

We and others have studied the effects of both age and potent inhalation agents on dose-response relationships of atracurium in infants, children, and adolescents.[142–146] On a weight basis (µg/kg) the ED95 for atracurium was similar in infants (1 to 6 months of age) and adolescents, whereas children had a higher dose requirement (Table 2–11). On a surface area basis (µg/m²) the ED95 for atracurium was similar in children and adolescents; the ED95 (µg/m²) for atracurium in infants was much lower (Fig. 2–8).

At equipotent doses (1 × ED95) the duration of effect (time from injection to 95 percent recovery) was 23 minutes in infants and 29 minutes in children and adolescents, compared with 44 minutes in adults. The time from injection to T25 (25 percent neuromuscular transmission) was 10 minutes in infants, 15 minutes in children and adolescents, and 16 minutes in adults. At T25 supplemental doses are needed to maintain relaxation for surgery. At higher multiples of the ED95 the duration of effect will be longer but the times from T5 to T25 will be the same. The shorter

Table 2–10. PHARMACOKINETIC AND PHARMACODYNAMIC VALUES OF D-TUBOCURARINE

Patient Group	N	t½ β (min)	VI (L/kg)	Vdss (L/kg)	Cl (mg/kg/min)	CPss50 (µg/ml)
Neonates	7	174±60	0.19±0.13	0.74±0.33	3.7±2.1	0.18±0.09
Infants	7	130±54	0.16±0.07	0.52±0.22	3.3±0.4	0.27±0.06
Children	9	90±23	0.14±0.05	0.41±0.12	4.0±1.1	0.42±0.14
Adults	8	89±18	0.11±0.02	0.30±0.10	3.0±0.8	0.53±0.14
Significance (p<0.05)		*	NS	†	NS	‡

Values are means ± 1 standard deviation.
NS = not significant.
*t½ β: Neonates > children and adults.
†Vdss: Neonates > infants, children, and adults.
‡CPss50: Neonates and infants < children and adults.

Table 2–11. MEAN ED50 AND ED95 VALUES FOR ATRACURIUM IN ANESTHETIZED CHILDREN

Anesthetic	ED50 µg/kg	ED95 µg/kg	ED50 µg/m²	ED95 µg/m²
Thiopental-fentanyl	170	350	3900	8200
Halothane	130	260	3300	6600
Isoflurane	120	280	3000	8600

Table 2–12. AGE-RELATED PHARMACOKINETICS OF ATRACURIUM

Parameter	Children	Infants
t 1/2 α	2.1 ± 0.56	1.04 ± 0.34*
t 1/2 β	19.1 ± 4.5	13.6 ± 1.4*
V_1 (ml/kg)	52.6 ± 5.66	50.55 ± 6.3
Vd (ml/kg)	139.0 ± 23.48	176.6 ± 22.2*
Cl (ml/kg/min)	5.1 ± 0.56	9.0 ± 1.65*

*$p < 0.05$.

duration of effect in the infant may represent a difference in pharmacokinetics.

The pharmacokinetics of atracurium differ between infants and children or adults. We have determined the kinetics of atracurium in infants and children; comparable data exist for adults.[147] The kinetic variables are shown in Table 2–12. The more striking differences are between infants and children. The volume of distribution is larger and the elimination half-life is shorter in infants than in children or adults. For both reasons clearance in infants is more rapid. Although there is little difference in the kinetics of atracurium among children aged 2 to 10, there are age-related differences in the volume of distribution and elimination half-life. The volume of distribution is higher in the younger patients and elimination half-life shorter; clearance is little different.

In children "light" isoflurane anesthesia (1 percent end-tidal) reduces the atracurium required by about 30 percent from that needed with thiopental-narcotic anesthesia. There was no statistically significant difference in the isoflurane or halothane dose response curve (Fig. 2–9). For clinical purposes both potent agents should be viewed as potentiating atracurium to the same degree.[144]

We have recently used a continuous infusion of dilute atracurium (200 µg/ml) following a bolus to maintain neuromuscular blockade at 95 ± 5 percent (Fig. 2–10).[144] To maintain this degree of steady-state block, an infusion rate of 4 to 5 µg/kg/min was required during halothane or isoflurane anesthesia and 8 to 10 µg/kg/min was required with thiopental-narcotic anesthesia following an initial bolus (Table 2–13). No cumulation was seen with prolonged infusion; recovery of neuromuscular transmission was prompt. The recovery of neuromuscular transmission from the same degree of blockade was similar with all three anesthetics. From these infusion data one can estimate the removal of atracurium. At steady state the infusion rate (Iss) equals the removal rate (Rss) of atracurium. Removal is directly related to the clearance and steady-state plasma concentration associated with 95 percent neuromuscular blockade. Hence:

$$Iss = Rss = Clearance \times CPss95$$

From this relationship one can estimate CPss95 from clearance and the steady-state infusion rate. In chil-

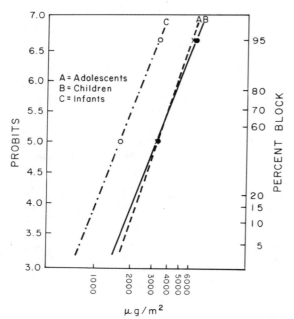

Figure 2–8. Mean dose-response curves for atracurium (µg/m²) for adolescents (A), children (B), and infants (C).

Figure 2–9. Mean dose-response curves for atracurium (µg/kg) during halothane (A), isoflurane (B), or nitrous oxide–narcotic (C).

Figure 2–10. Evolution of atracurium requirements calculated for 9-minute period (shaded area) to maintain neuromuscular blockade (solid dots) in a typical patient. The first 9-minute period represents in large part the bolus injection.

dren, during anesthesia induced by potent anesthetics CPss95 is about 1 μg/ml; during balanced anesthesia it is about 2 μg/ml. Comparable studies are in progress in infants. Atracurium infusion requirements in children during nitrous oxide–narcotic anesthesia are comparable to those noted in several age-groups of adults during similar anesthesia. D'Hollander and colleagues[148] noted that in patients 16 to 85 years old the steady-state atracurium infusion rate averaged 14.4 mg/m²/hr; this corresponds to 240 μg/m²/min. This value is similar to the 226 μg/m²/min we noted.

Vecuronium. Vecuronium, a steroidal relaxant related to pancuronium, is taken up largely by the liver, then excreted unchanged via the hepatobiliary system (40 to 50 percent) or alternatively excreted through the kidneys (4 to 14 percent). Limited biotransformation of vecuronium to the 3-hydroxy, 17-hydroxy, and 3,17-dihydroxy metabolites occurs. Only 3-hydroxy-vecuronium is known to have neuromuscular blocking effects.[149] These routes of elimination may be affected by physiological changes at the extremes of life.[150, 151]

The ED95 for vecuronium is somewhat higher in children than in infants and adults (Table 2–14).[150, 152] At equipotent doses (2 × ED95) of vecuronium the duration of effect (time from injection to 90 percent recovery) was longest for infants (73 minutes), compared with 35 minutes for children and 53 minutes for adults. Thus, vecuronium does not have interme-

diate duration in infants. Vecuronium is potentiated by potent inhalation anesthetics but not in a dose-dependent manner.[153, 154]

Fisher[155] has recently determined the pharmacodynamics and pharmacokinetics of vecuronium in infants and children (Table 2–15). The volume of distribution and mean residence time were greater in infants than in children. Clearance was similar in the two groups; the CPss50 was lower in infants than in children. The combination of a large volume of distribution in infants and fixed clearance results in a longer mean residence time. After a single dose of relaxant, recovery of neuromuscular transmission depends on both distribution and elimination. The combination of a longer mean residence time and a lower sensitivity for vecuronium explains the prolongation of neuromuscular blockade in infants.

Reversal of Neuromuscular Blocking Drugs

Fisher and associates[156, 157] have recently examined the dose of neostigmine and edrophonium required in infants, children, and adults to reverse a 90 percent block from a continuous D-tubocurarine infusion. In infants and children 15.0 μg/kg of neostigmine produced a 50 percent antagonism of the D-tubocurarine block; in adults 23 μg/kg was required. It was claimed that the duration of antagonism was equal in all three groups although the elimination half-life was clearly shorter for infants. A larger dose than that seemingly

Table 2–13. ATRACURIUM INFUSION REQUIREMENTS FOR SURGICAL RELAXATION DURING ANESTHESIA INDUCED BY VARIOUS DRUGS IN CHILDREN

Anesthetic	Infusion Rate* (μg/kg/min)	Infusion Rate* (μg/m²/min)
Thiopental-fentanyl	9.3 ± 0.8 (6.6–13.6)	226 ± 15 (171–309)
Halothane	6.8 ± 0.5 (4.8–9.3)	175 ± 19 (104–274)
Isoflurane	5.9 ± 0.7 (4.4–9.3)	147 ± 16 (94–217)

*Mean ± SE (Range).
Different from thiopental-fentanyl p < 0.05.

Table 2–14. AGE-RELATED POTENCY AND TIME COURSE FOR VECURONIUM

	Potency			Time Course (70 μg/kg)	
	ED50 (μg/kg)	ED95 (μg/kg)	ED95 Multiple	Onset Time (min)	Duration (min)
Infants	16.5	27.7	2.5	1.5 ± 0.6	73 ± 27
Children	19.0	45.5	1.5	2.4 ± 1.4	35 ± 6
Adults	15.0	33.8	2	2.9 ± 0.2	53 ± 21

Table 2–15. PHARMACOKINETICS AND PHARMACODYNAMICS OF VECURONIUM

	ED95 μg/kg	t 1/2 β (min)	CI (ml/kg/min)	Vdss (ml/kg)	CPss50 (ng/ml)
Infants	27.7	64.7 ± 30.2	5.6 ± 1	357 ± 70	57.3 ± 17.7
Children	45.5	41.0 ± 15.1	5.9 ± 2.4	204 ± 116	109.8 ± 28.1
Adult	33.8	70.7 ± 20.4	5.2 ± 0.7	269 ± 42	93.7 ± 33.5

recommended would give a higher sustained blood concentration. Whether this is of pharmacological benefit in the absence of a continuous infusion of relaxant is doubtful. The dissociation between the elimination half-life and the duration of antagonism may result from the carbamylation of cholinesterase by neostigmine.

In infants 145 μg/kg of edrophonium produced a 50 percent antagonism of the D-tubocurarine block, in children 233 μg/kg was required, and in adults 128 μg/kg was required. The volume of distribution of edrophonium was similar in all age groups. The elimination half-life of edrophonium was shorter in infants than in children or adults; hence, clearance was more rapid in infants. Since the molecular interaction between edrophonium and cholinesterase is readily reversible, Fisher and associates suggest that the shorter elimination half-life for edrophonium might limit the value of edrophonium in pediatric patients. This is doubtful.

Meakin and coworkers[158] compared the rate of recovery from pancuronium-induced neuromuscular blockade with several doses of neostigmine (0.036 or 0.07 mg/kg) or edrophonium (0.7 or 1.43 mg/kg) in infants and children. In the first 5 minutes recovery of neuromuscular transmission was more rapid after edrophonium than neostigmine in all age groups; the speed of recovery was faster in infants and children than in adults. By 10 minutes there was no difference in neuromuscular transmission achieved in infants and children with either reversal agent (at either dose); adults had lower neuromuscular transmission at the lower dose (0.036 mg/kg) of neostigmine. Thus, if speed of initial recovery is a critical issue then edrophonium is better than neostigmine and a high dose of neostigmine is better than a low dose. At 30 minutes after injection of either reversal agent (at any dose) there was no difference in neuromuscular transmission between age groups.

REFERENCES

1. Sereni F: Developmental pharmacology. Ann Rev Pharm 8:453, 1968.
2. Jusko WJ: Pharmacokinetic principles in pediatric pharmacology. Pediatr Clin Am 19:81, 1972.
3. Brown TCK: Pediatric pharmacology. Anaesth Intens Care 1:473, 1973.
4. Cook DR: Neonatal anesthetic pharmacology: a review. Anesth Analg 53:544, 1974.
5. Yaffe SJ, Juchau MR: Perinatal pharmacology. Ann Rev Pharmacol 14:219, 1974.
6. Cook DR: Pediatric anesthesia: pharmacological considerations. Drugs 12:212, 1976.
7. Rylance G: Clinical pharmacology: drugs in children. Br Med J 282:50, 1981.
8. Orme M: Drug absorption in the gut. Br J Anaesth 56:59, 1984.
9. DeBoer AG, DeLeede LGJ, Breimer DD: Drug absorption by sublingual and rectal routes. Br J Anaesth 56:69, 1984.
10. Huang NN, High RH: Comparison of serum levels following the adminstration of oral and parenteral preparations of penicillin to infants and children of various age groups. J Pediatr 42:567, 1958.
11. Borga O, Piafsky KM, Nilsen OG: Plasma protein binding of basic drugs. I. Selective displacement from alpha-1 acid glycoprotein by tris-butoxyethyl phosphate. Clin Pharmacol Ther 22:539, 1977.
12. Brem RF, Giardina EGV, Bigger JT: Time course of alpha-1 acid glycoprotein and its relationship to imipramine plasma protein binding. Clin Pharmacol Ther 31:206, 1982.
13. Edwards DJ, Lalka D, Cerra G, et al.: Alpha-1 acid glycoprotein concentration and protein binding in trauma. Clin Pharmacol Ther 31:62, 1982.
14. Grossman SH, Davis D, Kitchell BB, et al.: Diazepam and lidocaine plasma protein binding in renal disease. Clin Pharmacol Ther 31:350, 1982.
15. Kornguth ML, Hutchins LG, Eichelman BS: Binding of psychotropic drugs to isolated alpha-1 acid glycoprotein. Biochem Pharmacol 30:2435, 1981.
16. Piafsky KM: Disease-induced changes in the plasma binding of basic drugs. Clin Pharmacokinet 5:246, 1980.
17. Piafsky KM, Borga O, Odar-Cederlog I, et al.: Increased plasma protein binding of propanolol and chlorpromazine mediated by disease-induced elevations of plasma acid glycoprotein. N Engl J Med 299:1435, 1978.
18. Pike E, Skuterud B, Kierugg P, et al.: Binding and displacement of basic, acidic and neutral drugs in normal and orosomucoid-deficient plasma. Clin Pharmacokinet 6:367, 1981.
19. Nation RL: Meperidine binding in maternal and fetal plasma. Clin Pharmacol Ther 29:472, 1981.
20. Pruitt AW, Dayton PG: A comparison of the binding of drugs to adult and cord plasma. Eur J Clin Pharmacol 4:59, 1971.
21. Wood J, Wood AJJ: Changes in plasma drug binding and alpha-1 acid glycoprotein in mother and newborn infant. Clin Pharmacol Ther 29:522, 1981.
22. Dayton PG, Stiller RL, Cook DR, et al.: The binding of ketamine to plasma proteins: emphasis on human plasma. Eur J Clin Pharmacol 24:825, 1983.
23. Friss-Hansen B: Body composition during growth. Pediatrics 47:264, 1971.
24. Widdowson EM: Changes in body proportions and composite during growth. In Davis JA, Dobbing J (Eds.): Scientific Foundations of Pediatrics. Philadelphia, W. B. Saunders Co., 1974, pp 153–163.
25. Smith CA, Nelson NM: The Physiology of the Newborn Infant. 4th ed. Springfield, Illinois, Charles C Thomas, 1976, pp 179, 181, 188, 209.
26. Guignard JP, Torrado A, Cunha OD, et al.: Glomerular filtration rate in the first three weeks of life. J Pediatr 87:268, 1975.
27. Altman PL, Dittmer DS: Respiration and circulation handbook (revised edition). Bethesda, MD, Federation of American Societies for Experimental Biology, 1971, pp 426–427.
28. Oldendorf WH: The blood-brain barrier. In Bito LZ, Davson H, Fenstermacher JD (Eds.): The Ocular and Cerebrospinal Fluids. London and New York, Academic Press, 1977, pp 177–190.
29. Behnsen G: Farbstoffversuche mit Trypanblau an der

Schranke zwischen Blut und Zentralnervensystem der wach-senden Maus. Munch Med Wschr 73:1143, 1926.

30. Behnsen G: Uber die Farbstoffspeicherung im Zentralnerven-system der weissen Maus in verschiedenen Alterszugstanden. Z Zellforsch 4:515, 1927.

31. Barlow CF, Domek NS, Goldberg MA, et al.: Extracellular brain space measured by ^{35}S-sulphate. Arch Neurol 5:102, 1961.

32. Davson H: Physiology of the Cerebral Spinal Fluid. London, Churchill, 1967.

33. Ferguson RK, Woodbury DM: Penetration of ^{14}C-inulin and ^{14}C-sucrose into brain, cerebrospinal fluid, and skeletal mus-cle in developing rats. Exp Brain Res 7:181, 1969.

34. Evans CAN, Reynolds JM, Reynolds ML, et al.: The development of a blood-brain barrier mechanism in foetal sheep. J Physiol 238:371, 1974.

35. Evans CAN, Reynolds JM, Reynolds ML: The effect of hypercapnia on a blood brain barrier mechanism in foetal and newborn sheep. J Physiol 255:701, 1976.

36. Oldendorf WH: Measurement of brain uptake of radio-labelled substances using a tritiated water internal standard. Brain Res 24:372, 1970.

37. Oldendorf WH, Braun LD: [^{3}H]-Tryptamine and ^{3}H water as diffusible internal standard for measuring brain extraction of radio-labelled substances following carotid injection. Brain Res 113:219, 1976.

38. Oldendorf WH, Hyman S, Braun L et al.: Blood-brain barrier: Penetration of morphine, codeine, heroin and meth-adone after carotid injection. Science 178:984, 1972.

39. Gladtke E, Heimann G: The rate of development of elimi-nation functions in kidney and liver of young infants. In Morselli PC, Garattini S, Sereni F (Eds.): Basic and Thera-peutic Aspects of Perinatal Pharmacology. New York, Raven Press, 1975, pp 377–392.

40. Brown AK, Zwelzin WW, Burnett HH: Studies on the neonatal development of the glucuronide conjugating system. J Clin Invest 37:332, 1958.

41. Greene NM: The metabolism of drugs employed in anes-thesia. Anesthesiology 29:127, 1968.

42. Yaffe SJ: Neonatal pharmacology. Pediatr Clin N A 13:527, 1966.

43. Somogyi A, Gugler R: Drug interactions with cimetidine. Clin Pharmacokinet 7:23, 1982.

44. Katzung GB: Basic and Clinical Pharmacology. Los Altos, Lange Medical Publications, 1984.

45. Eger EI II: Anesthesia Uptake and Action. Baltimore, Williams and Wilkins, 1974.

46. Salanitre E, Rackow H: The pulmonary exchange of nitrous oxide and halothane in infants and children. Anesthesiology 30:388, 1969.

47. Rackow H, Salanitre E: The pulmonary equilibration of cyclopropane in infants and children. Br J Anaesth 46:35, 1974.

48. Steward DJ, Creighton RE: The uptake and excretion of nitrous oxide in the newborn. Can Anaesth Soc J 25:215, 1978.

49. Eger EI II, Bahlman SH, Munson ES: The effect of age on the rate of increase of alveolar anesthetic concentration. Anesthesiology 35:365, 1971.

50. Brandom BW, Brandom RB, Cook DR: Uptake and distri-bution of halothane in infants: in vivo measurements and computer simulations. Anesth Analg 62:404, 1983.

51. Gibbs CP, Munson ES, Tham MK: Anesthetic solubility coefficients for maternal and fetal blood. Anesthesiology 43:100, 1975.

52. Lerman J, Gregory GA, Willis MM, et al.: Age and solubility of volatile anesthetics in blood. Anesthesiology 61:139, 1984.

53. Cook DR, Brandom BW, Shiu G, et al.: The inspired median effective dose, brain concentration at anesthesia, and cardiovascular index for halothane in young rats. Anesth Analg 60:182, 1981.

54. Stoelting RK, Longnecker DE: Effect of right-to-left shunt on rate of increase in arterial anesthetic concentration. Anesthesiology 36:352, 1972.

55. Tanner G, Angers D, Barash PG, et al.: Does a left-to-right shunt speed the induction of inhalational anesthesia in congenital heart disease? Anesthesiology 57:A427, 1982.

56. Deming MV: Agents and techniques for induction of anes-thesia in infants and young children. Anesth Analg 31:113, 1952.

57. Gregory GA, Eger EI II, Munson ES: the relationship between age and halothane requirements in man. Anesthe-siology 30:488, 1969.

58. Nicodemus HF, Nassiri-Rahimi C, Bachman L: Median effective dose (ED$_{50}$) of halothane in adults and children. Anesthesiology 31:344, 1969.

59. Lerman J, Robinson S, Willis MM, et al.: Anesthetic requirements for halothane in young children 0–1 month and 1–6 months of age. Anesthesiology 59:421, 1983.

60. Gregory GA, Wade JG, Beihl DR, et al.: Fetal anesthetic requirement (MAC) for halothane. Anesth Analg 62:9, 1983.

61. Moss IR, Conner H, Yee WFH, et al.: Human β-endorphin in the neonatal period. J Pediatr 101:443, 1982.

62. Bayon A, Shoemaker WJ, Bloom FE, et al.: Perinatal development of the endorphin- and enkephalin-containing systems in rat brain. Brain Res 179:93, 1979.

63. Miller KM, Paton WDM, Smith EB, et al.: Physiochemical approaches to the mode of action of general anesthetics. Anesthesiology 36:339, 1972.

64. Rackow H, Salinitre E, Green LT: Frequency of cardiac arrest associated with anesthesia in infants and children. Pediatrics 28:697, 1961.

65. Friesen RH, Lichtor JL: Cardiovascular depression during halothane anesthesia in infants: a study of three induction techniques. Anesth Analg 61:42, 1982.

66. Friesen RH, Lichtor JL: Cardiovascular effects of inhalation induction with isoflurane in infants. Anesth Analg 62:411, 1983.

67. Rao CC, Bayer M, Krishna G, et al.: Effects of halothane, isoflurane and enflurane on the isometric contraction of the neonatal isolated rat atria. Anesthesiology 61:A424, 1984.

68. Boudreaux JP, Schieber RA, Cook DR: Hemodynamic effects of halothane in the newborn piglet. Anesth Analg 63:731, 1984.

69. Bailie MD, Alward CT, Sawyer DC, et al.: Effect of anesthesia on cardiovascular and renal function in the new-born piglet. J Pharmacol Exp Ther 208:298, 1979.

70. Merin RG, Verdouw PD, deJong JW: Dose-dependent depression of cardiac function and metabolism by halothane in swine (Sus scrofa). Anesthesiology 46:417, 1977.

71. Gootman PM, Gootman N, Buckley BJ: Maturation of central autonomic control of the circulation. Fed Proc 42:1648, 1983.

72. Gregory GA: The baroresponses of preterm infants during halothane anesthesia. Can Anaesth Soc J 29:105, 1982.

73. Duncan P, Gregory GA, Wade JA: The effects of nitrous oxide on the baroreceptor response of newborn and adult rabbits. Can Anaesth Soc J 18:339, 1981.

74. Wear R, Robinson S, Gregory GA: The effect of halothane on the baroresponse of adult and baby rabbits. Anesthesiology 56:188, 1982.

75. Wolfson B, Kielar CM, Lake C, et al.: Anesthetic index—a new approach. Anesthesiology 38:583, 1973.

76. Wolfson B, Hetrick WD, Lake C, et al.: Anesthetic in-dices—further data. Anesthesiology 48:187, 1978.

77. Kissen I, Morgan PL, Smith LR: Comparison of isoflurane and halothane safety margins in rats. Anesthesiology 58:556, 1983.

78. Uehleke H, Werner T: Postnatal development of halothane and other haloalkane metabolism and covalent binding in rat liver microsomes. In Morselli PL, Garattini S, Sereni F (Eds.): Basic and Therapeutic Aspects of Perinatal Pharma-cology. New York, Raven Press, 1975, pp 277–287.

79. Stoelting RK, Peterson C: Methoxyflurane anesthesia in pediatric patients: evaluation of anesthetic metabolism and renal function. Anesthesiology 42:26, 1975.

80. Goldenthal EI: A compilation of LD$_{50}$ values in newborn and adult animals. Toxicol Appl Pharmacol 18:185, 1971.

81. Marcucci F, Mussini E, Airoldi L, et al.: Diazepam metabolism and anticonvulsant activity in newborn animals. Biochem Pharmacol 22:3051, 1973.

82. Morselli PL, Mandelli M, Tognoni G, et al.: Drug interactions in the human fetus and in the newborn infant. In Morselli PL, Cohen SN (Eds.): Drug Interactions. New York, Drug Interactions, 1974, pp 320–333.

83. Carmichael EB: The median lethal dose (LD$_{50}$) of pentothal sodium for both young and old guinea pigs and rats. Anesthesiology 8:589, 1947.

84. Carmichael EB: The median lethal dose of Nembutal (pentobarbital sodium) for young and old rats. J Pharmacol Exp Ther 62:284, 1938.

85. Weatherall JA: Anaesthesia in newborn animals. Br J Pharmacol 15:454, 1960.

86. Domek NS, Barlow CF, Roth LJ: An octogenetic study of phenobarbital C-14 in cat brain. J Pharmacol Exp Ther 130:285, 1960.

87. Mirkin BL: Perinatal pharmacology. Anesthesiology 43:156, 1975.

88. Boreus LO, Jalling B, Kallberg N: Clinical pharmacology of phenobarbital in the neonatal period. In Morselli PL, Garattini S, Sereni F (Eds.): Basic and Therapeutic Aspects of Perinatal Pharmacology. New York, Raven Press, 1975, pp 331–340.

89. Knauer B, Draffen GA, Williams FM: Elimination kinetics of amobarbital in mothers and their newborn infants. Clin Pharmacol Ther 14:442, 1973.

90. Sorbo S, Hudson RJ, Loomis JC: The pharmacokinetics of thiopental in pediatric surgical patients. Anesthesiology 61:666, 1984.

91. Kosaka Y, Takahashi T, Mark LC: Intravenous thiobarbiturate anesthesia for cesarean section. Anesthesiology 31:489, 1969.

92. Lockhart CH, Nelson WL: The relationship of ketamine requirements to age in pediatric patients. Anesthesiology 40:507, 1974.

93. Chang T, Glazko T: Biotransformation and distribution of ketamine. Int Anesthesiol Clin 12:157, 1974.

94. Waterman AE, Livingston A: Effects of age and sex on ketamine anesthesia in the rat. Br J Anaesth 50:885, 1978.

95. Eng M, Bonica JJ, Akamatsu TJ, et al.: Respiratory depression in newborn monkeys at cesarean section following ketamine administration. Br J Anaesth 47:917, 1975.

96. Radney PA, Badola RP: Generalized extensor spasm in infants following ketamine anesthesia. Anesthesiology 39:459, 1973.

97. Lockhart CH, Jenkins JJ: Ketamine-induced apnea in patients with increased intracranial pressure. Anesthesiology 37:92, 1972.

98. Gassner S, Cohen M, Aygen M: The effect of ketamine on pulmonary artery pressure. Anaesthesia 29:141, 1974.

99. Morray JP, Lynn AM, Stamm SJ, et al.: Hemodynamic effects of ketamine in children with congenital heart disease. Anesth Analg 63:895, 1984.

100. Hickey PR, Hansen DD, Cramolini GM: Pulmonary and systemic hemodynamic responses to ketamine in infants with normal and elevated pulmonary vascular resistance. Anesthesiology 61:A438, 1984.

101. Way WL, Costley EC, Way EL: Respiratory sensitivity of the newborn infant to meperidine and morphine. Clin Pharmacol Ther 6:454, 1965.

102. Kupferberg HJ, Way EL: Pharmacologic basis for the increased sensitivity of the newborn rat to morphine. J Pharmacol Exp Ther 141:105, 1963.

103. Mirkin BL: Developmental pharmacology. Ann Review Pharmacol 10:255, 1970.

104. Hickey PR, Hansen DD: Fentanyl- and sufentanil-oxygen-pancuronium anesthesia for cardiac surgery in infants. Anesth Analg 63:117, 1984.

105. Hickey PR, Hansen DD, Wessell D: Responses to high dose fentanyl in infants: pulmonary and systemic hemodynamics. Anesthesiology 61:A445, 1984.

106. Schieber RA, Stiller RL, Cook DR: Cardiovascular and pharmacodynamic effects of high-dose fentanyl in newborn piglets. Anesthesiology, 63:166, 1985.

107. Koren G, Crean P, Goresky G, et al.: Fentanyl anesthesia for cardiac surgery in children: a) fentanyl-oxygen vs. fentanyl-N$_2$O; b) relationship between drug concentrations and pharmacodynamics. Anesthesiology 61:A444, 1984.

108. Koehntop D, Rodman J, Brundage D, et al.: Pharmacokinetics of fentanyl in neonates. Anesthesiology 61:A439, 1984.

109. Singleton MA, Rosen JI, Fisher DM: Pharmacokinetics of fentanyl for infants and adults. Anesthesiology 61:A440, 1984.

110. Johnson KL, Erickson JP, Holley FO, et al.: Fentanyl pharmacokinetics in the pediatric population. Anesthesiology 61:A441, 1984.

111. Collins G, Koren G, Crean P, et al.: The correlation between fentanyl pharmacokinetics and pharmacodynamics in preterm infants during PDA ligation. Anesthesiology 61:A442, 1984.

112. Ecobichon DJ, Stephen DS: Perinatal development of human blood esterases. Clin Pharmacol Ther 14:44, 1973.

113. Blankenbaker WL, DiFazio CA, Berry FA Jr: Lidocaine and its metabolites in the newborn. Anesthesiology 42:325, 1975.

114. Moore RG, Thomas J, Triggs DB, et al.: The pharmacokinetics and metabolism of anilide anesthetics in neonates. Eur J Clin Pharmacol 14:203, 1978.

115. Morgan D, McQuillan D, Thomas J: Pharmacokinetics and metabolism of the anilide local anesthetics in neonates. Eur J Clin Pharmacol 13:365, 1981.

116. Dauchot P, Gravenstein JS: Effects of atropine on the electrocardiogram in different age groups. Clin Pharmacol Exp Ther 12:274, 1971.

117. Gaviotaki A, Smith RM: Use of atropine in pediatric anesthesia. Int Anesthesiol Clin 1:97, 1962.

118. Cook DR: Clinical use of muscle relaxants in infants and children. Anesth Analg 60:335, 1981.

119. Anggard L, Ottoson D: Observations on the functional development of the neuromuscular apparatus in fetal sheep. Exp Neurol 7:294, 1963.

120. Close R: Dynamic properties of fast and slow skeletal muscles of the rat during development. J Physiol 173:74, 1964.

121. Close R: Force-velocity properties of mouse muscles. Nature 206:718, 1965.

122. Close R: Effects of cross-union of motor nerves to fast and slow skeletal muscles. Nature 206:831, 1965.

123. Buller AJ: Developmental physiology of the neuromuscular system. Br Med Bull 22:45, 1966.

124. Koenigsberger MR, Patten B, Lovelace RE: Studies of neuromuscular function in the newborn—a comparison of myoneural function in the full term and premature infant. Neuropadiatrie 4:350, 1973.

125. Goudsouzian NG: Maturation of neuromuscular transmission in the infant. Br J Anaesth 52:205, 1980.

126. Crumrine RS, Yodlowski EH: Assessment of neuromuscular function in infants. Anesthesiology 54:29, 1981.

127. Cook DR, Fischer CG: Neuromuscular blocking effects of succinylcholine in infants and children. Anesthesiology 42:662, 1975.

128. Cook DR, Fischer CG: Characteristics of succinylcholine neuromuscular blockade in infants. Anesth Analg 57:63, 1978.

129. Goudsouzian NG, Liu LMP: The neuromuscular response of infants to a continuous infusion of succinylcholine. Anesthesiology 60:97, 1984.

130. Walts LF, Dillon JB: The response of newborns to succinyl-choline and d-tubocurarine. Anesthesiology 31:35, 1969.
131. Churchill-Davidson HC, Wise RP: The response of the newborn infant to muscle relaxants. Can Anaesth Soc J 11:1, 1964.
132. Donlon JV, Ali HH, Savarese JJ: A new approach to the study of four non-depolarizing relaxants in man. Anesth Analg 53:924, 1974.
133. Goudsouzian NG, Liu LMP, Cote CJ: Comparison of equi-potent doses of non-depolarizing muscle relaxants in children. Anesth Analg 60:862, 1981.
134. Goudsouzian NG, Liu LMP, Savarese JJ: Metocurarine in infants and children: neuromuscular and clinical effects. Anesthesiology 49:266, 1978.
135. Goudsouzian NG, Ryan JF, Savarese JJ: The neuromuscular effects of pancuronium in infants and children. Anesthesiology 41:95, 1974.
136. Goudsouzian NG, Donlon JV, Savarese JJ, et al.: Re-evaluation of dosage and duration of action of d-tubocurarine in the pediatric age group. Anesthesiology 43:416, 1975.
137. Goudsouzian NG, Martyn JJA, Liu LMP: The dose response of long-acting non-depolarizing neuromuscular blocking agents in children. Can Anaesth Soc J 3:246, 1984.
138. Cook DR: Sensitivity of the newborn to tubocurarine. Br J Anaesth 53:320, 1981.
139. Fisher DM, O'Keefe C, Stanski DR, et al.: Pharmacokinetics and pharmacodynamics of d-tubocurarine in infants, children, and adults. Anesthesiology 57:203, 1982.
140. Stiller RL, Cook DR, Chakravorti S: In vitro degradation of atracur-ium in human plasma. Br J Anaesth, 57:1085, 1985.
141. Stiller RL, Brandom BW, Cook DR: Determinations of atracurium by high-performance liquid chromatography. Anesth Analg, 64:58, 1985.
142. Brandom BW, Woelfel SK, Cook DR, et al.: Clinical pharmacology of atracurium in infants. Anesth Analg 63:309, 1984.
143. Brandom BW, Rudd GD, Cook DR: Clinical pharmacology of atracurium in pediatric patients. Br J Anaesth 55:117s, 1983.
144. Brandom BW, Cook DR, Woelfel SK, et al.: Atracurium infusion in children during fentanyl, halothane, and isoflur-ane anesthesia. Anesth Analg, 64:471, 1985.
145. Goudsouzian NG, Liu L, Cote CJ, et al.: Safety and efficacy of atracurium in adolescents and children anesthetized with halothane. Anesthesiology 59:459, 1983.
146. Goudsouzian NG, Liu LMP, Gionfriddo M, et al.: Neuro-muscular effects of atracurium in infants and children. Anesthesiology, 62:75, 1985.
147. Brandom BW, Cook DR, Stiller RL, et al.: Pharmacokinetics of atracurium in infants and children. Clin Pharmacol Ther, in press.
148. D'Hollander AA, Luyckx C, Barvais L, et al.: Clinical evaluation of atracurium besylate requirement for a stable muscle relaxation during surgery: lack of age-related effects. Anesthesiology 59:237, 1983.
149. Durant NN: Norcuron, a new nondepolarizing neuromus-cular blocking agent. Semin Anesth 1:47. 1982.
150. Fisher DM, Miller RD: Neuromuscular effects of vecuronium (ORG NC45) in infants and children during N₂O, halothane anesthesia. Anesthesiology 58:519, 1983.
151. d'Hollander AA, Massaux F, Nevelsteen M, et al.: Age-dependent dose-response relationship of ORG NC45 in anaesthetized patients. Br J Anaesth 54:653, 1982.
152. Goudsouzian NG, Martyn J, Liu LMP, et al.: Safety and efficacy of vecuronium in adolescents and children. Anesth Analg 62:1083, 1983.
153. Rupp SM, Miller RD, Gencarelli PJ: Vecuronium-induced neuromuscular blockade during enflurane, halothane, and isoflurane in humans. Anesthesiology 60:102, 1984.
154. Miller RD, Rupp SM, Fisher DM, et al.: Clinical pharma-cology of vecuronium and atracurium. Anesthesiology 61:444, 1984.
155. Fisher DM: Pharmacodynamics of vecuronium in infants and children. Clin Pharmacol Ther, 37:402, 1985.
156. Fisher DM, Cronnelly R, Miller RD, et al.: The neuromus-cular pharmacology of neostigmine in infants and children. Anesthesiology 59:220, 1983.
157. Fisher DM, Cronnelly R, Sharma M, et al.: Clinical phar-macology of edrophonium in infants. Anesthesiology 61:428, 1984.
158. Meakin G, Sweet PT, Bevan JC, et al.: Neostigmine and edropho-nium as antagonists of pancuronium in infants and children. Anesthesiology 59:316, 1983.

3 | INFECTIOUS DISEASES

D. A. ZIDEMAN, M.B., B.S. • DAVID J. STEWARD, M.B.

Infections are common during infancy and childhood. The anesthesiologist may encounter infants and children who require surgical treatment related to infectious disease, or more often this disease may be present in a child who requires surgery for an unrelated lesion. In the latter case the risks of anesthesia in the presence of the infectious disease must be balanced against the urgency of the surgical procedure. Some of these judgments will be very difficult, and in all patients the anesthesia technique must be modified to accommodate any special aspects of the infectious disease.

Some childhood infectious diseases are extremely contagious, and the anesthesiologist must be familiar with the mode of transmission if he is to take adequate precautions to prevent the spread of infection to other patients and hospital staff. Many of the conditions to be discussed are now quite rare, and because of the rarity many physicians are less familiar with the special care that is required.

FEVER

Fever is defined as elevation of the body temperature above the normal. This elevation of body temperature, when it is associated with infection, is a part of the patient's response to that infection. Indeed, there is some evidence to suggest that fever may assist the body in combating the infective agent.[1] Certainly, during an infection the patient's thermoregulatory responses tend to maintain the elevated core temperature.

Low-birth-weight infants may not develop a fever in response to sepsis and, in fact, may become hypothermic. This lack of a febrile reaction might contribute to increased mortality from infection in newborn infants.[2]

The mechanism of production of fever is as follows. Infecting agents stimulate the production of pyrogen by leukocytes, macrophages, and other cells. This pyrogen, which is a polypeptide, acts upon the hypothalamus, either directly or via a prostaglandin, catecholamine, and cyclic AMP pathway. The result is a hypothalamic-induced increase in heat production centered principally in skeletal muscle in older children and adults. Young infants may become febrile as a result of non-shivering thermogenesis.[3]

The rise in body temperature during a fever is associated with an increased metabolic rate for oxygen. In adults this increase approximated 13 percent for each degree centigrade above normal body temperature.[4] The energy cost of fever in infants and small children will be higher as a result of greater heat loss from a relatively larger body surface area.[2]

The clinical manifestations of fever include chills, headache, rigors, and tachycardia. Sweating may occur as the fever resolves. Delirium and coma may occur during high fever, and convulsions may occur in children (see below). Fluid losses via the skin and respiratory tract are increased and may result in dehydration, particularly if fluid intake is reduced owing to anorexia or vomiting.

The treatment of fever should be directed at the underlying infective process. Active measures to reduce the body temperature of a febrile infected patient may cause harm; if the child is placed in a cool environment, heat losses will increase, but may be matched by increased thermogenesis unless the hypothalamic set-point is lowered. This increased thermogenesis will be accompanied by a further increase in the metabolic demand for oxygen. Antipyretic drugs may cause toxicity, but may be indicated where there is an urgent indication to lower the body temperature (for example, febrile convulsions or pre-existing heart disease.)[5]

Febrile Convulsions

Fever may be accompanied by convulsions in young children of 6 months to 6 years.[6] Fifty percent of all seizures in this age group may be due to fever. A simple febrile convulsion is characterized by a brief generalized (nonfocal) seizure during a fever. There is prompt recovery to a normal state of consciousness and no other signs of neurological or metabolic disease. There may be a family history or past history of febrile convulsions. It is most important that other causes of seizures be sought and excluded before accepting a diagnosis of seizure due to fever. Antecedent brain injury is often present in patients with febrile convulsions.

Treatment is directed at the cause of the fever, but must also ensure rapid termination of the seizure. Prompt reduction of the fever with antipyretics and tepid sponging is advised. Intravenous diazepam, 0.3 mg/kg administered at a rate of 1 mg/min, may be given until the seizure stops.[6] Appropriate steps should be taken to preserve the airway and minimize the risk of aspiration.

There is controversy as to the danger of neurological or intellectual sequelae of a febrile convulsion. Children who have repeated febrile convulsions may be placed on long-term anticonvulsant therapy, though this too is controversial.

Anesthesia for Patients with Fever

Patients with increased body temperature will have an increased metabolic rate for oxygen and carbon dioxide. The increase is directly related to the extent of pyrexia. Hence, special consideration should be given to ensuring a high concentration of inspired oxygen and an increased level of alveolar ventilation. Any interruption of oxygenation is very poorly tolerated by pyrexial patients; should hypoxia proceed to cardiac arrest, the neurological result may be very much worse than in normothermic patients. A perfect, continuous airway and very adequate oxygenation and ventilation must be absolutely assured.

Some other considerations also apply for the patient with pyrexia. Atropine should not be given as a premedicant as it will prevent sweating and hence may lead to further preoperative pyrexia. If necessary, atropine can be given once anesthesia is induced, as temperature management is more readily accomplished

during anesthesia. The patient should be placed on a cooling blanket and ice packs used if required to restore normothermia. Volatile anesthetic agents such as halothane and isoflurane may be useful to produce vasodilation of skin vessels and so increase heat loss from pyrexial patients. Neuromuscular blocking drugs should be given to prevent shivering, especially if active cooling measures are taken.

SEPTICEMIA

Septicemia (sepsis) implies a severe and overwhelming infection[7] with a bacteremia. The diagnosis is based on findings of fever, shock, debility, and possible disseminated intravascular coagulation in a patient who is susceptible to, or has a likely source of, infection.

Sepsis in pediatric patients is most commonly seen in the neonate, but fulminating sepsis may also occur in older children, especially with meningococcal, pneumococcal, staphylococcal, or streptococcal infections.

Neonatal Sepsis

This may affect 1 in 230 preterm infants and 1 in 1200 term infants.[8] Despite advances in antibiotic therapy, the mortality is high.

Several factors predispose the newborn to sepsis. Both cellular and humoral responses to infection are limited, especially in the preterm infant.[9] Leukocytes have impaired chemotaxis, phagocytosis, and bactericidal action. Immunoglobulin deficiency is also present, especially in the preterm infant, as transplacental transfer of globulins varies with the length of gestation.

This vulnerability to infection when associated with conditions that tend to introduce microorganisms into the infant's environment may result in severe sepsis. The risk of infection is high in the neonatal nursery.[10] Endotracheal intubation, venous infusions, and invasive monitoring lines all provide routes for infection. Preterm infants who undergo surgical procedures have a higher incidence of sepsis than others. Failure to observe strict hand washing prior to handling of infants is a leading cause of infection.

The organisms most commonly involved in neonatal sepsis are the gram positive group B streptococci and the gram negative Escherichia coli.[11]

The clinical picture of neonatal sepsis is very varied, and the early signs are frequently missed. Classic signs of sepsis are temperature instability, abdominal distention, jaundice, and apnea. In addition, changes in activity, feeding, and muscle tone may be noted. Later, cardiovascular changes result in hypotension, and mottling of the skin and a bleeding tendency may become apparent.

The diagnosis of sepsis is confirmed by blood, urine, and CSF culture, which may also identify the organism involved and its antibiotic sensitivities. Other laboratory tests may assist in diagnosis. Abnormal leukocyte counts and thrombocytopenia are often present. Gram stains of blood smears may reveal the presence of bacteria.

The treatment of neonatal sepsis must begin early (before culture results are available). Antibiotic therapy should be based on the likely organism involved. Various regimens have been used as initial therapy before the causative organism is identified. These are selected on the basis of the likely organism involved in the particular infant, with a knowledge of patterns of infection within the particular neonatal nursery. The reader is referred to texts of neonatal medicine for specific recommendations.[11, 12]

In addition to antibiotic therapy, the neonate with sepsis requires aggressive further treatment. The infant should be carefully maintained in a neutral thermal environment, electrolyte and acid-base disturbances corrected, and oxygenation ensured. The infant should be carefully monitored to detect apnea. Oral feedings should be discontinued and a gastric tube inserted to prevent gastric dilatation. Blood component therapy may be required to correct coagulopathy and anemia; platelet infusions and/or exchange transfusion may be required. Blood transfusions may reduce the mortality rate, especially in beta-streptococcal sepsis.[13] The seriously ill neonate with sepsis may require therapy with inotropic drugs.

The anesthesiologist may be involved in the surgical care of the infant with sepsis. It is important that the preoperative cardiorespiratory, metabolic, acid-base and electrolyte, and hematological status be accurately evaluated. Meticulous care during transport and intraoperatively must be directed at maintaining all therapy and avoiding further physiological stress. Cold stress, hypoglycemia, and fluid overload must be prevented. Asepsis must be assured in all anesthesia-related procedures (for example, venipuncture, endotracheal intubation).

Sepsis in Older Infants and Children

Sepsis after the neonatal period is most commonly due to meningococcal, pneumococcal, staphylococcal, or streptococcal infections.

Meningococcal Sepsis

The meningococcus, *Neisseria meningitidis,* is a gram negative diplococcus that is frequently found in the nasopharynx, where it may cause a mild pharyngitis or result in no symptoms. From such carriers the disease is spread and may be manifested as meningococcal meningitis, meningococcal bacteremia, or sepsis.

Meningococcal sepsis is a fulminating disease characterized by high fever and a petechial or purpuric rash. The rash may become widespread (purpura ful-

minans) with mucous membrane involvement. Meningitis may or may not be present. Arthritis is a common feature, and vomiting and diarrhea may occur.

Severe meningococcal sepsis in children may be complicated by adrenal insufficiency[14] due to bilateral adrenal hemorrhage (the Waterhouse-Friderichsen syndrome). The disease may proceed extremely rapidly with circulatory failure and death within a few hours. Myocarditis may complicate meningococcal sepsis, and disseminated intravascular coagulation may occur.

The first objective in treatment of meningococcal sepsis is to restore the circulating blood volume. Appropriate hemodynamic monitoring must be established to achieve this. An arterial line, central venous pressure line, and urinary catheter should be inserted. Plasma or 5 per cent albumin together with appropriate multiple electrolyte solutions should be infused to achieve an optimal filling pressure. If blood pressure remains low, inotropic drugs are required. A low urine output with adequate fluid intake and a normal blood pressure indicates the onset of renal failure.

The use of corticosteroids is controversial, but many authorities advise their use in the absence of any firm evidence of their lack of efficacy.[15]

The choice of antibiotics for serious meningococcal infections is penicillin or chloramphenicol. The sulfonamides have also been used, but some strains of the organism are resistant to these drugs.

Pneumococcal Sepsis

This disease is characteristically seen in patients with a nonfunctioning or absent spleen.[16, 17] The pneumococcus is especially dangerous to such children as it is an encapsulated bacterium; splenic function is thought to aid phagocytosis of such organisms by production of opsonins.[18] A critical illness with widespread purpura and disseminated intravascular coagulation may occur. The peripheral blood smear may demonstrate the bacteria on gram staining. The risk of sepsis is highest in infants under 2 years of age and in recently splenectomized children.

Prophylactic antibiotics are recommended for asplenic patients, but their value in preventing sepsis is unproven. A conservative approach to splenic trauma is recommended.[19] A pneumococcal vaccine is available and is advised for children over 2 years of age with impaired splenic function.

Staphylococcal Sepsis

Acute staphylococcal sepsis may occur without a previous focus of infection,[20] but usually can be related to a focal infection. Osteomyelitis, arthritis, and wound infections are common primary foci. Staphylococcal infections may appear as a complication of vascular cannulation.

The treatment of staphylococcal sepsis depends upon active fluid replacement and aggressive antibiotic therapy. Nafcillin and cefazolin are recommended drugs.

The patient with staphylococcal sepsis appears very ill and toxic. Skin rashes similar to those of meningococcal sepsis may occur. Hematuria, jaundice, seizures, and cardiac murmurs may occur as the disease progresses.[20] Disseminated intravascular coagulation is common.

Streptococcal Sepsis

Streptococcal sepsis may complicate cellulitis, chicken pox, or wound infections. Occasionally sepsis occurs without an obvious focal infection.

Septic Shock

Shock is a frequent manifestation of acute sepsis and is associated with a high mortality.[21] In fact, there has probably been an increase in the incidence of septic shock in children over the past decade. This is due to the increasing complexity of surgical procedures, widespread antibiotic use, prolongation of life of patients with defective immunity, and the use of invasive techniques that provide portals for infection.[21]

The common pathogens are gram negative organisms: *E. coli* and meningococcus (see above) are especially frequent. The initial disturbances of septic shock are mediated by endotoxins and result in changes in the microcirculation. Later the cardiovascular effects of secondary products (complement, kallikrein, and so forth) and other vasoactive agents become superimposed. In addition, there is failure of oxygen extraction at the cellular level, activation of compensatory mechanisms, and the effect of underlying host disease factors.[22]

The end result is an unpredictable pattern of circulatory insufficiency with inadequate tissue oxygenation. Three stages of the circulatory response to sepsis are generally recognized: hyperdynamic compensated, hyperdynamic uncompensated, and cardiogenic.[22] The early stages are characterized by tachycardia, tachypnea, bounding pulses, and normotension or hypertension, with a decreased systemic vascular resistance and a high cardiac index. Later the tachycardia persists, but is accompanied by hypotension, reduced cardiac index, and increased systemic vascular resistance. Hypoxemia is present throughout and in the last stages is accompanied by acidosis (respiratory and metabolic) and oliguria. A coagulopathy appears as the disease progresses. Multiple organ failure is the final outcome unless the process can be reversed.

The treatment of septic shock should aim to preserve the central nervous system, the myocardium, and renal function.[22] Intensive cardiovascular monitoring is essential to guide fluid therapy and drug administration. Cardiorespiratory support measures may be required from the outset. The important therapeutic steps are listed below.[23]

1. Appropriate cardiorespiratory support, which is directed at ensuring the best possible oxygenation and an adequate alveolar ventilation.

2. Intravenous fluid therapy to maintain the central venous pressure above 10 mm Hg and the hematocrit at 35 to 40 percent.

3. Aggressive intravenous antibiotic therapy.

4. Correction of acid-base and electrolyte disturbances, hypoglycemia, and hypocalcemia.

5. Dopamine infusion to reverse hypotension and oliguria when the CVP is above 10 mmHg. An infusion rate of 1 to 25 μg/kg/min may be required depending upon response.

6. Corticosteroids: methylprednisolone 30 to 60 mg/kg I.V. q4h until hypotension is corrected.

7. Appropriate surgical treatment of localized infections or other lesions.

Anesthesia for the Patient with Septic Shock

It may be necessary to anesthetize the patient in shock to drain localized infections or to resect infected or infarcted tissues. While it is important that optimal therapy for the shock state be in progress, surgical treatment should not be delayed unduly. The physical status of the patient may continue to deteriorate because of infected tissues. Hypovolemia and acidosis should be corrected and fever reduced prior to operation, hypoxia should be reversed as much as possible, and hypoventilation, if present, should be treated by controlled ventilation. Corticosteroid therapy should be augmented and inotropic therapy optimized.

Anesthesia techniques for the patient in septic shock should be selected to spare the cardiovascular system. Ketamine may be useful to induce anesthesia. Fentanyl and oxygen with neuromuscular blocking drugs is recommended for maintenance of anesthesia.[25]

PERINATAL INFECTIONS

There are several serious perinatal infections that may cause death or lasting damage to the child. The anesthesiologist should have some knowledge of the mode of transmission and the effects of these important diseases.

Cytomegalovirus

Cytomegalovirus (CMV) is a DNA virus of similar structure to the herpes virus. CMV is the most frequently recognized congenital infection and is a common cause of later mental retardation. In adults the infection is usually symptomless and innocuous. The virus is frequently found in cervical secretions and breast milk of the mother, but only some infants will acquire the infection and develop symptoms.

Cytomegalovirus is carried, probably in the leukocyte, in asymptomatic hosts and may be transmitted by blood transfusion. Transfusion-acquired CMV disease may occur in infants with serious sequelae. Blood transfused to infants should be screened for CMV.[26] The infant with CMV may infect the mother, and this may result in fetal CMV infection during subsequent pregnancies.[27]

The clinical manifestations of CMV disease depend upon the time of infection and the immune status of the infant: transplacental immunity may modify the disease. Intrauterine infection of the fetus may result in severe congenital deformity: microcephaly with mental retardation is common.[28] Intracranial periventricular calcification may be present. Other features of congenital CMV infection are hepatosplenomegaly, jaundice, thrombocytopenia, and eye disease (optic atrophy, chorioretinitis, coloboma, and cataracts).

Postnatal infection may result in pneumonia, hepatosplenomegaly, lymphadenopathy, and atypical lymphocytosis.

No specific treatment for congenital CMV has been shown to be effective. Antiviral agents have little effect on the course of the disease.

Congenital Rubella

In older children and adults, rubella is a mild infectious disease with an incubation period of 10 to 21 days. The systemic signs are very mild and are often missed. They include fever, sore throat, and lymphadenopathy in the sternomastoid and occipital regions. The maculopapular rash usually develops in the face and spreads to the trunk and limbs. Occasional complications include arthritis and encephalitis, which is rare. Thrombocytopenic purpura may occur with rubella.[29] The rubella syndrome that follows intrauterine infection is the most serious complication of the disease.[30]

Rubella Syndrome

Maternal rubella may cause severe fetal defects, especially if infection occurs during early gestation (less than 12 weeks). The classic rubella syndrome results in a low-birth-weight child with congenital heart disease (patent ductus arteriosus, pulmonary stenosis), eye defects (cataracts, glaucoma, and microphthalmia), and microcephaly. Deafness is also a common feature. In 1964 a severe epidemic of rubella in the United States resulted in other features of the syndrome being recognized. These include hepatosplenomegaly with jaundice, thrombocytopenic purpura, encephalitis, and myocarditis.[30]

A "late onset" rubella syndrome is also recognized. Affected infants show minimal signs at birth, but after 3 to 6 months develop multisystem disease. Pneumonia, skin rash, diarrhea, and hypogammaglobulinemia circulating immune complexes may be present.[32] Infants with rubella syndrome may develop hypotonia and convulsions later. Diabetes mellitus has also oc-

curred during childhood in patients with rubella syndrome.

Anesthetic Implications. The child with rubella syndrome may present for surgery of the various component defects of the syndrome, for complications thereof, or for any other surgical disease of childhood.

Special attention must be directed to the cardiovascular status, but other defects also demand consideration. Microcephaly may lead to difficulty with airway management and intubation, as may the presence of cleft palate and dental deformities. Anemia and thrombocytopenia may be present and require correction prior to anesthesia and surgery. The small size of the patient is frequently compounded by a generalized muscular weakness, and the response to and recovery from neuromuscular blocking drugs should be carefully assessed.

Finally it must be recognized that the rubella virus persists in some body fluids of the child for prolonged periods; thus, the possibility of cross infection must be considered and suitable isolation precautions taken.

Herpes Simplex Infection

Herpes simplex virus is a DNA structure very similar to cytomegalovirus. In the adult, infection characteristically produces cutaneous lesions about the mouth (Type 1 virus or HSV 1) or in the genital region (Type 2 virus or HSV 2). Oral lesions due to HSV 1 may be spread to other skin areas by direct contact, and digital infections are common in anesthesiologists.[33] HSV 2 infection is sexually transmitted.

The fetus may become infected in utero, but more commonly the neonate acquires the infection from the mother during birth. The extent of the disease in the infected neonate depends upon his immune status.[34] Neonatal herpes may also be acquired from other infants and hospital personnel.[35]

Neonatal herpes infection usually becomes apparent in the first month of life and may range from isolated skin lesions to widespread infection. The skin lesions typically are groups of vesicles. The disseminated infection presents with fever, pneumonia, hepatomegaly and jaundice, and coagulopathy.[36] Mortality is high in disseminated herpes and many survivors have neurological and/or ocular damage.

Treatment is with antiviral drugs such as acyclovir, but the long-term outcome is as yet uncertain. Prevention of maternal herpes and avoidance of nosocomial spread of the disease in the newborn are therefore of vital importance. Cesarean section is indicated in mothers with active genital herpes. Infants with suspected infection should be carefully isolated. The anesthesiologist who has a suspected active herpes infection should not become involved in the care of the neonate (or the immune-suppressed patient).[37]

Gown and gloves should be worn by all personnel when handling infected infants.

Neonatal Hepatitis

Acute hepatitis in the mother may result in premature birth and neonatal infection. Maternal hepatitis type A may also increase the risk of abortion.[38] The newborn may also become infected after delivery: hepatitis A infection usually results in a mild disease. Hepatitis B in newborns is more serious as it may proceed to chronic active hepatitis and even hepatoma later.[39]

Infected infants should be isolated. Those with type A hepatitis, which is spread by fecal contamination, should be in a single room with careful disposal of items that may be contaminated, such as used linens. Gowning, gloving, and meticulous hand washing by attendant staff are recommended. Hepatitis type B is spread primarily by blood and other secretions, and infected infants should be isolated and subject to precautions in handling blood and secretions. (For a full discussion of isolation requirements in hepatitis, see page 43.) Active and passive immunization is recommended for treatment of infants exposed to hepatitis B.[40]

Congenital Toxoplasmosis

Toxoplasma gondii is a protozoan parasite of mammals and birds. The intermediate stage oocyst forms only in the cat intestine. Human infection results from contact with infected material from household pets, or from ingestion of the organism in undercooked meats. Infection is often almost asymptomatic in adults, but may cause severe damage to the developing fetus.

Congenital toxoplasmosis may manifest with obstructive hydrocephalus, encephalitis, and scattered intracranial calcification.[41] These neurological signs may not appear until 2 to 3 months of age. Hepatosplenomegaly and anemia may be present. Chorioretinitis may develop later and cause blindness.

Infected infants are treated with pyrimethamine, sulfadiazine, and folinic acid for 3 weeks, and this regimen is repeated twice during the first year of life. This therapy is not thought to eliminate the organism completely, but it may halt progression of the disease. No isolation techniques are suggested for affected infants.

Congenital Syphilis

Syphilis is caused by the spiral bacterium *Treponema pallidum*. It is becoming more common in adults in the United States, and therefore an increase in congenital syphilis might be expected.

Intrauterine infection with syphilis may cause widespread damage to the fetus, but only rarely causes abortion. Most affected infants appear normal at birth and the classic features of the disease develop over the first months and years of life. Some infants may be small and premature, and some may show lymphadenopathy, hepatosplenomegaly, and jaundice at birth. A nasal discharge, sometimes bloodstained, may be present and may contain *Treponema pallidum* in high concentration. A maculopapular rash may develop over 2 to 3 weeks and may ulcerate, in which case the infectious organism is usually present in high concentration.

The clinical manifestations of congenital syphilis that appear in the first 2 years of life include bone lesions (panosteitis), central nervous system disease (meningitis, hydrocephalus, convulsions), iritis, and skin rashes.[42] Mucous patches may develop on the palate. Hepatosplenomegaly and a mild anemia are common. The later manifestations are bony abnormalities (deformed maxilla, frontal bossing); abnormal short, narrow, wide-spaced teeth (Hutchinson's teeth); interstitial keratitis, which may lead to blindness; nerve deafness; and chronic skin lesions.

The diagnosis of congenital syphilis is usually made on the serological testing of the mother and clinical signs in the infant. Serological testing of the infant is complicated by the fact that maternal antibody is passively acquired via the placenta. Isolation of the pathogen from lesions on the infant confirms the diagnosis. Treatment of the infant is with penicillin: a single dose of benzathine penicillin G 50,000 I.U. intramuscularly, or if neurosyphilis cannot be excluded aqueous penicillin G 50,000 I.U. intramuscularly per day for 10 days.

Lesions should become noninfectious after 48 hours of antibiotic therapy. The anesthesiologist who must handle an infant with active congenital syphilis (an ulcerating rash or nasal discharge) is advised to wear gloves.

Respiratory Infections of the Newborn

Pneumonia in the neonate may result from transplacental infection, intrauterine infection, infection during birth, or postnatal infection.[43] The newborn infant is especially vulnerable to infections of the lungs; since mucociliary clearance mechanisms are incompletely developed and IgA is relatively deficient in respiratory secretions.[44]

Congenital or intrauterine pneumonia is seen at autopsy of infants who die at or shortly after birth. Though there is a marked inflammatory reaction in the lungs, bacteria often are not seen and cultures may be negative. It is therefore not clear whether the changes seen are due to infection or hypoxia.[45] Indeed, it has been suggested that amniotic fluid may protect the fetus and newborn, as cases of bacterial pneumonia are rare.[44]

Pneumonia acquired during or after birth is similar to that seen in older patients. There is vascular congestion, hemorrhage, and areas of cellular infiltration and necrosis.[46] Bacteria are commonly present. The infecting agents are most usually *Streptococcus pneumoniae, Streptococcus pyogenes, Staphylococcus aureus, Haemophilis influenzae,* and the viruses.

Though some infants may be critically ill, the clinical manifestations of pneumonia in a newborn may be nonspecific: pallor, poor feeding, tachypnea, and tachycardia. Physical examination of the chest is unreliable as a means to diagnose the condition certainly, and chest x-rays are essential.

Symptoms in an infant who has a history of early rupture of the membranes and/or premature delivery, especially if the amniotic fluid appeared infected, should prompt a radiological investigation of the chest. Bacteriological diagnosis may be obtained by culture of tracheal aspirate, but this should be obtained at direct laryngoscopy to avoid contamination by upper respiratory tract flora. Blood or CSF, or, if present, pleural fluid culture may also indicate the pathogen. Lung puncture may be necessary to provide an immediate diagnosis in the critically ill neonate.

The management of infants with pneumonia must include immediate optimal antibiotic therapy, which should be modified as soon as cultures are completed. Initial therapy with penicillin, ampicillin, or, if staphylococcal infection is likely, a penicillinase-resistant penicillin together with an aminoglycoside is presently recommended.[43] Other measures should include appropriate oxygen therapy and respiratory care, maintenance of fluid, electrolyte, and acid-base status, and drainage of effusions if present.

INFECTIOUS DISEASES OF CHILDHOOD

Measles (Rubeola)

This is a very infectious viral disease spread by droplet infection. The incubation period is 7 to 12 days, but the child can infect others during the last few days of this time.

The clinical features of the disease include a high fever, severe cough, and conjunctivitis. After 3 to 4 days a rash appears, usually beginning on the face and neck and spreading to involve the whole body. An enanthem consisting of small white papules appears on the buccal mucosa 1 to 2 days before the typical maculopapular exanthem. The skin rash becomes confluent and lasts about 7 days.

The complications of measles can be severe. Respiratory infections are common and pneumonitis is present in 20 percent of patients.[48] In some children this may progress to a severe pneumonia, and this may occur in those who have received killed measles vaccine.[49] Pleural effusions may appear with atypical measles infection. Pneumomediastinum, pneumo-

thorax, and subcutaneous emphysema have occurred in association with measles.[50]

Laryngitis is a frequent complication of measles in some countries and is a leading cause of mortality in young malnourished children. Upper airway obstruction is often accompanied by lung disease, so tracheotomy or endotracheal intubation may not be followed by immediate improvement.[51] Myocarditis has been described in association with measles and may be diagnosed by ECG changes.[52]

Abdominal complications of measles include diarrhea, which may lead to severe fluid disturbances, especially if malnutrition is present. Lymphoid hyperplasia may result in abdominal pain and rarely may precipitate appendicitis.

Hematological changes occur with measles and include a marked leukopenia. Thrombocytopenia is much less common, but may result in severe episodes of bleeding.[53]

The most common neurological complication of measles is encephalitis.[54] This occurs within a few days of the onset of measles and has a clinical course of 1 to 2 weeks. The disease may be due to direct invasion by the virus or may be an allergic demyelinating disorder.[54] Symptoms include lethargy, irritability, tremors, and later convulsions and depressed consciousness. Meningeal signs are usually present. A later and rarer neurological complication is subacute sclerosing panencephalitis (SSPE). This is characterized by mental deterioration, myoclonic seizures, and eventual death and may follow several years after the initial measles infection. SSPE is thought to be due to persistent infection of the central nervous system by the measles virus and is usually seen in patients who had the initial infection in the first year of life.[55] There is no specific treatment.

Other neurological complications that may be associated with measles include the Guillain-Barré syndrome.[56] Muscle weakness and depressed tendon reflexes appear 1 to 2 weeks after the appearance of the measles rash and progress to the typical clinical picture of Guillain-Barré syndrome.

No specific isolation recommendations are made for children in the home, but those in the hospital should be isolated from the onset of the catarrhal stage until the third day of the rash to reduce possible exposure to those children at high risk (for example, immunosuppressed patients).

Varicella (Chicken Pox) and Herpes Zoster

Varicella is a common, extremely contagious disease. It is usually a relatively benign disease, but serious complications may develop in the very young or in immunosuppressed patients. Because of the highly contagious nature of the disease and the potential for severe complications in some patients (such as those on immunosuppressive drugs or with leukemia), it is most important that children who may have varicella are not inadvertently admitted to the hospital. Thus pediatric surgical patients who develop an illness or rash should be carefully examined prior to admission.

The first sign of varicella is usually the appearance of a "dewdrop" rash, mainly on the trunk. The prodromal symptoms are mild. The rash rapidly progresses through macular to papular to vesicular stages. The vesicles then dry and crust.

In the immunosuppressed patient, varicella may rapidly progress to a hemorrhagic disseminated infection. Death from pneumonia and/or encephalitis may ensue.[57]

Herpes zoster is caused by the same virus and is more common in adults, but can occur in children and even in infants.[58] There is usually a history of a previous attack of varicella. Herpes zoster presents with pain and a varicella-like rash along the course of a peripheral sensory nerve. The pain of herpes zoster is less in children than in older patients and the rash heals more rapidly. Postherpetic neuralgia is uncommon in children.

Varicella may be complicated by coagulopathy, which may be secondary to thrombocytopenia, factor V deficiency, low fibrinogen or prothrombin level, and an associated vasculitis. Another serious disease that has been associated with varicella is Reye syndrome (see page 61); as many as 15 percent of patients with this syndrome may give a history of an associated varicella infection.

Mumps (Epidemic Parotitis)

This is a viral infection that is most common in school-age children, though it may occur in adults. The disease is characterized by fever, malaise, and swelling of the parotid glands. The disease tends to cause milder symptoms in the younger age groups. The etiological agent is myxovirus parotidis, which is found in the saliva of patients with the disease.

The parotid glands become painful and enlarge within 24 hours of the onset of symptoms. The disease is sometimes limited to one side, but may involve both parotid glands and the submandibular and sublingual salivary glands.

The most common complication in older patients and adults is orchitis, which may occur in up to 35 percent of male adults with mumps. In the female oophoritis may occur, and if the right ovary is involved the symptoms may resemble appendicitis. Meningoencephalitis may occur with mumps and the virus may be found in the CSF in 10 percent of all patients. Neurological involvement is usually followed by complete recovery.

Other complications include deafness, possibly due to endolymphatic labyrinthitis, myocarditis, and possibly endocardial fibroelastosis (EFE).[59] The latter association is based on the finding of positive mumps antigen skin testing in children with EFE.[59] It has been suggested that mumps virus might be implicated in the etiology of juvenile diabetes mellitus.[60]

Roseola Infantum

This is a common infectious disease of infants. The disease results in a high fever (103 to 104°F) for a period of 3 to 4 days followed by a sudden fall to normal levels and the appearance of a measles-like rash. The patient usually does not appear as ill as the temperature would indicate, but convulsions may occur during the febrile period. No specific treatment is required and recovery is complete.

Infectious Mononucleosis

This disease of children, adolescents, and young adults is caused by Epstein-Barr virus (EBV) infection. The illness is characterized by lassitude, fever, pharyngitis, lymphadenopathy, and hepatosplenomegaly and usually runs a benign course, though serious complications can develop. EBV infection may cause serious disease or death in immunosuppressed patients.

Complications of EBV infection that may concern the anesthesiologist include airway obstruction due to massively enlarged tonsils, splenic rupture, and Guillain-Barré syndrome. Patients with impending airway obstruction may benefit from steroid therapy, though tracheotomy is sometimes required. Rupture of the spleen is a rare (0.2 percent) complication, but is extremely serious[61] and may occur up to 3 months after the development of the illness. Neurological complications of EBV infection may occur in 1 to 8 percent of cases and account for 50 percent of deaths from the disease. Guillain-Barré syndrome is seen in approximately 20 percent of those with nervous system involvement. The mortality rate with ascending polyneuritis is reported to be as high as 25 percent.[62]

Hepatic function may be impaired in patients with infectious mononucleosis, and jaundice may occur. Abnormal liver isoenzymes are found in the majority of patients.

Diphtheria

This is an acute infectious disease caused by *Corynebacterium diphtheriae*, which is a club-shaped gram positive rod. The organism invades the nose and throat causing a nasopharyngitis and also produces a powerful exotoxin that causes major myocardial and neurological damage.[63] Diphtheria is now a very rare disease in Western countries as a result of successful immunization programs. Sporadic cases do occur, however, and there is a continuing danger that recent immigrants might introduce the infection to unimmunized segments of the population. Because of airway, myocardial, and neurological involvements the disease is of importance to anesthesiologists.

The incubation period of diphtheria is 2 to 5 days, and the onset is insidious with a mild sore throat and pyrexia of 100 to 102°F. The pharynx is initially red, but within 24 hours whitish spots appear which coalesce to form a thin adherent membrane. The membrane becomes thicker and darker in color, with distinct margins. Attempts to remove the membrane result in bleeding and formation of a new membrane. The process subsides after 5 to 6 days, the membrane loosens, and symptoms resolve. However, cardiac and neurological damage may occur after even a mild infection.

In some patients infection and membrane formation is limited to the nasopharynx. The symptoms are then those of a mucoid or sanguineous nasal discharge. Systemic effects may be minimal owing to the poor absorption of toxin via the nasal mucosa. At the other extreme, the most severe form of diphtheria demonstrates rapid spread of the infection. The membrane spreads to cover pharynx, buccal cavity, and nasopharynx. There is marked cervical lymphadenopathy and swelling of the tissues of the neck, resulting in a "bull-neck" appearance. Such patients develop severe systemic symptoms of high fever, vomiting and diarrhea, muscle weakness, and central nervous system depression. Death may occur from respiratory obstruction or myocardial failure.

Laryngeal diphtheria occurs in up to 25 percent of cases. Voice changes occur early and the disease may progress rapidly to encroach on the airway. Sudden obstruction by a fragment of membrane is a constant potential threat. The patient must be kept under very close continuous observation by staff who are expert in emergency airway support.

Myocardial changes are due to a direct effect of the exotoxin and consist of cloudy swelling of muscle fibers that may proceed to complete degeneration.[63] Some degree of myocardial involvement is evident in up to 50 percent of patients with diphtheria. Early signs include tachycardia and a low pulse volume. Electrocardiographic changes include prolongation of the P-R interval, T wave inversion, and later bundle branch block or complete heart block.[64] As the myocardial involvement progresses, evidence of congestive cardiac failure appears. Myocarditis is likely to be most severe in patients who show evidence of this complication during the first 10 days of a diphtheria infection. Occasionally myocardial fibrosis may follow as a permanent complication of diphtheria.[65]

The neurological complications of diphtheria affect the cranial nerves and their nuclei and the spinal cord. Paralysis of some form is common, and muscles of the palate are most frequently affected. Paralysis, however, may be widespread and may affect the muscles of ventilation, requiring ventilatory therapy.[66]

The diagnosis of diphtheria is confirmed by isolation and culture of the infecting agent. Cultures should be taken before antibiotics are given. Treatment is with antitoxin and must be commenced early, usually before the diagnosis is confirmed by culture. Antitoxin is given intravenously in one dose diluted in normal saline. Penicillin or erythromycin should be given in addition. All patients should be carefully monitored to detect airway compromise or myocardial changes. Endotracheal intubation or tracheotomy may be required. Cardiac failure requires therapy with digitalis. Arrhythmias must be treated as appropriate and cardiac pacing may be necessary for heart block. Severe diphtheria interferes with oral feeding, and intravenous therapy is required.

Tetanus

Tetanus is caused by infection of a wound with the spore-bearing, anaerobic gram positive organism *Clostridium tetani,* which produces a powerful neurotoxin. This toxin is formed by the organism in the wound and spreads to the central nervous system via the motor nerves or bloodstream. The neurotoxic effects produce a characteristic clinical picture. The disease is now rare in developed countries as a result of immunization programs, but sporadic cases still occur in unprotected children. In developing countries the disease is still very common and often presents in the neonate following infection of the umbilicus. Tetanus is still a major cause of death worldwide.[67]

The clinical signs usually develop 3 to 21 days after infection. In general, the shorter the incubation period, the more severe is the disease. Trismus is the common presenting sign in older children. This is a result of the neurotoxin affecting the facial nerve centers in the region of the fourth cerebral ventricle. Muscle rigidity spreads to affect all the facial muscles, producing a classic fixed facial expression—risus sardonicus. Generalized painful tonic and clonic spasms of skeletal muscle follow as the disease progresses. Initially these spasms are intermittent and are triggered by sensory stimuli, including touch, noise, and bright light. Later the spasms become continuous. Muscle spasms occur as a result of the depressant effects of the neurotoxin on inhibitory internuncial neurons.

As the disease progresses spasms become more severe and continuous and eventually result in opisthotonos, flexion and adduction of the arms, and extension of the legs and feet. Spasms of the ventilatory muscles and/or laryngeal spasm may lead to respiratory failure and death.

The autonomic nervous system is also involved and this may lead to alterations in heart rate, labile hypertension, disordered temperature control, and serious cardiac arrhythmias.[68]

Neonatal tetanus has a short incubation period and presents as inability to suck.[67] This is rapidly followed by generalized stiffness and convulsions. Spasms of the muscles of ventilation may lead to apnea. Aspiration pneumonia is common. The differential diagnosis of neonatal tetany includes intracranial injury, hypocalcemia, sepsis, and meningitis.

The treatment of tetanus includes antitoxin and antibiotic therapy; penicillin and tetracycline* are effective against *Clostridium tetani.* The child should be nursed in a quiet area and all external stimuli avoided to decrease reflex spasms. Diazepam has been widely used to control spasms, but many patients will require neuromuscular blocking drugs and mechanical ventilation. Ileus is common and hence patients will require intravenous alimentation. All general supportive and nursing care is essential during the period of weeks for which therapy may be required.

Cardiovascular instability secondary to autonomic involvement may require therapy with antihypertensives, and it is suggested that D-tubocurarine is preferable to pancuronium for neuromuscular blockade in such patients.[69] It is also suggested that isoflurane may be the inhalation agent of choice for the patient with tetanus.[70] Isoflurane can be administered to achieve good control of blood pressure, and arrhythmias may be less troublesome than with halothane.

Botulism

Botulism is a disease of the neuromuscular system caused by the exotoxin produced by the infecting agent *Clostridium botulinum.* The disease usually follows the ingestion of the organisms and preformed toxin in improperly preserved foods. In infants the disease is rare, but may be caused by toxin formed in the gastrointestinal tract following infection by the same organism.[71]

In older children and adults the disease results from ingestion of the toxin in uncooked foods—the toxin is destroyed by heat. The disease is characterized by muscle weakness, which results from the effect of the botulism toxin on neuromuscular transmission. The toxin has now been shown to interfere with acetylcholine release at the presynaptic motor nerve ending;[72] synthesized acetylcholine is blocked from release from its storage sites in the synaptic vesicles. The resulting progressive paralysis results in generalized weakness and ventilatory failure. Diplopia, dysarthria, dysphasia, dry mouth, and dilated pupils are constant early symptoms. Fever is usually absent.

In infants with botulism resulting from gastrointestinal colonization by *Clostridium botulinum* the onset of symptoms is more insidious. Constipation is a common early sign and may be present for 7 to 10 days prior to the onset of progressive muscle weakness, poor feeding, and lethargy.[71] Weakness of the respiratory

muscles may lead to ventilatory failure. The diagnosis of infantile botulism can be furthered by the demonstration of the "staircase phenomenon" on electrical stimulation of a peripheral nerve.[73] Evoked muscle action potentials show a positive incremental response at stimulation frequencies above 10 Hz. This response may also be seen in antibiotic toxicity, the Eaton-Lambert syndrome, and snakebite by some species.

Treatment of infantile botulism must include respiratory and nutritional support as is indicated. The only recorded deaths have followed failure to maintain adequate artificial ventilation. Penicillin is effective against the organism, but may not clear the infection. Purgatives may be indicated to hasten excretion of toxin. The use of antitoxin is successful in only some patients. Artificial ventilation may be required for weeks, but may be followed by complete recovery.

Viral Hepatitis

Viral hepatitis may occur in children in three different forms: hepatitis A, hepatitis B, and non A/non B hepatitis.

Hepatitis A infections are common in school-age children, often as a cyclical epidemic disease. The usual mode of transmission is by ingestion of the virus in contaminated food. Parenteral transmission is rare. The incubation period of the disease is 2 to 6 weeks and the clinical course tends to be milder in children than in adults. Asymptomatic infection and anicteric disease are common in children.[74] Hepatitis A does not usually lead to chronic liver disease or a carrier state.

Hepatitis B virus causes a variety of responses in infected persons. Some maintain an asymptomatic carrier state with little or no liver damage. Others display varying degrees of liver dysfunction and may proceed to chronic active hepatitis. Hepatitis B is accompanied by a number of important extrahepatic manifestations that may concern the anesthesiologist. Glomerulonephritis, purpura, aplastic anemia, and polyarteritis may occur. Pleural effusion, pericarditis, and myocarditis have been described in children.[75]

A principal concern for the anesthesiologist caring for the child with hepatitis B infection is to avoid communicating the infection to other patients or to himself. Transmission of hepatitis B is principally via parenteral inoculation, but the virus can be found in urine, saliva, and other body fluids. Disposable equipment should be used for infected patients and be safely disposed. The anesthesiologist should be careful to avoid self-inoculation and should avail himself of appropriate prophylactic immunization against hepatitis B.[76]

Non A/non B hepatitis is a disease that is similar to hepatitis B in transmission and symptomatology, though it is usually not as severe.[74] It is most commonly transmitted during blood transfusion.

---

*Because of the risk of discoloration of permanent teeth, tetracyclines should not be used in children less than 8 years of age unless other drugs are contraindicated or would be ineffective.

Gastrointestinal Infections

Gastrointestinal infections are second only to respiratory tract infections as a cause of morbidity and mortality in children. The peak incidence of gastroenteritis is in the first year of life and at this age, infants are particularly vulnerable to the dehydrating and debilitating effects of diarrhea and vomiting. As in respiratory infections the most common pathogens are viruses, such as rotavirus, Norwalk virus, and enteroviruses. Bacteria that are commonly involved are *Salmonella, Shigella, Campylobacter* and *E. coli.*

Of particular concern to the anesthesiologist is the gastroenteritis that spreads in the infant wards of a hospital. Many infants who are admitted for surgery run the risk of such a hospital-acquired infection. The anesthesiologist must adhere strictly to the procedures for isolation of infected infants and contacts, so that he does not become a vector for the disease.

Rotavirus infection is a common cause of diarrhea in hospitalized infants, but adults may also become infected. In infants the gastrointestinal symptoms of rotavirus infection are often accompanied by an upper respiratory infection.[77] Most infections are self-limiting, but the disease may be serious in immunodeficient patients and others who are debilitated. Complications of rotavirus infection include intussusception and encephalitis. The most important prophylactic measures to prevent the spread of rotavirus infection are those of meticulous hand washing and proper disposal of soiled diapers and other linens.

Salmonella infections are also common in the infant wards of hospitals, and infants of under 3 months of age are particularly at risk.[78] Such infants commonly excrete *Salmonella* organisms from the bowel for several weeks after the symptoms of gastroenteritis have resolved.

Tuberculosis

Tuberculosis is still a major cause of childhood disease worldwide. In developed nations the disease is rarer and confined mainly to children in the lower socioeconomic groups. Because of the comparative rarity of the disease, there is a danger that tuberculosis will be missed as a diagnosis. The infective agent is *Mycobacterium tuberculosis* in most cases, though *Mycobacterium bovis* is also pathogenic in humans. These bacteria are relatively resistant to drugs, can survive in a dried state for prolonged periods, and remain viable in tissues for prolonged periods but are destroyed by direct sunlight or ultraviolet light.

Most tuberculous infections are due to airborne spread of the bacillus,[79] and pulmonary infection follows inspiration of infected air. The most contagious patients are those with an intrapulmonary infected cavity and large numbers of organisms in the sputum. Children with pulmonary or extrapulmonary tuberculosis are usually not contagious and need not be isolated.[80]

Primary tuberculosis infection involves the lungs and appears several weeks after infection. Many children are asymptomatic and the infection is apparent only on tuberculin testing. Most infected children will show enlarged hilar lymph nodes and some have pulmonary infiltrates and a pleural effusion. Most patients heal spontaneously without therapy, but if the disease is diagnosed, treatment may be ordered to prevent progression to other tissues or relapses. In a minority of patients the disease progresses to cavity formation in the lungs or extrapulmonary infections. The other tissues most commonly involved are the cervical lymph glands, bone, meninges, and kidneys.

The children that progress to chronic tuberculous infection commonly do so as a result of altered resistance to the disease. Factors that may predispose to chronic disease include young age, poor nutrition, other infections (for example, measles, pertussis), and surgical trauma.

The anesthesiologist may be involved with many aspects of the treatment of children with tuberculosis. The multiplicity of tissues that may be involved and require surgical intervention dictates that a great variety of critical problems may present. Each child must therefore be very fully assessed to determine the full effects of his disease. Contamination of anesthesia equipment is a possible hazard, so disposable items should be used whenever possible. Anesthetic and ventilator circuits should be protected by bacterial filters. All equipment that is not disposable should be treated by boiling for 3 minutes or placing in an antiseptic solution (such as 0.1 percent chlorhexidene) for 1 hour. All other items that might have become infected and cannot be treated as above should be gas sterilized using ethylene oxide. Large items of equipment in the operating room should be washed with a chemical disinfectant (such as 70 percent alcohol).[81]

PARASITIC DISEASES

Roundworms (Ascariasis)

Ascaris lumbricoides is a large roundworm, 20 to 45 cm in length and up to 6 mm in diameter. Ascariasis is common in the tropics and extends to the temperate climates. Infection usually occurs as a result of ingesting *Ascaris* eggs from soil that later hatch in the duodenum. The larvae migrate through the intestinal wall and pass via the lymphatics or venules into the liver and thence via the bloodstream to the lungs. In the lungs the larvae grow and later migrate via the glottis into the esophagus. They are then swallowed to infest the small intestine.

During the lung phase, large numbers of larvae may produce an atypical pneumonia (Löffler syndrome). The larvae at this stage may also induce an allergic response which is characterized by bronchospasm, urticaria, and eosinophilia.

As the mature worms grow in the intestine the most common symptom in children is colic. Occasionally a mass of worms may cause intestinal obstruction, intussusception, or ileus; perforation of the intestine has occurred.

The treatment of roundworm infestation is with piperazine citrate. This drug may cause further gastrointestinal disturbance and rarely visual effects and ataxia.

Hookworms

The hookworm *Ancylostoma duodenale* is an intestinal parasite that is widespread in tropical and subtropical countries. *Necator americanus* is a similar species found in many countries of the Western hemisphere. Hookworm embryos develop into a larva in warm moist soil and gain access to the body through the skin of feet or hands. The larvae migrate to the lungs, where they may cause hemorrhagic pneumonia. The larvae then pass via the glottis into the gastrointestinal tract, where they grow to maturity.

The most important symptoms of hookworm disease are those that result from chronic blood loss.[82] The resultant anemia is hypochromic and microcytic and may result eventually in cardiomegaly, congestive heart failure, and severe weakness.

Treatment of hookworm infections is with mebendazole, which may also cause diarrhea and abdominal pain. In addition the anemia must be treated with oral or parenteral iron. Patients who require urgent surgery should have packed cell infusions to increase the hemoglobin level preoperatively.

Trichinosis

The parasite *Trichinella spiralis,* which causes an intestinal and tissue infection, is ingested usually in uncooked pork or bear meat. The adult worm inhabits the intestine, causing abdominal pain and diarrhea. The larvae invade other tissues, particularly skeletal muscle, causing edema, myalgia, and eosinophilia. Eventually calcification of encysted larvae occurs. Occasionally the larvae enter cardiac muscle, causing myocarditis with chest pain, tachycardia, hypotension and ECG changes. Steroid theapy is indicated for patients with myocardial involvement.

Echinococcosis and Hydatid Disease

Echinococcus granulosus is a tapeworm that infests the intestine of the dog; humans and sheep are among the species that serve as intermediate hosts. If eggs are ingested by humans, the embryo hatches and pene-

trates the abdominal wall, enters lymphatic or venous channels, and is transported to one of several organs. Here it develops into the hydatid cyst. This cyst is fluid-filled and unilocular and is surrounded by an outer laminated layer and an inner germinal layer. The germinal layer produces protoscoleces, which may number up to 2 million and are capable of infecting the primary host if ingested.

The symptoms produced by the hydatid cyst vary according to the site. The structure most commonly affected is the liver (63 percent), followed by lung (25 percent), muscle (5 percent), bone (3 percent), and brain (1 percent). Hepatic cysts may be asymptomatic for years before presenting with abdominal pain and a palpable mass. Lung cysts are usually found on routine x-ray, but may cause cough, chest pain, and hemoptysis. The diagnosis is made from the history of a slow-growing mass, an eosinophilia which is usual but not constant, and sometimes by intradermal testing (Casoni test). The latter test is not reliable and has a high false positive rate.[83] The definitive diagnosis is made after excision of the cyst.

The treatment of hydatid cyst is surgical excision of the intact cyst. Aspiration for diagnosis or treatment is contraindicated owing to the potential danger of leakage of fluid into body cavities. Rupture of the cyst, whether spontaneous or during attempted removal, may be followed by an anaphylactic reaction. In some cases intraoperative aspiration of the cyst and injection of 20 percent saline, or absolute alcohol has been performed to prevent possible seeding of the contents.[84] If rupture and anaphylaxis occur during surgery, vasopressors such as epinephrine, a bronchodilator such as isoproterenol, and large doses of corticosteroid drugs are indicated.[85]

ANTIBIOTIC THERAPY AND ANESTHESIA

Many patients who present for general anesthesia are on antibiotic therapy, and in some instances it may be necessary to administer antibiotics during the course of an anesthetic. It is therefore necessary that the anesthesiologist have some knowledge of the side effects and possible interactions of these drugs. The antibiotics in general use will be discussed together with their potential side effects and interactions with anesthetic drugs.

Penicillins

These drugs may cause hypersensitivity reactions. Penicillin is now one of the most common causes of anaphylaxis with an incidence of 0.015 to 0.04 percent.[86] There is no evidence to suggest that patients with a history of atopy are at greater risk. Anaphylaxis develops within seconds of injection of the drug, with bronchospasm, hypotension, and an erythematous rash.

Prompt therapy is essential for survival. Epinephrine administration, endotracheal intubation, and ventilation with oxygen must be immediately performed. Bronchodilators, corticosteroids, and antihistamines may help to further reverse the anaphylactic state. Despite therapy the mortality rate may be as high as 10 percent; therefore, prevention of the state is highly desirable. Meticulous history-taking for evidence of antibiotic allergies is essential. Though penicillin is most commonly involved, anaphylaxis may also follow administration of ampicillin, streptomycin, vancomycin, and the sulfonamide drugs.[87]

Penicillin is also sometimes followed by less acute hypersensitivity reactions. Skin rashes, including urticaria and angioedema, may form immediately or appear a few days after the drug is given. More rarely severe dermatological conditions, including Stevens-Johnson syndrome, exfoliative dermatitis, and epidermal necrolysis may occur. Serum sickness, characterized by fever, rash, arthritis, and lymphadenopathy, may develop, usually appearing after an interval of 4 to 12 days.

Penicillin therapy has been associated with central nervous system complications, particularly when the drug is given in large doses. Grand mal seizures may occur,[88] and depression of consciousness and coma may develop.[89]

Hemopoietic disease may result from penicillin therapy.[90] Hemolytic anemia, neutropenia, and thrombocytopenic purpura may occur. The semisynthetic penicillins are more often a cause of hematological disease than are the naturally occurring penicillins.

Renal diseases, including glomerulonephritis and interstitial nephritis, are rare complications, particularly of methicillin therapy. This complication is more likely to occur in those with pre-existing renal disease.

Cephalosporins

Allergic reactions to cephalosporins (cefamandole, cephaloridine, cefazolin, and so forth) may occur and there is probably a cross-reactivity with penicillin. Thus patients known to be allergic to penicillin, especially if urticaria or anaphlylaxis occurs, should not receive cephalosporins. Cephalosporins may also induce allergic reactions in patients who are not allergic to penicillin.

Hematological reactions to cephalosporins are uncommon, but hypoprothrombinemia may occur following moxalactam therapy and may be corrected with vitamin K.[91] Cephaloridine administration in high dosage may rarely cause renal damage.[92]

Aminoglycosides

Aminoglycosides may cause serious side effects, and therefore their use should be limited to infections for which they are essential therapy. Renal damage and ototoxicity are the most important complications, but these drugs are also recognized to cause neuromuscular blockade. Patients with hypocalcemia or myasthenia gravis and those given other neuromuscular blocking drugs are particularly likely to develop skeletal muscle weakness.[93] If abnormal weakness persists in patients on aminoglycoside therapy following surgery, artificial ventilation and all appropriate respiratory care should be continued until the condition resolves. Attempts to reverse neuromuscular blocks caused by antibiotics using pharmacological agents are not usually fully successful.

Hypersensitivity reactions with aminoglycosides are rare, but fever and a skin rash may occur in a small percentage of patients.

Chloramphenicol

Very rarely chloramphenicol may cause aplastic anemia. Much more commonly the drug results in a predictable degree of reversible bone marrow suppression. Thus blood studies should be performed at regular intervals.

The gray-baby syndrome affects preterm and term neonates who are treated with large doses of chloramphenicol (more than 100 mg/kg/day) for several days. The condition is characterized by rapid onset of abdominal distention, cyanosis, tachycardia, hypotonia, and eventual cardiovascular collapse.[94] This condition is thought to be due to the inadequacy of neonatal liver function to metabolize the drug and the inability of the newborn's kidneys to excrete unconjugated drug.

Hypersensitivity reactions to chloramphenicol are extremely rare.

Vancomycin

The most common side effect of this drug is ototoxicity, which is dose-related. There are some other rarer, but important complications.

The "red neck" syndrome is an anaphylactoid reaction associated with rapid intravenous infusion of the drug. It is a histamine-like reaction with erythematous rash, bronchospasm, and hypotension, which may lead to death.[95] Slow administration of the drug will prevent this reaction.

Erythromycin

Erythromycin is widely regarded as one of the safest antibiotics. Gastrointestinal reactions, including pseudomembranous enterocolitis, may occur, and cholestatic hepatitis may develop in children over 12 years of age.

Rapid intravenous infusion of erythromycin may result in very severe hypotension.

Lincomycin and Clindamycin

Lincomycin and clindamycin may cause myocardial depression, and cardiac arrest has been reported following a rapid infusion of lincomycin.[96] It is suggested that the principal effects of lincomycin may be on conduction mechanisms in the heart rather than contractility.

Hepatotoxicity is common with lincomycin, but hepatic failure rarely develops. Interactions of lincomycin with neuromuscular blocking drugs have occurred.

True anaphylaxis to lincomycin may occur, but is rare. Severe skin rashes, including the Stevens-Johnson syndrome, have occurred.

In summary, all antibiotics are capable of producing severe side effects. The anesthesiologist must diligently seek a history of antibiotic drug allergy and must observe appropriate caution in the use of these drugs. Rapid intravenous injections must be avoided as they are associated with the highest incidence of severe reactions.

REFERENCES

1. Kluger MJ, Ringler DH, Anver MR: Fever and survival. Science 188:166, 1975.
2. Heim T: Homeothermy and its metabolic cost. In Davis JA, Dobbing J (eds.): Scientific Foundations of Pediatrics. 2nd ed. London, Heinemann, 1981, p 118.
3. Mathsaniotis N, Pastelis V, Agathopoulos A, et al.: Fever and biochemical thermogenesis. Pediatrics 47:571, 1971.
4. Dubois EF: The Mechanism of Heat Loss and Temperature Regulation. Lance Memorial Lectures. Palo Alto, CA, Stanford University Press, 1937.
5. Alessandri RM: Fever. In Waldmann RH, Kluge RM (Eds.): Infectious Diseases. New York, Medical Examination Publishing Co., 1984, pp 9–13.
6. Ouellette EM: The child who convulses with fever. Pediatr Clin N Am 21:467, 1974.
7. Moffet HL: Pediatric Infectious Diseases. 2nd ed. Philadelphia, J.B. Lippincott Co., 1981, p 263.
8. McCracken G, Shinefeld H: Changes in the pattern of neonatal septicemia and meningitis. Am J Dis Child 112:33, 1966.
9. Miller E: Chemotactic function in the human neonate: humoral and cellular aspects. Pediatr Res 5:487, 1971.
10. Keay AS, Simpson R: Prevention of infection in nurseries for the newborn. Postgrad Med J 53:583, 1977.
11. Klaus MH, Fanaroff AA: Care of the High Risk Neonate. Philadelphia, W.B. Saunders Co., 1979, p 275.
12. Remington JS, Klein JO: Infectious Diseases of the Fetus and Newborn Infant. Philadelphia, W.B. Saunders Co., 1983.
13. Sheoka A, Hall R, Hill H: Blood transfusion in group B streptococcal sepsis. Lancet 1:636, 1978.
14. Bosworth, DC: Reversible adrenocortical insufficiency in fulminant meningococcemia. Arch Intern Med 139:823, 1979.
15. Reichgott MJ, Melmon KL: Should corticosteroids be used in shock? Med Clin N Am 57:1211, 1983.
16. Coonrod JD, Leach RP: Antigenemia in fulminant pneumococcemia. Ann Intern Med 84:561, 1976.
17. Dickerman JD: Splenectomy and sepsis: a warning. Pediatrics 63:638, 1979.
18. Trigg ME: Immune function of the spleen. South Med J 72:593, 1979.
19. Sherman NJ, Aach MJ: Conservative surgery for splenic injuries. Pediatrics 61:267, 1978.
20. Hieber JP, Nelson AJ, McCracken GH: Acute disseminated staphylococcal disease in childhood. Am J Dis Child 131:181, 1977.
21. Hierro FR, Palomequee A, Calvo M, et al.: Septic shock in pediatrics. Paediatrician 8:93, 1979.
22. Perkin RM, Levin DL: Shock in the pediatric patient. Part I. J Pediatr 101:163, 1982.
23. Marks MI:, Pediatric Infectious Diseases. New York, Springer Verlag, 1985, pp 731–735.
24. Wilson RF, Chiscano AD, Quadros E, et al.: Some observations on 132 patients with septic shock. Anesth Analg 46:751, 1967.
25. Stanley TH, Reddy P: Fentanyl oxygen in septic shock. Anesthesiology 51:S100, 1979.
26. Adler SP, Chandrika T, Lawrence L, et al.: Cytomegalovirus infections in neonates acquired by blood transfusions. Pediatr Infect Dis 2:114, 1983.
27. Yeager AJ: Transmission of cytomegalovirus to mothers by infected infants: another reason to prevent transfusion acquired infections. Pediatr Infect Dis 2:295, 1983.
28. Pass RF, Stagno, S, Myers GJ, et al.: Outcome of symptomatic congenital cytomegalovirus infection: results of long-term longitudinal follow-up. Pediatrics 66:758, 1980.
29. Ozsoylu S, Kanra G, Savas G: Thrombocytopenic purpura related to rubella infection. Pediatrics 62:567, 1978.
30. Korones SB, Ainger LE, Monif GRG: Congenital rubella syndrome: a study of 22 infants. Am J Dis Child 110:434, 1965.
31. Miller E, Cradock-Watson JE, Pollock TM: Consequences of confirmed maternal rubella at successive stages of pregnancy. Lancet 2:781, 1982.
32. Tradieu M, Grospierre B, Durandy A, et al.: Circulating immune complexes containing rubella antigens in late onset rubella syndrome. J Pediatr 97:370, 1980.
33. Louis DS, Silva J: Herpetic whitlow: herpetic infections of the digits. J Hand Surg 4:90, 1979.
34. Yeager AS, Arvin AM, Urbani LJ, et al.: Relationship of antibody to outcome in neonatal herpes simplex virus infections. Infect Immun 29:532, 1980.
35. Light IJ: Postnatal acquisition of herpes simplex virus by the newborn infant: a review of the literature. Pediatrics 63:480, 1971.
36. Miller DR, Hanshaw JB, O'Leary DS, et al.: Fatal disseminated herpes simplex virus infection and hemorrhage in the neonate. J Pediatr 76: 409, 1970.
37. Adams G, Stover BH, Kennlyside RA, et al.: Nosocomial herpetic infections in a pediatric intensive care unit. Am J Epidemiol 113:126, 1981.
38. Stevens CE, Krugman S, Szmuness W, et al.: Viral hepatitis in pregnancy: problems for the clinician dealing with the infant. Pediatr Rev 2:121, 1980.
39. Dupey JM, Giraudd P, Dupey C, et al.: Hepatitis B in children. J Pediatr 92:200, 1978.
40. Chin J: Prevention of chronic hepatitis B virus infection from mothers to infants in the United States. Pediatrics 71:289, 1983.
41. Desmonts G, Couvrer J: Toxoplasmosis in pregnancy and its transmission to the fetus. Bull NY Acad Med 50:146, 1974.
42. Fiumara NJ: Syphilis in newborn children. Clin Obstet Gynecol 18:183, 1975.
43. Klein JO: Bacterial infections of the respiratory tract. In Remington JS, Klein JO (Eds.): Infectious Diseases of the Fetus and Newborn Infant. Philadelphia, W.B. Saunders Co., 1983, p 744.
44. Marks MI: Pediatric Infectious Diseases for the Practitioner. New York, Springer-Verlag, 1985, p 179.

45. Barter RA: Congenital pneumonia. Lancet 1:165, 1962.
46. Berstein J, Wang J: The pathology of neonatal pneumonia. Am J Dis Child 101:350, 1961.
47. Klein JO: Diagnostic lung puncture in the pneumonias of infants and children. Pediatrics 44:486, 1969.
48. Kohn JL, Koiransky H: Successive roentgenograms of the chest of children during measles. Am J Dis Child 28:258, 1929.
49. Gokiert JC, Beamish WE: Altered reactivity to measles virus in previously vaccinated children. Can Med Ass J 103:724, 1970.
50. Bloch A, Vardy P: Pneumomediastinum and subcutaneous emphysema in measles. Clin Pediatr 7:7, 1968.
51. O'Donovan C: Measles in Kenyan children. East Afr Med J 48:526, 1971.
52. Ross LJ: Electrocardiographic findings in measles. Am J Dis Child 83:282, 1952.
53. Hudson JB, Weinstein L, Chang T: Thrombocytopenic purpura in measles. J Pediatr 48:48, 1956.
54. Kipps A, Dick G, Moodie JW: Measles and the central nervous system. Lancet 2:1406, 1983.
55. Modlin JF, Halsey NA, Eddins DL, et al.: Epidemiology of subacute panencephalitis. J Pediatr 94:231, 1979.
56. Lidin-Janson G, Strannegard O: Two cases of Guillain-Barré syndrome and encephalitis after measles. Br Med J 2:572, 1972.
57. Feldman S, Hughes WT, Daniel CB: Varicella in children with cancer: seventy seven cases. Pediatrics 56:388, 1975.
58. Winkleman RK, Perry HO: Herpes zoster in children. JAMA 171:876, 1959.
59. Noren GR, Adams P, Anderson RC: Positive skin reactivity to mumps virus antigen in endocardial fibroelastosis. J Pediatr 62:604, 1963.
60. Sultz HA, Hart BA, Zielezny M: Is mumps virus an etiologic factor in juvenile diabetes mellitus? J Pediatr 86:654, 1975.
61. Rutkow IM: Rupture of the spleen in infectious mononucleosis. Arch Surg 113:718, 1978.
62. Grose C, Feorino PM: Epstein-Barr virus and Guillain-Barré syndrome. Lancet 2:1285, 1972.
63. Hodes HL: Diphtheria. Pediatr Clin N Am 26:445, 1979.
64. Nihoyannopoulos J, Agoroyannis S: Disorders of cardiac rhythm in diphtheria fascicular blocks and their prognostic value. Proc Assoc Evr Pediatr Cardiol 8:61, 1972.
65. Sayers EG: Diphtheritic myocarditis with permanent heart damage. Ann Intern Med 48:146, 1958.
66. Bowler DP: Post-diphtheritic polyneuritis with respiratory paralysis. Med J Aust 47:733, 1960.
67. Stoll BJ: Tetanus. Pediatr Clin N Am 26:415, 1979.
68. Hollow VM, Clark GN: Autonomic manifestations of tetanus. Anaesth Intens Care 3:142, 1975.
69. De Michele DJ, Da Silva AMT: Cardiovascular findings in a patient with severe tetanus. Crit Care Med 11:828, 1983.
70. Haselby KA: Infectious diseases. In Stoelting RK, Dierdorf SF (Eds.): Anesthesia and Co-existing Disease. New York, Churchill-Livingstone, 1983.
71. Polin RA, Brown LW: Infant botulism. Pediatr Clin N Am 26:345, 1979.
72. Kao I, Drachman DB, Price DL: Botulinum toxin: mechanism of presynaptic blockade. Science 193:1256, 1976.

73. Arnon SS, Midura TF, Clay AS, et al.: Infant botulism: epidemiological, clinical and laboratory aspects. JAMA 237:1946, 1977.
74. Seto DSY: Viral hepatitis. Pediatr Clin N Am 26:305, 1979.
75. Adler R, Takahashi M, Wright HT: Acute pericarditis associated with hepatitis B infection. Pediatrics 61:716, 1978.
76. du Moulin GC, Hedley-Whyte J: Hospital-associated viral infection and the anesthesiologist. Anesthesiology 59:51, 1983.
77. Steinhoff MC: Rotavirus: the first five years. J Pediatr 96:611, 1980.
78. Nelson SJ, Granoff D: Salmonella gastroenteritis in the first three months of life: a review of management and complications. Clin Pediatr 21:709, 1982.
79. Riley RL, Mills CC, O'Grady F, et al.: Infectiousness of air from a tuberculosis ward. Am Rev Respir Dis 85:511, 1962.
80. Davis SD, Rosenzweig DY: Tuberculosis: diseases due to Mycobacterium tuberculosis and atypical mycobacteria. In Wedgewood RJ, Davis SD, Ray CF, et al. (Eds.): Infections in Children. Philadelphia, J.B. Lippincott Co., 1982, p. 978.
81. The experts opine. Surv Anesth 22:587, 1978.
82. Roche M, Layusse M: The nature and causes of hookworm anemia. Am J Trop Med Hyg 15:1031, 1966.
83. Kagan IG, Osiman JJ, Varela JC, et al.: Evaluation of intradermal and serologic tests for the diagnosis of hydatid disease. Am J Trop Med Hyg 15:172, 1966.
84. Lewis JW, Koss N, Kerstein MD: A review of echinococcal disease. Ann Surg 181:390, 1975.
85. Jakubowski MS, Barnard DE: Anaphylactic shock during operation for hydatid disease. Anesthesiology 34:197, 1971.
86. Idsoe E, Guthe T, Willcox RR, et al.: Nature and extent of penicillin side-reactions, with particular reference to fatalities from anaphylactic shock. Bull WHO 38:159, 1968.
87. Martin MJ, Wellman WE: Clinically useful antimicrobial agents. Postgrad Med J 33:327, 1963.
88. Weinstein L, Lerner PI, Chew WH: Clinical and bacteriological studies of the effect of massive doses of penicillin G on infections caused by gram negative bacilli. N Engl J Med 271:525, 1964.
89. Smith H, Lerner PI, Weinstein L: Neurotoxicity and massive intravenous therapy with penicillin. Arch Intern Med 120:47, 1967.
90. Wilkowske CJ: The penicillins. Mayo Clin Proc 52:616, 1977.
91. Weinstein AJ: The new cephalosporins and penicillins. Compr Ther 8:26, 1982.
92. Fleming PC, Jaffe D: The nephrotoxic effect of cephaloridine. Postgrad Med J (Suppl) 43:89, 1967.
93. Pittinger C, Adamson R: Antibiotic blockage of neuromuscular function. Ann Rev Pharmacol 12:169, 1972.
94. Weiss CF, Glazko AJ, Weston JK: Chloramphenicol in the newborn infant. A physiologic explanation of its toxicity when given in excessive doses. N Engl J Med 262:787, 1960.
95. Newfield P, Roizen MF: Hazards of rapid administration of vancomycin. Ann Intern Med 91:581, 1979.
96. Daubeck JL, Daugherty MJ, Petty C: Lincomycin induced cardiac arrest: a case report. Anesth Analg 53:563, 1974.

CENTRAL NERVOUS SYSTEM DISEASES

4

M. E. McLEOD, M.D. • R. E. CREIGHTON, M.D.

GENERAL CONSIDERATIONS

During neurosurgical operations in children, both the anesthetist and the surgeon have great influence over the conditions at the operative site and must work together to optimize these and facilitate surgery. The dynamics of intracranial pressure (ICP) changes must be considered in planning the anesthetic management of the neurosurgical patient.

In the infant, the open fontanelle not only increases cranial compliance but also provides a means of assessing intracranial pressure noninvasively. In the older child, as in the adult, the skull must be considered as a rigid and essentially closed container in which the pressure depends on the total volume of brain substance, interstitial fluid, cerebrospinal fluid (CSF), and blood. The familiar pressure-volume curve of intracranial compliance shows that with initial volume changes in one compartment, compensation is possible and only a small pressure change results (Fig. 4–1).[1] This is achieved by displacement of CSF into the relatively distensible spinal dural sac as well as by changes in the volume of the intracranial vascular bed.[2] Once the limits of compensation are reached, a small change in intracranial volume results in a more dramatic change in intracranial pressure.

Since manipulations of CSF are possible only if access to the ventricular system is available, the control of ICP by the anesthesiologist usually depends on producing changes in cerebral blood volume or the volume of intracellular and interstitial fluid. Modifications to the nitrous oxide method of measuring cerebral blood flow (CBF) have allowed measurement in small children, and it is evident that both cerebral blood flow and cerebral metabolic rate (CMR O_2) are significantly higher in children while cerebrovascular resistance is significantly lower.[34]

Changes in cerebral blood flow, and therefore cerebral blood volume, can produce rapid changes in intracranial pressure. Normally, CBF is controlled by $PaCO_2$, PaO_2, and mean arterial pressure (Fig. 4–2). In the normal adult, cerebral blood flow remains relatively constant between mean arterial pressures of 50 to 150 torr, provided changes are not abrupt.[1] This autoregulation, however, can be abolished by trauma, acidosis, and various drugs.[5] The exact limits of autoregulation in infants and children have not been established. In the distressed newborn, it has been shown that autoregulation may be entirely absent.[6] The cerebral circulation may become pressure-passive in the neonate with birth asphyxia or respiratory distress syndrome with the increased risk of intraventricular hemorrhage if wide fluctuations in arterial pressure occur.

Except at extremes, arterial oxygen tension has little influence on cerebral blood flow. However, below a threshold level (PaO_2 of 50 torr) cerebral blood flow increases rapidly.[7]

The $PaCO_2$ is one of the most important regulators of cerebrovascular resistance and cerebral blood flow in man. A significant linear relationship exists such that

Figure 4–1. Idealized intracranial volume-pressure relationship. (*From* Shapiro HM: Intracranial hypertension: therapeutic and anesthetic considerations. Anesthesiology 43:445, 1975.)

Figure 4–2. Changes in cerebral blood flow secondary to PaCO₂ (---), PaO₂ (····), and blood pressure (——). (*From* Shapiro HM: Intracranial hypertension: therapeutic and anesthetic considerations. Anesthesiology 43:445, 1975.)

for each torr change in $PaCO_2$ the cerebral blood volume (CBV) changes 0.041 ml/100 gm perfused tissue and the CBF changes 1.8 ml/100 gm/min over the range of 15 to 76 torr.[8] Hyperventilation is therefore an important aspect of the management of the patient with raised intracranial pressure and allows the neuroanesthesiologist to shrink the intracranial contents prior to surgical intervention.

Reductions in ICP can also be achieved by reducing the cerebral interstitial volume with diuretics. Osmotic agents, in particular mannitol, have proved to be effective in lowering ICP.[9] The ICP lowering effects of mannitol depend on increasing plasma osmolality and drawing fluid from the intracellular and interstitial spaces. This action may result in transient increases in cerebral blood volume and ICP prior to the onset of diuresis.[10]

In attempts to avoid this initial elevation in intracranial pressure, nonosmotic diuretics have been used to reduce cerebral volume. Furosemide, in doses of about 1 mg/kg, will reduce intracranial pressure in the clinical situation without producing significant changes in serum osmolality or electrolytes.[10, 11] It provides a reasonable alternative to mannitol for the patient undergoing craniotomy. The precise mechanism by which furosemide lowers ICP is unclear, but it is thought to be due to effects on brain sodium levels and water transport.[12]

The use of mannitol and furosemide together may be even more effective than either agent alone. Pollay[13] has shown that a combination of mannitol 1 g/kg and furosemide 0.7 mg/kg results in a greater and more prolonged drop in ICP than that achieved with single drug therapy.

The use of steroids in neurosurgery has long been a subject of controversy. While there is evidence for the effectiveness of steroid pretreatment in reducing cerebral edema, and glucocorticoids have been shown to reduce CSF production,[14, 15] the efficacy of steroids in

reducing edema in patients with cerebral trauma or encephalopathy remains unconfirmed.

In the elective situation, when dexamethasone therapy precedes the surgical treatment of tumors or vascular lesions, experimental evidence suggests that steroids should be of value.[14] The head-injured patient, who is treated after the insult, is less likely to derive the same benefit.

ANESTHETIC DRUGS

Intravenous Agents

Various drugs have a deleterious or beneficial effect on intracranial pressure, and this factor determines their usefulness in the neurosurgical patient.

The time of induction of anesthesia and securing of the airway is one of the most hazardous for the patient with respect to elevations in ICP. The effectiveness of barbiturates in reducing intracranial pressure has long been recognized.[16] The dose-dependent decreases in both cerebral blood flow and metabolism make thiopentone an ideal induction agent for the patient with raised intracranial pressure.

The use of ketamine as an induction agent in neurosurgical patients in general should be avoided. In dogs, an 80 percent increase in CBF and a 16 percent increase in CMR O_2 occur after ketamine injection, and these values remain above control for 30 minutes.[17] In hydrocephalic children, ketamine has been shown to produce two- to threefold increases in CSF pressure when given either intramuscularly or intravenously.[18]

In spite of induction of anesthesia with thiopentone, laryngoscopy and intubation produce significant changes in mean arterial pressure and in intracranial pressure in patients with space-occupying lesions. The use of lidocaine, 1.5 mg/kg intravenously at induction, attenuates the blood pressure response and protects against increases in ICP.[19, 20] This technique has advantages over lidocaine aerosol in that blood levels are achieved prior to laryngoscopy and accurate doses can be given to small children. Lidocaine, like thiopentone, is also effective in lowering ICP when acute elevations occur intraoperatively.[21]

Narcotics are useful for the maintenance of anesthesia in neurosurgical patients although they are rarely used for premedication because of the danger of respiratory depression. Intravenous morphine has been shown to have little effect on cerebral blood flow, and autoregulation remains intact.[22] The high-dose fentanyl technique has also been used successfully in neuroanesthesia, but the need for postoperative naloxone infusion makes it impractical for the average patient.[23] Fentanyl in combination with droperidol results in small decreases in ICP,[24] making both neuroleptanesthesia and neuroleptanalgesia useful techniques.

Diazepam, in addition to its beneficial effects in controlling seizures, produces decreases in both cerebral blood flow and cerebral oxygen consumption.[25] Its effects on the electroencephalogram make its use undesirable in the child undergoing temporal lobectomy with cortical mapping to correct a seizure disorder.

Muscle relaxants have not been shown to have any direct effects on cerebral blood flow. They may possibly have indirect effects on the intracranial pressure either through histamine release (D-tubocurarine) or by increases in venous pressure due to fasciculation (succinylcholine).

Inhalation Agents

The effect of nitrous oxide on cerebral blood flow generally is considered to be minimal, although some authors have reported increases in both cerebral blood flow and cerebral metabolism.[26] The effect on the electroencephalogram is that of progressive loss of alpha rhythm as the concentration is increased above 30 percent.[27]

The commonly used volatile anesthetics are known to be cerebral vasodilators and must therefore be used with caution in the patient with raised intracranial pressure. Although both halothane and enflurane abolish autoregulation at 1.0 MAC, the cerebral vasculature remains responsive to changes in $PaCO_2$.[28] It has been shown that the prior establishment of hypocapnia minimizes the increase in ICP associated with halothane[29] and that cerebral blood flow begins to return toward control values after 30 minutes of halothane anesthesia.[30] The induction of anesthesia with inhalation agents is not recommended for patients with significantly elevated ICP. However, the use of the inhalation agents for the maintenance of anesthesia can result in a wide-awake child at the end of a short procedure without the postoperative respiratory depression that is associated with narcotics.

Enflurane, because of its effects on the EEG, should generally be avoided in neurosurgical patients. Isoflurane is a useful agent for neuroanesthesia and may have advantages over the more commonly used halothane. While cerebral blood flow is increased at levels greater than 1.1 MAC, this is less than occurs with halothane,[31] and the ICP returns to control levels more rapidly after the establishment of hypocapnia.[32] At higher inspired concentrations, the decrease in $CMR O_2$ may provide some measure of protection against ischemic insult.[33] In addition, its relatively rapid elimination permits early postoperative neurological assessment.

POSITIONING

Patient positioning is important in neuroanesthesia because of the effects on the airway, circulation, and intracranial pressure. In some centers, the sitting position is commonly used for procedures in the posterior fossa. The major disadvantages in this position are the increased risk of air embolism and the cardiovascular changes. A widely varying incidence of air embolism has been reported in patients undergoing surgery in the sitting position and is probably not significantly different in children when compared with adults.[34] Although the frequency of air embolism detected by precordial Doppler in children was found by Cucchiara and Bowers[34] to be only 33 percent, the incidence of hypotension associated with the air embolism was 69 percent compared with only 36 percent in the adult group. The precordial Doppler has been shown to be more sensitive than pulmonary artery pressure and end-tidal carbon dioxide concentrations in detecting air embolism,[35] but the use of electrocautery may render it less informative. The high incidence of hypotension associated with air embolism in children necessitates an immediate response by the anesthesiologist when air embolism is suspected. Nitrous oxide must be discontinued, the surgeon must flood the operative site with saline, and the head must be lowered. Attempts to aspirate air from a right atrial catheter are reported to be less successful in children.[34]

Elevation of the head is one means of decreasing ICP in the patient with brain injury. Elevations of 15 to 30 degrees have been shown to be beneficial; increases beyond 30 degrees may result in decreases in cardiac output and cerebral perfusion pressure.[36] This suggests that the sitting position may be undesirable in patients with intracranial hypertension.

The prone position provides an alternative to the sitting position for posterior fossa surgery and is also commonly used for surgery on the back and spinal cord. As the head is elevated no farther than in the supine position, the risk of air embolism is diminished. Care must be taken to secure the airway and support the circuit so that accidental extubation or disconnection cannot occur. A nasotracheal tube is more easily anchored in this position since the fixative tape is less likely to be loosened by secretions. Depending on the size of the child, either a U-shaped bolster or a Hall-Relton frame can be used to ensure free excursion of the diaphragm without obstruction of abdominal venous return. If a horseshoe headrest is used, careful padding and positioning of the face are required to avoid pressure on the eyes.

When patients are operated on in the supine position, a 15- to 30-degree anti-Trendelenberg tilt is often used, as this amount of elevation does decrease ICP.[36] If the head is to be turned to either side to an excessive degree, the lateral decubitus position is preferable, as this avoids obstruction of the jugular venous system by keeping the head in a neutral position. Regardless of the position chosen when the patient is placed on the operating table, the chest must be carefully auscultated after final positioning to ensure that turning or flexing the head has not resulted in either kinking of the endotracheal tube or endo-bronchial intubation. Use of an armored endotracheal tube will decrease the problems of tube kinking. Many children will need an armored tube with an internal diameter that is half a size smaller than expected for age because of the wall thickness of these tubes.

CRANIOSYNOSTOSIS

Craniosynostosis results from the premature fusion of cranial sutures. It may involve single, bilateral, or multiple sutures and may be part of a syndrome involving other anomalies. The bones of the calvarium arise from widely separated primary centers of ossification that spread centrifugally toward each other. The separation of adjacent bones is a result of expansion of underlying cranial contents and is compensated for by the addition of new bone at the sutural edges. Premature fusion (synostosis) will result in inhibition of the normal direction of growth of the neurocranial capsule.[37]

The premature fusion of the sagittal suture is the most common. It affects males more frequently than females.[38] Other sutures are involved much less commonly (Table 4–1).[39]

The many craniosynostosis syndromes can be classified on the basis of inheritance patterns and clinical similarities. The Crouzon syndrome, one of the more common, is inherited as an autosomal dominant condition and consists of craniosynostosis, maxillary hypoplasia, and shallow orbits with proptosis. In Apert syndrome, also an autosomal dominant condition, craniosynostosis is associated with syndactyly of the hands and feet.[40] Mental retardation can occur in any of the craniosynostosis syndromes, although it is more common in some.[40]

Anesthetic Considerations

The surgical correction of these defects ranges from simple craniectomy in the case of single suture involvement to the major craniofacial reconstructions required in patients with complex syndromes. In the patient presenting for sagittal craniectomy, the most common of these procedures, the major anesthetic concerns are those of positioning (usually prone), blood loss (due to the size of the incision and the vascularity of the bone), and the fact that the patient is a small infant.

Patients for craniofacial reconstruction require careful preoperative assessment to rule out associated anomalies and to evaluate the airway with regard to the difficulty of fitting a mask or visualizing the larynx. Preservation of CNS homeostasis, blood and fluid replacement, and temperature maintenance are the major intraoperative concerns.

To provide access to the facial structures from above, a relaxed brain is essential. This can be achieved by hyperventilation, diuresis, and adequate venous drainage.

Table 4–1. INCIDENCE OF CONGENITAL SYNOSTOSES

Suture	Percent
Sagittal	56
Single coronal	11
Bilateral coronal	11
Metopic	7
Lambdoid	1
Three or more	14

Reproduced by permission from Hardwood-Nash DC, Fitz CR: Neuroradiology in Infants and Children. Volume 1. St. Louis, 1976, The C.V. Mosby Co.

Blood loss may be considerable owing to the extent of the surgery and the vascularity of the structures. As losses are difficult to measure during these procedures, monitoring of central venous and intra-arterial pressures is important, as is measurement of urine output. The use of hypotensive techniques should be considered in primarily facial procedures but is less desirable in intracranial procedures, where the risk of cerebral ischemia is increased when hypotension is combined with the brain retraction required to gain access to the facial structures.[41]

The large volumes of blood and fluid administered as well as the large surgical field exposed by a coronal incision result in heat loss by the patient. A blood warmer, warming blanket, and heated humidifier are therefore important components of the anesthetic equipment. Rib grafts are often taken during these procedures to provide bone for vault reconstruction. This adds the potential for intraoperative complication in the form of pneumothorax, or occult blood loss from hemothorax. In addition, ventilation may be compromised in the postoperative period if several adjacent ribs are resected.

At the end of the procedure, patients must be wide awake so that neurological function, in particular vision, can be assessed. Any patient with a difficult airway should be left intubated until any risk of obstruction due to postoperative swelling has passed, and all patients should be monitored in an acute care setting.

NEURAL TUBE DEFECTS

Although the neural tube defects—anencephalus, spina bifida, and encephalocele—are among the most widely studied of birth defects, the etiology of these malformations is unknown. Most investigators have concluded that both genetic and environmental factors play a role.[42]

Encephalocele

Encephalocele, also known as cranium bifidum, is a herniation of cerebral tissue and meninges through a defect in the skull that may occur anywhere in the

Figure 4–3. Infant with nasopharyngeal encephalocele.

midline from the foramen magnum to the nasal cavity.[38] The incidence of encephalocele is between 1 and 3 per 10,000 live births.[43]

Anterior encephalocele commonly presents as a mass in the nasopharynx (Fig. 4–3). Although small lesions may go unnoticed for many years, patients with larger masses may present with continuous nasal discharge or recurrent meningitis. In the case of basal encephalocele, there may be associated feeding difficulties or respiratory obstruction. The size of the defect and the contents of the sac (potentially hypothalamus and pituitary) may preclude resection. Operative mortality for treatment of basal encephalocele has been reported to be as high as 50 percent.[44]

More commonly encountered in the neonatal period is the posterior encephalocele. In addition to the obvious occipital abnormality, Karch has demonstrated anomalies throughout the neuraxis in these infants. Hydrocephalus, epilepsy, paraplegia, spasticity, and blindness have been reported in survivors.[43] The Klippel-Feil deformity and cleft lip and palate are also frequently associated with encephalocele.[45] In addition, defects in thermoregulation have been demonstrated in infants with central nervous system abnormalities.[46]

Anesthetic Considerations

In the patient with a large anterior encephalocele and facial clefts, intubation may prove to be difficult,

and appropriate precautions should be taken. Securing the airway may also pose some problems in the infant with a large occipital encephalocele as the patient cannot be placed supine (Fig. 4–4). Intubation is best accomplished awake in the left lateral position in the neonate. If difficulty with intubation is not anticipated, a smooth intravenous induction is preferred to awake intubation in the older infant. Spontaneous ventilation has often been used as a monitor of brain stem integrity. However, in the neonate there is a significant risk of depression by anesthetic agents, and controlled ventilation is advisable. Changes in heart rate and rhythm will serve to warn of brain stem compromise. There is a danger that brain stem centers will be within the occipital encephalocele.

As these patients present in the neonatal period, particular care must be taken to maintain temperature homeostasis. Large volumes of blood and fluid may have to be given to replace losses from the vascular occipital structures, and these fluids should be warmed. Warming blankets, radiant heaters, and a heated humidifier will help to maintain normothermia in these patients, who may have abnormalities of thermoregulation.

Myelomeningocele

The commonly used term spina bifida merely refers to a failure of fusion of the vertebral arches. It occurs in 5 to 10 percent of cases as spina bifida occulta, in which skin and soft tissues cover the defect, usually at L5.[47] The alternative form is spina bifida aperta, in which the defect communicates with the outside either as a meningocele (sac covered by meninges but containing no neural elements) or a myelomeningocele in which the sac contains distended nerve roots and often part of the spinal cord. There usually is no function of roots below the lesion, resulting in paralysis and a neurogenic bladder and bowel. The incidence of myelomeningocele is estimated at 0.2 to 4 per 1000 live births with an increased risk in caucasians and females.[48] The defect is thought to occur early in intrauterine life and can be detected by amniocentesis during the second trimester. Most of these infants will have associated hydrocephalus. In O'Brien and McLanahan's review, none of 33 patients had a normal CT scan at birth.[48]

The urgency for surgery in these patients is related to the risk of infection in the central nervous system. Closure within the first 24 hours of life is preferred. This first trip to the operating room is usually one of many for these children. The average incidence of shunt revision is 0.44 revisions per year or about one every 2 years.[48] Multiple orthopedic and urological procedures may also be required to treat the complications of the neurogenic bladder. Those patients with thoracic lesions develop progressive spinal deformity with varying degrees of kyphosis, scoliosis, and lor-

Figure 4–4. Neonate with large occipital encephalocele. B, Occipital encephalocele following positioning and surgical preparation.

dosis, which may result in eventual cardiorespiratory compromise. Some of these children will present for instrumentation and spinal fusion to halt the progression of the spinal curve. Patients with lumbar lesions may also develop spinal deformity.

Anesthetic Considerations

The problems of anesthetizing these patients for closure of the myelomeningocele include those of anesthetizing any newborn infant. In addition, there are the problems of positioning and the large blood and fluid losses from the operative site resulting in heat loss from the patient.

In order to minimize the risk of trauma to the sac, these infants are best intubated in the lateral position. Because this is an unusual position for securing the airway, an awake intubation is prudent. If the patient must be placed supine to facilitate airway management, the sac can be protected by a cushioned ring.

A reliable intravenous line is essential as blood loss may be great 'if extensive undermining of skin is required to close the defect. Actual losses are usually difficult to estimate because of the use of irrigation and moist sponges. Changes in vital signs, especially systolic blood pressure, will closely parallel blood volume changes in the neonate. Warming of intravenous fluids and inspired gases will help to maintain body temperature.

When these patients return to the operating room in later life, anesthetic considerations become those of the specific procedure planned. They do, however, require special attention to their emotional needs, as their many trips to the hospital may result in an increased anxiety level. Venous access may become difficult after multiple surgical procedures.

HYDROCEPHALUS

Hydrocephalus is a condition in which there is a disproportionately large volume of cerebrospinal fluid relative to other cranial contents. It may arise because of a congenital abnormality or may be secondary to obstruction caused by neoplasm, infection, or trauma. In noncommunicating hydrocephalus the CSF is excluded from the subarachnoid space. In communicating hydrocephalus CSF flows unimpeded to the spinal subarachnoid space but is either excluded from the cerebral subarachnoid space or cannot be absorbed into the cerebral venous sinuses via the arachnoid villi.

A large portion of the CSF is formed by the choroid plexuses, and it has been shown that the formation of CSF is not dependent on hydrostatic pressure.[49] CSF continues to be produced in spite of increasing intracranial pressure, and the ventricles gradually dilate, usually between the plexus and the obstruction. As the process continues, the ventricles enlarge in conjunction with cortical thinning. In the infant in whom the sutures are not yet fused, the head gradually increases in size.

Hydrocephalus is associated with a variety of congenital anomalies. Eighty percent or more infants with myelomeningocele have hydrocephalus.[47] If these infants are excluded, the most common abnormalities found in infants with congenital hydrocephalus are aqueduct stenosis, intracranial tumor, arachnoid cyst, and porencephaly. The Arnold-Chiari and Dandy-Walker syndromes are less common.[38] Hydrocephalus is not invariably a progressive disorder, but signs of increased intracranial pressure or rapid increase in head circumference are indications for surgical intervention.

Surgery for hydrocephalus involves correction of the precipitating cause if possible and/or CSF shunting procedures. Ventriculoperitoneal shunt is the operation most commonly performed in noncommunicating hydrocephalus. Either the pleural cavity or the right atrium can be used in cases in which adhesive peritonitis makes the peritoneal route undesirable. Ventriculoatrial shunts are inserted using electrocardiographic control to ensure placement within the atrium.[50] This shunting technique, while being very effective, is less commonly employed than previously because of the risk of thrombus formation, multiple microemboli from the catheter tip, and superior vena cava obstruction.[51, 52] In communicating hydrocephalus, a lumboperitoneal shunt is often inserted.

With present therapy, infants with hydrocephalus at birth have approximately an 85 percent chance of survival and a 72 percent probability of normal or borderline intellectual function.[53]

Anesthetic Considerations

As a general rule preoperative sedation should not be used, as narcotics and sedatives may depress ventilation, resulting in further increases in ICP. Induction and maintenance of anesthesia are as for any patient with raised intracranial pressure. These are relatively short procedures, and a volatile agent is therefore often preferable to a narcotic-relaxant technique provided that the lowest concentration that maintains anesthesia is used and the $PaCO_2$ is maintained at approximately 30 mmHg.

These patients may be positioned in the supine position with the neck extended and the head turned, in the lateral decubitus position, or even face down with the body rotated (fourth ventricle-peritoneal shunt). Appropriate precautions should be taken to protect the face and airway and to maintain ventilation, depending on the position.

Arnold-Chiari Malformation and Syringomyelia

The Arnold-Chiari malformation is the most common anomaly involving the cerebellum. It is present in most children with myelomeningocele but is frequently asymptomatic. The malformation consists of an elongation of the cerebellar vermis that results in herniation of the caudal vermis and choroid plexus through the foramen magnum with kinking of the medulla and upper cervical cord.[54]

More than half of those children with myelomen-

ingocele who require treatment of an Arnold-Chiari malformation will present before the age of 3 months. The usual presenting signs and symptoms are swallowing difficulty, apneic episodes, stridor, aspiration, arm weakness, opisthotonos, or a combination.[55] Swallowing difficulties are manifested by feeding problems and pooling of oral secretions. In these infants, the gag reflex may be diminished or absent. Mortality is increased in those infants who progress to vocal cord paralysis, arm weakness, or cardiorespiratory arrest within 2 weeks of initial presentation.

Anesthetic Considerations

Surgical therapy involves laminectomy and opening of the dura to decompress the herniated cerebellar tongue. This procedure is performed with the patient prone and the neck in flexion. Particular care must be taken with positioning of the nasotracheal tube, as the flexed posture may result in endobronchial intubation. Controlled ventilation is recommended for these small infants; changes in heart rate or rhythm will warn of further brain stem compromise.

In those infants with vocal cord paresis and depressed gag reflex, it may be necessary to leave an endotracheal tube in place postoperatively. Some will eventually require tracheotomy and some will need a gastrostomy to decrease the risk of aspiration. Although stridor is frequently improved in the postoperative period, all patients require close monitoring for the first few days after surgery.

Syringomyelia

In older children and adults, the Arnold-Chiari malformation is commonly associated with syringomyelia. These patients typically present with upper extremity weakness with or without sensory abnormalities. The diagnosis is made when a thickened cord is seen on CT scan in conjunction with an Arnold-Chiari malformation or adhesions around the foramen magnum. Occasionally, a delayed scan will actually show dye entering the syrinx from the fourth ventricle.[56]

Surgical therapy of this condition consists of either plugging the obex or draining the hydromyelia, in addition to decompressive cervical laminectomy. It is important to assess these patients for bulbar symptoms preoperatively as these may influence the postoperative airway management.

ARTERIOVENOUS MALFORMATION AND ANEURYSM

Cerebral arteriovenous malformations (AVMs) are congenital lesions arising from an abnormality of development of the primitive arteriolar-capillary network normally interposed between the arteries and veins of the brain.[57] Signs and symptoms may not arise until later childhood or early adult life: only about 18 percent of AVMs that become symptomatic do so before the age of 15.[58] Intracranial hemorrhage is the most common form of presentation, occurring in about 70 percent of children.[59, 60] Seizure disorder is also a frequent sign at the time of diagnosis of the AVM.

The risk of rebleeding after the initial event is significant. Graf and colleagues, in their review, estimated the risk of recurrent hemorrhage at 2 percent per year after the first year, in which the rate was 6 percent.[61] In So's series, the risk of rebleeding within 5 years was 25 percent.[59] Surgical treatment is therefore indicated if the lesion is accessible.

Anesthetic Considerations

The anesthetic management of children with cerebral arteriovenous malformations will be determined by the preoperative condition. Of the patients who present with hemorrhage, some will be unconscious and require immediate resuscitative therapy prior to transfer to the operating room and others will have only signs of subarachnoid bleeding and can be scheduled for surgery after a period of stabilization. The first group requires airway support and should be considered to have an expanding space-occupying lesion in the form of an intracerebral clot. The sympathetic stimulation associated with intubation may result in a recurrence of bleeding from the lesion. These patients therefore require sedation and lidocaine prior to intubation. The usual precautions for elevated ICP and the potentially full stomach should be taken. Hyperventilation should be instituted as soon as the endotracheal tube is in place.

Patients scheduled for elective surgery of an AVM should be sedated preoperatively with the aim of achieving as smooth an induction as possible. A combination of fentanyl citrate and droperidol is useful in this situation.

In some cases induced hypotension will be of benefit in the surgical management of the AVM, particularly if the lesion is deep-seated and difficult to approach. The safe level and duration of controlled hypotension in children has not been defined, although their normally lower blood pressures and the absence of cerebrovascular disease lead one to expect children to tolerate pressures at least as low as those tolerated by adults.

The ideal method of inducing hypotension is yet to be found. A variety of methods, including oligemia, ganglionic blockade, deep inhalational anesthesia, and direct vasodilatation, have been employed.

In baboons, cerebral autoregulation is lost at a mean arterial pressure of approximately 65 mmHg whether sodium nitroprusside, trimethaphan, or hypovolemia is used to achieve the fall in pressure.[62] Effects on CMR O_2, however, differ. Hemorrhage results in an increase in cerebral metabolism as long as autoregulation is intact, but below the limits of autoregulation, CMR O_2 falls. With trimethaphan-induced hypotension, cerebral oxygen requirements decrease, likely owing in part to the sympathetic blockade, while the use of nitroprusside results in significant increases in CMR O_2.[62] Other studies, done in dogs, have demonstrated less deleterious metabolic effects with nitroprusside and halothane than with trimethaphan.[63]

The disadvantages of sodium nitroprusside, in addition to its potential for increasing CMR O_2, are difficulty in controlling pressure, resistance to the drug in some patients, cyanide toxicity, elevation of ICP,[64] and the possibility of rebound hypertension.[65] Trimethaphan, too, presents the difficulties of controlling an infusion and also has the problem of early tachyphylaxis. Pentolinium, a longer-acting ganglion blocker, eliminates both the above problems but does not allow minute-to-minute control of mean arterial pressure without the addition of another agent.

Intravenous nitroglycerin has the advantage over nitroprusside of being easier to control and having no reported toxicity. It too has been shown to increase intracranial pressure and also to decrease intracranial compliance in patients with hydrocephalus.[66]

Isoflurane has been used as a hypotensive agent for aneurysm surgery in adults and appears to be effective and easy to control.[67] Rebound hypertension does not occur, and increases in cerebral blood flow are minimal with this agent provided hypocapnia is maintained.[67] This may prove to be the most useful hypotensive agent in neurosurgical procedures.

Aneurysm

Ruptured intracranial aneurysm occurs less commonly in children than in adults, the incidence of rupture being about 3 percent under the age of 20 and 1 percent under the age of 15.[68] Many children with intracranial aneurysms will have had significant signs or symptoms, such as syncopal episodes, focal headache, or neurological deficit, prior to the event that precipitates hospital admission.[69] Cerebral aneurysms are more common in males, and lesions in children may occur in different locations than in the adult population.[68, 69, 70] As with arteriovenous malformations, most children will present with an acute hemorrhage, and subsequent morbidity and mortality are related to the neurological signs at the time of initial presentation.[68, 69, 70] Perioperative mortality is 22 percent overall, but only 8 percent in those patients who present with good preservation of neurological function (Botterell grades I and II).[70, 71]

Anesthetic considerations in these patients are similar to those for children with arteriovenous malformations. Hypotensive techniques usually will be required, but the duration of hypotension will be shorter.

Another uncommon vascular lesion in children is the arteriovenous malformation or aneurysm of the great cerebral vein of Galen. The age at which patients with this disease present is related to the size of the lesion, and patients can be divided into four groups clinically. Neonates have the poorest prognosis and present with a cranial bruit and severe congestive heart failure. Many die of cardiovascular complications before surgical therapy can be undertaken and others die in the early postoperative period.[72] Subendocardial damage due to pressure and volume overload of the neonatal heart combined with impaired myocardial perfusion contributes to the high mortality.[73] The second group of patients present later in infancy with craniomegaly and a cranial bruit, and some will have mild congestive heart failure. Slightly older children, the third group, will also have an enlarged head at the time of presentation and may have a bruit, but heart failure is unusual.[72] In the fourth and rarest group, patients with this lesion come to medical attention in late childhood or early adult life with headache, exercise syncope, and a calcified rim in the pineal region.[74]

The neonates present the greatest problem with respect to anesthetic management because they have compromised cardiac function and greater risk of massive hemorrhage as their lesions tend to be larger. Cardiopulmonary bypass and deep hypothermia have been used successfully in older infants,[75] but in the neonate this technique has not been of benefit.[76] Controlled hypotension has also been recommended and has been effective in the older infant.[77] In the neonate, however, there is a risk that the use of hypotensive techniques will decrease the already low diastolic pressure and further compromise blood flow to the myocardium. Maintenance of normotension during surgery is recommended.

CNS TUMORS

Tumors of the central nervous system are the second most common malignancy of childhood, with an incidence reported to range between 1.3 and 5 percent.[78] In the first year of life, supratentorial tumors are more common than infratentorial lesions, but the overall incidence throughout childhood is approximately equal.[39, 78]

Astrocytoma, choroid plexus papilloma, and teratoma are the most commonly reported neoplasms of the CNS in children under 1 year of age, while in older children astrocytoma, medulloblastoma, and ependymoma are most frequently seen. Choroid plexus papilloma and teratoma are very uncommon after the first 12 months of life.[79]

Hydrocephalus is a common finding at the time of presentation, as about half of all brain tumors in children are located near the midline.[80] In infants, the most common signs of tumors are a full fontanelle, rapidly increasing head size, vomiting, abducens palsy, lethargy, and irritability.[78] In the older child, headache and vomiting signal the increase in intracranial pressure and are often the presenting symptoms of tumor followed in frequency by unsteadiness of gait and impaired consciousness.[36]

Supratentorial Tumors

Children undergoing surgery for supratentorial lesions may or may not have raised intracranial pressure. The most important presenting signs in these patients are seizures, hemiparesis, visual impairment, and changes in behavior.[80]

Even if intracranial pressure is not elevated, heavy narcotic premedication is best avoided in these children. A smooth intravenous induction with thiopentone and a muscle relaxant allows placement of an oral armored tube and the rapid institution of hyperventilation to a $PaCO_2$ of 30 mmHg. If signs of raised ICP are present, lidocaine should be added to the induction sequence. These patients are frequently receiving dexamethasone to reduce edema around the tumor. A repeat dose should be given prior to any manipulation of the brain. In many cases diuretic will also be required to reduce brain bulk. An intra-arterial catheter and a central venous line are useful if considerable blood loss or a prolonged procedure is anticipated. Maintenance of anesthesia with either a nitrous-narcotic-relaxant technique or a low dose of isoflurane will provide a good surgical field.

The patient usually will be placed in the supine or lateral position with the head elevated 10 to 15 degrees. In positioning the head, care must be taken that venous return is not obstructed.

Infratentorial Tumors

Surgery for infratentorial neoplasm poses some additional problems to the anesthesiologist. Many of these patients will present with hydrocephalus, as the lesions are frequently midline. In order to improve the patient's fluid and nutritional status and reduce congestion of the operative site, it is sometimes advisable to insert a ventriculoperitoneal shunt prior to the definitive surgery.[81]

For excision of the tumor these patients will be placed in either the prone or the sitting position. (The advantages of the prone position have already been discussed.) The use of a nasal tube in prone patients allows secure fixation without the risk of loosening of tape by oral secretions. As with supratentorial tumors, a smooth intravenous induction is the method of choice, and controlled ventilation is commenced immediately. Anesthesia can be maintained with any of the commonly used techniques.

Air embolism and cardiac arrhythmias are the intraoperative complications encountered most frequently in posterior fossa surgery. The use of the prone position decreases the risk of embolism, and monitors such as precordial Dopplers and end-tidal carbon dioxide measurement assist in early diagnosis. Arrhythmia is often a result of tumor manipulation and may indicate proximity to brain stem centers.[82] In some cases brain stem reflexes may be impaired by the surgery, and this should be carefully assessed prior to extubation.

Suprasellar Tumors

These tumors are considered separately because of the associated endocrine abnormalities. This group of lesions includes craniopharyngiomas, optic chiasmal gliomas, and germ cell tumors and represents 15 percent of brain tumors in children.[83]

The most common sign in these patients at the time of presentation is decreasing visual acuity or a visual field defect. Sixty percent of patients with craniopharyngioma have evidence of optic atrophy at the time of diagnosis, and approximately 65 percent have papilledema.[84] With germ cell tumors symptoms of diabetes insipidus appear early, while this is uncommon in craniopharyngioma. About thirty percent of both groups have stunting of growth or delayed puberty.[83] Thomsett and associates found that 24 percent of patients had decreased levels of ACTH preoperatively and 72 percent had decreased levels of growth hormone.[85] It is therefore essential to undertake endocrinological assessment preoperatively and to treat patients with steroids if necessary.

There are two major approaches to surgical resection of suprasellar tumors, the transsphenoidal approach and the frontal craniotomy. The former is rarely used in small children. The anesthetic considerations are therefore similar to those for any other supratentorial lesion once the endocrine status has been assessed. Cardiac arrhythmias, in particular bradycardia, are common during dissection around the optic nerves. This bradycardia may be reversed with a small dose of atropine intravenously.

In the postoperative period these patients require close monitoring of fluid and electrolyte balance. Grant and Lyen found that 46 of 58 children undergoing resection of a craniopharyngioma had postoperative diabetes insipidus and 23 of 35 had ACTH deficiency.[86] It is important that pitressin therapy be started early, as attempts to replace urinary water losses with 5 percent dextrose in water may lead to hyperglycemic coma.[87]

NEUROBLASTOMA

Neuroblastoma is the most common soft tissue malignant tumor found in children.[88] Arising from postganglionic adrenergic cells of the sympathetic nervous system, neuroblastoma and ganglioneuroblastoma occur with an incidence of 9 to 10 per million children per year.[89] The adrenal glands and the cervical, thoracic, and abdominal sympathetic ganglia are the most frequent primary locations. Metastases are present at the time of initial presentation in two thirds of patients.[96] Prognosis is related to age, site of tumor, and stage of the disease at the time of diagnosis.[91] Survival decreases with increasing age at first diagnosis. Nonadrenal locations of the primary tumor have a better prognosis.[89]

Neuroblastoma sometimes occurs as a "dumbbell" with a primary in the mediastinum or retroperitoneum and extension into the spinal canal. The two components are joined via the intervertebral foramen. Compression of the spinal cord by tumor often results in neurologic abnormalities in these patients.[92] Surgery is carried out in two stages. Laminectomy and excision of the spinal portion usually precedes resection of the mediastinal component, as manipulation of the extraspinal tumor could result in edema or hemorrhage in the intraspinal component.[92]

Increased excretion of catechol metabolites is detectable in most of these patients.[89, 90] Hypertension generally is not considered to be a problem,[90, 93] but as many as 19 percent of patients with neurogenic tumors may have hypertension at some stage of the disease process.[94] Arrhythmias are very rare.

Coagulation abnormalities are common in children with metastatic neuroblastoma, and disseminated intravascular coagulation has been reported.[95, 96]

Anesthetic Considerations

Potential problems in these patients will depend on the size and location of the tumor, the stage of the disease, and the extent of the planned surgical excision. When radical excision of a large tumor is planned, blood loss may be very large. Appropriate monitors, large-bore intravenous lines, and blood warming devices should be used for these children. As the possibility of intraoperative hypertension exists, particularly when the tumor is handled, antihypertensive agents should be available in the operating room.[97] In patients with advanced disease, preoperative coagulation studies are essential.

NEUROFIBROMATOSIS

Neurofibromatosis is a disorder of neural crest derivation with proliferation of nerve fibers and Schwann cells and associated anomalies induced by the abnormal growth of neural tissue.[98] It occurs with a frequency of 1 in 2500 to 3300 births, and a positive family history is obtained in approximately 50 percent of cases.[99] Physical signs of this condition may be present at birth and tend to increase with age. Diagnosis usually is made before puberty.

Associated anomalies are frequently multiple. The central nervous system is involved in many cases, with clinical manifestations varying from mental retardation or seizure disorder to signs of a space-occupying lesion in the cranium or spinal cord.[99] Bony abnormalities are also common, and scoliosis may develop in 20 to 25 percent of patients.[98, 99] Malignant change is reported to occur in 2 to 16 percent of patients with neurofibromatosis.[98]

Giant plexiform neurofibromas may occur in the head and neck and result in ptosis, hemifacial gigantism, and visual problems if the lesion is in or around the orbit.[100] Attempts to excise these tumors may involve major craniofacial reconstructions.

The incidence of vascular anomalies has been reported to be as high as 9 percent, and hypertension may be more common with advanced age as neurofibromatous change produces more extensive small vessel disease.[98] In addition, hypertension may be present as a result of another tumor of neural crest origin. Pheochromocytoma occurs with increased frequency in patients with neurofibromatosis.[101]

Anesthetic Considerations

In patients with neurofibromatosis and intracranial space-occupying lesions, the usual precautions should be taken. When the neurofibroma involves the head and neck, careful assessment of the airway with regard to potential intubation difficulty is mandatory. There is also a risk of cervical instability. Tumor infiltration or abnormalities of spinal ligaments in neurofibromatosis will occasionally result in atlantoaxial dislocation.[102]

Major vessel anomaly and pheochromocytoma should be ruled out preoperatively in the patient with neurofibromatosis who is hypertensive at the time of presentation. Increased sensitivity to muscle relaxants has also been reported.[103, 104, 105]

TEMPORAL LOBE EPILEPSY

Temporal lobe epilepsy may present as psychomotor seizures or complex partial seizures. The latter form usually begins with an aura and is most often followed by a fixation of movements or by automatic, semi-purposeful movements such as mastication, swallowing, or repetitive gestures. This form of epilepsy is frequently refractory to medical therapy and may require cortical resection or temporal lobectomy.

In order to plan surgical therapy, laterality of seizure activity must be established. Electroencephalography (EEG) is the mainstay of diagnosis, as clinical signs are often unreliable. Cable telemetry, which provides a computer record of the EEG immediately before and during seizure activity, has been shown to be of value in determining the laterality of the lesion.[106] Depth EEG electrodes, placed with the patient under anesthesia, have also been used to demonstrate a predominant focus in cases in which the surface EEG was inconclusive.[106, 107]

When the dominant hemisphere is involved, the laterality of language function and independent memory capability of the contralateral temporal lobe should be assessed with the Wada test. While this may not be possible in the very young child, the child 8 or more years of age should be able to cooperate for this investigation. Intracarotid injection of amobarbital inactivates the anterior two thirds of one hemisphere and permits assessment of language and memory function in the opposite hemisphere.[107, 108] Since arterial

catheterization is required, sedation and supervision by an anesthesiologist usually are necessary. Once the Wada test is completed, general anesthesia is induced for completion of the arteriogram, as it is unreasonable to expect the child to remain still throughout arteriography.

Anesthetic Considerations

To minimize the risk of producing a neurological deficit, craniotomy is performed under a neuroleptic technique when the patient is old enough to cooperate. It is important to develop rapport with the child preoperatively so that verbal responses will be obtained when required during cortical mapping. Diazepam and barbiturates should be avoided as premedicants since these drugs may suppress epileptogenic foci. Steroid therapy usually is begun prior to surgery and should be continued in the perioperative period.

These patients will require all the usual monitors. In addition, an intra-arterial catheter placed with the patient under local anesthesia, which eliminates the need for frequent inflation of a blood pressure cuff, and a urinary catheter will help the patient to remain comfortable during the procedure.

Sedation is achieved by giving incremental doses of fentanyl and droperidol intravenously so that the patient is comfortable but responsive to questions and maintains a $PaCO_2$ less than 50 mmHg.[109] A mixture of 0.5 percent lidocaine and 0.375 percent bupivacaine with epinephrine 1:200,000 is used for local infiltration of the pin sites of the head rest and the incision line.[109] Maximum doses should be calculated prior to injection, as the possibility of inducing seizures exists. An oxygen mask is placed over the face prior to draping. Further sedation is added as required during painful parts of the procedure.

In patients too young to cooperate or for those in whom the speech areas are not at risk, a general anesthetic technique can be employed. Methohexital, unlike other barbiturates, is said to activate interictal electroencephalographic evidence of epileptic foci and may therefore improve intraoperative electrocorticographic mapping.[110] Ford and coworkers have employed a continuous infusion technique of 0.1 percent methohexital in combination with nondepolarizing relaxant, morphine, and droperidol for temporal lobectomy.[109] Rasmussen has also reported combination of light methohexital anesthesia, fentanyl, and ventilation with air and oxygen.[111] Nitrous oxide is avoided or discontinued before cortical recording because of its potential effects on the cortical EEG.[27, 111] Somatosensory evoked potentials are also of use in predicting potential neurological deficits when general anesthesia is employed.[109]

Anticonvulsants should be continued intravenously in the postoperative period, as seizures are common in the first 7 to 10 days after surgery and are not necessarily predictive of final outcome.[111] An elevated temperature is common in these patients postoperatively, presumably owing to the irritant effect of breakdown products of blood.[111]

HEAD INJURY

The term head injury is one that is difficult to define adequately, and the true incidence of significant head injury in children is therefore unknown. The treatment of the child with an acute head injury is often resuscitation rather than the actual administration of an anesthetic. Although young children appear to have greater capacity for recovery after a protracted period of coma, mortality is greater in patients under the age of 5 than in patients in the 5 to 19 year age group.[112] The use of the Glasgow Coma Scale (Table 4–2), which assesses eye opening, best verbal, and best motor responses, permits meaningful sequential assessment of patients with severe head injuries.[113]

Radiological investigation to rule out a surgically treatable lesion is necessary in most patients with severe head injury, and this procedure will require anesthetic supervision. Many children with cerebral trauma will not require operative treatment, as mass lesions are found in less than one third.[114] Some, however, will require anesthesia for the treatment of associated injuries. Comatose patients will require intervention by an anesthesiologist to protect the airway and begin resuscitative measures.

The aim of anesthetic management of the child with severe cerebral trauma is to prevent secondary physiological injury to the traumatized brain by hypoxemia, hypercarbia, intracranial hypertension, or systemic hypotension. Oxygen therapy should be started immediately, as more than 30 percent of patients with head injury have a PaO_2 less than 60 mmHg. This has been associated with poor outcome.[115] The presence of systemic hypotension in the head-injured adult indicates associated injury or brain stem failure. In an infant, a subdural hematoma containing a significant proportion of the blood volume can be responsible for systemic hypotension.[116]

Diffuse cerebral swelling is the most common initial finding with computerized tomography (CT) in children, occurring in 20 to 34 percent,[114, 117] and most frequently is associated with a Glasgow Coma Score (GCS) less than 8.[117] Children who deteriorate following an initial lucid interval are more often suffering from progressive brain edema than from an enlarging hematoma.[117] This severe cerebral swelling is associated with a marked increase in cerebral blood flow in the presence of a decreased cerebral metabolic rate.[117, 118] Aggressive therapy of brain edema can decrease the mortality associated with severe head injury.[114]

A patient with cerebral trauma, in addition to elevated ICP, must be assumed to have a full stomach. Intubation without sedation might therefore seem the safest course to take, and in the hemodynamically unstable patient this is certainly true. The response to intubation in the head-injured patient, however, may result in dangerous increases in intracranial pressure. If the blood pressure is stable and hypovolemia is not suspected, a rapid-sequence induction technique with lidocaine, atropine, thiopentone, and succinylcholine offers the best protection to the brain. When cervical spine injury cannot be ruled out, the surgeon should place traction on the head to prevent manipulation of the neck during laryngoscopy.

Continuous recording of ICP in comatose patients in the intensive care unit permits intervention as soon as severe intracranial hypertension occurs. Once the airway is controlled, therapy to reduce cerebral swelling can be instituted. The simplest and one of the most effective measures is hyperventilation. High-dose steroids have been found to have no effect on the outcome in severely injured patients who are comatose at the time of admission,[119] although this treatment is still recommended by some.[114] Once a mass lesion has been ruled out by CT scan, further therapy such as paralysis or barbiturate coma can be undertaken without the concern that focal neurological signs may be missed. Once the patient is paralyzed and hyperventilated, further elevations in intracranial pressure above 20 mmHg can be treated with intermittent doses of hypertonic mannitol and the intravenous use of pentobarbital. In spite of this aggressive management, mortality remains 21 to 40 percent.[114]

CEREBRAL PALSY

Cerebral palsy is a term used to describe a variety of disabilities, usually motor dysfunction or a movement disorder, that result from developmental problems or perinatal injury of the central nervous system. The incidence is approximately 7 per 1000 live

Table 4–2. GLASGOW COMA SCALE

	Observation	Score
Eye opening	spontaneous	4
	to speech	3
	to pain	2
	nil	1
Best motor response	obeys	6
	localizes	5
	withdraws	4
	abnormal flexion	3
	extends	2
	nil	1
Verbal response	orientated	5
	confused conversation	4
	inappropriate words	3
	incomprehensible sounds	2
	nil	1

Total score: 3–15 points.
From Jennet B, Teasdale G: Aspects of coma after severe head injury. Lancet *1*:878, 1977.

births.[120] Hemiplegia, spastic diplegia, and quadriplegia are the most common manifestations. Swallowing disorders, manifested by poor sucking, nasopharyngeal regurgitation, coughing, and gagging during feeding frequently are seen in patients with severe cerebral palsy.[121] The most common etiological factor is prematurity.[122]

Patients with cerebral palsy may require multiple surgical procedures. Orthopedic operations to improve function in extremities are common, and some patients will require surgical correction of progressive spinal deformity. In children with cerebral palsy and scoliosis the degree of pulmonary compromise may be difficult to assess, as children may be unable to cooperate for pulmonary function testing. In addition, severe contractures may make both venous access and positioning for surgery difficult.

Spasticity is sometimes disabling in these children and may require surgical as well as medical treatment. Improvement in spasticity can be obtained by posterior rhizotomy.[123] This technique involves stimulation of the dorsal roots intraoperatively with observation of muscle response. Ketamine has proved to be an effective anesthetic for this procedure, providing analgesia while maintaining muscle tone.[123]

In patients with swallowing difficulties, drooling may be a significant disability. Surgical therapy for this problem consists of salivary gland excision, duct relocation or ligation, or neurectomy of parasympathetic secretomotor fibers.[124] Duct relocation is one of the most effective of these procedures, as it maintains salivary gland function while improving drooling.[125] A nasotracheal tube is required for this procedure, and throat packing is advisable in the early stages of the dissection to minimize the risk of aspiration of blood and secretions. When duct relocation is performed, close postoperative observation is essential because of the possibility of airway compromise by excessive swelling in the floor of the mouth. In addition, swallowing may prove difficult in the early postoperative period, and patients will require intravenous hydration and assistance with secretions.

REYE SYNDROME

Reye syndrome, first described in 1963, is a disease of unknown etiology that occurs in children, usually following a viral illness.[126] The syndrome is characterized by encephalopathy and fatty degneration of the viscera, in particular the liver. Although described following upper respiratory tract infection, it has since been associated with other viral infections, in particular varicella and influenza A and B infections.[127]

In the recovery phase of a viral illness, the child develops vomiting and subsequently alteration of consciousness. The clinical criteria for diagnosis include the typical hisory of an antecedent viral infection, neurological abnormality, elevation of liver enzymes, increased ammonia levels, and the exclusion of other disease processes and specific toxins.[126] Diagnosis can also be made pathologically if the history is atypical. If obtained early in the course of the disease, liver biopsies show a distinctive pattern with 20 to 30 percent triglyceride infiltration and evidence of mitochondrial injury.[129]

As a means of assessing the severity of the disease and to follow its progression, Lovejoy has described staging in Reye syndrome (Table 4–3). The reported mortality in recent series ranges from 22 to 54 percent and is higher in patients whose therapy is started at later stages of the disease.[130–133] Mortality is also higher in children under the age of 6.[127]

As death is usually related to intracranial hypertension, treatment of the disease is directed toward control of intracranial pressure. The brain lesion appears to be a result of acute cytotoxic injury with astrocyte swelling, myelin bleb formation, and mitochondrial abnormality.[129] In the early stages, these changes are reversible. As brain swelling progresses, irreversible brain injury occurs and death may ensue even though liver function is returning to normal.

In order to control intracranial pressure, intubation and ventilation are recommended at the onset of Lovejoy stage III.[128] This therapy may be of greater benefit if instituted earlier when patients are combative and hyperventilating in stage II.[133] Continuous monitoring of ICP is useful in determining the need for further therapeutic intervention.[134] In addition to treatment with mannitol and dexamethasone to reduce cerebral edema, pentobarbital coma and hypothermia have been used to control intracranial pressure in Reye syndrome.[135] The latter therapy has been associated with increased pulmonary complications.[135] Both exchange transfusion and peritoneal dialysis have been employed in Reye syndrome in attempts to decrease the mortality and minimize the neurological sequelae. Neither of these treatment modalities has proved to be of more benefit than supportive therapy alone.[136] Early recognition of the condition remains one of the most important factors in the treatment of Reye syndrome.

Table 4–3. STAGING IN REYE SYNDROME

Stage I	Vomiting, lethargy, extensor plantar response, liver dysfunction
Stage II	Disorientation, combativeness, semicoma, hyperventilation, progressive liver dysfunction
Stage III	Coma, hyperventilation, decortication, continued liver dysfunction
Stage IV	Deepening coma, decerebration, continued liver function abnormalities
Stage V	Coma, medullary dysfunction, respiratory arrest, possible improvement in liver function abnormalities

From Lovejoy FH, Bresnan MJ, Lombroso CT, et al.: Anticerebral oedema therapy in Reye's syndrome. Arch Dis Child 50:933, 1975.

REFERENCES

1. Shapiro HM: Intracranial hypertension: therapeutic and anesthetic considerations. Anesthesiology 43:445, 1975.
2. Lofgren J, Zwetnow NN: Cranial and spinal components of the cerebrospinal pressure-volume curve. Acta Neurol Scand 49:575, 1973.
3. Kennedy C, Sokoloff L: An adaptation of the nitrous oxide method to the study of the cerebral circulation in children; normal values for cerebral blood flow and cerebral metabolic rate in childhood. J Clin Invest 36:1130, 1957.
4. Swedlow DB, Lewis LE: Measurement of cerebral blood flow in children. Anesthesiology 53:S160, 1980.
5. Lassen NA, Christensen MS: Physiology of cerebral blood flow. Br J Anaesth 48:719, 1976.
6. Lou HC, Lassen NA, Friis-Hansen B: Impaired autoregulation of cerebral blood flow in the distressed newborn infant. J Pediatr 94:118, 1979.
7. Lassen NA: Control of cerebral circulation in health and disease. Circ Res 34:749, 1974.
8. Grubb RL Jr, Raichle ME, Eichling JO, et al.: The effects of changes in PaCO$_2$ on cerebral blood volume, blood flow, and vascular mean transit time. Stroke 5:630, 1974.
9. Harbaugh RD, James HE, Marshall LF, et al.: Acute therapeutic modalities for experimental vasogenic cerebral edema. Neurosurgery 5:656, 1979.
10. Cottrell JE, Robustelli A, Post K, et al.: Furosemide- and mannitol-induced changes in intracranial pressure and serum osmolality and electrolytes. Anesthesiology 47:28, 1977.
11. Samson D, Beyer CW Jr: Furosemide in the intraoperative reduction of intracranial pressure in the patient with subarachnoid hemorrhage. Neurosurgery 10:167, 1982.
12. Buhrley LE, Reed DJ: The effect of furosemide on sodium-22 uptake into cerebrospinal fluid and brain. Exp Brain Res 14:503, 1972.
13. Pollay M, Fullenwider C, Roberts A, et al.: Effect of mannitol and furosemide on blood-brain osmotic gradient and intracranial pressure. J Neurosurg 59:945, 1983.
14. Eisenberg HM, Barlow CF, Lorenzo AV: Effect of dexamethasone on altered brain vascular permeability. Arch Neurol 23:18, 1970.
15. Weiss MH, Nulsen, FE: The effect of glucocorticoids on CSF flow in dogs. J Neurosurg 32:452, 1970.
16. Shapiro HM, Galindo A, Wyte SR, et al.: Rapid intraoperative reduction of intracranial pressure with thiopentone. Br J Anaesth 45:1057, 1973.
17. Dawson B, Michenfelder JD, Theye RA: Effects of ketamine on canine cerebral flow and metabolism: modification by prior administration of thiopental. Anesth Analg 50:443, 1971.
18. Crumrine RS, Nulsen FE, Weiss MH: Alterations in ventricular fluid pressure during ketamine anesthesia in hydrocephalic children. Anesthesiology 42:758, 1975.
19. Bedford RF, Winn HR, Tyson G, et al.: Lidocaine prevents increased ICP after endotracheal intubation. In Shulman K, et al. (Eds.): Intracranial Pressure. 4th ed. New York, Springer Verlag, 1980.
20. Abou-Madi MN, Keszler H, Yacoub JM: Cardiovascular reactions to laryngoscopy and tracheal intubation following small and large intravenous doses of lidocaine. Can Anaesth Soc J 24:12, 1977.
21. Bedford RF, Persing JA, Pobereskin L, et al.: Lidocaine or thiopental for rapid control of intracranial hypertension. Anesth Analg 59:435, 1980.
22. Jobes DR, Kennell E, Bitner R, et al.: Effects of morphine–nitrous oxide anesthesia on cerebral autoregulation. Anesthesiology 42:30, 1975.
23. Shupak RC, Harp JR, Stevenson-Smith W, et al.: High-dose fentanyl for neuroanesthesia. Anesthesiology 58:579, 1983.
24. Fitch W, Barker J, Jennett, WB, et al.: The influence of neuroleptanalgesic drugs on cerebrospinal fluid pressure. Br J Anaesth 41:800, 1969.
25. Cotev S, Shalit MN: Effects of diazepam on cerebral blood flow and oxygen uptake after head injury. Anesthesiology 43:117, 1975.
26. Theye RA, Michenfelder JD: The effect of nitrous oxide on canine cerebral metabolism. Anesthesiology 29:1119, 1968.
27. Clark DL, Rosner BS: Neurophysiologic effects of general anesthetics. Anesthesiology 38:564, 1973.
28. Miletich DJ, Ivankovich AD, Albrecht RF, et al.: Absence of autoregulation of cerebral blood flow during halothane and enflurane anesthesia. Anesth Analg 55:100, 1976.
29. Adams RW, Gronert GA, Sundt TM, et al.: Halothane, hypocapnia, and cerebrospinal fluid pressure in neurosurgery. Anesthesiology 37:510, 1972.
30. Albrecht RF, Miletich DJ, Madala LR: Normalization of cerebral blood flow during prolonged halothane anesthesia. Anesthesiology 58:26, 1983.
31. Eger EI II: Isoflurane: a review. Anesthesiology 55:559, 1981.
32. Adams RW, Cucchiara RF, Gronert GA, et al.: Isoflurane and cerebrospinal fluid pressure in neurosurgical patients. Anesthesiology 54:97, 1981.
33. Newberg LA, Michenfelder JD: Cerebral protection by isoflurane during hypoxemia or ischemia. Anesthesiology 59:29, 1983.
34. Cucchiara RF, Bowers B: Air embolism in children undergoing suboccipital craniotomy. Anesthesiology 57:338, 1982.
35. Furuya H, Suzuki T, Okumura F, et al.: Detection of air embolism by transesophageal echocardiography. Anesthesiology 58:124, 1983.
36. Durward QJ, Amacher AL, Del Maestro RF, et al.: Cerebral and cardiovascular responses to changes in head position in patients with intracranial hypertension. J Neurosurg 59:938, 1983.
37. Moss ML: Functional anatomy of cranial synostosis. Child's Brain 1:22, 1975.
38. Till K: Paediatric Neurosurgery. Oxford, Blackwell Scientific, 1975.
39. Harwood-Nash DC, Fitz DR: Neuroradiology in Infants and Children. Vol. 1. St. Louis, C. V. Mosby Co., 1976.
40. Cohen MM Jr: An etiologic and nosologic overview of craniosynostosis syndromes. Birth Defects 11:137, 1975.
41. Bennett MH, Albin MS, Bunegin L, et al.: Evoked potential changes during brain retraction in dogs. Stroke 8:487, 1977.
42. Sever LE: An epidemiologic study of neural tube defects in Los Angeles County. II. Etiologic factors in an area with low prevalence at birth. Teratology 25:323, 1982.
43. Karch SB, Urich H: Occipital encephalocele: a morphological study. J Neurol Sci 15:89, 1972.
44. Modesti LM, Glasauer FE, Terplan KL: Sphenoethmoidal encephalocele. Child's Brain 3:140, 1977.
45. Hendrick EB: Neurosurgery of congenital malformations. In Thompson RA, Green JR (Eds.): Pediatric Neurology and Neurosurgery. New York, Spectrum Publications, 1978.
46. Cross KW, Hey EN, Kennaird DL, et al.: Lack of temperature control in infants with abnormalities of central nervous system. Arch Dis Child 46:437, 1971.
47. Bahnson DH: Myelomeningocele and its problems. Pediatr Ann 11:528, 1982.
48. O'Brien MS, McLanahan CS: Review of the neurosurgical management of myelomeningocele at a regional pediatric medical center. In Concepts in Pediatric Neurosurgery. No. 1. 1981, p 202.
49. Bering EA Jr, Sato O: Hydrocephalus: changes in formation and absorption of cerebrospinal fluid within the cerebral ventricles. J Neurosurg 20:1050, 1963.
50. Creighton RE: Paedriatric neuroanaesthesia. In Steward DJ (Ed.): Some Aspects of Paediatric Anaesthesia. Amsterdam, Elsevier/North-Holland, 1982.
51. Nugent GR, Lucas R, Judy M, et al.: Thrombo-embolic

complications of ventriculo-atrial shunts. Angiocardiographic and pathologic correlations. J Neurosurg 24:34, 1966.

52. Hammon WM: Evaluation and use of the ventriculoperitoneal shunt in hydrocephalus. J Neurosurg 34:792, 1971.

53. McCullough DC, Balzer-Martin LA: Current prognosis in overt neonatal hydrocephalus. J Neurosurg 57:378, 1982.

54. Ellsworth CA, Shaw C-M, Sumi SM: Central nervous system developmental abnormalities. In Thompson RA, Green JR (Eds.): Pediatric Neurology and Neurosurgery. New York, Spectrum, 1978.

55. Park TS, Hoffman HJ, Hendrick EB, et al.: Experience with surgical decompression of the Arnold-Chiari malformation in young infants with myelomeningocele. Neurosurgery 13:147, 1983.

56. Cahan LD, Bentson JR: Considerations in the diagnosis and treatment of syringomyelia and the Chiari malformation. J Neurosurg 57:24, 1982.

57. Drake CG: Cerebral arteriovenous malformations: considerations for and experience with surgical treatment in 166 cases. In Carmel PW (Ed.): Clinical Neurosurgery. Baltimore, Williams and Wilkins, 1979.

58. Mori K, Murata T, Hashimoto N, et al.: Clinical analysis of aerteriovenous malformations in children. Child's Brain 6:13, 1980.

59. So SC: Cerebral arteriovenous malformations in children. Child's Brain 4:242, 1978.

60. McLeod ME, Creighton RE, Humphreys RP: Anaesthesia for cerebral arteriovenous malformations in children. Can Anaesth Soc J 29:299, 1982.

61. Graf CJ, Perrett GE, Torner JC: Bleeding from arteriovenous malformations as part of their natural history. J Neurosurg 58:331, 1983.

62. Grubb RL, Raichie ME: Effects of hemorrhagic and pharmacologic hypotension on cerebral oxygen utilization and blood flow. Anesthesiology 56:3, 1982.

63. Michenfelder JD, Theye RA: Canine systemic and cerebral effects of hypotension induced by hemorrhage, trimethaphan or nitroprusside. Anesthesiology 46:188, 1977.

64. Turner JM, Powell D, Gibsone RM, et al.: Intracranial pressure changes in neurosurgical patients during hypotension induced with sodium nitroprusside or trimethaphan. Br J Anaesth 49:419, 1977.

65. Rhambatta HJ, Stone JG, Khan E: Hypertension during anesthesia on discontinuation of sodium nitroprusside—induced hypotension. Anesthesiology 51:127, 1979.

66. Ghani GA, Sung YF, Weinstein MS, et al.: Effects of intravenous nitroglycerin on the intracranial pressure and volume pressure response. J Neurosurg 58:562, 1983.

67. Lam AM, Gelb AW: Cardiovascular effects of isoflurane-induced hypotension for cerebral aneurysm surgery. Anesth Analg 62:742, 1983.

68. Østergaard JR, Voldby, B: Intracranial arterial aneurysms in children and adolescents. J Neurosurg 58:832, 1983.

69. Storrs BB, Humphreys RP, Hendrick EB, et al.: Intracranial aneurysms in the pediatric age-group. Child's Brain 9:358, 1982.

70. Amacher AL, Drake CG: The results of operating upon cerebral aneurysms and angiomas in children and adolescents. Child's Brain 5:151, 1979.

71. Botterell EH, Lougheed WM, Scott JW, et al.: Hypothermia and interruption of carotid or carotid and vertebral circulation in the surgical management of intracranial aneurysms. J Neurosurg 13:1, 1956.

72. Amacher AL, Shillito J Jr: The syndromes and surgical treatment of aneurysms of the great vein of Galen. J Neurosurg 39:89, 1973.

73. Jedeikin R, Rowe RD, Freedom RM, et al.: Cerebral arteriovenous malformation in neonates. The role of myocardial ischemia. J Cardiol 4:29, 1983.

74. Russell W, Newton TH: Aneurysm of the vein of Galen. Am J Roentgenol 92:756, 1964.

75. Hood JB, Wallace CT, Mahaffey JE: Anesthetic management of an intracranial arteriovenous malformation in infancy. Anesth Analg 56:236, 1977.

76. Hoffman HJ, Chuang S, Hendrick EB, et al.: Aneurysms of the vein of Galen. J Neurosurg 57:316, 1982.

77. Takehara Y, Araki S, Motomatsu K, et al.: Anesthesia for Galen aneurysm. Jpn J Anesthesiol 28:737, 1979 (English abstract).

78. Raimondi AJ, Tomita T: Brain tumors during the first year of life. Child's Brain 10:193, 1983.

79. Schreiber D, Janisch W, Gerlach H: CNS tumours in infancy, childhood and adolescence. In Voth D, Gutjahr P, Langmaid C (Eds.): Tumours of the Central Nervous System in Infancy and Childhood. Berlin, Springer-Verlag, 1982.

80. Jacobi G: Clinical presentation of space-occupying lesions of the central nervous system. In Voth D, Gutjahr P, Langmaid C (Eds.): Tumours of the Central Nervous System in Infancy and Childhood. Berlin, Springer-Verlag, 1982.

81. Park TS, Hoffman HJ, Hendrick EB, et al.: Medulloblastoma: clinical presentation and management. J Neurosurg 58:543, 1983.

82. Meridy HW, Creighton RE, Humphreys RP: Complications during neurosurgery in the prone position in children. Can Anaesth Soc J 21:445, 1974.

83. Sung DI: Suprasellar tumors in children. Cancer 50:1420, 1982.

84. McLone DG, Raimondi AJ, Naidich TP: Craniopharyngiomas. Child's Brain 9:188, 1982.

85. Thomsett MJ, Conte FA, Kaplan SL, et al.: Endocrine and neurologic outcome in childhood craniopharyngioma: review of effect of treatment in 42 patients, J Pediatr 97:728, 1980.

86. Grant DB, Lyen K: Hypopituitarism after surgery for craniopharyngioma. Child's Brain 9:201, 1982.

87. Friedenberg GR, Kosnik EJ, Sotos JF: Hyperglycemic coma after suprasellar surgery. N Engl J Med 303:863, 1981.

88. Fortner J, Nicastri A, Murphy ML: Neuroblastoma: natural history and results of treating 133 cases. Ann Surg 167:132, 1968.

89. Wagner HP, Kaser H: The role of surgery, radio- and chemotherapy in the treatment of neuroblastoma and ganglioneuroblastoma. Prog Pediatr Surg 16:1, 1983.

90. Evans AE, D'Angio GJ, Koop CE: Diagnosis and treatment of neuroblastoma. Pediatr Clin North Am 23:161, 1976.

91. Coldman AJ, Fryer CJH, Elwood JM, et al.: Neuroblastoma: influence of age at diagnosis, stage, tumor site, and sex on prognosis. Cancer 46:1896, 1980.

92. King D, Goodman J, Hawk T, et al.: Dumbbell neuroblastomas in children. Arch Surg 110:888, 1975.

93. Duckett JW, Koop CE: Neuroblastoma. Urol Clin North Am 4:285, 1977.

94. Weinblatt ME, Heisel MA, Siegel SE: Hypertension in children with neurogenic tumors. Pediatrics 71:947, 1983.

95. Thompson EN, Bosley A: Disseminated intravascular coagulation in association with congenital neuroblastoma. Postgrad Med J 55:814, 1979.

96. Scott JP, Morgan E: Coagulopathy of disseminated neuroblastoma. J Pediatr 103:219, 1983.

97. Farman JV: Neuroblastomas and anaesthesia. Br J Anaesth 37:866, 1965.

98. Griffith BH, McKinney P, Monroe CW, et al.: Von Recklinghausen's disease in children. Plast Reconstr Surg 49:647, 1972.

99. Fienman NL, Yakovac WC: Neurofibromatosis in childhood. Pediatrics 76:339, 1970.

100. Jackson IT, Laws ER, Martin RD: The surgical management of orbital neurofibromatosis. Plast Reconstr Surg 71:751, 1983.

101. Griffiths DFR, Williams GT, Williams ED: Multiple endocrine neoplasia associated with von Recklinghausen's disease. Br Med J 287:1341, 1983.

102. Isu T, Miyasaka K, Abe H, et al.: Atlantoaxial dislocation associated with neurofibromatosis. J Neurosurg 58:451, 1983.

103. Manser J: Abnormal responses in von Recklinghausen's disease. Br J Anaesth 42:183, 1970.

104. Magbagbeola JAO: Abnormal responses to muscle relaxants in a patient with von Recklinghausen's disease. Br J Anaesth 42:710, 1970.

105. Nagao H, Yamashita M, Shinozaki Y, et al.: Hypersensitivity to pancuronium in a patient with von Recklinghausen's disease. Br J Anaesth 55:253, 1983.

106. Olivier A: Surgical management of complex partial seizures. In Nistico G, et al. (Eds.): Epilepsy: An Update on Research and Therapy. New York, Alan R. Liss, Inc., 1983.

107. Fisher RS, Uematsu S: Surgical therapy of complex partial epilepsy. Johns Hopkins Med J 151:332, 1982.

108. Blume WT, Grabow JD, Darley FL, et al.: Intracarotid amobarbital test of language and memory before temporal lobectomy for seizure control. Neurology 23:812, 1973.

109. Ford EW, Morrell F, Whisler WW: Methohexital anesthesia in the surgical treatment of uncontrollable epilepsy. Anesth Analg 61:997, 1982.

110. Musella L, Wilder BJ, Schmidt RP: Electroencephalographic activation with intravenous methohexital in psychomotor epilepsy. Neurology 21:594, 1971.

111. Rasmussen T: Cortical resection in the treatment of focal epilepsy. Adv Neurol 8:197, 1975.

112. Jennet B, Teasdale G: Aspects of coma after severe head injury. Lancet 1:878, 1977.

113. Jennet B, Teasdale G: Management of Head Injuries. Philadelphia, F. A. Davis, 1981.

114. Humphreys RP, Jaimovich R, et al.: Severe head injuries in children. In Humphreys RP (Ed.): Concepts in Pediatric Neurosurg. No. 4. Basel, S. Karger, 1983, p 230.

115. Lewelt W, Jenkins LW, Miller JD: Effects of fluid-percussion injury of the brain on cerebrovascular reactivity to hypoxia and hypercapnia. J Neurosurg 56:332, 1982.

116. Uchida M, Yamaoka H, Imanishi Y: Hypotension during surgery for subdural hematoma and effusion in infants. Crit Care Med 10:5, 1982.

117. Bruce DA, Alavi A, Bilaniuk L, et al.: Diffuse cerebral swelling following head injuries in children: the syndrome of "malignant brain edema." J Neurosurg 54:170, 1981.

118. Obrist WD, Gennarelli TA, Segawa H, et al.: Relation of cerebral blood flow to neurological status and outcome in head-injured patients. J Neurosurg 51:292, 1979.

119. Braakman R, Schouten HJA, Blaauw–van Dishoeck M, et al.: Megadose steroids in severe head injury—results of a prospective double-blind clinical trial. J Neurosurg 58:326, 1983.

120. Eiben RM, Crocker AC: Cerebral palsy within the spectrum of developmental disabilities. In Thompson GH (Ed.): Comprehensive Management of Cerebral Palsy. New York, Grune and Stratton, 1982.

121. Alvarez N: Neurologic examination. In Thompson GH (Ed.): Comprehensive Management of Cerebral Palsy. New York, Grune and Stratton, 1982.

122. O'Reilly DE, Walentynowicz JE: Etiological factors in cerebral palsy: an historical review. Dev Med Child Neurol 23:633, 1981.

123. Fasano VA, Broggi G, Barolat-Romana G, et al.: Surgical treatment of spasticity in cerebral palsy. Child's Brain 4:289, 1978.

124. Crysdale WS: The drooling patient: evaluation and current surgical options. Laryngoscope 90:775, 1980.

125. Crysdale WS: Submandibular duct relocation for drooling. J Otolaryngol 11:286, 1982.

126. Reye RDK, Morgan G, Baral J: Encephalopathy and fatty degeneration of the viscera. A disease entity in childhood. Lancet 2:749, 1963.

127. Luscombe FA, Monto AS, Baublis JV: Mortality due to Reye's syndrome in Michigan: Distribution and longitudinal trends. J Infect Dis 142:363, 1980.

128. Lovejoy FH, Bresnan MJ, Lombroso CT, et al.: Anticerebral oedema therapy in Reye's syndrome. Arch Dis Child 50:933, 1975.

129. Partin JC, Partin JS, Schubert WK, et al.: Brain ultrastructure in Reye's syndrome. J Neuropathol Exp Neurol 34:425, 1975.

130. Lovejoy FH, Smith AL, Bresnan MJ, et al.: Clinical staging in Reye's syndrome. Am J Dis Child 128:36, 1974.

131. Huttenlocher RP: Reye's syndrome: relation of outcome to therapy. Pediatr Pharm Ther 80:845, 1972.

132. Samaha FJ, Blau E, Berardinelli JL: Reye's syndrome: clinical diagnosis and treatment with peritoneal dialysis. Pediatrics 53:336, 1974.

133. Glascow JFT: Clinical features and prognosis of Reye's syndrome. Arch Dis Child 59:230, 1984.

134. Shaywitz BA, Leventhal JM, Kramer MS, et al.: Prolonged continuous monitoring of intracranial pressure in Reye's syndrome. Pediatrics 59:595, 1977.

135. Frewen TC, Swedlow DB, Watcha M, et al.: Outcome in severe Reye syndrome with early pentobarbital coma and hypothermia. J Pediatr 100:663, 1982.

136. Corey L, Rubin RJ, Hattwick MAW: Reye's syndrome: clinical progression and evaluation of therapy. Pediatrics 60:708, 1977.

DISEASES OF THE RESPIRATORY SYSTEM | 5

I. DAVID TODRES, M.D.

This chapter reviews the clinical presentation and diagnosis of diseases of the respiratory system and details specific anesthetic implications for each condition. The basic principles of thoracic anesthesia that apply in every situation are summarized in Table 5–1. Some uncommon conditions are discussed in more detail because of their important anesthetic implications.

LUNG GROWTH AND DEVELOPMENT

The respiratory system is frequently diseased at birth. Because it is essential for independent existence, compromise of the system may lead to significant morbidity and mortality. An appreciation of normal lung development in utero will provide an understanding of the pathological processes that may occur in the respiratory system following birth.

Normal lung growth is governed by three laws relating to the development of the airways, alveoli, and blood supply. Disturbances of growth and the gestational age at which this disturbance occurs may be appreciated from an understanding of these laws.[1-3]

Airways. The bronchial tree is fully developed by the 16th week of intrauterine life. Respiratory airways are formed between 16 weeks and birth and also in infancy.

Alveoli. Alveoli develop mainly after birth, increasing in number until approximately 8 years of age. Alveolar size increases until growth of the chest cage is complete.

Blood Supply. The arteries and veins (preacinar vessels) follow the development of the airways. The intra-acinar vessels follow the alveoli.

Embryonic and Fetal Development

By the 5th week of the embryonic period the lobar bronchi to each lung have formed, and by the 6th week all subsegmental bronchi are present. Following the embryonic period the fetal period consists of three stages of development.[4]

The glandular period (6 weeks to 16 weeks) consists of the formation of the preacinar airways, which are blind-ending tubes lined by epithelium and lying within loose mesenchymal stroma.

This period is followed by the canalicular stage (16 to 24 weeks) with increase in the caliber of the peripheral airways. At this stage the pulmonary capillaries invade the mesenchyme and develop with the

Table 5–1. GENERAL PRINCIPLES OF THORACIC ANESTHESIA

Preoperative

Complete history, physical examination, chest roentgenograms, assessment of arterial blood gases, pulmonary function tests

Optimize medical condition of child, with attention to special problems of the neonate

Avoid respiratory depressant drugs

Anticipate possible major hemorrhage in surgery, and order adequate blood for transfusion

Psychological preparation: what to expect postoperatively in the form of pain relief, intubation, and mechanical ventilation

Emergency surgery: do not compromise efforts to optimize medical condition, but recognize priorities and modify plan accordingly

Work out plan for surgery with team approach: surgeon, anesthesiologist, pediatrician, appropriate consultants

Operative

Recognize effect on $\dot{V}/\dot{Q}$ ratios with thoracotomy and lung surgery leading to potential hypoxemia; therefore increase FIO_2 and monitor oxygen saturation and PaO_2

Ensure reliable and adequate venous access to permit urgent and rapid transfusions

Anesthetic agents will depend upon the underlying physical condition of the patient and postoperative needs (inhalational or N_2O plus relaxants); avoid N_2O when there is a potential for increase in size of a life-threatening air space, e.g., congenital lobar emphysema

Recheck proper tube position following positioning of patient

Secretions and blood easily obstruct the endotracheal tube and airways; keep airway clear at all times

Retractions of lung may obstruct airway, impair ventilation, and compress heart and great veins, reducing venous return and causing a decrease in cardiac output and blood pressure; therefore, monitor ventilation continuously

Operative (*Continued*)

Monitor blood loss closely

Perform intermittent reexpansion of collapsed lung to optimize oxygenation; this requires close coordination between surgeon and anesthesiologist

Mechanical ventilation must be optimal, maintaining the $PaCO_2$ in the normal range (end-tidal carbon dioxide monitoring, blood gases); manual ventilation at times helpful in detecting changes in airway resistance and lung compliance

Intraoperative Monitoring

Precordial stethoscope to monitor heart and breath sounds

Esophageal stethoscope

Oscilloscope display of the ECG with audible signal

Blood pressure: Doppler probe, oscillometric, intra-arterial catheter

Oxygen saturation: pulse oximetry

Blood gases, pH: intra-arterial catheter

Temperature probe (esophageal when possible)

Central venous pressure in selected cases

Urine output via Foley catheter (should be at least 1 ml/kg/hr)

Postoperative

Extubate when patient is alert, muscle relaxation has been adequately reversed as determined by clinical evaluation and blockade monitor, and patient is able to cough effectively

Postoperative pain relief with intercostal blocks, cryopexy, or appropriate narcotic dosages

Monitor blood gases

Look for atelectasis or pneumothorax on chest roentgenograms

Monitor chest drains

Data from Bland JW Jr, Reedy JC, Williams WH: Pediatric and neonatal thoracic surgery. *In* Kaplan JA (Ed.): Thoracic Anesthesia. New York, Churchill Livingstone, 1983, pp 505–574; and Steward DJ: Manual of Pediatric Anesthesia. 2nd ed. New York, Churchill Livingstone, 1985, pp 181–203.

airways to form the beginnings of the blood-air interface. Toward the end of this stage, types I and II lining cells appear. Type II cells, or granular pneumocytes, have cytoplasmic lamellar bodies that appear at about 25 weeks and are associated with the production of surface active material (surfactant).

The alveolar period, from 24 weeks to term (40 weeks), represents the time during which there is further differentiation into respiratory bronchioles, alveolar sacs, and primitive alveoli. Of the 27 generations of airways, the first 19 generations (two main bronchi, lobar bronchi, segmental bronchi, lobular bronchi) are nonrespiratory airways. These are followed by 8 generations that form the respiratory bronchioles and alveolar ducts, which participate in gas exchange. Further growth of these structures is in part determined by a direct effect of growth hormone on the lung. During the alveolar period the amount of surfactant increases with duration of gestation. Surfactant is

critical in the prevention of respiratory distress syndrome (hyaline membrane disease). Glucocorticoids administered to the mother pass into the fetus and accelerate the production of surfactant as well as enhancing structural maturation of the lung.

The lung develops as a hollow fluid-filled organ from the canalicular phase to term. Fluid is secreted into the airways and contributes to amniotic fluid. The presence of the lung fluid appears to be important for lung growth to occur.[5]

In the respiratory epithelium, specialized cells secrete the lung liquid and also produce hormones that may affect lung growth. Sympathetic stimulation appears to be a factor in terminating secretion of lung liquid at birth.[6]

Respiratory movements in the fetus are noted early in the second trimester and particularly involve the diaphragm. These movements are depressed by barbiturates, hypoxia, and hypoglycemia. Fetal respiratory movements appear to be important for normal lung growth.[7]

At birth the "alveoli" are primitive spaces or saccules that will eventually develop into well-formed alveoli. There are approximately 20 million "alveoli" at birth, and by 8 years of age there are approximately 300 million.[8] It should be appreciated that the lung of the premature infant not only is smaller than that of the full-term infant but has less than the normal number of respiratory units.[9]

As stated in the third law the arteries and veins (preacinar vessels) follow the development of the airways so that by the 16th week of gestation all preacinar vessels are present. In utero the pulmonary artery trunk is exposed to systemic pressures and thus has relatively thick muscle within its wall. In more peripheral vessels also the muscle layer is relatively well developed, consistent with the high pulmonary vascular resistance in utero. This muscle layer thins out and eventually disappears at a level proximal to the terminal bronchioles. Thus the arteries to the acinus are nonmuscular. However, in persistent pulmonary hypertension found in conditions such as meconium aspiration, the alveolar wall arteries are all muscularized. This degree of muscularization represents the normal state in the adult but surprisingly may develop even before birth in certain pathological situations.

Abnormal Airway Growth

For abnormal airway growth—that is, reduction in bronchial airway generations—to have occurred, impairment of lung growth must have taken place before the 16th week of intrauterine life. Examples include congenital diaphragmatic hernia and renal agenesis. Should the pathological process follow the period of airway development, then alveolar multiplication receives the brunt of the insult, as seen, for example, in kyphoscoliosis.

Compensatory Growth

Following resection of a portion of the lung there is a compensatory increase in weight, volume, and alveolar size in the remaining lung.[10] If resection occurs during the period of alveolar multiplication, there is a more rapid multiplication of alveoli but the total number of alveoli that develops is not greater than normal.[11, 12]

With this basic understanding of the normal process of lung growth and development, deviations from the normal may be better appreciated. An outline of selected pathological processes of the respiratory system is given with emphasis on the clinical presentation and specific implications for the anesthesiologist dealing with the problem.

Association of Congenital Lung Abnormalities with Other Anomalies

Congenital abnormalities of the lung may be associated with other anomalies. This is especially important when medical and surgical treatment is undertaken for the specific pulmonary abnormality, as the associated anomaly may add significantly to the morbidity risks. Any infant or child who rapidly develops severe respiratory distress in a matter of hours following a mild respiratory illness should be rapidly evaluated for an underlying pulmonary malformation.

PULMONARY AGENESIS AND PULMONARY APLASIA

Arrested lung bud development early in pregnancy will result in either pulmonary agenesis or pulmonary aplasia. Arrested development later in pregnancy will result in failure of alveolar differentiation leading to pulmonary hypoplasia.

Unilateral pulmonary agenesis, that is, failure of the lung to develop, is compatible with normal life. The contralateral lung is larger owing to hypertrophy. Other anomalies involving particularly the cardiovascular, gastrointestinal, and genitourinary systems may be present in greater than 50 percent of cases and will significantly affect morbidity.

A small mainstem bronchial stump arising from a recognizable carina may exist with absence of lung tissue. When this occurs it is referred to as pulmonary aplasia, which is more commonly seen than pulmonary agenesis. Sexes are affected equally.[13-15]

Clinical Presentation

Recurrent pulmonary infections occur. These may be severe, as the bronchial stump acts as a nidus for infection. Severe respiratory distress may occur because of a marked shift of mediastinal structures and inadequate respiratory reserve, but clinical examination may reveal few signs. In agenesis of the right lung the heart sounds may be best heard in the right chest.[16]

Chest roentgenograms show marked deviation of the mediastinal structures, and the normal lung may be seen herniating across the mediastinum to the opposite side.

Diagnosis may be confirmed by bronchoscopy, bronchography, and radionuclide perfusion scans. Associated cardiac anomalies may be present.

Right-sided agenesis has twice the mortality of left-sided agenesis, probably as a result of greater mediastinal shift with cardiac displacement.

Treatment

Surgical treatment is occasionally required because of repeated infections of the bronchial stump. Excision of the stump will relieve the symptoms.

Anesthetic Implications

Standard thoracotomy procedures are required. Accidental intubation of the bronchial stump in right lung agenesis may lead to life-threatening hypoxemia.

PULMONARY HYPOPLASIA

Failure of the lung to develop to its normal size while containing essential anatomical ingredients for function represents pulmonary hypoplasia. The condition is associated with a decrease in lung volume and weight. The pulmonary function will be decreased to a degree commensurate with the degree of hypoplasia. A smaller than normal pulmonary artery may supply the hypoplastic lung. Perfusion scans have largely replaced pulmonary angiography for study of the vascular supply. A severe form of hypoplasia is seen in Potter syndrome, which consists of bilateral pulmonary hypoplasia associated with renal agenesis or dysplasia. A history of oligohydramnios in the mother is characteristic. Pathologically the lungs show reduced airway generations. The alveoli are small and fewer in number. The oligohydramnios appears to be the result of lung hypoplasia rather than its cause.[3, 17] Thus, pathologically it should be considered a form of primary hypoplasia. When pulmonary hypoplasia of undetermined origin is found a search for renal abnormalities should be made. Secondary hypoplasia occurs when the intrathoracic volume is reduced. This may be unilateral or bilateral. Causes include congenital diaphragmatic hernia (the most common cause), thoracic or skeletal dystrophy, and large pleural effusions.

Clinical Presentation

This condition is frequently misdiagnosed. Clinical symptoms will depend upon the degree of hypoplasia and associated anomalies. The normal lung herniates to the opposite side and the mediastinal shift displaces the normal position of the heart. In some cases the child is asymptomatic and the pathology is recognized as an incidental finding on a chest roentgenogram. Symptoms of pulmonary infection and occasional hemoptysis are clinically presenting signs in the second and third decades of life. With secondary hypoplasia the contralateral lung compression seen in congenital diaphragmatic hernia will further aggravate the respiratory distress because of the infant's inability to establish an adequate functional residual capacity (FRC).

Anesthetic Implications

The anesthesiologist should be particularly careful in the use of positive-pressure ventilation, as the hypoplastic lung tends to resist expansion. Excessive positive pressure may lead to bronchiolar rupture with interstitial emphysema and tension pneumothorax.

The treatment for the hypoplastic lung is basically conservative. However, if the lung should contain malformed bronchial tissue, recurring infections may necessitate resection.

Scimitar Syndrome

The scimitar syndrome is a special form of pulmonary hypoplasia occurring mostly in females.[18] Its name derives from the radiological picture showing a curvilinear shadow on the right lower lung field; this represents an anomalous pulmonary vein draining the right lung, usually into the inferior vena cava (Fig. 5–1). Occasionally it drains into the portal or hepatic veins. The condition may be asymptomatic or associated with frequent pulmonary infections. It may be associated with serious congenital anomalies, especially of the heart (ventricular septal defect, patent ductus arteriosus, coarctation of the aorta, and tetralogy of Fallot). Vertebral anomalies are usually present.

Pulmonary Hypoplasia with Horseshoe Lung

In this condition right and left lungs are joined behind the pericardial sac.[19] Embryologically a delay or failure in the formation and fusion of the pleuropericardial and pleuroperitoneal folds occurs. Hypoplasia of the right lung contributes to the cardiac dextroversion. Surgical removal of the hypoplastic lung may be necessary because of recurrent pulmonary infections.

PULMONARY SEQUESTRATION

In this condition embryonic and nonfunctioning lung tissue is sequestered from normal lung.[20–22] The abnormal lung receives its blood supply via systemic arteries. Embryologically, at 5 weeks of gestation the lung bud appears as an outgrowth from the ventral wall of the primitive foregut and gives rise to the tracheobronchial tree. Abnormal development of a supernumerary lung bud or buds caudal to the normal position is thought to be the underlying cause for pulmonary sequestration. Two forms of sequestration occur:

1. Intralobar sequestration results when there is early incorporation of the abnormal lung bud within the normal lung and its visceral pleura.[23]

2. Extralobar sequestration results when the abnormal lung bud development occurs after the pleura has already formed; thus, the extralobar lung is separated from the normal lung but related to it.[23, 24]

The sequestered lung tissue is embryonic, with multiple cysts and a disorganized arrangement of airless alveoli, bronchi, and cartilage receiving its blood supply via a systemic artery. The tissue is frequently infected and bronchiectatic. Occasionally the sequestered lung tissue may communicate with the alimen-

Figure 5–1. Scimitar syndrome. *A,* Anomalous pulmonary vein (*arrow*) with hypoplastic right lung. *B,* Angiogram defining the anomalous pulmonary vein. Note also the presence of right pulmonary artery hypoplasia. (Courtesy of Thomas Herman, M.D.)

tary tract. Most commonly such a communication involves the esophagus, in which case it is known as a bronchopulmonary foregut malformation.[25] This occurs more frequently on the right side. More commonly, the communication obliterates and disappears completely or remains as a fibrous stalk. The sequestered lung tissue receives its blood supply from a systemic artery, the aorta or one of its branches. It is associated with other foregut anomalies such as ectopic pancreas and foregut duplication cysts.

Intralobar Sequestration

This is a relatively common abnormality. It usually occurs in the lower lobes, mostly in the left posterior basal segment. It is rarely associated with other abnormalities. The sequestered lobe is made up of multiple cysts of varying size and filled with mucus, mucopurulent material, and air. Normal lung tissue is present in a disorganized fashion. Inflammatory changes and fibrosis are present. Arterial supply to the sequestered lobe is from an anomalous systemic artery from the descending thoracic aorta. In 10 to 15 percent of patients the arterial supply comes from below the diaphragm. Venous drainage is via the pulmonary veins. Patent communications with the gastrointestinal tract are rare.

Clinical Presentation

In neonates and infants the condition is frequently asymptomatic. Over half the cases are diagnosed after adolescence. Sex incidence is equal. The intralobar

form usually presents with signs of pulmonary infection in the first two decades of life. Onset of symptoms, however, may occur many years later. With an esophageal or gastric communication there may be severe respiratory distress and gastrointestinal symptoms. Pulmonary infections are progressive and recurrent with pneumonitis or lung abscess. The child will have fever, cough, weight loss, and possibly hemoptysis.

A chest roentgenogram shows intralobar sequestration as a dense mass that may contain cysts with fluid levels occurring usually in the posterior basal portion of the left lobe. An upper GI series will exclude a communication between the sequestration and gastrointestinal tract. Aortography and selective arteriography and pulmonary perfusion scans will identify the aberrant systemic arterial supply and aid the surgeon in approaching the resection of the sequestered lobe.

Extralobar Sequestration

This consists of bronchial and alveolar structures often found behind the lung. It occurs more commonly in males (80 percent). The majority of extralobar sequestration (90 percent) are found on the left at any level from the thoracic inlet to the upper part of the abdomen. More than half the cases are diagnosed before 1 year of age. Extralobar sequestration occurs in males three times more commonly than in females. It is frequently associated with diaphragmatic hernias or other congenital malformations. The arterial supply is from the aorta and the venous drainage is via the azygos vein. Pathologically there is interstitial fibrosis with cystic spaces, destroyed lung tissue, and dilated bronchioles.

Clinical Presentation

Extralobar sequestration is more commonly associated with congenital anomalies, most commonly congenital diaphragmatic hernia. Other associated anomalies include congenital heart disease and pulmonary arteriovenous malformations. Clinically extralobar sequestration presents in infancy with recurrent infections with an area of infiltrate identifiable in the same location. Cystic changes with air-fluid levels may be superimposed. Severe systemic arteriovenous shunting through aberrant vessels may cause cardiomegaly and high-output congestive heart failure with dyspnea and wheezing.[26]

On chest roentgenogram extralobar sequestrations are usually identified as triangular densities in the posterior and medial left base, with upper lobe presentation being rare. The diagnosis should be suspected when repeated clinical episodes of infection are associated with restriction and localization of roentgenographic findings to the same area. With abscess formation there may be a fluid level with surrounding pneumonitis. The sequestered lung may appear quite normal before changes of chronic infection set in.

Arteriography will define the abnormal systemic supply, which can be helpful at the time of surgery. Computed tomography or radionuclide hemodynamic studies with induction of pneumoperitoneum may be useful in identifying the aberrant artery.

Treatment and Anesthetic Implications

The sequestered lung tissue is usually resected with excellent results. The extralobar sequestration is excised, and the intralobar sequestration is removed by lobectomy. Communication with the gastrointestinal tract, if present, is severed. The aberrant artery or arteries may bleed readily, necessitating close monitoring of blood loss and its replacement. The sequestered tissue may contain significant amounts of purulent material, making excision a slow and deliberate process. Antibiotics are given for infection. Mortality and morbidity are low, especially when surgery is performed before repeated infections have occurred.

CYSTIC DISEASE OF THE LUNG

Congenital Pulmonary Cysts

Congenital pulmonary cysts have been classified in a number of ways. One classification separates them into (1) bronchogenic type, (2) alveolar type, and (3) a combination of bronchogenic and alveolar. It should be noted, however, that acquired cystic disease is much more common. Embryologically congenital cystic disease is thought to arise as an anomalous development

of the bronchopulmonary system at the stage of terminal bronchiolar or early alveolar development.[27, 28] The cyst arises on the basis of expiratory obstruction through bronchiolar narrowing. The more common form is a single peripheral air-filled cyst with a tracheobronchial communication. Cysts may be multiple. With infection it is difficult to distinguish histologically between a congenital cyst and an acquired cyst such as staphylococcal pneumatocele or a lung abscess. The cyst is filled with air either directly or through the pores of Kohn. Increase in size of the cyst leads to tension and distress in the newborn. Compression of normal lung occurs with shift of the mediastinum and a decrease in functioning lung tissue. Contralateral atelectasis occurs. Suppuration develops in the cyst.

Clinical Presentation

The clinical findings will depend upon the degree of distention of the cyst with air. Tension pneumothorax may develop and result in severe cardiopulmonary distress demanding emergency treatment. In late infancy and childhood, infection of the cyst usually occurs with symptoms of fever, cough, sputum, and possibly hemoptysis with the cyst developing into a lung abscess.

Chest roentgenogram shows a large distended cyst with mediastinal shift. There is compression atelectasis of upper and lower lobes, and the roentgenographic picture may resemble lobar emphysema. Diaphragmatic hernia may occasionally resemble multiple lung cysts. A staphylococcal pneumatocele will undergo resolution with treatment.

Treatment

Thoracotomy is indicated because of the potential for serious complications, namely, tension pneumothorax, abscess formation, bronchopleural fistula, and progressive and dangerous enlargement of the cyst. Elective lobectomy is therefore carried out. At times, however, emergency resection is required.[29] Antibiotics are administered in the perioperative period. Note that aberrant systemic arteries may exist, especially with lower lobe cysts.

Anesthetic Implications

Excision of the cyst may be difficult because of recurrent infection, and hence there may be significant blood loss.

Congenital Pulmonary Lymphangiectasis

This condition presents with respiratory distress in the newborn and is frequently fatal within the first 24 hours of life. Males are affected more than females. Other congenital anomalies may be associated. The condition is most often seen with congenital anomalies of the cardiovascular system, specifically total anomalous pulmonary venous drainage and cor triatriatum. On rare occasions it is part of a generalized lymphangiectasis. The etiology is thought to involve obstruction of pulmonary lymphatics or venous flow or malformation in the development of the lymphatic network. Both lungs are affected. The lung shows a nodular surface. Multiple fluid-containing cystic cavities are seen beneath the pleural surface of the lungs.

Clinical Presentation

The infant is in severe respiratory distress with cyanosis. Symptoms may be aggravated by the presence of a pneumothorax.

Chest roentgenogram shows a diffuse involvement of both lung fields resembling hyaline membrane disease. The normal areas of lung may show emphysematous changes.

Treatment

The prognosis is grave with diffuse involvement of both lungs. No specific treatment is available.

INFANTILE LOBAR EMPHYSEMA

This condition is characterized by overinflation and air trapping in the affected lobe with compression atelectasis of the adjacent lung parenchyma and displacement of the mediastinum. The left upper lobe is most often affected, followed by right middle and right upper lobes.

Males are affected twice as often as females. The cause is unknown in 50 percent of cases. In others bronchial obstruction appears to be due to some factors such as congenital deficiency of bronchial cartilages, bronchial stenosis, or extrinsic vascular compression from the pulmonary artery. Over 50 percent of cases show evidence of bronchial cartilage deficiency. It may be a manifestation of generalized lung disease resulting from loss of static recoil of the lungs. Ten percent of patients also have congenital heart disease.

Clinical Presentation

Progressive respiratory distress occurs in the newborn period or early infancy. The respiratory distress may be intermittent and is aggravated by feeding and crying. Tachypnea, retractions, wheezing, and cyanosis occur. Rapid deterioration may occur, requiring urgent surgery. The emphysematous lobe displaces the mediastinum to the opposite side and causes compression atelectasis of the contralateral lung. The shift of the mediastinum causes increased intrathoracic pressure, impeding venous return and leading to decreased cardiac output. The emphysematous lobe does not participate in gas exchange; this, combined with atelectasis of the opposite lung, results in severe compromise of gas exchange. The infant may present with failure to gain weight and respiratory infections with cough, wheezing, and tachypnea. Associated congeni-

tal heart disease occurs in a significant number of children.

Chest roentgenogram shows the emphysematous lobe (overdistention of alveoli) with basilar atelectasis of the lower lobe. There is diaphragmatic displacement and mediastinal shift with contralateral lung atelectasis. The emphysematous lobe appears to herniate across the mediastinum. Congenital lobar emphysema must be differentiated from postpneumonic pneumatocele, pulmonary cystic disease, and tension pneumothorax. Note that bronchovascular markings are present in congenital lobar emphysema, in contrast to a pneumothorax or lung cyst.

Treatment

Bronchoscopy for the older infant is indicated if there is a possibility of intraluminal obstruction causing emphysema of a lobe. Treatment consists of removal of the affected lobe. Surgical excision in the neonate may be urgent if the lobe is expanding rapidly.[30] Outcome after surgery is good, with compensation for loss of lung parenchyma by expansion of the remaining lung. In the older infant with few symptoms, nonsurgical treatment may be considered.[31] For example, conservative therapy including a bronchoscopy may relieve obstruction due to a mucous plug. However, it should be stressed that the condition usually progresses, and lobectomy is indicated to avoid the high mortality rate in the symptomatic patient.

Anesthetic Implications

An associated cardiac anomaly needs to be considered in the anesthetic and surgical management. During induction of anesthesia vigorous positive pressure may inflate the emphysematous lobe still further with increase in cardiopulmonary distress. Therefore, spontaneous ventilation is preferred until the chest is open and the thorax decompressed. Nitrous oxide is avoided because of its potential for increasing the size of the emphysematous lobe.[32]

CONGENITAL CYSTIC ADENOMATOID MALFORMATION

This is a very rare condition. It may be associated with other congenital anomalies. It usually is unilateral and affects one or more lobes, usually the lower lobe. Differentiation from cystic disease of the lung is not always clear (Fig. 5–2). The condition has been classified into types I, II, and III based on gross and histological criteria.[33]

Clinical Presentation

The child presents either in (1) acute respiratory distress in the newborn period or (2) pulmonary infections running a chronic course. Type I lesions have large cysts which may expand rapidly after birth and cause increasing respiratory distress. The cysts

Figure 5–2. Chest roentgenogram showing cystic adenomatoid malformation of the right lung. Note the lower lobe inflation and the upper lobe herniating across the midline (*arrow*). The radiological picture resembles that of congenital lobar emphysema. (Courtesy of David Kushner, M.D.)

communicate with each other and with the bronchus. Lack of bronchial cartilage leads to bronchial collapse during expiration. Type II and III lesions are usually not compatible with survival because of associated anomalies seen with type II lesions and the gross extent of the lesions with type III.

The differential diagnosis on chest roentgenogram includes congenital and acquired cystic disease, lobar emphysema, and congenital diaphragmatic hernia.

Treatment

In the newborn, operation may be urgent because of tension from enlarging cysts causing severe cardiopulmonary distress similar to that seen in obstructive emphysema. Lobectomy is performed. In older children chronic infection, which is inevitable, will require a thoracotomy and lobectomy.

BRONCHOGENIC CYST

Bronchogenic cysts occur at any age but usually in older children. They are unilocular cysts lined with respiratory epithelium and may have cartilage and bronchial glands in the wall. They usually do not communicate with the tracheobronchial tree.

Clinical Presentation

Bronchogenic cysts may be asymptomatic and discovered on a routine chest roentgenogram. Clinically

they may present with respiratory infections and cough. However, the cyst may cause severe respiratory distress through compression of a mainstem bronchus, in which case the cyst is commonly situated beneath the carina and compresses the left mainstem bronchus.[34] The cysts contain mucus and frequently become infected. Barium swallow, bronchography, and CT scanning help to delineate the pathology.

CHYLOTHORAX

In this condition a pleural chylous effusion forms. The fluid will have a lipid concentration greater than 400 mg/ml. In the newborn it occurs owing to a congenital abnormality or following traumatic rupture of the thoracic duct during the birth process.[35] It has been described as a complication of chest tube placement in the newborn.[36] The congenital abnormality is thought to be due to a failure of the proper fusion of mediastinal and pulmonary lymphatics and the production of multiple lymphatic fistulas. It is usually right-sided. The condition may rarely be bilateral.[37] Chylothorax may exist alone or be part of a generalized lymphangiectasia. The fluid fills the hemithorax and displaces the mediastinum.

Clinically the infant is in severe respiratory distress within a few hours after birth. The distress is progressive unless relieved urgently through a thoracentesis. Large fluid, protein, and fat loss occurs through this effusion. The fluid aspirated is straw-colored before feedings are started, after which the fluid becomes milky in color. There is also a high concentration of lymphocytes in the fluid. Prolonged loss of fluid may lead to hypoproteinemia and fluid imbalance. Metabolic acidosis from loss of lymph has been described.[38]

In later childhood chylothorax occurs from trauma or following surgical procedures, especially repair of patent ductus arteriosus, coarctation of the aorta, or the Blalock-Taussig shunt.[39] Chylothorax may be seen secondary to superior vena caval obstruction.[40] Occasionally the chylous fluid enters the pericardial sac and causes chylopericardial tamponade, in which case it is important to assess the respiratory difficulty in terms of a cardiac versus a pulmonary basis.[39, 41]

Clinical Presentation

Chylothorax is a rare cause of neonatal respiratory distress. The infant is tachypneic with chest retractions and is cyanotic. On examination of the chest there is dullness to percussion and diminished breath sounds on the affected side.

Chest roentgenogram shows opacification on the affected side, usually the right, with mediastinal shift and compression of the underlying lung.

Treatment

Thoracentesis or chest tube drainage will relieve the problem of respiratory distress.[42, 43] Drainage usually ceases in 1 to 2 weeks. In the meantime the infant should receive nutrition in the form of medium-chain triglycerides. With appropriate diet and if necessary total parenteral nutrition, operation is rarely necessary. Should operation be required, thoracotomy is performed and ligation of the thoracic duct is carried out.[44, 45] In some cases identification of the thoracic duct is helped by feeding neutral fats stained with dyes to outline lymphatic channels. The overall prognosis is very good. In some cases, however, there may be significant morbidity from infection and malnutrition.

ESOPHAGEAL ATRESIA AND TRACHEOESOPHAGEAL FISTULA

In the first month of the developing human embryo the dorsal foregut (the forerunner of the esophagus) separates from the ventral trachea. This separation starts at the carina and extends in a cephalad direction. By the 26th day of gestation the trachea and esophagus have separated as two parallel tubes up to the level of the larynx. When this separation is interrupted a tracheoesophageal fistula (TEF) arises. Esophageal atresia results when the lateral esophageal grooves continue distally in the process of separating the dorsal esophagus from the ventral trachea.

Tracheoesophageal fistula is one of the lesions found in the "VATER syndrome" where a disturbance in embryogenesis produces a well recognized association of anomalies, namely, *v*ertebral anomalies, *a*nal malformations, *t*racheoesophageal fistula, *r*adial limb dysplasia, and *r*enal deformities.

The esophageal atresia and TEF malformations can be classified into five categories with their respective incidence.

1. Esophageal atresia (7 percent). In this condition the upper esophageal pouch ends blindly. The distal esophageal segment may be widely separated from the upper pouch, but there is no fistula.

2. Esophageal atresia with proximal TEF (2 percent).

3. Esophageal atresia with proximal and distal TEFs (1 percent).

4. Esophageal atresia with distal TEF (86 percent). This is the most common form. The distal esophageal segment is usually separated from the upper pouch by a distance of 1 to 2 cm and communicates with the airway just above the carina and posteriorly.

5. Tracheoesophageal fistula without atresia (4 percent). The fistula is most often located at the thoracic inlet.

Clinical Presentation

There is an incidence of 1 in 3000 live births. Polyhydramnios is frequently present in the mother. Prematurity occurs in about one third of cases of esophageal atresia and TEF. Associated anomalies occurring in 50 percent of cases are presently the most significant cause of morbidity and mortality; particu-

larly important are cardiac anomalies, which occur in 14 percent of cases.[46] Combined esophageal and duodenal atresia has been described.[47]

Pulmonary complications are a potentially serious consequence of esophageal atresia. The infants appear to salivate excessively because of their inability to swallow. Choking, coughing, and regurgitation classically occur with the first feeding. Cyanosis and apnea may occur.

In esophageal atresia the distended upper pouch compresses the cartilage of the tracheal wall, weakening its structure and causing tracheomalacia.[48, 49] The degree of tracheomalacia usually results in airway obstruction associated with a characteristic "barking" cough. The degree of obstruction may be severe enough to compromise the airway such that a tracheostomy is required. Aspiration into the tracheobronchial tree occurs from the fluid in the pharynx which cannot be swallowed because of the esophageal atresia. The distal TEF allows air to distend the stomach, especially with the infant crying. With gastric distention the diaphragm is markedly elevated and ventilatory effort may be severely impeded. Reflux occurs readily and gastric juice is aspirated into the lungs, producing pneumonitis.

The diagnosis is made by passing a large rigid tube through the mouth or nose to the stomach. Obstruction is met at approximately 11 cm from the infant's nares. A roentgenogram will confirm the diagnosis with the tube held up in the upper pouch. The presence of air in the stomach and intestines is indicative of a distal TEF. Isolated TEF without atresia is more difficult to diagnose. Choking, coughing with feeding, and pneumonitis should suggest the diagnosis. Symptoms may be subtle, however. A contrast esophageal study usually shows the communication. If the study is negative, however, bronchoscopy is necessary to identify the fistula in the posterior tracheal wall. A significant number of cases have associated anomalies. They vary from minor to life-threatening. Cardiac and gastrointestinal anomalies occur most commonly. Cardiac anomalies are particularly significant in determining the outcome.

Treatment

Preoperative. Pulmonary complications preoperatively contribute to morbidity and mortality. These should be prevented until surgery can be performed. The infant is kept NPO and positioned semi-upright to minimize regurgitation of gastric juice through the fistula. The proximal segment is suctioned continually through a Replogle tube to prevent aspiration of nasopharyngeal secretions. Atelectasis and pneumonitis occur, particularly in the right upper lobe.

With severe hypoxemia and respiratory failure, endotracheal intubation and ventilation is required. Other aspects of newborn care must be optimized, namely, maintaining body temperature and treatment of hypoglycemia and other problems such as respiratory distress syndrome and hyperbilirubinemia. If the infant is critically ill a gastrostomy is performed (sometimes using local anesthesia) and thoracotomy is postponed until respiratory function has improved. Usually the respiratory status will not improve until the fistula is ligated, however. A careful search is made for associated anomalies, such as cardiac anomalies, anal atresia, and renal anomalies—that is, those anomalies associated with the Vater syndrome. The electrolyte status is assessed and corrected as necessary. A type and cross match is performed for packed red blood cells. Broad-spectrum antibiotics are administered if pneumonitis is suspected.

Operative. Primary definitive repair is performed when the infant is more than 1800 grams in weight without pneumonitis and other serious congenital anomalies. With very low birth weight or critically ill infants the operative procedure is staged.[50] Gastrostomy for feeding and division of the distal tracheo-esophageal fistula is performed. The proximal pouch is suctioned continuously to prevent pneumonitis. When the infant has gained weight and is physically stable, definitive repair—anastomosis of the upper and lower portions of the esophagus—is carried out. Parenteral nutrition has contributed significantly to improving the outcome by optimizing the caloric intake and thus having the infant in the best possible condition both pre- and postoperatively. With esophageal atresia without a fistula, bougienage stretching of the upper pouch is carried out over several weeks to prepare for a primary anastomosis.

Anesthetic Implications

A precordial stethoscope is placed in the left axilla to help detect intraoperative airway obstruction and to monitor the heart sounds. An arterial catheter to monitor pressure and blood gases is set up. The infant is premedicated with atropine 0.02 mg/kg intravenously at the time of induction.

Tracheal intubation is carried out with the patient awake after the esophageal pouch has been suctioned. The endotracheal tube is positioned to avoid gaseous distention of the stomach, that is, just distal to the fistula. Gastric distention will impede ventilatory efforts and venous return and if severe may lead to cardiopulmonary arrest or gastric rupture.[51-53] The fistula is usually located just proximal to the carina on the posterior aspect of the trachea. Thus the endotracheal tube is advanced into the right mainstem bronchus and withdrawn to a position just above the carina when breath sounds are heard on both sides.

Anesthesia is carried out with nitrous oxide, oxygen, and low concentrations of halothane or isoflurane, to avoid cardiovascular depression. Positive pressure should be avoided if possible. It may, however, be necessary to employ positive pressure in order to prevent hypoxemia and hypercarbia, in which case it must be performed in a very gentle manner so as to avoid the danger of gastric distention. In performing a gastrostomy the addition of local anesthesia is helpful because it eliminates the need to use high concentrations of volatile anesthetic agents. A nondepolarizing muscle relaxant is added for optimal operating conditions.

Hyperoxia in premature infants should be avoided because of the potential for retinopathy of prematurity and its possible sequela, retrolental fibroplasia. Serial blood gas analysis for PaO_2 and $PaCO_2$ is carried out. The recent addition of pulse oximetry to monitor oxygen saturation provides a continuous assessment of safe levels of oxygen. Suctioning of the endotracheal tube and airways is critical because of the likelihood of secretions and blood obstructing the airway. Airway obstruction may occur at any time from surgical manipulation of the trachea.

Maintaining the infant's body temperature at normal levels is critical and a number of factors that help to do so are implemented, namely, the use of a warming blanket, delivery of warmed humidified gases, and keeping the operating room environment appropriately warmed. Warm intravenous fluids with dextrose are given at 4 ml/kg/hr, and an additional 6 to 8 ml/kg/hr is given for intraoperative evaporative and "third space" losses. Blood loss is measured in the suction bottle and by weighing sponges, and replacement is provided if necessary with warmed blood.

Postoperative Care and Complications

Postoperative care is carried out in the intensive care unit with special attention to the possible development of atelectasis and pneumonitis from retained secretions in the tracheobronchial tree. Careful suctioning should avoid introducing the catheter too far into the esophagus so as not to disturb the anastomosis. The infant may require tracheal intubation to help reexpand the lung and may need to remain intubated and ventilated.

The most important complications relevant to the surgery include anastomotic leaks and strictures. The latter require repeated dilatation procedures.[54] Recurrent TEF after division and suture occurs in approximately 12 percent of children.[55] Total parenteral hyperalimentation is carried out while the anastomotic leak is allowed to heal. The anastomotic stricture problem may be compounded and aggravated by the presence of gastroesophageal reflux, in which case a fundoplication procedure may be necessary.[56] This results in marked decreases in symptoms and frequency of dilatation procedures.

Tracheomalacia occurs postoperatively in about 25 percent of cases. Symptoms vary from mild to severe. Characteristically in the mild forms, there is a "barking" cough for months to years. Some infants with severe airway obstruction may require a tracheostomy. The airway obstruction due to tracheomalacia may in some cases be resolved by fixing the aortic arch to the sternum and in this way preventing continued tracheal pressure.[57] All infants following repair of the esophageal atresia have some degree of dysphagia due to disordered peristalsis.[58]

Overall survival rate is 82 percent including all categories, with excellent results in those infants who have no associated life-threatening congenital anomalies. Supportive measures in addition to skilled anesthesia in surgery are crucial in affecting survival.[59] Follow-up lung function studies have shown a high incidence of lung damage and hypersensitive airways, which probably results from continuing subclinical aspiration of esophageal contents.[60]

CONGENITAL LARYNGOTRACHEOESOPHAGEAL CLEFT

This is a rare anomaly with a high mortality rate. It has been classified according to extent. Type I cleft is limited to the larynx; type II is a partial cleft and type III is a complete cleft from the larynx to the carina. Donahoe recently reported the first successful management and repair of an infant with complete laryngoesophageal cleft.[61]

Embryologically at 28 days of gestation, bilateral indentations of the mesoderm begin to separate the foregut tube into anterior trachea and posterior esophagus. The separation begins caudally and proceeds in a cephalad direction, reaching the larynx by 33 days. Interference with this advance will determine the extent of the defect.[62]

Clinical Presentation

Clinical presentation will depend on severity of the lesion and the presence of associated anomalies. Mild forms of cleft often escape detection in the first few weeks of life. The physician should suspect the diagnosis when presented with a history of a hoarse or muffled cry, excess mucus production, and cyanotic spells with exacerbation of these symptoms during feeding. Episodes of coughing and apnea and atelectasis or pneumonitis may occur from recurrent aspiration of feedings. Severe defects are usually discovered soon after birth because of the severe respiratory distress in the infant.[63]

The clinical picture should make one suspect the diagnosis, and further studies must be carried out to confirm it, namely, radiological studies, laryngoscopy, and bronchoscopy.[64] A definitive diagnosis is made at the time of bronchoscopy. Note that smaller clefts that involve the larynx and cricoid only are easily missed on laryngoscopy and bronchoscopy because the edges of the cleft are approximated. Chest roentgenogram may show areas of infiltrate, atelectasis, and overaeration. Contrast studies with barium will demonstrate overflow of contrast into the distal tracheobronchial tree.

Anesthetic Implications

Preoperative preparation includes antibiotics for probable aspiration pneumonia. Prior to definitive repair gastrostomy is performed and tracheostomy may be necessary. Parenteral hyperalimentation is given via a central vein. A specially modified endotracheal tube is used. This tube has endobronchial bifurcations, which are placed in each mainstem bronchus to ensure ventilation of both lungs and thus avoid the danger of gastric inflation.[61]

From the anesthetic point of view stabilization of the airway is the most crucial.[65] Surgical technique is crucial in preventing recurrences following repair.[66] The surgical procedure in the type III cleft involves both cervical and thoracic approaches and requires close teamwork between anesthesiologists and surgeons. Postoperatively the anesthesiologist should be involved in caring for the infant's airway, which will involve keeping the infant paralyzed and ventilated to eliminate motion and high swings in intraluminal pressure. The postoperative care requires the highest standards in integrated teamwork involving intensive care specialists, surgeons, anesthesiologists, and nursing staff.

TRACHEAL STENOSIS

Tracheal stenosis in infants and children may be congenital or acquired.

Congenital Tracheal Stenosis

This is a rare life-threatening condition.[67] Pathologically the luminal narrowing is due to the presence of complete tracheal rings. This lesion may occur alone or exist with other anomalies. This is seen in the condition of an aberrant left pulmonary artery or pulmonary artery sling in which compression and narrowing of the posterior tracheal wall is due to an anomalous origin of the left pulmonary artery from the right pulmonary artery near its origin. The anomalous left pulmonary artery passes behind the trachea to supply the left lung.[68] Surgical correction of this defect still leaves the child with tracheal stenosis because of the underlying tracheal defect. With other vascular anomalies—for example, double aortic arch—compression of the trachea may also occur. Here correction of the vascular anomaly will largely improve the airway problem. Innominate artery compression of the trachea is a much disputed pathological entity.

Acquired Tracheal Stenosis

Tracheal stenosis may be acquired in a number of different circumstances, for example: (1) postintubation (endotracheal tube or tracheostomy), (2) posttraumatic, (3) thermal and chemical burns, or (4) primary tumors.[70, 71] Of special concern to the anesthesiologist is the iatrogenic complication of tracheal stenosis following prolonged endotracheal intubation or tracheostomy.

In neonates stenosis is uncommon. However, in older children the problem is more frequently encountered. Pressure necrosis from the tube leads to the formation of granulation tissue, perichondritis, and finally scar formation with stricture. Symptoms of obstruction are delayed following the removal of the tube. Increasing respiratory distress from further stricture becomes life-threatening.

Clinical Presentation

Mucus plugs and inflammatory reaction following upper respiratory infection may acutely precipitate respiratory failure. Respiratory distress, stridor, and chest retractions increase with agitation and crying in the child as a result of dynamic collapse of the airway associated with increased respiratory efforts. Airway obstruction is aggravated from inability to clear mucus. Depending on the site of the tracheal obstruction, wheezing may be heard and may be misdiagnosed as "allergic asthma." Thus, a thorough history is necessary and a suspicion of this complication should exist if a history of recent intubation or tracheostomy is given, particularly if the patient's condition has been diagnosed as asthma and has not responded well to standard therapeutic maneuvers. Physical examination will reveal diffuse inspiratory and expiratory wheezing that may resemble asthma. Otherwise, the physical examination is not very revealing.

Roentgenograms of the posteroanterior, lateral cervical, and chest views with the aid of a copper filter will provide excellent visualization of the location and extent of the tracheal pathology. Airway fluoroscopy will show the dynamic movements of the airway with respirations and the degree of tracheomalacia associated. These studies are followed by laminogram views to obtain a clear definition of the lesion. Bronchograms and tracheograms are potentially dangerous because of possible reaction to the contrast material causing further obstruction of the airway. Computed tomography (CT) is a useful technique to demonstrate the extent and severity of the lesion. Patients who require these studies and have an endotracheal tube in place for a safe airway are at potentially grave risk when extubated for the radiological study. If this procedure is to be carried out in the x-ray facility, an anesthesiologist should be in attendance to replace the endotracheal tube if necessary.

Bronchoscopy is performed to provide the definitive diagnosis. The bronchoscopy may be attended by some bleeding and edema and provoke increasing airway difficulty. This should be anticipated and the child carefully observed in the intensive care unit following the procedure. Inhalation of racemic epinephrine may alleviate some obstruction due to edema. In an emergency prior to intubation if this is required, positive pressure with a face mask, 100 percent oxygen, and an adjustable "pop-off" valve can force oxygen into the lungs by counteracting the dynamic airway collapse that occurs with increasing respiratory efforts.

Anesthetic Implications

The anesthesiologist must have a clear understanding of (1) the nature of the airway obstruction and its effect on the patient and (2) the general medical condition, especially the cardiopulmonary status, because of the possibility of associated anomalies.[72–76]

Preoperatively the child should be in an intensive care unit, where airway compromise may be carefully monitored and treated should deterioration occur. The use of premedication will be dictated by the underlying condition of the patient. If significant airway obstruction is present, narcotics and sedatives should not be given, as they may cause central respiratory depression and respiratory failure.

Atropine may produce drying of secretions, which can lead to further airway obstruction. Atropine should be used only at the time of induction, and then its primary purpose would be to prevent bradycardia from vagal stimuli. Blood gas analysis is not particularly helpful, as values may be normal despite significant airway obstruction.

Standard monitoring for a thoracotomy is employed, including esophageal stethoscope, ECG, blood pressure monitoring, and arterial cannulation. The right radial artery should not be used. During surgery the innominate artery, which is in close proximity to the trachea, is compressed and thus the radial artery pulse is lost. Oxygenation can be measured with pulse oximetry, and carbon dioxide elimination with analysis of end-tidal gases. An assortment of airway equipment, including different sizes of endotracheal tubes, is essential to deal with unanticipated degrees of airway obstruction.

Induction of anesthesia is best carried out with spontaneous ventilation and assisted breaths with nitrous oxide, oxygen, and increasing concentrations of halothane. Relaxants should be avoided, as it may be impossible to ventilate the patient with a face mask and positive pressure under these conditions. At an adequate depth of inhaled anesthesia, topical anesthesia with lidocaine (2 percent) provides optimal conditions for the bronchoscopy that usually precedes the surgical resection.

An appropriate size endotracheal tube is passed to a point either above the obstruction or through and beyond it. Tube position and patency are critical at all times. Anesthesia is maintained with nitrous oxide, oxygen, and halothane, and ventilation is controlled by hand. When the trachea is exposed and the resection procedure commences, a close understanding between the anesthesiologist and the surgeon is essential. Once the trachea is transected below the lesion, the lower trachea is intubated by the surgeon and sterile connecting equipment is passed to the anesthesiologist for continuation of the anesthesia. This procedure must be well orchestrated to avoid the potential for hypoxemia.

The lesion is resected and the upper and lower ends are brought together with removal of the distal armored tube.[70] The original endotracheal tube is then passed beyond the anastomosis into the distal trachea under direct vision. Position of the distal end of the tube is critical, as flexion of the neck to bring the ends of the anastomosis together may lead to accidental mainstem bronchial intubation. A technique using high-frequency jet ventilation for tracheal resection in a child has been described.[77]

At the conclusion of the procedure the child is allowed to breathe spontaneously. Extubation at the conclusion is preferred, as the presence of a foreign body in the trachea may predispose to breakdown of the anastomosis. Extubation is attempted in the operating room with the patient under moderate to deep anesthesia to avoid marked increase in intraluminal pressures and tension on the sutures. Reintubation, however, may be necessary. If it is anticipated that reintubation would be a very potentially hazardous procedure, the infant is allowed to awake from anesthesia before extubation, with every effort made to restrain the child and avoid excessive movement. The child is then transferred to the intensive care unit for postoperative care. Should the child have to remain intubated, endotracheal tube positioning is critical because the infant's shortened trachea and flexed head may predispose to accidental mainstem intubation or extubation with minimal movement.

A variety of techniques have been utilized before undertaking resection in selected cases. These include dilatations, diathermic resection, cryosurgery, laser therapy, and steroid injections. These techniques may be helpful while granulation tissue is present or while the scar is still in the early stages. Once the scar tissue becomes hard and fibrous, resection would appear to offer the best chance for success. Resection of tracheal stenosis is possible even in small infants.[78] Conservative treatment is favored if it will tide the child over the difficulty to an age at which resection would be considered to be a safer undertaking. Where possible, primary anastomosis is carried out. However, with extensive tracheal stenosis newer techniques, such as the use of cartilage grafts or pericardial patch, are being explored.[79–81]

LARYNGOMALACIA

This congenital abnormality is best referred to as a "flabby larynx."[82] The fibrous and cartilaginous support of the supraglottic larynx is flaccid as a result of immaturity in development.[83] Laryngomalacia is the most common cause of stridor in the newborn and infant.

Clinical Presentation

The stridor commences at birth or in the first few days or weeks following birth. It is an inspiratory stridor caused by an infolding of the supraglottic structures (epiglottic and aryepiglottic folds) leading to obstruction of the glottic opening. The inspiratory stridor may be intense, yet the child is not clinically ill. The infant's cry is normal. The stridor is markedly improved during sleep and with the infant in the prone position. The condition resolves spontaneously within 12 to 24 months.

The history and clinical picture are often diagnostic. Fluoroscopy of the upper airway will demonstrate the supraglottic structures drawing in with inspiration. Laryngoscopy will confirm the diagnosis. Fiberoptic visualization at the bedside is less traumatic and provides a dynamic visualization free of the stress of direct laryngoscopy.

Anesthetic Implications

These infants are usually clinically well. The inspiratory stridor and airway obstruction clear as anesthesia is induced. Hence, diagnostic laryngoscopy should be performed when the infant is awake or recovering from anesthesia. The use of continuous positive airway pressure (CPAP) may help in stabilizing a clear airway. Very rarely, intubation or tracheostomy is required.

TRACHEOMALACIA

Tracheomalacia is a condition of abnormal flaccidity of the tracheal wall leading to tracheal collapse during respiration.[82] Congenital tracheomalacia as a primary defect is very rare. The condition is found associated with tracheoesophageal fistula when there is deficiency of tracheal cartilage or when extrinsic compression occurs with vascular anomalies and mediastinal masses.[84] It may occur with systemic disease that affects cartilage and connective tissue, namely, Ehlers-Danlos syndrome. Acquired tracheomalacia follows tracheostomy and prolonged tracheal intubation, especially with cuffed endotracheal tubes.

Clinical Presentation

The clinical history of previous intubation or tracheostomy may suggest the diagnosis in a child who has symptoms of airway obstruction that are particularly aggravated by stress, crying, and agitation.

Airway fluoroscopy defines the dynamic aspects of tracheomalacia, with constriction and dilatation of the tracheal wall related to phases of respirations. Bronchoscopy at light levels of anesthesia with spontaneous ventilation confirms the radiological findings.

Treatment

The natural tendency for the trachea is to stiffen with age, and thus surgery is rarely indicated. However, underlying causes for the secondary tracheomalacia should be identified and treated. Occasionally tracheostomy may be required until the trachea has firmed up and stabilized. In some cases vascular suspension of the aorta or innominate artery relieves the problem. Surgical treatment using an implanted splint has been successfully carried out.[85]

CONGENITAL DIAPHRAGMATIC HERNIA

Congenital diaphragmatic hernia (CDH) has an incidence of 1 per 2500 live births. The condition is the result of the premature return of the midgut to the abdominal cavity during its embryonic development before the diaphragm has completely formed. As a result the abdominal viscera appear in the chest. This usually includes the stomach, the small or large intestine, and occasionally the liver and spleen.[86] There may be an associated malrotation of the gut.

The herniation occurs most often through the pleuroperitoneal sinus (foramen of Bochdalek) on the left; much less commonly the herniation occurs through the substernal sinus (foramen of Morgagni). Pulmonary hypoplasia occurs on the affected side and in many cases in the opposite lung as well. Severe pulmonary hypoplasia is usually the cause of death in these infants.[87] However, if the herniation occurs later in the development of the lungs, there is more functional lung tissue and the outcome is more favorable. Approximately one in four newborns with CDH has associated congenital anomalies.

Clinical Presentation

Immediately after birth the infant is cyanotic and is tachypneic with marked chest retractions. There is decreased chest movement on the affected side, with a shift of the cardiac impulse to the opposite side. The abdomen is scaphoid as a result of the bowel being displaced into the chest. Breath sounds are absent on the affected side, while bowel sounds may be heard in the chest.

Roentgenographic studies are diagnostic, showing gas-filled loops of bowel in the chest with marked shift of the mediastinum to the opposite side and compression of the contralateral lung. This may be confused with congenital cystic lung disease (Fig. 5–3).

The infant is severely hypoxemic as reflected in the blood gases. Hypercarbia and acidemia may also be prominent. Hypercarbia occurring within 2 hours of surgery that is unresponsive to vigorous hyperventilation is associated with a mortality rate of 90 percent. Pathologically these infants have bilateral pulmonary hypoplasia and severe preductal shunting. Those who respond well to hyperventilation with a reduction in $PaCO_2$ have a more favorable outcome.[88] Further respiratory compromise may be the result of a pneumo-

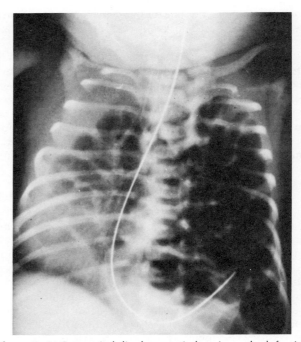

Figure 5–3. Congenital diaphragmatic hernia on the left with shift of the mediastinum to the right and atelectasis of the contralateral lung. Note presence of nasogastric tube in the chest.

thorax from the contralateral lung which may occur pre-, intra-, or postoperatively and is frequently unsuspected. This possibility should always be uppermost in the mind of the anesthesiologist. A decreasing incidence of pneumothorax has been correlated with improving survival with CDH.[89]

Treatment and Anesthetic Implications

Congenital diaphragmatic hernia remains one of the most challenging problems for the surgeon and the anesthesiologist. The urgency of operation is related to the degree of cardiorespiratory distress. In the severely distressed infant the first priority in management consists of decompression of the stomach through insertion of a nasogastric tube. Establishing an airway through awake oral intubation and instituting rapid, low-volume, controlled respirations to avoid high peak inflation pressures are essential. A reliable intravenous line is secured, and sodium bicarbonate (2 mEq/kg) is administered to buffer existing metabolic acidosis. Monitoring includes electrocardiography, use of an esophageal stethoscope, and blood pressure monitoring with a Doppler flow probe. Monitoring blood oxygen tension using pulse oximetry or a transcutaneous electrode, and end-tidal carbon dioxide measurements are recent helpful additions.

The surgical procedure should not be delayed to place an arterial line, but after decompression is accomplished, a right radial arterial line will aid in postoperative management. Anesthetic agents should include a narcotic, such as fentanyl, to provide adequate analgesia and suppress autonomic responses, which may increase pulmonary vascular resistance. Nondepolarizing muscle relaxants are administered. Nitrous oxide is avoided because of its potential for increasing bowel distention. Initially, potent inhalational agents should be avoided because myocardial depression may occur and further potentiate any existing cardiovascular compromise. Once the chest is decompressed, inhalational agents may be used to supplement the anesthesia.

Postoperative Care

Pulmonary artery hypertension is a major factor in the postoperative period. Relentless and progressive pulmonary hypertension with periods of improvement ("flip-flop") is frequently seen. Thus, efforts to reduce pulmonary artery hypertension caused by a hyperactive pulmonary vasculature are the keystones of postoperative care. During the period of increased pulmonary artery pressure, blood flow is rerouted away from the lungs through the ductus arteriosus and foramen ovale. This leads to progressive hypoxemia and acidemia. Unless this deterioration is rapidly checked, death ensues.

Factors that provoke pulmonary artery vasoconstriction, namely, hypoxemia, hypercarbia, acidemia, and hypopthermia, must therefore be avoided.[90] Changes in plasma concentrations of thromboxane have been associated with changes in pulmonary vascular resistance.[91] Noxious stimuli such as pain and endotracheal tube suctioning may contribute to the development of pulmonary artery hypertension. Therefore, to minimize these effects, a prolonged "anesthetic state" is maintained with the use of infusions of narcotics, such as fentanyl, and muscle relaxants.[92] Hyperventilation to a pH of 7.5 to 7.6 is used to augment pulmonary vasodilation.[93]

Pharmacological vasodilator therapy remains controversial. Reports of early successes with vasodilators such as tolazoline, isoproterenol, PGE_1, and nitroglycerin have not always been followed with consistently good results. In addition to its alpha-adrenergic blocking effect, tolazoline inhibits platelet thromboxane synthesis. Dopamine is frequently used for its inotropic effects and maintenance of systemic vascular resistance. Recently, extracorporeal membrane oxygenation (ECMO) has been used with some success in selected infants with severe ductal and foramen ovale shunting following repair of the diaphragmatic hernia and in other conditions with underlying persistent pulmonary hypertension.[94] This technique requires further evaluation, but early results are encouraging for treatment of a condition that, despite advances in medical therapy, still has an unacceptably high mortality. A recent follow-up of 20 patients with CDH showed that functional impairment from pulmonary hypoplasia was insignificant as evidenced by the existence of a normal working capacity and maintenance of a normal alveolar gas exchange during exercise on a high work load.[95]

EVENTRATION OF THE DIAPHRAGM

This is a condition in which an entire hemidiaphragm bulges into the chest. It may resemble a diaphragmatic hernia with a sac. In some cases the eventration may be bilateral.[96, 97]

Clinical Presentation

The condition may be asymptomatic or associated with a history of respiratory infections and effort intolerance due to a reduced pulmonary functional reserve. Roentgenographic studies will show the elevated hemidiaphragm. It may resemble diaphragmatic paralysis. However, with paralysis there is paradoxical motion that is not seen with eventration. Special studies such as a diagnostic pneumoperitoneum or radionucleotide scans of the liver and spleen may be necessary to establish the diagnosis.

Treatment

Operative repair consists of plication of the diaphragm through either a thoracic or an abdominal approach. There are no specific or unusual problems related to anesthesia for this condition.

TRAUMATIC DIAPHRAGMATIC HERNIA

This condition is seen in children associated with severe trauma to the abdomen. Usually there are other associated injuries. The diaphragmatic hernia may be evident at the time of the injury or may be detected months later. A major concern with traumatic rupture of the diaphragm is the danger of bowel strangulation.[98, 99]

A chest roentgenogram will be abnormal and may show bowel in the chest. In selected cases diagnostic studies include pneumoperitoneum, gastrointestinal barium study, and liver and spleen scans.

Treatment

Treatment usually will involve operative repair of the ruptured diaphragm as well as associated injuries.

Anesthetic Implications

The anesthetic technique used will depend, to a large extent, upon the associated injuries of other organ systems.

PNEUMONIA

Pneumonia in infancy and childhood is an important cause of morbidity. The emphasis in this outline is on the clinical, diagnostic, and therapeutic approach to

Figure 5–4. Infant with staphylococcal pneumonia showing presence of pneumatoceles (*arrows*).

the problem. For a more detailed account of individual types of pneumonia, the reader is referred to standard texts in pediatrics.

Pneumonia in children may be caused by a wide variety of microorganisms and also by noninfectious processes.[100] The effect of the pneumonia on the physiology of the respiratory system of the child is important in applying a rational approach to therapy. Antibiotic therapy is essential in some situations to bring about resolution of the pneumonia.[101] It should be appreciated, however, that the majority of cases of pneumonia beyond the neonatal period are viral in origin, making antibiotic therapy unnecessary and potentially harmful. Staphylococcal pneumonia, although relatively uncommon, has reappeared and should be considered in the differential diagnosis.[102] A pneumatocele on the roentgenogram is characteristic (Fig. 5–4).

Pneumonia in the neonate can be a rapid and devastating disease. For example, group B streptococcal infection may mimic hyaline membrane disease both clinically and radiologically. Viral causes such as cytomegalovirus (CMV) and herpes are also significant in the neonate.[103]

Pneumonia may at times be part of a larger systemic illness involving other organ systems, for example, Goodpasture disease or Wegener granulomatosis. Goodpasture disease is an autoimmune disease that affects adolescents and presents with pulmonary hemorrhages followed by renal failure due to glomerulonephritis. Wegener granulomatosis presents with upper and lower airway disease due to necrotizing granulomas. Pulmonary destruction leads to respiratory failure. The kidneys are also involved and renal failure develops.

Classic symptoms of pneumonia seen in adults are often absent in children. The chest roentgenogram, however, is a vital part of the examination and may be suggestive. Pneumonia should be differentiated from atelectasis.

Lobar or Segmental Consolidation

This type of pneumonia is usually caused by the pneumococcus or Klebsiella organism, with pneumococcus accounting for the majority of cases.

Bronchopneumonia

The term bronchopneumonia is applied when the pneumonia is diffuse and not limited by lobar or segmental distribution. Causative organisms include viruses, bacteria, *Mycoplasma*, and less commonly *Pneumocystis* or *Rickettsia*. Viruses are responsible for the overwhelming majority. *Pneumocystis* is found in premature infants and older children with compromised immunological status.

The majority of children with viral infections have a mild self-limited disease. Adenovirus infection, however, usually causes a more significant respiratory infection and may cause a destructive pneumonia. Bacterial pneumonia, in contrast to viral pneumonia, is usually sudden in onset. In the infant and younger child symptoms may be minimal and physical examination may not show any positive signs. Chest auscultation may be entirely normal. A chest roentgenogram shows early obstructive emphysema with viral infections. Fever and tachypnea may be the only clues. This is not seen in bacterial infection. Bacterial pneumonia will clinically deteriorate rapidly with signs of severe dyspnea and cyanosis. The rapid progression is also evident on serial chest roentgenograms taken a few hours apart. Ordinarily pneumonia has a single cause, and this factor should be taken into account when considering appropriate antibiotic therapy.

A number of investigations apart from traditional sputum cultures may be considered to elucidate the underlying cause if the etiology is unclear or if the child fails to respond to drug therapy. Lung puncture is one such useful procedure. It is contraindicated, however, in a child with a major bleeding tendency or in the presence of emphysema. Note that viral pneumonias and *Mycoplasma* infections may be indistinguishable.

Aspiration Pneumonia

This may result from mechanical (e.g., foreign body), chemical, or bacterial causes. For a foreign body aspiration bronchoscopy provides the diagnosis and is therapeutic. Chemical aspiration into the lung occurs during swallowing or vomiting. Examples of this type are accidental ingestion of gasoline, furniture polish, or charcoal lighter fluid. Aspiration pneumonia in children commonly involves anaerobic bacteria,[104] as is seen when there are central nervous system disorders and tracheoesophageal malformations.

Pneumonia in a Compromised Host

This has recently become a significant problem. It is seen particularly in cystic fibrosis or in children with an immunodeficiency disease, or when immunosuppressive medication is used to treat a malignancy. Unusual organisms are involved and combinations of organisms may occur, for example, *Pseudomonas* with *Aspergillus* or *Pneumocystis*. Diagnosis is made on the basis of the clinical and physical examination together with blood and tracheal cultures and other special investigations, for example, lung biopsy.

Open lung biopsy is commonly performed for the diagnosis of diffuse pulmonary lesions.[105, 106] A recent study showed that clinical diagnosis gave a correct diagnosis in 55 percent of patients, but lung biopsy and histological examination gave the final answer in all patients.[107] *Pneumocystis carinii* was found to be the causative organism in 67 percent of the immunosuppressed patients. Open lung biopsy is recommended as a procedure that should be performed earlier in the clinical course than is often the practice. The benefits of biopsy would appear to outweigh the risks of its complications.[107]

Thoracoscopic evaluation of intrathoracic lesions in children has been advocated as a safe and valuable procedure carried out under local or light general anesthesia.[108]

Anesthetic Implications

General anesthesia is usually well tolerated. For this reason the open lung biopsy is preferred to thoracoscopy. General anesthesia with controlled ventilation will optimize oxygenation and carbon dioxide elimination. Also, it provides direct access for control of any bleeding or pulmonary air leaks. Postoperatively the potential for a tension pneumothorax exists.

Pneumonia Associated with Pleural Effusion and Empyema

The presence of a pleural effusion is generally indicative of a bacterial pneumonia. The organism responsible is most commonly the pneumococcus or a group A streptococcus. Viral infections of the lung usually do not give rise to a pleural effusion. Empyema may be a presenting sign of pneumonia due to *Haemophilus influenzae*. Staphylococcal pneumonia is frequently associated with empyema.

Empyema evolves in three stages: exudative, fibropurulent, and organizing. In the early part of its course that is the exudative phase the empyema may be drained by needle thoracentesis. Later in the course more aggressive therapy to drain the pus is necessary. Drainage of pus is a critical part of the treatment in addition to the administration of the appropriate antibiotics.

A recent study of the clinical course of empyema and long-term follow-up of empyema in 16 children showed the organisms responsible to be predominantly *Haemophilus influenzae*, *Staphylococcus aureus*, and *Streptococcus pneumoniae*. Chest tube drainage and antibiotic therapy was necessary in all patients. Three patients required an open thoracotomy because of an unsatisfactory clinical response. The long-term outcome was excellent.[109]

LUNG ABSCESS

This may be a primary event when it is due to a *Staphylococcus* or *Klebsiella* organism. It is secondary when it follows an event such as a foreign body aspiration. The condition is much less common today because of effective antibiotic therapy. Lung abscesses occur in children at any age but are rare in the neonate. Secondary abscesses occur more often in younger children.

The organisms responsible include bacteria, viruses, fungi, and protozoa. *Staphylococcus aureus* is the most common organism cultured. In the neonatal period, Group B streptococcus, *Klebsiella pneumoniae*, and *Escherichia coli* are implicated.

Pathologically a focus of inflammation is followed by central necrosis, with progressive fibrosis of the enclosing wall. Histologically there is suppurative destruction of the lung parenchyma with central cavitation. Large abscesses may affect ventilation and perfusion, causing hypoxemia.

Clinical Presentation

In older children fever, malaise, and weight loss occur. There may be a history of cough, dyspnea, sputum production, and hemoptysis. Putrid odor of the breath occurs as a result of invasion with anaerobic organisms, namely *Bacteroides* or microaerophilic streptococci. Chest physical signs may be minimal compared with the more overt signs in the adult, particularly following foreign body aspiration. Chest roentgenography may show solitary or multiple abscesses. An air-fluid level is often present. Computed tomography may be helpful in defining a cavity if present and distinguishing the abscess from an empyema.[110] Blood cultures may be positive in secondary lung abscesses. Determination of the organism is difficult because of the lack of sputum production in children.

Treatment

Antibiotics are crucial in the therapy. In children with a primary abscess antibiotic therapy alone causes resolution of the problem.[111] All secondary abscesses must be drained. Clinical resolution usually occurs in 2 weeks, but roentgenographic resolution may take months.

CYSTIC FIBROSIS

This is the most common cause of suppurative lung disease in children. Cystic fibrosis (CF) occurs in 1 in 2000 Caucasian live births. The disease is extremely rare in blacks and Orientals. The disease is inherited as an autosomal recessive. It is the most common lethal genetic disorder. Survival rates are improving with advances in therapy.[112] Up to 75 percent of affected individuals now reach adult life. There are newly recognized instances in which the condition has first been diagnosed in middle and later life.[113] The pathogenesis remains unknown. Multiple organs are involved with obstructive lesions and disordered mucus and electrolyte secretion. The increase in the levels of sodium and chloride in sweat is a feature of the disease and is the basis for the diagnostic test for CF. The pulmonary involvement leads to undue susceptibility to lower respiratory infection. Obstruction of bile canaliculi leads to biliary cirrhosis and portal hypertension.

Of special concern to the anesthesiologist is the involvement of the respiratory system. The basic pathological change in the lungs is suppurative bronchitis and bronchiolitis, which eventually produces permanent damage in the airways. Complete obliteration of some smaller airways is common, and varying degrees of bronchiectasis occur. *Staphylococcus aureus* is the most common organism in younger children. In infants under 24 months of age gram negative organisms, especially *Pseudomonas aeruginosa*, are prevalent. *Pseudomonas cepacia* is an emergent problem in CF.[114] Fibrosis occurs in areas of chronic infection. Localized areas of pneumonia are common and may progress to abscess formation. Lung abscess associated with aspiration may occur.[115] Respiratory viral infections have been associated with pulmonary deterioration in patients with CF.[116]

Increased airway resistance is associated with tra-

cheobronchial collapse, rendering expectoration of purulent sputum ineffective. As a result of airways disease, patchy areas of collapse and hyperinflation occur in the lungs. Partial obstruction of small airways leads to maldistribution of ventilation and perfusion, resulting in hypoxemia.[117] Hypercapnia develops when the airway obstruction becomes widespread.[118] Pulmonary hypertension develops with extensive pulmonary disease, probably as a result of hypoxemia. Right heart failure is a frequent terminal event. Spontaneous pneumothorax, pneumomediastinum, and hemoptysis are complications of pulmonary involvement in adolescents. Hemoptysis most commonly arises from bronchiectatic lesions but also occasionally from dilated bronchial arteries.[119, 120]

Clinical Presentation

Recurrent or persistent chest infection is the most common presentation. Digestive tract manifestations of the disease are the result of exocrine pancreatic insufficiency. Maldigestion of fat and protein are the major manifestations of exocrine pancreatic insufficiency.[121] The clinical manifestations are chronic diarrhea with bulky, foul, greasy, pale stools, abdominal distention, and malnutrition. In a significant number of patients hypoproteinemia leads to edema.

Rectal prolapse occurs in 20 to 30 percent of cases and usually occurs during the second year of life. Meconium ileus may be the presenting symptom as intestinal obstruction in the neonatal period. This occurs in 10 to 15 percent of newborn infants with cystic fibrosis. A significant number of infants with meconium ileus have other anomalies, such as intestinal atresia.

As a result of defective bile salt absorption, cholelithiasis develops in at least 10 percent of patients. This may lead to cholecystitis or biliary colic with obstructive jaundice.

Other aspects of the disease, apart from the pulmonary complications, add to the morbidity.

Hepatic involvement occurs in 20 to 50 percent of patients with CF. As the child grows the liver becomes hard and nodular. However, hepatic failure is rare. Clotting factors are reduced.

Biliary cirrhosis develops in a small number of older children and adolescents and may be complicated by portal hypertension with splenomegaly, hypersplenism, and bleeding esophageal varices. There are many emotional problems for patient and family that require understanding and support.

Anesthetic Implications

Increased airway resistance leads to gas trapping and an increase in FRC. There is an imbalance of ventilation and perfusion (V/Q) leading to significant hypoxemia. The $PaCO_2$ is usually normal. Should the $PaCO_2$ be elevated this would be an indication of advanced lung disease. With pulmonary fibrosis giving rise to low $\dot{V}/\dot{Q}$ areas, induction of anesthesia and emergence are therefore prolonged. It is important to appreciate that the patient may be responsive to a hypoxic respiratory drive, and thus with oxygen administration ventilatory assistance may be necessary.

Cor pulmonale may occur with or without heart failure.[122] The underlying basis for it is hypoxemia especially when the PaO_2 is less than 50 torr. In addition there is evidence of left ventricular enlargement. Cor pulmonale is invariably present in the late stages of CF, and digoxin and diuretic therapy are indicated.

Preoperative. These patients have excessive bronchial secretions and therefore their lung function should be optimized prior to surgery with appropriate chest physiotherapy.[123, 124] In addition, lung function tests are carried out if the child is of appropriate age. Narcotics are avoided because of their respiratory depressant effect. These patients may be on diuretic therapy, and therefore electrolyte imbalance should be checked for. Bronchoscopy and washout for cystic fibrosis to improve ventilation and oxygenation may be necessary. For this procedure transcutaneous oxygen monitoring or pulse oximetry is helpful in detecting dangerous hypoxemia.[125, 126]

Selective bronchial arteriography and bronchial artery embolization has been developed to control massive hemoptysis in children with CF.[127, 128] Thoracotomy and pleural stripping may be necessary to control recurrent pneumothorax.

Operative. Occasionally pulmonary resection, mainly lobectomy, is required for complications of the cystic fibrosis—namely, bronchiectasis, abscess, and hemoptysis—and when there has been an inadequate response to conservative medical therapy.[129]

The anesthetic management for patients with cystic fibrosis has been recently reviewed.[130] Regional anesthesia is preferred whenever this is possible. The most common operation performed is nasal polypectomy. Ketamine should be avoided because of its association with increased bronchial secretions. For pulmonary resection when a lung abscess is present, endobronchial blockers are necessary.[129] Nitrous oxide should be avoided when there is obstruction of bullae, pneumothorax, or intestinal obstruction.[131, 132] Anesthesia is effectively carried out with volatile anesthetic agents such as halothane or isoflurane or with a balanced technique (muscle relaxant and narcotic). The patient should be kept well hydrated, as dehydration leads to further inspissation of secretions.

Postoperative. Chest physiotherapy is vital in this phase of care, as is adequate control of pain. For this purpose intercostal nerve blocks or cryopexy is very suitable. Antibiotic needs must be carefully determined, and it should be appreciated that high doses may be needed because of an increase in renal clearance.[133] Significant deterioration in lung function occurs after general anesthesia in patients with cystic fibrosis.

BRONCHIECTASIS

Bronchiectasis is a permanent dilation of bronchi usually associated with inflammation. The condition is relatively uncommon and is associated with chronic and frequent repeated lung infections. The etiology and pathogenesis are controversial. The two types of bronchiectasis are (1) congenital, due to a malformation of the bronchial wall from absent or deficient cartilage plates, (2) acquired, associated with acute respiratory infections and damage to the lung. Acquired bronchiectasis accounts for a majority of cases. Obstruction of a bronchus may lead to bronchiectasis.

The disease usually follows bronchitis or pneumonia during the first or second year of life. Organisms associated with this development are respiratory syncytial virus (RSV), adenovirus, influenza virus, measles virus, *Bordetella pertussis*, and *Mycoplasma pneumoniae*. Severe adenovirus pneumonia is particularly likely to be followed by this complication. In spite of the prevalence of viral infections in children, only a very small percentage of infants are affected with bronchiectasis. It appears that different host and immunological factors contribute. Bronchiectasis may follow the aspiration of a foreign body if the patient has not been properly managed.

Small airways become obstructed with secretions and inflammation. The ciliated epithelium of the airway is destroyed, making it difficult to clear the airway of secretions. In addition there is an increase in secretions from hypertrophied glands. As a result atelectasis occurs distal to the obstruction. This is followed by abscess formation, which then leads to destruction and weakening of the bronchial wall. The result is dilatation of the airways from negative intrathoracic pressure and traction from surrounding fibrous tissue. Bronchiectasis is a complex disease, however, and simple mechanical forces may not be adequate as an explanation for the pathological picture. The volume of bronchial secretions and the presence of bronchial wall infection appear to be the most important etiological factors.[134] Pathologically, the dilated bronchi are saccular, cylindrical, or both.

The changes may affect one or both lungs. The bronchial arteries undergo hypertrophy of their walls. There is shunting of blood by bronchopulmonary anastomoses with pulmonary hypertension.

Clinical Presentation

The disease is characterized by chronic and frequent recurrent infections of the respiratory tract. Persistent cough and purulent sputum are classic symptoms, but bronchiectasis may still be present in the absence of sputum. Hemoptysis may also occur but is relatively uncommon. Wheezing is also uncommon. As the disease progresses the child becomes progressively more dyspneic on exercise. On physical examination there are bronchovesicular breath sounds over the affected area and inspiratory crackles.

Bronchiectasis occurs most commonly in the left lower lobe, lingula, and right middle lobe. However, most children have the disease more diffusely. There is clubbing of fingers. Failure to thrive occurs in the more chronic case.

A chest roentgenogram may show characteristic findings, especially in advanced cases.[135] However, the diagnosis rests upon the demonstration of bronchiectasis by bronchography. CT scanning has also been used for the diagnosis of bronchiectasis. More recently, ventilation and perfusion lung scanning has been performed in children.

Bronchiectasis has been observed with certain syndromes, especially the unilateral hyperlucent lung (Swyer-James syndrome or MacLeod syndrome)—a syndrome that follows various insults to the lung such as viral infections, tuberculosis, mycoplasmal pneumonia, foreign body aspiration, ingestion of hydrocarbons, and radiotherapy.[136] Bronchiectasis is also an integral part of Kartagener syndrome, a condition that also includes situs inversus and chronic paranasal sinusitis.[137]

Treatment and Anesthetic Implications

Treatment is aimed at the underlying infection by the use of appropriate antibiotics. In addition, mucous plugging of the airways is treated aggressively with chest physiotherapy and if necessary bronchoscopy. Bronchoscopy can be particularly helpful in obtaining appropriate sputum specimens for culture and sensitivity. Bronchography has traditionally been performed with the patient under general anesthesia.[138] A newer technique using the blind passage of an endotracheal catheter in lightly sedated children has been reported.[139] Fiberoptic bronchoscopy combined with selective bronchography appears to be an advance in diagnostic capabilities.[140]

General anesthesia in children requires endotracheal intubation. During anesthesia the child is closely monitored for potential hypoxemia both clinically and with the aid of a pulse oximeter for oxygen saturation. Wheezing following extubation may occur. Also, fever has been noted in one third of the patients.[141]

Pulmonary resection, that is, lobectomy, although relatively uncommon, may be necessary in selected cases. Improvement in symptoms, a decreasing need for medications, and improved social life are offered as advantages for surgery.[142–144] Surgery is usually delayed if possible until the child is 6 to 12 years of age to allow for resolution of the disease.

Anesthetic problems relate to the possible spread of purulent material to the healthy lung. For this reason use of bronchial blockers or one-lung anesthesia (in the adolescent) is necessary. Bronchoscopic aspiration of affected lobes immediately prior to surgical resection may also be useful in decreasing the risk of contamination of the remaining lungs.

TUMORS OF THE LUNG

Primary lung tumors are uncommon in infants and children. Metastatic tumors are more commonly seen.

Benign Tumors

Vascular tumors such as hemangiomas are extremely rare. In such cases, there may be other vascular anomalies in other organs (mucous membranes, skin, brain) as occurs in the syndrome of hereditary telangiectasia. The tumors usually occur in the lower lobes and are single or multiple.[145] On microscopic examination the tumor resembles a capillary or cavernous hemangioma. Sclerosing hemangiomas are usually found in the periphery of the lung in the lower lobes.[146, 147] The child is usually asymptomatic and the lesion is usually discovered on a chest roentgenogram.

Plasma cell granuloma is probably the most common benign tumor of the lung in childhood. It is regarded by some to be a postinflammatory pseudotumor. The tumor is composed primarily of plasma cells. Histiocytes filled with fat are also present and give the lesion a xanthomatous appearance.[148] Females are more often affected. The child is usually asymptomatic. However, the tumor may obstruct a bronchus and produce respiratory distress. Chest roentgenography shows a solitary circumscribed parenchymal lesion or coin lesion. Surgery is the treatment of choice with a good prognosis.

Other tumors are very rare and include multiple congenital leiomyomas, granular cell myoblastoma, fibromas, chondromas, and teratomas.

Malignant Tumors

Primary malignant tumors are rare in childhood. They include fibrosarcoma, leiomyosarcoma, and rhabdomyosarcoma. Bronchial adenomas include bronchial carcinoid, cylindroma, and mucoepidermoid tumors, with bronchial carcinoid being the most common.[149, 150] Primary carcinoma of the lung is very rare in childhood.

Metastatic Tumors

Metastasis to the lung is a significant problem in childhood cancer. The metastases are usually very large. They may be few or large in number. Metastases to the lung are common in Wilms tumor, osteosarcoma, Ewing sarcoma, hepatoblastoma, and neuroblastoma.[151] The lungs may also be involved in leukemia, non-Hodgkin lymphoma, and Hodgkin disease. Usually lung function is not compromised. However, if there are large showers of metastases, pulmonary function may be affected. Bronchial infiltration of the tumor may cause bronchial stenosis.

Treatment

An aggressive approach to resecting the metastatic tumors is favored. This may involve multiple thoracotomies.[152] Results appear best with Wilms tumor metastases.[153] The aggressive surgical approach has led to a reduction in the need for radiotherapy with its potential for long-term sequelae.

Anesthetic Implications

Biopsy of bronchial adenomas may lead to severe bleeding; the lesion should therefore be approached surgically. For tumors of the lung in children the surgical procedure is relatively safe with a standard anesthetic approach to thoracotomy. The potential for postoperative pneumothorax should be monitored.

FOREIGN BODIES

Foreign body aspiration causes airway obstruction that may be acutely life-threatening or if undetected result in severe lung damage. Children in the first 2 to 3 years of age are particularly prone to aspirate any of a wide array of foreign objects. A national study showed that 65 percent of food asphyxial deaths occurred in infants younger than 2 years of age.[154] Foreign body aspiration (of a balloon) has been reported even in a 3-month-old infant.[155] Therefore, foreign body aspiration must be considered in all cases of sudden respiratory distress regardless of age.

Intrabronchial Foreign Bodies

This is a common cause of respiratory illness in young children.[156–159] In two thirds of children the diagnosis is made within the first few days. In a significant number, however, there is a considerable delay. Males are involved more often than females by a ratio of 2 to 1, with 80 percent of cases in children under 4 years of age. Peanuts, hot dogs, candy, and grapes are among the most common offenders. Most lodge in a main or stem bronchus, right more often than the left. Sharp foreign bodies include plastic, egg shells, and pins. They impact in the larynx and produce symptoms of acute laryngeal edema. One should also suspect that a "foreign body aspiration" may be multiple foreign bodies. Foreign bodies may move from their original position.

Clinical Presentation

The clinical picture is modified by the interval that has elapsed from the time of foreign body aspiration.

With cases diagnosed within 24 hours, there is a history of violent coughing, gagging, and severe respiratory distress with cyanosis. Wheezing may be present. However, the diagnostic triad of wheezing, coughing, and decreased breath sounds over the affected side is more common in the case diagnosed later. A recent study showed that this diagnostic triad was incomplete in 61 percent of all patients.[160] After initial dramatic symptoms, an annoying cough and wheezing persist without respiratory distress.

Chest roentgenography and fluoroscopy are useful diagnostic procedures. It should be appreciated that the majority of aspirated foreign bodies are not radiopaque. One may see atelectasis (Fig. 5–5) or obstructive emphysema; an expiratory film is very often diagnostic (Fig. 5–6). In some situations the movement of the foreign body and its breaking up into fragments may produce atelectasis followed by hyperinflation.

If there has been delay in diagnosis, pneumonitis may be detected. Recurrent persistent localized pneumonitis that does not respond to standard medical therapy should make one suspicious that there may be an underlying foreign body. In the study by Wiseman more than half of the patients with aspirated foreign bodies were diagnosed later when there was evidence of significant airway obstruction.[160] Early diagnosis should be made from the history of choking. Also, the anesthesiologist must appreciate that children who wheeze are not necessarily "asthmatic" and a foreign body aspiration may well be the underlying cause.

Foreign bodies impacting on the esophagus, especially at sites of anatomical constriction—the postcricoid region and at the level of the aortic arch—may produce compression of the trachea and serious airway obstruction (Fig. 5–7).

Figure 5–5. Foreign body in right mainstem bronchus leading to right middle lobe collapse and right upper lobe overinflation.

Figure 5—6. Foreign body in right mainstem bronchus causing hyperaeration of the lung and shift of the mediastinum to the opposite side.

Anesthetic Implications

The anesthesiologist should be familiar with emergency room measures to dislodge a foreign body that is producing a life-threatening crisis. Debate continues over the various maneuvers.[161] The Academy of Pediatrics (Section of Accident and Poison Prevention) recommends back blows followed by chest thrusts. Back blows have been blamed by some investigators for causing further distal impaction of the foreign body. Abdominal thrusts (Heimlich maneuver) have been known to be effective. In small children, however, liver trauma is possible with abdominal thrusts and hence chest thrusts are preferred.

Anesthesia and bronchoscopy for removal of the foreign body should be carried out by skilled personnel with appropriate equipment.[162] The Storz pediatric bronchoscope with the Hopkins rod lens telescope

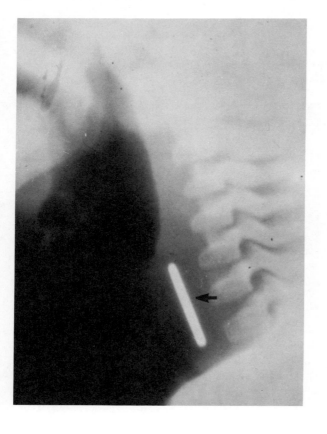

Figure 5—7. Coin in esophagus (*arrow*) impacting on trachea and causing airway obstruction.

provides excellent visualization of the foreign body and allows for the introduction of a forceps to remove the foreign body.[163, 164]

Preoperatively narcotics and sedatives are avoided. The child is calmed to prevent dynamic collapse of the airway from agitation, which can cause further obstruction. Electrocardiographic monitoring and a precordial stethoscope are set up to monitor cardiac activity.

Anesthesia is induced with halothane and oxygen with spontaneous respirations. Induction is slow because of airway obstruction. An intravenous line is placed when an analgesic level of anesthesia is achieved. Atropine is given intravenously to reduce the tendency to bradycardia with laryngeal and tracheobronchial stimulation. During induction of anesthesia, ventilation is spontaneous unless it is apparent that hypoventilation, reflected in decreased movement of the chest or cardiac arrhythmias, is occurring. In this situation ventilation must be assisted despite theoretical risks of forcing the foreign body further down. Once the bronchoscope is inserted, ventilation continues via the bronchoscope connected to the anesthetic circuit; if necessary, ventilation can be controlled. Removal of the foreign body is usually accomplished with a forceps. On occasion a Fogarty embolectomy balloon catheter is used to dislodge an impacted foreign body.[165] The catheter is pulled back together with the bronchoscope to the pharynx, from which the foreign body is removed. Rarely the foreign body, if deeply lodged in the bronchus, may have to be removed via a thoracotomy and bronchotomy.

In some situations following removal of the foreign body the child may still have symptoms because of the presence of residual foreign bodies. Flexible fiberoptic bronchoscopy appears to be a useful technique in this situation to screen for a possible residual foreign body.[166]

Following a difficult removal of a foreign body the child may have residual glottic and airway edema and require steroid therapy and racemic epinephrine inhalations. Early extraction through bronchoscopy will reduce local damage and distal parenchymal complications. Extraction may be difficult with foreign bodies that tend to crumble, such as peanuts.

MEDIASTINUM

Pneumomediastinum

Pneumomediastinum is a collection of air in the mediastinum that results from a pulmonary air leak, most often following trauma or associated with the use of mechanical ventilation, or that occurs in children with severe asthmatic attacks. The air usually tracks to the superior mediastinum. Generally the pneumomediastinum resolves spontaneously and does not produce significant pathophysiological effects. However, on rare occasions large collections of air may produce

circulatory tamponade, in which case urgent decompression is essential.

Pneumomediastinum may also predispose to intracranial hypertension from interference with venous drainage from the cranium. A recent case has been reported in which intracranial hypertension was refractory to therapy until the pneumomediastinum was decompressed by the placement of a mediastinal tube.[167]

Mediastinal Masses

Mediastinal masses occur in the anterior, middle, and posterior mediastinum, and their diagnosis is related to their anatomical position. The anesthesiologist is particularly concerned with the effect of the mediastinal masses on the airways, lungs, and cardiovascular system. Common mediastinal masses according to location are:

1. Anterior mediastinum: lymphoma, teratoma, cystic hygroma, thymoma, and pericardial cysts. A diaphragmatic hernia that has passed through the foramen of Morgagni is situated in the anterior mediastinum.

2. Middle mediastinum: lymphoma, tuberculous glands.

3. Posterior mediastinum: neurogenic tumors, esophageal duplication cysts. A diaphragmatic hernia via the foramen of Bochdalek is situated in the posterior mediastinum.

The details of the various mediastinal masses, with their clinical features, diagnosis, and management, may be found in standard pediatric texts. Of importance to the anesthesiologist is the recognition that anesthesia in these patients is hazardous and that thorough investigation and preparation is therefore mandatory.

Anterior Mediastinum

Anterior mediastinal masses may produce severe respiratory and cardiovascular complications. Obstruction of major airways, cardiac compression producing tamponade, and superior vena caval obstruction may occur.

Keon has described a 9-year-old child undergoing a cervical node biopsy who sustained a cardiopulmonary arrest during induction of anesthesia and in whom efforts at resuscitation were unsuccessful.[168] Autopsy revealed a massive malignant lymphoma in the anterior mediastinum that enveloped the heart with infiltration of the pericardium, producing a pericardial tamponade effect.

Most anterior mediastinal masses are lymphomatous in origin (Hodgkin and non-Hodgkin lymphoma). It is important to appreciate that cervical masses, for example, cystic hygroma, may have a deep extension into the mediastinum. Mediastinal masses may also go unsuspected and be found on a routine chest roentgenogram.

Figure 5–8. Neurogenic cyst exposed at thoracotomy. Airway compression gave rise to symptoms suggestive of "asthma." (Courtesy of Samuel Kim, M.D.)

Posterior Mediastinum

Posterior mediastinal masses, for example, an esophageal duplication cyst, may cause respiratory distress through encroachment on pulmonary reserve. In addition, compression of the esophagus leads to dysphagia and the possibility of reflux and aspiration on induction of anesthesia.

In some situations symptoms are attributed to more benign conditions. An 8-year-old child was referred with severe dyspnea unresponsive to treatment with antispasmodic medications. On further investigation the child was found to have a large mediastinal mass (neurogenic tumor) obstructing the airway (Fig. 5–8).

Anesthetic Implications

Children with mediastinal masses are at significant risk undergoing anesthesia and provide a special challenge.[169–172] Preoperative preparation of the child with a mediastinal mass includes a special focus on (1) evaluation of the degree of airway obstruction and (2) possible cardiovascular compromise. In addition to clinical evaluation of airway patency and hemodynamic stability, other special studies are carried out. Roentgenography of the airway might include tomography and fluoroscopy. CT scans of the airway also provide better definition of any obstruction. Pulmonary flow volume loop studies, in both the upright and supine positions, provide sensitive indicators of obstructive lesions of the major airways. The peak flow rate may show a significant decrease even when the CT scan has revealed no airway obstruction.[173]

In evaluating hemodynamic stability, the possibility of cardiac tamponade must be considered; thus, it is important to examine for pulsus paradoxus. Echocardiography is also performed with the patient in the upright and supine positions. Barium swallow examinations are performed in selected cases.

The position for induction of anesthesia must be one that produces the least cardiopulmonary compromise; this usually means having the child propped up. Drugs for resuscitation should be immediately available because of the high risks associated with induction of anesthesia. A rigid bronchoscope should be at hand. For this reason, too, the surgical team should be present at this time to assist in any crisis that may develop. Induction of anesthesia is best carried out under spontaneous ventilation, and assisted ventilation is performed should this become necessary. Muscle relaxants are best avoided at this time.

In some cases in which compression of the trachea and bronchi by the mediastinal mass is perceived as life-threatening, especially in Hodgkin disease, radiation to the tumor prior to anesthesia may ameliorate the degree of airway obstruction and provide for a safe induction. Local anesthesia in preference to general anesthesia should be used for the biopsy procedure if this is suitable in the particular patient. In rare situations standby cardiopulmonary bypass equipment is necessary. Thoracotomy is usually necessary to make the specific diagnosis. Excision of the entire mediastinal mass is undertaken if this is possible. Note that the extent of the pathology and its location may predispose to significant blood loss with excision.

Mediastinal Infection

Infections are today less of a problem than in the past, because of improved surgical techniques and antibiotic control. Acute suppurative mediastinitis results from postsurgical infections and tracheal or esophageal perforation. Neonatal tracheal perforation may result from nasotracheal intubation.[174]

Suppurative mediastinitis secondary to infected lymph nodes is extremely unusual and occurs with chronic diseases such as tuberculosis and histoplasmosis. Accurate and urgent diagnosis of acute suppurative mediastinitis is essential, and specific antibiotic therapy is instituted. Surgical drainage may be necessary. Caudal extension of cervical infections may lead to serious mediastinitis. Paratracheal lymph nodes compressing the trachea and producing obstruction may be due to atypical mycobacteria. The appearance of a right upper lobe collapse may be due to a paratracheal mass. At operation the etiology may be uncertain with the enlarged nodes resembling malignant nodes. Excision is therefore an important part of the treatment.

REFERENCES

1. Reid L: The lung: its growth and remodeling in health and disease. AJR *129*:777, 1977.
2. Reid L: The pulmonary circulation: remodeling in growth and disease. Am Rev Respir Dis *119*:531, 1979.

3. Reid L: Lung growth in health and disease. Br J Dis Chest 78:113, 1984.

4. Hislop A, Reid L: Growth and development of the respiratory system—anatomical development. *In* Davies J, Dobbin J (Eds.): Scientific Foundations of Paediatrics. London, Heinemann, 1974, pp 214–523.

5. Alcorn D, Adamson TM, Lambert TF, et al.: Effects of chronic tracheal ligation and drainage on the fetal lamb lung. J Anat 123:649, 1977.

6. Brown MJ, Oliver RE, Ramsden CA, et al.: Effects of adrenaline infusion and of spontaneous labor on lung liquid secretion and absorption in the fetal lamb. J Physiol 313:13, 1981.

7. Boddy K, Davies GS: Fetal breathing. Br Med Bull 31:3, 1975.

8. Thurlbeck WM: Postnatal growth of the lung. Am Rev Respir Dis 111:803, 1975.

9. Hislop A, Reid L: Development of the acinus in the human lung. Thorax 29:90, 1974.

10. McBride J, Wohl ME, Strieder DJ, et al.: Lung growth and airway function after lobectomy for congenital lobar emphysema. J Clin Invest 66:962, 1980.

11. Davies P, McBride J, Murray GF, et al.: Structural changes in canine lung and pulmonary arteries after pneumonectomy. J Appl Physiol 53:859, 1982.

12. Thurlbeck WM, Galaugher W, Mathers J: Adaptive response to pneumonectomy in puppies. Thorax 36:424, 1981.

13. Sbokos CG, McMillan IKR: Agenesis of the lung. Br J Dis Chest 71:183, 1977.

14. Borja AR, Ransdell HT, Villa S: Congenital developmental arrest of the lung. Ann Thorac Surg 10:317, 1970.

15. McCormick TL, Kuhns LR: Tracheal compression by a normal aorta associated with right lung agenesis. Radiology 130:659, 1979.

16. Maltz DL, Nadas AS: Agenesis of the lung: presentation of eight new cases and review of the literature. Pediatrics 42:175, 1968.

17. Hislop A, Hey E, Reid L: The lungs in congenital bilateral renal agenesis and dysplasia. Arch Dis Child 54:32, 1979.

18. Jue KL, Amplatz K, Adams P Jr, et al.: Anomalies of great vessels associated with lung hypoplasia. The scimitar syndrome. Am J Dis Child 111:35, 1966.

19. Orzam F, Angelini P, Oglieth J, et al.: Horseshoe lung: report of two cases. Am Heart J 93:501, 1977.

20. Buntain WC, Woolley MD, Mahour GH, et al.: Pulmonary sequestration in children. A twenty-five year experience. Surgery 81:413, 1977.

21. Khalik KG, Kilman JW: Pulmonary sequestration. J Thorac Cardiovasc Surg 70:928, 1975.

22. Savic G, Birtel FJ, Tholen W, et al.: Lung sequestration: report of seven cases and review of 540 published cases. Thorax 34:96, 1979.

23. Heifhoff KG, Sane SM, Williams HJ, et al.: Bronchopulmonary foregut malformations. A unifying etiological concept. Am J Roentgenol 126:46, 1976.

24. Stocker JT, Kagan-Hallet K: Extralobar pulmonary sequestration. Analysis of 15 cases and review of 540 published cases. Am J Clin Pathol 72:917, 1979.

25. Lewis JE, Murray RE: Pulmonary sequestration with bronchoesophageal fistula. J Pediatr Surg 3:575, 1968.

26. Ransom JM, Norton JB, Williams GD: Pulmonary sequestration presenting as congestive failure. J Thorac Surg 7:68, 1969.

27. Bientain WL, Isaacs H, Payne VC, et al.: Lobar emphysema, cystic adenomatoid malformation, pulmonary sequestration, and bronchogenic cysts in infancy and childhood: a clinical group. J Pediatr Surg 9:85, 1974.

28. Demos NJ, Teresi A: Congenital lung malformation, a unified concept and a case report. J Thorac Cardiovasc Surg 70:260, 1975.

29. Crawford TJ, Cahill JJ: The surgical treatment of pulmonary cystic disorders in infancy and childhood. J Pediatr Surg 6:251, 1971.

30. Leape LL, Longine LA: Infantile lobar emphysema. Pediatrics 34:246, 1964.

31. Eigen H, Lemon RJ, Waring WW: Congenital lobar emphysema: long term evaluation of surgically and conservatively treated children. Am Rev Respir Dis 113:823, 1976.

32. Côté CJ: Anesthetic management of congenital lobar emphysema. Anesthesiology 49:296, 1974.

33. Stocker JT, Madewell JE, Drake RM: Congenital cystic adenomatoid malformation of the lung. Classification and morphologic spectrum. Hum Pathol 8:155, 1977.

34. Eraklis AJ, Grisom NT, McGovern JB: Bronchogenic cysts of the mediastinum in infancy. N Engl J Med 281:1150, 1969.

35. Bensoussan AL, Braun P, Guttman FM: Bilateral spontaneous chylothorax of the newborn. Arch Surg 110:1243, 1975.

36. Kumar SP, Belik J: Chylothorax—a complication of chest-tube placement in a neonate. Crit Care Med 12:411, 1984.

37. Van Aerde J, Campbell AN, Smyth JA, et al.: Spontaneous chylothorax in newborns. Am J Dis Child 138:961, 1984.

38. Siegler RL, Pearce MB: Metabolic acidosis from loss of thoracic lymph. J Pediatr 93:465, 1978.

39. Hargus EP, Carson SC, McGrath RL, et al.: Chylothorax and chylopericardial tamponade following Blalock-Taussig anastomosis. J Thorac Cardiovasc Surg 75:642, 1978.

40. Seiber JJ, Golladay ES, Keller C: Chylothorax secondary to superior vena cava obstruction. Pediatr Radiol 12:252, 1982.

41. Ducharme JC, Belanger R, Simard P, et al.: Chylothorax, chylopericardium with multiple lymphangioma of bone. J Pediatr Surg 17:365, 1982.

42. Brodman RF: Congenital chylothorax: recommendations for treatment. NY State J Med 75:553, 1975.

43. Stringel G, Mercer S, Bass J: Surgical management of persistent postoperative chylothorax in children. Can J Surg 27:543, 1984.

44. Johnson DC, Cartmill TB: Low thoracic duct ligation for postoperative chylous effusions in infants and children. Aust NZ J Surg 47:94, 1977.

45. Milson JW, Kron IL, Rheuban KS, et al.: Chylothorax: an assessment of current surgical management. J Thorac Cardiovasc Surg 89:221, 1985.

46. Greenwood RD, Rosenthal A: Cardiovascular malformations associated with tracheoesophageal fistula and esophageal atresia. Pediatrics 57:87, 1976.

47. Spitz, L, Ali N, Brereton RJ: Combined esophageal and duodenal atresia: experience in 18 patients. J Pediatr Surg 16:4, 1981.

48. Benjamin B, Cohen D, Glasson M: Tracheomalacia in association with congenital tracheoesophageal fistula. Surgery 79:504, 1976.

49. Davies MRG, Cywes S: The flaccid trachea and tracheoesophageal congenital anomalies. J Pediatr Surg 13:363, 1978.

50. Iko T, Sugito T, Nagaya M: Delayed primary anastomosis in poor-risk patients with esophageal atresia associated with tracheoesophageal fistula. J Pediatr Surg 19:243, 1984.

51. Calverley RK, Johnston AE: The anesthetic management of tracheoesophageal fistula: a review of 10 years experience. Can Anaesth Soc J 19:270, 1972.

52. Jones TB, Kirchner SG, Lee FA, et al.: Stomach rupture associated with esophageal atresia, tracheoesophageal fistula and ventilatory assistance. Am J Radiol 134:675, 1980.

53. Salem MR, Wong AY, Lin YH, et al.: Prevention of gastric distension during anesthesia for newborns with tracheoesophageal fistulas. Anesthesiology 38:82, 1973.

54. Filler RM, Rossello PJ, Lebowitz RL: Life threatening anoxic spells caused by tracheal compression after repair of esophageal atresia: correction by surgery. J Pediatr Surg 11:739, 1976.

55. Kafrouni G, Baick CH, Woolley MM: Recurrent tracheoesophageal fistula: a diagnostic problem. Surgery 68:889, 1970.

56. Pieretti R, Shandling B, Stephens CA: Resistant esophageal

stenosis associated with reflux after repair of esophageal atresia: a therapeutic approach. J Pediatr Surg 9:355, 1974.

57. Schwartz MZ, Filler RM: Tracheal compression as a cause of apnea following repair of tracheoesophageal fistula: treatment by aortopexy. J Pediatr Surg 15:842, 1980.

58. Duranceau A, Fisher SR, Flye MW, et al.: Motor function of the esophagus after repair of esophageal atresia and tracheoesophageal fistula. Surgery 82:116, 1977.

59. Koop CE, Schnaufer L, Broennle AM: Esophageal atresia and tracheoesophageal fistula. Supportive measures that affect survival. Pediatrics 54:558, 1974.

60. Milligan DWA, Levison H: Lung function in children following repair of tracheoesophageal fistula. J Pediatr 95:24, 1979.

61. Donahoe PK, Gee PE: Complete laryngotracheoesophageal cleft: management and repair. J Pediatr Surg 19:143, 1984.

62. Felman AH, Talbert JL: Laryngotracheoesophageal cleft. Radiology 103:641, 1972.

63. Donahoe PK, Hendren WH: The surgical management of laryngotracheoesophageal cleft with tracheoesophageal fistula and esophageal atresia. Surgery 73:363, 1972.

64. Cotton RT, Schreiber JT: Management of laryngotracheoesophageal cleft. Ann Otol Rhinol Laryngol 90:401, 1981.

65. Ruder CB, Glaser LC: Anesthetic management of laryngotracheoesophageal cleft. Anesthesiology 47:65, 1977.

66. Hendren WH: Repair of laryngotracheoesophageal cleft using interposition of a strap muscle. J Pediatr Surg 11:425, 1976.

67. Cotton RT: Pediatric laryngotracheal stenosis. J Pediatr Surg 19:699, 1984.

68. Smith RJ, Smith MC, Glossop LP, et al.: Congenital vascular anomalies causing tracheoesophageal compression. Arch Otolaryngol 110:82, 1984.

69. Welz A, Reichert B, Weinhold C, et al.: Innominate artery compression of the trachea in infancy and childhood: is surgical therapy justified? Thorac Cardiovasc Surg 32:85, 1984.

70. Grillo HC, Zannini P: Management of obstructive tracheal disease in children. J Pediatr Surg 19:414, 1984.

71. O'Neill JA Jr: Experience with iatrogenic laryngeal and tracheal stenosis. J Pediatr Surg 19:235, 1984.

72. Clarkson WB, Davies JR: Anesthesia for carinal resection. Anesthesia 33:815, 1978.

73. Ellis RH, Hinds CJ, Gadd LT: Management of anesthesia during tracheal resection. Anesthesia 31:1076, 1976.

74. Geffin B, Bland J, Grillo HC: Anesthetic management of tracheal resection and reconstruction. Anesth Analg 48:844, 1969.

75. Lee P, English ICW: Management of anesthesia during tracheal resection. Anesthesia 29:305, 1974.

76. Wilson RS: Tracheostomy and tracheal reconstruction. In Kaplan JA (Ed.): Thoracic Anesthesia. New York, Churchill Livingstone, 1983, pp 426–445.

77. Neuman GG, Asher AS, Stern SB, et al.: High frequency jet ventilation for tracheal resection in a child. Anesth Analg 63:1039, 1984.

78. Sorensen HR, Holsteen V: Resection of congenital stenosis of the trachea in an infant. Acta Paediatr Scand 73:141, 1984.

79. Akl BF, Yahek SM, Berman W Jr: Total tracheal reconstruction in a three month old infant. J Thorac Cardiovasc Surg 87:543, 1984.

80. Idriss FS, DeLeon SY, Ilbawi MN, et al.: Tracheoplasty with pericardial patch for extensive tracheal stenosis in infants and children. J Thorac Cardiovasc Surg 19:527, 1984.

81. Majeski JA, Schreiber JT, Cotton R, et al.: Tracheoplasty for tracheal stenosis in the pediatric patient. J Trauma 20:81, 1981.

82. Benjamin B: Endoscopy in congenital tracheal abnormalities. J Pediatr Surg 15:164, 1980.

83. Holinger PH, Schild JA, Weprin L: Pediatric laryngology. Otolaryngol Clin North Am 3:625, 1970.

84. Wailoo MP, Emery JL: The trachea in children with tracheoesophageal fistula. Histopathology 3:329, 1979.

85. Filler RM, Buck JR, Bahoric A, et al.: Treatment of segmental tracheomalacia and bronchomalacia by implantation of an airway splint. J Pediatr Surg 17:597, 1982.

86. Reynolds M, Luck S, Lappen R: The "critical" neonate with diaphragmatic hernia: a 21 year perspective. J Pediatr Surg 19:364, 1984.

87. Nguyen L., Guttman FM, De Chadarevian JP, et al.: The mortality of congenital diaphragmatic hernia. Is total pulmonary mass inadequate, no matter what? Ann Surg 198:766, 1983.

88. Bohn DJ, James I, Filler RM, et al.: The relationship between $PaCO_2$ and ventilation parameters in predicting survival in congenital diaphragmatic hernia. J Pediatr Surg 19:666, 1984.

89. Hansen F, James S, Burrington J, et al.: The decreasing incidence of pneumothorax and improving survival of infants with congenital diaphragmatic hernia. J Pediatr Surg 19:383, 1984.

90. Rudolf AM, Yuan S: Response of the pulmonary vasculature to hypoxia and H^+ ion concentration changes. J Clin Invest 45:399, 1966.

91. Ford WD, James MJ, Walsh JA: Congenital diaphragmatic hernia: association between pulmonary vascular resistance and plasma thromboxane concentrations. Arch Dis Child 59:143, 1984.

92. Vacanti JP, Crone RK, Murphy JD, et al.: The pulmonary hemodynamic response to perioperative anesthesia in the treatment of high risk infants with congenital diaphragmatic hernia. J Pediatr Surg 19:672, 1984.

93. Drummond WH, Gregory GA, Heymann MA, et al.: The independent effects of hyperventilation, tolazoline, and dopamine on infants with persistent pulmonary hypertension. J Pediatr 98:603, 1981.

94. Bartlett RH, Roloff DW, Cornell RD, et al.: Extracorporeal circulation in neonatal respiratory failure: a prospective randomized study. Pediatrics 76:479, 1985.

95. Freyschuss U, Lannergren K, Freckner B: Lung function after repair of congenital diaphragmatic hernia. Acta Paediatr Scand 73:589, 1984.

96. Bishop HC, Koop CE: Acquired eventration of the diaphragm in infancy. Pediatrics 22:1088, 1958.

97. Othersen HB, Lorenzo RL: Diaphragmatic paralysis and eventration: new approaches to diagnosis and operative correction. J Pediatr Surg 12:309, 1977.

98. McElwee TB, Myers RT, Pennell TC: Diaphragmatic rupture from blunt trauma. Am Surg 50:143, 1984.

99. Sharma LK, Kennedy RF, Heneghan WD: Rupture of the diaphragm resulting from blunt trauma in children. Can J Surg 20:553, 1977.

100. Eichenwald HF: Pneumonia syndromes in children. Hosp Pract 2:89, 1976.

101. Nelson JD: Pocketbook of Pediatric Antimicrobial Therapy. 6th ed. Baltimore, Williams & Wilkins, 1985.

102. Chartrand SA, McCracken GH Jr: Staphylococcal pneumonia in infants and children. Pediatr Infect Dis 1:19, 1982.

103. Avery ME, Fletcher BD, Williams RG: The Lung and Its Disorders in the Newborn Infant. 4th ed. Philadelphia, W. B. Saunders Co., 1981.

104. Brook I, Finegold SM: Bacteriology of aspiration pneumonia in children. Pediatrics 65:1115, 1980.

105. Imoke E, Dudgeon DL, Colombani P, et al.: Open lung biopsy in the immunocompromised pediatric patient. J Pediatr Surg 18:816, 1983.

106. Prober CG, Whyte H, Smith CR: Open lung biopsy in immunocompromised children with pulmonary infiltrates. Am J Dis Child 138:60, 1984.

107. Leijala M, Louhimo I, Lindfors EL: Open lung biopsy in children with diffuse pulmonary lesions. Acta Paediatr Scand 71:717, 1982.

108. Janik JS, Nagaraj HS, Groff DB: Thoracoscopic evaluation

of intrathoracic lesions in children. J Thorac Cardiovasc Surg 83:408, 1982.

109. McLaughlin FJ, Goldmann DA, Rosenbaum DM, et al.: Empyema in children: clinical course and long-term follow up. Pediatrics 73:587, 1984.

110. Stark DD, Federle MP, Goodman PC, et al.: Differentiating lung abscess and empyema: radiography and computed tomography. AJR 141:163, 1983.

111. Asher MI, Spier S, Beland M, et al.: Primary lung abscess in childhood. The long-term outcome of conservative management. Am J Dis Child 136:491, 1982.

112. Wilmott RW, Tyson SL, Dinwiddie R, et al.: Survival rates in cystic fibrosis. Arch Dis Child 58:835, 1983.

113. Hunt B, Geddes DM: Newly diagnosed cystic fibrosis in middle and later life. Thorax 40:23, 1985.

114. Isles A, Maclusky I, Corey M, et al.: Pseudomonas cepacia infection in cystic fibrosis: an emerging problem. J Pediatr 104:206, 1984.

115. Lester LA, Egge A, Hubbard VS, et al.: Aspiration and lung abscess in cystic fibrosis. Am Rev Respir Dis 127:786, 1983.

116. Wang EEL, Prober CG, Manson B, et al.: Association of respiratory viral infections with pulmonary deterioration in patients with cystic fibrosis. N Engl J Med 311:165, 1984.

117. Gurwitz D, Corey M, Francis PWJ, et al.: Perspectives in cystic fibrosis. Pediatr Clin North Am 26:603, 1979.

118. Corey M, Levison, Crozier D: Five- to seven-year course of pulmonary function in cystic fibrosis. Am Rev Respir Dis: 114:1085, 1976.

119. Schuster SR, Fellows KE: Management of major hemoptysis in patients with cystic fibrosis. J Pediatr Surg 12:889, 1977.

120. Swersky RB, Chang JB, Wisoff BG, et al.: Endobronchial balloon tamponade of hemoptysis in patients with cystic fibrosis. Ann Thorac Surg 27:162, 1979.

121. Park RW, Grand RJ: Gastrointestinal manifestation of cystic fibrosis: a review. Gastroenterology 81:1143, 1981.

122. Moss AJ: The cardiovascular system in cystic fibrosis. Pediatrics 70:728, 1982.

123. Rossman CM, Waldes R, Sampson D, et al.: Effect of chest physiotherapy on the removal of mucus in patients with cystic fibrosis. Am Rev Respir Dis 126:131, 1982.

124. Sutton PP, Lopez-Vidriero M, Pavia D, et al.: Effect of chest physiotherapy on the removal of mucus in patients with cystic fibrosis. Am Rev Respir Dis 127:390, 1983.

125. Fanconi S, Doherty, P, Edmonds JF, et al.: Pulse oximetry in pediatric intensive care. Comparisons with measured saturations and transcutaneous oxygen tension. J Pediatr 107:362, 1985.

126. Harnick E, Kulezycki L, Gomes MN: Transcutaneous oxygen monitoring during bronchoscopy and washout for cystic fibrosis. Anesth Analg 62:357, 1983.

127. Fellows KE, Khaw KT, Schuster S, et al.: Bronchial artery embolization in cystic fibrosis. Technique and long term results. J Pediatr 95:959, 1979.

128. Fellows KE, Stigol L, Shuster S, et al.: Selective bronchial arteriography in patients with cystic fibrosis and massive hemoptysis. Radiology 114:551, 1975.

129. Marmon L, Schidlow D, Palmer J, et al.: Pulmonary resection for complications of cystic fibrosis. J Pediatr Surg 18:811, 1983.

130. Lamberty JM, Rubin BK: The management of anaesthesia for patients with cystic fibrosis. Anaesthesia 40:448, 1985.

131. Eger EI, Saidman LJ: Hazards of nitrous oxide anesthesia in bowel obstruction and pneumothorax. Anesthesiology 26:61, 1965.

132. Schuster SR, McLaughlin FJ, Mathews WJ Jr, et al.: Management of pneumothorax in cystic fibrosis. J Pediatr Surg 18:492, 1983.

133. MacDonald NE, Anas NS, Peterson RG, et al.: Renal clearance of gentamicin in cystic fibrosis. J Pediatr 103:985, 1983.

134. Lewiston NJ: Bronchiectasis in childhood. Pediatr Clin North Am 31:865, 1984.

135. Vandevivere J, Spehl M, Dab I, et al.: Bronchiectasis in childhood. Comparison of chest roentgenograms, bronchoscopy and lung scintigraphy. Pediatr Radiol 9:193, 1980.

136. Stokes D, Sigler A, Khouri NF, et al.: Unilateral hyperlucent lung (Swyer-James syndrome) after severe Mycoplasma pneumoniae infections. Am Rev Respir Dis 117:145, 1978.

137. Resouly A: Kartagener's syndrome: a case report and review of the literature. J Laryngol Otol 86:1237, 1972.

138. Levy M, Gick B, Springer C, et al.: Bronchoscopy and bronchography in children. Am J Dis Child 137:14, 1983.

139. Wilson JF, Peters GN, Fleshman JK: A technique for bronchography in children. Am Rev Respir Dis 105:564, 1972.

140. Lundgren R, Hietala S, Adelroght E: Diagnosis of bronchial lesions by fiber-optic bronchoscopy combined with bronchography. Acta Radiol (Diagn) 23:231, 1982.

141. Cameron EW, Holloway AM: Bronchography in children aged 3 years and under. Anesthetic techniques and results. S Afr Med J 54:271, 1978.

142. Annest LS, Kratz JM, Crawford FA Jr: Current results of treatment of bronchiectasis. J Thorac Cardiovasc Surg 83:546, 1982.

143. Campbell DN, Lilly JR: The changing spectrum of pulmonary operations in infants and children. J Thorac Cardiovasc Surg 83:680, 1983.

144. Wilson JF, Decker AM: The surgical management of childhood bronchiectasis. Ann Surg 195:354, 1982.

145. Wagenvoort CA, Beetstra A, Spijker J: Capillary hemangiomatosis of the lungs. Histopathology 2:401, 1978.

146. Katzenstein ALA, Gmelich JT, Carrington CB: Sclerosing hemangioma of the lung. A clinicopathologic study of 51 cases. Am J Surg Pathol 4:343, 1980.

147. Liebow AA, Hubbell DS: Sclerosing hemangioma (histocytoma, xanthoma of the lung). Cancer 9:53, 1956.

148. Pearl M, Woolley MM: Pulmonary xanthomatous postinflammatory pseudotumors in children. J Pediatr Surg 8:255, 1973.

149. Brandt B, Heintz SE, Rose EF, et al.: Bronchial carcinoid tumors. Ann Thorac Surg 38:63, 1984.

150. McCaughan BC, Martini N, Bains MS, et al.: Bronchial carcinoids. Review of 124 cases. J Thorac Cardiovasc Surg 89:8, 1985.

151. Price CHG, Zhuker K, Saezer-Kuntschik M, et al.: Osteosarcoma in children. A study of 125 cases. J Bone Joint Surg 57:341, 1975.

152. Beattie EJ: Surgical treatment of pulmonary metastases. Cancer 54:2729, 1984.

153. Baldeyrou P, Lemoine G, Zucker GM, et al.: Pulmonary metastases in children: the place of surgery. A study of 134 patients. J Pediatr Surg 19:121, 1984.

154. Harris CS, Baker SP, Smith GA, et al.: Childhood asphyxiation by food. 251:2231, 1984.

155. Anas NG, Perkin MD: Aspiration of a balloon by a 3 month old. JAMA 250:285, 1983.

156. Aytac A, Yardakl Y, Ikizler C, et al.: Inhalation of foreign bodies in children: report of 500 cases. J Thorac Cardiovasc Surg 74:145, 1977.

157. Blazer S, Navelo Y, Friedman A: Foreign body in the airway. Am J Dis Child 134:68, 1980.

158. Cotton E, Yasuda K: Foreign body aspiration. Pediatr Clin North Am 31:937, 1984.

159. Majd NS, Mofenson HC, Greensher J: Lower airway foreign body aspiration in children. Clin Pediatr 16:13, 1977.

160. Wiseman NE: The diagnosis of foreign body aspiration in childhood. J Pediatr Surg 19:531, 1984.

161. Abman SH, Fan LL, Colton EK: Emergency treatment of foreign body obstruction of the upper airway in children. J Emerg Med 2:7, 1984.

162. Hight EW, Phillipart AI, Hertzler JH: The treatment of retained foreign bodies in the pediatric airway. J Pediatr Surg 16:694, 1981.

163. Black RE, Choi KJ, Syme WC, et al.: Bronchoscopic removal

of aspirated foreign bodies in children. Am J Surg *14*:77, 1984.

164. Cohen SR, Herbert WI, Lewis GB Jr, et al.: Foreign bodies in the airway: five year retrospective study with special reference to management. Ann Otol Rhinol Laryngol *89*:437, 1980.

165. Hunsicker RC, Gartner WS: Fogarty catheter technique for removal of endobronchial foreign body. Arch Otolaryngol *103*:103, 1977.

166. Wood RE, Gauderer MW: Flexible fiberoptic bronchoscopy in the management of tracheobronchial foreign bodies in children: the value of a combined approach with open tube bronchoscopy. J Pediatr Surg *19*:693, 1984.

167. Tyler DC, Redding G, Hall D, et al.: Increased intracranial pressure: an indication to decompress a tension pneumomediastinum. Crit Care Med *12*:467, 1984.

168. Keon TP: Death on induction of anesthesia for cervical node biopsy. Anesthesiology *55*:399, 1975.

169. Amaha K, Okutsu Y, Nakamura Y: Major airway obstruction by a mediastinal tumor: a case report. Br J Anaesth *45*:1082, 1973.

170. Bittar D: Respiratory obstruction associated with induction of general anesthesia in a patient with mediastinal Hodgkin's disease. Anesth Analg *54*:399, 1975.

171. Piro AH, Weiss DR, Hellman S: Mediastinal Hodgkin's disease: a possible danger for intubation anesthesia. Int J Radiat Oncol Phys *1*:415, 1976.

172. Todres ID, Reppert G, Hall D, et al.: Management of critical airway obstruction in a child with a mediastinal tumor. Anesthesiology *45*:1000, 1976.

173. Neuman GG, Weingarten AE, Abramowitz RM, et al.: The anesthetic management of the patient with an anterior mediastinal mass. Anesthesiology *60*:144, 1984.

174. Talbert JL, Rogers BM, Felman AH, et al.: Traumatic perforation of the hypopharynx in infants. J Thorac Cardiovasc Surg *74*:152, 1977.

DISEASES OF THE CARDIOVASCULAR SYSTEM ‖ 6

INGRID B. HOLLINGER, M.D.

Safe anesthetic management of the infant or child with heart disease requires not only familiarity with anesthetic techniques and agents used in the pediatric age group but also a thorough understanding of the specific cardiac lesion, its pathophysiological consequences, and the possible effects of anesthetic techniques on these. In addition, the requirements of the proposed surgery have to be considered.

The purpose of this chapter is to review common and uncommon cardiac lesions, their current management, the results of therapy, and their implications for anesthetic management in noncardiac surgery.

Heart disease in infancy and childhood is due to congenital cardiac lesions in 90 percent of cases. These may be caused by deficiency of tissue leaving open communications between cardiac chambers, formation of excessive tissue causing obstruction at or near cardiac valves, persistence or development of anomalous connections between arteries or veins and cardiac chambers, or combinations of these problems. However, the most common congenital cardiac lesions, the floppy mitral valve and bicuspid aortic valve, are caused by improperly formed tissue that usually functions normally during infancy and childhood and generally does not lead to cardiac dysfunction until the later decades of life.

The incidence of congenital heart disease, with the exclusion of mitral valve prolapse and congenital bicuspid aortic valve, is approximately 6 to 8 per 1000 live births. This means that 24,500 children are born each year with congenital heart disease. In prematures, the incidence of congenital heart disease is two to three times higher, even if persistent patency of the ductus arteriosus is excluded. Certain genetic syndromes and infectious or chemical teratogens can change the incidence of congenital heart disease. A listing of syndromes and teratogens and the commonly associated lesions is provided in Table 6–1.

Associated extracardiac defects may be present in children with congenital heart disease. Genitourinary tract anomalies may be present in 4 to 15 percent of patients with congenital heart disease and should be sought at angiography. Approximately half of all infants with congenital heart disease require hospital admission for either medical or surgical therapy during the first year of life, the majority within the first 2 months. The mortality for this group as a whole, despite therapy, is approximately 40 percent. Since only patients with the more severe and life-threatening anomalies present for therapy during infancy, the relative frequency of various cardiac lesions changes if analyzed in a prospective study of unselected births rather than from admission data of cardiac clinics (Table 6–2). Nevertheless, one should realize that 80 percent of all congenital heart disease is distributed among only eight lesions: ventricular septal defect, atrial septal defect, pulmonary stenosis, patent ductus arteriosus, tetralogy of Fallot, aortic stenosis, coarctation of the aorta, and transposition of the great vessels. All other lesions are rare. Table 6–3 list the various cardiac lesions in an anatomical-functional classification that will be followed in the discussion of the individual defects.

INTRACARDIAC DEFECTS PRODUCING PREDOMINANT LEFT-TO-RIGHT SHUNT

Atrial Communications

Patent Foramen Ovale

Functional closure of the foramen ovale occurs after birth, but anatomical closure is not complete until 2 to 3 months of age. Patency of the foramen ovale on probing persists in 50 percent of children up to 5 years and in 20 to 30 percent of the adult population. Because of the flaplike closure of this communication by the left-sided septum primum, shunting can occur only right-to-left after an increase in right atrial pressure. However, if the foramen ovale is stretched by a distended left atrium or the flap valve is deficient, left-to-right shunting occurs through the opened communication. This latter situation is frequently observed in infants with a large patent ductus arteriosus or ventricular septal defect. Obstruction to left ventricular outflow, such as coarctation of the aorta or aortic stenosis, also may lead to large left-to-right shunts across a stretched foramen ovale, further aggravating pulmonary hyperperfusion and/or congestion.

Correction of the primary lesions will generally lead to a decrease in the size of the left atrium and disappearance of the left-to-right shunt across the foramen. If an intracardiac repair is performed, the foramen may be closed surgically. Systemic blood flow through a patent foramen ovale permits survival in certain congenital cardiac lesions, such as right ventricular obstruction, total anomalous pulmonary venous return, aortopulmonary transposition, and mitral atresia.

Isolated patency of the foramen ovale causes no clinical symptoms and cannot be diagnosed unless detected during cardiac catheterization.

Secundum Atrial Septal Defect (ASD)

Seventy-five percent of all atrial septal defects are of the secundum type, located at the fossa ovalis. This defect represents about 8 percent of all congenital heart disease. It is more common in females, with a male-to-female ratio of 1:2. The intra-atrial communication is usually large. The magnitude and direction of the shunt are related to the relative inflow resistance of the right and left ventricle, since the atria are low-pressure systems and have a very small pressure difference. In infancy and early childhood the right ventricle is relatively thicker and less compliant and offers more resistance to right atrial outflow. As pulmonary vascular resistance falls and the right ventricular wall becomes relatively thinner, right ventricular stroke volume and atrial shunt increase. This condition is usually not diagnosed before 2 or 3 years of age. Because of the difference in left and right atrial pressures, shunting is preferentially left-to-right, but a small right-to-left shunt of blood returning from the inferior vena cava is usually present. Immediately after a Valsava maneuver this venous blood flow is increased and may cause a drop in systemic arterial saturation. Pulmonary blood flow is usually markedly increased (often three to four time normal), but pulmonary artery pressure is normal until adult life and obstructive pulmonary vascular disease usually does not develop until the third or fourth decade of life. The main cause of deterioration of patients with secundum ASD in adult life is atrial arrhythmias, particularly atrial fibrillation and flutter. Children with secundum ASD are usually asymptomatic. With large shunts mild fatigue and dyspnea may be present. On auscultation there is fixed splitting of the second heart sound. A systolic ejection murmur is heard maximally over the upper left sternal border. With moderate to large shunts there is a short mid-diastolic murmur at the lower left sternal border. Echocardiography can distinguish secundum ASD from other lesions and eliminate the need for cardiac catheterization. Treatment consists of elective surgical repair before school age.

Sinus Venosus Defect

These defects account for about 5 to 10 percent of ASDs. They are located posterior to the fossa ovalis,

Text continued on page 101

Table 6–1. SYNDROMES WITH CONGENITAL CARDIAC DEFECTS

Chromosomal Abnormalities

	Incidence of Congenital Heart Disease (% of Patients)	Cardiac Lesions in Order of Frequency (%)
Trisomy 21 (Down)	40	ECD (32), VSD (29), ASD (11), TOF (8), PDA (7)
Trisomy 18	90	VSD (66), PDA (50), ASD (33), bicuspid PV (25), CoA (15), bicuspid AV (15)
Trisomy 13	80	PDA (63), VSD (43), ASD (40), abnormal valves (22), CoA (10)
5p⁻ (Cri du chat)	25	VSD, PDA, ASD, PS
4p⁻ (Wolf)	50	VSD, ASD, PDA, PS
XO (Turner)	10–30	CoA (50), AS, VSD, ASD

Teratogenic

	Incidence of Congenital Heart Disease (% of Patients)	Cardiac Lesions in Order of Frequency
Alcohol	25–30	VSD, PDA, ASD
Amphetamines	5–10	VSD, PDA, ASD, TGA
Hydantoin	2–3	PS, AS, CoA, PDA
Trimethadione	15–30	TGA, TOF, hypoplastic LH
Thalidomide	5–10	TOF, VSD, ASD, truncus arteriosus
Rubella	35	Peripheral PS, PDA, VSD, ASD
Maternal diabetes	3–5	TGA, VSD, CoA
Maternal phenylketonuria	25–50	TOF, VSD, ASD
Maternal systemic lupus erythematosus	20–40	Congenital complete heart block

Genetic or Unknown Etiology

	Etiology	Incidence of Congenital Heart Disease (% of Patients)	Characteristic Cardiac Defect
Skeletal Defects Predominant			
Ellis–van Crefeld	R	50–60	Single atrium, ECD, PDA
Laurence-Moon-Biedl	R		TOF, VSD
Carpenter	R		PDA, VSD
Holt-Oram	D	50	ASD, VSD, TOF, PS, PDA
Fanconi	R		PDA, VSD
Thrombocytopenia, absent radius	R	10–15	ASD, TOF
Rubinstein-Taybi		15–20	CAV, ASD
Vater			Variable
Characteristic Facies			
Noonan	D	50	PS (dysplastic PV), ASD
DiGeorge	?	90–100	Interrupted aortic arch type B, aberrant right subclavian, right aortic arch, truncus arteriosus, TOF
Smith-Lemli-Opitz	R	15–20	VSD, PDA
Facial dysmorphism	D	10	PDA
de Lange	?	20	VSD, PDA, ASD, TOF
Goldenhar	?	50	TOF, VSD, PDA, CoA
Williams elfin face	?	80	Supravalvular AS, peripheral AS, peripheral PS, interrupted arch
Asymmetric crying facies			Variable
Skin Lesions Prominent			
Forney (deafness, freckles)	D		MI
Leopard (deafness, lentigines)	D		PS
Neurofibromatosis	D		PS, renal artery stenosis
Tuberous sclerosis	D		Rhabdomyoma
Situs Inversus			
Kartagener (bronchiectasis)	R		Dextrocardia
Ivemark asplenia or polysplenia	?		Complex cyanotic heart disease
Connective Tissue Disorders			
Marfan	D	30–100	Dilation of proximal aorta (AI, aneurysm), MVP, cystic medial necrosis

Table continued on following page

Table 6–1. SYNDROMES WITH CONGENITAL CARDIAC DEFECTS *Continued*

	Etiology	Incidence of Congenital Heart Disease (% of Patients)	Characteristic Cardiac Defect
		Genetic or Unknown Etiology		
Ehlers-Danlos	D	20–30	MVP, arterial rupture
Cutis laxa	R		Peripheral PS
Osteogenesis imperfecta	D, R		MVP, AI
Pseudoxanthoma elasticum	R		Coronary artery disease
Metabolic Disorders			
Glycogen storage disease II (Pompe)	R		Massive cardiac enlargement due to glycogen deposition
Homocystinuria	R		Thrombosis of arteries
Mucopolysaccharidoses			
Type I, Hurler	R		Pseudoatherosclerosis, AI, MI
Type II, Hunter	X-linked		AI
Types IV, V, VI	R		AI
Neuromuscular Disorders			
Friedreich ataxia	R		Cardiomyopathy
Myotonic dystrophy	D		MVP, cardiomyopathy
Muscular dystrophy	X-linked		Cardiomyopathy
Arrhythmias			
Jervell and Lange-Nielsen (deafness)	R		Prolonged Q–T and R–T intervals, VF
Romano Ward (no deafness)	D		Prolonged Q–T interval, VF
Refsum's (polyneuritis)	R		Arrhythmia, heart block
Familial periodic paralysis	D		Hypokalemia, SVT

Data from Noonan JA: Association of congenital heart disease with syndromes and their defects. Pediatr Clin North Am 25:797, 1978; and Steinberg AG, et al.: Progress in Medical Genetics. Vol. V. Genetics of Cardiovascular Disease. Philadelphia, W.B. Saunders Co., 1983.

ECG = endocardial cushion defect; VSD = ventricular septal defect; ASD = atrial septal defect; TOF = tetralogy of Fallot; PDA = patent ductus arteriosus; PV = pulmonary valve; CoA = coarctation of aorta; AV = aortic valve; PS = pulmonic stenosis; AS = aortic stenosis; TGA = transposition of great arteries; LH = left heart; CAV = canalis atrioventricularis; MI = mitral insufficiency; AI = aortic insufficiency; MVP = mitral valve prolapse; VF = ventricular fibrillation; SVT = supraventricular tachycardia; R = recessive; D = dominant; ? = unknown

Table 6–2. INCIDENCE OF VARIOUS CONGENITAL CARDIAC LESIONS (% OF TOTAL)

In Normal Births*		All Congenital Heart Disease Seen in Infancy and Childhood†		Symptomatic in First Year of Life‡	
VSD	29.1	VSD	25	VSD	15.7
PS	8.1	PDA	12.5	D-TGA	9.9
PDA	7.7	PS	8.7	TOF	8.9
ASD secundum	7.4	TOF	7.9	CoA	7.5
CoA	6.5	CoA	6.6	Hypoplastic L.H.	7.4
ECD	4.4	AS	6.3	PDA	6.1
TOF	3.5	ASD secundum	5.8	ECD	5.0
AS	3.5	D-TGA	4.5	Heterotaxia (dextrocardia,	4.0
Hypoplastic left heart	3.5	ECD	3.1	mesocardia, asplenia)	
VSD + PS	2.4	Hypoplastic left heart	1.5	PS	3.3
Peripheral PS	2.4	Dextrocardia	1.5	Pulmonary atresia	3.1
D-TGA	2.5	Vascular Ring	1.45	ASD secundum	2.9
EFE	2.2	PAPVR	1.4	TAPVR	2.6
Truncus arteriosus	2.0	TAPVR	1.3	Myocardial disease	2.6
Vascular ring	1.5	MI	1.15	Tricuspid atresia	2.6
Pulmonary atresia	1.5	Tricuspid atresia	1.14	Single ventricle	2.4
Tricuspid atresia	1.5	Single ventricle	1.0	AS	1.9
Anomalies of coronary arteries	1.5	EFE	1.0	DORV	1.5
DORV	1.1	Absent pulmonary	1.0	Truncus arteriosus	1.4
Single ventricle	0.9	AI	0.97	L-TGA	0.7
MI	0.7	Truncus arteriosus	0.74	Miscellaneous	10.4
EMF	0.7	L-TGA	d0.58		
Miscellaneous	6.1	Pulmonary atresia	0.5		
		Ebstein anomaly	0.5		
		Pulmonary atresia	0.5		
		Ebstein anomaly	0.5		
		Coronary anomalies	0.5		
		DORV	0.35		
		MS	0.3		
		Aortopulmonary window	0.24		
		Interrupted arch	0.175		
		Common atrium	0.17		
		Cor triatriatum	0.1		

*Data from Mitchell SC, et al.: Congenital heart disease in 56,109 births. Circulation 63:323, 1971.

†Data from Nadas AS, Fyler DC: Pediatric Cardiology. 3rd ed. Philadelphia, W. B. Saunders Co., 1972; and Keith JD, et al. (Eds.): Heart Disease in Infancy and Childhood. 3rd ed. New York, Macmillan, 1978.

‡Data from Fyler DC, et al.: Report of the New England Regional Infant Cardiac Program. Pediatrics 65(Suppl):388, 1980.

VSD = ventricular septal defect; PS = pulmonic stenosis; PDA = patent ductus arteriosus; ASD = atrial septal defect; CoA = coarctation of aorta; ECD = endocardial cushion defect; TOF = tetralogy of Fallot; AS = aortic stenosis; TGA = transposition of great arteries; EFE = endocardial fibroelastosis; DORV = double outlet right ventricle; MI = mitral insufficiency; EMF = endomyocardial fibrosis; PAPVR = partial anomalous pulmonary venous return; TAPVR = total anomalous pulmonary venous return; AI = aortic insufficiency; MS = mitral stenosis; LH = left heart.

Table 6–3. CARDIOVASCULAR DEFECTS IN INFANTS AND CHILDREN

Types of Lesions	Special Considerations
Intracardiac Defects	
A. Lesions producing dominant L–R shunt	
1. Intra-atrial communications	
a. Patent foramen ovale	Volume overload
b. Atrial septal defect	Paradoxical embolization
c. Endocardial cushion defect	Atrial arrhythmias
i. Partial	
ii. Complete	Congestive heart failure
	Mitral regurgitation
2. Interventricular communications	
a. VSD, simple	Volume and pressure overload
b. VSD, complicated (other associated cardiac lesions)	Pulmonary hypertension
c. Single ventricle	Shunt reversal with increased RV pressure
d. Left ventricle to right atrium	Congestive heart failure
e. L-Transposition of the great vessels	Dependent shunting
	Delayed intravenous induction
f. Eisenmenger syndrome	Fixed elevated pulmonary vascular resistance
	Reversed shunt
B. Lesions producing dominant R–L shunt with cyanosis	
1. Lesions with decreased pulmonary blood flow	
a. Tetralogy of Fallot	Dynamic RV outflow obstruction
b. Pulmonary atresia with VSD	Low SVR increases R–L shunt
c. Double-outlet right ventricle with pulmonic stenosis	Systemic embolization
d. Single ventricle with PS	Polycythemia and thrombosis
e. L-Transposition with VSD and PS	Reduced myocardial function postoperatively
	Tachyarrhythmias late postoperatively
	Rapid intravenous induction
	Delayed inhalation induction
2. Lesions with increased pulmonary blood flow	
a. D-Transposition of the great vessels	Congestive heart failure
b. Double-outlet right ventricle	Pulmonary hypertension
	Systemic embolization
	Atrial dysrhythmias
C. Obstructive lesions	
1. LV outflow	
a. Aortic stenosis	
i. Valvular	Pressure overload—left ventricle
ii. Supravalvular	High endocarditis risk
iii. Subvalvular	Tachycardia causes ischemia
iv. Obstructive cardiomyopathy	Cardiac output fixed
	Peripheral vasodilation poorly tolerated
	Maintain preload and afterload
	Sudden death
2. RV outflow	
a. Pulmonic stenosis	
i. Valvular	Pressure overload—right ventricle
ii. Infundibular	Shunting across patent foramen ovale
iii. Anomalous right ventricular bands	Syncope with stress in severe stenosis
iv. Peripheral pulmonic stenosis	Myocardial fibrosis and limited cardiac reserve may persist
v. Pulmonary atresia	postoperatively
3. LV inflow	
a. Mitral stenosis	Increased left atrial pressure
b. Parachute mitral valve (Shone syndrome)	Pulmonary congestion
c. Cor triatriatum	Ventilatory abnormalities
d. Supravalvular ring	Tachycardia worsens symptoms
e. Hypoplastic left heart syndrome	Maintain preload and afterload
4. RV inflow	
a. Tricuspid atresia	R–L shunting
b. Tricuspid stenosis	Systemic embolization
c. Ebstein anomaly of tricuspid valve	High endocarditis risk
	Maintain preload and afterload
	Maintain sinus rhythm
	Maintain low pulmonary vascular resistance

Table continued on opposite page

Table 6–3. CARDIOVASCULAR DEFECTS IN INFANTS AND CHILDREN *Continued*

Types of Lesions	Special Considerations
Intracardiac Defects Continued	
D. Regurgitant lesions	

1. Aortic
     a. Aortic insufficiency
     b. Fenestration of aortic leaflets
     c. Aneurysm of sinus of Valsalva
     d. Aorto–left ventricular tunnel
     e. VSD with aortic insufficiency
	Volume overload—left ventricle
	Regurgitation reduced by tachycardia and low peripheral vascular resistance
	Maintain myocardial contractility

2. Mitral
     a. Anomalous
     b. Cleft anterior or posterior leaflet
     c. Mitral valve prolapse
     d. Obstructive cardiomyopathy
	Volume overload—left ventricle
	Regurgitation reduced by tachycardia and low peripheral vascular resistance
	Pulmonary congestion and ventilation abnormalities
	Monitor for arrhythmias with mitral valve prolapse

3. Pulmonic	
a. Pulmonary valve insufficiency	Usually well tolerated in the absence of pulmonary vascular disease
b. Absent pulmonary valve	Dilatation of pulmonary arteries leading to tracheal and bronchial compression Associated with VSD, may present as tetralogy of Fallot

4. Tricuspid
     a. Ebstein anomaly
     b. Tricuspid insufficiency
     c. Uhl anomaly
	Volume overload—right ventricle
	R–L shunt at atrial level common
	Maintain right-sided filling pressures
	Tachycardia reduces regurgitation
	Maintain low pulmonary vascular resistance
	Intravenous induction prolonged

Malformations Involving the Great Vessels	
A. Arterial	
1. Systemic arteries	
a. Patent ductus arteriosus	Endocarditis risk preoperatively
b. Aortopulmonary window	Congestive failure L–R shunting Shunt reversal
c. Truncus arteriosus	Congestive failure L–R shunting Shunt reversal RV–PA conduit postoperatively
d. Coarctation of aorta e. Interrupted aortic arch	Hypertension in upper extremity, may persist postoperatively

f. Vascular ring anomalies
       i. Double aortic arch
       ii. Aberrant right subclavian artery
       iii. Anomalous innominate artery
       iv. Right aortic arch
       v. Anomalous left carotid artery
       vi. Anomalous left pulmonary artery (vascular sling)
	Tracheal or bronchial compression
	Esophageal compression
	Tracheomalacia may persist postoperatively

g. Congenital subclavian steal	Cerebral ischemia with exercise of affected arm Usually associated with coarctation or interrupted arch
2. Pulmonary arteries	
a. Anomalous origin of one pulmonary artery from the aorta	Severe pulmonary hypertension Development of obstructive pulmonary vascular disease
b. Congenital absence of one pulmonary artery	Associated pulmonary anomalies Recurrent infections Bronchiectasis Increased dead space
c. Congenital pulmonary arteriovenous fistula	Intrapulmonary R–L shunt Paradoxical embolization Polycythemia and systemic thrombosis

Table continued on following page

Table 6–3. CARDIOVASCULAR DEFECTS IN INFANTS AND CHILDREN *Continued*

Types of Lesions	Special Considerations
Malformations Involving the Great Vessels Continued	
B. Venous	
1. Pulmonary veins	
a. Total anomalous pulmonary venous return	
i. Supracardiac	Pulmonary venous obstruction
ii. Cardiac	L–R shunt at atrial level
iii. Infracardiac	Volume overload—right ventricle
iv. Mixed	
b. Partial anomalous pulmonary venous return	
i. Superior vena cava	Present similar to ASD
ii. Right atrium	Pulmonary infections common
iii. Inferior vena cava (scimitar syndrome)	
2. Systemic veins	
a. Anomalous systemic venous return	
i. Persistent left superior vena cava to left atrium	Problems with cardiac catheterization
ii. Absence of inferior vena cava	Problems with cardiac catheterization and venous cannulation for bypass
C. Anomalies of the coronary arteries	
1. Aberrant left coronary artery (Bland-White-Garland syndrome)	Left ventricular ischemia and failure
2. Coronary arteriovenous fistula	L–R shunt through fistula Failure and ischemia rare
Cardiomyopathies: See Table 6–4.	
Tumors of the Heart	Obstruction to filling and blood flow
A. Benign	Embolization of tumor fragments
1. Rhabdomyoma	
2. Fibroma	
3. Myxoma	
4. Benign teratoma	
B. Malignant	
1. Malignant teratoma	
2. Rhabdomyosarcoma	
Conduction Defects	
A. Congenital atrioventricular block	Usually well tolerated past infancy
B. Supraventricular tachycardia	May require temporary pacing for surgery
C. Wolff-Parkinson-White syndrome	Abnormal conduction pathway (Kent)
D. Lown-Ganong-Levine syndrome	Reentry tachycardia May be triggered by sympathetic stimulation Patients on digoxin
E. Prolonged Q–T interval	Imbalance of cardiac sympathetics Patients on beta blockers Syncope due to ventricular fibrillation triggered by sympathetic stimulation Bradycardia may result in escape beats and ventricular fibrillation
Diseases of the Pericardium	
A. Pericardial defect	Restriction to ventricular filling
B. Pericarditis	Pulsus paradoxus
C. Constrictive pericarditis	Fixed cardiac output
D. Pericardial tumors	Maintain heart rate, preload, afterload
Malpositions of the Heart	
A. Dextrocardia (asplenia syndrome)	Associated congenital cardiac lesions common
B. Ectopia cordis	
Acquired Heart Disease	
A. Rheumatic heart disease	Valvular involvement usually mild in pediatric age group Penicillin prophylaxis and prevention of bacterial endocarditis
B. Kawasaki syndrome	Coronary artery disease Aspirin therapy
C. Takayasu disease	Hypertension

with the vena cava frequently overriding the defect and the pulmonary veins from the right upper lobe, and less commonly the entire right lung connected to either the right atrium or the superior vena cava.

Coronary Sinus ASD

The least common of all ASDs lies at the site of the anticipated coronary sinus ostium. It is usually associated with absence of the coronary sinus and a persistent left superior vena cava draining into the roof of the left atrium. It may be associated with a complete atrioventricular (AV) canal defect and the asplenia syndrome.

Clinical manifestations of both sinus venosus defect and coronary sinus ASD when isolated are similar to those of secundum ASD. Partial anomalous pulmonary return requires construction of a baffle to divert the anomalous pulmonary blood flow to the left atrium. Surgery is usually performed during childhood.

Endocardial Cushion Defect

Defects in the development and fusion of the endocardial cushions lead to incomplete septation of the primitive AV canal and various forms of atrial and/or ventricular communications described as partial or complete endocardial cushion defect or AV canal. Endocardial cushion defects occur in 3 to 4 percent of children with congenital heart disease who are otherwise normal, but are the predominant cardiac lesion (30 to 50 percent) in children with trisomy 21. At least 25 percent of children with endocardial cushion defect have Down syndrome. Almost all patients with asplenia syndrome have some form of endocardial cushion defect. About half of the patients with Ellis—van Crefeld syndrome have congenital heart disease, with the most frequent defect (40 percent) being single atrium, considered a form of endocardial cushion defect. Endocardial cushion defect is equally distributed between the sexes.

Partial AV canal is one fourth as frequent as secundum ASD and is characterized by nearly complete central fusion of the anterior and posterior cushions so that the mitral and tricuspid annuli are well formed (Fig. 6–1). The most common type is the ostium primum ASD with a cleft anterior mitral leaflet. The defect lies anterior and inferior to the fossa ovalis and is usually quite large. The lesion is frequently discovered during infancy because of the prominence of the cardiac murmur. Symptoms, including heart failure, may occur early, most commonly if the defect is associated with mitral insufficiency. Dyspnea, fatigue, and susceptibility to frequent respiratory infections may be present. Mitral insufficiency is rarely seen in infants but may become apparent by age 4 to 5 years.

Shunting in ostium primum defect occurs through two mechanisms; one similar to secundum defect depends on the difference in the inflow resistance of the right and left ventricle. With high pulmonary vascular resistance there is minimal right-to-left shunt, whereas with low pulmonary vascular resistance there

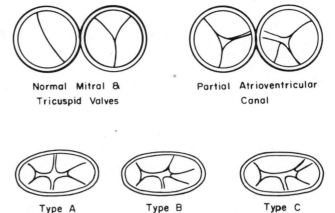

Figure 6–1. Schematic representation of partial and complete atrioventricular canal. Classification after Rastelli.

is left-to-right shunting proportional to the difference in pulmonary and systemic vascular resistances. This represents dependent shunting. Obligatory shunting occurs from a high-pressure to a low-pressure chamber, in this lesion from the left ventricle to the right atrium across the cleft mitral valve and ostium primum defect.

Pulmonary vascular disease rarely develops before adolescence. The ECG typically shows left axis deviation, AV conduction abnormalities (usually first degree block), and right ventricular conduction defect with or without hypertrophy. The heart is usually large on plain chest films and there may be evidence of pulmonary hyperperfusion. Treatment consists of surgical repair of the defect with a patch of pericardium or prosthetic material and repair of the mitral cleft with sutures in cases with mitral incompetence.

Mitral insufficiency may persist postoperatively and ultimately require mitral valve replacement. If no symptoms are present, repair is generally performed when the patient is between 5 and 7 years of age.

Anesthetic Considerations. Children with uncomplicated ASD pose no unusual anesthetic risks. In noncardiac surgery the major concern has to be directed toward prevention of systemic air embolization, especially in coronary sinus ASD. Although the dominant direction of the shunt in ASD is from left to right atrium, reversal of the shunt direction can occur with sudden increases in right ventricular outflow resistance. This has been observed with embolization of air, as in neurosurgical procedures in the sitting position, and with marked increases in intrathoracic pressure during bronchoscopy with jet ventilation. Paradoxical embolization of air can occur through a persistent foramen ovale. Application of positive end-expiratory pressure (PEEP) under these circumstance may increase right-to-left shunting by increasing pulmonary vascular resistance. Hypoxia, hypercarbia, and acidosis all increase pulmonary vascular resistance and may lead to shunt reversal in ASD. Airway maintenance and prevention of hypoventilation during anesthesia are therefore particularly important. In small children and patients with Down syndrome, endotracheal intubation should be considered for all but the most trivial procedures.

Endocarditis prophylaxis is necessary for patients with primum and sinus venosus defects pre- and postoperatively but not for patients with simple secundum defects pre- or postoperatively (if closed without prosthetic material).

Complete Endocardial Cushion Defect. Complete AV canal is the lesion most commonly associated with Down syndrome. It is characterized by a large combined AV defect and a single AV valve with five to six leaflets and commissures (Fig. 6–1). Angiography demonstrates the characteristic goose-neck deformity of the left ventricular outflow tract.

Symptoms invariably occur early in infancy owing to the large increase in pulmonary blood flow and pressure, which leads to pulmonary hypertension. Mitral regurgitation is present in at least 50 percent of patients. Congestive heart failure, pneumonia, and failure to thrive are the common presenting features. Pulmonary vascular obstructive disease develops in two thirds of cases within the first year of life. With medical management more than 50 percent of infants die within the first 12 months and 85 per cent by the end of the second year of life. Left-to-right shunting occurs at the atrial and ventricular levels and becomes bidirectional or reversed with progressive increase in pulmonary vascular resistance.

Treatment of choice at present is complete repair whenever unmanageable symptoms occur before 1 year of age. Pulmonary artery banding is ineffective in the presence of AV valve incompetence and carries over 30 percent mortality in complete AV canal. Late postoperative complications of complete AV canal repair in infancy include mitral valve insufficiency in 10 to 30 percent of patients and AV conduction disturbances including complete heart block.

Anesthetic Considerations. Infants with uncorrected AV canal defects rarely undergo elective surgical procedures. Anesthetic management has to be directed toward maintenance of cardiac output with a failing myocardium. Patients are usually digitalized and on diuretic therapy. Congestive failure and electrolyte abnormalities should be controlled and monitoring of intravascular volume and pressure should be established for major surgery. Anesthetic agents that are known to cause myocardial depression should be avoided.

Chronic pulmonary congestion may lead to airway closure and atelectasis. Large bronchi may be compressed by the pulmonary arteries or left atrium, small airway resistance is increased, compliance is decreased, and intrapulmonary right-to-left shunting occurs. Patients may be on the verge of respiratory failure. The airway should always be secured by endotracheal intubation, and ventilation controlled to assure adequate gas exchange. In the presence of obstructive pulmonary vascular disease, pulmonary interstitial and alveolar edema may occur with fluid shifts because of the reduced pulmonary vascular bed.

Patients may require postoperative ventilation. Use of unnecessary high oxygen concentration may aggravate congestive heart failure by increasing left-to-right shunting because of a reduction in pulmonary vascular resistance. Hyperventilation, hypokalemia, and alkalosis may lead to ventricular arrhythmias in the digitalized patient. Serum potassium should be maintained above 4 mEq/L perioperatively and digitalis discontinued 12 hours preoperatively. If cardiovascular deterioration occurs, use of intravenous inotropic agents (dopamine, dobutamine) should be considered. Patients require careful endocarditis prophylaxis.

Two thirds of patients who have undergone complete AV canal repair are in functional class I (NYHA classification). Anesthetic management should be directed toward the general management of the patient with Down syndrome and the prevention of bacterial endocarditis. If mitral regurgitation is present, maintenance of an adequate heart rate and low systemic vascular resistance is important. Myocardial depression can readily lead to congestive failure, especially when combined with operative fluid overload. Patients require very careful monitoring.

Common Atrium

Common atrium is characterized by virtually complete absence of the atrial septum. It is frequently combined with other cardiac anomalies such as transposition, double outlet right ventricle, univentricular heart, and anomalous pulmonary venous connection in association with asplenia or polysplenia syndrome. Nearly complete mixing of systemic and pulmonary blood occurs but pulmonary blood flow exceeds systemic blood flow. Cyanosis may be constantly present or apparent only during exercise. Surgical repair is performed early in life to prevent development of pulmonary vascular disease. Endocarditis prophylaxis, prevention of systemic embolization, and shunt reversal are considerations in anesthetic management.

Interventricular Communications

Simple Ventricular Septal Defect

Isolated ventricular septal defect (VSD) is the most common congenital cardiac lesion causing symptoms in infants and children and is seen in 20 to 25 percent of all patients with congenital heart disease. It is slightly more common in females (56 percent) than in males (44 percent). Eighty percent of defects are located in the membranous portion of the ventricular septum beneath the crista interventricularis. Supracristal defects located beneath the pulmonic valve constitute approximately 5 to 7 percent of VSDs except in Japan or other Far Eastern countries, where they may constitute close to 30 percent. Defects may also be located in the muscular septum (frequently multiple) or beneath the septal leaflet of the tricuspid valve (AV canal type defect).

The size of the defect largely determines the degree of pathophysiological derangement. With small to medium lesions the size limits left-to-right shunting. With large defects (approximately the size of the aortic orifice), there is no restriction to flow and shunting depends largely on differences between systemic resistance and resistance of the pulmonary vascular bed. Symptoms of left-to-right shunting usually develop between the second and third week of life with the normal decline in pulmonary vascular resistance. With very large defects and systemic pressures in the pulmonary arteries, the resistance of the pulmonary vascular bed declines more slowly and congestive failure due to volume overload of the left ventricle may not occur until 2 to 3 months postnatally.

Spontaneous closure of the VSD is estimated to occur in 25 to 50 percent of small to moderate-sized defects, generally during the first year of life. Probably less than 5 percent of large VSDs undergo spontaneous closure. These infants are severely ill with congestive heart failure and pulmonary hypertension; if treated only medically, 25 percent die within the first 6 months. The high pulmonary artery pressures lead to progressive pulmonary vascular obstructive disease, particularly after the second year. Pulmonary artery banding has been performed in small infants in the past to protect the pulmonary vasculature, but the combined mortality of the initial procedure and the subsequent repair of the VSD with debanding approaches 25 percent. For this reason primary surgical closure of the defect is presently recommended in the first year of life in infants with intractable congestive heart failure and failure to thrive, with a mortality quoted at 5 percent or less. All defects with significant pulmonary artery hypertension are generally closed before 24 months to prevent development of obstructive pulmonary vascular disease.

In moderate-size defects with only mild elevation of pulmonary artery pressures medical management is preferred during infancy; only if a large left-to-right shunt (greater than twice systemic blood flow) persists by 4 to 5 years of age is the defect then closed surgically. Surgery is not recommended for small VSDs.

Patients who had their defects closed during infancy show normal growth and development. Pulmonary artery pressures return to normal, as does left ventricular function. In patients operated upon during childhood, left ventricular function may remain mildly depressed and show abnormality with intense exercise, despite lack of clinical symptoms. Patients may have conduction defects after surgical closure, most commonly right bundle branch block or a combination of right bundle branch block with left anterior hemiblock. Complete heart block is fortunately rare.

Ventricular Septal Defect with Pulmonic Stenosis

Hypertrophy of the infundibulum of the right ventricle may occur in patients with large ventricular septal defects (particularly those with right aortic arch). This obstruction leads to progressive decrease in left-to-right shunting and protection of the pulmonary vascular bed from systemic pressures. If the muscle hypertrophy becomes severe enough, right-to-left shunting may eventually occur, initially only during exercise, and patients may have the same clinical features as in tetralogy of Fallot.

Pulmonary stenosis rarely becomes prominent before 4 to 5 years of age. Treatment is surgical repair during childhood with closure of the septal defect and resection of the infundibular muscle bands.

Ventricular Septal Defect with Aortic Insufficiency

Approximately 5 percent of patients with a VSD develop signs of aortic valve incompetence, which may become the predominant problem. It occurs more commonly in males. Supracristal VSD is especially prone to this complication. The right coronary cusp tends to herniate through the VSD in these patients and may cause some degree of right ventricular outflow obstruction. Aortic insufficiency in infracristal VSD is rare and usually is associated with anomalies of the aortic commissures and infundibular pulmonic stenosis. Mild aortic insufficiency may be treated by closure of the VSD alone. With more severe insufficiency, aortic valvuloplasty is performed at the time of VSD closure. The aortic regurgitation appears not to progress after repair. Surgery is carried out as soon as prolapse of a cusp is noticed on angiography or if signs of aortic insufficiency occur.

Left Ventricular to Right Atrial Shunt

Communications between the left ventricle and right atrium constitute less than 1 percent of all congenital cardiac defects. There is a slight female preponderance. Approximately one third of the defects are located above the tricuspid valve, the remainder below in association with malformation of the septal leaflet. The shunt is always large because of the marked pressure difference between the left ventricle and right atrium during systole, which is present from birth. Volume overload of the right ventricle and enlargement of the pulmonary artery occur. The increased pulmonary venous return leads to volume overload of the left side, and heart failure may occur in the first months of life. There is always marked enlargement of the right atrium. The lesion may decrease in size, but spontaneous closure has not been observed.

There is a high incidence of endocarditis (6 percent of recorded cases) and atrial dysrhythmias (5 percent of recorded cases). Because of the large shunt and high endocarditis risk, surgical correction should be performed in early childhood. Long-term postoperative complications include complete heart block (4 percent) and atrial dysrhythmias (3 percent).

Single Ventricle

Connection of both atria usually via two AV valves to a single ventricular chamber is a rare anomaly, accounting for approximately 1 to 1.5 percent of all congenital heart disease. There is a slight male preponderance. In nearly 80 percent of cases the single ventricle is a morphological left ventricle and the relationship of the great vessels is either D-transposed or L-transposed. All patients with D-transposition have some degree of subaortic stenosis, while more than 50 percent of those with L-transposition tend to have subaortic and subpulmonary obstruction.

Half the patients are seen within the first month of life and close to 90 percent within the first 6 months. Without surgical intervention three quarters of these infants die within this period.

Patients without obstruction to pulmonary blood flow present in early infancy with signs of a large left-to-right shunt in congestive failure with growth retardation and frequent respiratory infections. Despite nearly complete mixing of systemic and pulmonary venous blood in the systemic ventricle, cyanosis is not prominent in these children. In patients with obstruction to pulmonary outflow, cyanosis is present and heart failure rare. With pulmonary atresia pulmonary blood flow may be ductus-dependent.

Palliative procedures carried out during infancy consist of pulmonary artery banding in patients without pulmonary stenosis who have unremitting congestive heart failure. Development of secondary subaortic stenosis following this procedure may make a later septation operation impossible. In patients with pulmonary outflow obstruction a systemic to pulmonary shunt is created. The mortality rate for banding ranges from 25 to 50 percent; for shunting it is less than 20 percent. Long-term survival is poor with palliative operations because of development of progressive myocardial fibrosis, secondary subaortic obstruction, or insufficient pulmonary blood flow.

Patients with favorable anatomy should undergo a septation procedure between 4 and 5 years of age. Those with a small ventricle or outlet foramen obstruction should have a modified Fontan procedure with connection of the right atrium to the pulmonary artery, closure of the right-sided inlet valve, and diversion of all ventricular output to the aorta. In infants in the first year of life with refractory congestive heart failure and favorable anatomy, an initial septation procedure should be considered because of the poor results of septation following pulmonary artery banding. Mortality for "corrective" procedures ranges around 40 percent.

Long-term follow-up of patients after septation or the Fontan operation indicates that septation is more likely to result in normal cardiac function. Only half of patients after the Fontan operation were asymptomatic and all patients were still on digitalis and/or diuretics, compared with only 10 percent of patients after septation.

L-Transposition of the Great Arteries

Abnormal rotation of the bulboventricular loop results in ventricular inversion and transposition of the great arteries. The anatomical left ventricle receives the systemic venous return and ejects into the pulmonary artery, and the anatomical right ventricle receives the pulmonary venous return and ejects into the aorta (Fig. 6-2). If no additional anomalies exist, a hemodynamically normal heart is the result; hence the name corrected transposition.

This malformation is rare, occurring in less than 1.5 percent of all congenital heart disease with slight male preponderance. Only 1 percent of patients have physiologically normal hearts. Because of the ventricular inversion the AV valves, the coronary arteries, and the conduction system are also inverted (Fig. 6-3). The left-sided tricuspid valve is frequently insufficient. The left anterior descending coronary artery, originating on the right, traverses the pulmonary outflow tract. The bundle of His has a much longer course, which may explain the very high incidence of heart block, both spontaneously and following surgery. Eighty percent of patients have a large VSD and 70 percent of patients have pulmonary outflow obstruction. Malposition of the heart (dextrocardia or mesocardia) is frequently present.

The majority of patients present in the first month of life with signs of congestive failure in the presence of a large left-to-right shunt through the VSD and with cyanosis and hypercyanotic spells with pulmonary outflow obstruction. Prognosis depends on the degree of hemodynamic abnormality. Patients with a large VSD and no pulmonary stenosis have a higher mortality (35 percent) during the first year of life than those with pulmonary outflow obstruction (20 percent).

Heart failure is initially treated with digitalis and diuretics, and if this is unsuccessful, banding of the

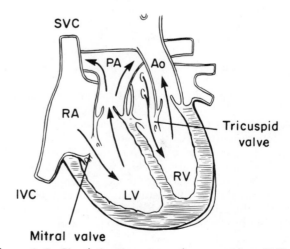

Figure 6-2. Circulation in corrected transposition. SVC = superior vena cava; IVC = inferior vena cava; RA = right atrium; PA = pulmonary artery; Ao = Aorta; RV = right ventricle; LV = left ventricle. (Redrawn from Kidd BSL: Transposition of the great arteries. *In* Keith JD, et al. [Eds.]: Heart Disease in Infancy and Childhood. 3rd ed. New York, Macmillan, 1978.)

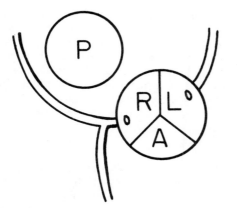

Figure 6–3. Coronary anatomy in corrected transposition. The right coronary artery gives off the anterior descending branch. The left coronary artery has only the circumflex distribution.

pulmonary artery may be performed to relieve failure and protect the pulmonary vascular bed. Nearly 50 percent of children with pulmonary obstruction will require a systemic-to-pulmonary shunt for palliation of cyanosis. Total correction in corrected transposition is surgically difficult and carries a high mortality (40 percent). Because of the abnormal coronary arterial anatomy a conduit repair is required for correction of severe pulmonic stenosis. Systemic AV valve insufficiency may require repair or replacement at the time of VSD closure. Conduction disturbance is present in 40 to 50 percent of patients postoperatively. Patients may develop sudden complete heart block after the age of 20.

Anesthetic Considerations

Uptake of inhalational anesthetic agents is only minimally influenced by a left-to-right shunt unless peripheral perfusion is poorly maintained. Under these circumstances induction with a poorly soluble agent may be accelerated. Induction with intravenous agents, however, may be quite delayed, since a considerable portion of the drug will be recirculated through the lung. If the amount of drug injected is increased to achieve the desired effect more rapidly, side effects of overdose may appear after all drug finally reaches the brain and peripheral circulation.

Increases in peripheral vascular resistance tend to increase left-to-right shunting because of the obstruction to left ventricular outflow. Increases in pulmonary resistance tend to decrease the shunt. With marked obstruction to right ventricular outflow (for example, by embolization), however, reversal of the shunt and cyanosis can occur. In patients with a dynamic increase in pulmonary vascular resistance and a nonrestrictive VSD, administration of oxygen (a potent pulmonary vasodilator) may cause a very large increase in the left-to-right shunt owing to the reduction in pulmonary vascular resistance, resulting in congestive failure and peripheral collapse due to insufficient systemic perfu-

sion. Therefore, in patients with reactive pulmonary vascular resistance, oxygenation during anesthesia must be monitored carefully to avoid flooding of the lung due to a marked reduction in pulmonary vascular resistance. Hypoxia may lead to shunt reversal through an increase in pulmonary vascular resistance.

Patients with small to moderate-sized VSDs most commonly may require anesthesia for elective surgery with the defect still open. If no signs of heart failure are present, they should not have any undue anesthetic risk. The main concern has to be directed toward prevention of endocarditis and air embolization.

In patients with large VSDs, heart failure should be optimally controlled prior to surgery by the use of digitalis, diuretics, and if necessary a peripheral vasodilator (hydralazine). Because chronic pulmonary congestion leads to small airway disease, the airway should be secured by intubation and oxygenation should be carefully monitored to avoid changes in pulmonary vascular resistance. Potent inhalation anesthetics are poorly tolerated by a failing myocardium and may cause severe hypotension. Narcotic-relaxant techniques are better for such patients coming for repair of their cardiac lesion. Nitrous oxide increases pulmonary vascular resistance and may decrease the shunt. High-dose narcotics and ketamine appear to blunt the stress response in the pulmonary vascular bed. Ketamine, because of its indirect sympathomimetic effect, appears to also be well tolerated by patients with borderline myocardial reserve.

In patients with pulmonic obstruction, agents that cause a marked increase in inotropy (such as ketamine) should be avoided. Any increase in right ventricular outflow resistance may easily reverse the shunt. In patients with signs of aortic insufficiency, bradycardia and increases in peripheral vascular resistance may cause significant increase in regurgitation. Mild tachycardia is desirable, as is mild reduction in left ventricular afterload. Isoflurane may be a useful agent under these circumstances, although no cases have been reported. Patients who have undergone repair of their lesion during infancy should be normal postoperatively. They do, however, require endocarditis prophylaxis. Careful electrocardiographic monitoring is required in patients with postoperative conduction defects, although no instance of complete heart block occurring during anesthesia has been reported. Patients whose defects were closed later during childhood may not be able to respond to stress as well as normal controls. Invasive hemodynamic monitoring to assess ventricular function and pulmonary artery pressures probably should be established early for surgery involving large and/or rapid fluid shifts. Patients may require mechanical ventilation postoperatively until fully recovered from anesthesia and surgery, to minimize the work of breathing and optimize pulmonary vascular resistance.

Anesthetic management of patients with corrected transposition will be influenced by the existing hemodynamic abnormality. The alteration in blood flow is similar to that in patients with a large VSD without pulmonary obstruction or to that in patients with tetralogy of Fallot. All patients have to be carefully monitored for conduction disturbances. Endocarditis prophylaxis is indicated in all patients with associated defects. The hemodynamic effect in patients with single ventricle who have undergone Fontan-type repair is physiologically similar to that in patients with "repaired" tricuspid atresia. Anesthetic considerations for these patients will be discussed later.

Eisenmenger Complex and Syndrome

The development of markedly elevated pulmonary vascular resistance with reversal of the shunt in the presence of a large VSD, first described by Victor Eisenmenger, has been termed the Eisenmenger complex. The designation Eisenmenger syndrome describes a pathophysiological entity in which pulmonary hypertension at systemic level due to a high pulmonary vascular resistance leads to a bidirectional or predominantly right-to-left shunt at the aortopulmonary, atrial, or ventricular level. Less than 10 percent of children with a large VSD develop this problem, but it is present in over 50 percent of adults with large aortopulmonary or ventricular communications. Because the underlying defect must allow for equalization of pressures between the ventricles, there is usually a history of congestive failure in infancy which improves as pulmonary vascular resistance increases. Obstructive pulmonary vascular disease may be present after the age of 2 years, and presence of a fixed elevation in pulmonary vascular resistance renders the underlying defect inoperable. Children usually show few symptoms except for occasional exertional dyspnea and fatigue. Cyanosis and failure are rare. Symptoms become increasingly prominent during the late twenties and early thirties. Average age at death, which frequently occurred suddenly, ranged between 33 and 36 years in various series.

Anesthetic Management. Perioperative dehydration should be avoided in patients who are cyanotic, since it may cause an increase in blood viscosity and result in thrombosis in the pulmonary and systemic vascular beds. Meticulous attention should be paid to intravenous lines to prevent embolization of air or clot to the systemic circulation. Since the pulmonary vascular resistance is fixed, shunting is largely determined by systemic vascular resistance. A fall in systemic vascular resistance will lead to increased cyanosis owing to increased right-to-left shunting. High ventilation pressures may cause further reduction in pulmonary blood flow. Pulmonary function in these patients is abnormal, with reductions in total lung capacity, vital capacity, and compliance. Residual and closing volumes are increased.

Various reports of anesthetic management of patients with Eisenmenger syndrome have been published. Recommendations include sedation to reduce preoperative anxiety and oxygen consumption, use of anesthetic agents with minimal effect on peripheral vascular resistance and myocardial contractility (narcotic or ketamine), prevention of hypoxia and hypoventilation intra- and postoperatively, and prevention of bradycardia by the use of anticholinergics. Regional anesthesia with attendant sympathetic blockade is relatively contraindicated in these patients. All patients require endocarditis prophylaxis.

INTRACARDIAC LESIONS PRODUCING PREDOMINANT RIGHT-TO-LEFT SHUNT WITH CYANOSIS

Lesions with Decreased Pulmonary Blood Flow

Tetralogy of Fallot

The combination of VSD, pulmonic valvular and/or infundibular stenosis, right ventricular hypertrophy, and straddling of the VSD by the aorta is known as tetralogy of Fallot. It is the most common cyanotic defect seen after the first year of life, contributing to 10 percent of all congenital cardiac lesions. Males are more often affected than females by a 3:2 ratio, and 25 to 30 percent of patients have a right-sided aortic arch.

The degree of pulmonic obstruction determines the onset and severity of cyanosis. With severe pulmonic stenosis, cyanosis appears with closure of the ductus arteriosus and death occurs within the first 2 to 3 months, unless pulmonary blood flow is improved surgically. Many infants do not develop symptoms until after 3 to 6 months and even then may not appear cyanotic at rest. However, episodes of severe cyanosis with hyperventilation and acidosis, known as hypercyanotic spells, may occur. They are caused by severe infundibular spasm, probably induced by changes in venous return and peripheral vascular resistance. Reduction in peripheral vascular tone leads to decreased pulmonary blood flow, since blood tends to be shunted to the systemic circulation. Fall in venous return further decreases pulmonary blood flow. Squatting may improve symptoms through an increase in venous return from the lower extremities and by increasing peripheral vascular resistance. Treatment consists of intravenous morphine 0.1 to 0.2 mg/kg or propranolol 0.05 to 0.1 mg/kg.

In tetralogy of Fallot both ventricles work at systemic pressure, but volume overload does not occur and congestive heart failure is rare. If pulmonary stenosis is moderate, the patient may be acyanotic and have signs of left-to-right shunt. With progression of infundibular stenosis cyanosis becomes apparent. Chronic hypoxemia leads to polycythemia and the development of collateral circulation to the lungs.

Mortality of untreated patients with tetralogy of Fallot approaches 50 percent by 5 years of age and 70 percent by the age of 10. Only 3 to 5 percent survive to adulthood. Complications occuring early in patients with tetralogy of Fallot are cerebrovascular accidents, probably due to venous thrombosis from polycythemia, cerebral abscesses, and subacute bacterial endocarditis. In infants and children with frequent spells, early corrective surgery is presently advocated and results in low operative mortality (<10 percent). Infants with hypoplasia of the pulmonary arteries are not candidates for early correction. A systemic to pulmonary artery shunt is created to improve pulmonary blood flow and allow growth of the pulmonary vasculature.

The Blalock-Taussig operation is preferred if vessel size is adequate, or a Gore-tex graft may be inserted. Alternatively, the right ventricular outflow tract may be enlarged without closing the VSD. Pulmonary artery growth then appears to be more rapid with forward flow, and repair of the VSD may be possible sooner. The Potts and Waterston-Cooley shunts have been associated with congestive failure and development of pulmonary vascular obstructive disease. Both significantly increase the risk of subsequent intracardiac repair.

Elective repair of tetralogy of Fallot is generally carried out after the age of 2. The right ventricular obstruction has to be completely relieved, if necessary with a large patch crossing the pulmonary valve annulus and extending into the main pulmonary artery. The resulting pulmonary insufficiency appears to be well tolerated. Complications of reparative surgery include residual pulmonic stenosis (10 to 20 percent), residual VSD (5 percent), and, rarely, complete heart block. Right bundle branch block is commonly observed after right ventriculotomy. Between 8 and 11 percent of patients develop supraventricular tachycardia postoperatively. Up to 23 percent of patients develop premature ventricular contractions that occur with exercise. The majority of these patients had elevation of right ventricular pressure preoperatively. In one series, 38 percent of patients with premature ventricular contractions on a resting electrocardiogram died

suddenly within 3 months to 8 years postoperatively. Approximately 7 percent of patients died within 15 years after intracardiac repair. Ventricular premature beats after intracardiac repair should be treated with propranolol or quinidine.

Left and right ventricular dysfunctions have been observed to persist after complete repair of tetralogy of Fallot even in the absence of residual hemodynamic defects. Response to maximal exercise is abnormal, with reduction in maximal oxygen uptake and a reduced cardiac index. Repair before the age of 2 appears to be associated with better preservation of myocardial function.

Pulmonary Atresia with Ventricular Septal Defect

Pulmonary atresia with VSD may be considered an extreme form of tetralogy of Fallot. The majority of infants born with this anomaly become cyanotic shortly after birth and may die within hours after the ductus arteriosus closes. They require a surgical shunt within the first few days of life. The remainder of patients in this group have large and multiple aortopulmonary collaterals and may not exhibit cyanosis until childhood, when the collateral vessels may become inadequate or stenotic. With very large collateral vessels obstructive pulmonary vascular disease may develop.

Definitive repair for these children consists of placement of a valved conduit between the right ventricle and pulmonary artery and closure of the VSD (Fig. 6–4). Large collateral vessels are ligated. Surgery is generally performed between 5 and 15 years of age.

Currently available conduits develop obstruction within 5 to 10 years following the procedure in a significant number of patients. Sixty percent of aortic homografts and probably 30 percent of Dacron conduits with a porcine valve become obstructed and necessitate reoperation within 10 years.

A number of anatomically different congenital cardiac lesions may present with clinical features similar

Figure 6–4. Pulmonary atresia before and after operation. Repair after Rastelli (conduit). Ao = Aorta; RPA = right pulmonary artery; LPA = left pulmonary artery; RV = right ventricle; LV = left ventricle.

to those of tetralogy of Fallot. These include double-outlet right ventricle with subaortic VSD and pulmonary stenosis, single ventricle with pulmonic stenosis, corrected transposition with VSD and pulmonic stenosis, and truncus arteriosus. The physiological considerations important for anesthetic management are similar.

Anesthetic Management. Patient should arrive in the operating room well sedated. Preoperative fluid restriction should be minimized and maintenance fluid given intravenously to prevent hemoconcentration and hypovolemia. Smooth induction is important to prevent increases in oxygen demand or hypercyanotic spells. The agents used should have minimal peripheral vasodilating effects. Mild myocardial depression may relieve infundibular obstruction. If intravenous agents are used, they should be carefully titrated to prevent relative overdose. Intravenous barbiturate requirements may be reduced by half. The airway should be secured by intubation. Excessive airway pressures should be avoided. Adequacy of ventilation should be ascertained by arterial blood gas measurements. Low-dose halothane or narcotic relaxant techniques may be used. Oxygenation is frequently improved under general anesthesia, probably by relaxation of the infundibular muscle, pulmonary vasodilation from higher oxygen concentrations, and reduced peripheral oxygen demands.

Monitoring blood pressure may become problematic in patients with previous shunting procedures using the subclavian arteries. For major surgery intra-arterial and intravenous pressures should be measured directly. This will also allow blood sampling for blood gas and acid-base measurements. Because the major stress rests on the right ventricle in these patients, central venous pressures can be used to assess cardiac performance.

Presence of a right-to-left shunt prolongs induction with poorly soluble inhalational anesthetics. This may be offset by the presence of a surgically created systemic-to-pulmonary shunt. Induction time with highly soluble agents may be nearly normal because these patients usually hyperventilate to maintain a normal arterial P_{CO_2}. Intravenous induction is rapid, but conventional doses may produce undesirable side effects because of high systemic concentrations, since the drugs enter the systemic circulation without passage through the lung.

With a fixed obstruction to pulmonary outflow, right-to-left shunting is influenced by changes in peripheral vascular resistance. A decline in systemic vascular resistance may lead to increasing cyanosis, acidosis, and myocardial depression, creating a vicious circle. In patients with dynamic infundibular stenosis, severe infundibular spasm may be triggered intraoperatively by hyperventilation, hypovolemia, relative anemia, manipulation of intracardiac monitoring lines, and inotropic agents. Prompt treatment is essential. Intravenous morphine (0.1 to 0.2 mg/kg) or propranolol (0.05 to 0.1 mg/kg) should be used. Oxygen may

have little effect in improving systemic oxygenation. Acidosis should be corrected and venous return improved by administration of fluids. If peripheral vasodilatation was a contributing factor, peripheral vascular resistance should be increased by a peripherally acting agent like phenylephrine (NeoSynephrine), (5 to 10 µg/kg IV).

Maintenance of cardiac output is essential since the oxygen content of the blood is low. Bradycardia is very poorly tolerated for this reason. In patients with systemic-to-pulmonary shunts, adequate systemic blood pressure is necessary to maintain pulmonary perfusion.

All patients with right-to-left shunts are at an increased risk of systemic embolization of air or blood clots from intravenous lines. In patients with severe polycythemia, hemodilution to a hematocrit of 55 to 60 should be performed prior to elective surgery. This will improve cardiac output, peripheral perfusion, and oxygen transport. It may also improve the coagulation defects commonly found in polycythemic patients. Hemodilution to normal levels may be very dangerous, however, as oxygen transport will then be seriously limited.

Endocarditis prophylaxis is essential for all surgery associated with bacteremia. Patients with systemic to pulmonary shunts are at particularly high risk.

Patients with cyanosis have a blunted response to hypoxia, which may persist after correction of the underlying lesion. In patients with reduced pulmonary blood flow marked ventilation/perfusion inequalities exist. Positive pressure ventilation may worsen this problem, leading to an increase in dead space ventilation and raised arterial P_{CO_2}.

Patients who have undergone correction present less of an anesthetic problem. They may, however, have some impairment of right and left ventricular function and have a tendency to develop arrhythmias. Ventricular extrasystoles should be treated, since they have been implicated in sudden death. Patients require endocarditis prophylaxis for their lifetime. Presence of residual defects should be determined prior to elective surgery in postcorrection patients.

Lesions with Increased Pulmonary Blood Flow

D-Transposition of the Great Arteries

In transposition of the great arteries the aorta arises above the right ventricle and the pulmonary artery above the left ventricle (Fig. 6–5). The pulmonary and systemic circulations therefore run in parallel instead of in series, and systemic oxygenation depends on mixing between the circulations through anatomical communications.

It is a common malformation. The overall incidence is 5 percent of all congenital heart disease but it is the most common lesion (17 percent) seen during the first

Figure 6–5. Transposition of the great vessels. Schematic representation of systemic and pulmonary blood flow in uncorrected transposition of the great vessels. SVs = systemic veins; PVs = pulmonary veins; Ao = aorta; PA = pulmonary artery. (Redrawn after Kidd BSL: Transposition of the great arteries. *In* Keith JD, et al. [Eds.]: Heart Disease in Infancy and Childhood. 3rd ed. New York, Macmillan, 1978.)

week of life. Without treatment, 50 percent of patients die within the first month, 70 percent within the first 6 months, and 90 percent within the first year of life. There is a marked male preponderance (60 to 70 percent).

Blood shunted anatomically from left to right constitutes the effective systemic blood flow and blood shunted right to left constitutes th effective pulmonary blood flow, while the very large blood volume that is being recirculated constitutes physiologic right or left shunting. Patients with transposition may be divided into groups depending on the presence of VSD and/or restriction of pulmonary blood flow. Transposition with an intact septum is the most common lesion (50 percent), followed by transposition with VSD (30 percent).

Patients present with hypoxemia, acidosis, and/or congestive heart failure in the newborn period or early infancy. If pulmonic stenosis is significant, signs of pulmonary underperfusion occur.

Patients with an intact septum usually are cyanotic within hours of birth as the ductus arteriosus closes, and develop progressive acidosis and failure. They require immediate cardiac catheterization, at which time a balloon atrial septostomy is carried out to allow mixing between the two circulations. The procedure permits survival until "corrective" surgery can be performed. From 10 to 40 percent of those in whom only a balloon septostomy has been performed die within the first year. Patients with an intact septum and a large patent ductus arteriosus (PDA) may be less cyanotic with reversal of flow through the ductus. The persistence of a large ductus is a lethal lesion in transposition, associated with a 90 percent mortality in the first 6 months with or without surgery.

Infants with a large VSD will have adequate mixing despite the transposition and are usually only mildly cyanotic. They do, however, develop severe congestive heart failure between 2 and 6 weeks of age, often resistant to medical management, and may require pulmonary artery banding or early correction for survival. Transposition is associated with the early development of pulmonary obstructive disease within the first year, even in the absence of VSD or patent ductus arteriosus. The high pressures and/or flows in the pulmonary artery combined with polycythemia may be responsible for these changes. Most patients demonstrate preferential perfusion to the right lung. Patients with VSD and pulmonic stenosis may present later, as heart failure is rare and cyanosis mild. With severe pulmonary stenosis, a shunting procedure to improve pulmonary circulation may become necessary.

Although babies with transposition are commonly well developed at birth, they subsequently develop severe growth retardation.

At present the trend in most surgical centers is toward early correction. The most commonly performed operations are the Mustard and Senning procedures (Fig. 6–6). These are only physiological corrections, directing systemic venous return through the mitral valve into the left ventricle and pulmonary artery and pulmonary venous return through the tricuspid valve into the right ventricle and aorta via placement of an intra-atrial baffle. An elective Mustard or Senning repair is commonly performed between 6 and 12 months to prevent pulmonary vascular disease. Mortality for this procedure ranges from 5 to 20 percent in patients in the first few weeks and months of life.

Anatomical correction by switching of the great

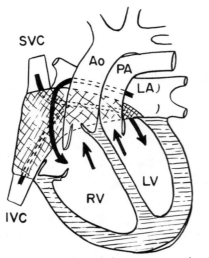

Figure 6–6. Transposition of the great vessels. Schematic representation of systemic and pulmonary blood flow after an atrial inversion procedure (Mustard or Senning). SVC = superior vena cava; IVC = inferior vena cava; Ao = Aorta; PA = pulmonary artery; LA = left atrium; RV = right ventricle; LV = left ventricle.

arteries with coronary reimplantation (Fig. 6–7) has recently been advocated by Jatene for newborns with an intact septum instead of balloon septostomy. It is also used in patients with a large VSD to avoid the high combined mortality of a banding operation followed by late intra-atrial baffle repair.

In the patient with left ventricular outflow obstruction a Rastelli procedure is performed between 2 and 4 years of age. If inadequate blood flow is present in infancy a systemic- to-pulmonary shunt is performed initially. In the Rastelli procedure, blood flow is diverted from the left ventricle via the VSD and a baffle to the aorta, and the pulmonary artery is divided and connected via prosthetic graft to the right ventricle. With normal pulmonary vascular resistance a valveless conduit is used because of the high incidence of conduit obstruction with valved grafts.

In patients with raised pulmonary vascular resistance a palliative Mustard operation without closure of the VSD improves systemic oxygenation. Late complications after Mustard or Senning repair include systemic and/or pulmonary venous obstruction, atrial dysrrhthmias including sick sinus syndrome, tricuspid incompetence, and systemic (right) ventricular dysfunction. Obstruction of valved conduits occurs in up to 60 percent of patients within 10 years, depending on the material used. Patients who have undergone arterial switch may be prone to developing early coronary vascular changes.

Anesthetic Management. Other than patients with severe pulmonic obstruction who are awaiting a Rastelli procedure, it is rare that a patient with D-transposition will be encountered who requires noncardiac surgery prior to intra-atrial repair. No experience with anesthesia for these patients who need noncardiac operations has been reported.

These patients are at a very high risk for systemic embolization. Patients with only balloon septostomy have a 10 to 20 percent incidence of cerebrovascular accidents, which are thought to be due to thrombosis. Perioperative dehydration increases the viscosity of the already hyperviscous polycythemic blood and may lead to thrombosis. Hematocrit should be kept below 60, if necessary by hemodilution. Endocarditis prophylaxis is mandatory.

Because of the low effective pulmonary blood flow, induction of anesthesia with inhalational agents is prolonged and adverse side effects may linger after the anesthetic is discontinued. Intravenous agents must be used with caution; they have a rapid onset of action, since most of the venous return enters the aorta. Chronic congestive failure is often present with congestion of the lung and low ventilatory volumes, which predispose the patient to atelectasis. Myocardial depression is poorly tolerated, and bradycardia is usu-

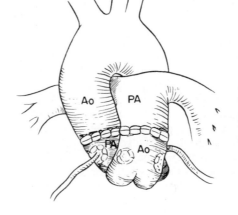

Figure 6–7. Repair of transposition of the great vessels, by arterial switch. *Left,* Before operation. *Right,* After operation. Ao = Aorta; PA = pulmonary artery. (Redrawn after Jatene AD, Iontes VF, Paulista PP: Anatomical correction of transposition of the great vessels. J Thorac Cardiovasc Surg 72:364, 1976.)

ally associated with acidosis. Because of the compromised cardiac and ventilatory function, postoperative mechanical ventilation may be advisable.

Anesthetic agents should have minimal cardiovascular side effects. Narcotic-relaxant techniques, particularly with fentanyl and/or ketamine, have been used with minimal side effects. Low concentrations (0.5 to 0.75 percent) of isoflurane may be used to supplement relaxant techniques. In patients with limited pulmonary blood flow, increases in pulmonary vascular resistance through coughing and struggling should be avoided. In the presence of a systemic-to-pulmonary shunt, maintenance of blood pressure is essential to allow pulmonary perfusion.

An ever-increasing number of children who have survived reparative procedures may present for noncardiac surgery in later years. Although they appear clinically normal without evidence of cyanosis or failure, they may not tolerate anesthesia and surgery well. Atrial dysrhythmias are common after intra-atrial repairs and may become more frequent with time. The most serious of these is sick sinus syndrome, which may necessitate placement of a temporary pacemaker for surgery if a permanent pacemaker is not already in place. There may be systemic venous obstruction at the baffle site, leading to signs of venous congestion. Significant baffle obstruction usually requires reoperation. Left-sided baffle obstruction (more common after the Senning procedure) may lead to pulmonary hypertension. Increases in peripheral vascular resistance will worsen the condition of the patient under these circumstances.

Insertion of pulmonary artery catheters in these patients is technically difficult because of the tortuous pathway of the venous blood flow and may cause arrhythmias and/or baffle disruption. The right ventricle, carrying the systemic load, has limited reserve and may fail if stressed by rapid fluid shifts or use of myocardial depressing agents. Patients are still at risk for endocarditis, and patients with conduits are at a higher risk postoperatively than before. Arterial switching operations are relatively recent, and therefore very little is known about the long-term effects of this procedure. Coronary artery disease may appear early in these patients. ECG monitoring for ischemia and an anesthetic technique that reduces myocardial oxygen demand are essential choices.

Asplenia and Polysplenia Syndrome

Agenesis of the spleen is associated with malposition of the abdominal viscera and complex cyanotic congenital heart disease (Ivemark syndrome). A combination of the following defects is usually present: L- or D-transposition of the great vessels, pulmonary atresia or severe stenosis, large defects or absence of the atrial and ventricular septa, atrioventricular canal, total anomalous pulmonary venous return, persistence of the left superior vena cava, and absence of the coronary sinus. In the majority of cases there are bilateral trilobed lungs. Dextrocardia is present in 50 percent of cases.

The condition is extremely rare (0.1 percent of congenital heart disease) and because of the complexity of the lesions, surgical correction at present is not feasible. Males are affected more frequently, by a 2:1 ratio. Two thirds of patients die within the first 2 months of life. Survivors may be aided by palliative surgery to improve pulmonary blood flow. These patients are extremely susceptible to overwhelming infection, and prophylatic antibiotics and bacterial vaccines may have to be used. Patients have Howell-Jolly bodies in the peripheral blood smear.

Polysplenia is defined as the presence of two or more spleens of nearly equal size and is nearly always associated with complex cardiac malformation. The syndrome is extremely rare. The lesions most commonly associated with polysplenia are total anomalous pulmonary venous return, absence of the hepatic portion of the inferior vena cava with azygos continuation, atrial septal defect, and situs inversus. The lungs are bilaterally bilobed. Symptoms of heart failure usually develop in infancy. Cyanosis is uncommon. Prognosis depends on the underlying defect but is in general better than in asplenia. The lesions are frequently operable. The patients do not appear to be more susceptible to infection.

Anesthetic Management. No experience with anesthesia in asplenic or polysplenic patients has been reported. Choice of technique and degree of monitoring will depend on the presentation of the dominant hemodynamic derangement and the proposed procedure. Prevention of embolization and endocarditis is essential.

Double-Outlet Right Ventricle

In double-outlet right ventricle (DORV) both great vessels arise from the morphological right ventricle. There is always an associated VSD. This malformation accounts for less than 0.5 percent of all congenital heart disease and shows no predilection for either sex or race. Prematurity is common, as is the presence of coarctation and mitral valve disease. Clinical presentation is largely determined by the location of the ventricular septal defect in relation to the great vessels and the presence or absence of pulmonic stenosis (Fig. 6–8).

Patients with subaortic VSD clinically resemble those with a large VSD and are acyanotic until pulmonary vascular disease develops. The majority of these patients, however, have associated pulmonic stenosis, and their clinical presentation is similar to that in tetralogy of Fallot. They compose the majority of patients with DORV. Patients with subpulmonic VSD compose the so-called Taussig-Bing group of DORV, which is rarely associated with pulmonic stenosis. They clinically resemble patients with D-transposition and are cyanotic from birth. In rare cases the VSD is either beneath both great vessels or completely remote. The

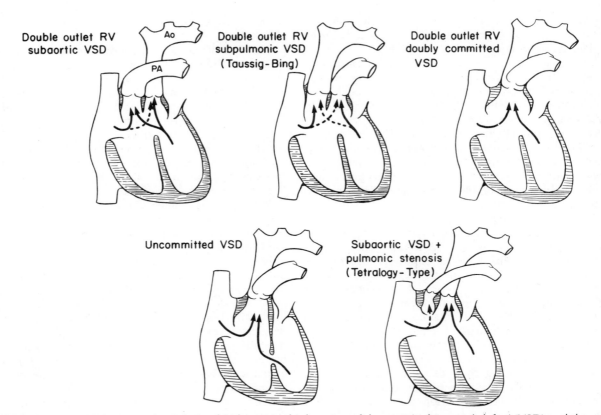

Figure 6–8. Double outlet ventricle. Relationship between the location of the ventricular septal defect (VSD) and the great vessels. The first diagram represents the most common form of double outlet right ventricle. Ao = Aorta; PA = pulmonary artery.

latter anatomy is usually associated with other complex anomalies like AV canal and the asplenia syndrome.

Patients with unrestricted blood flow to the lung present with congestive heart failure and/or cyanosis in early infancy. Presence of associated coarctation (25 to 30 percent of Taussig-Bing group) or mitral valve disease (30 percent of subaortic VSD without pulmonary stenosis) is an ominous prognostic feature; mortality approaches 100 percent within the first 6 months.

Patients with pulmonic stenosis usually present later and generally have no other associated defects, appearing clinically similar to those with tetralogy of Fallot. They have the best prognosis of all groups of patients with DORV, as 75 percent survive to adulthood, while only 50 percent of patients with only subaortic VSD and unrestricted pulmonary blood flow and 35 percent of patients with the Taussig-Bing malformation survive early childhood.

Medical treatment in patients with volume and pressure overload consists of control of congestive heart failure by digitalis and diuretics. Because of the complex anatomy normally present, surgical correction is generally delayed until 2 to 4 years of age and only palliative operations are performed in infancy. These include pulmonary artery (PA) banding to control congestive heart failure and prevent development of pulmonary vascular obstructive disease, and creation of a systemic-to-pulmonary shunt in the patient with pulmonic stenosis and insufficient pulmonary blood flows. Surgical correction consists of diverting the left ventricular output via an intracardiac tunnel to the aorta, which may necessitate enlargement of the VSD. Blood from the right ventricle flows around the tunnel to the pulmonary artery. Enlargement of the right ventricular outflow tract or interposition of a prosthesis may be necessary in patients with pulmonic stenosis. Repair of a Taussig-Bing anomaly may necessitate conversion of the lesion to D-transposition with subsequent atrial inversion (Mustard or Senning procedure) or arterial switch.

Anesthetic Consideration. Cardiac function in DORV patients who have had palliative surgery will be similar to that in patients who have VSD with PA banding, D-transposition with PA banding, or tetralogy of Fallot with or without a systemic-to-pulmonary shunt. Prevention of systemic embolization and endocarditis prophylaxis are important.

Myocardial depression, excessive peripheral vasodilatation, and increases in pulmonary vascular resistance should be avoided. After correction patients may appear normal clinically, but they may exhibit reduced myocardial reserve under stress and may develop conduction disturbances in later life. Endocarditis prophylaxis is particularly important in patients with external valved conduits.

Double-Outlet Left Ventricle

In double-outlet left ventricle both great arteries arise entirely or predominantly above the left ventricle. Fourteen diferent anatomical types of this malformation have been described. Patients may present with signs of tetralogy of Fallot, transposition, large VSD, Ebstein anomaly, or tricuspid atresia. Surgical palliation and either anatomical or physiological correction are usually possible with acceptable risk if patients survive infancy. Anesthetic management should be guided by the predominant physiological derangement. Endocarditis prophylaxis is required pre- and postoperatively.

OBSTRUCTIVE CARDIAC LESIONS

Lesions Causing Left Ventricular Outflow Obstruction

Valvular Aortic Stenosis

Valvular aortic stenosis represents one of the more common congenital defects, accounting for 3 to 6 percent of all congenital heart disease. It is much more common in males, by a 4:1 ratio. Twenty percent of patients have associated defects, most commonly patent ductus arteriosus and coarctation of the aorta. A bicuspid aortic valve is present in approximately 1 percent of the population but will generally not cause aortic stenosis or insufficiency until after childhood. Thickening and increased rigidity of the valve tissue and varying degrees of commissural fusion constitute the basic malformation in valvular aortic stenosis. Only severe stenosis, usually with unicuspid valve and hypoplastic aortic valve ring, is symptomatic in infancy. The vast majority of children with aortic stenosis are clinically asymptomatic.

The essential hemodynamic abnormality consists of a pressure gradient between the left ventricle and the aorta during the systolic ejection period. Blood flow is turbulent and the pressure gradient is proportional to the square of the flow rate across the valve. The left ventricle develops concentric hypertrophy, which offers resistance to filling. The mean left atrial pressure does not rise, except in severe stenosis, but the left atrium develops vigorous contractions that prevent elevation of the pulmonary venous pressure while at the same time elevating left ventricular end-diastolic pressure sufficient for effective left ventricular action.

Left ventricular myocardial fibrosis may develop over time. Left ventricular ejection is prolonged, which leads to changes in the second heart sound (narrow splitting or single). Myocardial blood supply may be compromised owing to myocardial hypertrophy and raised end-diastolic intracavitary pressure. Shortened diastole, as in tachycardia, will worsen this situation.

Most children have only a murmur and are otherwise normal. The major threats to these children are from endocarditis and sudden death, especially with exercise. The risk of endocarditis, which may occur in more than 4 percent of patients, is unrelated to the severity of obstruction. The risk of sudden death is reported to be between 4 and 18 percent.

Critical aortic stenosis is present when the pressure gradient across the valve is greater than 75 mmHg in the presence of a normal cardiac output, or the valve area is less than 0.5 cm^2 per m^2 of body surface area. These patients are always symptomatic and require surgery. Infants present with dyspnea and congestive failure. Older children may show dyspnea, syncope, or anginal pains.

Surgery consists of open valvotomy. This procedure usually can palliate the symptoms with significant reduction in the pressure gradient. Percutaneous balloon valvuloplasty may also be used in cases of moderate to severe stenosis. Since the valve is malformed, however, re-stenosis, calcification, or aortic insufficiency may develop with time in a large number of these children. Valve replacement is usually postponed as long as possible, since it will require repeat operations to replace the valve for inadequate size or malfunction. Critical aortic stenosis in newborns and infants is frequently associated with endocardial fibroelastosis from myocardial ischemia and mitral insufficiency from papillary muscle dysfunction. Operative mortality is greater than 50 percent among these patients.

Supravalvular Aortic Stenosis

In supravalvular aortic stenosis the aorta is locally or diffusely narrowed above the level of the coronary arteries. This is most commonly associated with Williams syndrome—idiopathic infantile hypercalcemia. Patients are often retarded. Since the coronary arteries are located proximal to the obstruction, they are subjected to the high pressures of the left ventricle, are frequently tortuous, and may develop premature coronary arteriosclerosis. Clinical symptoms are similar to those of valvular aortic stenosis. Treatment consists of patch enlargement of the narrowed segment if localized stenosis is present.

Discrete Subvalvular Aortic Stenosis

In this lesion a membranous diaphragm or ring encircling the left ventricular outflow tract is present. The malformation accounts for 8 to 10 percent of all cases of congenital aortic stenosis. Jet lesions of the aortic cusps occur with this type of aortic stenosis, causing valve degeneration with development of aortic insufficiency. There is a very high risk of infective endocarditis. Clinical presentation is similar to that of valvular aortic stenosis and depends on the severity of obstruction. Because of the likelihood of development of progressive obstruction and aortic insufficiency, surgery is recommended even for mild to moderate stenosis. It consists of excision of the membranous or fibrous ridge. Because of the existing jet lesion and scarring following manipulation of the valve during surgery, children with this malformation may eventually require valve replacement.

Anesthetic Considerations in Aortic Stenosis

Increases in the inotropic state of the heart or increases in peripheral vascular resistance tend to increase the pressure gradient across the stenotic area. Tachycardia shortens the duration of diastole more than systole and may cause myocardial ischemia in these patients. The stroke volume is limited by the size of the aortic orifice and ejection time. Peripheral vasodilatation may critically lower blood pressure because cardiac output is fixed. This reduces myocardial perfusion dangerously.

Anesthetic agents with minimal effects on myocardial performance and heart rate should be chosen. Prevention of anxiety and stress and the resulting tachycardia are important. Low-dose inhalation anesthesia or narcotic relaxant techniques may be useful. For major surgery, invasive monitoring should be established. Endocarditis prophylaxis is of utmost importance. Patients who have undergone valvuloplasty usually have a residual defect that should be assessed prior to elective surgery. They are still at high risk for endocarditis. Patients with critical stenosis should not undergo elective noncardiac surgery.

Hypoplastic Left Heart Syndrome

Atresia of the aortic valve, associated with atresia or severe stenosis of the mitral valve, hypoplasia or absence of the left ventricle, and hypoplasia of the ascending aorta or interrupted aortic arch constitute the hypoplastic left heart syndrome. It is more common in males and affects 7 to 9 percent of all infants seen with cardiac disease. Systemic perfusion is maintained via a patent ductus arteriosus and an atrial septal defect. Severe heart failure is always present. Mortality approaches 95 percent within the first month.

Surgical palliation is possible in selected patients (Fig. 6–9). The heart is converted physiologically to a single-ventricle system with the proximal pulmonary artery connected to the aorta and supplying systemic perfusion. The distal pulmonary artery is banded or pulmonary blood flow is supplied via an aortopulmonary graft. Eventual physiological correction consists of a modified Fontan procedure with redirection of pulmonary venous return to the right ventricle, which supplies the aorta.

Anesthetic Considerations. Only palliated patients will ever be seen for noncardiac surgery. They are at risk for systemic embolization and endocarditis. Patients will exhibit various degrees of cyanosis depending on atrial mixing and pulmonary blood flow. Pulmonary venous return has to pass across an ASD to the right atrium and right ventricle to reach the aorta. Maintenance of normal pulmonary and systemic vas-

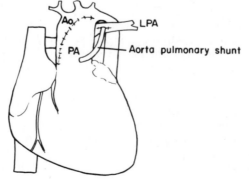

Figure 6–9. Palliation of hypoplastic left heart syndrome. RA = right atrium; Ao = Aorta; RV = right ventricle; MPA = main pulmonary artery; PDA = patent ductus arteriosus. (After Norwood WI, Lang P: N Engl J Med 308:23, 1983.)

cular resistance are essential. After physiological correction patients need sufficient venous pressure to maintain pulmonary and hence systemic perfusion, as the right atrium becomes the systemic venous chamber.

Lesions Causing Right Ventricular Outflow Obstruction

Pulmonary Stenosis

The presence of a pressure gradient between the right ventricle and the pulmonary artery constitutes the main physiological derangement in pulmonary stenosis. It is an associated feature in 25 to 30 percent of congenital cardiac lesions but occurs as an isolated defect in about 10 percent of patients with congenital heart disease. It is the lesion most commonly associated with Noonan syndrome. Most commonly, the stenosis is at the valve level with fusion of the leaflets producing a dome-shaped valve with a small central opening. The severity of clinical symptoms depends on the degree of obstruction to right ventricular outflow. Patients with mild to moderate obstruction are generally asymptomatic, and the stenosis is usually discovered during a routine examination because of the presence of a systolic murmur.

Secondary changes include hypertrophy of the right ventricle (which may produce infundibular stenosis) and poststenotic dilatation of the pulmonary trunk.

In severe stenosis, right ventricular pressure may exceed the pressure in the left ventricle. Right atrial pressure is elevated and right-to-left shunting occurs across a patent foramen ovale or atrial septal defect. If no communication between the right and left heart exists, syncope may occur during exercise because of inability to increase cardiac output. Right ventricular ischemic changes with myocardial fibrosis and coronary artery occlusions may develop in these patients, leading to right ventricular failure.

All symptomatic patients, or those with right ventricular to pulmonary artery gradients exceeding 70 mmHg, require relief of their obstruction. Patients with gradients of less than 50 mmHg usually do not become worse over time. Obstruction may be relieved by open or closed valvotomy or percutaneous valvuloplasty. The latter is not recommended for patients with associated infundibular stenosis. Successful valvotomy will lead to a reduction in right ventricular pressure to half of preoperative values or lower. Infundibular stenosis will usually improve with time. In the presence of a dysplastic valve, enlargement of the valve ring may be necessary, leading to postoperative pulmonary valve insufficiency.

Infants with critical pulmonic stenosis usually present within 24 to 48 hours of birth with cyanosis and metabolic acidosis. Pulmonary blood flow is ductus-dependent. These patients frequently have hypoplasia of the right ventricle associated with endomyocardial fibrosis. Relief of the right ventricular outflow obstruction has to be performed on an emergency basis, frequently combined with a systemic-to-pulmonary shunt, since pulmonary blood flow may still be insufficient. Right-to-left shunting, even with adequate relief, may persist for some time postoperatively owing to the stiff, noncompliant right ventricle maintaining elevated right-sided pressures and patency of the foramen ovale. Infusion of prostaglandin E_1 may maintain pulmonary perfusion via the ductus until the right ventricle has adapted to forward flow. Surgical mortality ranges from 15 to 40 percent. Without surgical intervention patients do not survive infancy.

Primary Infundibular Stenosis. This lesion is rare as an isolated malformation. If the stenosis is discrete, immediately below the valve, the clinical symptoms are similar to those of valvular stenosis and depend on the degree of obstruction. If, however, there is a long narrow segment, the obstruction behaves more dynamically and may vary with the degree of muscular activity. It becomes worse during exercise or with positive inotropic drugs. Treatment is surgical if symptoms and/or significant pressure gradients exist.

Anomalous Right Ventricular Muscle Bands. Aberrant right ventricular muscle bands cause division of the right ventricle into a proximal high-pressure chamber and a distal low-pressure chamber. Clinical presentation is similar to that of valvular or infundibular stenosis. Treatment is surgical.

Peripheral Pulmonic Stenosis. Stenosis of the pulmonary arteries, either proximal or distal, occurs in 2 to 3 percent of all patients with congenital heart disease. This and patency of the ductus arteriosus are the lesions most commonly associated with the congenital rubella syndrome. Patients with mild to moderate bilateral stenosis or unilateral disease are usually asymptomatic. Patients with severe obstruction present with dyspnea, fatigue, and signs of right heart failure. Treatment is surgical if the obstruction is located proximally. Multiple distal stenoses may improve with growth of the patient; otherwise, death occurs during infancy or early childhood.

Anesthetic Considerations. All patients with pulmonic stenosis (pre- or postoperatively) need endocarditis prophylaxis. Patients with mild degrees of obstruction should otherwise experience no anesthetic problems. Patients with moderate degrees of obstruction or those who have had relief of severe pulmonic obstruction and appear clinically normal may have limited myocardial reserve. Increase in pulmonary vascular resistance may cause right heart failure. During stressful surgery, right heart function should be carefully monitored. Patients with infundibular stenosis may benefit from mild reduction in myocardial contractility, such as is induced by 0.5 percent halothane.

Pulmonary Atresia. Absence of the pulmonary valve with an intact ventricular septum and varying degrees of right ventricular hypoplasia accounts for about 1 percent of all congenital heart disease. Pulmonary blood flow is completely dependent on the ductus arteriosus, which is frequently hypoplastic.

Symptoms appear shortly after birth with cyanosis and tachypnea. Metabolic acidosis and signs of heart failure may develop rapidly. Patients require palliation or correction within the first few days of life. Patency of the ductus arteriosus is maintained with prostaglandin E_1 or E_2. In the presence of severe hypoplasia of the right ventricle or atresia of the main pulmonary artery, a systemic-to-pulmonary shunt is performed, combined with balloon atrioseptostomy. If the right ventricle is normal, open or closed valvotomy is performed and the patient is maintained on a prostaglandin infusion until the right ventricle has adapted to increasing forward flow. In patients with questionable hypoplasia, a systemic-to-pulmonary shunt in addition to valvotomy may have to be performed to maintain pulmonary perfusion and systemic oxygenation.

Prognosis without surgery is dismal: Most patients die within the first few weeks of life. Even with surgery these patients do poorly because of their abnormal right ventricular anatomy and function. Surgical mortality may approach 50 percent, and three quarters of palliated patients do not survive the first year of life. In patients with a severely hypoplastic thickened right ventricle, insufficient growth of the right ventricle occurs even after successful valvotomy. These patients are clinically similar to those with tricuspid atresia, and their pulmonary atresia may be "corrected" with a Fontan-type operation. In patients with atresia of the pulmonary trunk, a Rastelli operation can be performed in later childhood if the right ventricle is of adequate size.

Anesthetic Considerations. Patients presenting for elective surgery should have a functioning systemic-to-pulmonary shunt or should have undergone relief of the obstruction by valvotomy, patch graft, conduit insertion, or right ventricular bypass. Endocarditis prophylaxis is necessary in all patients. Anesthetic management has to be tailored to the specific hemodynamic sequelae of the corrective or palliative procedure. Maintenance of acceptable systemic pressure, preload, and pulmonary vascular resistance are essential. The right ventricle in these patients may function abnormally permanently and may fail with surgical stress or use of myocardial depressing agents.

Lesions Causing Left Ventricular Inflow Obstruction

Mitral Stenosis

Isolated mitral stenosis is one of the rarest forms of congenital heart disease, occuring in 0.6 percent of autopsied and 0.2 to 0.4 percent of clinically diagnosed patients with congenital heart disease. It is more common in males.

Developmental abnormalities of the mitral valve leaflets, commissures, chordae tendineae, annulus, supravalvular area, or papillary muscles may lead to obstruction of left ventricular filling. Left atrial pressure rises as a compensatory mechanism to maintain blood flow across the stenotic area. With further reduction in valve orifice, blood flow becomes turbulent, which increases resistance to total flow and leads to a higher pressure gradient. Pulmonary venous pressure becomes secondarily elevated, eventually leading to elevation of pulmonary artery and right ventricular pressures. The vascular congestion results in a decrease in static and dynamic compliance. Bronchial venous congestion leads to edema of the bronchial mucosa and increased airway resistance. The work of breathing is increased and abnormalities in gas exchange are common with significant disease. Pulmonary interstitial or alveolar edema occurs if pulmonary capillary hydrostatic pressures exceeds plasma oncotic pressure and the maximal transport capacity of the pulmonary lymphatics.

Left ventricular filling depends on the size of the valve orifice and diastolic filling time. Tachycardia will lead to marked elevation in atrial pressure and reduction in cardiac output. Left ventricular dysfunction from ischemia and fibrosis frequently complicates severe stenosis. Approximately 50 percent of patients with congenital mitral stenosis have other congenital cardiac anomalies.

Patients commonly present with exertional dyspnea and recurrent pulmonary infections. Infants may show failure to thrive, and episodes of congestive heart failure may occur. The diagnosis is frequently established late. Patients with mild to moderate stenosis (gradient less than 25 mmHg across the mitral valve) are managed medically with control of failure and attention to pulmonary infections and endocarditis. Survival appears to be related mostly to the presence of associated cardiac lesions, and the median survival is 3 years.

Patients with intractable congestive failure, pulmonary edema, or pulmonary artery hypertension at systemic level require surgical intervention. Unrelieved left atrial hypertension will lead to progressive obstructive pulmonary vascular disease. Mitral valvotomy or fenestration of the mitral valve is generally carried out in infants or small children. With severely deformed valves, radical valvuloplasty is recommended to avoid replacement. These procedures will generally palliate these patients sufficiently to allow for growth and development and relief of clinical symptoms. Eventually mitral valve replacement will become necessary in the majority of cases.

Prognosis of symptomatic infants is poor. Forty percent die within the first 6 months irrespective of therapy. Surgical mortality is reported between 30 and 40 percent, with 50 percent of patients surviving beyond 5 to 10 years. Presently less than 20 percent of patients survive to adulthood.

Supravalvular Ring

Accumulation of connective tissue arising from the atrial surface of the mitral valve produces a supravalvular ring, reducing the effective mitral orifice. It rarely occurs as an isolated malformation but is usually associated with some degree of valvular mitral stenosis. The clinical presentation is indistinguishable from valvular stenosis. Treatment consists of surgical excision of the ring tissue.

Parachute Mitral Valve—Shone Syndrome

Insertion of all chordae tendineae into a single papillary muscle leads to a parachute deformity of the mitral valve. Blood flow from the left atrium must pass through the interchordal spaces, and various degrees of functional mitral stenosis are the result. The lesion is commonly associated with other forms of left-sided obstruction, for example, supravalvular mitral ring, subvalvular or valvular aortic stenosis, and coarctation of the aorta. Presence of all four obstructive lesions together constitutes the Shone syndrome. Median survival approaches 10 years of age and correlates best with left ventricular size. Patients are managed medically with control of heart failure and pulmonary infections throughout childhood, since relief of the obstruction requires mitral valve replacement.

Anesthetic Considerations

Because of the rarity of the lesion and the poor prognosis, no experience with anesthesia in patients with any form of congenital mitral stenosis has been reported. Extrapolating from experience with adults, the following management suggestions could be made. All preoperative and the majority of postoperative patients will have a pressure gradient across the mitral valve. Flow through the valve occurs during diastole, and shortening diastole will decrease ventricular filling. Hypovolemia and reduction in preload may decrease left atrial pressure below the pressure necessary to pump blood across the stenotic valve. With reduction in afterload, the heart may be unable to compensate by increasing stroke volume or cardiac output, since both are limited by the amount of blood that can pass across the stenotic area. Overzealous administration of fluids or alterations in position may increase central blood volume and cause a rapid rise in left atrial pressure; this may lead to pulmonary edema, since the volume cannot be transported rapidly across the stenosis. Patients are at risk for bacterial endocarditis. Patients may have marked alterations in gas exchange.

The anesthetic technique chosen should cause no tachycardia, minimal vasodilatation, and no depression of myocardial function. Preload must be maintained. Tachycardia, if it occurs, requires prompt treatment with digitalis, propranolol, or verapamil. Atrial fibrillation is extremely uncommon in children with mitral stenosis, as is systemic embolization. Congestive failure should be controlled, but without excessive depletion of intravascular volume, since induction of anesthesia may lead to severe hypotension under these circumstances. Hypotension, if due to peripheral vasodilatation, should be treated with judicious use of a peripheral vasoconstrictor like phenylephrine.

Because of frequently seen disturbances in pulmonary gas exchange, the airway should be secured and positive pressure ventilation, which tends to counteract pulmonary edema, should be utilized. Patients require higher inspired oxygen concentrations. Hypoxia may lead to acute right heart failure through a further increase in pulmonary vascular resistance.

Circulatory and fluid status for any major surgery should be assessed by intravascular monitoring. Electrolyte abnormalities caused by diuretic therapy should be normalized prior to elective surgery. Pulmonary artery monitoring will reflect only filling status of the left atrium, with left ventricular end-diastolic pressure dependent on the gradient across the valve and the outflow resistance of the left ventricle. Acute elevations in left atrial pressure may be treated with an increase in positive pressure ventilation and venodilatation (nitroglycerin, low-dose nitroprusside, and reverse Trendelenburg position) to promote venous pooling. Patients who decompensate during surgery may need inotropic support.

A narcotic-relaxant technique may be a prudent choice. Induction of anesthesia may be markedly prolonged secondary to low cardiac output. Ketamine causes less tachycardia in infants and children and will maintain vascular tone. Inhalation anesthetics may be poorly tolerated in the presence of a low, fixed cardiac output. Regional techniques may cause extensive sympathetic blockade, which will readily lead to hypotension and necessitate the use of vasopressors. Fluid therapy may cause left atrial hypertension and pulmonary edema when the sympathetic block wears off.

Cor Triatriatum

In cor triatriatum the left atrium is abnormally portioned into two chambers, the upper one receiving the pulmonary veins and the lower containing the mitral valve. Communication between the two chambers is through fenestrations in the dividing membrane. The hemodynamic consequence is pulmonary venous obstruction similar to that in mitral stenosis. The malformation occurs in about 0.5 percent of all congenital heart disease. Males are slightly more affected.

In classic cor triatriatum, no communication exists between the two left atrial chambers and the right atrium. Consequent to the obstruction of pulmonary venous return, pulmonary artery hypertension develops with right ventricular hypertrophy. Onset of symptoms is usually within the first few years of life, characterized by breathlessness and frequent respiratory infections. Patients with severe obstruction present with pulmonary edema and right heart failure and are often considered to have primary pulmonary disease. Death occurs within months if the obstruction is not relieved by surgical excision of the membrane dividing the atrium. Patients who survive the operation (40 percent mortality) have an excellent prognosis. The pulmonary vascular changes appear to be reversible.

Some patients with subdivided left atria have connections between the upper chamber and the right atrium via a patent foramen ovale or atrial septal defect. The clinical presentation is similar to that of total anomalous pulmonary venous return. Correct diagnosis is often established only at surgery or autopsy. Treatment consists of excision of the obstructing membrane and closure of the intra-atrial communication. Surgical enlargement of the left atrium may be required.

Anesthetic Considerations. Patients with classic cor triatriatum have clinical signs and symptoms similar to those of mitral stenosis and should be managed accordingly. Patients who have undergone surgical repair should be normal clinically but require endocarditis prophylaxis.

Lesions Causing Right Ventricular Inflow Obstruction

Tricuspid Atresia

Atresia of the tricuspid valve is always associated with an ASD (usually a patent foramen ovale). The mitral valve and left ventricle are hyperplastic and the right ventricle is hypoplastic or absent. Tricuspid atresia occurs in 1.5 to 3 percent of all patients with congenital heart disease and is slightly more common in males.

Tricuspid atresia can be divided into three different types (I, II, and III), depending on the relationship of the great vessel (normal, D-transposed, or L-transposed) (Fig. 6–10). Further subclassification relates to the presence of pulmonic stenosis and/or a ventricular septal defect. Fifty percent of all patients with tricuspid atresia have normally related great vessels, a small VSD, and pulmonary atresia and stenosis. Only 10 to

Tricuspid Atresia With No Transposition (69 percent)

Pulmonary atresia

Pulmonary hypoplasia, small ventricular septal defect

No pulmonary hypoplasia, large ventricular septal defect

Tricuspid Atresia With D Transposition (27 percent)

Pulmonary atresia

Pulmonary or subpulmonary stenosis

Large pulmonary artery

Figure 6–10. Classification of tricuspid atresia. (After Vlad P: Tricuspid atresia. *In* Keith JD, et al. [Eds.]: Heart Disease in Infancy and Childhood. 3rd ed. New York, Macmillan, 1978.)

Tricuspid Atresia With L Transposition (3 percent)

Pulmonary or subpulmonary stenosis

Subaortic stenosis

15 percent have no obstruction to pulmonary blood flow.

Cyanosis occurs often on the first day of life and is due to the obligatory right-to-left shunt across the ASD. The intensity varies with the degree of pulmonary outflow obstruction and is most intense in patients with intact septum. Patients with transposition and a large VSD may have only mild cyanosis and present with congestive heart failure in the first few months. Diagnosis of tricuspid atresia should be suspected in the presence of cyanosis with left axis deviation on the ECG and a left ventricular hypertrophy pattern in the precordial leads.

Prognosis without surgical intervention is poor; 50 percent die within the first 6 months, and only 10 percent survive past the age of 10 years. Tricuspid atresia is an incorrectable lesion, and only palliative surgery is available. With surgical management more than 50 percent of patients survive past the second decade of life.

Patients with excessive pulmonary blood flow may develop pulmonary obstructive disease within the first year of life. Patients with a Potts or Waterston shunt may develp the same problem.

Patients have delayed growth. If the foramen ovale is restrictive, signs of venous congestion with a prominent "a" wave in the jugular pulse may become apparent. This is unusual in infants and more common in children and adolescents. Life-threatening atrial dysrhythmias tend to develop in older patients, probably owing to the distention of the atrium. They tend to aggravate existing heart failure and reduce pulmonary blood flow.

Severely cyanotic newborns whose pulmonary blood flow depends on patency of the ductus require urgent shunting. Infusion of prostaglandin E_1 may maintain oxygenation by preventing ductal closure. A Blalock-Taussig shunt is preferred whenever technically feasible since it is not associated with the development of obstructive pulmonary vascular disease. A shunt from the superior vena cava to the right pulmonary artery (Glenn) can be created in older children. It has a very high failure rate over time and may not function if pulmonary vascular resistance rises. Patients with increased pulmonary blood flow require pulmonary artery banding in the first 6 months of life for control of failure and to protect the pulmonary vasculature. Thirty-eight percent of patients with VSDs undergo spontaneous closure of the defect, at which point cyanosis intensifies and a shunt procedure becomes necessary.

Twenty-five to 30 percent of patients with tricuspid atresia and shunts develop endocarditis. Between 1 and 5 percent develop brain abscesses.

During the past decade, physiological correction of tricuspid atresia has gained popularity. The procedures were first described by Fontan and Kreutzer and consist of connection of the right atrium to the pulmonary artery or right ventricular infundibulum and closure of the septal defects (Fig. 6–11). This separates the pulmonary and systemic circulations, with relief of cyanosis and left ventricular volume overload. The procedure can be performed only in patients with normal pulmonary vascular resistance. In some centers it is performed instead of a shunting procedure in children past early infancy. Pulmonary blood flow is dependent on a pressure difference between the right atrium and the pulmonary artery. Right atrial pressures are mild to moderately elevated postoperatively. Chronic liver congestion and ascites may be present and patients may be unable to increase cardiac output appropriately. Maintenance of sinus rhythm is important to maintain pulmonary blood flow and low systemic venous pressures.

Anesthetic Considerations. Most patients with tricuspid atresia requiring anesthesia for noncardiac surgery will have a functioning systemic-to-pulmonary shunt. Anesthetic management is similar to that of patients with tetralogy of Fallot and a shunt. Rigorous endocarditis prophylaxis, prevention of systemic embolization, maintenance of cardiac output, peripheral vascular resistance, and venous return are paramount. Perioperative dehydration should be avoided to prevent increase in blood viscosity and intravascular thrombosis. Hematocrit should not exceed 60 percent.

Patients with increased pulmonary blood flow should have their failure well controlled with digitalis and diuretics. They have a high incidence of pulmonary infections and require careful ventilatory management perioperatively. After a Fontan-type correction patients require maintenance of right-sided filling pressures for pulmonary perfusion. Increases in pulmonary vascular resistance may lead to an acute drop in systemic cardiac output and cyanosis.

Maintenance of sinus rhythm is important, since atrial dysrhythmias may also lead to deterioration in cardiac performance. Venous pooling should be counteracted.

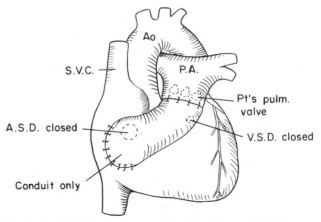

Figure 6–11. Schematic representation of a modified Fontan repair for tricuspid atresia. SVC = superior vena cava; Ao = Aorta; PA = pulmonary artery; ASD = atrial septal defect; VSD = ventricular septal defect.

Ketamine may be a useful anesthestic agent for these patients, while regional techniques causing sympathetic blockade are probably contraindicated. Cardiac output should be monitored carefully, and positive pressure ventilation should be used cautiously, since it may interfere with venous return and pulmonary perfusion and thereby lead to reduction in systemic cardiac output.

Ebstein Anomaly of the Tricuspid Valve

Ebstein anomaly consists of malformation of the posterior and septal leaflets of the tricuspid valve, which are adherent to the right ventricular wall, resulting in downward displacement of the free edge of the valves into the right ventricle away from the atrioventricular junction. The portion of the right ventricle above the downwardly displaced valve is thin-walled and forms a common chamber with the right atrium. The right ventricle below the displaced valve is normal but markedly reduced in size, with a patent foramen ovale in 75 percent of cases. The malformation is rare, with an incidence of 0.5 percent of all congenital heart disease, and affects both sexes equally. Familial occurrence has been reported.

Tricuspid valve stenosis and insufficiency coexist in most cases. Cyanosis due to intra-atrial shunting may be present to various degrees and tends to become more pronounced with age. With severe tricuspid malformation, cyanosis may be present in the neonate and improves with the fall in pulmonary vascular resistance postnatally. Tachycardia causes increased cyanosis owing to impaired right ventricular filling. Atrial emptying is delayed, blood being shunted back and forth between the right atrium and the atrialized portion of the right ventricle between atrial and ventricular systole (ping-pong effect). Paroxysmal atrial tachycardias occur in 25 percent of patients and may lead to syncope. Death during childhood is due to congestive heart failure or cardiac arrhythmias. About one third of patients die before the age of 10, and less than 20 percent survive beyond adolescence.

If exercise intolerance, heart failure, and progressive cyanosis appear in patients with this anomaly, surgical intervention should be considered. The abnormal valve may be replaced, or plication of the atrialized portion of the ventricle together with tricuspid annuloplasty may be carried out. The latter procedure appears to have better results.

Anesthetic Management. Prevention of endocarditis and systemic embolization is important. Patients frequently are marginally compensated hemodynamically and may develop frank failure with myocardial depression or volume overload. Intravenous induction may be markedly delayed owing to pooling of blood in the right atrium. Tachycardia is very poorly tolerated and tachyarrhythmias should be treated promptly. Intracardiac lines may trigger serious arrhythmias and are probably contraindicated, since right heart failure is the dominant feature and measurement of central venous pressure should be an adequate guide to volume replacement. Agents producing myocardial depression or tachycardia should be avoided.

Tricuspid Stenosis

Isolated stenosis of the tricuspid valve is extremely rare. Usually, severe stenosis or atresia of the pulmonary valve with right ventricular hypoplasia is present. The lesion is more common in females and has a strong tendency to occur in families. Signs of right heart failure with a prominent "a" wave on the jugular pulse tracing, liver congestion, and ascites are present with severe obstruction. Cyanosis occurs through shunting via a patent foramen ovale. The clinical presentation may be indistinguishable from that of tricuspid atresia. Some cases are amenable to corrective surgery through valvuloplasty or replacement of the tricuspid valve if an adequately sized right ventricle is present and there is no pulmonary outflow obstruction. Patients without intra-atrial communications will demonstrate signs of right heart failure without cyanosis unless pulmonary blood flow is insufficient. Patients with severely deformed valves may require shunting to increase pulmonary blood flow.

Anesthetic management is similar to that for patients with tricuspid atresia and reduced pulmonary perfusion. Increases in pulmonary vascular resistance may worsen cyanosis and signs of right heart failure. Maintenance of adequate venous pressure is essential to permit flow across the stenotic area. Reduction in left ventricular outflow resistance will increase right-to-left shunting. Endocarditis prophylaxis is required pre- and postoperatively. Patients are at risk for systemic embolization if an intra-atrial communication is present.

REGURGITANT CARDIAC LESIONS

Aortic Regurgitation

Isolated aortic valvular insufficiency does not occur in infancy except in Marfan syndrome, in which it is associated with annuloaortic ectasia. A variety of congenital defects, however, are associated with development of aortic insufficiency, usually during childhood. Five percent of patients with ventricular septal defects develop signs of aortic insufficiency, which is progressive unless the underlying defect is closed. The jet lesion of discrete subaortic stenosis may cause extensive damage to the aortic cusps, but aortic insufficiency is generally not recognized until after excision of the obstruction. Patients with truncus arteriosus may show signs of truncal valve insufficiency prior to surgery, but can also develop truncal valve insufficiency some time after corrective surgery. The congenital bicuspid aortic valve becomes insufficient in approximately one third of affected patients past the age of 20.

The main physiological derangement is left ventricular volume overload by the diastolic regurgitation of blood across the incompetent valve. Net forward blood flow is decreased, unless left ventricular stroke volume and work are increased. The left ventricle initially dilates to accommodate the regurgitated volume, and maximum force is generated by the Frank-Starling mechanism. In chronic regurgitation, left ventricular hypertrophy develops, but compliance remains high, maintaining left ventricular end-diastolic pressures. Because of the regurgitation and low peripheral vascular resistance that are commonly present, diastolic pressure is low and coronary ischemia may occur, a problem not seen in the pediatric population. Patients have a wide pulse pressure and a characteristic diastolic murmur. With severe regurgitation, particulary if acute in onset, congestive heart failure may occur. Children with mild to moderate degrees of regurgitation may be asymptomatic.

If signs of congestive failure or angina occur, surgery becomes necessary. In infants with aortic regurgitation and failure, valvuloplasty is performed whenever possible, while valve replacement is usually necessary in symptomatic children.

Aorto–Left Ventricular Tunnel

This represents an extremely rare congenital malformation, with fewer than 50 cases reported. An endothelialized vascular tunnel arises above the right coronary ostium, traverses the right infundibular portion of the ventricular septum, and enters the left ventricle just below the right and left aortic cusps. Severe aortic regurgitation is produced, with left ventricular enlargement, congestive failure, dilatation of the aortic valve ring, and secondary valvar insufficiency occurring with time. Symptoms occur early in life, usually within the first weeks; medical therapy of heart failure is generally ineffective. Early surgical repair is indicated to prevent deformity of the aortic valve and consists of patching of the aortic orifice of the tunnel.

Aneurysm of the Sinus of Valsalva

Congenital weakness of the tissue of one sinus of Valsalva results in gradual downward bulging of this structure, which eventually herniates into an atrium or ventricle and may rupture. It is a rare problem in infancy and chilhood and occurs more commonly in adults. Seventy-five percent of reported cases occurred in males. Aneurysms of the sinus of Valsalva are most commonly associated with a ventricular septal defect. The rupture usually occurs into the right ventricle, but may occur into the left ventricle or right atrium. Patients exhibit a wide pulse pressure from diastolic runoff; volume overload of the right and left ventricle, with a left-to-right shunt with rupture to the right heart; and severe aortic insufficiency with rupture into the left ventricle. Heart failure is acute and severe. Diagnosis should be established and corrective surgery performed as soon as possible, since most patients follow a progressive downhill course if the defect is not corrected. Residual aortic insufficiency is common after surgical repair.

Anesthetic Considerations. In children with mild to moderate aortic insufficiency, anesthetic techniques that have minimal influence on myocardial contractility should be chosen to maintain left ventricular stroke volume. Tachycardia causes shortening of diastole, thereby decreasing regurgitant flow. High peripheral vascular resistance increases regurgitation, and the usual low peripheral vascular tone should be maintained. Isoflurane and narcotic-relaxant techniques combined with adequate atropination may be useful choices. Intravascular monitoring is indicated for major or traumatic surgery. In patients with impaired ventricular function due to severe regurgitation, ketamine may be indicated in combination with a butyrophenone such as droperidol, which counteracts the peripheral constricting effect of ketamine. These patients will generally undergo repair of their lesions prior to elective surgery. All patients require endocarditis prophylaxis. Postoperative patients with non-tissue prosthetic valves are treated with anticoagulants and require reversal of anticoagulation prior to further surgery.

Mitral Regurgitation

Congenital Mitral Regurgitation

Insufficiency of the mitral valve as an isolated defect is an extremely rare condition. It is generally associated with other congenital cardiac defects, like endocardial cushion defect, corrected transposition, or anomalous origin of the left coronary artery. Lesions causing dilatation of the left ventricle may cause dilatation of the valve ring with secondary mitral incompetence. These include patent ductus arteriosus, VSD, ASD, aortic stenosis or incompetence, endocardial fibroelastosis, and obstructive cardiomyopathy. Insufficiency of the mitral valve may accompany congenital metabolic disorders and is the most common presenting feature of Marfan syndrome in childhood.

Isolated insufficiency is generally caused by abnormal clefting of either the anterior or posterior leaflet, anomalous chordae, or deformed valve tissue. In the complex of anomalous mitral arcade, the free margins of the valve are thickened and the chordae shortened and fused. Together they form an arcade-like structure connecting directly to the papillary muscle.

The obvious hemodynamic defect in mitral insufficiency is the regurgiration of blood into the left atrium during ventricular systole. This augments the volume of the left atrium that empties into the left ventricle during the next diastole, leading to diastolic overload. Since regurgitation occurs into a low-pressure system, left ventricular wall tension during systole is decreased. In order to allow for sufficient stroke output into the systemic circulation, left ventricular volume increases. The left ventricle slowly increases in size, both in systole and in diastole. Eventually congestive heart failure due to volume overload occurs. The left atrium adapts to the increased volume by enlargement in chronic regurgitation, and left atrial pressure is maintained close to normal.

Infants with congenital mitral insufficiency are generally symptomatic within the first year of life, whereas older patients tend to tolerate the condition for many years. There is a history of fatigue, frequent respiratory infections, and failure to grow. Congestive heart failure is a common feature. The maximally dilated left atrium in severe regurgitation may encroach on the left mainstem bronchus, leading to signs of airway obstruction and/or recurrent atelectasis. Mild to moderate pulmonary hypertension is frequently present. In severe or rapidly occurring mitral incompetence, left atrial pressure may be markedly elevated and pulmonary venous congestion and edema may be present. Mitral insufficiency complicating any congenital cardiac lesion considerably worsens the prognosis of the underlying defect. Mild to moderate degrees of central regurgitation can generally be managed medically with control of failure through childhood. Progress of the lesion has to be assessed at regular intervals. In cases with severe regurgitation or persistent congestive failure, plication or annuloplasty of the mitral valve is performed. Prosthetic replacement is delayed if at all possible because of the problems of anticoagulation, valve size, and prosthetic failure.

Anesthetic Considerations. Volume overload of the left ventricle is the major problem. Myocardial depression may cause congestive failure. Regurgitation is less with fast heart rates, and tachycardia is therefore desirable. An increase in peripheral vascular resistance will increase impedance to left ventricular output, leading to an increase in regurgitated volume and a fall in systemic cardiac output.

Agents with minimal myocardial depressing side effects should be used. Maintenance of heart rate and drying of excessive secretions may be achieved by generous atropinization. Adequate oxygenation should be assured by securing the airway and controlled ventilation. Infants may show the pulmonary sequelae of congestive failure with ventilation-perfusion inequalities, small airway disease, and pulmonary congestion. Intravascular monitoring should guide fluid replacement in all major surgical cases. A low peripheral vascular resistance should be maintained by adequate depth of anesthesia and the use of appropriate anesthetic agents (isoflurane, droperidol with narcotic or ketamine).

Electrolyte abnormalities should be corrected preoperatively and digitalis therapy discontinued for the immediate perioperative period to avoid occurrence of digitalis toxicity. When possible, regional techniques may be reasonable alternatives to general anesthesia. Endocarditis prophylaxis is mandatory. Patients who have undergone valvuloplasty or annuloplasty are generally only palliated and still have some degree of regurgitation. Patients with non-tissue prosthetic valves receive anticoagulant treatment, which must be reversed prior to further surgery.

Mitral Valve Prolapse

Mitral valve prolapse or the clinical constellation of mid-systolic click and late systolic murmur represents the most common congenital anomaly. It is present probably in 6 percent of the pediatric population, similar to the incidence reported in adults, with a marked female preponderance of 2:1. Mitral valve prolapse may be an associated feature of various other congenital cardiac lesions, most frequently secundum ASD (up to 40 percent), Ebstein anomaly, and corrected transposition. It is commonly associated with Marfan syndrome.

The mitral valve contains redundant tissue and is generally markedly enlarged, and the chordae are lengthened. The leaflets show focal myxomatous degeneration. Apposition of the leaflets during ventricular systole is incomplete, with slippage and ballooning of the affected leaflet, which exposes leaflets and chordae to the full stress of ventricular contraction. During diastole, dumping of the blood-filled leaflet into the left ventricular cavity subjects the valve tissue to additional trauma. The traumatized endothelium provides a nidus for thrombi and sterile or infected vegetation.

The disease is relatively benign during childhood, with a mean age at diagnosis of 10 years. The presenting feature is generally an atypical murmur, and some patients complain of exertional chest pain. Arrhythmia or fatigue is extremely uncommon. Most patients show the characteristic electrocardiographic pattern of isolated T-wave inversion, but diagnosis is generally established by the characteristic auscultatory findings.

Serious but infrequent complications of mitral valve prolapse are infective endocarditis, development of severe mitral regurgitation, and ventricular arrhythmias with episodes of ventricular tachycardia and/or fibrillation. Cerebrovascular accidents due to embolization have been described. Long-term studies in adults, with a mean follow-up period of 14 years, have revealed a 15 percent incidence of serious complications. In children, cardiac dysrhythmias at rest or during exercise are uncommon. They generally respond to therapy with propranolol. Progressive mitral regurgitation develops in at least 2 percent of pediatric patients and can be treated with annuloplasty or valvuloplasty.

Anesthetic Considerations. Most pediatric patients with mitral valve prolapse are asymptomatic, and no particular anesthetic technique appears superior. Careful electrocardiographic monitoring in the perioperative period is indicated because of the reported tendency to ventricular ectopy in these patients, particularly under stress. Endocarditis prophylaxis is necessary for all operations causing bacteremia. Patients with signs of mitral insufficiency should be managed according to the degree of hemodynamic derangement.

Pulmonary Regurgitation

Isolated pulmonary valve regurgitation is an uncommon congenital lesion, accounting for less than 1 percent of all congenital heart disease. More commonly, pulmonary insufficiency is the result of pulmonary artery hypertension or of surgery to relieve pulmonary outflow obstruction. In congenital pulmonary insufficiency the plumonary valve is hypoplastic or deformed and the main pulmonary artery trunk is dilated.

Patients with congenital pulmonary insufficiency are generally asymptomatic. The normally low diastolic pressure in the pulmonary artery precludes the regurgitation of large volumes of blood during ventricular diastole. Patients are usually diagnosed because of the presence of a harsh, early diastolic murmur and main pulmonary artery dilatation.

If, however, a patient develops secondary pulmonary hypertension as a sequela of lung disease or left heart failure, pulmonary regurgitation worsens and may lead to right ventricular volume overload and failure. This generally does not occur until the later decades of life.

A few isolated cases of neonatal pulmonary insufficiency complicated by severe heart failure have been described. The high pulmonary vascular resistance of persistent fetal circulation in these infants leads to massive regurgitation. Therapy of heart failure and the natural regression of pulmonary vascular resistance will lead to improvement with time if the patient does not succumb in the initial stage of the disease from heart failure and hypoxia.

Anesthetic Considerations. Since patients are generally asymptomatic, no special anesthetic problems should arise. Because of the malformed pulmonary valve, patients are susceptible to infectious endocarditis and appropriate prophylaxis is necessary. Acute elevation in pulmonary vascular resistance due to hypoxia or pulmonary embolization may cause massive and acute right heart failure.

Absent Pulmonary Valve Syndrome

Congenital absence of the pulmonary valve is a very rare congenital anomaly. It is always associated with a VSD; some right ventricular outflow tract obstruction, either infundibular or at the site of the pulmonary annulus; and massive dilatation of the pulmonary arteries. Branching of the pulmonary arteries is abnormal at the segmental artery level. The condition appears to be more common in males and has been reported with a variety of other congenital cardiac lesions.

Severely affected infants present shortly after birth with symptoms of respiratory distress due to tracheobronchial compression by the massively dilated pulmonary arteries leading to atelectasis and obstructive emphysema. Patients with little right-sided obstruction may show, in addition, signs of congestive heart failure due to a large left-to-right shunt, while patients with significant right ventricular outflow tract obstruction are cyanotic and appear clinically similar to those with tetralogy of Fallot. Prognosis is related to the degree of bronchial obstruction, with the majority of patients dying within the first year of life from pulmonary obstructive disease or intractable congestive failure.

Various surgical approaches have been used to correct the abnormality of the pulmonary arteries, including aneurysmectomy, plication of the pulmonary arteries, and interposition of a prosthetic valve or valved conduit in addition to closure of the VSD. Results of surgery in infants are relatively poor and depend primarily on whether or not bronchial obstruction has been relieved. Patients who survive infancy usually improve spontaneously, probably owing to maturational changes with stiffening and enlargement of the tracheobronchial tree, rendering it less susceptible to collapse from outside compression. In addition, pulmonary artery pressure may decrease owing to a relative increase in valve ring stenosis. Definitive repair is carried out in older children, with good results. Insertion of a valve at the pulmonary annulus appears to lead to better hemodynamic performance.

Anesthetic Considerations. Recommendations regarding anesthesia can be made only on a theoretical basis. Symptomatic infants will need meticulous respiratory care. Positive intratracheal pressure may counteract the external bronchial compression. Pulmonary vascular resistance should be kept low to avoid increases in regurgitation and right-to-left shunting. Myocardial depression may lead to worsening congestive failure. Maintenance of heart rate is essential. Reduction in peripheral vascular resistance should benefit patients with predominant left-to-right shunt, while it may worsen cyanosis in patients with severe right ventricular outflow obstruction.

Infundibular spasm may occur and should be treated promptly with either morphine or propranolol. Perioperative mechanical ventilation is probably indicated. Older children may have less respiratory problems and should be managed according to the predominant hemodynamic presentation—ventricular septal defect with or without pulmonic stenosis or tetralogy of Fallot. Endocarditis prophylaxis is indicated in all patients, particularly in patients with prosthetic valves or conduits.

Tricuspid Insufficiency

Isolated congenital tricuspid incompetency is extremely rare. More commonly it is associated with Ebstein anomaly, right ventricular hypertension due to right-sided outflow obstruction, obstructive pulmonary vascular disease, or a cleft tricuspid valve due to an endocardial cushion defect. Occasionally, transient tricuspid insufficincy may follow perinatal asphyxiation. The proposed etiology is myocardial ischemia leading to papillary muscle dysfunction, which is reversible.

In isolated congenital tricuspid insufficiency the valve leaflets and chordae tendineae are dysplastic. Affected patients present as neonates or young infants with extreme cardiomegaly, heart failure, and cyanosis. The free regurgitation across the tricuspid annulus may make it impossible for the right ventricle to generate enough pressure to open the pulmonary valve in the presence of the high perinatal pulmonary vascular resistance. With the normal fall in pulmonary vascular resistance, the tricuspid insufficiency improves.

Treatment in infancy is supportive with judicious use of digoxin and diuretics. In older patients, tricuspid annuloplasty or replacement may be performed. Infants with severe tricuspid regurgitation and right ventricular outflow obstruction have a very poor prognosis. Mortality approaches 100 percent with or without surgery.

Patients who survive infancy and still have tricuspid insufficiency will eventually develop right ventricular and atrial hypertrophy with dilatation due to volume overload and signs of right ventricular failure in later life, unless the lesion is corrected surgically.

Uhl Anomaly

Partial or complete absence of the myocardium of the right ventricle, also known as parchment right ventricle, is an extremely rare congenital anomaly usually not recognized during life. Pulmonary atresia or stenosis and atrial septal defect can occur concurrently. Clinical presentation is similar to that of Ebstein anomaly and tricuspid insufficiency, with signs of right heart failure, massive cardiomegaly (caused by dilatation of the right atrium and ventricle), cyanosis, and growth failure, usually within the first years of life. Patients respond poorly to conservative management. Complete heart block may occur spontaneously and is unresponsive to transvenous pacing because of the lack of excitable tissue in the right ventricle, which serves only as a venous reservoir.

The characteristic catheterization findings are equal pressures in the right atrium, ventricle, and pulmonary artery. Creation of an anastomosis of the superior vena cava to the right pulmonary artery has been recommended to increase pulmonary blood flow and relieve venous congestion. The majority of patients die within the first 2 years of life, although survival to late adulthood with only mild symptoms has been described.

Anesthetic Considerations

Only patients who survive infancy will present for elective surgery. The primary physiological derangement in tricuspid insufficiency is volume overload of the right ventricle, which is usually well tolerated past infancy. Right atrial pressure remains low since the regurgitation volume dissipates in the very compliant venous vascular bed. Right ventricular filling volume has to be high to maintain cardiac output in the presence of regurgitation. Increase in pulmonary vascular resistance may lead to decrease in forward output of the right ventricle, increased regurgitation, and cardiovascular collapse. Tachycardia decreases regurgitation, as it does in mitral insufficiency. Induction with intravenous agents may be delayed because of pooling in a large right atrium and regurgitation from the right ventricle. Maintenance of right-sided filling volume, low pulmonary vascular resistance, and adequate heart rate should be essential and can be achieved by a variety of anesthetic techniques. Antibiotic prophylaxis is necessary.

MALFORMATIONS INVOLVING THE GREAT VESSELS

Patent Ductus Arteriosus (PDA)

During fetal life 55 to 60 percent of the combined ventricular output is carried by the ductus arteriosus, which develops from the distal portion of the sixth aortic arch and connects the main pulmonary artery to the descending aorta. This avoids unnecessary perfusion of the nonventilated lung. Within 10 to 15 hours after birth, closure of the ductus occurs through contraction of medial smooth muscle and intimal protrusion. The main stimulus to ductal closure appears to be the increase in arterial oxygen tension. Permanent closure through intimal fibrosis and connective tissue formation generally is completed by 2 to 3 weeks of age.

Persistent patency of the ductus arteriosus occurs in about 1 in 2000 live full-term births, accounting for 5 to 10 percent of all congenital heart disease. It is more common in females by a ratio of 2:1. In these infants failure to close is due to structural abnormality. This is commonly associated with congenital rubella syndrome together with stenosis of the peripheral pulmonary arteries and of the systemic arteries, especially the renal arteries. Persistent patency of the ductus is essential for postnatal survival in patients with congenital cardiac lesions with right ventricular outflow obstruction or in those with aortic atresia or interrupted arch. Patency may have to be maintained by infusion of prostaglandin E_1 until surgical palliation or correction can be performed.

In premature infants, closure of the ductus arteriosus may be markedly delayed. This may be due to immature ductal musculature, which responds poorly to the constricting effect of oxygen but is very sensitive to the vasodilating effect of prostaglandins (PGE_2 and PGI_2), which are produced intramurally in the ductus. Persistent patency is inversely related to the maturity of the infant. More than 80 percent of infants of less than 1000 gm birth weight have a significant PDA.

This frequency decreases to 15 to 45 percent in infants between 1000 and 1750 gm birth weight.

Clinical symptoms depend on the degree of shunting across the ductus. Because of the higher postnatal systemic vascular resistance, the systemic arterial pressure exceeds pulmonary artery pressure and shunting occurs from left to right. The magnitude of shunting depends on the diameter of the ductus, the pressure gradient between the aorta and pulmonary artery, and the difference between systemic and pulmonary vascular resistances. With a small ductus, resistance to flow is high and only a small shunt will occur despite a large pressure gradient. With a large ductus, pressures may become equalized and shunting is determined by the difference in vascular resistance between systemic and pulmonary circulations.

Left-to-right shunting leads to an increased volume load for the left ventricle. Left ventricular diastolic volume is increased, leading to increased ventricular stroke volume through the Frank-Starling mechanism. In newborns and particularly in prematures, the myocardium is not fully developed; it contains fewer contractile elements, and sympathetic innervation is incomplete. Volume loads are less well tolerated than later in life, and left ventricular failure occurs readily. As a result of increased left ventricular end-diastolic pressure, left atrial pressure rises, leading to overt pulmonary edema through pulmonary venous congestion. Eventually, pulmonary hypertension and right ventricular failure may occur. With a dilated left atrium, stretching of the foramen ovale may occur with subsequent shunting at the atrial level. Aortic diastolic pressure is low with a large ductus, owing to runoff into the low-pressure pulmonary circulation. This may lead to myocardial ischemia in the presence of elevated left ventricular end-diastolic pressures, further aggravating heart failure. Systemic perfusion and oxygen delivery may become compromised, particularly if anemia is also present with a high percentage of fetal hemoglobin.

Symptoms of left-to-right shunting due to PDA generally appear at 3 to 5 days of age, most commonly in infants recovering from respiratory distress syndrome. Patients develop a systolic or continuous murmur, bounding pulses, and a hyperactive precordium. Tachycardia and tachypnea are signs of early left ventricular failure. Respiratory function deteriorates with increasing oxygen requirements and elevation of arterial PCO_2. Patients without lung disease may have symptoms of mild heart failure, while infants with severe lung disease present with deteriorating ventilatory function and failure to wean. Diagnosis can usually be made clinically and confirmed by echocardiography.

Medical therapy with fluid restriction, maintenance of a hematocrit above 45 percent, and administration of indomethacin 0.2 mg/kg (maximum 3 doses 12 to 24 hours apart intravenously or via nasogastric tube) are usually sufficient to control symptoms and effect functional closure of the ductus. Digitalis is generally ineffective in premature infants and may cause toxicity. If after 48 to 72 hours of medical management symptoms persist, surgical ligation is performed. Indomethacin is contraindicated in patients with impaired renal function or elevated bilirubin levels.

Manifestations of PDA in term infants and older children are similar to the ones described for prematures and are dependent on the degree of shunting. With a small ductus, patients are generally asymptomatic and the characteristic machinery murmur is detected on routine physical examination. Development of bacterial endocarditis is the main risk for this group. With a moderate-sized ductus, symptoms may include poor feeding and tachypnea. Compensatory ventricular hypertrophy develops in these patients and symptoms improve. General physical development is usually retarded, however, and easy fatigability is noted in older children. Infants with a large ductus are always symptomatic with failure to grow, poor feeding, sweating, tachypnea, and recurrent respiratory infections. Without surgery, patients eventually develop obstructive pulmonary vascular disease with progression to Eisenmenger syndrome.

Surgical repair of the ductus should be performed in all patients to prevent long-term complications (endocarditis with a small to moderate ductus, irreversible pulmonary vascular disease with a large one). Indomethacin is ineffective in term infants and children. Life expectancy of patients with PDA after the age of 17 is half that of the general population.

Anesthetic Considerations. Presence of a small ductus does not interfere with general anesthetic management, since cardiovascular function is normal. The main risk is bacterial endocarditis. With a large ductus chronic pulmonary congestion may be present and heart failure may occur with rapid fluid administration or increase in pulmonary vascular resistance. The latter may cause shunt reversal and systemic embolization of air or debris. These patients should generally undergo ductus repair prior to elective surgery. Their anesthetic management is similar to that of patients with a large left-to-right shunt at the ventricular level. Avoidance of agents with a myocardial depressant effect, careful ventilatory management to avoid hypoventilation and atelectasis, and monitoring of fluid administration are important. Endocarditis prophylaxis should be maintained. Premature infants have been successfully managed with narcotic-relaxant techniques and air-oxygen mixtures. Prevention of retinopathy of prematurity is an added concern in this age group.

Infants and children are normal after closure of an isolated ductus arteriosus and have no specific anesthetic requirements. Endocarditis prophylaxis is not necessary postoperatively.

Aortopulmonary Window

Failure of aortopulmonary septation during early fetal life leaves an open communication between the

Figure 6–12. Truncus arteriosus. Classification according to Colett and Edwards. Ao = Aorta; PA = pulmonary artery; RPA = right pulmonary artery; LPA = left pulmonary artery; RV = right ventricle; LV = left ventricle.

great arteries just above their valve origins. This lesion is exceedingly rare and is isolated in over 50 percent of cases. The clinical presentation is indistinguishable from that of a large PDA, since the defect is usually large. Congestive heart failure in infancy is generally the presenting symptom. Pulmonary and right ventricular pressures are at or near systemic levels. Prognosis without surgical repair is poor, with death occurring from congestive failure in infancy or obstructive pulmonary vascular disease developing after the first year of life. If possible, failure should be medically controlled in early infancy and the defect closed electively in the second half of the first year. If medical therapy fails, surgery is performed earlier. Repair consists of transaortic closure of the defect with a patch, requiring cardiopulmonary bypass.

Less than 10 percent of patients with this anomaly have a small defect and can be treated as if they have a small ductus. Since the surgical approach is radically different for these two lesions, definite diagnosis has to be established prior to attempts at correction.

Anesthetic considerations are similar to those that apply to patients with a large ventricular septal defect in infancy. Elective noncardiac surgery should preferably be postponed until the lesion has been repaired. Endocarditis prophylaxis is necessary pre- and postoperatively. Closure of the defect should lead to normalization of physiological parameters.

Truncus Arteriosus

Truncus arteriosus is an uncommon congenital anomaly in which one great vessel arises from both ventricles above a large VSD, giving rise to the pulmonary and coronary arteries. This malformation represents 4 percent of congenital cardiac lesions. At present three forms of truncus are differentiated (Fig. 6–12). In type I a short pulmonary trunk arises from the truncus and divides into both pulmonary arteries;

in type II the pulmonary arteries arise separately but in close proximity to each other from the posterior aspect of the truncus; and in type III both pulmonary arteries arise separately from the respective lateral aspects of the truncal artery.

In early infancy patients show signs of congestive heart failure and pulmonary overperfusion. Truncal valve insufficiency may also be present. Heart failure is severe and resistant to therapy. Unless surgical correction is performed, death occurs in the first year of life in over 80 percent of patients. Survivors develop obstructive pulmonary vascular disease, rendering them inoperable. These patients all deteriorate progressively, with signs of pulmonary hypertension and right heart failure.

Because of the dismal natural history of this disease, correction is generally performed between 6 and 9 months of age or earlier if heart failure cannot be controlled. It consists of closure of the VSD with the left ventricular output diverted to the truncal artery and positioning of a valved graft between the right ventricle and pulmonary artery (or arteries) (Fig. 6–13). Surgical mortality ranges from 9 to 25 percent. Since only a small conduit can be used during infancy, at least one other operation will become necessary with growth of the patient once the size of the conduit becomes inadequate. Currently available conduits still have the problem of valve deterioration and secondary obstruction, and replacement of the conduit for this reason may become necessary during later life. Truncal valve insufficiency may necessitate valve replacement at either initial or subsequent surgery.

Anesthetic Considerations. Elective surgery is unlikely to be performed prior to the correction of the cardiac lesion in the first year of life. Patients with truncus arteriosus that is considered inoperable may present with this lesion and Eisenmenger syndrome. After successful correction patients may appear asymptomatic but nevertheless have a considerable pressure gradient across the right ventricular to pulmonary

Figure 6–13. Truncus arteriosus before and after operation. Repair with insertion of a conduit between the right ventricle and pulmonary artery and closure of the ventricular septal defect. Ao = Aorta; RPA = right pulmonary artery; LPA = let pulmonary artery; RV = right ventricle; LV = left ventricle.

artery conduit. Right ventricular failure and ventricular arrhythmias may develop with stress or large and rapid fluid shifts. Central venous monitoring will be essential under these circumstances to assess right ventricular function. Increases in pulmonary vascular resistance will worsen the condition of these patients, and acute preload reduction may lead to systemic cardiovascular collapse.

Selection of anesthetic agents should center on drugs with minimal effect on vasomotor tone and myocardial performance. Maintenance of heart rate is essential, as is endocarditis prophylaxis. Use of invasive monitoring should be considered early for extensive surgery. Because of the presence of a prosthetic valve in the pulmonary outflow tract, use of a Swan-Ganz catheter is contraindicated.

Coarctation of the Aorta

Isolated coarctation of the aorta is the fifth or sixth most common congenital cardiac defect, accounting for 6 to 7 percent of all congenital heart disease. It affects males twice as frequently as females. It is the lesion most commonly associated with the Turner syndrome of XO karyotype. A bicuspid aortic valve is found in 50 to 80 percent of patients with coarctation.

The coarctation occurs as a constriction of the aorta, at or near the junction of the ductus arteriosus and the aortic arch and distal to the left subclavian artery. The involved segment may be discrete or of significant length. The narrowing of the aorta may occur above the entrance of the ductus (preductal or infantile type of coarctation), usually as a long segmental narrowing, or at or below the ductus (postductal or adult type of coarctation), usually localized (Fig. 6–14). Forty percent of patients with preductal coarctation have associated severe intracardiac anomalies, compared with only 14 percent of patients with postductal coarctation.

The physiological problem in coarctation is the maintenance of blood flow to the lower half of the body in the presence of an aortic obstruction. Adaptive mechanisms result in elevation of the systolic blood pressure in the proximal aorta to increase the pressure gradient, arteriolar constriction to maintain diastolic pressure, and development of collaterals to bypass the obstruction. In the preductal form of coarctation blood flow to the lower half of the body occurs via a patent ductus arteriosus.

Coarctation of the aorta is the second most common cause of congestive heart failure in infancy and childhood, with more than half of patients becoming symptomatic within the first years of life. Eighty percent of these patients have an associated defect, most commonly PDA (two thirds) or VSD (30 to 35 percent). In two thirds of these infants the coarctation is preductal.

Elevation of the systolic blood pressure in the upper

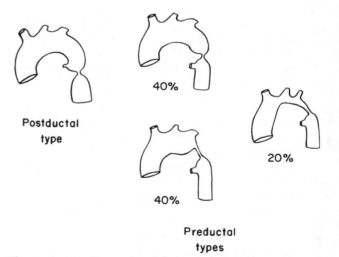

Postductal type

40%

40%

20%

Preductal types

Figure 6–14. Coarctation of the aorta. (After Keith JD: Coarctation of the aorta. *In* Keith JD, et al. [Eds.]: Heart Disease in Infancy and Childhood. 3rd ed. New York, Macmillan, 1978.)

Figure 6–15. Methods of repair for coarctation of the aorta. *A,* Resection and end-to-end anastomosis. *B,* Patch aortoplasty. *C,* Subclavian flap repair.

extremity, particularly the right arm, above the systolic pressure in the lower extremity is generally present except in patients with a low output state or with a large ductus supplying blood flow to the lower extremity. The latter is frequently associated with a VSD and systemic pressures in the pulmonary artery.

Medical therapy is frequently unsuccessful, necessitating surgical repair of the coarctation by resection and end-to-end anastomosis, patch aortoplasty, or subclavian flap (Fig. 6–15). The last procedure appears to be associated with a low surgical mortality and low risk of recoarctation. Reduction of left ventricular afterload by coarctation repair will generally lead to improvement in patients with associated VSD. Repair of these defects can be postponed, since 50 percent become smaller or close spontaneously. In patients with complex lesions that could result in pulmonary hypertension and are not amenable to correction in infancy, pulmonary artery banding is carried out at the time of coarctation repair. A PDA is always ligated.

The majority of patients with isolated postductal coarctation are not diagnosed until later in life, most commonly because of the incidental finding of a heart murmur or systolic hypertension between 4 and 5 years of age. Systolic pressure is higher in the upper extremity than in the lower extremity in all patients, and systolic hypertension in the upper extremity is present in 90 percent. The children are otherwise normal, without signs of congestive failure.

Surgical repair is performed during early childhood, preferably between 2 and 4 years of age if diagnosis is made that early. Repair in later childhood and adolescence is associated with a 10 to 20 percent incidence of persistent hypertension despite adequate relief of the obstruction. This leads to premature death from cardiovascular disease.

Patients with coarctation have an increased incidence of cerebral aneurysm, which may lead to cerebrovascular accidents even in the presence of a normal postoperative blood pressure. The risk of endocarditis is not eliminated with coarctation repair. Infection may occur at the anastomotic site, with mycotic aneurysm formation and aortic rupture, or at the aortic or mitral valve; these valves are frequently abnormal (bicuspid aortic valve, mitral valve prolapse). Aneurysmatic dilatation of the site of the coarctation repair has been described as a long-term sequela of patch aortoplasty. In childhood it has been seen only in patients with hypertension. A very rare but catastrophic sequela of coarctation repair is spinal cord injury with paraplegia.

The prognosis for unrepaired coarctation is poor. Twenty percent die in the second decade of life and 90 percent before the age of 50 as a consequence of severe hypertension.

Two percent of patients with coarctation have associated coarctation of the abdominal aorta. This is most commonly seen in females. Hypertension is usually pronounced, and renal involvement is common. Corrective surgery is usually performed after childhood, with resection of the lesions or interposition of a graft.

Anesthetic Considerations. Symptomatic infants usually undergo coarctation repair prior to any elective noncardiac surgery. Heart failure should be relieved and blood pressure should be normal postoperatively. Persistent hypertension despite relief of the obstruction is not generally seen after repair in infancy. Recurrence of a pressure gradient is indicative of recoarctation. These patients may show an exaggerated blood pressure response with stress and require sufficient anesthetic depth to prevent this problem. Inhalation anesthetics and muscle relaxants without sympathomimetic side effects appear to be wise choices. The presence of associated cardiac defects and their physiological consequences should be taken into consideration. Patients with associated Turner syndrome may present difficulties with intubation. Hypertension is commonly seen in older patients prior to coarctation repair and persists in a considerable percentage of patients postoperatively. With stress, two thirds of patients after coarctation repair may show marked systolic hypertension. Since cerebral aneurysms are more common in these patients, subarachnoid hemorrhage may occur.

Resting hypertension should be controlled medically prior to elective surgery. Blood pressure should be monitored carefully perioperatively, and early, direct monitoring should be established for major surgery. Pressure should always be measured in the right arm, since blood pressures may still differ between the upper extremities postoperatively, even if the subclavian artery was not sacrificed. Sufficient depth of anesthesia should be achieved prior to stressful manipulations. Topical anesthesia, superior laryngeal nerve block, or intravenous lidocaine should be used to attenuate the sympathetic response to laryngoscopy and intubation. Inhalation anesthesia lowers blood pressure and allows for rapid changes in anesthetic depth. Relaxants should also be chosen according to their cardiovascular side effects.

All patients require endocarditis prophylaxis pre- and postoperatively.

Interrupted Aortic Arch

Interrupted aortic arch is an uncommon congenital lesion accounting for approximately 1.4 percent of all infants seen with congenital heart disease. A segment of the aortic arch is absent or atretic, leading to complete aortic discontinuity. The embryogenetic basis is failure of fusion of the fourth and sixth aortic arches. The defect may be located distal to the left subclavian artery (type A), between the left carotid and left subclavian arteries (type B), or distal to the innominate and proximal to the left carotid arteries (type C) (Fig. 6–16). The lesion is commonly associated with VSD and PDA, the latter suppplying the blood flow to the distal aorta. Type B interruption is most commonly seen. Symptoms of a large left-to-right shunt with heart failure and pulmonary hyperperfusion are present shortly after birth. Physiologic closure of the ductus leads to systemic underperfusion with metabolic acidosis and renal failure. Without surgical intervention, death occurs in 90 percent of patients within the first month of life. Bypassing the interruption by using the carotid or subclavian artery, tube graft interposition, and direct anastomosis have been utilized. Pulmonary artery banding or primary repair of an associated VSD has been performed simultaneously.

Prostaglandin E_1 is used preoperatively to maintain patency of the ductus and systemic perfusion. Surgical mortality between 23 and 45 percent is reported. No long-term follow-up of survivors has been reported. Subaortic stenosis appears to be more common in these patients, requiring further surgery. With growth, relative coarctation at the graft site may occur, necessitating surgical revision.

Anesthetic Management. Survivors should pose problems similar to those in patients after coarctation repair. Aortic interruption may be associated with DiGeorge syndrome* and patients may develop severe hypocalcemia. Calcium levels should be monitored perioperatively.

Vascular Ring Anomalies

Anomalies in the development of the aortic arch system may lead to the formation of anomalous vascular structures compressing the trachea and/or esophagus (Fig. 6–17). The incidence of aortic arch malformation is not known. Symptomatic patients comprise approximately 1.5 percent of patients seen with congenital heart disease.

The heart is generally normal in these patients and symptoms usually relate to the degree of respiratory obstruction. In patients with severe tracheal compression stridor, wheezing, recurrent pneumonia, and emphysematous pulmonary changes are present within the first few months of life. Respiratory distress is aggravated by feeding and lessened by hyperextension of the head. Severely affected infants show failure to thrive. Other causes of stridor or frequent pneumonia (for example, laryngeal web, tracheomalacia, tracheoesophageal fistula, gastric reflux, Pierre-Robin anomaly, choanal atresia) have to be excluded. The airway obstruction may be life-threatening. The compressed area is frequently located in the lower trachea but may be located distally in one of the main bronchi. Esophageal obstruction may occur, with swallowing difficulties and frequent vomiting. However, symptoms are generally less severe and the condition may remain undiagnosed for many years.

Medical management consists of careful positioning to minimize tracheal compression, feeding with liquids or soft foods, and prompt treatment of pulmonary infections. As the infant grows the trachea becomes stiffer and less easily compressed. In patients with severe symptoms and significant tracheal narrowing, surgery to relieve the vascular obstruction must be performed.

---

*Absence of thymus and parathyroid glands associated with impaired immunity, neonatal tetany, hypocalcemia, and facial abnormalities.

Figure 6–16. Interrupted aortic arch. Classification after Celoria and Patton. Ao = Aorta; MPA = main pulmonary artery; RPA = right pulmonary artery; PDA = patent ductus arteriosus; LPA = left pulmonary artery; RS = right subclavian artery; LS = left subclavian artery; RCC = right common carotid artery; LCC = left common carotid artery.

Figure 6–17. Vascular ring anomalies: *a,* double aortic arch; *b,* right aortic arch with left ligamentum arteriosum; *c,* anomalous right subclavian artery; *d,* anomalous right innominate artery; *e,* anomalous left common carotid. Ao = aorta; PA = pulmonary artery; RCC = right common carotid; LCC = left common carotid; LS = left subclavian; RS = right subclavian. (Redrawn from Gross RE: The Surgery of Infancy and Childhood. Philadelphia, W. B. Saunders Co., 1953.)

Double Aortic Arch

This is the most common vascular ring anomaly and usually occurs as an isolated entity. A right and a left aortic arch arise from the ascending aorta, encircle the trachea and esophagus, and unite to form a single descending aorta. Symptoms of tracheal compression are usually present in early infancy. Surgical treatment consists of division of the smaller of the two arches, usually the left.

Right Aortic Arch with Left Ligamentum Arteriosus

In this anomaly a vascular ring is formed by the right aortic arch, the left subclavian artery, and a left-sided ductus or ligamentum arteriosus connecting the left subclavian artery to the left pulmonary artery. This anomaly is only rarely associated with intracardiac defects. In contrast, with right aortic arch with mirror image branching of the brachiocephalic vessels and no vascular ring malformation, intracardiac defects are present in over 90 percent of patients. Symptoms of tracheal compression are often less severe and surgical treatment is not usually necessary. Division of the ligamentatum arteriosus and/or division of the subclavian artery will relieve the obstruction.

Anomalous Innominate Artery

In this anomaly, the innominate artery arises more posteriorly and may be congenitally short. Symptoms of tracheal compression occur in early infancy and may include apneic spells. With severe symptomatology, surgery is indicated and consists of mobilizing the offending vessels and suturing them to the posterior aspect of the sternum. An anomalous left carotid artery arising more posteriorly may cause similar symptoms. Relief is provided through fixation of the vessel to the sternum.

Aberrant Right Subclavian Artery

In this lesion, the right subclavian artery arises as the last branch of the aortic arch and courses to the right arm at an oblique angle behind the esophagus. It is frequently associated with tetralogy of Fallot and may be present in over one third of patients with Down syndrome. It has been observed in 0.5 to 0.7 percent of postmortem examinations. Dysphagia lusoria has long been attributed to this lesion, while respiratory symptoms have only rarely been associated. Most patients are asymptomatic and require no treatment. In symptomatic infants the artery can be divided surgically; however, in older patients reconstruction of the vessel is recommended to prevent ischemic changes and/or the subclavian steal syndrome.

Anomalous Origin of the Left Pulmonary Artery (Vascular Sling)

In this anomaly, the left pulmonary artery arises from an elongated main pulmonary artery on the right, encircles the right main stem bronchus, and passes to the left between the trachea and esophagus. Constriction of the right main bronchus, the trachea, or both may occur. Congenital tracheal stenosis or tracheal rings are frequently associated. Symptoms of tracheal compression are usually severe and begin within the first few weeks of life. Prognosis without surgical intervention is extremely poor, with death occurring within the first few months. The surgical procedure consists of detachment of the anomalous pulmonary artery at its origin and reanastomosis to the main pulmonary artery anterior to the trachea. Mortality for this procedure approaches 50 percent. If tracheal stenosis is also present, symptoms may be only partially relieved.

Anesthetic Considerations

Various degrees of airway compromise are the prominent feature of these anomalies; securing and maintaining an adequate airway is the main anesthetic problem. Secondary pulmonary changes of atelectasis or emphysema may complicate the respiratory impairment.

Smooth induction of anesthesia, preferably with a nonirritating inhalational anesthetic like halothane, should be attempted. Struggling on induction, which increases negative intrathoracic pressure, may cause considerable worsening of the symptoms and even complete tracheal or bronchial obstruction. The head should be kept extended and continuous positive airway pressure applied, which tends to maintain the patency of the airway by passive distention. Relaxants or intravenous agents should not be given unless controlled ventilation can be performed adequately. If secondary pulmonary changes are present, higher than normal inspired oxygen concentrations may be necessary to insure adequate oxygenation. The smallest diameter endotracheal tube permitting adequate ventilation should be chosen to minimize mechanical trauma to the compressed area. Adequacy of gas exchange and ventilation of both lungs should be monitored closely throughout surgery. Controlled ventilation with constant positive airway pressure should be maintained.

If no audible leak is present, worsening of the respiratory impairment should be expected postoperatively and the patient closely monitored. Mechanical ventilation may be necessary until tracheal edema subsides.

Postoperatively, the trachea may remain weakened for a considerable time and symptoms may recur with tracheal narrowing due to inflammatory or reactive edema. All patients should be closely observed for signs of airway obstruction for several hours.

Except in patients who have undergone repair of pulmonary artery sling, endocarditis risk is not increased in these patients unless other cardiovascular anomalies are present.

Congenital Subclavian Steal

Obstruction of blood flow into the subclavian artery proximal to the origin of the vertebral artery may cause reversal of flow in the latter vessel, draining blood from the cerebral circulation into the arm. This is a very rare congenital anomaly usually occurring together with either severe coarctation or interrupted aortic arch with one or both subclavian arteries originating distal to the obstruction. Isolated stenosis or atresia of the origin of the subclavian artery has also been observed. Symptoms of cerebral ischemia include dizziness, vertigo, blurred vision, headaches, and syncope and may be brought on by exercise of the affected arm. Pain, numbness, or fatigue of the arm may also be present, and blood pressure is decreased on the side of the subclavian obstruction. Diagnosis is established angiographically. In symptomatic patients, bypassing the obstruction with a shunt is the preferred procedure.

Anesthetic Considerations. Patients should pose no unusual anesthetic problems if the lesion is isolated, except that systemic blood pressure should not be monitored on the affected side. Since most patients have other cardiac anomalies, anesthetic management should be guided by the predominant physiological derangement.

Anomalies of the Pulmonary Arterial Tree

Anomalous Origin of the Pulmonary Artery from the Aorta

Origin of one pulmonary artery from the ascending aorta is a rare congenital malformation usually affecting the right pulmonary artery. The anomalous vessels may originate anywhere on the aortic arch.

The pathophysiological consequences result from a large left-to-right shunt at systemic pressures with consequent pulmonary hypertension in one or both lungs and the development of obstructive pulmonary vascular disease. Patients are uniformly symptomatic within the first few weeks of life, and most die within the first 6 months if surgical correction is not performed. The symptoms are those of congestive heart failure, respiratory distress, and poor weight gain. Early diagnosis and correction are imperative to prevent development of irreversible pulmonary vascular disease. Surgical correction consists of anastomosing the aberrant vessel to the main pulmonary artery and correcting associated defects (usually PDA). Prognosis after surgery is good.

Anesthetic Considerations. No particular anesthetic technique can be recommended. Patients should be asymptomatic postoperatively but require endocarditis prophylaxis.

Congenital Absence of One Pulmonary Artery

Unilateral absence of one pulmonary artery is a rare congenital malformation and may be associated with tetralogy of Fallot. Blood flow to the affected lung is provided through bronchial collaterals or an abnormal vessel arising from the ductus arteriosus. In isolated cases pulmonary hypertension is present in the unaffected lung. If an intracardiac defect with left-to-right shunt coexists, pulmonary hypertension is nearly always present.

The majority of patients are asymptomatic in childhood. They may develop recurrent pulmonary infections, with associated malformations of the tracheobronchial tree, bronchiectasis, and hemoptysis. If severe pulmonary symptoms are present, pneumonectomy should be considered. In patients with left-to-right shunt, early correction of the lesion should be performed to prevent development of pulmonary vascular disease.

Anesthetic Considerations. Patients are generally asymptomatic but have pulmonary function abnormalities consistent with a ventilated but underperfused lung. Since patients are also prone to respiratory infections, particular attention should be paid to adequacy of ventilation and tracheobronchial toilet. In the presence of unilateral bronchiectasis, contamination of the healthy lung during surgery should be prevented by the use of endobronchial intubation or a bronchus blocker such as a Fogarty catheter.

Congenital Pulmonary Arteriovenous Fistula or Aneurysm

Direct communication between branches of the pulmonary artery and pulmonary veins without interposition of capillaries is a relatively uncommon lesion. It may occur as single or multiple communications or extremely rarely as a communication of an aneurysmal

dilatation of the right pulmonary artery and left atrium. Both sexes are equally affected. In 60 percent of multiple fistulas, the condition is associated with hereditary hemorrhagic telangiectasia (Rendu-Osler-Weber syndrome).

The essential physiological disturbance is a shunt of venous blood into the systemic circulation producing various degrees of arterial desaturation. Although between 18 and 89 percent of the right ventricular output may pass through the fistula, cardiac output is usually not increased and pulmonary pressures remain normal.

Clinical symptoms present in childhood and consist of cyanosis and exertional dyspnea. There are usually abnormal shadows on the chest roentgenogram. Neurological symptoms due to paradoxical embolization or thrombosis from polycythemia or brain abscesses occur in at least 25 percent of patients. Hemoptysis may occur either from telangiectatic lesions of the bronchial mucosa or from rupture of the aneurysmatic fistula. Because of the frequency of fatal complications past childhood, repair should be performed in all symptomatic patients. Resection of the involved lung segment or resection of the aneurysm in cases with left atrial communication is performed.

Anesthetic Considerations. Cyanosis is due to the direct pulmonary arteriovenous connection and is influenced little by the addition of oxygen. Normal arterial PCO_2 is maintained by hyperventilation if the shunt is large. In low flow states causing low venous saturation, systemic desaturation may worsen. Meticulous attention should be paid to the prevention of systemic air embolization from venous lines. Polycythemia should be controlled to a hematocrit of less than 60 percent perioperately to prevent systemic thrombosis. Manipulation of the airway should be performed atraumatically to prevent bleeding from telangiectatic lesions. Patients should be protected against endocarditis.

After resection of the fistula, patients should pose no special anesthetic problems unless familial telangiectasia is also present. Since the heart is normal in these patients, no particular anesthetic technique can be recommended.

Anomalies of the Pulmonary Venous Bed

Total Anomalous Pulmonary Venous Return

Connection of all pulmonary veins to either the right atrium or one of the systemic veins is a relatively rare congenital anomaly present in less than 1.5 percent of all patients with congenital heart disease, but is the twelfth most common lesion seen during the first year of life. It is seen more frequently in males. Four anatomical sites of anomalous vein insertion are usually differentiated: *supracardiac*, into either a left or right superior vena cava; *cardiac*, into the coronary sinus or right atrium; *infracardiac*, into the portal or hepatic

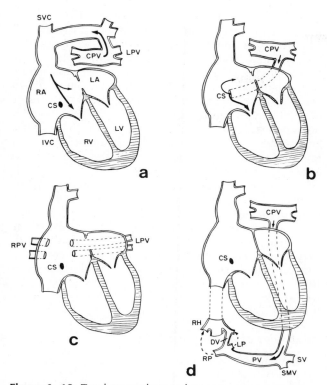

Figure 6–18. Total anomalous pulmonary venous return: *a,* to left innominate vein; *b,* to coronary sinus; *c,* to right atrium; *d,* infradiaphragmatic to portal vein. SVC = superior vena cava; IVC = inferior vena cava; CPV = common pulmonary vein; LPV left pulmonary vein; RPV = right pulmonary vein; LA = left atrium; RA = right atrium; CS = coronary sinus; RV = right ventricle; LV = left ventricle; SV = splenic vein; PV = portal vein; DV = ductus venosus; RH = right hepatic vein; SMV = superior mesenteric vein. (Redrawn from Lucas RV: Anomalous venous connections, pulmonary and systemic. *In* Adams FH, Emmanouilides GC [Eds.]: Heart Disease in Infants, Children, and Adolescents. 3rd ed. Baltimore, Williams and Wilkins, 1983.)

veins or ductus venosus; and *mixed*, with insertion at more than one level (Fig. 6–18). Drainage into the left superior vena cava is seen most frequently. Twenty-five to 30 percent of patients have associated cardiac anomalies, particularly of the asplenia type. Presence of an intra-atrial communication is necessary for survival, and an atrial septal defect or patent foramen ovale is part of the complex.

The right heart carries an increased volume load from a large left-to-right shunt, similar to the physiology of a secundum atrial septal defect. Systemic saturation and output depend on the degree of mixing at the atrial level. Pulmonary arterial hypertension is present in the majority of supracardiac and cardiac connections and in all infradiaphragmatic connections owing to obstruction to pulmonary venous return. It may also develop in later life secondary to high pulmonary blood flow in patients without venous obstruction but with a large intra-atrial communication, which allows survival into adulthood.

The majority of patients are symptomatic within the first month of life. If no pulmonary venous obstruction is present, signs of congestive heart failure from volume overload and only mild cyanosis are seen. Tachypnea, frequent respiratory infections, and failure to thrive are the common presenting features. Without surgical treatment mortality of these infants approaches 80 percent by 1 year of age. In the presence of pulmonary venous obstruction, cyanosis and tachypnea are present at birth or shortly thereafter. Cardiac failure occurs from obstruction to right heart output relatively early, and patients die within days to a few months from hypoxia and pulmonary edema unless surgical relief can be achieved. At surgery, a connection between the common pulmonary venous trunk and the left atrium is created and the intra-atrial connection is closed. Surgical mortality ranges from 30 to 60 percent.

Anesthetic Considerations. The majority of patients with this anomaly who present for elective noncardiac surgery will have undergone a corrective procedure. Since adequate surgical survival has occurred only in recent years, no long-term observations are yet available. In patients with pulmonary vascular disease at the time of surgery, progression of the pulmonary arteriolar obstruction may occur despite repair. This is unlikely to occur in patients operated upon in infancy. As the child grows, stenosis of the pulmonary venous to left atrial anastomosis may occur, leading to secondary pulmonary venous and arterial hypertension. Such patients will present with a clinical picture somewhat similar to that seen in patients with mitral stenosis. Patients with a widely patent intra-atrial connection, no venous obstruction, and an increase in pulmonary arteriolar resistance restricting pulmonary blood flow may have few clinical symptoms and present with signs similar to those of an atrial septal defect. Endocarditis prophylaxis and prevention of systemic embolization are important anesthetic considerations.

Common Pulmonary Vein Atresia

Complete absence of a connection between the pulmonary veins and the left atrium is an extremely rare and nearly uniformly fatal congenital cardiac lesion. Cyanosis, tachypnea, and heart failure occur shortly after birth. The lesion is generally isolated. Surgical connection has been successfully performed only recently. Patients should be normal postoperatively unless stenosis of the pulmonary venous–left atrial connection occurs.

Partial Anomalous Pulmonary Venous Return

Connection of one or more, but not all, of the pulmonary veins to either the right atrium or a systemic vein is a fairly common condition observed in 0.7 percent of all routine postmortem examinations. It is present in 9 percent of patients with atrial septal defects. Both sexes are equally affected. Most commonly the right pulmonary veins drain into the superior vena cava or right atrium with an associated sinus venosus defect. The physiological consequences and clinical symptomatology are similar to those of a secundum ASD.

Drainage of the right pulmonary veins to the inferior vena cava constitutes part of the scimitar syndrome. The atrial septum is usually intact. Anomalies of the bronchial system of the right lung, including hypoplasia of the lung and right pulmonary artery, and abnormal systemic arterial connections are generally present. Respiratory infections are commonly seen owing to the abnormal pulmonary structure. The abnormal venous connection produces a crescent- or scimitar-shaped shadow in the right lower lung field on the chest x-ray. The clinical presentation is similar to that seen in the patient with an ASD.

Surgical correction is recommended during childhood in all patients with partial anomalous pulmonary venous connection to prevent development of obstructive pulmonary vascular disease. Those with the scimitar syndrome may require pulmonary resection. Diversion of the abnormal venous return to the left atrium can be a technically difficult surgical problem.

Postoperative prognosis when surgery has been successful is excellent unless pulmonary vascular obstruction is present.

Anesthetic Considerations. Patients should be managed similarly to patients with secundum ASD. Endocarditis prophylaxis is necessary pre- and postoperatively.

Anomalies of the Systemic Venous Return

Aberrations in the embryological development of the cardinal venous system result in either persistence of two superior venae cavae, or anomalies of the coronary sinus. They frequently are associated with other congenital cardiac anomalies, most commonly tetralogy of Fallot. These anomalies are usually important only with regard to difficulties during cardiac catheterization and cardiac surgery.

Persistent Left Superior Vena Cava

The most common anomaly of systemic venous return is persistence of a left superior vena cava draining into the coronary sinus and the right atrium. It is found in 0.3 percent of routine postmortems but is present in 20 percent of patients with tetralogy of Fallot and 3 to 5 percent of all patients with congenital heart disease. Since venous drainage is physiologically normal, no clinical manifestations are present. Patients with this anomaly who undergo central venous catheterization from the left may demonstrate an abnormal pathway of the catheter on the follow-up chest x-ray. This is probably the only important anesthetic implication of this syndrome.

In 8 percent of cases with persistent left superior vena cava the vessel connects directly to the left atrium. This lesion is almost always associated with complex cardiac anomalies. Occasionally the right superior vena cava is absent. The anomaly results in various degrees of right-to-left shunting, depending on blood return through the abnormal vessel, from 20 to 40 percent of total venous return. Cyanosis may be prominent if no atrial communication is present, without cardiac enlargement or failure. Systemic embolization and brain abscesses may occur. Treatment is surgical with either ligation or transposition of the abnormal vessel.

Anesthetic Considerations. The physiological consequences of the associated lesions will generally be the prominent feature guiding anesthetic management. In isolated forms management should be similar to the management of cyanotic lesions with normal pulmonary blood flow and directed toward prevention of endocarditis, systemic embolization, and thrombosis from polycythemia. No particular anesthetic technique seems likely to be superior, since the myocardial function in these patients is normal.

Anomalies of the Coronary Sinus

Anomalies of the coronary sinus are rare and are infrequently diagnosed during life. Complete absence of the coronary sinus is always associated with a persistent left superior vena cava. The coronary sinus may be hypoplastic, stenosis of the ostium may be present, or drainage may occur to the inferior vena cava or left atrium. The latter will result in a small right-to-left shunt, which is of no clinical significance. No unusual anesthetic problems should be caused by these anomalies.

Anomalies of the Inferior Vena Cava

Complete absence of the inferior vena cava with drainage of infradiaphragmatic systemic venous return through an enlarged azygos vein is present in close to 3 percent of patients with congenital heart disease but extremely rare in those with normal hearts. The anomaly has no physiological consequences but may cause problems during cardiac catheterization and venous cannulation for cardiac surgery.

A very rare anomaly consists of drainage of the inferior vena cava to the left atrium. It may occur as an isolated lesion or in conjunction with persistence of the sinus venosus valve and/or an ASD. Signs of systemic venous obstruction and a right-to-left shunt are present. Fifty percent of patients have associated cardiac defects, most commonly right ventricular outflow obstruction. Treatment of this anomaly is surgical. Its presence may complicate surgical repair of associated cardiac lesions, particularly atrial septal defect. Anesthetic implications are similar to those in patients with persistent left superior vena cava drainage into the left atrium.

Anomalies of the Coronary Arteries

Anomalous Origin of the Left Coronary Artery

Anomalous origin of the left coronary artery from the righ sinus of Valsalva results in this vessel's running between the aorta and right ventricular outflow tract or pulmonary trunk. Compression of the vessel may occur during exercise and has been implicated as a cause of death in young healthy athletes. The anomaly is rare.

Origin of the left coronary artery from the pulmonary trunk is a rare but frequently lethal anomaly. It is usually referred to as Bland-White-Garland syndrome. Eighty to 90 percent of patients become symptomatic in infancy and the majority die from congestive heart failure. The physiological derangement consists of perfusion of the left coronary artery from a low-pressure system with reduced oxygen saturation. This occurs as pulmonary pressure falls postnatally, although pulmonary artery pressure may remain elevated subsequent to poor left ventricular output with elevated left atrial pressures and secondary pulmonary hypertension.

Development of collateral vessels from the right coronary artery may be life-saving but results in a left-to-right shunt and volume overload of the heart with coronary steal. More commonly, endocardial and myocardial ischemia and infarction result from the decreased left myocardial perfusion, leading to papillary muscle dysfunction and mitral regurgitation. With feeding infants may present with signs of anginal attacks. The electrocardiogram resembles that of an adult with coronary artery disease. Infants with ischemic attacks require urgent surgery because of the risk of sudden death, while patients with heart failure may be managed conservatively in the expectation that collateral circulation will develop and myocardial function will improve.

Eventually all patients with this anomaly require correction to prevent sudden death. Various surgical approaches have been used. Simple ligation of the vessel in cases with left-to-right shunting and good collaterals may effect cure, but the result is unpredictable and leaves the patient with a system with one coronary artery. Presently favored are procedures that preserve a system with two coronary arteries by anastomosing either a systemic artery or a vein graft to the anomalous vessel, redirecting aortic blood flow to the anomalous coronary ostium via transpulmonary arterial baffle, or reanastomosing the vessel with a cuff of pulmonary trunk to the aorta. Surgery results in resolution of ischemic attacks and improved myocardial performance. Long-term prognosis of infants after surgery is not yet known.

Anesthetic Considerations. Patients with classic Bland-White-Garland syndrome require early surgical correction. Elective noncardiac surgery should be performed only after cardiac surgery. Management will depend on the degree of residual cardiovascular abnormality. Patients may have reduced cardiac reserve owing to myocardial scarring or residual mitral insufficiency. Use of anesthetic agents causing minimal myocardial depression, maintenance of heart rate, and direct monitoring of systemic arterial and venous pressures for major surgery are indicated.

In older patients with the uncorrected anomaly, care should be taken to avoid increases in myocardial oxygen demand (tachycardia, hypertension) or decreases in myocardial oxygen supply (low diastolic pressure, high left ventricular end-diastolic pressure). A left-to-right shunt is often present but of only small to moderate size. Patients are at risk for bacterial endocarditis after corrective surgery.

Anomalous Origin of the Right Coronary Artery

Origin of the right coronary artery from the pulmonary artery causes no symptoms. The area supplied by the pulmonary artery is the low-pressure right ventricle and no ischemia results. The condition is extremely rare and has usually been seen only on routine postmortem.

Anomalous Origin of Both Coronary Arteries

Origin of both coronary arteries from the pulmonary artery is extremely rare and is uniformly fatal within the first weeks of life unless associated with a lesion causing pulmonary hypertension, such as truncus arteriosus. The latter lesion requires correction in infancy.

Coronary Arteriovenous Fistula

Communication between the arterial and venous coronary vasculature can occur singly or as numerous, aneurysmatically dilated loops. This anomaly is rare. Over 90 percent of fistulas drain into the right side of the heart, with the physiological consequence of a left-to-right shunt with runoff from the aorta and volume overload of the left heart and pulmonary vasculature. Presentation is similar to that of patients with PDA but with an atypical murmur. Signs of myocardial ischemia from coronary steal are very uncommon. In the presence of a large shunt, symptoms of congestive heart failure and pulmonary hyperperfusion may occur. With most fistulas symptoms are minimal and the shunt is small. Since patients are at risk for endocarditis, secondary atherosclerotic changes with rupture, and thromboembolic phenomena, surgical correction of the lesion is recommended. Usually the fistula can be clamped and ligated without the use of cardiopulmonary bypass, with very low surgical mortality. Patients should be normal postoperatively. Prior to surgical correction, patients should be managed similarly to patients with a small to moderate PDA. They require endocarditis prophylaxis.

CARDIOMYOPATHIES

Cardiomyopathies are diseases of the myocardium not caused by structural abnormalities of the heart. They can be divided into primary cardiomyopathies, not associated with other disease and usually of unknown etiology, and secondary cardiomyopathies, associated with other diseases or known etiological agents. Pediatric cardiomyopathies are characterized by a high degree of morbidity and mortality. Primary cardiomyopathies are relatively uncommon. They can be classified according to the main physiological derangement into congestive cardiomyopathy, characterized by poor systolic ejection function; restrictive, with poor ventricular compliance or reduced ventricular volume; and obstructive, with obstruction to left ventricular output and/or obliteration of the ventricular cavities (Table 6–4).

Congestive Cardiomyopathies

The physiological derangement in congestive cardiomyopathy is a reduction in contractile force of the heart muscle. The initial compensatory mechanism consists of increased filling volumes, which maintain stroke volume via the Frank-Starling mechanism. As the ventricle dilates, wall tension and end-diastolic pressure increase, adversely affecting myocardial oxygenation. As stroke output falls, reflex sympathetic stimulation occurs, increasing impedance to left ventricular output, which increases myocardial oxygen demand. The elevated end-diastolic pressures are transmitted to the left atrium and pulmonary vascular bed, leading to pulmonary venous engorgement, pulmonary arterial hypertension, and eventually right heart failure. The elevated pulmonary vascular pressures result in transudation of fluid, interstitial and/or alveolar

Table 6–4. PEDIATRIC CARDIOMYOPATHIES

	Clinical Symptoms	Associated Features
Primary Cardiomyopathies		
Congestive nonobstructive		
Endocardial fibroelastosis of infancy	Mitral and aortic insufficiency	Long-term digitalis therapy
Idiopathic nonobstructive cardiomyopathy	Left ventricular thrombi	
	Pulsus alternans	
Restrictive		
Endomyocardial fibrosis	Atrial fibrillation, marked	Common in Africa
Hypertrophic form with ventricular hypertrophy and small ventricular cavities	cardiomegaly, ventilation-perfusion abnormalities, restriction to cardiac filling, A-V valve incompetence	
Loeffler endocarditis	Restriction to ventricular filling	
	Eosinophilia	Steroid therapy
Obstructive		
Idiopathic hypertrophic subaortic stenosis	Obstruction increased by inotropic agents or reduction in preload or afterload	Familial
		Uncommon in pediatric age groups
	Sudden death	
Secondary Cardiomyopathies		
Infective		
Virus	Congestive failure	
Trypanosoma	Congestive failure	May progress to chronic cardiopathy
Myocardial abscess in bacterial endocarditis	Congestive failure	
Diphtheria	Congestive failure	Heart block
Rheumatic carditis	Conduction defects common	Sensitive to digitalis
Metabolic		
Glycogenous Type II (Pompe)	Massive cardiomegaly	Unremitting failure
	Outflow tract obstruction	
Associated with neurological or vascular disease		
Friedreich ataxia	Conduction defects	Replacement of muscle fibers by connective tissue
Duchenne muscular dystrophy	Tachyarrhythmias	
Collagen disorders		
Disseminated lupus erythematosus	Pericarditis and pericardial effusion	
Dermatomyositis		
Neoplastic		
Leiomyofibroma		
Lymphoma	Mechanical obstruction	
Myxoma		
Miscellaneous		
Radiation		
Phosphorus		
Lead		
Antineoplastic drugs	Myocarditis	Congestive failure
Snake venom		
Scorpion venom		

pulmonary edema, and ventilation-perfusion abnormalities through small airway disease caused by bronchial cuffing and reduced compliance. Low cardiac output results in poor peripheral perfusion with metabolic acidosis and salt and water retention secondary to poor renal blood flow. Nutritional status deteriorates owing to reduced caloric intake and increased metabolic demand from respiratory distress.

Signs and symptoms of congestive heart failure in infancy are the same irrespective of etiology. Tachycardia and tachypnea are commonly present. Patients have a history of feeding difficulties, poor weight gain, frequent respiratory infections, excessive sweating (particularly with feeding), grunting, and wheezing. Rales may be heard together with pallor and peripheral cyanosis secondary to poor output. Older children may have tachycardia on exertion, orthopnea, chest discomfort or abdominal pain from a distended liver, a persistent dry cough, and anorexia. Pulses may be normal or reduced with cold extremities.

Therapy consists of digitalization, fluid restriction, diuresis, and reduction of cardiac afterload with an oral vasodilator (hydralazine). In the acutely decompensated patient, intravenous inotropic support with isoproterenol or dopamine infusion may be necessary. Isoproterenol reduces afterload by peripheral vasodilatation and is a pulmonary vasodilatator. Its undesirable side effects are tachycardia and ventricular dysrhythmias. It is the preferred agent in patients with pulmonary hypertension requiring afterload reduction and an increase in peripheral perfusion and in whom tachycardia or arrhythmias are not problems. Patients with arrhythmias or in whom tachycardia is undesirable should be treated with dopamine or dobutamine. Dopamine will not influence left ventricular afterload but causes renal arteriolar dilatation. Nitroprusside or nitroglycerin may be added for preload and afterload reduction.

Anesthetic Considerations. Elective surgery should be carried out only in compensated patients. Since myocardial reserve may be very limited, filling pressures of the right and left sides of the heart and continuous intra-arterial blood pressure should be monitored during major surgery to allow better assessment of the circulatory status as well as blood gases. Electrocardiographic monitoring is essential, since arrhythmias or conduction defects may readily occur. Electrolyte abnormalities should be corrected and alkalosis avoided in these patients, since they may precipitate digitalis toxicity.

Anesthetic agents with minimal effects on myocardial contractility should be used to avoid precipitating heart failure. Inhalation anesthetics are probably best avoided. Narcotics, particularly fentanyl, and ketamine are useful alternatives. Heart rate should be maintained so that cardiac output does not decrease, since stroke volume is generally limited. The generous use of atropine and the appropriate choice of muscle relaxants are important. Because of the ventilatory impairment

commonly present, the airway and ventilation should be controlled. Regional techniques may be a useful alternative to general anesthesia where possible.

Primary Endocardial Fibroelastosis

Primary endocardial fibroelastosis occurs in approximately 2 to 4 percent of patients with congenital heart disease and constitutes the most common cause of heart failure and death in children with heart disease between 2 months and 1 year of age. It occurs equally in both sexes. Secondary fibroelastosis is a common complication of cardiac lesions producing left ventricular wall stress (aortic stenosis, coarctation, mitral valve disease, hypoplastic left heart, anomalous origin of the left coronary artery).

The disease affects the left ventricle and usually extends into the left atrium. The right side of the heart is only rarely affected. Heart size is markedly increased, because of enlargement of the left ventricle and left atrium. The endocardium is diffusely thickened and is of milky-white appearance. Chordae tendineae and papillary muscles are involved in the fibrotic process.

The disease typically leads to rapid cardiac decompensation in a previously healthy infant. One third of patients become symptomatic within the first 3 months and 80 percent within the first year of life, with classic signs of left ventricular failure. Thrombi may form in the dilated ventricle and cause systemic embolization. One third of patients develop mitral insufficiency in later stages of the disease.

The clinical course of patients with early onset of the disease is poor. Death commonly occurs between 2 and 6 months of age despite vigorous anticongestive therapy. Patients who present in late infancy and early childhood may recover completely from their symptoms. The mainstay of therapy for endocardial fibroelastosis is prompt and prolonged administration of digitalis. Digitalis therapy should be maintained for a minimum of 2 years after symptoms have disappeared.

Premature discontinuation of digitalis may lead to recurrence of heart failure, which may not respond to renewed digitalis administration. If heart failure recurs on cessation of digitalis therapy, patients usually progress to chronic cardiac failure and ultimately death. Mitral insufficiency may progress and necessitate valve replacement in childhood or adolescence.

Anesthetic Considerations. Patients should be managed according to the recommendations outlined earlier for congestive failure. Maintenance of digitalis therapy is essential. Patients need close monitoring for signs of digitalis toxicity.

Idiopathic Nonobstructive Cardiomyopathy

This form of congestive cardiomyopathy is characterized by dilatation of both ventricular cavities, reduced ejection fraction, and increased end-systolic volume. This disease is very common in South Africa, accounting for 25 to 35 percent of cases of heart disease, but rare elsewhere. The increased end-systolic volume leads to relative stasis of the blood in the apical portion of the ventricles, resulting in intracavitary thrombosis. Patients present with signs of congestive failure and usually pulsus alternans. The disease may be present in infants but more commonly occurs in children and adolescents. Treatment consists of anti-congestive therapy and anticoagulation until symptoms resolve. The majority of patients have a slow downhill course over a number of years.

Anesthetic management should be tailored to the degree of myocardial failure.

Restrictive Cardiomyopathies

Restrictive cardiomyopathies are characterized by abnormal diastolic function while ventricular contractile function is unimpaired or even greater than normal. The resistance to diastolic filling from the nonelastic ventricles results in elevation of ventricular end-diastolic pressures, leading to elevation in atrial and systemic and pulmonary venous pressures. Pulmonary hypertension is usually observed. Left-sided filling pressures are generally higher than right-sided pressures, in contrast to constrictive pericarditis. Eventually signs of right-sided failure with systemic venous distention and hepatic congestion and ascites occur. Stroke volume may be limited and cardiac output maintained by increases in heart rate. The most common clinical symptoms are dyspnea and exercise intolerance. Atrial fibrillation may occur in patients with marked atrial enlargment and usually leads to clinical deterioration because of further impairment in left ventricular filling. Patients may respond poorly to digitalis. Diuretic therapy may control symptoms temporarily.

Anesthetic Management. Maintenance of cardiac contractility and heart rate is essential. Preload must be adequate to maintain filling pressures and cardiac output. Patients may be unable to compensate for reduction in afterload, which should be kept close to normal. Direct monitoring of filling and systemic arterial pressures should be established for all major procedures. Because pulmonary congestion is frequently present, ventilation-perfusion abnormalities should be expected and treated with higher oxygen concentrations and controlled ventilation. Reliable electrocardiographic monitoring is necessary, and every effort should be made to maintain sinus rhythm.

Patients with the hypertrophic form of restrictive myocarditis may benefit from use of an inhalational anesthetic agent, such as halothane, that causes reduction in the hypercontractile state of the left ventricular muscle unless congestive heart failure is present. All other forms of restrictive myocarditis require maintenance of myocardial contractility, and narcotics and ketamine are probably better choices for anesthetic management.

Patients require endocarditis prophylaxis.

Endomyocardial Fibrosis

Endomyocardial fibrosis is an unusual form of cardiomyopathy characterized by restriction to ventricular filling and obliteration of the inflow portion of the ventricles by dense fibrosis and thrombus formation. The fibrosis involves the papillary muscles, leading to secondary AV valve incompetence. The right heart is usually more affected, and signs of right-sided obstruction are present. In addition, pleural and pericardial effusion are common. Atrial fibrillation is commonly seen in advanced disease. The disease is most prevalent in tropical Africa, where it affects up to 20 percent of patients with heart disease. It is a disease of children and young adults; 70 percent of patients are under 20 years of age.

Medical therapy in symptomatic patients is generally unsuccessful, with a reported average 2-year survival. Surgical therapy consists of pericardiectomy or pericardioperitoneal shunt in patients with recurrent massive pericardial effusion. A Glenn shunt may be performed to improve pulmonary perfusion. Corrective surgery consists of stripping of the endocardium with or without AV valve replacement.

Loeffler Endocarditis

This is a form of myocardiopathy similar to tropical endomyocardial fibrosis but is seen in temperate climates and more commonly in males. It is associated with marked eosinophilia without identifiable cause. Multiple organs may be affected in addition. The disease occurs in adolescents and young adults. Concentric left ventricular wall thickening occurs with intracavitary thrombosis and systemic embolization. In addition, scarring of the mitral valve with adhesion of the posterior leaflet to the ventricular wall results in mitral insufficiency. The disease causes a high morbidity and mortality, but the prognosis appears to have improved recently with corticosteroid and/or hydroxyurea therapy.

Obstructive Cardiomyopathies

Idiopathic Hypertrophic Cardiomyopathy

Hypertrophic cardiomyopathy is a primary disease of cardiac muscle characterized by a hypertrophied, nondilated left ventricle. Histologically, marked disorganization of myocardial cells, particularly of the ventricular septum, is present. The disease is genetically transmitted in the majority of cases as an autosomal dominant trait and affects both sexes equally. It is rare in Africans and black Americans. It appears to be associated with lentiginosis, neurofibromatosis, pheochromocytoma, and Friedreich ataxia.

Obstructive hypertrophic cardiomyopathy represents 0.7 percent of all congenital heart disease and 10 percent of all cases of aortic stenosis. Septal hypertrophy of at least 1.3 times the thickness of the left ventricular free wall is an invariable feature. Although the disease was originally described in the context of dynamic left ventricular outflow obstruction (idiopathic subaortic stenosis), in reality this obstruction is absent in a large proportion of patients with this disease.

Clinical manifestations are generally not present until adolescence or adulthood. The most frequent presentation is in the third or fourth decade of life. The predominant complaint is exertional dyspnea or fatigue; in childhood the usual presenting finding is a murmur. When the disease presents during infancy, which is rare, a high incidence of congestive heart failure and right and left ventricular outflow obstruction is noted. Heart failure in these infants occurs in the presence of a nondilated ventricle with normal or increased systolic function and appears to be a sign of poor prognosis. The majority of affected infants die from their congestive failure within the first year of life. Congestive heart failure is uncommon in older children and adolescents with this disease.

The major abnormality in hypertrophic cardiomyopathy is a diminution in left ventricular compliance causing increased resistance to left ventricular filling. Left ventricular outflow tract obstruction is caused by the hypertrophied septum and an abnormal forward movement of the anterior mitral leaflet during systole. The latter frequently also results in some mitral valve incompetence. The obstruction is dynamic in nature and may be reduced by increased ventricular volume, reduced contractility, and increased systemic vascular resistance. Hypovolemia, low peripheral vascular resistance, and increased contractility (as in sympathetic stimulation) will lead to worsening of the gradient across the left ventricular outflow tract. Patients with hypertrophic cardiomyopathy have a high incidence of serious ventricular arrhythmias despite lack of symptoms.

Sudden death occurs in 3 to 4 percent of affected patients and is particularly common in young patients between 12 and 30 years, frequently in association with strenuous exercise. Half of these patients are asymptomatic prior to sudden death. Sudden death appears to be more common in some families.

Atrial fibrillation may occur in later stages, probably owing to left atrial enlargement caused by a poorly compliant left ventricle. It generally leads to clinical deterioration, since it interferes with left ventricular filling.

The mainstay of medical therapy for hypertrophic cardiomyopathy is beta-adrenergic blockade. Calcium channel blockers may prove beneficial by improving left ventricular filling. Excessive use of diuretics, preload and afterload reducing agents, beta-agonistic drugs, and digitalis may lead to worsening of symptoms because of an increase in subaortic obstruction. Paroxysmal atrial fibrillation may require use of digitalis to control the dysrhythmia, and patients require anticoagulation to prevent systemic embolization.

Surgical therapy is of only limited use. Septal myotomy or myectomy is usually recommended for patients with severe symptoms refractory to medical therapy and outflow gradients of 50 mmHg or more. Operative mortality ranges from 5 to 10 percent. Surgery usually results in relief of the obstruction when the patient is at rest, although a mild to moderate gradient may recur with provocation. Aortic insufficiency due to damage of the cusps at surgery may develop later. The mortality for patients with hypertrophic cardiomyopathy not treated surgically ranges around 3 percent per year, but mortality appears to be somewhat lower for patients after surgery (1.9 percent).

Anesthetic Considerations. Preoperative anxiety should be reduced by generous sedation. In addition to reliable electrocardiographic monitoring, close monitoring of systemic and right or left filling pressures is indicated for all major surgery. Changes in filling volume, distending pressure of the left ventricle, heart rate and rhythm, and left ventricular afterload and contractility may adversely influence left ventricular outflow obstruction and decrease cardiac output. In addition, these patients exhibit a high propensity for ventricular arrhythmias.

Hypovolemia, vasodilation, and hypotension should be prevented. Use of the Trendelenburg position and phenylephrine may be helpful for acute therapy. Tachycardia and sympathetic stimulation may accompany light anesthesia and lead to increased contractility and decreased filling, increasing obstruction. Reduction in peripheral vascular resistance, as with sympathetic blockade, may also result in an increased outflow gradient.

Inhalation anesthetics (particularly halothane) appear to be well tolerated together with adequate volume replacement, since they tend to decrease myocardial contractility and permit rapid changes in anesthetic depth. A smooth induction is essential. In older children a barbiturate induction may be useful. Excessive positive-pressure ventilation should be avoided since it interferes with venous return and may cause a decrease in left ventricular volume and subsequent worsening of the outflow gradient.

Sinus rhythm should be maintained. Tachyarrhythmias may require treatment with propranolol or verapamil. Positive inotropic agents and vasodilators should be avoided. Fentanyl, which causes mild bradycardia and has little cardiovascular effect, may prove useful, whereas ketamine is relatively contraindicated.

Major regional anesthesia is probably contraindicated since it results in widespread sympathetic blockade. Peripheral vascular resistance should be maintained, if necessary with a peripherally acting vasoconstrictor like phenylephrine. Patients require endocarditis prophylaxis.

TUMORS OF THE HEART

Primary tumors of the heart and pericardium are rare, with an incidence between 0.001 and 0.28 percent in reported autopsy series.

In infants and children rhabdomyoma is the most common cardiac tumor. Seventy-five percent of all cardiac tumors in infants less than 1 year old are rhabdomyomas or teratomas. In children from 1 to 15 years of age rhabdomyomas, fibromas, and myxomas account for 80 percent of benign cardiac tumors and 60 percent of all tumors and cysts of the heart and pericardium. Malignant tumors account for less than 10 percent of all tumors and cysts in this age group.

The manifestations of cardiac tumors depend on the location of the tumor. Involvement of the conduction tissue may lead to dysrhythmias. Intracavitary tumors may result in obstruction to blood flow and filling of the affected chamber, obstruction of valves, or embolization of fragmented tumor material. Involvement of the myocardium may lead to myocardial failure.

Benign Tumors

Rhabdomyoma

This is the most common tumor in infancy and childhood, occurring in 80 percent of patients with cardiac tumors who are less than 1 year old. The tumors commonly are multiple, occurring in the right and left ventricles or less often in the atria. The largest mass is usually located in the ventricular septum, but over half of the tumors are intracavitary and lead to obstruction of blood flow. Thirty percent of patients have tuberous sclerosis and adenomas of the sebaceous glands. Presenting symptoms are arrhythmias, congestive failure, or signs of valvular obstruction, usually of the inlet type. The natural history of patients with cardiac rhabdomyoma is poor. Fifty percent die within the first 6 months and 80 percent before 1 year unless surgical excision of the tumor is performed. Survival after excision appears excellent, with resolution of cardiac symptoms.

Fibroma

Cardiac fibromas are almost always solitary and constitute the second most common cardiac tumor in childhood. Symptoms generally occur within the first decade. The tumors compress surrounding structures because of their size. They frequently occur in the ventricular septum and invade the conduction system, leading to ventricular dysrhythmias and sudden death. With large tumors intractable heart failure or signs of cardiac obstruction are common.

Tumors located in the free ventricular wall are usually amenable to resection, while septal tumors often cannot be completely removed but can be sufficiently debulked to result in improvement in clinical symptoms. Prognosis after debulking is guarded. Patients often die from ventricular arrhythmias.

Myxoma

Intracavitary myxomas constitute about half of all benign cardiac tumors in adults but occur rarely in children. The tumor commonly arises as a pedunculated mass from the atrial septum; 75 percent occur in the left atrium. Patients present with changing signs of mitral valve disease, either stenosis or insufficiency, and a history of fainting spells. Because the tumor is soft it fragments easily, with resulting pulmonary and/or systemic embolization, depending on the primary location of the myxoma. Signs of mitral stenosis in a child should lead the physician to suspect left atrial myxoma.

Therapy consists of surgical excision of the tumor and the attached atrial wall to prevent recurrence. Prognosis postoperatively is generally excellent. Patients with systemic embolization prior to surgery may develop coronary and cerebral aneurysms in later years from myxomatous degeneration at the embolic site.

Teratoma

The majority of teratomas of the heart are extracardiac but intrapericardial, arising from the origin of the great vessels. These tumors are very rare, are usually seen in infancy or childhood, and more commonly affect females. The tumors cause cardiac compression with dyspnea and cyanosis. Surgical excision is the only effective therapy.

Malignant Tumors

Primary malignant tumors of the heart are very uncommon in infants and children. They are most commonly malignant teratomas or rhabdomyosarcomas. Clinical presentation depends on the degree of intracavitary obstruction and the involvment of the conduction system. The cardiac valves are often invaded by the tumor in rhabdomyosarcoma. Prognosis is poor, with most patients dying within a year of diagnosis.

Anesthetic Considerations

Patients with benign lesions should undergo excision prior to elective surgery. Reliable electrocardiographic monitoring is essential and should be continued postoperatively, since conduction defects may persist. Agents causing increased ventricular irritability should be avoided in patients with known propensity for ventricular arrhythmias. Blood pressure control may be important after myxoma excision, since patients may have unrecognized cerebral aneurysms. Those with myocardial fibromas may have a residual defect similar to a restrictive cardiomyopathy with decreased diastolic function and require careful fluid management and maintenance of myocardial contractility.

CONGENITAL CONDUCTION DEFECTS

Congenital Complete Heart Block

Congenital complete heart block is a rare anomaly, occurring in less than 1 percent of patients with congenital heart disease. It is, however, very common in children of mothers with lupus erythematosus even if the mother is clinically asymptomatic. The defect is commonly a singular one but may be associated with other congenital cardiac anomalies, particularly corrected transposition or atrial septal defects. Heart block in infancy and childhood most commonly arises following repair of intracardiac lesions.

Congenital complete heart block is characterized by complete absence of conduction between the atria and ventricles. The heart rate is usually less than 80 in infants and around 50 in children. The diagnosis may be suspected prenatally if there is a fetal heart rate of less than 100 in the absence of any etiology for fetal distress. Most patients have a block located high in the septum between the AV node and the His bundle. The QRS complexes are narrow (less than 0.1 sec) and normally configurated. The heart rate characteristically can be increased by exercise, atropine, and sympathomimetics. In contrast to acquired complete heart block, cardiac output is maintained by an increased stroke volume. Clinically, patients exhibit bounding pulses, a low diastolic pressure from diastolic runoff with a slow heart rate, and cannon waves in the jugular pulse when the atrium contracts against the closed tricuspid valve.

A small subgroup of patients with congenital heart block have the block located distal to the bundle of His. In these patients the QRS complex is widened and abnormal, and the heart rate is usually slower; most such patients are symptomatic.

Congestive heart failure is the usual presenting symptom in infancy, while older children with congenital heart block who become symptomatic usually have exercise intolerance and a history of syncopal attacks, which are frequently caused by ventricular dysrhythmias and not bradycardia.

Death from congenital heart block usually occurs within the first year, generally in infants with heart rates below 55 and wide QRS complexes. Older children tend to be asyptomatic. They may exhibit episodic supraventricular dyshythmias without untoward side effects. Asymptomatic patients need continued follow-up to evaluate exercise tolerance and search for development of ventricular ectopy.

Symptomatic infants and children with a history of congestive failure, syncope, or marked exercise intolerance, as well as patients with block below the bundle of His and those with associated cardiac defects and heart rates below 65 to 70, require pacing. Occurrence of frequent or complex ventricular dysrhythmias may also be an indication for pacing. Permanent pacemakers in infants and children are fraught with technical problems. Infants usually require placement of epicardial pacer leads, while transvenous pacing is reserved for older children. The mortality rate for pediatric patients with pacemakers is reported as 15 percent, with half of the deaths due to pacemaker failure. Infection, erosion, and breakage or failure of leads, particularly with growth, are common problems. Av-

erage duration of pacing in one study was 20 to 30 months, with frequent reoperations to maintain pacing (at least one procedure per patient per year).

The most common indication for implantation of a permanent pacemaker is acquired heart block below the bundle of His following repair of an intracardiac congenital lesion.

Anesthetic Considerations. Because of the relatively high risk of death from congenital heart block in infants, a temporary pacemaker should be inserted in these patients prior to any anesthetic. In older children who are asymptomatic and have a narrow QRS complex, anesthesia and surgery have been carried out without problems and without temporary pacing. Adequate vagolysis and the use of anesthetic agents without negative chronotropic or inotropic side effects (atropine, ketamine, narcotics, isoflurane, pancuronium, or gallamine) is recommended. An isoproterenol infusion and temporary external or transvenous pacing should be readily available in the operating room.

Local anesthetics may be used for selected procedures if low blood levels are maintained, but high blood levels of local anethetics may cause further slowing of ventricular conduction.

Patients with wide QRS complexes, a history of syncope or congestive heart failure, moderate to severe exercise intolerance, associated cardiac anomalies, and/or absence of chronotropic response to atropine and all patients with acquired heart block require at least temporary pacing prior to administration of any anesthetic, since perioperative stress may cause life-threatening dysrhythmias.

Reentry Tachycardias

Supraventricular Tachycardia

Supraventricular tachycardia (SVT) is a common pediatric disorder. It is estimated to occur in 1 in 25,000 children and is more common in males and in the first few months of life. Recognition of the anomaly is important, since congestive heart failure develops in a significant number of infants with sustained SVT of longer than 24 hours' duration.

The etiology in most cases is unknown and may be related to abnormal postnatal development of the specialized tissue in the atrioventricular node and His bundle. Twenty-five to 50 percent of infants with SVT will manifest Wolff-Parkinson-White syndrome on their ECG after conversion. Most cases of SVT in children are due to a reentry mechanism with antegrade conduction through a slow pathway and retrograde conduction through a fast pathway. In this form of tachycardia, P waves are not visible on the surface ECG, since atrial activation and ventricular depolarization occur simultaneously.

Infants who present with SVT and fast heart rates are usually in heart failure or cardiogenic shock, either of which represents a medical emergency. Normal cardiac rhythm should be restored by direct synchronized cardioversion. Digitalization should be carried out immediately after cardioversion. In infants with less cardiac impairment vagal stimulation by the diving reflex may be successful in converting the tachycardia. A small plastic bag filled with ice and covering the face may be used instead of dunking the face in ice water. If the diving reflex is not successful, rapid intravenous digitalization or direct current cardioversion is advocated. If these maneuvers fail, intravenous propranolol or overdrive pacing may be attempted.

The majority of infants with SVT readily respond to digoxin, have few recurrences, and may have digoxin therapy withdrawn after 1 year of age. Patients unresponsive to digoxin should be treated with propranolol. Older children who develop supraventricular tachycardia have a higher incidence of Wolff-Parkinson-White syndrome and usually do not present in heart failure. Besides vagal stimulation, treatment with verapamil 0.1 mg/kg as an intravenous bolus is currently recommended. Verapamil should not be given to patients on propranolol therapy or patients suspected of sick sinus syndrome. With relatively slow tachycardias, chronic digitalization should be started. All patients are maintained on digitalis to prevent recurrence of tachycardia.

Wolff-Parkinson-White Syndrome

This form of reentry tachycardia is characterized by the presence of an accessory atrioventricular conduction pathway (Kent bundle), represented on the normal electrocardiogram with a short P–R interval, widened QRS complex, and presence of a delta wave in the initial portion of the QRS complex.

The syndrome is probably present in 0.1 percent of unselected children, but more frequent in children with congenital heart disease. About 70 percent of patients are male. Forty percent of children with Wolff-Parkinson-White syndrome have associated congenital heart disease, most commonly Ebstein anomaly. Corrected transposition, primary cardiomyopathies, atrial septal defect, and floppy mitral valve have also been described. Wolff-Parkinson-White syndrome may be subdivided into type A, with abnormal conduction along the left bundle, and type B, with conduction along the right bundle. Seventy percent of patients with Wolff-Parkinson-White syndrome develop premature beats and tachyarrhythmias. The episodes may be triggered by sympathetic stimulation. Digoxin is effective in controlling arrhythmias in the majority of cases. Propranolol, quinidine, and recently amiodarone have been used in refractory cases. If no control of tachyarrhythmias can be achieved, overdrive pacing or surgical division of the accessory pathway can be performed. The latter procedure has been reported with a 90 percent success rate in infants and children. Transvenous electrical or cryoablation of the abnormal pathways can be performed in older children or adolescents.

Lown-Ganong-Levine Syndrome

A rare cause of supraventricular tachycardia is the presence of an AV nodal bypass (James fiber). The ECG is characterized by a short P–R interval and a normal QRS complex. Patients have a high incidence of atrial flutter-fibrillation. It is more common in females. Therapy is similar to that for the Wolff-Parkinson-White syndrome. Quinidine and procainamide may slow conduction through the abnormal bypass tract.

Anesthetic Considerations

Prevention of reentry tachycardias, which may lead to very rapid ventricular response and cardiovascular collapse, is the major anesthetic problem. Since sympathetic stimulation may trigger a tachyarrhythmia, adequate preoperative sedation and sufficient depth of anesthesia are important. Antiarrhythmic therapy should be continued preoperatively. Anesthetic agents without positive chronotropic or sympathomimetic side effects should be used. Halothane, although it causes sinus bradycardia, may predispose to occurrence of atrial extrasystoles, which may trigger reentry tachycardias. Enflurane and isoflurane appear to have a mild dysrhythmic effect and may be preferable. Barbiturates, narcotics, nitrous oxide, and muscle relaxants other than pancuronium and gallamine have been successfully used. Increased sympathetic activity, exogenous epinephrine, hypoxia, hypercarbia, and metabolic acidosis may all cause increased atrial or ventricular automaticity and trigger SVT.

If SVT occurs during anesthesia, vagal stimulation by a Valsalva maneuver, stimulation of the gag reflex, ice application to the face, or unilateral carotid massage should be tried initially. If these measures are unsuccessful, verapamil, propranolol, direct current cardioversion, or esophageal overdrive pacing can be used to restore sinus rhythm. In patients with junctional ectopic tachycardia, verapamil should not be used, since it may lead to acceleration of the ventricular rate with cardiovascular collapse. Should this problem occur it may be treated with intravenous calcium chloride. Propranolol and verapamil should not be given concurrently, since complete heart block and severe myocardial depression may result. Patients on amiodarone may develop pulmonary fibrosis or thyroid dysfunction. Amiodarone causes beta receptor blockade and has a half-life of 25 to 55 days. Patients on this drug need careful monitoring to prevent undue cardiovascular side effects.

Prolonged Q–T Interval

The association of a prolonged Q–T interval, congenital deafness, syncopal attacks, and a high incidence of sudden death is known as Jervell and Lange-Nielsen syndrome. It affects approximately 0.3 percent of children with congenital neural deafness and is transmitted as an autosomal reccessive gene. An identical condition without congenital deafness is about three times more frequent and is known as Romano-Ward syndrome. It is transmitted as an autosomal dominant gene. Familial ventricular tachycardia, also transmitted as an autosomal dominant gene, is an atypical form of prolonged Q–T interval with prolongation occurring during exercise. The syncopal attacks in all three conditions are due to paroxysmal ventricular fibrillation of the type known as torsades de pointes and typically are triggered by exercise or physical or emotional stress. All these factors result in increased sympathetic activity, and the arrhythmias appear to be caused by an imbalance of the outflows of the right and left cardiac sympathetics. The mortality in untreated cases is high, between 30 and 70 percent. Attacks usually begin in childhood and become less frequent with increasing age.

Treatment of choice consists of adequate beta blockade. Therapeutic levels have to be maintained. In resistant cases a combination of beta blockade and phenytoin is usually successful. If medical treatment fails, left stellate ganglionectomy should be performed, which generally results in complete suppression of the attacks although the Q–T interval may not be normalized. Left stellate ganglion block may also result in shortening of the Q–T interval and abolition of the arrhythmia. Right-sided stellate ganglion block results in worsening of the condition.

Anesthetic Management. Reliable electrocardiographic monitoring is essential. A defibrillator should be immediately available. All conditions causing excitement and anxiety should be avoided. Heavy preanesthetic sedation is useful, as is adequate perioperative pain relief. Bradycardia should be avoided, since it may lead to escape beats and trigger a ventricular arrhythmia in these susceptible patients. Maintenance of adequate beta blockade is essential. Anesthetic agents that sensitize the myocardium to endogenous catecholamines or have sympathomimetic side effects should be avoided, as should all drugs causing prolongation of the Q–T interval. These include the phenothiazines, quinidine, lidocaine, and procainamide. Hypokalemia, hypomagnesemia, and hypocalcemia have the same undesirable effect. Barbiturates, narcotics, enflurane, and isoflurane have all been used successfully in combination with nitrous oxide in patients with prolonged Q–T interval.

DISEASES OF THE PERICARDIUM

Absent Pericardium

Partial or complete absence of the pericardium is an extremely rare congenital defect. The defect is usually left-sided. Most cases have no symptoms but may demonstrate an abnormal shift of the heart on x-ray. Complete absence of the pericardium does not interfere with a normal life if no other malformations are present. Partial absence may allow herniation followed by strangulation of the atria or part of the ventricles, which can cause death. Patients with defects large enough to allow herniation require pericardioplasty or enlargement of the defect to prevent strangulation. Small defects require no treatment.

Pericardial Cyst

Pericardial cysts usually are solitary and lie against the parietal pericardium, and rarely communicate with the pericardial sac. They may be confused with cardiac tumors. They commonly are located at the costophrenic angles, usually on the right. They generally are asymptomatic but give rise to a tremendously enlarged heart on radiological examination without evidence of heart failure or electrocardiographic changes. Treatment consists of surgical removal.

Pericarditis

Except for the two conditions already discussed, pericardial disease is a manifestation of some other systemic disease that leads to either fluid accumulation in the pericardial sac, resulting in cardiac tamponade, or scarring and fibrosis of the pericardium, leading to constrictive pericarditis. The latter condition is extremely rare in pediatric patients.

The most common cause of pericarditis in children is rheumatic pericarditis. Pericarditis can otherwise be due to pyogenic organisms, rheumatoid arthritis, or viral, uremic, or neoplastic disease or can be part of the post-pericardiotomy syndrome. Lupus, tuberculosis, congenital hypoplastic anemia, Mediterranean anemia, Friedreich ataxia, ulcerative colitis, and radiation are rare causes of pericardial disease in children.

The physiological disturbance in pericardial disease is due to impairment of cardiac filling caused by either compression from accumulated fluid or restriction of myocardial movement. The restriction of cardiac filling leads to elevation of the venous pressure and a fall in stroke volume and cardiac output. Compensatory mechanisms include increases in heart rate, contractility, and peripheral vasoconstriction. Decreased renal perfusion leads to aldosterone secretion and salt and fluid retention. Coronary perfusion may be decreased secondary to reduced diastolic time and increased intraventricular pressure. Myocardial dysfunction is more commonly seen with pericardial tamponade. The raised diastolic pressure in both ventricles results in equality of all filling pressures. Right atrial, pulmonary artery diastolic, and left atrial pressures are equal. Normal respiratory variation in systemic blood pressure due to pooling of blood in the pulmonary vascular bed is markedly increased with the restriction of cardiac filling, leading to pulsus paradoxus (a fall of greater than 10 mmHg in systolic blood pressure with inspiration).

Most patients with acute pericardial disease respond to medical management. Anti-inflammatory agents, steroids, or antibiotics are used, depending on the etiology. Patients with cardiac tamponade may require pericardiocentesis under local anesthesia to improve cardiac performance. With recurrent fluid accumulation a pericardial window may have to be constructed. Patients with symptomatic constrictive pericarditis require surgical pericardiectomy.

Anesthetic Considerations. Patients with acute pericarditis will be seen only on an emergency basis for relief of cardiac tamponade. Patients with mild constrictive pericarditis not requiring surgical intervention should be treated similarly to patients with restrictive cardiomyopathy. Electrocardiographic monitoring and direct measurement of filling and systemic pressure are indicated for most procedures. Right-sided pressures and volume are more seriously affected in pericardial effusion, and central venous pressure measurements are usually sufficient. Patients require maintenance of adequate filling pressures and heart rate. Anesthetic agents causing minimal myocardial depression should be used. Peripheral vascular resistance should be maintained. Positive-pressure ventilation may seriously interfere with cardiac filling, and spontaneous ventilation should be maintained if possible. Ketamine, narcotics, and relaxants with sympathomimetic side effects may be advantageous.

MALPOSITIONS OF THE HEART

The heart may be located on the right, on the left with the viscera inverted, in the middle of the thorax, or outside the thorax.

Dextrocardia

Dextrocardia is the most common malposition of the heart. It may occur with or without situs inversus and is commonly associated with asplenia or polysplenia syndrome. In most cases other cardiac anomalies are present, most commonly transposition and septation defects. Isolated dextrocardia is usually associated with other congenital malformations, particularly hypoplasia or aplasia of the right lung. In patients with dextrocardia and asplenia syndrome, complex cardiac malformations are the rule. Fifty to 80 percent of patients with dextrocardia and situs inversus, however, have normal hearts. In Kartagener syndrome this form of dextrocardia is associated with bronchiectasis and sinusitis.

Levocardia

Levocardia is associated with either asplenia or polysplenia and visceral heterotaxy in 80 percent of cases and with situs inversus in only 20 percent. Complex cyanotic heart disease is frequently present, and the majority of patients die in infancy.

Mesocardia

Mesocardia is extremely rare, and congenital cardiac lesions are present in 75 percent of patients.

Anesthetic Considerations

The associated cardiac defects and the physiological derangement caused thereby will generally influence the anesthetic management. Patients with asplenia syndrome need prophylaxis against encapsulated bacteria like *Klebsiella*, *Escherichia*, and *Haemophilus* with either amoxicillin or ampicillin. Patients with isolated dextrocardia may have marked ventilatory impairment owing to reduced lung tissue and tracheal compression from the aortic arch. Bronchiectasis may be present in patients with "mirror image" dextrocardia (dextrocardia and situs inversus).

Ectopia Cordis

Position of the heart partially or completely outside the thorax represents ectopia cordis. The malformation is extremely rare. The classical form of ectopic cordis is the thoracic type with a sternal defect; absence of the parietal pericardium; cephalic orientation of the apex, which beats against the infant's chin; epigastric omphalocele or diastasis recti; and a small thoracic cavity. Other cardiac lesions are usually present. Patients require immediate surgery to correct their cardiac lesion and reconstruct the chest wall defect. Initially the heart cannot usually be positioned inside the small thoracic cavity without causing kinking of the vessels or tamponade.

Thoracoabdominal Ectopia Cordis

The heart is displaced inferiorly through an anterior diaphragmatic defect into the epigastrium. Partial cleft of the lower sternum, a defect of the diaphragmatic pericardium, and omphalocele or diastasis recti are always present. Most patients have congenital heart disease. Repair has been achieved by closure of the diaphragmatic defect and repair of the abdominal wall defect. Thoracic ectopia has a high mortality with or without surgery. Survival into adulthood with abdominal ectopia cordis without surgical intervention has been described.

ACQUIRED HEART DISEASE

Rheumatic Heart Disease

Acute rheumatic fever remains the leading pediatric acquired heart disease in the United States and Western Europe. In the developing countries rheumatic fever represents the predominant cause of all heart disease in the pediatric age group.

Rheumatic fever is closely associated with group A beta-hemolytic streptococcal infections of the upper respiratory tract. Approximately 3 percent of infected patients will develop acute rheumatic fever within 7 to 35 days. The disease most commonly occurs in the young school-age child from a low socioeconomic group in winter or spring. The pathogenetic basis of the disease is still not fully understood but may involve hypersensitivity reactions, an autoimmune process, direct toxic effects of bacterial lysins, or direct bacterial infection.

Rheumatic heart disease is present in approximately 0.7 to 1.6 per 1000 school children in the United States. The fatality rate is estimated to be 2 to 3 percent. The disease is by nature recurrent, and chronic disability and death are related to recurrent attacks. Recurrence is invariably preceded by streptococcal infection, with the highest risk of recurrence in the first few years after the initial event. Adequate prolonged penicillin treatment and continuous sulfadiazine or low-dose penicillin prophylaxis is highly effective in protecting from recurrent attacks. The most effective form of prophylaxis appears to be benzathine penicillin G 1.2 million units intramuscularly once a month, which should be continued throughout childhood.

The diagnosis of acute rheumatic fever is still based on the Jones criteria. The major criteria are fever, polyarthritis, carditis, chorea, erythema marginatum, and subcutaneous nodules. Evidence of preceding streptococcal infection (antistreptolysin titer) strengthens the diagnosis. Carditis may be silent in its appearance until heart failure or a murmur appears or a pericardial effusion is manifested. It is noted in 76 percent of cases within the first week of onset of the disease.

Aspirin and corticosteroids are dramatically effective in suppressing the acute manifestations of rheumatic fever. Aspirin does not appear to alter the frequency of residual rheumatic heart disease. Steroids appear to improve the prognosis of patients with moderate to severe carditis but their dosage should be tapered as soon as the acute disease is under control and the patient is changed over to aspirin therapy. Aspirin in daily doses of 90 to 120 mg/kg is usually sufficient to achieve therapeutic blood levels of 20 to 25 mg/100 ml. Higher doses may produce hepatic injury. Residual streptococcal infection is eradicated with therapeutic doses of penicillin, with prophylaxis started subsequently. Patients with carditis may require prolonged bed rest and should not be ambulatory until all signs of heart failure have disappeared. Heart failure may be treated with digitalis and diuretics.

The patient with severe carditis or frequent recurrences may develop rheumatic heart disease. This complication occurs with high frequency in economically underprivileged areas, particularly in Africa and Asia, and most often in childhood. In 85 percent of cases the mitral valve is involved, in 54 percent the aortic valve, and in less than 5 per cent the tricuspid or pulmonary valve.

Rheumatic carditis may heal with residual interstitial fibrosis and some fibrosis of the endocardium. These lesions do not appear to be progressive and produce no hemodynamic abnormalities, but predispose patients to endocarditis. The interstitial fibrosis may lead to intensified myocardial dilatation resulting from valvular defects.

Mitral Insufficiency

Valvular rheumatic heart disease in childhood and adolescence is most commonly present as mitral insufficiency. Because the left ventricle is subject to only diastolic volume overload, most defects are well tolerated for many years. Pressure and volume of the left atrium are elevated, and chronic pulmonary congestion, pulmonary hypertension, and right ventricular hypertrophy and dilatation develop with time. In most children and adolescents the lesion is mild, with absence of symptoms and only a murmur of mitral regurgitation. The main emphasis is placed on long-term prophylaxis. Patients with signs of heart failure should be managed conservatively. Surgery is seldom indicated for children and adolescents. If surgery is necessary an annuloplasty or valvuloplasty is performed if possible to avoid the long-term problems of prosthetic valves.

Mitral Stenosis

Many years are usually necessary to develop narrowing of the mitral orifice sufficient to produce symptoms. For this reason, significant rheumatic mitral stenosis is extremely uncommon in the pediatric age group. However, in some parts of the world, particularly Asia and Africa, tight mitral stenosis occurs relatively frequently in children less than 15 years old. Mitral stenosis is more common in females.

The physiological derangement, as described in the discussion of congenital mitral stenosis earlier in the chapter, consists of an obstruction to ventricular filling at the mitral valve. To overcome the obstruction, left atrial pressure is raised and a gradient is established between left atrial mean and left ventricular end-diastolic pressures. Filling depends on orifice size, pressure gradient, and diastolic interval. With a fast heart rate, diastolic filling time is reduced and cardiac output may fall. Elevated left atrial pressure leads to pulmonary venous congestion and secondary pulmonary hypertension. Pulmonary edema may occur. With progressive disease pulmonary function becomes markedly abnormal with decreased total lung volume and vital capacity, reduced compliance, and increased work of breathing.

Mitral stenosis in children is generally asymptomatic except for the characteristic mid-diastolic–presystolic murmur. In rare instances affected children show some exertional dyspnea or fatigue. If cardiac symptoms occur, acute carditis should be suspected.

The management of children with rheumatic mitral stenosis centers on prevention of recurrent attacks of rheumatic fever and prevention of bacterial endocarditis. In the rare child with progressive severe mitral stenosis, mitral commissurotomy may have to be performed to pallitate the obstruction. Calcific mitral stenosis is extremely rare in children. Mitral valve replacement is avoided if at all possible because of the long-term problems with prosthetic valves in this age group.

Anesthetic Management. Anesthetic considerations have been discussed in the section on congenital mitral stenosis. Prevention of tachycardia, maintenance of cardiac contractility, avoidance of peripheral vasodilatation, and careful ventilation and fluid management are essential. Endocarditis prophylaxis is indicated.

Aortic Insufficiency

Rheumatic aortic valve disease presents as isolated or dominant aortic insufficiency with mild or moderate aortic stenosis. Males are more commonly affected.

The physiological derangement of aortic insufficiency consists of volume overload of the left ventricle with resultant dilatation of the chambers. Stroke volume is increased, but end-diastolic pressure is maintained near normal. Aortic impedance is usually low because peripheral vasodilatation reduces regurgitation, resulting in a wide pulse pressure. Regurgitation occurs during diastole and is reduced with fast heart rates. The characteristic finding is an early blowing diastolic murmur.

Aortic regurgitation is less common than mitral regurgitation with rheumatic fever but may also occur early in the disease. It is generally well tolerated throughout childhood, since the left ventricle is able to compensate well. The average life expectancy in patients with aortic insufficiency is 20 to 30 years after the onset of the disease. Death usually occurs suddenly and is due to arrhythmias or heart failure.

Treatment of rheumatic aortic insufficiency in childhood consists mostly of prevention of recurrence of rheumatic carditis. If signs of congestive heart failure, ventricular arrhythmias, or anginal attacks occur, sur-

gical therapy is indicated. Surgery should be performed before serious left ventricular dysfunction occurs. Aortic valve replacement is usually required, with the inherent problems of anticoagulation, thromboembolism, and valve dysfunction. Patients present high endocarditis risks after surgery and continue to require prophylaxis against rheumatic fever.

Anesthetic Considerations. Anesthetic management of aortic insufficiency is discussed earlier in this chapter. Regurgitation is decreased by fast heart rates and low peripheral vascular resistance. Vasodilatation and tachycardia are desirable and can be achieved by various anesthetic techniques. Depression of myocardial contractility should be avoided. Children with rheumatic aortic insufficiency usually have adequate cardiac reserve. They require endocarditis prophylaxis. After valve replacement patients should be asymptomatic but require reversal of anticoagulation if they are being treated with vitamin K antagonists.

Kawasaki Disease

Mucocutaneous lymph node syndrome or Kawasaki disease is an acute febrile erythematous disease with desquamative conjunctivitis, stomatitis, and nonsuppurative lymphadenitis, accompanied by myocarditis in 25 to 50 percent of cases. The disease is most common between 6 months and 5 years, with a median age of 2.3 years, and occurs primarily in Asian males. It is most prevalent in Japan.

The pathological basis for the disease consists of widespread microvasculitis. Involvement of the coronary vessels results in development of coronary aneurysms, coronary artery stenoses, thromboses, or rupture. A coronary artery lesion occurs in about 17 percent of affected patients. Involvement of the heart accounts for the 1.2 to 2.5 percent mortality reported for this disease. The coronary arteritis is usually silent until infarction or angina occurs.

Treatment consists of therapy with aspirin until all symptoms have subsided. In patients with coronary aneurysms aspirin therapy should be continued for at least 12 months. The aneurysms usually regress spontaneously. If no improvement occurs and severe coronary artery disease persists, bypass grafting or coronary aneurysmectomy must be performed. Prognosis for patency of bypass grafts appears to be less favorable in this young group of patients.

Anesthetic Considerations. Anesthetic management should take into consideration the predominant cardiac derangement. Heart failure or dysrhythmias may be present. With significant coronary artery disease, maintenance of myocardial oxygen balance is necessary. Monitoring for arrhythmias and myocardial ischemia is essential. For major surgery, direct monitoring of systemic and filling pressures is indicated. Vasoactive and antiarrhythmic drugs should be readily available.

Takayasu Disease

Takayasu disease is a relatively rare form of arteritis that predominantly occurs in Japanese and Korean females in the second and third decades. It involves the aorta and the proximal segments of its branches, leading to progressive destruction and occlusion. The disease may begin during childhood. Symptoms in this age group include hypertension, dyspnea, cardiomegaly, and absent pulses. Treatment with steroids and cytotoxic drugs is recommended, but the disease is nevertheless slowly progressive. Survival ranges from 1 to 20 years after onset of symptoms.

Anesthetic Management. Control of blood pressure is probably the major anesthetic problem. Patients should be observed for signs of myocardial ischemia. Steroid supplementation may be indicated.

REFERENCES

Congenital Heart Disease: Incidence, Etiology, Classification

Editorial: Congenital heart disease: incidence and etiology. Lancet 2:692, 1975.

Fyler DC, Buckley LP, Hellenbrand WE, et al.: Report of the New England Regional Infant Cardiac Program. Pediatrics 65(Suppl):376, 1980.

Keith JD: Congenital heart disease: Prevalence, incidence and epidemiology. In Keith JD, Rowe RD, Vlad P (eds.): Heart Disease in Infancy and Childhood. New York, Macmillan, 1978.

Mitchell SC, Korones SB, Berendes HW: Congenital heart disease in 56,109 births. Circulation 63:323, 1971.

Mitchell SC, Sellman RH, Westphal MC, et al.: Etiologic correlates in a study of congenital heart disease in 56,109 births. Am J Cardiol 28:653, 1971.

Morgan BC: Incidence, etiology and classification of congenital heart disease. Pediatr Clin North Am 25:721, 1978.

Nadas AS, Fyler DC: Pediatric Cardiology. 3rd ed. Philadelphia, W.B. Saunders Co., 1972.

Noonan JA: Association of congenital heart disease with syndromes or other defects. Pediatr Clin North Am 25:797, 1978.

Nora JJ: Etiologic aspects of heart disease. In Adams FH, Emmanouilides GC (Eds.): Heart Disease in Infants, Children, and Adolescents. 3rd ed. Baltimore, Williams and Wilkins, 1983.

Roberts WC: Congenital cardiovascular anomalies usually silent until adulthood. Cardiovasc Clin 10:407, 1979.

Steinberg AG, Bearn AG, Motulsky AG, et al.: Progress in Medical Genetics. Vol. V. Genetics of Cardiovascular Disease. Philadelphia, W.B. Saunders Co., 1983.

Van Mierop LHS, Gessner IH: Pathogenetic mechanisms in congenital cardiovascular malformations. Prog Cardiovasc Dis 15:67, 1972.

Wagner HR: Cardiac disease in congenital infections. Clin Perinatol 8:481, 1981.

Congenital Heart Disease: Long-Term Prognosis

Fyler DC, Rothmann KJ, Buckley LP, et al.: The determinants of five year survival of infants with critical congenital heart disease. Cardiovasc Clin 12:393, 1981.

Kidd LS, Rowe RD (Eds.): The Child with Congenital Heart Disease After Surgery. Mount Kisco, Futura Publ. Co., 1976.

McNamara DG, Latson LA: Long-term follow-up of patients with malformations for which definite surgical repair has been available for 25 years or more. Am J Cardiol 50:560, 1982.

Pacifico AD, McKay R: Advances in the surgical management of congenital heart disease in infants and children. Cardiovasc Clin 12:127, 1981.

Roberts WC: Cardiac valvular residua and sequelae after operation for congenital heart disease. Am Heart J 106:1181, 1983.

Roberts WC (Ed.): Congenital heart disease in the adult. Cardiovasc Clin 10, No. 1, 1979.

Wilkinson JJ: Changing patterns of congenital heart disease. J Roy Soc Med 72:432, 1979.

Anesthesia and Congenital Heart Disease

Allen HD: Anesthesia and congenital heart disease. In Brown B (Ed.): Contemporary Anesthesia Practice. Vol 2. Philadelphia, F. A. Davis Co., 1980.

Arens JF: Anesthesia for congenital cardiac disease. ASA Refresher Course Abstracts, No. 124, 1984.

Beynen FM, Tarhan S: Anesthesia for surgical repair of congenital heart defects in children. In Tarhan S (Ed.): Cardiovascular Anesthesia and Postoperative Care. Chicago, Year Book Medical, 1982.

Bland JW, Williams WH: Anesthesia for treatment of congenital heart defects. In Kaplan JA (Ed.): Cardiac Anesthesia. New York, Grune and Stratton, 1979.

Bull AP: The anesthetic evaluation and management of the surgical patient with heart disease. Surg Clin North Am 63:1035, 1983.

Crean P, Goresky G, Koren G, et al.: Fentanyl pharmacokinetics in children with congenital heart disease. Anesthesiology 59:A448, 1983.

Duncan PG: Anesthesia for patients with congenital heart disease. Can Anesth Soc J 30:S20, 1983.

Eger EI: Effect of shunting on alveolar anesthetic rise. In Eger EI: Anesthetic Uptake and Action. Baltimore, Williams and Wilkins, 1974.

Hickey PR, Hansen DD, Cranolini GM: Pulmonary and systemic hemodynamic responses to ketamine in infants with normal and elevated pulmonary vascular resistance. Anesthesiology 61:438, 1984.

Hickey PR, Hansen DD, Wessel D: Response to high dose fentanyl in infants. Anesthesiology 61:A445, 1984.

Hickey PR, Hansen DD: Fentanyl- and sufentanil-oxygen-pancuronium anesthesia for cardiac surgery in infants Anesth Analg 63:117, 1983.

Lowenstein E, Walker HL, Zaroff LI: The effect of a standard cyanotic circulatory lesion on the induction dose of methohexital in the dog. Anesthesiology 26:254, 1965.

Radnay PA, Nagashima H (Eds.): Anesthetic Considerations for Pediatric Cardiac Surgery. Int Anesth Clin 18, No. 1, 1980.

Stolting RK, Longnecker DE: The effect of right-to-left shunt on the rate of increase of arterial anesthetic concentration. Anesthesiology 36:352, 1972.

Tanner GE, Anger DG, Barash PG, et al.: Effects of left-to-right, mixed left-to-right and right-to-left shunts on inhalational anesthetic induction in children. Anesth Analg 64:101, 1985.

Werner JC, Fripp RR, Whitman V: Evaluation of the pediatric surgical patient with congenital heart disease. Surg Clin North Am 63:1003, 1983.

Ventilatory Function in Congenital Heart Disease

Bancalari E, Jesse MJ, Gelband H, et al.: Lung mechanics in congenital heart disease with increased and decreased pulmonary blood flow. J Pediatr 90:192, 1977.

Blesa MI, Lahiri S, Rashkind WT, et al.: Normalization of the blunted ventilatory response to acute hypoxia in congenital cyanotic heart disease. N Engl J Med 296:237, 1977.

Hoffman JI, Rudolph AM, Heymann MA: Pulmonary vascular disease with congenital heart lesions: pathologic features and causes. Circulation 64:873, 1981.

Jenkins J, Lynn A, Edmonds J, et al.: Effects of mechanical ventilation on cardiopulmonary function in children after open-heart surgery. Crit Care Med 13:77, 1985.

Lister G, Pitt BR: Cardiopulmonary interactions in the infant with congenital cardiac disease. Clin Chest Med 4:219, 1983.

Shannon DC, Kazemi H: Distribution of lung function in patients with anomalies of the pulmonary circulation. J Thorac Cardiovasc Surg 64:26, 1972.

Intracardiac Defects Producing Predominant Left-to-Right Shunt

Feldt AH, Edwards WD, Page FJ, et al.: Atrial septal defects and atrioventricular canal. *In* Adams FH, Emmanouilides GC (Eds.): Heart Disease in Infants, Children, and Adolescents. 3rd ed. Baltimore, Williams and Wilkins, 1983.

Graham TP, Bender HW: Preoperative diagnosis and management of infants with critical congenital heart disease. Ann Thorac Surg 29:272, 1980.

Graham TP, Bender HW, Spach MS: Ventricular septal defect. *In* Adams FH, Emmanouilides GC: Heart Disease in Infants, Children, and Adolescents. 3rd ed. Baltimore, Williams and Wilkins, 1983.

Gronert GA, Messick JM, Cucchiara RF, et al.: Paradoxical air embolism from a patent foramen ovale. Anesthesiology 50:548, 1979.

Keith JD: Ventricular septal defect and atrial septal defect. *In* Keith JD, Rowe RD, Vlad P (Ed.): Heart Disease in Infancy and Childhood. 3rd ed. New York. MacMillan, 1978.

Kidd LBS: Single ventricle. *In* Keith JD, Rowe RD, Vlad P (Eds.): Heart Disease in Infancy and Childhood. 3rd ed. New York, Macmillian, 1978.

Nadsas AS, Fyler DC: Communications between systemic and pulmonary circuits with predominantly left to right shunt. *In* Nasas AS, Fyler DC: Pediatric Cardiology. Philadelphia, W.B. Saunders Co., 1972.

Rao TLK, Mathou M, Azad C, et al.: Bronchoscopy and reversal of intracardiac shunt. Anesthesiology 51:558, 1979.

Riemenschneider TA: Left ventricular–right atrial communication. *In* Adams FH, Emmanouilides GC: Heart Disease in Infants, Children, and Adolescents. 3rd ed. Baltimore, Williams & Wilkins, 1983.

Rudolph AM: Ventricular septal defect. *In* Rudolph AM: Congenital Diseases of the Heart. Chicago, Year Book Medical, 1974.

Rudolph AM: Endocardial cushion defect. *In* Rudolph AM: Congenital Diseases of the Heart. Chicago, Year Book Medical, 1974.

Rudolph AM: Atrial septal defect: partial anomalous drainage of pulmonary veins. *In* Rudolph AM: Congenital Diseases of the Heart. Chicago, Year Book Medical, 1974.

Stevenson GJ: Acyanotic lesions with increased pulmonary blood flow. Pediatr Clin N Am 25:743, 1978.

Eisenmenger Complex and Syndrome

Bird TM, Strybub L: Anesthesia for a patient with Down's syndrome and Eisenmenger's complex. Anesthesia 39:48, 1984.

Graham, TP: The Eisenmenger reaction and its management. Cardiovasc Clin 10:531, 1979.

Lumley J, Whitwan JG, Morgan M: General anesthesia in the presence of Eisenmenger's syndrome. Anesth Analg 56:543, 1977.

MacArthur CGC, Hunter D, Gibson GJ: Ventilatory function in the Eisenmenger syndrome. Thorax 34:348, 1979.

Weber RK, Buda AJ, Levene DL: General anesthesia in Eisenmenger's syndrome. Can Med Assoc J 117:1413, 1977.

Young D, Mark H: Fate of the patient with Eisenmenger syndrome. Am J Cardiol 28:653, 1971.

Intracardiac Lesions Producing Predominant Right-to-Left Shunt with Cyanosis

Arciniegas E, Farokin ZR, Hakimi M, et al.: Classic shunting operations for congenital cyanotic heart defects. J Thorac Cardiovasc Surg, 84:88, 1982.

Elliot JP, Anderson RH, Bargeron LM, et al.: Single or univentricular heart. *In* Adams FH, Emmanouilides GC (Eds.): Heart Disease in Infants, Children, and Adolescents. 3rd ed. Baltimore, Williams and Wilkins, 1983.

Freed MD, Heyman MA, Lewis AB, et al.: Prostaglandin E₁ in infants with ductus arteriosus–dependent congenital heart disease. Circulation 64:899, 1981.

Graham TP, Bender HW: Preoperative diagnosis and management of infants with critical congenital heart disease. Ann Thorac Surg 29:272, 1980.

Gunteroth WG, Kawabori J, Baun D: Tetralogy of Fallot. *In* Adams FH, Emmanouilides GC (Eds.): Heart Disease in Infants, Children, and Adolescents. 3rd ed. Baltimore, Williams and Wilkins, 1983.

Gutgesell HP, Garson A, McNamara DG: Prognosis for the newborn with transposition of the great arteries. Am J Cardiol 44:96, 1979.

Hagler DJ, Ritter DG, Puga FJ: Double outlet right ventricle. *In* Adams FH, Emmanouilides GC (Eds.): Heart Disease in Infants, Children, and Adolescents. 3rd ed. Baltimore, William and Wilkins, 1983.

Jatene AD, Iontes VF, Paulista PP: Anatomical correction of transposition of the great vessels. J Thorac Cardiovasc Surg 72:364, 1976.

Kam CA: Infundibular spasm in Fallot's tetralogy. An account and its management in anesthesia. Anaesth Intens Care 6:138, 1978.

Kidd BSL: Transpositions of the great arteries. *In* Keith JD, Rowe RD, Vlad P: Heart Disease in Infancy and Childhood. 3rd ed. New York, Macmillan, 1978.

Lev M, Bharati S, Meng CCL et al.: A concept of double outlet right ventricle. J Thorac Cardiovasc Surg 44:271, 1972.

Nadas AS, Fyler DC: Valvular and vascular lesions with a right to left shunt or no shunt at all. *In* Nadas AS, Fyler DC: Pediatric Cardiology. Philadelphia, W.B. Saunders Co., 1972.

Nadas AS, Fyler DC: The transpositions. *In* Nadas AS, Fyler DC: Pediatric Cardiology. Philadelphia, W.B. Saunders Co., 1972.

Paul MH: Transposition of the great arteries. *In* Adams FH, Emmanouilides GC (Eds.): Heart Disease in Infants, Children, and Adolescents. 3rd ed. Baltimore, Williams and Wilkins, 1983.

Rosenthal A, Nathan DG, Marty AT, et al.: Acute hemodynamic effects of red cell volume reduction in polycythemia of cyanotic congenital heart disease. Circulation 42:297, 1970.

Rowe RD: Tetralogy of Fallot. *In* Keith JD, Rowe RD, Vlad P (Eds.): Heart Disease in Infancy and Childhood. 3rd ed. New York, Macmillan, 1978.

Rudolph AM: Pulmonic stenosis with ventricular septal defect and aortopulmonary transposition. *In* Rudolph AM: Congenital Diseases of the Heart. Chicago, Year Book Medical, 1974.

Ruttenberg HD: Corrected transposition of the great arteries and splenic syndromes. *In* Adams FH, Emmanouilides GC (Eds.): Heart Disease in Infants, Children, and Adolescents. 3rd ed. Baltimore, Williams and Wilkins, 1983.

Sondheimer HM, Freedom RM, Olley PM: Double outlet right ventricle. *In* Keith JD, Rowe RD, Vlad P (Eds.): Heart Disease in Infancy and Childhood 3rd ed. New York, Macmillan, 1978.

Van Praagh R, Weinberg PM: Double outlet left ventricle. *In* Adams FH, Emmanouilides GC: Heart Disease in Infants, Children, and Adolescents. 3rd ed. Baltimore, Williams and Wilkins, 1983.

Valvular Lesions

Bisset GS, Schwartz DC, Meyer RA, et al.: Clinical spectrum and long-term follow up of isolated mitral valve prolapse in 119 children. Circulation 62:423, 1980.

Bloom KR: Mitral valve and tricuspid valve stenosis. *In* Keith JD, Rowe RD, Vlad P (Eds.): Heart Disease in Infancy and Childhood. 3rd ed. New York, Macmillan, 1978.

Braunwald E.: Mitral regurgitation. N Engl J Med 281:425, 1969.

Brooks JL, Kaplan JA: Valvular lesions. *In* Katz J, Benumof J, Kadis LB (Eds.): Anesthesia and Uncommon Diseases. 2nd ed. Philadelphia, W.B. Saunders Co., 1981.

Brown LM: Mitral valve prolapse in children. Adv Pediatr 25:327, 1978.

Collins-Nakai RL, Rosenthal A, Castaneda AR, et al.: Congenital mitral stenosis. Circulation 56:1039, 1977.

Dobell ARC, Bloss RS, Gibbons JE, et al.: Congenital valvular aortic stenosis. J Thorac Cardiovasc Surg 81:916, 1981.

Elsten JL, Kim YD, Hanowell JT, et al.: Prolonged induction with exaggerated chamber enlargement in Ebstein's anomaly. Anesth Analg 60:909, 1981.

Emmanouilides GC, Baylen BG: Congenital absence of the pulmonary valve, pulmonary stenosis and pulmonary atresia with intact ventricular septum. In Adams FH, Emmanoulides GC (Eds.): Heart Disease in Infants, Children, and Adolescents. 3rd ed. Baltimore, Williams and Wilkins, 1983.

Freedom RM: Congenital valvar regurgitation. In Keith JD, Rowe RD, Vlad P (Eds.): Heart Disease in Infancy and Childhood. 3rd ed. New York, Macmillan, 1978.

Freedom RM: Hypoplastic left heart syndrome. In Adams FH, Emmanouilides GC: Heart Disease in Infants, Children, and Adolescents. 3rd ed. Baltimore, Williams and Wilkins, 1983.

Freedom RM, Keith JD: Pulmonary atresia. Aortic atresia. In Keith JD, Rowe RD, Vlad P (Eds.): Heart Disease in Infancy and Childhood. 3rd ed. New York, Macmillan, 1978.

Friedman WF, Benson LN: Aortic stenosis. In Adams FH, Emmanouilides GC (Eds.): Heart Disease in Infants, Children, and Adolescents. 3rd ed. Baltimore, Williams and Wilkins, 1983.

Fulton DR, Hongen TJ, Keane JF, et al.: Repeat aortic valvotomy in children. Am Heart J 106:60, 1983.

Gardner TJ, Roland JM, Neill CA, et al.: Valve replacement in children. J Thorac Cardiovasc Surg 83:178, 1982.

Guigell RL, Vlad P: Mitral valve prolapse. In Keith JD, Rowe RD, Vlad P (Eds.): Heart Disease in Infancy and Childhood. New York, Macmillan, 1978.

Ishikawa T, Neutze JM, Brandt PWT, et al.: Hemodynamics following the Kreutzer procedure for tricuspid atresia in patients under two years of age J Thorac Cardiovasc Surg 88:373, 1984.

Keith JD: Biscuspid aortic valve. In Keith JD, Rowe RD, Vlad P (Eds.): Heart Disease in Infancy and Childhood. 3rd ed. New York, Macmillan, 1978.

Keith JD: Congenital mitral atresia. In Keith JD, Rowe RD, Vlad P (Eds.): Heart Disease in Infancy and Childhood. 3rd ed. New York, Macmillan, 1978.

Keith JD: Ebstein's disease. In Keith JD, Rowe RD, Vlad P (Eds.): Heart Disease in Infancy and Childhood. 3rd ed. New York, Macmillan, 1978.

Levy MJ, Schachner A, Blieden, LC: Aortico-left ventricular tunnel. J Thorac Cardiovasc Surg 84:102, 1982.

Nadas AS, Fyler DC: Valvular and vascular lesions with a right-to-left shunt or no shunt at all. In Nadas AS, Fyler DC: Pediatric Cardiology. 3rd ed. Philadelphia, W.B. Saunders Co., 1972.

Norwood WI, Lang P, Hansen DD: Physiology repair of aortic atresia—hypoplastic left heart syndrome. N Engl J Med 308:23, 1983.

Olley PM, Bloom KR, Rowe RD: Aortic stenosis. In Keith JD, Rowe RD, Vlad P (Eds.): Heart Disease in Infancy and Childhood. 3rd ed. New York, Macmillan, 1978.

Perez Diaz L, Quero Jimenez M, Moreno Granados F, et al.: Congenital absence of myocardium of right ventricle: Uhl's anomaly. Br Heart J 35:570, 1973.

Richardson JV, Doty DB, Siewers RD, et al.: Cor triatriatum. J Thorac Cardiovasc Surg 81:232, 1981.

Rosenthal H, Dick M: Tricuspid atresia. In Adams FH, Emmanouilides GC, (Eds.): Heart Disease in Infants, Children, and Adolescents. 3rd ed. Baltimore, Williams and Wilkins, 1983.

Roth SL, Thomas SJ, Tunick P, et al.: Mitral valve prolapse: risk of dysrhythmias in the perioperative period. Anesthesiology, 55:A57, 1981.

Rowe RD: Pulmonary stenosis and pulmonary arterial stenosis. In Keith JD, Rowe RD, Vlad P (Eds.): Heart Disease in Infancy and Childhood. 3rd ed. New York, Macmillan, 1978.

Rudolph AM: Aortic atresia, mitral atresia and hypoplastic left ventricle. In Rudolph AM: Congenital Disease of the Heart. Chicago, Year Book Medical, 1974.

Rudolph AM: Aortic stenosis. In Rudolph AM: Congenital Diseases of the Heart. Chicago, Year Book Medical, 1974.

Rudolph AM: Pulmonary stenosis and atresia with intact ventricular septum. In Rudolph AM: Congenital Diseases of the Heart. Chicago, Year Book Medical, 1974.

Rudolph AM: Tricuspid atresia and hypoplastic right ventricle. In

Rudolph AM: Congenital Diseases of the Heart. Chicago, Year Book Medical, 1974.

Sanders SP, Wright GB, Keane JF, et al.: Clinical and hemodynamic results of the Fontan operation for tricuspid atresia. Am J Cardiol 49:1733, 1982.

Schaff HV, DiDonato RM, Danielson GK, et al.: Reoperation for obstructed pulmonary ventricle—pulmonary artery conduits. J Thorac Cardiovasc Surg 88:334, 1984.

Shone JD, Sellers RD, Anderson RC, et al.: The developmental complex of parachute mitral valve, supravalvular ring of left atrium, subaortic stenosis and coarctation of the aorta. Am J Cardiol 11:714, 1963.

Thomas SJ Lowenstein E: Anesthetic management of the patient with valvular heart disease. Int Anesthesiol Clin 17:67, 1979.

Uhl HS: A previously undescribed congenital malformation of the heart: almost total absence of the myocardium of the right ventricle. Bull Johns Hopkins Hosp 91:197, 1952.

Van Mierop L, Schiebler GC, Victorica BE: Ebstein's anomaly. In Adams FH, Emmanouilides GC (Eds.): Heart Disease in Infants, Children, and Adolescents. 3rd ed, Baltimore, Williams and Wilkins, 1983.

Vlad P: Tricuspid atresia. In Keith JD, Rowe RD, Vlad P (Eds.): Heart Disease in Infancy and Childhood. 3rd ed. New York, Macmillan, 1978.

Malformations Involving the Great Vessels

Abe T, Kuribayashi R, Sato M, et al.: Direct communication of the right pulmonary artery with the left atrium. J Thorac Cardiovasc Surg 64:38, 1972.

Asch AJ: Turner's syndrome occurring with Horner's syndrome seen with coarctation of the aorta and aortic aneurysm. Am J Dis Child 133:817, 1979.

Bergdahl LAL, Blackstone EH, Kirklin JW, et al.: Determinants of early success in repair of aortic coarctation in infants. J Thorac Cardiovasc Surg 83:736, 1982.

Bhat R, Fisher E, Raju TNK, et al.: Patent ductus arteriosus: recent advances in diagnosis and management. Pediatr Clin North Am 29:1117, 1982.

Culham JAG: Congenital anomalies of the coronary arteries. In Keith JD, Rowe RD, Vlad P (Eds.): Heart Disease in Infancy and Childhood. 3rd ed. New York, Macmillan, 1978.

Dalal FY, Bennett EJ, Salen MR, et al.: Anesthesia for coarctation. Anaesthesia 29:704, 1974.

Editorial: Patent ductus arteriosus: current clinical status. Arch Dis Child 55:106, 1980.

Emmanouilides GC, Baylen BG: Congenital absence of the pulmonary valve. In Adams FH, Emmanouilides GC (Eds.): Heart Disease in Infants, Children, and Adolescents. 3rd ed. Baltimore, Williams and Wilkins, 1983.

Ergin MA, Jayaram N, La Corte M: Left aortic arch and right descending aorta: diagnostic and therapeutic implications of a rare type of vascular ring. Ann Thorac Surg 31:82, 1981.

Fishman NH, Bronstein MH, Berman W, et al.: Surgical management of severe aortic coarctation and interrupted aortic arch in neonates. J Thorac Cardiovasc Surg 71:35, 1976.

Friedman WF, Fitzpatrick KM, Merritt TA, et al.: The patent ductus arteriosus. Clin Perinatol 5:283, 1978.

Garcia OL, Hernandez FA, Tamer G, et al.: Congenital bilateral subclavian steal. Am J Cardiol 44:101, 1979.

Gersony WM: Coarctation of the aorta. In Adams FH, Emmanouilides GC (Eds.): Heart Disease in Infants, Children, and Adolescents. 3rd ed. Baltimore, Williams and Wilkins, 1983.

Hayward RH, Martt JM, Brewer LM, et al.: Surgical correction of the vena cava bronchovascular complex. J Thorac Cardiovasc Surg 64:203, 1972.

Jimenert MQ, Guillen FA: Arteriovenous fistulas. In Adams FH, Emmanouilides GC (Eds.): Heart Disease in Infants, Children, and Adolescents. 3rd ed. Baltimore, Williams and Wilkins, 1983.

Keith JD: Coarctation of the aorta. In Keith JD, Rowe RD, Vlad P (Eds.): Heart Disease in Infancy and Childhood. 3rd ed. New York, Macmillan, 1978.

Keith JD: Congenital pulmonary arteriovenous aneurysm. *In* Keith JD, Rowe RD, Vlad P (Eds.): Heart Disease in Infancy and Childhood. 3rd ed. New York, Macmillan, 1978.

Khousari B, Saunders PW, Lees MH, et al.: Common pulmonary vein atresia. J Thorac Cardiovasc Surg 83:443, 1982.

Lucas RV: Anomalous venous connections, pulmonary and systemic. *In* Adams FH, Emmanouilides GC (Eds.): Heart Disease in Infants, Children, and Adolescents. 3rd ed. Baltimore, Williams and Wilkins, 1983.

Lurie PR, Takahashi M: Abnormalities and diseases of the coronary vessels. *In* Adams FH, Emmanouilides GC (Eds.): Heart Disease in Infants, and Children, and Adolescents. 3rd ed. Baltimore, Williams and Wilkins, 1983.

Mair DD, Edwards WD, Fuster V, et al.: Truncus arteriosus. *In* Adams FH, Emmanouilides GC (Eds.): Heart Disease in Infants, Children, and Adolescents. 3rd ed. Baltimore, Williams and Wilkins, 1983.

McLeskey CH, Martin WE: Anesthesia for repair of a pulmonary artery sling in an infant with severe tracheal stenosis. Anesthesiology 46:368, 1977.

Moes CAF: Vascular rings and anomalies of the aortic arch. *In* Keith JD, Rowe RD, Vlad P (Eds.): Heart Disease in Infancy and Childhood. 3rd ed. New York, Macmillan, 1978.

Moodie DS, Fyfe D, Gill CC, et al.: Anomalous origin of the left coronary artery from the pulonary artery (Bland-White-Garland syndrome) in adult patients: long-term follow-up after surgery. Am Heart J 100:381, 1983.

Nadas AS, Fyler, DC: Coarctation of the aorta. *In* Nadas AS, Fyler DC: Pediatric Cardiology. Philadelphia, W.B. Saunders Co., 1972.

Nadas AS, Fyler DC: Communications between great arteries. *In* Nadas AS, Fyler DC: Pediatric Cardiology. 3rd ed. Philadelphia, W.B. Saunders Co., 1972.

Nadas AS, Fyler DC: Venous anomalies. *In* Nadas AS, Fyler DC: Pediatric Cardiology. 3rd ed. Philadelphia, W.B. Saunders Co., 1972.

Neuman GG, Hansen DD: The anesthetic management of preterm infants undergoing ligation of a patent ductus arteriosus. Can Anaesth Soc J 27:248, 1980.

Robinson S, Gregory GA: Fentanyl-air-oxygen anesthesia for ligation of patent ductus arteriosus in preterm infants. Anesth Analg 60:331, 1981.

Rowe RD: Anomalies of venous return. *In* Keith JD, Rowe RD, Vlad P (Eds.): Heart Disease in Infancy and Childhood. 3rd ed. New York, Macmillan, 1978.

Rudolph AM: Aortic coarctation and isthmus narrowing. *In* Rudolph AM: Congenital Diseases of the Heart. Chicago, Year Book Medical, 1974.

Rudolph AM: The ductus arteriosus and persistent patency of the ductus arteriosus. *In* Rudolph AM: Congenital Diseases of the Heart. Chicago, Year Book Medical, 1974.

Rudolph AM: Truncus arteriosus. *In* Rudolph AM: Congenital Diseases of the Heart. Chicago, Year Book Medical, 1974.

Rudolph AM: Total anomalous pulmonary venous drainage. *In* Rudolph AM: Congenital Diseases of the Heart. Chicago, Year Book Medical, 1974.

Sissman NJ: Anomalies of the aortic arch complex. *In* Adams FH, Emmanouilides GC (Eds.): Heart Disease in Infants, Children, and Adolescents. 3rd ed. Baltimore, Williams and Wilkins, 1983.

Stelein G, Jonas RA, Goh TH et al.: Surgical treatment of absent pulmonary valve syndrome in infants: relief of bronchial obstruction. Ann Thorac Surg 36:468, 1983.

Cardiomyopathies

Artman M, Graham TP: Congestive heart failure in infancy. Am Heart J 103:1040, 1982.

Artman M, Parrish MD, Graham TP: Congestive heart failure in childhood and adolesence. Am Heart J 105:471, 1983.

Bowers JR: Anesthesia and cardiomyopathies. Anesth Analg 50:1013, 1971.

Brooks JL, Kaplan JA: Cardiac diseases. *In* Katz J, Benumof J,

Kadis LB (Eds.): Anesthesia and Uncommon Diseases. 2nd ed. Philadelphia, W.B. Saunders Co., 1981.

Cherian G, Vijayaragharan G, Krishnaswami S, et al.: Endomyocardial fibrosis. Am Heart J 105:659, 1983.

Epstein SE, Maron BJ: Hypertrophic cardiomyopathy. Clin Invest Med 3:185, 1980.

Harris LC, Nghiem RX: Cardiomyopathies in infants and children. Prog Cardiovasc Dis 15:255, 1972.

Hirota Y, Furubayashi K, Kaku K, et al.: Hypertrophic nonobstructive cardiomyopathy. Am J Cardiol 50:990, 1982.

Keith JD, Rose V, Manning JA: Endocardial fibroelastosis. *In* Keith JD, Rowe RD, Vlad P (Eds.): Heart Disease in Infancy and Childhood. 3rd ed. New York, Macmillan, 1978.

Kowey PR, Eisenberg R, Engel TR: Sustained arrhythmias in hypertrophic obstructive cardiomyopathy. N Engl J Med 310:1566, 1984.

Maron BJ: Cardiomyopathies. *In* Adams TH, Emmanouilides GC (Eds.): Heart Disease in Infants, Children, and Adolescents. 3rd ed. Baltimore, Williams and Wilkins, 1983.

Maron B, Epstein SE: Hypertrophic cardiomyopathy. Am J Cardiol 45:141, 1980.

Maron BJ, Tajik AJ, Ruttenberg HD, et al.: Hypertrophic cardiomyopathy in infants. Circulation 65:7, 1982.

Nadas AS, Fyler DC: Myocardial diseases. *In* Nadas AS, Fyler DC: Pediatric Cardiology. 3rd ed. Philadelphia, W.B. Saunders Co., 1972.

Reitan JA, Wright RG: The use of halothane in a patient with asymmetric septal hypertrophy. Can Anaesth Soc J 29:154, 1982.

Seward JB, Tajik AJ: Primary cardiomyopathies: classification, pathophysiology, clinical recognition and management. Cardiovasc Clin 10:199, 1980.

Jaiyesimi F: Controversies and advances in endomyocardial fibrosis. Afr J Med Sci 11:37, 1982.

Wiberg-Jorgensen F, Skovsted P, Fischer Hansen J, et al.: Cardiovascular haemodynamics during fluroxene anaesthesia in patients with muscular subaortic stenosis. Acta Anaesth Scand 17:142, 1973.

Tumors of the Heart

Edwards JE: Cardiac tumors. *In* Adams FH, Emmanouilides GC (Eds.): Heart Disease in Infants, Children and Adolescents. 3rd ed. Baltimore, Williams and Wilkins, 1978.

Fowler RS, Keith JD: Cardiac tumors. *In* Keith JD, Rowe RD, Vlad P (Eds.): Heart disease in Infancy and Childhood. 3rd ed. New York, Macmillan, 1978.

McAllister HA: Primary tumors and cysts of the heart. Curr Probl Cardiol 4:1, 1979.

Reece IJ, Cooley DA, Frazier OH, et al.: Cardiac tumors. J Thorac Cardiovasc Surg 88:439, 1984.

Semb BKH: Surgical consideration in the treatment of cardiac myoxoma. J Thorac Cardiovasc Surg 87:251, 1984.

Congenital Conduction Defects

Burchell HB: The QT interval historically treated. Pediatr Cardiol 4:139, 1983.

Callaghan ML, Nichols AB, Sweet RB: Anaesthetic management of prolonged QT interval syndrome. Anesthesiology 47:67, 1977.

Carlock FJ, Brown M, Brown EM: Isoflurane anaesthesia for a patient with long QT syndrome. Can Anaesth Soc J 31:83, 1984.

Diaz JH, Friesen RH: Anesthetic management of congenital complete heart block in childhood. Anesth Analg 58:334, 1979.

Duffy BL: Congenital complete heart block. Anesthesia 36:956, 1981.

Gillette PC: Advances in the diagnosis and treatment of tachydysrhythmias in children. Am Heart J 102:111, 1981.

Gillette PC, Carson A, Porter CJ, et al.: Dysthythmias. *In* Adams FH, Emmanouilides GC (Eds.): Heart Disease in Infants, Children, and Adolescents. Williams and Wilkins, 1983.

Jones RM, Broadbent MP, Adams P: Anaesthetic considerations

in patients with paroxysmal supraventricular tachycardia. Anaesthesia 39:307, 1984.

Nadas AS, Fyler DC: Arrhythmias. *In* Nadas AS, Fyler DC: Pediatric Cardiology. Philadelphia, W.B. Saunders Co., 1972.

O'Callaghan AC, Normandale JP, Morgan M: The prolonged QT syndrome. A review with anesthetic implications. Anaesth Intens Care 10:50, 1982.

O'Gara JP, Edelman JD: Anesthesia and the patient with complete congenital heart block. Anesth Analg 60:906, 1981.

Olley PM: Cardiac arrhythmias. *In* Keith JD, Rowe, RD, Vlad P (Eds.): Heart Disease in Infancy and Childhood. 3rd ed. New York, Macmillan, 1978.

Pickoff AS, Wolff GS, Tamer D, et al.: Arrhythmias and conduction system disturbances in infants and children. Cardiovasc Clin 11:203, 1980.

Sadowski AR, Moyers JR, Anesthetic management of the Wolff-Parkinson-White Syndrome. Anesthesiology 51:553, 1979.

Steward DJ, Izukawa T: Congenital complete heart block. Anesth Analg 59:81, 1980.

Van der Starre PJ: Wolff-Parkinson-White syndrome during anesthesia. Anesthesiology 48:369, 1978.

Vetter VL, Raskhind WJ: Congenital complete heart block and connective tissue disease. N Engl J Med 309:236, 1983.

Yanagida H, Kemi C, Suwa K: The effects of stellate ganglion block on idiopathic prolongation of the Q–T interval with cardiac arrhythmia (the Romano-Ward syndrome). Anesth Analg 55:782, 1976.

Diseases of the Pericardium

Brooks JL, Kaplan JA: Cardiac diseases. *In* Katz J, Benumof J, Kadis LB (Eds.): Anesthesia and Uncommon Diseases. W.B. Saunders Co., 1981.

Keith JD: Pericarditis. *In* Keith JD, Rowe RD, Vlad P (Eds.): Heart Disease in Infancy and Childhood. 3rd ed. New York, Macmillan, 1978.

Lake CL: Anesthesia and pericardial disease. Anesth Analg 62:431, 1983.

Nadas AS, Fyler DC: Diseases of the pericardium. *In* Nadas AS, Fyler DC: Pediatric Cardiology. 3rd ed. Philadelphia, W.B. Saunders Co., 1972.

Malpositions of the Heart

Keith JD: Ectopia cordis. *In* Keith JD, Rowe RD, Vlad P (Eds.): Heart Disease in Infancy and Childhood. 3rd ed. New York, Macmillan, 1978.

Nadas AS, Fyler DC: The transpositions. *In* Nadas AS, Fyler DC: Pediatric Cardiology. 3rd ed. Philadelphia, W.B. Saunders Co., 1972.

Rao PS: Dextrocardia. Am Heart J 102:389, 1981.

Van Praagh R, Weinberg PM, Matsuoka R, et al.: Malpositions of the heart. *In* Adams FH, Emmanouilides GC (Eds.): Heart Disease in Infants, Children, and Adolescents. 3rd ed. Baltimore, Williams and Wilkins, 1983.

Acquired Heart Disease

Bell DM, Moorens DM, Holman RC, et al.: Kawasaki syndrome in the United States. Am J Dis Child 137:211, 1983.

Kaplan E, Shulman ST: Endocarditis. *In* Adams FH, Emmanouilides GC (Eds.): Heart Disease in Infants, Children, and Adolescents. 3rd ed. Baltimore, Williams and Wilkins, 1983.

Kaplan EL: Acute rheumatic fever. Pediatr Clin North Am 25:817, 1978.

Kaplan EL, Anthony BF, Bisno A, et al.: AHA Committee report on prevention of bacterial endocarditis. Circulation 56:139A, 1977.

Kaplan S: Chronic rheumatic heart disease. In Adams FH, Emmanouilides GC (Eds.): Heart Disease in Infants, Children, and Adolescents. 3rd ed. Baltimore, Williams and Wilkins, 1983.

Keith JD: Rheumatic fever and rheumatic heart disease. *In* Keith JD, Rowe RD, Vlad P (Eds.): Heart Disease in Infancy and Childhood. 3rd ed. New York, Macmillan, 1978.

Lurie PR, Takahashi M: Abnormalities and diseases of the coronary vessels. *In* Adams FH, Emmanouilides GC (Eds.): Heart Disease in Infants, Children, and Adolescents. 3rd ed. Baltimore, Williams and Wilkins, 1983.

McNiece WL, Krishna G: Kawasaki disease. A disease with anesthetic implications. Anesthesiology 58:269, 1983.

Nadas AS, Fyler DC: Acute rheumatic fever and rheumatic heart disease. *In* Nadas AS, Fyler DC: Pediatric Cardiology. 3rd ed. Philadelphia, W.B. Saunders Co., 1972.

Nadas AS, Fyler DC: Bacterial endocarditis. *In* Nadas AS, Fyler DC: Pediatric Cardiology. 3rd ed. Philadelphia, W.B. Saunders Co., 1972.

Shulman ST, Amren DP, Bisno AL, et al.: Prevention of bacterial endocarditis. Circulation 70:1123A, 1984.

Shulman ST, Amren DP, Bisno Al, et al.: Prevention of rheumatic fever. Circulation 70:1118A, 1984.

Sum K, Takeuchi Y, Shiroma K, et al.: Early and late postoperative studies in coronary arterial lesions resulting from Kawasaki's disease in children. J Thorac Cardio Vasc Surg 84:224, 1982.

Stinson EB: Surgical treatment of infective endocarditis. Prog Cardiovasc Dis 22:145, 1979.

Wannamaker LW, Kaplan EL: Acute rheumatic fever. *In* Adams FH, Emmanouilides GC. Heart Disease in Infants, Children, and Adolescents. 3rd ed. Baltimore, Williams and Wilkins, 1983.

Appendix A

CARDIOVASCULAR SIDE EFFECTS OF COMMONLY USED ANESTHETIC AGENTS

	Heart Rate	Myocardial Contractility	SVR	PVR	Ventricular Irritability
Halothane	↓	↓↓	↓	↓	↑
Enflurane	↑	↓↓	↓	↓	↑/↓
Isoflurane	↑	↓	↓↓	↓	—
Narcotics	↓	—/↓	—/↓	—	—
Barbiturates	↑	↓	↓	—	—/↓
Benzodiazepines	—	—	—/↓	—	—
Ketamine	↑	↓	↑	—	—
D-Tubocurarine	↓	—	↑	—	—
Pancuronium	↑	—	↑	—	—
Succinylcholine	↓	—	—	—	↑

Appendix B

ENDOCARDITIS PROPHYLAXIS

Endocarditis prophylaxis is at present recommended for all congenital heart disease with the exception of uncomplicated secundum atrial septal defect. It should also be used in all postoperative congenital heart disease except secundum atrial septal defect repaired without patch (after 6 months), and in ligated ductus arteriosus. The incidence of bacterial endocarditis in children is highest in postoperative congenital aortic stenosis and systemic-to-pulmonary arterial shunts. Endocarditis prophylaxis is also required in patients with prosthetic heart valves; rheumatic, calcific, or other acquired valvular heart disease; idiopathic hypertrophic subaortic stenosis; mitral valve prolapse syndrome; or a transvenous pacemaker. Endocarditis prophylaxis in those with ventriculoatrial shunts for hydrocephalus or dialysis shunts or fistulas is not clearly necessary but is probably helpful.

Prophylaxis against recurrence of acute rheumatic fever is insufficient for the prevention of bacterial endocarditis. These patients have to be treated with recommended antibiotic therapy for prevention of bacterial endocarditis. Endocarditis prophylaxis should be initiated shortly (less than 1 hour) before the procedure and not prolonged beyond 48 hours to prevent selection of resistant bacterial flora.

Antibiotic Regimen
(American Heart Association)

For dental, otolaryngological (e.g. tonsillectomy, adenoidectomy) and bronchoscopic procedures.
A. Standard regimen
  1. *Oral*
     Penicillin V 2.0 gm orally 60 minutes prior to the procedure and then 1.0 gm orally 6 hr later. Children less than 60 lb receive half the above doses.
  2. *Parenteral*
     Aqueous penicillin G 50,000 units/kg IV or IM 30–60 minutes before the procedure, followed by aqueous penicillin G 25,000 units/kg 6 hours later.
  3. *For patients allergic to penicillin*
     a. Erythromycin 20 mg/kg orally 1 hour prior to the procedure, followed by 10 mg/kg orally 6 hours later.
     b. Vancomycin 20 mg/kg intravenously slowly over 60 minutes, beginning 60 minutes prior to the procedure. Because of the long half-life of vancomycin, a repeat dose is not necessary.
B. Special regimen (recommended for all patients with prosthetic heart valves)
  1. Ampicillin 50 mg/kg IM or IV *plus* gentamicin 1.5 mg/kg IM or IV 30 minutes before the procedure, followed by penicillin V 1.0 gm (500 mg if less than 60 lb) orally 6 hours later or by the initial parenteral dose once 8 hours later.
  2. *For patients allergic to penicillin* oral regimen
     Erythromycin 20 mg/kg orally 1 hour before the procedure followed by half the dose 6 hours later.
  3. *For patients allergic to penicillin* parenteral regimen
     Vancomycin 20 mg/kg intravenously over 30–60 minutes, beginning 30–60 minutes before the procedure.
C. Oral regimen for minor or repetitive procedure with low risk
  Amoxicillin 50 mg/kg orally 1 hour before the procedure followed by 25 mg/kg 6 hours later.

For genitourinary or gastrointestinal surgery or instrumentation (or any surgery of infected or contaminated tissue)

A. Standard regimen

Ampicillin 50 mg/kg IM or IV plus gentamicin 2.0 mg/kg IM or IV 30–60 minutes prior to the procedure. One follow-up dose may be given 8 hours later.

B. *For patients allergic to penicillin*

Vancomycin 20 mg/kg slowly IV over 1 hour plus gentamycin 2.0 mg/kg IV or IM 1 hour prior to the procedure. May be repeated once 8–12 hours later.

Maximal single dose of drugs: aqueous penicillin G 2 million units, amoxicillin 3 gm, vancomycin 1 gm, erythromycin 1 gm, ampicillin 1 gm, gentamycin 80 mg, vancomycin maximal 44 mg/kg/24 hours. In patients with compromised renal function the dose of antibiotics may need modification.

Appendix C

COMMONLY USED PEDIATRIC CARDIAC DRUGS

Drug	Route	Dose	Onset of Action	Indications (I), Precautions (P), and Complications (C)
Digoxin	P.O.	*Initial:* <2 yr 0.04–0.06 mg/kg >2 yr 0.02–0.04 mg/kg	1–2 hr	I: Congestive failure, supraventricular arrhythmias
	P.O.	*Maintenance:* ¼–⅓ initial dose divided in 2 doses		C: Toxicity may appear with fluid shifts and hypokalemia perioperatively
	IM IV	75% of P.O. dose	15–60 min 5–30 min	P: Give 50% of total digitalizing dose, then 2 doses of 25% q 6–8 hr
Furosemide	IV P.O.	1–2 mg/kg 1–4 mg/kg/day	5–15 min	I: Congestive failure with fluid retention C: Causes hypokalemia and metabolic alkalosis
Propranolol	IV	0.01–0.015 mg/kg over 10 min, repeat q 6–8 min 0.1–0.2 mg/kg maximum repeat q 6–8 hr	2–5 min	I: Hypertrophic myopathy, beta blockade, atrial arrhythmias
	P.O.	0.5–1.0 mg/kg q 6 hr	30–60 min	I: Hypercyanotic spells C: May cause failure and heart block
Lidocaine	IV IV cont. infusion	0.5–1.0 mg/kg 0.01–0.05 mg/kg/min	15–90 sec	I: Ventricular dysrhythmia C: Causes heart block, hypotension, convulsion
Dopamine	IV cont. infusion	5–25 µg/kg/min	Minutes	I: Hypotension due to reduced contractility P: Low dose improves renal perfusion C: May cause tachyarrhythmias, tissue necrosis
Dobutamine	IV cont. infusion	5–20 µg/kg/min	Minutes	I: Heart failure, cardiogenic shock
Epinephrine	IV IV cont. infusion	10 µg/kg 1–10 µg/kg/min, start with 0.1 µg/kg/min	Seconds	I: Cardiac arrest, bradycardia, hypotension C: Causes ventricular arrhythmias
Phenylephrine	IV	5–10 µg/kg		I: To counteract sudden decrease in peripheral vascular resistance in cyanotic lesion; paroxysmal tachycardia C: May cause bradycardia and hypertension
Norepinephrine	IV cont. infusion	0.1 µg/kg/min, titrate to desired effect		I: Hypotension without peripheral vasoconstriction C: May cause hypertension and tissue necrosis
Calcium chloride	IV	10–15 mg/kg		I: Slow and weak cardiac action C: May cause cardiac arrest and tissue necrosis
Isoproterenol	IV cont. infusion	0.05–0.4 µg/kg/min, titrate to desired effect	30–60 sec	I: Bradycardia and failure C: Causes ventricular irritability
Sodium nitroprusside	IV cont. infusion	0.5–0.8 µg/kg/min	Minutes	I: Afterload reduction, lowering of blood pressure C: Hypotension, cyanide toxicity
Tolazoline	IV	1–2 mg/kg over 15–20 min, then 2.0 mg/kg/hr	Minutes	I: Pulmonary vasodilation C: Systemic hypotension
Prostaglandin E₁	IV cont. infusion	0.01–0.1 µg/kg/min	Minutes	I: Prevention of ductal closure C: Apnea, fever, hypotension
Nitroglycerin	IV cont. infusion	0.2–0.6 µg/kg/min, titrate to desired effect	Minutes	I: Preload reduction C: Hypotension tachycardia

Appendix D

REVERSAL OF ANTICOAGULATION

In order to avoid bleeding problems during surgery, anticoagulation with vitamin K antagonists is generally discontinued 36 hours prior to elective surgery; anticoagulation is then maintained with intravenous heparin, which can be more readily reversed if necessary. For emergency procedures, 10 ml/kg of fresh frozen plasma is administered pre- and postoperatively along with vitamin K_1, 10 mg IM or slowly IV, as soon as possible preoperatively to reverse the effect of warfarin (Coumadin).

DISEASES OF THE RENAL SYSTEM

7

G. MARK CRAMOLINI, M. D.

Normal renal physiology in the preterm, full-term, and older infant differs significantly from that of the normal adult. Differences in total body water content and distribution, glomerular filtration rate, electrolyte and solute excretion, concentrating ability, and drug distribution and clearance are well known to the anesthesiologist caring for children, and are thoroughly discussed elsewhere.[1, 2] Likewise, the effect of anesthesia on renal function is a topic unto itself and will be discussed here only in the context of interactions with specific renal diseases.

There are many hereditary, congenital, and acquired diseases affecting the kidney, ureter, bladder, urethra, and genitalia in infants and children. Structural abnormalities often require early surgical intervention for correction. Functional abnormalities may be intrinsic or the result of structural abnormalities or other diseases. The resulting pathophysiological manifestations have implications for anesthesia, whether or not surgery is directed at the genitourinary problem.

Many of these disorders lead to chronic renal failure and ultimately to end-stage renal disease. The manifestations of uremia are widespread, involving almost every organ system, and have a myriad of anesthetic implications. An understanding of the pathophysiological changes in renal failure and the resulting anesthetic considerations forms the basis for the detailed anesthetic management of these complex patients. It also provides a background against which the anesthetic implications of specific, less severe renal and genitourinary abnormalities can be readily discussed. We will therefore begin with a discussion of renal failure in pediatric patients and the consequent anesthetic implications for diagnostic, palliative, and therapeutic surgical interventions, including pediatric renal transplantation.

CHRONIC RENAL FAILURE

Adequate renal function is essential for the functional integrity of the other organ systems. The newborn is provided with approximately one million nephrons per kidney. Symptoms do not appear until there is destruction of almost 80 percent of the nephrons, and survival is possible with only 2 to 3 percent.[3, 4] Thus renal homeostasis may not be threatened until genitourinary disease is well advanced; on the other hand, by preventing the appearance of symptoms this adaptive capability may cause treatment to be delayed until significant loss has occurred.

Incidence and Etiologies

More than 50 different renal diseases may progress to renal failure over time spans of months to decades.[3] The incidence of renal failure in adults shows a striking racial difference with an incidence of 188 per million blacks and 44 per million whites.[5, 6] Table 7–1 shows the causes of chronic renal failure (CRF) in adults in the United States according to race. Fewer data exist on the incidence and causes of chronic renal failure in children. The entry rate of children into chronic renal failure treatment programs ranges from 1 to 2.4 per million total population per year; of new children

155

Table 7–1. CAUSES OF CHRONIC RENAL FAILURE IN ADULTS IN THE UNITED STATES

Disease	White (%)	Black (%)	Total (%)
Glomerulonephritis	36	26	31
Hypertension	10	46	28
Diabetes	13	12	13
Interstitial nephropathy	17	5	11
Polycystic disease	9	2	6
Undetermined	7	4	6
Collagen disorders	4	3	4
Others*	4	2	1

*Hereditary disease, neoplasms, other cystic diseases, congenital diseases, gout, amyloidosis, sickle cell disease, radiation, cortical necrosis, trauma.

From Kuruvila KC, Schrier RW: Chronic renal failure. Int Anesthesiol Clin 22:101, 1984.

entering such programs, 5 percent are under 5 years of age, 26 percent between 5 and 10 years of age, and 69 percent between 10 and 15 years of age.[7] These data reflect only those children who enter a treatment program; those who die without undergoing dialysis are not included. In particular, very few data exist on the mortality from chronic renal failure in children under 5 years of age.[8] Table 7–2 shows the distribution of underlying renal diseases in children entering renal failure treatment programs in Europe in 1978. When the underlying cause is glomerular disease, renal failure in children may progress very rapidly, while CRF due to urological abnormalities tends to have a more prolonged course. The progression of CRF in infants and children is difficult to predict, but a plot of their glomerular filtration rate (GFR) versus age can give some indication of this rate. Table 7–3 lists the clinical status and need for intervention at different degrees of renal failure as assessed by the GFR.[8] When evaluating plasma creatinine and GFR in infants and children, one must recall that normal values vary with age as shown in Figure 7–1 and Table 7–4. An empirical approximation for the normal predicted GFR for different-sized patients[9, 10] is given by:

$$GFR = K \frac{L}{P_{creat.}}$$

Table 7–2. PRIMARY RENAL DISEASE IN CHILDREN ENTERING RENAL FAILURE PROGRAMS IN EUROPE, 1978

Disease	Incidence (%)
Glomerulonephritis	34
Pyelonephritis	22
Cystic disease	8
Hereditary nephropathy	8
Renal hypoplasia/dysplasia	11
Renal vascular disease	2
Cortical/tubular necrosis	1
Other*	14

*Principally kidney tumors and the hemolytic-uremic syndrome.

From Barratt TM, Baillod RA: Chronic renal failure and regular dialysis. *In* Williams DI, Johnston JH (Eds.): Paediatric Urology. London, Butterworth Scientific, 1982.

Table 7–3. GFR VERSUS CRF STATUS AND INTERVENTION

GFR (ml/min 1.73m²)	CRF Status	Intervention
80 to 40	Mild, asymptomatic	Follow growth status
		Detect and treat hypertension
40 to 20	Moderately severe, growth failure probable, risk of osteodystrophy	Careful medical supervision
		Initiate dietary management
20 to 10	Severe, uremic symptomatology	Tight dietary management to optimize growth
		Control infection, hypertension, edema, cardiac failure
		Psychological, social, medical preparation for dialysis and/or transplant
10 or less	Extreme	Need for dialysis or transplantation is imminent

Data from Barratt TM, Baillod RA: Chronic renal failure and regular dialysis. *In* Williams DI, Johnston JH (Eds.): Paediatric Urology. London, Butterworth Scientific, 1982.

where GFR = glomerular filtration rate in ml/min per 1.73 m², L = length (height) in cm, $P_{creat.}$ = plasma creatinine in mg/100 ml, and K = 0.55 in children (age 1 year and older) or 0.45 in infants (full term to 1 year). (Studies are in progress to determine K in premature infants.[9]) It is important to note that this empirical formula is for patients who are not growth-retarded.

Physiological Adaptation to Renal Failure

As there is progressive renal destruction, each remaining nephron must assume a larger workload in order to maintain homeostasis. In the "intact nephron" hypothesis, as nephrons are destroyed, surviving neph-

Table 7–4. Normal Glomerular Filtration Rate by Age

Age	GFR Mean	GFR Range ± 2 SD
Premature	47	29–65
2–8 days	38	26–60
4–28 days	48	28–68
35–95 days	58	30–86
1–5.9 months	77	41–103
6–11.9 months	103	49–157
12–19 months	127	63–191
2–12 years	127	89–165
Adult male	131	88–174
Adult female	117	87–147

GFR measured in ml/min/1.73 m².

From Barratt TM: Renal function. *In* Williams DI, Johnston JH (Eds.): Paediatric Urology. London, Butterworth Scientific, 1982.

Figure 7–1. Normal plasma creatinine concentrations in neonates, infants, and children. Mean plasma creatinine concentration on ordinate is plotted for specific age group denoted on abscissa. Figures within each bar represent numbers of patients studied. Length of vertical line above bar corresponds to 1 standard error. (*From* Schwartz GJ, Feld LG, Langford DJ: A simple estimate of glomerular filtration rate in full term infants during the first year of life. J Pediatr *104*:849, 1984.)

rons continue to function normally or "supranormally."[12] The renal function as a whole resembles that of a normal kidney, but with an increased requirement of solute and water diuresis. As a result, the kidney demonstrates a diminished ability to adapt to changes in plasma volume and composition.[12]

The "trade off" hypothesis proposes that the improved efficiency of individual surviving nephrons comes only at a cost.[13] This cost expresses itself as the clinical manifestations of uremia and renal failure. Examples would be raised plasma urea levels, which rise until excretion again matches production; hypertension, which results from an overexpansion of extracellular fluid needed to drive sodium excretion; and hyperparathyroid bone disease, which is a result of increased secretion of parathyroid hormone needed to decrease tubular reabsorption of phosphate.[13]

Anesthetic Implications of the Pathophysiological Manifestations of Renal Failure

The clinical manifestations of renal failure involve almost every organ system (Table 7–5). Since most of these manifestations have implications for anesthesia, we will detail them individually and follow with the anesthetic considerations for each.

Sodium and Water Excretion

As GFR decreases, less sodium and water are filtered and available for excretion. To compensate for this the fractional excretion (the portion filtered which is excreted) of sodium and water increases. This occurs because of Na^+ and H_2O retention leading to an expanded extracellular fluid (ECF) volume and effective arterial volume. Volume receptors that modulate Na^+ reabsorption then cause a decrease in reabsoption of the filtered Na^+ and thus an increase in Na^+ excretion. The detector and effector mechanisms involved in this natriuresis are still debated but may include the juxtaglomerular apparatus and the renin-angiotensin-aldosterone system,[15, 16] redistribution of renal blood flow and glomerular filtrate,[16, 17] intrarenal hemodynamic changes,[18] and a proposed "natriuretic hormone."[19-21] Volume-mediated hypertension may result as a "trade off" for this adaption.[22, 23]

Several patterns of abnormal sodium and water excretion exist in infants and children in renal failure, and these are somewhat characteristic for the underlying renal lesion.[14] In congenital renal dysplasia and urinary obstructive diseases, the renal medullary concentrating mechanism may be poorly developed or damaged. A state resembling nephrogenic diabetes insipidus may ensue in which there is excretion of large volumes of dilute urine low in sodium content. Such infants will often cry until provided fluids, but since babies are generally assumed to be frequently "wet," their large volumes of urinary output may not be obvious unless measured. If fluid intake is decreased owing to illness, these infants are at high risk for severe dehydration. Routine NPO orders preoperatively may be particularly dangerous. Serial weights and accurate intake and output measurements are necessary to manage fluids properly in these children.

In chronic glomerulonephritis there may be a greater reduction in glomerular filtration than in tubular reabsorption, causing glomerulotubular imbalance.[14] Sodium and water retention may lead to hypertension, congestive failure, and pulmonary edema. Peripheral edema may be exacerbated by hypoproteinemia secondary to marked proteinuria. The volume of urinary production is normal but with a fixed osmolality that may be equal to (isosthenuria) or, in advanced renal

Table 7–5. FEATURES OF CHRONIC RENAL FAILURE AND UREMIA IN CHILDREN

Fatigue, lethargy, somnolence, coma
Anorexia, nausea, vomiting, hematemesis, gastric ulcers
Uremic colitis, diarrhea, melena
Pericarditis, myocardiopathy, cardiac failure
Pleuritis, pulmonary edema, pulmonary hemorrhage
Anemia, thrombasthenia, purpura
Edema, hypertension
Rickets/osteomalacia, osteitis fibrosa, hyperphosphatemia, hypocalcemia, hyperparathyroidism, pruritus
Hyperkalemia, metabolic acidosis, hyperuricemia
Glucose intolerance
Peripheral neuropathy
Impaired immunologic competence
Retardation of growth and maturation

From Lewy PR, Hurley JK: Chronic renal insufficiency. Pediatr Clin North Am *23*:829, 1976.

failure, less than (hyposthenuria) plasma osmolality.[24] Sodium restriction, diuretics, and antihypertensives are useful in limiting edema and ameliorating hypertension.[25]

A third pattern of abnormal salt and water excretion is that of salt wasting, accompanied by an inability to concentrate or dilute the urine. This is seen in some children with chronic pyelonephritis, sickle cell nephropathy, hydronephrosis, or medullary cystic disease.[14] Sodium reabsorption is defective primarily in the distal nephron, resulting in large volumes of urine high in sodium content (60 to 120 mEq/liter). These children will spontaneously ingest large amounts of sodium, and sodium restriction can quickly lead to severe hyponatremic dehydration. Proper fluid management is based on careful measurement of the obligatory urinary loss and urine sodium content.

With end-stage renal disease, GFR has decreased to the point that excretion of normal sodium and water loads is not possible. Sodium and water retention leads to edema and vascular congestion and may result in pulmonary edema, hypertension, and congestive heart failure. These symptoms can be controlled with careful water and sodium restriction. When problems in fluid management are severe, peritoneal dialysis or hemodialysis may be necessary. Special attention to the management of sodium intake is needed in all these patients. Even in end-stage renal failure, if there is urine output, then there is an obligate urinary sodium loss. This is attributable to the increased filtered load of sulfates and phosphates which require excretion of Na^+ as the primary accompanying cation, and to the osmotic diuresis of solutes per remaining nephron.[26] Because of edema and hypertension, the diagnosis of excessive sodium intake is easily made. Inadequate sodium intake, on the other hand, results in symptoms that are subtle and may be overlooked in the absence of a high index of suspicion. This diagnosis is important to make, however, since overzealous sodium restriction or sudden sodium losses may result in a contracted extracellular fluid volume, a decreased GFR, and an exacerbation of uremia.[27] The relative hypovolemia that exists represents an unexpected hazard at the time of anesthetic induction.

The pathophysiological abnormalities of sodium and water homeostasis described above hold several implications for the anesthetic management of these children. They cannot compensate for incorrect sodium and water administration pre-, intra-, or post-operatively. The preoperative evaluation of exact volume status is essential. Edema and hypertension are signs of sodium and water overload that will require preoperative sodium and fluid restriction, diuretics, antihypertensives, and/or dialysis. As noted above, a high index of suspicion is needed to detect a state of sodium depletion. Clues to this are a worsening in uremic symptoms and signs of hypovolemia, such as orthostatic changes in pulse and blood pressure or a decreased requirement for antihypertensives. Children

with obligate urinary losses due to renal disease, who present with an acute illness preventing intake or causing large sodium and water losses (for example, bowel obstruction or gastroenteritis) may suffer profound hypovolemia. They will require preoperative fluid resuscitation, based on clinical signs (as given in Table 7–6) and/or a knowledge of the magnitude of an acute weight loss. This may be accomplished with normal saline[29] or Ringer's lactate, but a solution of the following composition has been suggested as being one that simulates ECF more exactly: isotonic sodium chloride 800 ml plus 22 mEq of sodium bicarbonate, plus 5 percent dextrose in water to a total volume of 1 liter (Na^+ = 140 mEq/L, Cl^- = 118 mEq/L, HCO_3 = 22 mEq/L)[27]. Careful monitoring during ECF expansion is necessary to avoid causing fluid overload.

Even if volume status is normal, it is important to determine which pattern of abnormal sodium and water excretion the child demonstrates, since this will influence perioperative fluid management. The underlying lesion causing renal failure may provide a clue to the pattern of sodium and water excretion, but a more accurate method is to assess ongoing intake and output, urine and serum osmolalities and electrolytes, and serial weights. If an obligate large urinary water and/or sodium loss exists, then an intravenous fluid and electrolyte regimen based on the above assessment should be instituted prior to making the patient NPO preoperatively. One such regimen, which is useful for most situations, including anuria, is as follows. Insensible losses (based on 45 ml per 100 kcal metabolized[28] or approximately 30 ml/kg/day for infants up to 1 year of age and 20 ml/kg/day to a maximum of 500 ml in older children[14]) are replaced IV with 10 percent dextrose in water. (Caloric expenditure may be calculated as 100 kcal/kg for the first 10 kg, 50 kcal/kg for the next 10 kg, and 20 kcal/kg for each additional kilogram.)[28] "Piggy-backed" into this is an IV solution that is equal in electrolyte composition to the urine produced and is run ml for ml to replace urinary losses. Important to remember when utilizing this regimen is that any other fluid losses (such as NG, CSF, or stool) must also be quantified in volume and electrolyte composition and replaced. Adjustment to

Table 7–6. CLINICAL ESTIMATES OF VOLUME DEFICITS IN INFANTS AND YOUNG CHILDREN

Sign	Percent Deficit	Volume of Deficit per Kilogram of Body Weight
Dry oral mucous membranes	5	50 ml
Absent tears		
Decreased skin turgor ("tenting")	10	100 ml
Depressed fontanelle		
Shock	15	150 ml

From Nash MA: Water and solute homeostasis. *In* Edelmann CM Jr (Ed.): Pediatric Kidney Disease. Boston, Little, Brown, 1978.

Table 7–7. MODIFICATION OF FLUID REQUIREMENT DUE TO PHYSIOLOGICAL ALTERATIONS

Reason for Modification	Modification Required
Altered Metabolic Rate	
Fever	Increase water allowance by 12% per °C increase in body temperature
Hypermetabolic states	Increase water allowance by 25–75%
Decreased Metabolic Rate	
Hypothermia	Decrease water allowance by 12% per °C decrease in body temperature
Hypometabolic states	Decrease water allowance by 10–25%
Sweating	
Mild to moderate sweating	Add 10–25 ml/100 kcal for water loss and an additional 0.5–1.0 mEq sodium and chloride per 100 kcal
Sweating in cystic fibrosis	Increase water allowance by same amount as in normal subjects but allow 1–2 mEq/100 kcal additional sodium and chloride

Modified from Nash MA: Water and solute homeostasis. *In* Edelmann CM Jr (Ed.): Pediatric Kidney Disease. Boston, Little, Brown, 1978. Adapted from Winters RW: Principles of Pediatric Fluid Therapy. North Chicago, Abbott Laboratories, 1975.

the rate for insensible losses may need to be made, based on whether inspired gases are dry (increasing the losses) or humidified (decreasing the losses), as well as for other variables shown in Table 7–7. Serial determinations of serum and urine electrolytes and osmolality, with appropriate modification of IV therapy, is a cornerstone of fluid management of these patients while NPO pre-, intra-, and postoperatively. Intraoperative blood losses and fluid shifts may further complicate fluid management. It is imperative to remember that when urinary output is obligatory, it is *not* a reflection of the child's volume status. For this reason, central venous pressure assessment of volume status is frequently a useful tool both intra- and postoperatively.

Hyperkalemia

The chronically failing kidney has the capacity to increase K^+ secretion by the distal tubule, decrease fractional reabsorption of K^+ and thereby increase K^+ excretion per nephron as much as sixfold.[14] This, coupled with increased fecal loss of K^+, makes hyperkalemia rare until very late in chronic renal failure. Hyperkalemia in a child with renal failure with a usual GFR of more than 10 ml/min/1.73m² should alert one to an acute deterioration. Alternatively, hyperkalemia could be due to increased catabolism, metabolic acidosis, dietary K^+ excess, GI hemorrhage with absorption of K^+, potassium-sparing diuretics, angiotensin antagonists, converting enzyme inhibitors which de-

crease aldosterone availability, K^+ salts of drugs (such as penicillin), constipation due to phosphate binders which decrease fecal K^+ excretion and so forth.[4, 26]

With anuria, potassium accumulates at a rate of 0.4 to 0.8 mEq/L/day and the rate may be increased by acidosis, infection, hemolysis, and malnutrition.[30] The major concern with hyperkalemia is its effects on cardiac rhythm and function. These are mediated by the effect of the intra- to extracellular concentration gradient of K^+ ions on transmembrane potential, and may occur at different serum K^+ levels depending on the rate of potassium accumulation. For this reason, different authors recommend different serum K^+ levels at which to be concerned (serum K^+ = 7.0 mEq/L,[30] serum K^+ = 6.5 mEq/L,[14] serum K^+ = 5.5 mEq/L[31]). All agree however, that ECG monitoring provides insight into the status of the transmembrane potential and that ECG changes are an indication for aggressive therapy. Figure 7–2 shows the ECG changes associated with progressive hyperkalemia, and Table 7–8 lists the therapeutic regimens used to treat hyperkalemia in children aggressively. In treating children, one must

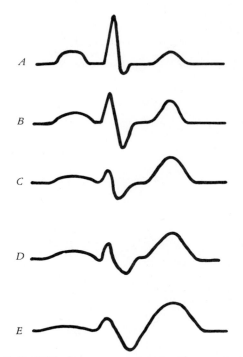

Figure 7–2. ECG changes associated with progressive hyperkalemia. *A,* Normal pattern. *B,* Slight prolongation of P wave, decrease in R wave, and increase in amplitude and peaking of T wave. *C,* Flattening of P wave, widening of QRS, and further increase in T wave amplitude. *D,* Marked flattening and prolongation of P wave; wide, low-voltage QRS; and wide, tall T wave. *E,* Sine wave pattern due to marked widening and slowing of QRS, depression of S–T segment, and increased amplitude of T wave. (*From* Rudolph AM: Disturbances of the cardiovascular system. *In* Edelmann CM Jr [Ed.]: Pediatric Kidney Disease. Boston, Little, Brown, 1978.)

Table 7–8. REGIMENS FOR THE TREATMENT OF HYPERKALEMIA

Regimen	Dosage and Route	Onset and Duration	Mode of Action	Comments
Calcium gluconate 10% (100 mg/ml = 9 mg elemental Ca/ml) Calcium chloride 10% (100 mg/ml = 27 mg elemental Ca/ml)	5 to 10 mg elemental Ca/kg IV slowly	Immediate onset Transient duration	Stabilizes myocardial membrane, no change in serum K^+	Monitor ECG May cause bradycadia if given as bolus Tissue damage with extravasation Precipitates with $NaHCO_3$
$NaHCO_3$ 8.4% (1 mEqHCO_3^-/ml)	1–3 mEq/kg IV bolus (Dilute 1:1 with sterile water and give slowly in prematures and newborns)	Rapid onset Short-term duration	K^+ enters cells in exchange for H^+	Monitor ECG Large osmotic shift with IV bolus associated with intraventricular hemorrhage in prematures Tissue damage with extravasation Precipitates with CA^{++}
Regular insulin and glucose	Give 3 gm glucose/L of ECF to lower K^+ by 1 mEq/L Insulin: glucose ratio of 1 unit: 3 grams. Give ½ dose to achieve desired serum K^+ IV over 10 min or by infusion	Moderate onset Longer duration	Promotes K^+ entry into cells with glucose	Monitor ECG Monitor for hypoglycemia with serial glucoses. Monitor serial serum K^+ Adjust insulin: glucose ratio based on serum glucose
Sodium polystyrene sulfonate (Kayexelate) Mix 1 gm/4 ml of 70% sorbitol for oral use (non-constipating) and 1 gm/4 ml of $D_{10}W$ for rectal use	1 gm/kg (each gram will exchange ~ 1 mEq K^+) (Warm the enemas, especially in small infants)	Slow onset Enema needs to be retained at least 50 minutes, the longer the better Initial results in 2–4 hours, may repeat q 4 hr	Na^+ on resin is exchanged for K^+ in large bowel	1–2 mEq Na^+ absorbed/gm of resin. Observe for overload Also exchanges Ca^{++} and Mg^{++} Constipating (sorbitol 70% helps) Concretions with aluminum hydroxide may cause intestinal obstruction Monitor serum K^+, Ca^{++}, Mg^{++}, Na^+ Total body depletion of K^+ may not be reflected in serum K^+. Observe for weakness, ECG changes of prolonged QT, wide, flat or inverted T, prominent U waves, with prolonged use
Dialysis (peritoneal dialysis and hemodialysis)		May take time to arrange, especially if peritoneal catheter or hemodialysis access sites are not already available	Ion exchange across peritoneal membrane or dialysis membrane	BP, ECG, electrolyte monitors Done under supervision of pediatric nephrologist and experienced nursing and technical personnel Most effective means of decreasing total body K^+ Serum K^+ may not reflect total body K^+ immediately post dialysis Monitor ECG

Data from Levy and Hurley,[14] Trainin and Spitzer,[30] and Jordan and Lemire.[427]

be careful not to be misled by false elevations in serum K^+. This is not an uncommon occurrence because of the difficulty in obtaining blood samples and may result from hemolysis induced by small sampling needles or from tissue breakdown products contaminating "heel-stick" samples.

Most authors recommend preoperative treatment of serum K^+ in excess of 5.5 mEq/L.[31, 33] This conservative value is chosen out of a concern about intraoperative rises in serum K^+ due to tissue catabolism, further intraoperative renal deterioration (due to hypovolemia, hypotension, or surgical misadventure), transfusion, acidosis, or infection. Succinylcholine will raise serum K^+ by 0.5 to 0.7 mEq/L in normal subjects when given as a bolus dose of 1 mg/kg, and this increase is not ameliorated by pretreatment with curare.[34, 35] This increase is not made larger by the presence of renal failure and for this reason a single dose of succinylcholine in patients in renal failure whose serum K^+ is less than 5.5 mEq/L has been considered safe.[36, 37] On the other hand, increases by as much as 2.4 mEq/L have been reported, with repeated doses of succinylcholine.[34, 38] Although one controlled study could only demonstrate a rise of less than 0.6 mEq/L in serum K^+,[39] the safety of multiple doses of succinylcholine is debated. The effects of succinylcholine on serum K^+ in patients with uremic neuropathy are unpredictable, and perhaps this explains the difference in the above observations. It has been suggested that in the presence of uremic neuropathy succinylcholine should be avoided altogether.[36, 40]

Acidosis

Children produce 1.5 to 2.0 mEq/kg/day of acid (almost twice that of adults[41, 42]) and 20 mEq of hydrogen ion is released for each gram of calcium deposition in new bone.[43] With a decrease in the GFR to about 20 ml/min/1.73 m^2 retention of fixed acid occurs[44] resulting in a fall in serum HCO_3 by as much as 1 to 2 mEq/L/day.[45] Renal compensatory mechanisms include tubular hydrogen ion secretion and urinary acidification, proximal and distal tubular reabsorption of HCO_3^-, excretion of titratable acid, and ammonium production and excretion.[46, 48, 49] All of these may be defective in CRF. The primary cause of metabolic acidosis, however, is thought to be a deficiency in total ammonia production, which decreases in proportion to the fall in GFR even though each remaining nephron secretes more than normally.[44, 46] In a few children with CRF, bicarbonate wasting may also add to acidosis.[47] Other compensatory mechanisms that come into play are buffering by calcium phosphate of bone, resulting in bone dissolution and increased urinary excretion of Ca^{++},[50] secondary hyperparathyroidism, which increases the tubular excretion of titratable acids and mobilizes extrarenal buffer in bone,[51] and respiratory alkalosis. Large anion gap metabolic acidosis is seen with retention of sulfates and phosphates. Hyperchloremic acidosis may also be seen,

especially if a sodium deficit has been corrected with sodium chloride alone (see Sodium and Water Excretion above). Chronic acidosis has been shown to be deleterious in children, especially in retarding growth.[52]

For the anesthesiologist the major concern is that a child with a low P_{CO_2} and serum HCO_3^- is extremely vulnerable to any further metabolic insult. Diarrhea with HCO_3^- loss, catabolic states, hypoglycemia, cold and hypotension with poor tissue perfusion, and lactic acidosis may cause a precipitous and life-threatening fall in arterial pH.[4] Hyperkalemia may also be seriously increased by acidosis.[53] Serum levels of bicarbonate less than 15 should be corrected preoperatively by dialysis if time allows,[51] or by administration of sodium bicarbonate (8.4 percent = 1 mEq/ml), where 1 mEq/kg of HCO_3 can be expected to raise the serum HCO_3 acutely by approximately 2 mEq/L.[30] It has been recommended that the same degree of hyperventilation should be maintained intraoperatively as was present preoperatively.[55]

Hypocalcemia, Hyperphosphatemia, and Renal Osteodystrophy

The normal homeostasis of serum calcium, phosphate, and bone metabolism depends on a complex interplay of many factors: dietary intake; gastrointestinal and renal reabsorption and secretion; acid-base balance; parathyroid hormone; calcitonin; vitamin D intake and metabolic conversion in skin, liver, and kidney; and the influence of other hormones such as somatomedin, thyroid hormone, estrogens, and androgens.[51, 56] The interaction and feedback control in this complex system is only partially understood, but it is known that the kidney plays a central role as a primary controller of calcium and phosphate excretion and reabsorption, as a target organ for endocrine control systems, as a metabolic activator of vitamin D, and as the site of degradation of parathyroid hormone and calcitonin. It is not surprising, therefore, that renal failure has a profound effect on calcium, phosphate, and bone metabolism. It is a tribute to the feedback control mechanism, given the central role of Ca^{++} in so many processes essential to life, that a fatal outcome is delayed.

It is also not surprising that in growing children renal osteodystrophy occurs more frequently than in adults. In one study, almost half of the children receiving hemodialysis in preparation for transplantation met radiological criteria for renal osteodystrophy, twice the figure for adults.[57] Renal osteodystrophy is more frequent and severe in children whose renal failure has occurred early in life as a result of congenital nephropathies or obstructive uropathies and has persisted many years before treatment of the bone disease. Abnormalities in renal osteodystrophy include osteopenia or generalized demineralization, osteitis fibrosa, osteosclerosis, rickets, and metastatic calcification. Secondary hyperparathyroidism may occur when GFR falls to 45 ml/min/1.73 m².[58] Although symptoms may appear at any age, the peak incidence is in the 5 to 10 year age range.[51]

The pathogenesis of renal osteodystrophy is as complex as the normal homeostatic mechanisms outlined above; a simplified overview is shown in Figure 7–3. As the filtered load of phosphate falls, remaining nephrons are unable to increase their fractional excretion of phosphate adequately and hyperphosphatemia occurs. Serum calcium falls in a reciprocal manner causing increased parathyroid hormone secretion. Concomitantly, the conversion of 25-hydroxy vitamin D to 1,25-hydroxy vitamin D in the kidney is impaired by the renal disease and possibly by the metabolic acidosis in renal failure.[59] The result is hypocalcemia, hyperphosphatemia, and renal osteodystrophy.

The first step in treatment is to lower serum phosphate. Dietary restriction and oral administration of aluminum hydroxide (60 mg/kg/day) is effective,[60] although there is some evidence that aluminum toxicity may be contributory in renal osteodystrophy.[61] Calcium administration in the face of hyperphosphatemia is ineffective and may cause metastatic calcification.[30] Once serum phosphate is in an acceptable range (3 to 5 mg/100 ml), dietary supplementation with calcium carbonate not only supplies additional calcium but aids in correcting acidosis.[51] Vitamin D therapy may then be instituted with careful monitoring of serum Ca^{++} levels. 1,25-hydroxy vitamin D_3 is frequently used, not only because lower doses of this end product are needed, but because of the very rapid turnover which allows more rapid resolution of hypercalcemic toxicity when overdose occurs.[56] If the above measures fail to lower parathyroid hormone, subtotal parathyroidectomy is considered.[62] With renal transplantation vitamin D metabolism, parathyroid hormone, and somatomedin levels normalize and osteodystrophy heals, but growth may continue to be

impaired due to immunosuppressive steroid therapy,[51] which may also weaken bone.

For the anesthesiologist the above problems have several implications. Hypocalcemia may be present, although it is usually not symptomatic. Treatment should be directed at lowering serum phosphorus, and if this is urgent, dialysis is indicated. In emergent cases in which symptoms of hypocalcemia are present or when it is difficult to rule out hypocalcemia as a cause of seizures, intravenous calcium may be given slowly, although its effectiveness may be short-term and repeated doses may result in metastatic calcification.[30] Hypocalcemia has been reported to prolong postoperative curarization,[63] but there are many other reasons why this might occur in renal failure patients (see below).

Anesthesia for parathyroidectomy must include consideration of the manifestations of the renal disease as well as consideration of surgery in the region of the airway.[64] Hypocalcemic seizures and tetany may occur postoperatively if serum Ca^{++} is not closely followed. Hypocalcemia is treated with Ca^{++} supplements and vitamin D.[4] In children with severe osteodystrophy and/or a history of chronic steroid therapy (see Chapter 12), the anesthetist must take care with intraoperative positioning to avoid fractures.

Hypermagnesemia

Infants and children with chronic renal failure usually have serum magnesium levels in the normal range (1.9 to 2.5 mg/100 ml). Hypermagnesemia is a rare finding,[32] but it may occur when the GFR falls below 10 ml/min/1.73 m², especially if the patient is receiving magnesium-containing antacids.[65] Very high magnesium levels may lead to neuromuscular weakness, respiratory depression, refractory hypotension, and coma[66] and will potentiate the neuromuscular blockade of both depolarizing and nondepolarizing muscle re-

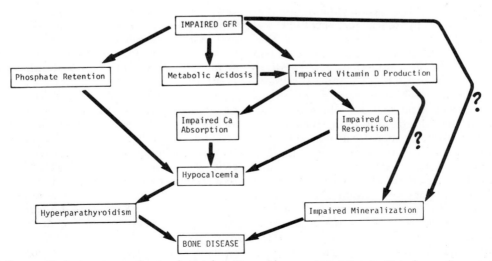

Figure 7–3. Pathogenetic factors in renal osteodystrophy. (*From* Norman ME: Vitamin D in bone disease. Pediatr Clin N Amer 29:947, 1982.)

laxants.[67] Dialysis will effectively lower serum magnesium, and intravenous calcium administration will acutely antagonize the neuromuscular effects.[54]

Anemia

Anemia is a consistent finding in CRF when the serum creatinine rises above 3 mg/100 ml[68] and is poorly correlated to the degree of uremia.[69] The degree of anemia varies with hemoglobin levels ranging from 5 to 10 gm/100 ml. It is usually a normocytic and normochromic anemia with a normal reticulocyte count.[70] Slowed erythropoiesis is attributed to decreased renal production of erythropoietin[71] and to circulating inhibitors that may be removed by dialysis.[72, 73]

Red cell survival is also decreased.[74] In vitro autohemolysis studies[75] and human cross-transfusion studies show that it is the uremic plasma and not a defect of the red blood cell that causes the short survival.[76] Several byproducts of the urea cycle (for example, guanidines) are elevated in uremia and have been implicated as toxins, possibly inhibiting normal red blood cell enzymes (such as transketolase and various glucolytic enzymes needed for energy production).[78-80] The acquired abnormalities of the pentose phosphate pathway put these patients at risk for increased hemolysis when exposed to oxidizing drugs such as quinidine, primaquine and sulfonamides.[4]

Microangiopathic changes are seen only when CRF is severe.[81] It is important to remember that anemia from blood loss (gastrointestinal, frequent venipuncture, dialysis) and from nutritional deficiencies (due to anorexia or removal by dialysis) may be superimposed on the chronic anemia in growing children. These additional factors should be diagnosed and treated with iron, folate, and vitamin B_6 supplementation.[14]

Compensatory mechanisms for anemia include an increased cardiac output and a shift in the oxygen hemoglobin dissociation curve to improve tissue O_2 delivery. 2,3-Diphosphoglycerate (2,3-DPG) levels do increase in CRF, but not to the degree expected for the anemia present.[82] This may be because metabolic acidosis, although directly shifting the oxygen-hemoglobin dissociation curve to the right by the Bohr effect, also decreases 2,3-DPG levels.[54] A study of the hemoglobin P_{50} values in anemic, dialyzed patients showed no significant difference from normals.[83]

Infants and children with CRF tolerate their anemia remarkably well, and routine transfusions are rarely required.[70] It was once feared that transfusion would cause sensitization to histocompatibility antigens and threaten future graft survival. The opposite has now been shown to be true.[83a] Repeated, pretransplant transfusions improve graft survival slightly with frozen washed cells, significantly with packed red blood cells (from 50 to 68 percent), and remarkably with whole blood (from 49 to 89 percent).[84, 85]

Therapy for anemia in chronic renal failure includes dialysis and treatment of deficiencies in iron, folate,

and vitamin B_6.[86] Exogenous erythropoietin administration is not yet available for human use, and animal studies suggest that the erythropoietic response is subnormal and dependent on the severity of uremia.[87] Renal transplantation dramatically raises serum erythropoietin, reticulocytes, and hemoglobin.[88] Except for pretransplantation, multiple transfusions are not advisable because of risks of hemosiderosis, suppression of erythropoiesis, developement of anti–red blood cell antibodies, hemolytic reactions, volume overload, and blood-borne infection. If transfusion is urgently required to raise the hematocrit, packed red blood cells (pRBCs) achieve this with the lowest volume. Frozen pRBCs have the lowest potassium content (1 to 2 mEq/L for frozen pRBCs as opposed to 18 to 26 mEq/L in citrated pRBCs).[89] Citrated cells may also further lower serum Ca^{++} in an already hypocalcemic patient. The decision to transfuse preoperatively depends on the child's overall condition, associated problems such as the presence of cardiac or pulmonary disease, and the anticipated risk of surgical blood loss. It has been suggested that no patient should be anesthetized with a hemoglobin level of less than 5 gm/100 ml.[33]

It is also important to remember that anemic children with CRF, because of their low hemoglobin levels, appear pale rather that cyanotic when hypoxic. Arterial blood gas measurement is the best way to document adequate arterial oxygenation. Increased inspired O_2 concentrations will help guard against subtle hypoxemia in these children whose O_2 transport capability is diminished.

The blood gas partition coefficient of halothane is decreased by 15 to 25 percent with anemia, and alveolar concentrations approach inspired concentrations more quickly, leading to more rapid induction and emergence.[90] The need to maintain an increased cardiac output to compensate for the decreased oxygen-carrying capacity, as well as impaired myocardial function in chronic renal failure, contraindicate the use of high inspired halothane concentration and controlled ventilation during a mask induction. Spontaneous ventilation with gradual titration of halothane concentration will help preserve venous return and cardiac output if this induction technique is chosen. Frequently, concerns about regurgitation and aspiration call for an intravenous induction (see below). Regardless of the technique chosen, anesthetics and positive-pressure ventilation should be utilized in a manner that ensures adequate venous return and cardiac output.

Coagulopathy

Bleeding in chronic renal failure may be a result of capillary fragility due to malnutrition or steroid therapy, irritation of mucosal and serosal surfaces by uremic toxins, and abnormal platelet number and function. Depression of specific clotting factors and prolongation of prothrombin time (PT) and partial thromboplastin times (PTT) have been reported but are rare.[70] Prolongation of coagulation times preoperatively should alert one to the possibility of residual or rebound heparinization, which can occur up to 10 hours after dialysis.[91] The incidence of this may be greatly reduced with regional heparinization, and any residual heparin effect may be reversed with protamine.[120]

Platelets are sometimes decreased in number, but rarely below 50,000/μl, and platelet survival is normal, indicating that the problem is reduced production.[92] The most significant hemostatic defect, however, is a reversible platelet malfunction attributed to dialyzable uremic compounds. Guanidinosuccinic acid concentrations are elevated enough in uremia to inhibit ADP-induced activation of platelet factor III, which normally promotes platelet adhesion.[93] Phenol and phenolic acids have also been implicated.[94] Defects of clot retraction, decreased adhesiveness, impaired aggregation, and diminished platelet factor III have all been demonstrated[95, 96] and fortunately seem to be induced by plasma factors that are removable by hemodialysis or peritoneal dialysis.[97]

Patients with creatinine levels that are still below 6 mg/100 ml usually have normal platelet function.[98] However, if the child is dialyzed, it is wise to check coagulation studies for platelet function and heparin effect. If the PT and PTT are elevated, the thrombin time is a more specific test to elucidate residual heparin effect.[99] This may be reversed with protamine. The bleeding time correlates well with the danger of hemorrhage and should be measured preoperatively.

Dialysis reverses the platelet dysfunction and is advisable preoperatively. Platelet transfusions should be reserved for the treatment of symptomatic deficits, since they otherwise produce only transient improvement.[100] This is not surprising, since the plasma factors causing the reversible platelet dysfunction persist and presumably have a similar pathological effect on the freshly transfused platelets. On the other hand, transfusion of cryoprecipitate has been shown to shorten the bleeding time for about 12 hours with return to original prolonged times by 24 to 36 hours.[101]

Recently, infusion of deamino-8-D-arginine vasopressin (DDAVP) at a rate of 0.3 μ/kg in normal saline over 30 minutes, has been shown to shorten the bleeding time. The effect occurs 90 minutes after infusion and lasts about 4 hours.[102, 103] DDAVP given by nasal insufflation is also being studied for this effect.[4]

In emergency cases in which preoperative dialysis is not possible, these measures may be helpful. More study of the mode of action, the time course and efficacy, and side effects of vasopressin is needed before its routine use can be recommended. If major intraoperative bleeding is anticipated, then warmed platelet concentrate, packed red cells and fresh frozen plasma, or fresh whole blood should be available. Adequate intravenous lines should be established to administer these products; in the infant or small child this may require a saphenous or antecubital cut-down.

Regional anesthesia, spinal or epidural, has been advocated for adults with renal failure, including those undergoing transplantation.[104-106] Regional techniques are not frequently used in children, and if contemplated for the older child, must raise consideration of the risk of bleeding, as well as of possible infection and psychological trauma (see below).

Infection

Infection and sepsis are serious problems in patients with renal failure and may lead to death.[107, 108] In vitro studies demonstrate an impaired immunological status in uremia.[109] Infection may increase caloric requirements and worsen azotemia, hyperkalemia, hyperphosphatemia, and acidosis. It may delay wound healing, lead to pyelonephritis, and further impair renal function. Septic shock may decrease renal perfusion and GFR with grave consequences. The most common site of infection is the urinary tract followed by the lungs, surgical wounds, and blood. The organisms most often isolated are *Staphylococcus aureus* and various gram negative bacilli. Treatment may be hampered by poor urinary excretion of bactericidal drugs and because of drug resistance.[30, 117] Care must be taken to use aseptic technique when placing intravenous cannulas or invasive monitors in these children.

Up to 55 percent of patients on hemodialysis are hepatitis B antigen carriers.[110] This appears to be due not only to their frequent exposure to dialysis equipment and blood products but also to depressed interferon production, which predisposes them to becoming chronic carriers.[111] Because transmission can occur with mucosal as well as percutaneous exposure to infected secretions or blood, anesthesiologists should protect themselves appropriately and treat needle sticks seriously.[112] Hepatitis B immune globulin is effective for protection after known inoculation. Because the hepatitis B risk to anesthesiologists is five to eight times that of the general population and similar to that of other medical personnel frequently exposed to blood, vaccination against hepatitis B has been recommended.[113, 114] Hepatitis B vaccination has also been tried in chronic dialysis patients, with 80 percent developing antibodies after a booster dose 6 months later (as compared with 98 percent in persons not on dialysis).[115]

Cardiovascular Manifestations

Hypertension. A major manifestation of renal failure is hypertension, which affects many children with advanced CRF.[116, 118] Eight separate but interacting mechanisms for the autoregulation of blood pressure have been proposed: baroreceptors (in the aorta and carotid sinus), chemoreceptors (carotid and aortic arteries), the CNS (the vasomotor center), the renin-angiotensin-aldosterone system (involving kidney, plasma, liver, adrenals, and lung), a stretch receptor mechanism (in arteriolar muscle), a capillary transudation mechanism (with transudation decreasing circulating volume), the renal-ECF mechanism (involving renal water and salt retention, independent of aldosterone effects) and a vasodilation mechanism (an ill-defined blood pressure–lowering role of the kidney).[119] Although hypertension may involve any of these interacting control mechanisms to some degree, it has been attributed primarily to abnormalities in renal ECF regulation. Fluid overload, the renin-angiotensin-aldosterone system (Figure 7–4) and perhaps the deficiency of a vasodilator substance released by normal kidneys may also be involved.[121–123]

Diagnosis of hypertension (BP > 95th percentile) is important in children with renal failure. Treatment is effective in preventing cerebral and cardiac involvement and in slowing the progression of renal failure due to hypertension, independent of the original disease.[118, 124, 128]

Figures 7–5, 7–6, 7–7 show normal blood pressures and percentile ranges in neonates, infants, children, and adolescents.[125-127] Proper equipment and technique are required for reliable measurements. The cuff should be appropriate for the size of the child's arm, covering two thirds of the length of the upper arm. The bladder should encircle more than half the arm over the brachial artery.[124, 127, 128] In infants, flush pressure (the cuff pressure at which capillary refilling occurs) approximates mean arterial pressure,[129] but Doppler ultrasound provides systolic pressure more accurately and reproducibly[130, 133] and should be used intraoperatively. If blood pressure is measured using Korotkoff sounds, the best index of diastolic pressure in children is the onset of muffling rather than the disappearance of sounds, which is the index used in monitoring

adults.[127, 131] Provided appropriate techniques and equipment are used, blood pressure measurements made on the thigh, lower leg, and forearm approximate upper arm measurement fairly well.[132]

Treatment of hypertension is directed at the pathophysiological mechanism that predominates. ECF sodium and water overload is the most common problem and is thought to increase cardiac output and peripheral vascular resistance.[123] It is often successfully treated with salt restriction (taking care not to over-restrict and decrease GFR; see Sodium and Water Excretion above), diuretics, and dialysis.[118, 124, 128] Those who do not respond have a major component of vasoconstriction mediated by increased autonomic tone, circulating catecholamines, and angiotensin II.[118, 123, 128] These children are treated with antihypertensive medication. These are vasodilators or have an anti–renin-angiotensin effect. Care must be exercised to eliminate foods and drugs (for example, licorice or decongestants) that can exacerbate hypertension.[128, 134] When even with dialysis these measures fail to control the hypertension, determination of elevated plasma renin activity may distinguish those children whose blood pressure will improve with bilateral nephrectomy.[135, 136]

As mentioned above, evidence exists for an antihypertensive renal function which has been variously attributed to renal production of prostaglandins,[135, 136] a nonprostaglandin neutral lipid,[139] and/or kallidin—an active kinin produced by renal kallikrein.[140] It is hypothesized that these may become deficient, but too little is known to provide a basis for speculation about therapeutic replacement.

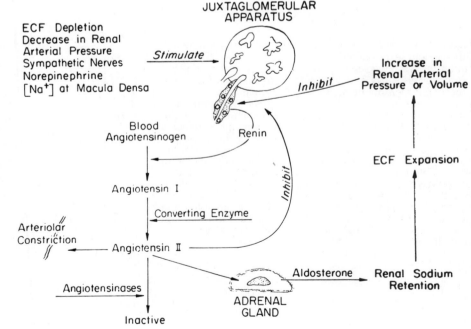

Figure 7–4. The juxtaglomerular apparatus and control of renin secretion. (*From* Mulrow PJ, Siegel NJ: Mechanisms in hypertension. Edelmann CM Jr [Ed.]: Pediatric Kidney Disease. Boston, Little, Brown, 1978.)

Figure 7–5. Linear regressions (*broken lines*) and 95 percent confidence limits (*solid lines*) of systolic and diastolic aortic blood pressures on birth weight in 61 healthy newborn infants during the first 12 hours after birth. For systolic pressure, $y = 7.13x + 40.45$; $r = 0.79$. For diastolic pressure, $y = 4.81x + 22.18$; $r = .71$. For both, n = 413 and p<.001. (*From* Versmold HT, Kitterman JA, Phibbs RH, et al.: Aortic blood pressure during the first 12 hours of life in infants with birth weight 610 to 4,220 grams. Pediatrics 67:607, 1981. Reproduced by permission of Pediatrics.)

Figure 7–6. Percentiles of systolic blood pressure in awake infants (both sexes pooled) at age 4 days to 1 year (Brompton study). At age 6 weeks the percentile values were calculated from the 594 boys and 538 girls who were awake at the time of BP measurement. At ages 6 months and 1 year all infants were awake. At age 4 days there were only 174 infants awake at the time of BP measurement, and the percentile values were therefore taken from measurements made on sleeping infants and corrected for wakefulness. The percentiles for ages 2 to 14 years have been taken from the values for 29 to 45 boys from the Miami study and from 453 to 592 boys from the Muscatine and Rochester studies (Iowa-Mayo pool), as summarized by the Task Force for Blood Pressure Control in Children. (*From* DeSwiet M, Fayers P, Shinebourne EA: Systolic blood pressure in a population of infants in the first years of life: the Brompton study. Pediatrics 65:1028, 1980. Reproduced by permission of Pediatrics.)

Percentiles of blood pressure measurement in boys
(right arm, seated).

Percentiles of blood pressure measurement in girls
(right arm, seated).

Figure 7–7. Systolic and diastolic blood pressure in children and adolescents. (*From* Report of the Task Force on Blood Pressure Control in Children. Pediatrics 59[Suppl]:803, 1977. Reproduced by permission of Pediatrics.)

Table 7–9 lists the medications commonly employed for treatment of hypertension in children with renal disease.[128] Several caveats and specifics should be mentioned. The pharmacokinetics of renal excretion of many drugs (for example, methyldopa) are altered in CRF, so that their dosage and dosing interval must be adjusted accordingly, and their elimination may be delayed when they are discontinued (see Drug Pharmacokinetics and Pharmacodynamics later in this chapter). Conversely, the pharmacodynamics of some of these drugs are such that abrupt discontinuation may cause severe rebound hypertension (for example, minoxidil[141] and clonidine[142]) or tachycardia (for example, propranolol[143]). It is important to recognize this preoperatively, especially for drugs such as minoxidil and clonidine for which IV preparations are not readily available. Ideally, these drugs should be carefully tapered preoperatively and replaced with drugs available in IV preparation.

The most commonly used drugs are the thiazide diuretics (chlorothiazide and hydrochlorothiazide), which are effective in mild hypertension. They work initially by diuretic and natriuretic effects, and volume, salt, and potassium depletion must be anticipated. Their sustained antihypertensive effect is most likely a result of decreased peripheral vascular resistance.[144] In severe renal failure the thiazide diuretics are usually ineffective and may actually be harmful since they may decrease GFR and increase the level of azotemia and hyperuricemia.[128] The potent "loop" diuretics, furosemide and ethacrynic acid, are more effective in severe renal failure, although they may also cause hypokalemia, volume depletion, and hyperuricemia. Furosemide has been shown to increase renal blood flow and GFR transiently in acute glomerulonephritis and is especially indicated for this condition.[145] The doses required in severe renal failure may be very large, and have been associated with transient hearing loss. Ethacrynic acid has been associated with permanent nerve deafness.[128]

Vasodilators are frequently added to diuretic therapy to control hypertension in children with CRF. Even though mental status changes and a possible association with breast cancer have limited the use of reserpine in children,[118, 128] some nephrologists feel that it is more effective at controlling hypertension in children than in adults.[146] Anesthesiologists may still encounter children on this drug. Bradycardia and nasal congestion may occur with use of reserpine; this drug is contraindicated in infants whose cardiac output is very rate-dependent and who are obligate nasal breathers.[128] Reserpine, like guanethidine, acts by depleting catecholamine stores. Treatment of intraoperative hypotension with directly acting pressor amines (such as

Table 7–9. ORAL MEDICATIONS USED IN THE MANAGEMENT OF HYPERTENSION IN CHILDREN AND ADOLESCENTS WITH RENAL DISEASE

Drug	Oral Dose Initial (per kg/day)	Maximum (per kg/day)	Action	Comment
Propranolol	1–2 mg	15 mg	Beta-blocker	Drug of choice; contraindicated in asthma and cardiac failure
Hydralazine	1–2 mg	8 mg	Direct vasodilator	Drug of choice; occasionally causes reversible lupus syndrome; reflex tachycardia is avoided by use of a beta-blocker as well
Chlorothiazide	10 mg	40 mg	Diuretic	Useful for mild hypertension; may need potassium supplementation
Furosemide	0.5–1.0 mg	15 mg	Diuretic	Often necessary with vasodilator drugs and in renal failure; potassium supplementation necessary
Prazosin	0.05–0.1 mg	0.4 mg	Direct vasodilator and alpha-blocker	Well tolerated; introduce carefully since hypotension can occur with a large initial dose
Minoxidil	0.1–0.2 mg	1–2 mg	Direct vasodilator	Extremely effective refractory hypertension; side effects hirsutism and saline retention
Captopril	0.3 mg	5 mg	Converting enzyme inhibitor	Remarkably effective in renin-dependent hypertension
Methyldopa	5 mg	40 mg	Central alpha-adrenergic stimulator	Main problem is sedation and depression
Bethanidine	0.4 mg	10 mg	Postganglionic adrenergic blocker	Marked postural hypotension
Diazoxide	5 mg	25 mg	Direct vasodilator	Saline retention, hyperglycemia and hirsutism
Clonidine	5 μg	30 μg	Central alpha-adrenergic stimulator	Depression; reflex hypertension on withdrawal
Phenoxybenzamine	1 mg	4 mg	Alpha-sympathetic blocker	Useful for oral control of blood pressure in pheochromocytoma before surgery; often needs a beta-blocker because of reflex tachycardia
Spironolactone	1 mg	3 mg	Competitive aldosterone antagonist	Potassium retention and gynecomastia

Modified from Dillon MJ: Hypertension. *In* Williams DI, Johnston JH (Eds.): Paediatric Urology. London, Butterworth Scientific, 1982.

norepinephrine, phenylephrine, methoxamine, or metaraminol) may evoke a greatly exaggerated increase in blood pressure. Indirectly acting pressor amines, which rely in part on the secondary release of norepinephrine from nerve terminals (such as ephedrine), may have a disappointingly small effect.[147] In addition to catecholamine depletion, guanethidine causes alpha-adrenergic block with resultant symptomatic postural hypotension. A decrease in cardiac output occurs, leading to a decrease in renal blood flow and GFR with possible worsening of azotemia.[128] Methyldopa, a "false neurotransmitter," is thought to have no deleterious effects on renal blood flow or GFR and lowers serum renin levels.[148]

Propranolol, a nonspecific beta blocker, is useful for its antirenin effects[149] as well as direct effects on the central vasomotor center.[150] Beta-adrenergic blocking agents may reduce cardiac output, renal blood flow, and GFR and should be used with caution in heart failure, asthma, and diabetes. Patients receiving up to 7 mg/kg/day of propranolol show a normal increase in heart rate with atropine administration, but those receiving larger doses in the treatment of renal hypertension have an impaired chronotropic response and

may require large doses of isoproterenol to overcome bradycardia due to beta blockade.[155] Severe bradycardia following administration of neostigmine to patients on propranolol has been reported.[155, 156] This may be much less responsive to atropine administration. Excessive negative inotropic effects of propranolol may be overcome without resorting to beta agonists by using intravenous calcium or glucagon, which bypass the beta receptor mechanism.[157]

Hydralazine directly relaxes arteriolar smooth muscle, thereby decreasing peripheral vascular resistance and blood pressure.[151] Tolerance to its antihypertensive effects occurs less frequently in children, in whom the side effect of tachycardia is well tolerated and easily controlled with propranolol. Parenteral administration can cause nausea, vomiting, flushing, and headache, and this may be confusing when the possibility of hypertensive encephalopathy exists.[128]

Minoxidil, also a peripheral vasodilator, is extremely potent and reserved for severe hypertension resistant to usual drug therapy. It causes sodium and water retention, necessitating concurrent use of diuretics or dialysis, and may lead to pericardial effusions and severe rebound hypertension if abruptly discontinued.[141, 152] It has been used with success in children with severe, uncontrollable hypertension.[153]

Clonidine, (a central alpha agonist) and prazosin (a direct peripheral vasodilator with alpha blockade properties) do not seem to have any major advantages in children over the above-mentioned drugs and are rarely used.[124] Abrupt withdrawal of clonidine may cause severe rebound hypertension,[143] and this can be treated with combined alpha and beta receptor blockade or nonspecific arterial vasodilators.[154]

Captopril reduces blood pressure by inhibiting angiotensin I converting enzyme and thus blocking the conversion of angiotensin I to angiotensin II, as well as by indirectly elevating bradykinin and suppressing aldosterone secretion.[158] It has also been used effectively in children with severe, resistant hypertension and is currently reserved for this use, with major side effects being hyperkalemia, leukopenia, proteinuria and rashes.[159]

The treatment of a hypertensive crisis is an emergency in which anesthesiologists may be involved, either in the perioperative period or in the ICU setting. Diazoxide given as an IV bolus at a dose of 5 mg/kg (up to 300 mg) has a rapid onset of action and a dramatic and predictable vasodilator effect with prompt lowering of blood pressure.[160, 163] Care must be taken to avoid extravasation, which may result in tissue necrosis, but otherwise a single bolus dose is relatively safe and rarely results in hypotension.[161] Its effect may be expected in seconds to minutes, and a dose may be repeated in 60 minutes if the desired effect has not been achieved. Once controlled, the blood pressure will usually stay down for several hours to a day, during which time other antihypertensives may be instituted.[128] Repeated doses may be associated with sodium and water retention requiring diuretic therapy and may also lead to severe hyperglycemia and elevation of serum amylase.[161]

Sodium nitroprusside is a potent vasodilator familiar to anesthesiologists that acts rapidly and is a very effective parenterally administered antihypertensive.[162, 164] Its rapid onset and cessation of action allows a continuous infusion to be readily titrated to the desired effect. This offers advantages in the perioperative setting where other factors (volume status, anesthetics) may rapidly alter blood pressure. Continuous infusion in the 0.5 to 8 μg/kg/min dosage range is almost always effective and usually avoids cumulative cyanide toxicity.[165] The renal clearance of thiocyanate is normally low (2.2 ml/min) and is reduced by almost half in patients with renal disease (1.3 ml/min).[166] Thiocyanate levels should be measured during prolonged nitroprusside administration in patients with renal failure. At levels of 10 mg/100 ml weakness, nausea, tinnitus, and behavioral changes are manifest.[128, 165, 166] Excessive levels can be lowered by discontinuing nitroprusside and by peritoneal dialysis or hemodialysis.[166] Intraoperatively, adding or increasing the concentration of halothane or isoflurane may effectively reduce the nitroprusside dose requirement.[167] Interestingly, cyanide toxicity is rarely a problem in renal failure patients, probably because decreased renal excretion of thiosulfate provides additional substrate for the conversion of cyanide to thiocyanate, which then accumulates as described above. An increased resistance to nitroprusside-induced cyanide toxicity has been demonstrated in anuric dogs.[168]

Labetalol, a new alpha and beta blocker given by infusion, may replace diazoxide as the drug of choice in hypertensive crises.[169, 170, 170a] Table 7–10 lists the dosages and route of administration of drugs used in hypertensive crises.[170]

Congestive Heart Failure and Pericarditis. Children with marked hypertension due to renal failure may develop left ventricular failure. Mitral valve insufficiency (due to cardiac distention), dyspnea, rales, and later right ventricular failure with hepatomegaly, venous congestion, and worsening edema may occur.[38] Volume overload, anemia, hypoproteinemia, shunting through arteriovenous connections, negative inotropic effects of electrolyte disturbances, and acidosis may all contribute to congestive cardiac failure.[4, 171] Recent echocardiographic assessment of cardiac function in children with chronic renal failure suggests that while

Table 7–10. DRUGS USED IN THE TREATMENT OF ACUTE HYPERTENSIVE CRISES

Drug	Dose	Action	Comment
Labetalol	1–3 mg/kg per h IV (total 0.5–5.0 mg/kg)	Alpha-blocker and beta-blocker	Use alone; stop infusate when blood pressure is controlled; effective 4–6 hours
Sodium nitroprusside	0.5–0.8 μg/kg per min IV	Direct vasodilator	Very short duration of action; effective only while being infused
Diazoxide	2–10 mg/kg IV bolus	Direct vasodilator	Can cause hyperglycemia, hypotension, and salt and water retention
Hydralazine	0.1–0.2 mg/kg IV or IM	Direct vasodilator	Can cause tachycardia, headache, and flushing
Minoxidil	0.1–0.2 mg/kg PO	Direct vasodilator	Rapidly effective even though orally administered
Furosemide	1–2 mg/kg IV	Diuretic	Avoid unless saline overload is obvious
Phentolamine	0.1–0.2 mg/kg IV	Alpha-blocker	Hypertensive crisis of pheochromocytomas

Modified from Dillon MJ: Hypertension. *In* Williams DI, Johnston JH (Eds.): Paediatric Urology. London, Butterworth Scientific, 1982.

only a minority of children with advanced CRF develop severe congestive heart failure, this is probably a result of a cardiodepressant substance in uremia.[185] Hemodialysis transiently improves this cardiac dysfunction, whereas successful transplantation reverses it.[185]

Immediate therapy is directed at the control of hypertension, volume overload, anemia, and the correction of acidosis and electrolyte abnormalities. Dialysis is the most effective means of achieving these ends.

Digitalis therapy in children with renal disease may be difficult to regulate, because of electrolyte abnormalities and markedly reduced urinary excretion.[32] Recent evidence suggests that inotropic support with dopamine (up to 15 μg/kg/min) in infants does not lead to a reduction in GFR.[172] This may be preferred to digitalis in the rare case when control of hypertension and fluid overload does not improve cardiac output.

The possibility of pericardial effusion and tamponade must be considered.[32] Up to 60 percent of patients with untreated uremia may develop pericardial disease.[171] Twenty percent may develop pericarditis in spite of hemodialysis,[173] and 30 percent of these may develop cardiac tamponade.[174] Although dialysis, steroids, and indomethacin are beneficial, surgical intervention with pericardiocentesis, pericardiotomy, or pericardiectomy may be necessary.[175] Although a recent report suggests that chronic percutaneous pericardial drainage in children is safe,[186] past experience in uremic patients has shown that pericardiocentesis carries a significant mortality.[175] Repeated pericardiocentesis increases the subsequent operative risk substantially,[176] therefore it should be reserved for the emergency relief of acute tamponade. The use of local anesthesia for subxiphoid pericardiotomy has been recommended as safe,[176, 177] and this may be acceptable in older, cooperative children. In such cases intra-arterial and central venous pressure lines are useful to monitor blood pressure and to insure optimal volume status and cardiac preload.

Sedative premedicants are contraindicated.[54] However, anticholinergics are indicated to prevent vagally induced bradycardia upon induction and laryngoscopy, since cardiac output may be critically dependent on heart rate (because of a restricted stroke volume). This is especially important in infants and small children. Extreme caution should be exercised with inhalational agents, which may lead to vasodilatation, decreased preload and afterload, hypotension, bradycardia, and even cardiac arrest.[178]

Positive-pressure ventilation may decrease venous return, cardiac output and blood pressure. Spontaneous ventilation preserves venous return and obviates these concerns. Controlled ventilation can be safely accomplished with shortened inspiratory times, low peak pressures, avoidance of PEEP, and slower rates. This will decrease mean intrathoracic pressure and minimize effects on venous return.

In adults with uremic pericardial effusions undergoing pericardiectomy, ketamine has been recommended because of its effects of preserving peripheral vascular resistance and increasing heart rate and cardiac output.[179] It is also very useful for children, although recent evidence suggests that the salutary effects of ketamine on heart rate and cardiac output may not be present.[180]

Pulmonary Manifestations

Fluid may accumulate in the lungs of children with renal failure as a result of congestive failure and fluid overload, hypoproteinemia (resulting in decreased intravascular oncotic pressure), and increased pulmonary vascular permeability.[4] Decreased vital capacity and diffusion capacity and mild restrictive defects may be the result.[181] Pleuritis and both transudative and exudative pleural effusions may occur, and organizing fibrous exudates can cause adhesions and restrictive pleuritis.[181] Although acute exacerbations of pulmonary edema may be palliated with positive airway pressure and ventilation, forced diuresis and dialysis are the most effective treatments. Metabolic acidosis, which induces pulmonary vasoconstriction and may exacerbate cardiac failure and contribute to pulmonary edema, can concomitantly be corrected with dialysis.

Neurological Manifestations

Many neurological complications may occur in children with chronic renal failure. These include uremic encephalopathy, hypertensive encephalopathy, seizures, peripheral neuropathy, autonomic nervous system dysfunction, and neurological complications of dialysis (dialysis disequilibrium syndrome).[182-184] Uremic encephalopathy is characterized by a global depression of cerebral function, although focal neurological signs may occur. These include transient loss of vision (uremic amaurosis), abducens nerve palsy, hearing loss, cerebellar ataxia, transient monoplegia, and hemiplegia.[182, 187] Focal neurological deficits and EEG changes are more commonly characteristic of hypertensive encephalopathy and may include focal weakness, asymmetrical reflexes, unilateral Babinski sign, nystagmus, oculomotor palsies, and visual disturbances that may progress to cortical blindness.[188] Acute funduscopic changes with a hypertensive crisis are rarer in children than in adults,[146] and children may have seizures without manifesting papilledema, retinal hemorrhages, or exudates. Subarachnoid or intracerebral hemorrhage or other rapidly expanding mass lesions must also be considered in the differential diagnosis of hypertensive encephalopathy.

The management of uremic encephalopathy consists of adequate dialysis. Hypertensive encephalopathy requires urgent reduction of blood pressure (as detailed above) and, if severe, the institution of measures aimed at the reduction of cerebral edema and increased intracranial pressure. In patients with renal failure, and oliguria or anuria, the use of hyperosmotic agents to achieve this must be controlled as determined by continual assessment of their effects on intravascular volume and electrolytes.[197, 198]

Generalized seizures occur frequently in renal failure, sometimes as a result of uremic or hypertensive encephalopathy, but more frequently owing to rapid metabolic changes in pH, calcium, and electrolytes. Hyponatremia may occur owing to water overload, or to transient cerebral edema in association with the dialysis disequilibrium syndrome.[182] While correction of the inciting etiology of the seizure is essential, intravenous diazepam at 0.1 mg/kg (up to 0.25 mg/kg) is the drug of choice for its initial control. Subsequent seizure control is maintained with longer-acting anticonvulsants such as phenobarbital or phenytoin.[182] A significant portion of administered phenobarbital is normally excreted unchanged in the urine,[189] and dosage modification may be required in renal failure.[190] The initial loading dose of phenobarbital in children is 10 mg/kg IV slowly, with a maintenance dose of 5 mg/day divided b.i.d., striving for a therapeutic level of 20 to 40 μg/ml. Twenty to 40 percent of phenobarbital is bound to plasma protein,[190] but in renal failure the ratio of free to bound barbiturate may be increased. Thus sensitivity is increased compared with that in normals at the same serum levels.[182] This is also true of phenytoin. Only 5 percent is excreted in the urine and the half-life is actually shortened in end-stage renal disease,[190] yet renal failure has a marked influence on effective plasma levels.[182, 191] Ninety percent of phenytoin is protein-bound, and the remaining 10 percent is pharmacologically active.[190, 191] In uremia, protein binding is markedly diminished[192, 193] so that the effective plasma level is less than the normal of 10 to 20 μg/ml.[184] The loading dose of phenytoin is 10 to 15 mg/kg IV slowly, followed by lower maintenance doses of 3 to 5 mg/kg/day divided b.i.d. Measurement and proper interpretation of plasma levels are necessary for control of therapy.

Peripheral neuropathy is a common manifestation of chronic renal failure with which the anesthesiologist should be familiar. The pathological lesion is axonal degeneration with segmental demyelination, which may be caused by uremic inhibition of the enzyme transketolase.[196] This is often reversible with dialysis or transplantation.[182, 195] The common peroneal and median nerves are frequently involved,[194] and distal, symmetrical lesions first involving the lower, then the upper extremities are usually seen.[182] The "restless leg syndrome" and the "burning feet syndrome" are initial manifestations that may herald progressive sensory, motor, and sympathetic neuropathy, which may progress to paraplegia. Unilateral pressure palsies, secondary to sensory neuropathy, may occur.[182] Sensory and motor deficits, such as foot drop, should be carefully documented preoperatively especially if positioning (stirrups for GU surgery) or surgery (such as the creation of a shunt in an arm or leg) will involve an affected extremity.

The possibility of progression to paraplegia may influence the anesthesiologist's choice of conduction versus general anesthesia. Diagnosis of overt clinical neuropathy is rare under 10 years of age, yet prolonged nerve conduction velocities in young children[195] suggest that in this group the lesions are simply not recognized until advanced.[182] When uremic neuropathy has led to immobilization, succinylcholine has unpredictable effects on serum K^+ and is best avoided.[36, 40]

Children with end-stage renal failure may also develop an autonomic neuropathy with impairment of sweating and baroreceptor activity. Hypotension that is unresponsive to volume but responds to norepinephrine infusion may occur during dialysis.[201, 202] This possibility should be kept in mind intraoperatively when unexplained hypotension unresponsive to volume is encountered.[54]

Finally, "dialysis dementia" has been attributed to chronic aluminum intoxication in adults on chronic dialysis.[204, 205] This is characterized by progressive dementia, speech disturbances, bizarre involuntary movements, facial grimacing, and myoclonic seizures and sometimes progresses to coma and death.[203] This syndrome has recently been described in children,[341, 342] and elevated serum and bone aluminum levels have been documented in those undergoing continuous ambulatory peritoneal dialysis who were taking aluminum hydroxide.[343]

Gastrointestinal Manifestations

Anorexia, nausea, vomiting, hiccoughs, gastrointestinal bleeding, diarrhea, and constipation may all accompany chronic renal failure and uremia.[206] Autonomic neuropathy as described above may account for delayed gastric emptying in renal failure, and this may double in association with hemodialysis.[207] Metoclopramide (0.1mg/kg) has been suggested to improve gastric motility, although caution must be exercised when it is used in children. Extrapyramidal side effects occur more frequently in children than in adults, and are especially common in patients with known seizure disorders.

Despite earlier suggestions of decreased gastric acid secretions in uremia,[4, 208] gastric acid hypersecretion, thought to be due to decreased renal removal of gastrin in renal failure,[209, 212] is known to occur.[210] It is suggested as the cause of peptic ulceration in renal failure.[211, 212] Cimetidine (5 mg/kg every 12 hours in severe renal failure) may be given preoperatively.[194, 213]

Persistent hiccoughs may be a particularly distressing gastrointestinal symptom which may not always yield to treatment with vagal maneuvers, nasopharyngeal stimulations, or phenothiazines.[4] Profound neuromuscular blockade may be required intraoperatively in order to eliminate bothersome movement during intra-abdominal surgery.

Endocrine, Nutritional, and Psychological Manifestations

Chronic renal failure in children leads to a myriad of abnormalities in endocrine control systems.[216] Disturbances of nitrogen, carbohydrate, and lipid metabolism[215] may occur and affect growth and development.[216] Peptide hormones, such as vasopressin, prolactin, growth hormone, calcitonin, somatostatin, parathyroid hormone, glucagon, and insulin, all tend to be elevated, although the end organ effects are variable.[217] Other hormones are decreased, such as erythropoietin and 1,25-dihydroxycholecalciferol, resulting in some of the common clinical manifestations of renal disease, such as anemia and renal osteodystrophy. Carbohydrate metabolism is altered in end-stage renal failure. Some patients develop hypoglycemia but most have a mildly elevated fasting glucose and abnormal glucose tolerance test.[215, 281] It is interesting that while diabetic patients tend to require less insulin as renal failure progresses, the nondiabetic patient with CRF develops peripheral insulin resistances and glucose intolerance.[218] In addition, exogenously administered corticosteroids may further contribute to endocrine, carbohydrate metabolism, and growth disturbances. Because of potential adrenal insufficiency, perioperative steroid coverage is recommended.[194]

Finally, the impairment of growth, development, and sexual maturation coupled with the psychological stress of a limiting, chronic illness may lead to severe psychological disturbance in children with CRF and in their family members.[219] Extra time and effort will be required of the anesthesiologist in order to establish optimal communication and understanding during the perioperative period.

Drug Pharmacokinetics and Pharmacodynamics

The pharmacokinetics and pharmacodynamics of most drugs are altered in chronic renal failure. This results from decreased renal excretion of the drug and/or its metabolites, decreased renal metabolism, altered volume of distribution, altered protein binding, altered lipid solubility, and altered end organ sensitivity and/or response.[220, 221] The effects of these pharmacological alterations on drugs used in the treatment of the specific clinical manifestations of renal failure, have already been discussed. For additional information about the use of specific drugs in the presence of renal failure, readers are referred to the excellent reviews available in the literature.[190, 220-222]

Anesthetic drugs also are altered in their pharmacokinetics and pharmacodynamics by renal failure and have significant effects on renal function.

The use of succinylcholine in renal failure is well studied [34-40] and has been discussed in detail above under "Hyperkalemia." Concern over lowered plasma cholinesterase levels with the older cellophane-type dialysis membrane no longer exists with current hemodialysis membrane materials.[224]

Reduced muscle mass, reduced renal blood flow, and alterations in the distribution volume of nondepolarizing muscle relaxants may result in a lower dosage requirement.[194, 225] Furthermore, neuromuscular blockade may be potentiated in renal failure by acidosis, hypokalemia, hypocalcemia, hypermagnesemia, diuretics, and antibiotics (Table 7–11).[67, 194, 226, 227] Gallamine is excreted exclusively by the kidney.[54, 194]

Renal excretion plays a major role in the excretion of pancuronium and metocurine, although biliary and other routes of elimination may increase in the face of renal failure.[225, 228] D-Tubocurarine has been the nondepolarizing drug of choice because its protein binding and potency are unchanged in renal failure,[229, 230] and hepatic excretion appears to be significantly increased.[230, 231] Curare may cause hypotension through ganglionic blockade and vasodilatation due to histamine release.[194]

Atracurium and vecuronium are newer nondepolarizing muscle relaxants with great promise for use in renal failure. Atracurium is cleared by Hoffman elimination and nonspecific esterases and is not dependent on renal excretion.[233] Early experience with its use in renal failure is encouraging,[232, 234] and experience is being gained with its use in infants and children.[235-237] Concerns have been raised about accumulation of

Table 7–11. INTERACTION OF ANTIBIOTICS, MUSCLE RELAXANTS, NEOSTIGMINE, AND CALCIUM

Antibiotic	Neuromuscular Block from Antibiotic Alone Antagonized by		Increase in Neuromuscular Block of		Neuromuscular Block from Antibiotic-dTc Antagonized by	
	Neostigmine	*Calcium*	*dTc*	*SCh*	*Neostigmine*	*Calcium*
Neomycin	Sometimes	Sometimes	Yes	Yes	Usually	Usually
Streptomycin	Sometimes	Sometimes	Yes	Yes	Yes	Usually
Gentamycin	Sometimes	Yes	Yes	*	Sometimes	Yes
Kanamycin	Sometimes	Sometimes	Yes	Yes	Sometimes	Sometimes
Paromomycin	Yes	Yes	Yes	*	Yes	Yes
Viomycin	Yes	Yes	Yes	*	Yes	Yes
Polymyxin A	No	No	Yes	*	No	No
Polymyxin B	No†	No	Yes	Yes	No†	No
Colistin	No	Sometimes	Yes	Yes	No	Sometimes
Tetracycline	No	*	Yes	No	Partially	Partially
Lincomycin	Partially	Partially	Yes	*	Partially	Partially
Clindamycin	Partially	Partially	Yes	*	Partially	Partially

*Not studied.
†Block augmented by neostigmine.
From Miller RD: Reversal of Muscle Relaxants. 32nd Annual Refresher Course Lectures, American Society of Anesthesiologists, Lecture 222, pp 1–6, October 1981.

the degradation products laudanosine[239] and acryl-ates,[238] especially in renal failure where uremia may predispose to an abnormal blood-brain barrier[240] and seizures. Vecuronium relies primarily on biliary elimination,[241] and has been studied in patients with end-stage renal failure,[242] and in infants and children.[243] "Re-curarization" should not be a problem with either of these agents. Reversal of nondepolarizing neuromuscular blockade may be accomplished with pyridostigmine or neostigmine, the elimination of which are prolonged with renal failure to the same degree as that of D-tubocurarine.[244, 245]

Inhalational agents are taken up and eliminated rapidly via the lungs, independent of renal function. This, in addition to their usefulness in potentiating neuromuscular relaxation and controlling hypertension, have made them popular agents for anesthesia in patients with renal failure.[194] All potent inhalational agents may depress renal function if cardiovascular depression leads to a reduction in renal blood flow and glomerular filtration rate.[246] Metabolism of these agents and release of inorganic fluoride with resultant nephrotoxicity is another problem. At a GFR below 16 ml/min/m^2, normal excretion of inorganic fluoride is impaired,[247] and accumulation will depend on the degree of metabolic degradation versus the rate of elimination. Methoxyflurane is no longer used as a result of these concerns.[248] Enflurane is metabolized less than methoxyflurane,[249] but there have been several reports of renal failure associated with elevated inorganic fluoride levels.[250-252] For this reason enflurane is generally not used in patients with renal failure.[54, 194] In one recent study, however, enflurane administered in the presence of mild renal failure (serum creatinine of 1.5 to 3.0 mg/100 ml) was associated with a slight improvement in postoperative renal function.[253] In the total absence of renal function, the question of nephrotoxicity is moot. Enflurane has been used in this setting without excessive serum fluoride accumulation because of deposition of fluoride in bone.[256] The availability of isoflurane, which is less metabolized[254] and results in lower fluoride levels,[255] or halothane generally obviates the need to use enflurane.

Narcotics should be used with caution in renal failure. Increased secretion of ADH and decreased urine output was originally thought to be a direct effect of morphine,[257] but is now thought to be a result of surgical stimulation.[258] Although narcotics are metabolized in the liver, urinary output can markedly influence the duration of their effect.[259] Prolonged respiratory depression has been reported in anuric patients.[260] The repeated use of meperidine may lead to the accumulation of the active metabolite, normeperidine, and can result in seizures.[261] Unlike other plasma protein–bound drugs, the magnitude of change in the free fraction of fentanyl found in uremic patients is not clinically significant.[262] In high doses, fentanyl significantly attenuates the catecholamine response to surgery and preserves renal function.[263] Fentanyl in combination with droperidol for "neuroleptanalgesia"

has been used with success in patients with renal failure.[264, 265] Neuroleptanalgesia causes minimal hemodynamic changes and little effect on renal function.[266, 267] Droperidol when given alone to patients with renal failure causes a small decrement in blood pressure and an increased cardiac output.[268]

Pentothal is normally 75 percent plasma protein–bound, but in uremia the free fraction increases significantly owing to reduced albumin levels and to displacement by uremic products.[270] Clinically, the required induction dose may be significantly decreased (as much as 75 percent) and the duration of action prolonged depending on the severity of the azotemia.[269] This may also be due to an abnormal blood-brain barrier in uremia.[240]

Ketamine is largely metabolized in the liver. Following intravenous administration only 4 percent is recoverable in the urine either unchanged or as norketamine, and 16 percent as hydroxylated derivatives.[272] Animal studies suggest that ketamine causes little or no change in renal blood flow and urine output.[273, 274] It has been used in pediatric patients for intramuscular induction, but caution must be exercised in the presence of uncontrolled hypertension.[271]

Little is known about the effect of renal failure on the pharmacokinetics and pharmacodynamics of local anesthetics in infants and children. Lack of acceptance along with concerns about coagulopathy, peripheral and autonomic uremic neuropathy, uncertain volume status, poor acid/base status, and alterations of the blood-brain barrier in uremia has limited the experience with regional techniques in uremic children. Epidural and spinal anesthesia has been used successfully in adults with renal failure.[104-106, 223] It has been shown in patients with normal renal function that if blood pressure is maintained, GFR and renal hemodynamics are only minimally altered.[275, 276] Brachial plexus block has been considered a useful anesthetic for the creation of an arteriovenous fistula in the arm because of the attendant sympathetic blockade.[265, 277] It is also a technique used with success in children.[278] Duration of the block in renal failure patients has been noted to be significantly shorter (38 percent), and this has been attributed to faster tissue washout due to an increased cardiac output.[277] One study in adults showed that plasma levels of etidocaine after axillary block were significantly higher in renal failure patients.[279] This, in connection with a report of bupivicaine cardiotoxicity with regional anesthesia in a patient with renal failure,[280] suggests that the ratio of effective to toxic dose may be decreased and dosage of regional anesthetics should be reduced in patients with renal failure.

Anesthesia for Children with Renal Failure

Multiple reviews describing various successful anesthetic techniques in renal failure have been published,[31, 33, 54, 104-106, 194, 265, 282, 283] demonstrating that no particular technique is best.[54] The foregoing discussion details the anesthetic implications of the manifestations of renal failure in children. This information provides the basis for the preoperative evaluation and the design of an anesthetic tailored to the individual needs of the uremic child and the particular surgery planned. Although surgery of any kind may be necessary, an operation in the child with renal failure will usually be related to the child's renal disease. Renal biopsy, diagnostic or radiotherapeutic procedures, peritoneal catheter insertion, arteriovenous fistula creation, parathyroidectomy, pericardial drainage or pericardiectomy, nephrectomy, and renal transplantation may be indicated. The best method of anesthesia for a child having a particular procedure will depend on the child's status, age, and state of cooperation, and the procedure contemplated. Techniques may include local or regional blocks, intramuscular or intravenous sedation, or general anesthesia requiring invasive monitoring. Comments on appropriate monitoring and anesthetic choices for given problems have been included earlier in this chapter in the discussions of the anesthetic implications of the manifestations of renal failure.

Renal Transplantation in Infants and Children

Renal transplantation is the ultimate therapeutic procedure for end-stage renal failure. This operation is being undertaken with increasing frequency in infants and children.[83a, 281, 284-286, 294] It presents an anesthetic challenge in which all of the problems of renal failure may complicate the usual concerns about anesthesia in seriously ill infants and small children. Many reviews of anesthesia for renal transplantation, with a focus on adults, have been published,[105, 106, 287-293] and the considerations presented are equally relevant when the child is the kidney recipient. The usual retroperitoneal approach and right iliac fossa placement of the kidney graft may be satisfactory in children over 20 kg in body weight.[294] However, in infants and smaller children (under 20 kg) the surgery needs to be modified. In these small patients a long midline incision and a transperitoneal approach are necessary. This large exposure necessitates special consideration of heat loss and fluid balance.

A large kidney placed in a small infant's abdomen may require maximal abdominal relaxation to facilitate closure. Nasogastric tube decompression of the bowel and discontinuation of nitrous oxide to reduce intestinal distention are helpful. Increased intra-abdominal pressure may result in respiratory compromise necessitating prolonged postoperative assisted ventilation, particularly in infants, in whom much of the respiratory excursion is diaphragmatic. Other problems arising from the transperitoneal approach and tight abdominal closure are prolonged ileus, compromised venous return, and kinking of vascular anastomoses, which may threaten graft survival.[281, 294]

Because of the discrepancy in size between the donor graft (often an adult kidney) and the recipient's small vasculature, anastomoses to the bifurcations of the aorta and inferior vena cava, rather than to the iliac vessels are used (Fig. 7–8).[281] As a result, there is the potential for major hemorrhage and the need for cross clamping of the aorta and inferior vena cava. Large-bore intravenous catheters must be placed in the upper body so that transfused volume may reach the heart via the patent superior vena cava. A central venous catheter, placed from an antecubital fossa or an external jugular vein, may be useful to evaluate trends in central venous pressure and volume status. If these lines are long, the additional resistance may make rapid transfusion of viscous blood products through them difficult. Percutaneous placement of internal jugular and subclavian lines is difficult in infants and carries the attendant risk of pneumothorax and occult bleeding, especially if clotting parameters are abnormal. In the very small child destined to receive a large kidney, it is not unreasonable as a first step to surgically place a large-bore central venous line, such as a Hickman or Broviac catheter. This may then be used intraoperatively for assessment of volume status, blood transfusion, and medications, and postoperatively for hyperalimentation if required. Infection is always a concern in uremic patients who will receive immunosuppressive therapy, and all lines must be placed aseptically.

An arterial line is necessary for continuous blood pressure monitoring as well as for serial blood gas, hematocrit, and electrolyte determinations. Concern about graft failure and the future need for hemodialysis has led some to strongly discourage the use of any artery at a potential shunt site.[295] This has led others

Figure 7–8. Placement of a large donor kidney in a small recipient. (*From* Fernando ON: Renal transplantation in children. *In* Williams DI, Johnston JH [Eds.]: London, Butterworth Scientific, 1982.)

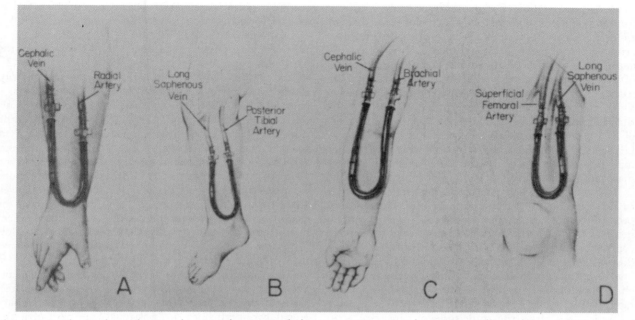

Figure 7–9. The Scribner shunt and various locations of placement. (*From* Buselmeier TJ, Kjellstrand CM: A-V shunts and fistulas for hemodialysis in neonates, infants, and small children. Proc E.D.T.A. *10*:511–515, 1973, with permission.)

to recommend cannulation of the dorsalis pedis or temporal artery.[54, 265] In small children in whom the need to cross clamp the abdominal aorta is likely, lower extremity arterial lines are of limited value. Furthermore, temporal artery cannulation in infants has been shown to carry a high risk of retrograde cerebral embolization.[296-298] Studies of radial artery cannulation in adults[299] have suggested that the risk of arterial obstruction increases with increasing catheter size, decreasing patient age, duration of cannulation, and cutdown versus percutaneous insertion. In a study of 53 cannulations in 47 pediatric patients, radial artery obstruction occurred in 27 cases (51 percent), but all obstructed vessels eventually became patent again, most within 1 to 2 weeks.[300] The placement of a small nontapered catheter, preferably percutaneously, into a radial artery for as short a period as possible would seem to be justified. For the child who presents with a Scribner dialysis shunt already in place in an upper extremity (Fig. 7–9), an excellent solution is to remove the external connecting catheter, as is routinely done at the time of dialysis. The venous end can then be used to infuse blood, plasma, or fluids, and the arterial end to monitor blood pressure and arterial blood gases and electrolytes.[294] Subcutaneous arteriovenous fistulas have been used for infusions and for blood gas sampling,[295, 301] but this should probably be reserved for extreme access problems and emergencies. When not in use the fistula should be padded, and one should refrain from taking blood pressures in that extremity, if possible. Fistula patency may be continuously monitored with an overlying Doppler flow probe.[194]

A final problem associated with a large kidney in a small child is the volume of blood "stolen" from the circulation to fill the new kidney,[294] and the consid-

erable proportion of the patient's cardiac output that is diverted to the new organ.[281] Cardiac arrest has been reported following anastomosis and release of the arterial clamp in the potassium-preserved kidney and upon unclamping of the iliac artery in adults.[302, 303] This has been attributed to hyperkalemia from the graft preservative and acidosis from the ischemic leg. This is exacerbated in the small child, in whom the volume of preservative relative to the patient's size is larger, and aortic cross clamping causes the whole lower body to become ischemic and acidotic. It has been recommended to transfuse 75 to 100 ml of blood prior to releasing the vascular clamps in order to accommodate the increased vascular volume and flow required by the new graft.[294] Likewise, it is advisable to administer 1 mEq/kg of sodium bicarbonate prior to release of the vascular clamp, in order to combat the predictable lactic acidosis and hyperkalemia.[294] Hypotension occurring intraoperatively or immediately postoperatively may be a result of poor cardiac output and depressed myocardial performance as a result of acidosis or hyperkalemia. However, in small uremic patients with potential coagulopathies, immunosuppression, and high ventilatory pressures due to a tight abdominal closure, other complications that must be considered include hemorrhage, hypocalcemia, sepsis, adrenal insufficiency, pericardial effusion with tamponade, and pneumothorax.

ACUTE RENAL FAILURE

Incidence and Etiologies

A major intra- and postoperative concern in transplant recipients or other children with marginal renal function is the onset of an acute deterioration in renal function. Even in children without prior renal disease, trauma, surgery (especially cardiac surgery), intraoperative hemoglobinuria or myoglobinuria, drug toxicity, and the use of radiocontrast media are significant causes of perioperative acute renal failure.[304-308] Trauma, infection, muscle ischemia, succinylcholine administration, and malignant hyperthermia may all lead to rhabdomyolysis,[45, 311, 315] and at serum concentrations of 0.15 gm/L myoglobin appears in the urine.[310] Likewise, hemolysis and transfusion reactions (which may be delayed up to several days after transfusion) may cause serum levels of hemoglobin as high as 0.5 to 1.4 gm/L, at which time it appears in urine.[309] Up to 12 percent of patients undergoing radiocontrast procedures may develop signs of renal injury, and the incidence is higher after angiography than after other contrast studies, probably because the occurrence is dose-dependent.[307, 316] Excretory urography can be a low-yield and high-risk procedure in the infant or child with oliguria, and therefore ultrasonography and radionuclide studies are preferred.[312-314]

Table 7-12 lists the multitude of causes of acute renal failure (ARF) in infants and children.[30, 304, 317, 318] Some of these, such as renovascular defects and obstructive uropathies, are amenable to surgical intervention, and the implications for anesthesia for these entities are discussed below.

Prognosis

Despite early institution of dialysis and parenteral hyperalimentation, the mortality rate of postsurgical patients with ARF remains 25 to 65 percent.[304, 305, 318] Although the underlying illness is a major determinant of mortality in ARF, infection accounts for one third to two thirds of all deaths.[319, 320, 322] Gastrointestinal hemorrhage is also a frequent complication and can contribute significantly to mortality.[320, 321] Use of antacids for prophylaxis against gastritis and peptic ulcer may be difficult because of the danger of magnesium toxicity.[304] Mental confusion may result from cimetidine therapy in renal failure.[323] There is encouraging evidence in children, however, that when the underlying cause of ARF is reversible and appropriate treatment is instituted early, the child has an excellent chance of survival and recovery of renal function.[324] Hence, early recognition and treatment of ARF is essential.

Diagnosis

Oliguria is usually the first sign of ARF. However, azotemia and signs of tubular dysfunction may be present in spite of a normal urine output or even polyuria, particularly in burn patients or when ARF is induced by toxins.[325, 326] Fortunately, this insidious

form of "nonoliguric" ARF is easier to manage and is associated with a more favorable prognosis.[326, 327, 338]

It should be noted that up to 16 percent of newborns, regardless of gestational age, will not void for 16 hours postnatally, but that all should void by 24 hours of age.[328] After that time, oliguria is variably defined as a urine output of less than 1.5 to 1 ml/kg/hr.[329-331] Glomerulogenesis occurs up to the 36th week of gestation[332] and infants of low birth weight normally have higher plasma creatinine levels than term neonates or older children.[333-336] Likewise, normal GFR and renal blood flow measurements vary for term infants, healthy premature infants, and premature infants with respiratory distress syndrome and are lower than for older children.[332, 333, 335, 337] Evaluation of parameters of renal function must take into consideration these age and developmental differences. Figure 7-1 and Table 7-4 give normal values for plasma creatinine and GFR by age.

The evaluation of the acute onset of oliguria and azotemia should proceed in a rapid but organized fashion to eliminate the possibilities of "prerenal" (renal hypoperfusion) or "postrenal" (urinary obstructive) causes. One systematic approach is shown in Figure 7-10.[304] Underlying, insidious, chronic renal failure exacerbated by an acute deterioration will usually be diagnosed by a careful review of the child's history, physical findings, and laboratory examinations prior to and during the acute deterioration.[304] A cause for the acute exacerbation must be aggressively sought and treated, in order to preserve maximal residual renal function. Physical exam and imaging techniques (preferably ultrasound, radionuclide scans, and computed tomography scans rather than radiocontrast studies, as discussed above) are usually successful at ruling out obstructive uropathy.[304, 312] Acute obstruction causes intratubular backflow pressure which diminishes GFR and leads to decreased urine flow and increased sodium and water reabsorption by functional tubules.[339] This may yield a concentrated urine low in sodium, similar to the urine produced with diminished renal blood flow. On the other hand, prolonged partial obstruction in which the GFR is maintained and tubular function fails may yield an isotonic or hypotonic urine. This is high in sodium, with low potassium and hydrogen ion content suggestive of nonoliguric acute parenchymal renal failure.[304, 339]

In addition to oliguria and azotemia due to obstructive lesions, "prerenal" or "functional" renal failure arising from inadequate renal perfusion needs to be ruled out. This should begin with an accurate assessment of the child's volume status and effective cardiac output, and may require central venous pressure measurement and Doppler echocardiography or invasive assessment of cardiac function, in addition to clinical examination. If the volume status is normal or has been returned to normal, and there is no evidence for fluid overload or congestive failure, then urine and serum samples should be obtained for analysis, and a

Table 7–12. CAUSES OF ACUTE RENAL FAILURE IN INFANTS AND CHILDREN

Renal Ischemia
Hypovolemia
  Hemorrhage
  Dehydration
  Burns
  Hypoproteinemia
  Peritonitis
  Sepsis
Cardiogenic shock
  Cardiomyopathy
  Myocarditis
  Congenital heart disease
  Cardiac surgery
Renovascular
  Bilateral renal artery thrombosis (rare, usually associated with umbilical artery lines)
  Renal artery stenosis/dysplasia and hypertension
  Renal vein thrombosis (associated with birth asphyxia, maternal diabetes mellitus, cyanotic congenital heart disease, hyperosmolar dehydration, trauma, nephrotic syndrome)
  Microvascular occlusion (DIC, sickle cell disease, thrombotic thrombocytopenic purpura, hemolytic-uremic syndrome, Shwartzman reaction—endotoxic cortical necrosis)
  Prolonged use of vasoconstrictive drugs
  Malignant hypertension
  Prolonged aortic cross-clamping (coarctation repair)

Inflammatory and Immunological Processes
Infectious
  Pyelonephritis
  Bacterial endocarditis
  Shwartzman reaction—endotoxic cortical necrosis
Immune-related
  Postinfectious glomerulonephritis (including poststreptococcal)
  Idiopathic crescentic glomerulonephritis
  Membranoproliferative glomerulonephritis
  Tubulointerstitial nephritis
  Membranous nephropathy
  IgA-IgG (Berger) nephropathy
  Henoch-Schönlein purpura (anaphylactoid purpura)
  Systemic lupus erythematosus
  Wegener granulomatosis
  Periarteritis nodosa, scleroderma
Specifically directed autoimmunity
  Anti–glomerular basement membrane disease
  Goodpasture syndrome
  Renal transplant rejection
Hypersensitivity reactions
  Penicillins, sulfonamides, cephalosporins, rifampin
  Anticonvulsants

Direct Nephrotoxicity
Uricosuric or hyperuricemic agents
  Antineoplastic agents
  X-ray contrast media
  Salicylates
  Furosemide, ethacrynic acid
  Pancreatic enzymes
Other medications
  Aminoglycosides
  Amphotericin B
  Cyclosporin A
  Salicylates
  Methoxyflurane, enflurane
Heavy metals
  Mercurials, lead, bismuth, gold, iron, copper, arsenic, thallium, cadmium, uranium
Glycols and organic solvents
  Carbon tetrachloride
  Turpentine
  Methanol
Organic toxins
  Mushrooms (*Amanita phalloides*)
  Snake bites (especially sea snakes)
  Phosphorus
Hemoglobinuria, myoglobinuria
  Burns
  Crush injury
  Myonecrosis (electric shock, snake bites)
  Hemolysis

Obstructive Uropathy
Ureteral obstruction
  Retroperitoneal masses or fibrosis
  Solitary kidney with obstruction
  Renal calculi
  Ureteral debris
  Bilateral ureteral pelvic junction obstruction
Urethral obstruction
  Posterior urethral valves
  Urethral stenosis
  Periurethral abscess
  Pelvic hematoma
  Neoplasm
  Trauma

Hepatorenal syndrome

Data from Trainin and Spitzer,[30] Ruley and Bock,[304] Oken,[317] and Ellis et al.[318]

Figure 7–10. Systematic approach to the child with renal failure. (*From* Ruley EJ, Bock GH: Acute renal failure in infants and children. *In* Shoemaker WC, Thompson WL, Holbrook PR [Eds.]: The Society of Critical Care Medicine: Textbook of Critical Care. Philadelphia, W. B. Saunders Company, 1984.)

diagnostic challenge with 20 ml/kg of saline or lactated Ringer's solution should be administered.[30, 340] If this does not increase urine output, then examination of urinary sediment and laboratory tests to assess tubular function, as outlined in Table 7–13, are helpful in distinguishing prerenal azotemia from acute parenchymal renal failure.[318] Early in "prerenal" oliguria, tubular function remains intact and increased tubular reabsorption of urea, sodium, and water occurs in the face of diminished glomerular filtration and reduced tubular flow.[304] All of the indices in Table 7–13 make use of these facts in order to assess tubular function. The single best test appears to be the fractional excretion of sodium (FE_{Na}) which is 90 percent accurate.[329, 330, 344, 345] In the newborn the ratio of urine to plasma osmolality is also a good index.[330]

A challenge with mannitol or potent loop diuretics has also been used in an effort to distinguish prerenal

Table 7–13. LABORATORY STUDIES USED TO DIFFERENTIATE PRERENAL AZOTEMIA FROM PARENCHYMAL ACUTE RENAL FAILURE IN CHILDREN AND NEONATES

	Study	Prerenal azotemia	ARF	Comment
Children	FE_{Na} (%)	<1	>3	FE_{Na} may be low in acute glomerulonephritis and in cases of early obstructive uropathy
	RFI	<1	>1	
	U_{Na} (mEq/L)	<20	>40	Considerable overlap exists
	U osmolarity (mOsm/kg H_2O)	>500	<350	For patients with in between values for U_{Na}, U osmolarity, U/P creatinine, and U/P urea
	U/P creatinine	>40	<20	
	U/P urea	>8	<3	
	U/P osmolarity	>1.3	<1.3	Unreliable in malnourished children
Neonates	FE_{Na} (%)	<2.5	>2.5	
	RFI	<2.5	>2.5	
		<3	>3	
	U/P osmolarity	>1	<1	As good as Fe_{Na} in newborns
	U/P urea	>4.8	<4.8	
	U/P creatinine	Variable	Variable	Not reliable

Indices should not be obtained after a sodium load or after administration of diuretic agents. Indices are more reliable in oliguric patients. They are not valid in infants less than 32 weeks gestational age.

FE_{Na} = fractional excretion of filtered sodium = (U/P)Na/(U/P) creatinine × 100.

U = urinary; P = plasma.

RFI = renal failure index = U_{Na}(U/P) creatinine.

Modified from Ellis D, Gartner JC, Galvis AG: Acute renal failure in infants and children: diagnosis, complications, and treatment. Crit Care Med 9:607, 1981 © 1981, The Williams and Wilkins Co., Baltimore.

from parenchymal acute renal failure,[346-350] but this particular diagnostic maneuver may be fraught with several hazards. First, this challenge yields confounding information if obstruction has not been ruled out. Likewise, it may exacerbate renal ischemia and azotemia if an adequate volume status has not been established prior to the challenge, and significant hypotension may result.[318, 349, 351] Also, if parenchymal renal failure is present, an increased urine output may be falsely reassuring, since it may only represent a conversion from oliguric to nonoliguric renal failure.[327, 350, 391] While this may be favorable from the standpoint of prognosis and ease of management, it may not obviate the problem of ongoing azotemia and should not be interpreted as signalling resolution of renal decompensation.[326] Finally, the administration of diuretic agents, by impairing tubular reabsorption in the normal kidney, invalidates subsequent urinary index studies as outlined in Table 7–13, for at least 6 to 8 hours.[318] It is important to remember that if obstructive or prerenal insults are prolonged, renal parenchymal injury will ensue and amelioration of the extrarenal factors at that point will not result in the rapid restoration of renal function.[304, 318]

Pathophysiology

The pathophysiology of acute parenchymal renal failure remains controversial, but important concepts have emerged.[352, 353] Several of the theories of the pathogenesis of acute parenchymal renal failure are incorporated into Figure 7–11.[318] Renal ischemia is a consistent finding even in toxin-induced models of ARF,[354] and may initiate ARF by lowering glomerular capillary pressure to such a degree that filtration ceases. Ischemia may also injure tubular cells, which swell and cause further ischemia, which contributes to the continuation of ARF.[45, 382] The term "vasomotor nephropathy" refers to this pathogenetic sequence of events.[317] Likewise, tubular injury, with functional and often morphological changes, is a hallmark of ARF and may be a primary event.[45, 355] The term "acute tubular necrosis" is used to describe this pathogenetic theory.[352] As indicated by the bidirectional arrows in Figure 7–11, tubular injury, tubular obstruction, and renal ischemia may all interrelate, regardless of the initial insult, and contribute to the initiation and maintenance of acute parenchymal renal failure.[315]

A unifying hypothesis has recently evolved from an understanding of the role of mitochondria and calcium ions in ischemic and toxic cellular injury.[356, 357] An ischemic or toxic insult may lead to decreased cellular energy production and increased calcium entry into the cellular cytoplasm and mitochondria. The resulting arteriolar vasoconstriction and vascular endothelial swelling perpetuates the ischemia and alters glomerular permeability. Likewise, tubular cellular metabolism is impaired, leading to tubular swelling, dysfunction,

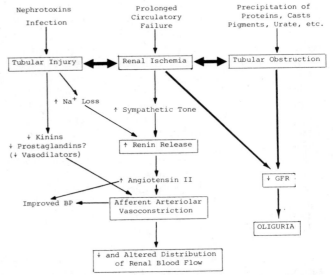

Figure 7–11. Pathogenesis of acute parenchymal renal failure. According to this schema, renal ischemia is the central event but *bidirectional arrows* indicate important interaction between tubular obstruction, tubular injury, and renal ischemia in the development of renal insufficiency and oliguria. Note that renal ischemia may continue despite correction of prerenal events that initiated ARF, owing to persistence of tubular damage, tubular obstruction, or altered intrarenal hemodynamics. Undernutrition (not shown) may prolong the oliguric phase by contributing to hypoperfusion and delayed healing of damaged tissue. (*From* Ellis D, Gartner JC, Galvis AG: Acute renal failure in infants and children: diagnosis, complications and treatment. Crit Care Med 9:607, 1981. © 1981, The Williams and Wilkins Co., Baltimore.)

back-leak, and obstruction.[45] The end result of both is the clinical manifestation of acute parenchymal renal failure.

Prevention and Treatment

The theories of the mechanism of renal injury have led to several proposals for the prevention of acute parenchymal renal failure. Postischemic infusion of adenine nucleotide energy substrate and magnesium chloride as a calcium antagonist results in significant renal protection in experimental models.[358] The administration of verapamil at the time of hypoxemia or norepinephrine-induced renal ischemia protects the glomerular filtration rate and prevents the morphological changes usually seen in the proximal tubular cells.[45, 578] Interruption of the renin-angiotensin-aldosterone cascade with captopril, an inhibitor of angiotensin-converting enzyme, improves systemic and renal hemodynamics, renal blood flow, and GFR in adults with azotemia and heart failure.[368, 369] Likewise, hydralazine and nitroprusside have been shown to improve renal perfusion in the face of severely depressed left ventricular function, provided filling pressures are optimized and the decrease in systemic arterial pressure is not excessive.[373, 374] Propranolol has been shown to attenuate experimentally induced postischemic renal failure, perhaps as a result of depression of renin release.[359] Thus, this is not in apparent contradiction to the salutary effects seen with administration of low-dose dopamine in acute parenchymal renal failure.[360, 361]

Dopamine at low doses (<5 μg/kg/min) is primarily a dopaminergic receptor stimulant which causes selective renal arteriolar dilatation plus inhibition of aldosterone secretion to increase renal blood flow, GFR, sodium excretion, and total urine output.[362, 363] In addition, low-dose dopamine may well have direct diuretic and natriuretic effects and may inhibit norepinephrine release and norepinephrine-induced vasoconstriction.[365, 366] Finally, low-dose dopamine has been experimentally shown to increase renal blood flow, GFR, and urinary flow in transplanted kidneys despite beta receptor blockade, when a constant cardiac output, heart rate, and mean arterial pressure are maintained.[367] Certainly, decreased cardiac output and hypotension induced by beta blockers or calcium channel blockers would be extremely deleterious, and much more clinical work needs to be done before these experimental findings will become clinically applicable. Other experimentally successful regimens that fall into this category include infusions of acetylcholine, prostaglandin E, and bradykinin as renal vasodilators.[370-372]

Simple volume loading with optimization of preload is known to help prevent parenchymal ARF in high-risk patients.[375, 376] In addition to improving cardiac output, this may result because left atrial hypotension is a potent stimulus of renal vasoconstriction, whereas left atrial hypertension causes renal vasodilatation.[378-380] This effect occurs independently of the volume-induced decrease in renin secretion.[377]

Mannitol (0.25 to 0.5 gm/kg) has been used to prevent or attenuate parenchymal ARF in almost every setting, but has been especially useful with post-traumatic, hemoglobinuric, and myoglobinuric renal insults.[347, 348, 381, 384, 387] By acting as an intratubular osmotic agent, mannitol may maintain GFR at or above control values in the hypoperfused kidney.[385] It may also prevent cellular swelling and continued ischemia while the forced osmotic tubular diuresis may prevent tubular obstruction.[383-385] Renal arteriolar vasodilatation has also been shown,[386, 392] and the volume expansion accompanying administration may also be beneficial.[388] The risks of excessive mannitol administration include the possibility of decreased renal perfusion if volume is not replaced during vigorous diuresis, or if volume overload and ventricular failure ensue. Hyponatremia, acidosis, and hyperkalemia may also be exacerbated.[197-200]

Furosemide has also been used in parenchymal ARF in moderate (1 to 2 mg/kg) to large (8 to 10 mg/kg) doses.[389, 395] Several beneficial effects of potent diuretics in ARF have been documented. They are renal arteriolar vasodilatation and an increase in renal blood

flow,[350, 390] an increase in urinary flow,[389] a conversion from oliguric to nonoliguric parenchymal ARF,[327, 350, 391] and a decrease in the need for dialysis.[389, 394] Furosemide appears to be particularly useful in parenchymal ARF of acute childhood glomerulonephritis.[145] On the other hand, prospective, controlled studies have shown a questionable value in preventing parenchymal ARF,[351] no benefit in established parenchymal ARF in medical patients,[395] and no change in duration of ARF or in overall mortality.[393-395] The timing of diuretic therapy seems to be important. Administration just prior to the insult is twice as effective as just after, and mannitol alone is ineffective after a renal insult, as is furosemide once parenchymal ARF is established.[395, 400] Combinations of drug therapy may be more effective, as shown by the synergistic protection afforded by dopamine in combination with furosemide in experimental nephrotoxic ARF.[361]

Although conversion to nonoliguric ARF and a decreased need for dialysis are important benefits, the use of furosemide or ethacrynic acid in the doses required is not without risk. These risks include causing hypovolemic cardiac instability, exacerbating renal failure, and producing ototoxicity, especially if acidosis or other ototoxins (for example, aminoglycosides) are present.[318, 396-398]

Anesthetic Implications

A practical approach for the anesthesiologist faced with a child with early, acute parenchymal renal failure is to eliminate all potential nephrotoxins and to ameliorate renal ischemia by optimizing preload and cardiac output. This may require invasive monitoring (arterial and central venous lines and rarely pulmonary artery catheter and cardiac output thermistor) in order to diagnose and treat hypovolemia, septic shock, or cardiac failure. When administering dopamine to infants to optimize hemodynamics, one must recall that significantly higher doses may be required than those needed in the adult, presumably owing to catecholamine receptor immaturity or deficiency.[399] Fortunately, at these higher doses (15 μg/kg/min as compared to 5 μg/kg/min in the adult) there seem to be no adverse effects on GFR or urinary output.[172] Following hemodynamic optimization, mannitol and/or furosemide may be administered in an attempt to prevent tubular obstruction and to convert oliguric ARF to nonoliguric parenchymal ARF. Diuretic administration should never be a substitute for hemodynamic optimization, and great care should be taken to avoid worsening the hemodynamic status. This means that careful monitoring and replacement of obligatory urinary fluid and electrolyte losses are mandatory.[400]

Once ARF is established, the major pathophysiological changes are impaired fluid and electrolyte balance, abnormal acid-base status, altered excretion of protein catabolytes and drugs, the appearance of hypertension, bleeding diatheses and anemia, and decreased resistance to infection.[317, 318, 401] The anesthetic implications and management of these problems are discussed in detail earlier in this chapter (see Anesthetic Implications of the Pathophysiologic Manifestations of Renal Failure). Caloric and nutritional balance seems to be an important factor in acute renal failure, and aggressive enteral or parenteral alimentation has been shown to be one of the few interventions that may hasten the recovery of renal function and improve the prognosis of ARF.[402-404, 406, 408] The beneficial effects seem to accrue from a decrease in urea nitrogen production,[405, 409] from a decreased incidence of and improved recovery from infection,[402, 403, 405] and from direct enhancement of tubular regeneration.[407] Because infection is a frequent life-threatening occurrence in ARF, meticulous care must be exercised in handling hyperalimentation and all other intravascular lines in these children.

Finally, dialysis during the course of ARF may become necessary to allow adequate volume for hyperalimentation, to treat acute volume overload resulting in intractable hypertension or congestive failure, to treat hyperkalemia unresponsive to other treatment regimens, to correct acidosis, and to remove nitrogenous wastes, which may rise suddenly during times of metabolic stress and result in encephalopathy.[30, 318, 401] Early institution of dialysis has been reported to reduce the overall incidence of serious complications, such as gastrointestinal hemorrhage and infection.[320, 321, 410-412] Because children have a high ratio of peritoneal to total body surface area, peritoneal dialysis achieves 50 percent of the efficiency of hemodialysis. This is in contrast to adults, in whom peritoneal dialysis is only 20 percent as efficient.[413] In addition, peritoneal dialysis is immediately available after catheter placement (often done with the patient under local anesthesia), is easier for ICU staff to administer, and requires no heparinization. It can be administered continuously and is less hemodynamically destabilizing, especially in infants, in whom a hemodialysis machine's volume may be large compared with the total blood volume of the infant and thus may require priming with blood. It also does not require large vessels for access, sparing them for other uses.[318, 414-416] On the other hand, peritoneal dialysis may not be as rapidly effective as hemodialysis in the removal of potassium and certain toxins and drugs,[318, 411] and it is not without its own risks. These include hemorrhage, infection (peritonitis, pneumonia, sepsis), respiratory compromise (from subdiaphragmatic pressure or acute hydrothorax), hollow viscus perforation, increased protein loss and a reduction in exchange efficiency if splanchnic blood flow is compromised.[417]

Anesthesiologists called upon to anesthetize children who are also undergoing peritoneal dialysis need to be aware of these potential hazards. It is also important to recognize that when hypertonic dialysate is used to remove excess intravascular volume, what appears to be only a moderate amount of peritoneal volume at the beginning may increase to the point of compromising ventilation, venous return, and cardiac output by the end of the dwell period. Positioning that might improve venous return (Trendelenburg positioning) may then further impair ventilation, and vice versa. Positive-pressure ventilation in and of itself may decrease renal blood flow and GFR, and this effect may be augmented if higher ventilatory pressures are required (Fig. 7–12).[420, 421] These considerations, along with the increased risks of regurgitation and aspiration associated with intra-abdominal distention, are strong arguments for the anesthesiologist to resist the suggestion that an intraoperative peritoneal dialysate dwell would optimize the patient's intraoperative and postoperative metabolic status. Preoperative dialysis should be completed and the dialysate drained from the peritoneal cavity (except for a small, isotonic volume to help prevent catheter adherence to omentum or bowel) before the patient is brought to the operating room. In adults with severe heart disease and renal failure, intraoperative hemodialysis has been utilized while the patient has been on cardiopulmonary

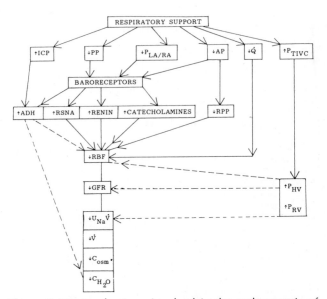

Figure 7–12. Mechanisms involved in the pathogenesis of renal dysfunction during respiratory support. ICP = intracranial pressure; PP = pulse pressure; $P_{LA/RA}$ = transmural left and right atrial pressures; AP = systemic arterial pressure; $\dot{Q}$ = cardiac output; P_{TIVC} = thoracic inferior vena caval pressure; ADH = antidiuretic hormone; RSNA = renal sympathetic nerve activity; RPP = renal perfusion pressure; RBF = renal blood flow; GFR = glomerular filtration rate; P_{HV} = hepatic venous pressure; P_{RV} = renal venous pressure; $U_{NA}V$ = urinary sodium excretion; $\dot{V}$ = urinary output; C_{Osm} = osmolal clearance; C_{H_2O} = free water clearance. Dotted lines indicate that the mechanism is unlikely to be of significance. (*From* Priebe HJ, Hedley-White J: Respiratory support and renal function. Int Anesthesiol Clin 22:203, 1984.)

bypass[418, 419] but this has not been described in children.

DISEASES OF RENAL PARENCHYMA

As noted previously, there are multitudes of congenital, hereditary, and acquired renal diseases, as well as systemic illnesses not usually considered primarily renal, that may result in renal parenchymal injury and failure (see Tables 7–1, 7–2, and 7–12). As shown in Table 7–14, classification of these illnesses is further complicated by the fact that each distinct histopathological finding on renal biopsy may be associated with many very different clinical entities and syndromes.[422, 425] Conversely, distinct clinical syndromes (such as acute nephritis or the nephrotic syndrome) may demonstrate many different histopathological findings and have many etiologies (Table 7–15). Because of these difficulties in classification, information about etiology, epidemiology, and prognosis is often conflicting and confusing. From the standpoint of anesthetic care, it is therefore more important to evaluate each of the particular clinical components of renal impairment

Table 7–14. HETEROGENEITY OF CLINICAL SYNDROMES WITHIN DISTINCT HISTOPATHOLOGICAL CATEGORIES

Proliferative Glomerulonephritis
Nephrotic syndrome
Acute glomerulonephritis
Rapidly progressive (oliguric) glomerulonephritis
Chronic glomerulonephritis
Persistent hematuria and proteinuria
Schönlein-Henoch purpura
Systemic lupus erythematosus
Periarteritis nodosa and hypersensitivity angiitis
Bacterial endocarditis
Mixed essential cryoglobulinemia
Rheumatic fever
Narcotic abuse
Hereditary progressive nephritis (Alport syndrome)
Hereditary deficiency of complement
Tumor-associated nephropathy
Sarcoidosis
Bee-sting nephrotic syndrome

Necrotizing and Crescentic Glomerulonephritis
Acute glomerulonephritis
Rapidly progressive glomerulonephritis
Membranoproliferative glomerulonephritis
Chronic glomerulonephritis
Schönlein-Henoch purpura
Periarteritis nodosa and hypersensitivity angiitis
Goodpasture syndrome
Wegener granulomatosis
Systemic lupus erythematosus
Mixed essential cryoglobulinemia
Bacterial endocarditis
Hereditary progressive nephritis (Alport syndrome)

Membranous Glomerulonephropathy
Nephrotic syndrome
Chronic glomerulonephritis
Renal vein thrombosis
Systemic lupus erythematosus
Diabetes mellitus
Tumor-associated nephropathy
Sarcoidosis
Rheumatoid arthritis
Bullous dermatoses
Chronic infection
    Syphilis, schistosomiasis
    Filariasis, Guillain-Barré
    Hepatitis B antigenemia
Drug-associated nephrotic syndrome
    Trimethadione, D-penicillamine
    Gold, mercury
Slowly progressive glomerulonephritis

Membranoproliferative Glomerulonephritis
Nephrotic syndrome
Acute glomerulonephritis
Rapidly progressive (oliguric) glomerulonephritis
Chronic glomerulonephritis
Slowly progressive glomerulonephritis
Persistent hematuria and proteinuria
Schönlein-Henoch purpura
Systemic lupus erythematosus
Allograft rejection
Progressive and partial lipodystrophy
Sickle cell disease
Hereditary deficiency of complement
Hepatic cirrhosis and chronic hepatitis
Quartan malaria
Chronic staphylococcal bacteremia ("shunt nephritis")

Focal Glomerulonephritis
Nephrotic syndrome
Acute glomerulonephritis
Chronic glomerulonephritis
Chronic hematuria
Bacterial endocarditis
Schönlein-Henoch purpura
Systemic lupus erythematosus
Goodpasture syndrome
Periarteritis nodosa and hypersensitivity angiitis
Wegener granulomatosis
Hereditary deficiency of complement

Focal Segmental Glomerulosclerosis
Nephrotic syndrome
Chronic glomerulonephritis
Persistent hematuria
Asymptomatic proteinuria
Rheumatoid arthritis
Narcotic abuse (heroin)
Hereditary progressive nephritis (Alport and nail-patella syndromes)
Sickle cell disease
Massive obesity
Allograft rejection

From Bernstein J, Barnett HL, Edelmann CM Jr: Glomerular diseases: introduction and classification. *In* Edelmann CM Jr (Ed.): Pediatric Kidney Disease. Boston, Little, Brown, 1978.

Table 7–15. CLINICAL SYNDROMES OF RENAL PARENCHYMAL DISEASE AND THEIR MULTIPLE ETIOLOGIES

Persistent Microscopic and Recurrent Gross Hematuria
Benign recurrent hematuria
Hereditary progressive nephritis (Alport)
IgA nephropathy (Berger)
Schönlein-Henoch purpura
Systemic lupus erythematosus
Membranoproliferative glomerulonephritis
Postinfectious glomerulonephritis
Chronic glomerulonephritis
Sickle cell disease
 	
Acute Glomerulonephritis
Acute postinfectious glomerulonephritis
  Following streptococcal infection
  Following other infections (staphylococcal, viral)
Membranoproliferative glomerulonephritis
Exacerbation of persistent glomerulonephritis
Recurrent hematuria and IgA nephropathy
Schönlein-Henoch purpura
Systemic lupus erythematosus
Familial nephritis (Alport)
 	
Rapidly Progressive Glomerulonephritis
Idiopathic crescentic and necrotizing glomerulonephritis
Acute postinfectious glomeruonephritis
Membranoproliferative glomerulonephritis
Goodpasture syndrome
Hemolytic-uremic syndrome
Schönlein-Henoch purpura
Systemic lupus erythematosus
Hypersensitivity angiitis
	Nephrotic Syndrome
	Corticosteroid-sensitive minimal change nephrotic syndrome
	Corticosteroid-resistant nephrotic syndrome with focal
	  segmental glomerulosclerosis
	Corticosteroid-resistant nephrotic syndrome with membranous
	  glomerulonephropathy
	Corticosteroid-resistant nephrotic syndrome with
	  membranoproliferative glomerulonephritis
	Congenital nephrotic syndrome
	Acute postinfectious glomerulonephritis
	Schönlein-Henoch purpura
	Systemic lupus erythematosus
	Narcotic addiction
	Sickle cell disease
	Familial nephritis (Alport)
	Diabetes mellitus
	Amyloidosis
	Renal vein thrombosis
	Quartan malaria
	Congenital syphilis
	Drug reaction
	Neoplasia
	Bee stings
	Poison oak dermatitis
	Bullous dermatoses

From Bernstein J, Barnett HL, Edelmann CM Jr.: Glomerular diseases: introduction and classification. *In* Edelmann CM Jr (Ed.): Pediatric Kidney Disease. Boston, Little, Brown, 1978.

that an individual child demonstrates than just to know the clinical or histopathological diagnosis. With this understanding, we will now consider some of the more distinct clinical syndromes of parenchymal renal disease, and the extrarenal manifestations with which the anesthesiologist should be familiar. Little has been published with regard to anesthetic recommendations for these entities, and especially for specific rare conditions in children. Anesthetic evaluation and care must therefore follow from theoretical considerations with regard to pathophysiology, and from anecdotal anesthetic experience with some of the rarer pediatric renal diseases.

Glomerulonephritis

As first described, *acute glomerulonephritis (Bright disease)* was any acute inflammatory process of the glomerulus and nephron resulting in hematuria and proteinuria.[426] It is now recognized to be a collection of many diseases (Tables 7–14 and 7–15) with varying presentations.[422, 427] Acute glomerulonephritis is thought to result from immunological injury to the kidney due to anti–glomerular basement membrane disease, tubulointerstitial disease, and immune complex deposition.[428-430] The antigen involved may be renal or nonrenal endogenous antigen, exogenous antigen, or foreign material that is haptogenic combining with endogenous protein to form the antigen (Table 7–16).[427, 431, 432] The immune complexes may be deposited from the circulation during glomerular filtration or may form in situ, or both.[427, 429, 430] Complement activation and platelet aggregation also seem to be involved in the mechanism of injury and have led to trials of anticoagulant and platelet inhibitory therapy.[434-437] Children with glomerulonephritis may also be treated with glucocorticoids and cytotoxic agents such as cyclophosphamide, and so in addition to having an induced abnormality in clotting, they may be relatively immunosuppressed and may require perioperative "stress" coverage with glucocorticoids. The inflammation and injury of acute glomerulonephritis manifests itself clinically as an acute nephritic episode, the nephrotic syndrome, or interstitial nephritis.[433] Although it frequently completely resolves, acute glomerulonephritis may progress to cause permanent damage and chronic renal failure.

Acute Nephritic Syndrome

The acute nephritic syndrome is characterized by the sudden onset of hematuria, frequently accompanied by proteinuria, hypertension, oliguria, and edema.[433]

Acute poststreptococcal glomerulonephritis is a prime example of this syndrome. It is the most common form of glomerulonephritis in children and follows a skin or upper respiratory tract infection with group A beta-hemolytic streptococci.[427, 438] The true

Table 7–16. ANTIGENIC FACTORS ASSOCIATED WITH ACUTE IMMUNE COMPLEX–MEDIATED GLOMERULONEPHRITIS

Glomerulonephritis mediated by anti-GBM antibodies. Also includes anti-GBM antibody nephritis with pulmonary hemorrhage (Goodpasture syndrome).

Glomerulonephritis mediated by immune complexes deposited from the circulation or possibly formed in situ.

Infectious agents associated AICGN
  Bacterial
    Group A β-hemolytic streptococci
    Streptococcus viridans
    Diplococcus pneumoniae
    Staphylococcus aureus
    Treponema pallidum
    Leptospirosis
    Salmonella typhosa
    Staphylococcus epidermidis
  Viral
    Hepatitis-B
    Cytomegalovirus
    Enteroviral infections
    Measles
    Guillain-Barré syndrome
    Oncornavirus
    Mumps virus

Parasitic
  Plasmodium malariae and *falciparum*
  Toxoplasmosis
  Schistosomiasis
  Filariasis
  Trypanosomiasis
Rickettsial
  Scrub typhus
Fungal
  Coccidioides immitis
Drugs, toxins and antisera
  Vaccinations, excessive DPT
  Antivenoms and antitoxins
  Organic gold compounds
  D-penicillamine
  Organic and inorganic mercurials
  Sulfonamides
  Captopril
Endogenous antigens
  Tumor-associated antigens
  Thyroglobulin
  Autologous immunoglobulin
  DNA

GBM = Glomerular basement membrane; AICGN = Acute immune complex–mediated glomerulonephritis; DPT = Diptheria, pertussis, tetanus toxoid vaccine.
From Jordan SC, Lemire JM: Acute glomerulonephritis: diagnosis and treatment. Pediatr Clin North Am 29:857, 1982.

incidence is unknown since the majority of cases are subclinical.[439, 440] It is most prevalent during the school-age years, with an average onset at ages 6 to 7 years, although cases have been described during infancy and it may occur during adolescence or adulthood.[427, 441] Most series report a prevalence in males of twice that in females, although this has been attributed to the tendency to diagnose mild cases in females as cystitis.[427] Analysis of the male-to-female ratio during epidemics shows no sex predilection.[427] A latent period of 8 to 21 days following infection usually precedes the onset of clinical glomerulonephritis, although cases with shorter or longer latency have been described.[428] In symptomatic patients the common presenting features are those of the acute nephritic syndrome: hematuria, proteinuria, hypertension, edema, and oliguria. Frequently there may also be circulatory congestion with pulmonary edema, exacerbated by mild anemia which is partially dilutional. In severe cases hypertensive encephalopathy and seizures may occur, and rarely renal impairment may progress to anuria.[427] Treatment follows the principles detailed above under Acute Renal Failure, and as mentioned previously, furosemide appears particularly useful in the management of fluid overload and hypertension in these children.[145] The development of poststreptococcal glomerulonephritis does not seem to be decreased with early antibiotic treatment of the streptococcal infection, but the severity of the disease may be attenuated.[427, 442] Improvement following immunosuppressive therapy in severe proliferative glomerulonephritis

following streptococcal infection has been reported, but a cause-and-effect relationship between the treatment and the improvement has not been established.[438] In general, corticosteroids and immunosuppressive drugs are not routinely used in acute poststreptococcal glomerulonephritis.[438, 442] The prognosis is remarkably good, with all but 2 to 5 percent of children recovering completely.[430] Sporadic rather than epidemic cases, as well as cases in the older child, seem to have a worse prognosis, with residual renal impairment.[427] Recurrence of poststreptococcal glomerulonephritis is fortunately rare.[430]

Differentiation of acute poststreptococcal glomerulonephritis from other causes of the nephritic syndrome is important from a treatment and prognostic standpoint. Detection of rising antibody titers to various streptococcal antigens (most commonly antistreptolysin O titers) together with a depression in complement C_3 levels aids greatly in the diagnosis.[427, 442] Included in the differential diagnosis are the infectious agents and disease entities listed in Tables 7–14 to 7–16. Although clinical presentation, clinical course, and response to treatment may distinguish between different entities, renal biopsy may be necessary.[430]

Chronic glomerulonephritis, made apparent by an acute exacerbation, *membranoproliferative glomerulonephritis*, *membranous or epimembranous glomerulonephritis*, and *rapidly progressive glomerulonephritis* are all primary renal diseases that may present with the nephrotic syndrome (see below), the acute nephritic syndrome, or both.

These may be even further subcategorized according to histopathological findings, rate of progression, response to immunosuppressants, and prognosis.[422, 430] Major manifestations are those of nephritis, nephrosis, and ARF.

Benign recurrent hematuria (familial and nonfamilial), *focal nephritis*, and *Berger disease (IgG-IgA mesangial nephropathy)* are benign diseases that are characterized by recurrent hematuria, which may be gross.[427, 443] Usually the occurrence of benign hematuria coincides with a febrile illness or exercise, but it may also occur with the stress of surgery and be unnecessarily alarming. In Berger disease, gross hematuria and moderate proteinuria occur simultaneously with a febrile illness, usually a nonstreptococcal rhinopharyngeal infection.[430]

Hereditary progressive nephritis is characterized by recurrent hematuria, progressive renal failure, and a frequent association with high-frequency neurosensory hearing loss and lenticular ocular abnormalities.[427, 430, 444] The distinction between *Alport disease* (hereditary nephritis with deafness) and *Guthrie disease* (hereditary nephritis alone) has no medical or historical basis, since these contemporary investigators studied and reported the same family.[444] The disease is thought to be due to an autosomally inherited defect in glomerular basement membrane, and immunofluorescent staining for immunocomplexes is negative.[422] Variable expression and penetrance are required to explain all patterns of inheritance, and one fifth of affected newborns may represent new mutations.[445] The prevalence of the disease is unknown, but men are affected more than women and blacks are rarely affected. It is estimated that Alport disease accounts for 3 percent of chronic renal failure in childhood.[444] Variants of Alport disease may have associated polyneuropathy, severe ichthyosis, diabetes, myopathy, or thrombocytopenia with giant platelets.[444] Each patient must be individually evaluated for these associated problems, which may affect anesthetic care. Presence of the nephrotic syndrome may also influence anesthetic management (see below).

Hereditary onycho-osteodysplasia, or *"nail-patella syndrome,"* is characterized by dystrophic and hypoplastic nails, iliac horns, malformed radial heads, and hypoplastic patellae.[444] Abnormal pigmentation of the iris and cutaneous manifestations may also occur. Forty percent of patients have renal disease, which progresses to renal failure in 25 percent. An abnormality of basement membrane is transmitted with an autosomal dominant inheritance, linked to the gene locus for ABO blood groups, and distinct from Alport disease.[444, 446]

Prolonged bacteremia associated with infected ventriculoatrial shunts or bacterial endocarditis may produce immune complex glomerulonephritis presenting as a persistent nephritic syndrome (*"endocarditis nephritis"* and *"shunt nephritis"*).[430, 447, 448] Antibiotic therapy may often be ineffective, requiring surgical removal of the infected shunt or valve.[430] The anesthesiologist is then faced with anesthetizing a child with ongoing nephritis and bacteremia, as well as the problems associated with either a malfunctioning ventriculoatrial shunt or an infected heart valve.

Henoch-Schönlein purpura (Schönlein-Henoch syndrome, anaphylactoid purpura, allergic purpura, purpura rheumatica) is a serious cause of nephritis and may account for up to 15 percent of glomerular nephropathies in children.[430, 499] Males are more commonly affected than females. The age of onset is usually between 6 months and 6 years of age, more severe renal involvement occurs in older children, and recurrent episodes are common.[430, 449, 453] It is a disease of unknown etiology, which usually presents 1 to 3 weeks after a nonspecific upper respiratory tract infection. A characteristic purpuric and symmetrical rash invariably appears over the lateral malleoli, and is frequently distributed over the extensor surfaces of the lower leg, arms, and buttocks.[449, 453] Painful edema of the scalp, hands, and feet along with ankle and knee joint pain may occur independently of the degree of renal involvement. Subcutaneous bleeding may occur in the conjunctiva, eyelids, scrotum (mimicking torsion of the testicle), and calves (mimicking deep venous thrombosis). Colicky abdominal pain is common, suggesting an acute abdominal emergency, and indeed may be accompanied by hematemesis, melena, and rarely intussusception, requiring surgical intervention.[449, 451] Other extrarenal manifestations of importance to the anesthesiologist are severe nosebleeds, hepatomegaly, and rare neuronal involvement including facial palsy, chorea, encephalopathy, and convulsions.[449] Hematological studies reveal an elevated white cell count and erythrocyte sedimentation rate, and a hemoglobin concentration which is normal or depressed in proportion to the degree of prior bleeding. Clotting studies, platelet count, and bleeding time are all normal. The bleeding, purpura, edema, and renal and gastrointestinal manifestations are all thought to be vascular in origin.[449] This may be particularly frustrating to the anesthesiologist and surgeon faced with diffuse intraoperative bleeding unresponsive to replacement therapy. The renal involvement usually begins within 4 weeks of onset of the illness, may be quite variable, and markedly influences the prognosis.[452, 454] Although the combination is fortunately uncommon, of those children who manifest both an acute nephritic syndrome and nephrosis, 50 percent at 10-year follow-up will demonstrate, or have died of, severe renal insufficiency.[449, 450, 452] Treatment has been attempted with corticosteroids, immunosuppressive drugs (such as cyclophosphamide and azathioprine), oral anticoagulants, and platelet inhibitors (dipyridamole). The anesthesiologist may encounter children on any one or combination of these drugs, with their attendant side effects. Although spectacular recoveries have been reported, there are no data from adequately controlled studies that this treatment favorably alters the course of either the disease or the renal involvement,[449, 453] and institution of such therapy represents a desperate effort in the severely affected child. Fortunately, most children have mild to moderate disease and require only symptomatic care. More severe illness may require supportive treatment according to the degree of renal failure and complications. Secondary nephrotic syndrome may become manifest with the attendant implications for anesthetic care (see below).

Goodpasture syndrome (hemorrhagic pulmonary-renal syndrome, lung purpura with nephritis, pulmonary hemosiderosis with glomerulonephritis, hemorrhagic and interstitial pneumonitis with nephritis) is a combination of pulmonary hemorrhage and glomerulonephritis, most commonly occurring in adolescent males.[455, 456] Most patients present with hemoptysis, which ranges from scant to massive and fatal. Extensive alveolar hemorrhage causes a decrease in pulmonary compliance, impaired gas exchange, and arterial hypoxemia. Compensatory hyperpnea may result in respiratory alkalosis.[455] Microcytic and hypochromic anemia results from the large quantity of blood chronically lost into the lung.[456] Glomerulonephritis causing hematuria, proteinuria, and hypertension may rarely precede the pulmonary symptoms, but usually occurs concomitantly or following pulmonary involvement by up to several months.[455, 457] Kidney biopsies antedating clinical signs of renal involvement will still show immunofluorescent and electron microscopic abnormalities. These are characteristic of the anti–basement membrane lesions that cause both the renal and pulmonary injury.[455, 457, 458]

The prognosis of Goodpasture syndrome is poor, with the usual acute, fulminant onset leading to pulmonary or renal failure within months of presentation. Reports of prolonged survival and spontaneous remission emphasize the unpredictability of the illness in any given patient, however, and make reports of apparent responses to therapy difficult to interpret.[455] Steroids and immunosuppressive drugs (such as azathioprine, 6-mercaptopurine, cyclophosphamide, and nitrogen mustard) have all been tried, with the pulmonary manifestations seemingly responding better than the renal lesions.[455, 457] Because of the pulmonary hemorrhage, anticoagulants have not been used. Plasmapheresis (undertaken to decrease anti–glomerular basement membrane antibody titers) in combination with steroid and alkylating agent therapy has shown promise.[454] The most aggressive and radical intervention has been bilateral nephrectomy, which has been associated with dramatic cessation of massive pulmonary hemorrhage.[460, 461] This treatment is not always effective, however.[457, 462] Advanced renal failure has been treated with transplantation, with a surprisingly low incidence of recurrence of anti–glomerular basement membrane lesions in the kidney allograft.[457, 463]

Considerations for anesthesia in these very ill patients include those for acute or chronic renal failure and renal transplantation as discussed previously. The severe pulmonary involvement, coupled with anemia, may result in severe hypoxemia, pulmonary hypertension, and a reduced oxygen carrying capacity. This places further demands on a cardiovascular system already compromised by systemic hypertension, fluid overload, electrolyte imbalance, and azotemia. When possible, these problems should be corrected preoperatively with dialysis, antihypertensives, and transfusion. Because of the severe pulmonary involvement and oliguria, intraoperative volume assessment necessitates the use of pulmonary capillary wedge pressures to estimate left atrial filling pressures.

The *hemolytic-uremic syndrome* (HUS) is characterized by acute renal failure, hemolytic anemia (with fragmented erythrocytes) and thrombocytopenia.[464, 465, 467] The syndrome occurs mainly in white infants and children, and rarely in neonates; there is no sex predilection.[467] Cases have also been reported in adults, often in association with pregnancy, and the similarity to *thrombotic thrombocytopenic purpura* has led to the suggestion that these syndromes are essentially the same, but occurring in different age groups.[464, 468] Recognition that the triad of acute renal failure, hemolytic anemia, and thrombocytopenia is a syndrome and not a distinct clinicopathological entity helps in understanding the geographical differences in reported incidence and age of onset. It has also been observed that there is a mild form, a severe acute form, a severe progressive form, and two distinct forms of familial involvement, one autosomal recessive, the other autosomal dominant, both with incomplete penetrance.[464, 467, 469] Severity and prognosis vary among these groups.

Many infectious agents (viral and bacterial) have been implicated as precipitating factors in epidemics and individual cases of HUS, and an association with *Shigella* and *Salmonella* infections has been particularly convincing.[464, 470] A universal finding is injury to the epithelial lining or arterioles in the kidney and elsewhere, leading to deposition of platelet and fibrin thrombi, which cause vascular occlusion.[471] A composite theory of the pathogenesis of the vascular endothelial injury is that bacterial neuraminidase, *Shigella* toxin, or circulating endotoxin precipitates localized intravascular coagulation and microangiopathic changes. This occurs in individuals genetically predisposed to microvascular thrombosis because of a congenital prostacyclin deficiency, increased thromboxane production and/or antithrombin III deficiency.[464, 472]

Widespread occlusion of arterioles is responsible for the acute renal deterioration and may lead to bilateral renal cortical necrosis. These microvascular lesions are not restricted to the kidneys. Microangiopathic hemolytic anemia and platelet consumption occurs diffusely and may involve other organ systems, most notably the central nervous system, heart, and gastrointestinal tract.[464, 466]

A prodromal illness usually precedes the onset of the hemolytic-uremic syndrome by a few days or weeks. This prodrome may consist of diarrhea, which may be frankly bloody, and vomiting with occasional hematemasis. Otherwise it may consist of an upper respiratory tract infection, urinary tract infection, varicella, or measles.[464, 465]

The onset of the full-blown syndrome may be heralded by any one or combination of severe gastrointestinal pain, oliguria, petechiae, striking pallor due to anemia, hypertension, volume overload, congestive heart failure, and convulsions.[464, 465, 467] In 20 percent of cases the symptoms may mimic an abdominal emergency. In a few, intestinal ulceration, obstruction, gangrene, perforation, or intussusception may require emergency surgery.[464] The liver may also be involved with hepatosplenomegaly and elevation of liver enzymes, but jaundice is rare. The anemia may be acute and severe, with hemoglobin concentrations falling by 2 gm/100 ml/hr, resulting in hemoglobin levels as low as 2 gm/100 ml on admission.[465] This degree of anemia, coupled with hypervolemia, azotemia, hypertension, and electrolyte abnormalities, as well as direct myocardial involvement, may lead to severe congestive heart failure.[465, 466, 473] Central nervous system involvement may occur, with drowsiness, irritability, coma, seizures, and hemiparesis. This may result from hypertensive or uremic encephalopathy, hyponatremia or hypocalcemia, hemorrhage due to thrombocytopenia or anticoagulant therapy, or direct microvascular involvement.[467, 474, 475] The majority of patients recover from the central nervous system involvement, although some suffer permanent neurological impairment, and a few infants may die as a result.[465]

The renal involvement in HUS is acute in onset and always present. It may vary from a transient decrease in urinary volume and renal function to fulminant acute renal failure with bilateral cortical necrosis, anuria, and progression to chronic renal failure.[465, 476] All of the systemic manifestations of renal failure may appear. Early diagnosis and aggressive treatment, including dialysis, have reduced the mortality to 4 to 7 percent in endemic areas, and revealed the importance of the nonrenal disease processes in the prognosis of HUS.[464, 466, 467]

In addition to therapy for renal failure, treatment of the anemia and thrombocytopenia may be necessary, especially in the event of bleeding or in preparation for surgery. Attempts to raise the platelet count may fail owing to ongoing consumption and may cause further microvascular occlusion. Therefore, platelet transfusion is usually reserved for extreme thrombocytopenia (platelet counts of less than 20,000 per μl) or to treat active bleeding.[465, 467] Transfusion of packed red blood cells to treat anemia must be carefully monitored, since the infusion of even a small volume of blood may induce, or severely exacerbate, hypertension or congestive heart failure.[467] There is also speculation that the hemolysis of relatively older transfused cells may release large amounts of adenosine disphosphate. This is a potent stimulant of platelet aggregation, resulting in increased microvascular thrombosis.[464]

Attempts have been made to interrupt the microvascular thrombosis with aspirin, dipyridamole, heparin and streptokinase. The results are mixed, and all of the attendant risks of anticoagulant therapy are present.[464, 477, 483] Other interventions have been directed at removing increased plasma thrombogenic factors (such as thromboxane) by exchange transfusion or plasmapheresis.[480-482] Replacement of deficient plasma inhibitors of platelet aggregation and coagulation by infusions of prostacyclin, antithrombin III, or fresh frozen plasma has also been tried.[464, 478, 479] Bilateral nephrectomy has resulted in a prompt return of the platelet count to normal.[464] Successful subsequent renal homotransplantation has been reported in infants, children, and adults, despite the occasional recurrence of HUS lesions in the transplanted kidney.[484, 485] Fortunately, HUS very rarely requires such aggressive intervention.

Anesthetic considerations for surgery in an infant or child with HUS primarily involve the presence of acute renal failure. The child's condition should be optimized with preoperative dialysis, and treatment of hypertension and anemia is desirable. This is frequently impossible when these children require exploratory laparotomy for a suspected intra-abdominal emergency. This contraindicates peritoneal dialysis. The anticipation of oliguria, a large operative blood loss, and dramatic hemodynamic responses to even small blood volume changes justifies invasive monitoring. Intra-arterial and central venous pressure lines, as well as large-bore intravenous catheters should be inserted by surgical placement if necessary. In small infants, large intraoperative blood loss requires diligent replacement with blood components or fresh whole blood and platelets, as well as careful monitoring and treatment of plasma calcium levels. The anesthesiologist may take solace in the knowledge that incidental intraoperative exchange transfusion may be beneficial to his patient.[480]

Nephrotic Syndrome

The nephrotic syndrome, as defined, consists of massive proteinuria, hypoalbuminemia, hyperlipidemia, and edema.[486-488] In children this means a urinary protein loss exceeding 0.05 gm/kg/day and serum albumin levels of less than 2.5 gm/100 ml.[486] Like the acute nephritic syndrome, it represents a particular pattern of response of the kidney, to one of many different insults and diseases. Many diseases that cause nephritis may also result in the nephrotic syndrome (see Table 7–15). Although varying with etiology, age, and subtype, the overall incidence of the nephrotic syndrome in children under 16 years of age is 2 in 100,000.[486] It results from primary glomerular disease in 90 percent of affected children, while in the remaining 10 percent the nephrotic syndrome arises secondary to a systemic disease.[487] The primary or "idiopathic" nephrotic syndrome may be divided into subtypes according to histopathological appearance.

Minimal change nephrotic syndrome (*minimal lesion, nil lesion, lipoid nephrosis, foot process disease,* or *idiopathic primary nephrotic syndrome*) is the most common lesion in children, accounting for up to 75 percent of cases, whereas it is associated with only 30 percent of adult nephrotic syndrome.[489] The onset is usually between 2 and 7 years of age, with a male to female predilection of 2 to 1.[489, 491] The course of the disease may vary with the initial response to treatment and the success of treating relapses, intercurrent infections, and complications, but in general the prognosis is excellent for the minimal change lesion.[490, 492, 494]

Focal segmental glomerulosclerosis (*focal glomerular sclerosis*) is found in about 10 percent of children with nephrotic syndrome. Clinical onset may be at any age, and there is no sex predilection.[493] It should be distinguished from *focal global glomerulosclerosis* or *congenital glomerulosclerosis,* which can be seen normally in kidneys during the first year of life and in which less than 1 percent of glomeruli are involved by total sclerosis. This probably represents an error in nephrogenesis, and is of little consequence to overall renal function.[493] The finding of focal *segmental* glomerulosclerosis is far more ominous, because a significant proportion of children with this condition are resistant to therapy and progress to end-stage renal disease.[487, 504] Therapy with high-dose steroids, azathioprine, cyclophosphamide, and chlorambucil has yielded occasional success but a poor overall response rate.[487] Preliminary trials with aspirin and dipyridamole have shown some success.[495, 496]

Diffuse proliferative glomerulonephritis can be divided into *membranoproliferative glomerulonephritis* (*mesangiocapillary, persistent hypocomplementemic,* or *lobular glomerulonephritis*) and *mesangial proliferative glomerulonephritis* (*pure endocapillary, endocapillary,* or *extracapillary proliferative glomerulonephritis*).[486] Mesangial proliferation occurs in 2 to 5 percent of children with the nephrotic syndrome.[487] Response to treatment and prognosis is difficult to determine because of confusion about classification of these lesions, but overall, the mesangial proliferative lesion carries a good prognosis. Nonresponders are subsequently found to have had, or to have developed, focal segmental glomerulosclerosis.[487] Membranoproliferative glomerulonephritis, on the other hand, has a poor long-term prognosis with no evidence of therapeutic benefit from corticosteroids, anticoagulants, or cytotoxic drugs.[497] In fact, administration of corticosteroids in high daily doses is associated with rapid deterioration of renal function and severe hypertension.[488, 497] Massive perioperative steroid coverage is not indicated and may be detrimental. Children who present with the acute nephritic syndrome and never develop nephrosis may have a better prognosis, but most children with membranoproliferative glomerulonephritis progress to end-stage renal failure over 8 to 15 years and are then candidates for renal transplantation.[497]

Membranous nephropathy (*membranous glomerulonephropathy, epimembranous nephropathy, extramembranous, perimembranous, transmembranous glomerulonephritis*) may occur at any age from infancy to adulthood, and shows a predilection for males.[498] The clinical course is extremely variable and is characterized by spontaneous remissions which have confused the evaluation of response to therapy. Steroids, anticoagulants, and immunosuppressant agents have all been used, but in one study remissions were most frequent in untreated patients.[498] Presence or persistence of the nephrotic syndrome is a poor prognostic sign and usually occurs in the 10 percent of children who progress to end-stage renal failure.[498]

Congenital nephrotic syndrome, presenting at birth or shortly thereafter, is usually secondary to congenital infection (syphilis, toxoplasmosis, cytomegalovirus), renal vein thrombosis (due to perinatal trauma, asphyxia, or shock), renal tumors, or toxins.[499]

Primary or "idiopathic" congenital nephrotic syndrome is usually a familial disease, inherited in an autosomal recessive pattern, and designated as *congenital nephrotic syndrome of the Finnish type.* It has been reported in various ethnic groups and races from many different geographical locations but occurs most commonly in Finland, where the incidence is 10 per 100,000 births (five times the incidence of nephrosis from all causes in children below the age of 16 in the United States).[486, 499] Affected infants are often nephrotic at birth, with edema and abdominal ascites, and do not respond to therapy. The disease is invariably fatal, with few patients surviving beyond 2 years of age. The immediate cause of death is usually gastrointestinal or pulmonary infection.[499]

Other idiopathic congenital nephrotic syndromes have been reported, one being an autosomal recessive familial form (*diffuse mesangial sclerosis*) which sometimes responds to corticosteroid therapy, but invariably progresses to renal failure and death at an age of 1 to 3 years.[499] It is important to remember that focal segmental glomerulosclerosis, minimal change nephrotic syndrome, and nephrotic syndrome secondary to infectious causes may all occur in the first year of life and are amenable to therapeutic intervention.[486, 500] The incidence and prognosis depend on the underlying etiology.

Regardless of the cause, the pathophysiology of the nephrotic syndrome appears to uniformly result from an increase in glomerular permeability to plasma protein.[486-488] Selective permeability is a remarkable attribute of normal glomerular capillary membrane which allows it to distinguish macromolecules on the basis of size, shape, and molecular charge.[501-503] Structural damage to the basement membrane may result in passage of high-molecular-weight proteins. This occurs in acute and chronic nephritis and focal segmental glomerulosclerosis.[487, 505] The disruption of selective permeability may be much more subtle, however. It has been proposed that in minimal change nephrotic syndrome the selectively increased permeability to low-molecular-weight polyanionic proteins such as albumin occurs solely because of a loss of fixed negative ions situated in the glomerular capillary membrane.[506, 507] The relative resistance to therapy of focal segmental glomerulosclerosis as compared with the responsiveness of minimal change nephrosis may represent a clinical correlation of the major structural damage in the former lesion, versus the minor electrostatic changes in the latter.[487]

Once glomerular permeability has been altered, the clinical manifestations of the nephrotic syndrome appear as a result of the pathophysiological mechanisms illustrated in Figure 7–13.[486] Hypoproteinemia and edema lead to other complications with implications for anesthesia. In spite of the edema and appearance of fluid overload, these children usually have depleted intravascular volume, especially when salt intake is restricted.[486, 515] Diuretics may induce severe volume contraction, hypokalemia, and azotemia, and induction of anesthesia may be associated with a marked fall in blood pressure.[486, 488, 515] Central venous pressure monitoring may be necessary for accurate volume assessment. Gastrointestinal disturbances are common, and diarrhea, attributed to edema of the intestinal mucosa, may further add to volume depletion.[486, 487] Ascites and abdominal distention may result in the appearance of umbilical or inguinal hernias.

Respiratory compromise may occur from increased intra-abdominal pressure or from pleural effusions, which further confuse the concept of fluid overload.[486, 487] Respiratory distress may increase in the supine position, and the risk of passive regurgitation from increased intra-abdominal pressure is always present.

In such cases, it is reasonable to delay surgery and administer salt-poor albumin intravenously in a dose of 0.5 to 1.0 gm/kg over 30 minutes while the patient is carefully monitored for hemodynamic changes. This will usually mobilize pleural, peritoneal, and peripheral edema fluid and often result in a diuresis.[508] If

after 30 to 60 minutes a diuresis has not occurred and intravascular volume is judged to be adequate, then a dose of furosemide, 1 to 2 mg/kg, may be given intravenously, with continued hemodynamic monitoring. This almost always result in diuresis and symptomatic improvement.[488] If necessary, the same regimen can be employed intraoperatively. This emphasizes the need for invasive monitoring to assess volume and hemodynamic status accurately.

An increased susceptibility to infection in the nephrotic child has been attributed to low immunoglobulin levels, generalized protein and nutritional deficiency, decreased bactericidal activity of leukocytes, and immunosuppressive therapy.[488] Pneumonia, peritonitis, and septicemia due to pneumococcus, *Escherichia coli*, *Pseudomonas*, and *Serratia* can be life-threatening.[509] Sterile technique during placement of invasive lines should be carefully observed.

An increased incidence of vascular thrombosis is observed in the nephrotic syndrome. It is known that renal vein or inferior vena caval thrombosis may cause nephrosis, but in children the nephrotic syndrome is usually the primary event.[488, 510, 511] Thromboses have occurred in the pulmonary, coronary, and mesenteric arteries. They are not infrequent in the femoral artery following femoral puncture, and have occurred in axillary and subclavian veins.[488, 511, 513, 514] The hypercoagulability has been attributed to hemoconcentration (due to intravascular volume depletion), thrombocytosis, increased platelet aggregation, elevated levels of coagulation factors V and VII, and low plasma levels of antithrombin III and plasminogen.[512, 516] Prophylactic anticoagulant therapy has not been adequately assessed and is not currently recommended.[488] It would seem prudent to be particularly vigilant of intravascular lines and to remove them as soon as they are no longer necessary or at the first signs of possible vascular compromise.

Preoperative laboratory assessment of renal function in nephrotic children will often show elevations of BUN and creatinine. This is presumably due to intra-

Figure 7–13. Pathophysiology of clinical manifestations of the nephrotic syndrome. PBI = protein-bound iodine; ADH = antidiuretic hormone; Aldo = aldosterone. (*From* Rance CP, Arbus GS, Balfe JW: Management of the Nephrotic Syndrome in Children. Pediatr Clin N Am 23:735, 1976. Modified from Earley LE, Havel RJ, Hopper J, et al.: Nephrotic Syndrome. Calif Med 115:23, 1971.)

vascular volume depletion and decreased GFR, since these tests normalize following resolution of proteinuria.[487, 490] Preservation of maximal renal function requires the restoration and maintenance of intravascular volume. In addition to albumin, whole blood, plasma, and dextran have been used, and have resulted in diuresis.[488] With a normal volume status and GFR, creatinine and urea clearance may actually be increased, possibly from leakage and loss into tubular fluid.[486, 518] Preoperative electolyte studies may demonstrate hypokalemia from aggressive diuretic and corticosteroid therapy, and the patient may require replacement therapy. Hypocalcemia is usually attributable to hypoproteinemia, but low ionized calcium levels may occur in chronically nephrotic patients owing to loss of vitamin D metabolites in the urine.[520]

Immunosuppressant, antihypertensive, and corticosteroid therapy should be continued in the perioperative period, with an increase in steroid dosage to provide "stress" coverage. The acute illness or surgical stress may nevertheless exacerbate the nephrotic syndrome, and children in remission may begin to spill protein intraoperatively. Urine should be monitored for protein content and, if the surgery is prolonged or the proteinuria massive, replacement with albumin will help prevent postoperative edema. Intraoperative steroids may also be given. Continued monitoring of hemodynamics and urine for protein in the postoperative period is necessary to detect sudden resolution of the albuminuria and avoid fluid overload from continued infusion of albumin. Finally, the dosage of highly protein-bound drugs, such as thiopental, may have to be reduced in presence of hypoproteinemia.[270] Children with nephrotic syndrome and progressive renal disease may develop increasing degrees of renal failure and their anesthetic management must also be tailored to these concerns.

Interstitial Nephritis, Pyelonephritis, and Focal Renal Scarring

Interstitial nephritis (interstitial renal inflammation) is another type of renal response to injury. It is characterized by inflammation in the interstitial space between nephrons and the renal vasculature. This leads to interstitial scarring, resulting in atrophy and loss of renal tubules.[521] Table 7–17 lists the many causes of interstitial renal inflammation. The incidence and population at risk varies with each etiology. Frank *papillary necrosis* is associated with diseases that cause renal papillary ischemia (shock, dehydration, aplastic and sickle cell anemia, diabetes mellitus, renal vascular compromise, and urinary obstruction) and a similar mechanism may be associated with the renal lesions of analgesic abuse.[522, 523]

Acute and chronic recurrent pyelonephritis have been implicated as major causes of interstitial renal inflammation. Whether the infection, associated reflux, or a combination of both is the primary cause of renal injury is still debated.[521, 524-526] The degree of renal

Table 7–17. CAUSES OF INTERSTITIAL NEPHRITIS

Group & Etiology	Group & Etiology
Group 1. Immunologic reactions	Aplastic anemia
Transplantation rejection	Hemorrhagic fever
Drug hypersensitivity	Balkan nephropathy
Methicillin	Analgesic mixture
Rifampin	abuse—phenacetin,
Penicillin	phenylbutazone,
Ampicillin	other
Other antibiotics	Transplantation
Anticonvulsant drugs	rejection
Glafenine	Aging
Diuretics	Alcoholism
Phenindione	Unilateral
Allopurinol	xanthogranulomatous
Lupus erythematosus	change with
Glomerulonephritis	pyelonephritis
Sjögren syndrome	
Sarcoidosis	B. Papillary injury
Granulomatous disease,	Uric acid deposition
unknown etiology	Gout
	Lesch-Nyhan
Group 2. Congenital lesions	syndrome
Cystinosis	Nephrocalcinosis
Oxalosis	Potassium depletion
Wilson's disease	Hyperphosphatemia
Alport's syndrome	Sulponamides
? Ask-Upmark kidney	Heavy metal poisoning
Medullary cystic disease	Amyloidosis
and/or nephronophthisis	
Other congenital lesions	Group 4. Miscellaneous causes
	Choline deficiency
Group 3. Association with	Irradiation
papillary damage	Disseminated intravascular
A. Papillary necrosis	coagulation
Urinary obstruction	Systemic infection
Vesicoureteral reflux	Scarlet fever
Diabetes mellitus	Typhoid fever
Vascular disease of the	Toxoplasmosis
kidney	Leptospirosis
Sickle cell disorders	Brucellosis
	Bacterial sepsis
	Viral infection
	? Syphilis
	Heat stroke
	Acute tubular necrosis
	Group 5. Bacterial infection of the kidney

From Freedman LR: The interstitial nephritides. *In* Edelmann CM Jr (Ed.): Pediatric Kidney Disease. Boston, Little, Brown, 1978.

damage appears to depend on the presence of obstruction, age (younger children suffer greater injury), delay in therapy, individual susceptibility, and bacterial virulence.[527, 528] A recent hypothesis of renal damage proposes that there are specific epithelial cell surface receptors to which pyelonephritogenic *E. coli* adhere.[527] Ascending ureteral infection occurs with transport of bacteria by turbulent flow and reflux, while ureteral receptors facilitate local bacterial replication. Structural damage to the ureter and endotoxic inhibition of peristalsis causes pyelorenal backflow at low pressure. Finally, bacterial attachment to tubular epithelial receptors results in acute interstitial inflammation.[527]

Children with interstitial nephritis may present with oliguria, hypertension, and renal insufficiency. Presenting symptoms may also be those of the underlying illness, such as urinary tract infection, pyelonephritis with flank pain and fever, diabetes, or sepsis. Damage to renal tubules may result in impairment of the ability to concentrate urine and cause tubular loss of bicarbonate, sodium, and potassium.[521] Medical management is directed at treatment of the underlying disease and the manifestations of renal failure. Discontinuation of analgesics is essential in nephropathy due to these drugs.

Sterilization of the urine is of great importance because interstitial nephritis with persistent infection may precipitate acute papillary necrosis, leading to life-threatening sepsis or renal insufficiency.[521]

Although sterile pyuria may result during the recovery phase of papillary necrosis and persist for weeks or months after antibiotic treatment, renal tuberculosis should be considered in children with persistent sterile pyuria.[521] Blood-borne extension from a primary focus establishes renal cortical tubercles, which, if untreated, may pass into the tubules, renal papillae, renal pelvis, ureter, and ultimately the bladder.[529] The ureteral orifice may become rigid and open, allowing vesicoureteral reflux, and exacerbate the interstitial nephritis. Inflammatory strictures may form at the pelviureteral junction, while severe scarring and contraction of the bladder may occur, requiring surgical intervention.[529]

Viral infections, such as infectious mononucleosis, may also cause interstitial nephritis with foci of tubular necrosis and result in sterile pyuria.[531] Though rare, many bacterial, rickettsial, viral, fungal, and parasitic agents have been identified as causing nephritis, sometimes by direct renal involvement, but more commonly through immunological mechanisms.[530] Proper diagnosis may require recognition of the systemic manifestation of the underlying illness.

Regardless of etiology, the manifestations of interstitial nephritis important to the anesthesiologist are those of impairment of renal function. Preoperative evaluation should determine the child's pattern of obligate urine output and bicarbonate and electrolyte loss, so that appropriate preoperative replacement can be accomplished. Severely ill children who have been unable to maintain oral intake may require volume replacement prior to anesthetic induction. Those children with hypertension, oliguria, and renal insufficiency merit the anesthetic considerations for acute renal failure detailed previously.

Renal Tubular Disorders

Disorders of tubular function may arise secondary to generalized renal parenchymal disease or may be present as inherited or acquired defects.[532]

Renal Tubular Acidosis

Renal tubular acidosis (RTA) is perhaps the prime example of disorders of renal tubular function. It may be broadly classified as proximal or distal. Table 7–18 details this classification together with some of the causes and characteristics of renal tubular acidosis.[533] Renal tubular acidosis may be further subdivided on the basis of serum electrolyte findings and the response to mineralocorticoids, and the incidence, prognosis, and pattern of presentation vary according to subtype.[532, 533] Some children share features of both proximal and distal RTA and are considered to have hybrid renal tubular acidosis. All forms, however, are characterized by renal tubular inability to adequately reabsorb bicarbonate, excrete hydrogen ions, or both.[533]

Normally almost all filtered bicarbonate is reabsorbed in the proximal tubule and appears in the urine only when plasma bicarbonate levels exceed the renal threshold. In adults this occurs at plasma bicarbonate concentrations above 25 mmol/L, but in normal infants the threshold is as low as 22 mmol/L.[534] In proximal renal tubular acidosis the threshold is depressed to as low as 16 mmol/L.[535] A distinguishing feature of proximal renal tubular acidosis is the continued ability of the distal tubule to excrete hydrogen ion and acidify the urine.[533] This prevents nephrocalcinosis. Biochemical manifestations are limited to a hyperchloremic metabolic acidosis, hypokalemia, and a decreased ability to concentrate the urine, and symptoms may be limited to excessive vomiting in early infancy and growth retardation.[532] Rickets and osteomalacia may occur with time. As opposed to the transient infantile proximal RTA, the permanent, hereditary infantile form may be associated with cataracts and mental retardation.[532, 536]

Therapy for proximal RTA requires frequent replacement of lost bicarbonate with 10 mEq/kg/day, or more, of bicarbonate. Potassium replacement is frequently necessary, especially when potassium loss increases with correction of acidosis and diuretic therapy.[537] In severe proximal RTA, the administration of hydrochlorothiazide 1 to 3 mg/kg/day increases the bicarbonate threshold and reduces the required dose of replacement bicarbonate.[538] Thiazide diuretics may produce this effect by increasing tubular reabsorption of phosphate and decreasing urinary calcium excretion, thereby decreasing parathyroid hormone levels and its bicarbonate wasting effect on the tubule.[533] This leads to improvement in osteomalacic lesions and would explain why thiazides, which decrease calcium excretion, raise the serum bicarbonate threshold, whereas furosemide, which increases calcium excretion, does not.[533] On the other hand, increased tubular reabsorption of bicarbonate may occasionally be achieved with sodium chloride restriction.[532] In both cases, the mechanism of action may be related to contraction of the extracellular fluid volume.[539] This explains why pre- or intraoperative expansion of a chronically reduced extracellular volume in some of these children may paradoxically induce acidosis.[532] Conversely, obligatory urine output, sodium wasting, and diuretic therapy may produce significant hypovolemia. Since urinary

Table 7–18. CLASSIFICATION, CAUSES, AND CHARACTERISTICS OF RENAL TUBULAR ACIDOSIS

Etiology Diagnosis, and Treatment	Renal Tubular Acidosis	
	Proximal	*Distal*
Etiology		
Primary	Permanent	Permanent
	Familial	Classic adult type
	Isolated (vitamin D deficiency?)	Incomplete RTA
	Transient	With bicarbonate wasting
	Infantile	With nerve deafness
		Transient (in infancy?)
Secondary	Fanconi syndrome	Primary hyperthyroidism with nephrocalcinosis
	Cystinosis	Primary hyperparathyroidism with nephrocalcinosis
	Lowe's syndrome	Idiopathic hypercalcemia
	Hereditary fructose intolerance	Vitamin D intoxication
	Primary and secondary hyperparathyroidism	Idiopathic hypercalciuria with nephrocalcinosis
	Vitamin D deficiency	Amphotericin B nephropathy
	Medullary cystic disease	Toxicity to lithium
	Renal transplantation	Hepatic cirrhosis
	Osteopetrosis	Hyperglobulinemic states
	Cyanotic congenital heart disease	Hereditary fructose intolerance with nephrocalcinosis
	Leigh's syndrome	Ehlers-Danlos syndrome
	Mineralocorticoid deficiency	Elliptocytosis
		Medullary sponge kidney
		Renal transplantation
Diagnosis		
Urine pH	4.5 to 7.8 depending on level of plasma bicarbonate	Always above 6.0 regardless of level of plasma bicarbonate
Bicarbonate threshold	Decreased	Normal
Hydrogen ion excretion	Normal, below bicarbonate threshold	Impaired, below bicarbonate threshold
Therapy	Resistant to alkali therapy; diuretics have effect	Sensitive to alkali therapy; no effect of diuretics

From Rodriguez-Soriano J: Renal tubular acidosis. *In* Edelmann CM Jr (Ed.): Pediatric Kidney Disease. Boston, Little, Brown, 1978.

output and metabolic acidosis may not reflect volume status, pre- and intraoperative measurement of central venous pressure is extremely useful. Restriction of oral intake preoperatively requires ongoing intravenous replacement of fluids, electrolytes, and diuretics.

In *distal renal tubular acidosis* the primary defect is the diminished ability to excrete hydrogen ions as ammonium and titratable acid in the distal tubule, despite a low plasma bicarbonate concentration.[532] Acidosis results primarily from the inability to excrete the full endogenous load of nonvolatile acid, and loss of bicarbonate is minimal. Correction with exogenously administered alkali must meet or exceed the rate of endogenous fixed acid production, which is 1 mEq/kg/day in adults and 2 to 3 mEq/kg/day in infants and children.[533] Clinical manifestations of distal RTA are more severe than those of proximal RTA and result from the inability to acidify the urine (Fig. 7–14).[533]

Permanent, primary distal renal tubular acidosis (Butler-Albright Syndrome, adult type distal RTA) is inherited in an autosomal dominant fashion, but frequently occurs sporadically. There is a slight predominance in females, and onset usually occurs after 2 years of age. It is distinguished from *transient, primary distal renal tubular acidosis (Lightwood syndrome, infantile type distal RTA)*, which is mild, transient, and observed only

within the first year of life.[533] Permanent distal RTA varies considerably in its degree of severity but usually presents with anorexia, vomiting, constipation, polyuria, dehydration, and growth retardation. Nephrocalcinosis is almost a constant finding and may lead to interstitial nephritis and renal failure.[532] Nephrolithiasis, urolithiasis, osteomalacia, and pathological fractures may occur with advancing age, if treatment is delayed. Potassium loss and hypokalemia may be so severe as to cause weakness and periodic paralysis. Severe polyuria, hypokalemia, acidosis, and vomiting may combine to cause life-threatening dehydration, respiratory difficulty, flaccid paralysis, coma, cardiac arrhythmias, and circulatory collapse.[532, 533]

Despite the potential severity of symptoms the prognosis of permanent distal RTA is good, provided that diagnosis and treatment are established early enough to prevent severe nephrocalcinosis, interstitial nephritis, and renal damage.[533] Because the proximal tubule is able to avidly reabsorb bicarbonate, sustained correction of acidosis may be achieved with less than 3 mEq/kg/day of bicarbonate and results in reversal of bony lesions and arrest of renal injury.[541] Potassium administration may also be necessary. It should begin prior to correction of acidosis if severe hypokalemia is present in order to prevent a further fall in serum potassium. Administration of thiazide diuretics is of

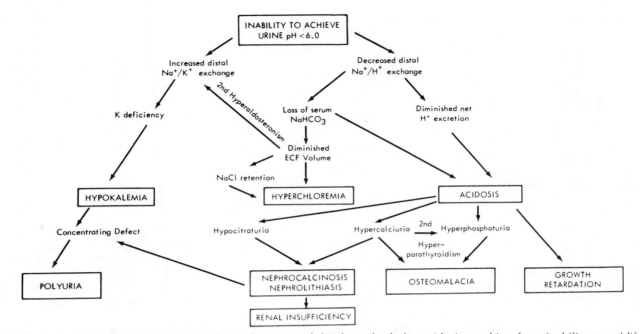

Figure 7–14. Pathophysiology of clinical manifestations of distal renal tubular acidosis resulting from inability to acidify urine. (*From* Rodriquez-Soriano J, Edelmann CM Jr: Renal Tubular Acidosis. Ann Rev Med *20*:363, 1969. Reproduced, with permission, from the Annual Review of Medicine, Vol. 20 © 1969 by Annual Reviews Inc.)

limited benefit and may aggravate the hypokalemia. As the name indicates, the distal tubular defect is permanent and interruption or attempts to withdraw therapy result in reappearance of metabolic acidosis and other clinical manifestations.[533] Any intercurrent illness that limits oral intake demands prompt intravenous replacement. Preanesthetic care requires evaluation of the adequacy of therapy and correction of volume, acid-base, and electrolyte abnormalities. Children with inadequate therapy over long periods of time may have varying degrees of nephrocalcinosis and renal failure. A central venous line is useful not only for evaluation of volume status but also as a secure port for perioperative administration of irritating electrolyte solutions. The usual precautions when delivering concentrated potassium solutions must be observed.

Finally, *hyperkalemic distal renal tubular acidosis (RTA type 4)* may result from aldosterone deficiency, from reduced tubular responsiveness to aldosterone, or from obstructive uropathy.[542-544] A primary defect in tubular secretion of potassium is the cause of acidosis in the *Spitzer-Weinstein syndrome.*[544, 560, 561] Interestingly, unilateral renal disease may induce a generalized state of tubular aldosterone unresponsiveness in both kidneys, amenable to oral bicarbonate and diuretic therapy and resolving with nephrectomy of the diseased kidney.[532, 543] *Pseudohypoaldosteronism* is a similar aldosterone-resistant lesion characterized by renal salt wasting, and effectively treated by sodium supplementation.[547, 561]

The Fanconi Syndrome

The *Fanconi syndrome (de Toni-Debré-Fanconi syndrome)* is characterized by impaired tubular reabsorption of

glucose, amino acids, phosphate, bicarbonate, uric acid, and potassium.[532] It is a generalized disorder of renal tubular transport, which may be congenital or acquired, either primary or secondary, as indicated in Table 7–19.[568] Children with the Fanconi syndrome present with metabolic acidosis, hypokalemia, hypophosphatemia, hypercalciuria, glucosuria, aminoaciduria, and polyuria. Rickets, osteomalacia, and pathological fractures may result, as well as the other

Table 7–19. CAUSES OF THE FANCONI SYNDROME

1. Heritable disorders
   A. Cystinosis
   B. Idiopathic
   C. Lowe syndrome (oculo-cerebro-renal syndrome)
   D. Tyrosinemia, type 1
   E. Familial nephrosis
   F. Galactosemia
   G. Glycogen storage disease
   H. Hereditary fructose intolerance
   I. Wilson disease
2. Other disorders
   A. Human kidney transplantation
   B. Myeloma or Bence-Jones proteinuria
   C. Amyloidosis
   D. Sjögren syndrome
   E. Nephrotic syndrome
   F. Pancreatic carcinoma
   G. Hyperparathyroidism
3. Exogenous toxins
   A. Heavy metals (especially lead, mercury; including organic mercurials)
   B. Nonmetals (Lysol, maleic acid, methyl-3-chromone, outdated tetracycline, streptozotocin, vitamin D)

From Shulman JD, Schneider JA: Cystinosis and the Fanconi syndrome. Pediatr Clin North Am *23*:779, 1976.

clinical manifestations of renal tubular acidosis discussed above.[532] Children with primary Fanconi syndrome progress slowly to chronic renal failure; the progression and prognosis of secondary Fanconi syndrome depends on the response of the underlying illness to specific therapy.

Symptomatic treatment consists of correction of acidosis and hypokalemia by bicarbonate, hydrochlorothiazide, and potassium therapy, together with supplementation with neutral phosphate and high-dose vitamin D to treat the bony involvement.[532, 545] Indomethacin has improved tubular function in patients with Fanconi syndrome due to *cystinosis* (*cystine storage disease*),[532] and renal transplantation has been successful in these patients.[532] Anesthetic recommendations for Fanconi syndrome have emphasized consideration of the characteristic fluid and electrolyte disorders, and are essentially the same as those for renal tubular acidosis discussed above.[548] Frequently anesthetic management is also influenced by the systemic manifestations of the precipitating illness. For example, children with Fanconi syndrome due to cystinosis may also suffer from recurrent epistaxis, portal hypertension, esophageal varices, hypothyroidism, and diabetes mellitus.[532] Finally, patients with end-stage illness with renal failure may present with any or all of the problems associated with azotemia, including cardiovascular impairment.[548]

Primary Hypophosphatemic Rickets

Primary hypophosphatemic rickets (*vitamin D–resistant rickets*) is characterized by reduced tubular reabsorption of phosphate leading to profound hypophosphatemia (less than 0.6 mEq/L), with normocalcemia, short stature, rickets, and osteomalacia.[532] It is usually transmitted via an X-linked dominant gene, although sporadic autosomal dominant and recessive patterns have been reported.[551] Clinical features appear at the end of the first year of life, and aside from the hyperphosphaturia, renal function is normal.[532] Treatment with inorganic phosphate supplementation and high-dose vitamin D (used to suppress parathyroid hormone hypersecretion) is usually able to achieve the therapeutic goal of raising serum phosphate levels to greater than 1.8 mEq/L (normals in growing children may be as high as 6 mEq/L).[533, 549, 551] Overzealous treatment can result in hypercalcemia, hypercalciuria, and nephrocalcinosis resulting in renal injury.[550] Appropriate early treatment may result in normal growth rates and avoidance of bony deformities.[549, 550] Anesthetic care should include preoperative evaluation of serum calcium levels and the degree of bony involvement. Precautions should be taken with positioning and intraoperative manipulation to avoid fractures in older children with severe osteomalacia.

Nephrogenic Diabetes Insipidus

Nephrogenic diabetes insipidus is characterized by persistent hyposthenuria due to a partial or complete inability of the renal tubules to respond to antidiuretic hormone.[532] The primary disorder is X-linked with variable expression in females. More commonly nephrogenic diabetes insipidus occurs secondary to a systemic disease (for example, *Sjögren syndrome* or *amyloidosis*) or drug therapy (lithium, propoxyphene, demeclocycline).[532, 552] ADH normally binds tubular receptors to activate adenylate cyclase increasing intracellular cyclic AMP.[553, 554] This leads to a cascade of enzymatic processes that result in increased tubular free water absorption along the medullary concentration gradient.[552, 555] Hypokalemia and hypercalcemia may interfere with tubular cellular cyclic-AMP production in response to ADH, and any disorder leading to hypokalemia or hypercalcemia may lead to renal concentrating defects.[552, 554, 556, 557]

Likewise, disorders that reduce the medullary concentration gradient will interfere with tubular reabsorption of water and urinary concentration, independent of ADH. Such disorders may include any osmotic diuresis, acute and chronic renal failure, obstructive nephropathy, interstitial nephritis, medullary cystic disease, polycystic renal disease, sickle cell anemia, and others.[552] Clinical manifestations are polydipsia, nocturia, and polyuria, all of which may go unnoticed in infants. Inadequate hydration may rapidly lead to severe hypernatremic dehydration, seizures, and coma.[532] Treatment consists of providing adequate fluids, reducing dietary solute intake, and administering thiazide diuretics (which increase proximal tubular fluid reabsorption by causing extracellular volume contraction).[559] Aspirin and indomethacin inhibition of prostaglandin synthetase may also help reduce urine output.[558] Anesthetic management must include preoperative evaluation of volume status, electrolyte abnormalities (hypokalemia and hypercalcemia may be induced by diuretics, and contribute to the urinary concentrating abnormality), and platelet function (for children on aspirin or indomethacin). Intraoperative evaluation of the volume status should be made independently of the large, obligate urinary output.

Liddle Syndrome

Liddle syndrome (*pseudohyperaldosteronism*) is an autosomal dominant disorder appearing as early as 10 months of age and characterized by hypertension, hypokalemic alkalosis, and hyperkaliuria with low aldosterone levels.[561] Hypertension, retinopathy, headaches, paresthesias, epigastric cramping, polyuria, weakness, acute paralysis, and occasionally tetany may occur. Apart from the failure to conserve potassium, renal function is normal. Spironolactone and aldosterone synthesis inhibitors have no effect on the disease, but triamterene (8 to 10 mg/kg/day) normalizes serum potassium and blood pressure by inhibiting the excessive distal tubular ion transport. This is aided by potassium supplementation and sodium restriction.[561]

Bartter Syndrome

Bartter syndrome is characterized by juxtaglomerular and renomedullary cell hyperplasia, hyperreninemia, hyperaldosteronemia, and hypokalemic metabolic alkalosis. Blood pressure is normal, however, and there is no hypertensive response to infused angiotensin II or norepinephrine.[562] Clinical features appearing in infancy or childhood include anorexia, failure to thrive, polyuria, polydipsia, and muscle weakness. Rarely hypercalcemia, hypophosphatemia, rickets, tetany, seizures, and distal renal tubular acidosis may be present. Renal failure may develop in a few patients.[561, 563] Elevated production of prostaglandins has been linked to the disease and had led to effective therapy with prostaglandin synthetase inhibitors such as aspirin, indomethacin, and ibuprofen.[564, 565] Treatment may also include potassium supplementation, spironolactone as an aldosterone antagonist, propranolol to block renin secretion, captopril to block angiotensin converting enzyme, and triamterene as a potassium-sparing diuretic. It is not yet known whether early detection and aggressive treatment will prevent development of the mental retardation seen in one third of patients.[532] Anesthetic considerations for patients with Bartter syndrome must focus on the status of renal function, the intravascular volume, serum electrolytes, and the side effects of medications used to treat the syndrome.[566] Hyperventilation and consequent respiratory alkalosis should be avoided in the presence of hypokalemic metabolic alkalosis. The diminished response to angiotensin and norepinephrine, the use of diuretics, and the presence of hypovolemia and beta blockade may all predispose the patient to hypotension and a reduced response to vasopressors. Prostaglandin synthetase inhibitors may impair platelet function. If renal impairment is significant, systemic manifestations of azotemia must also influence anesthetic care.

Idiopathic Hypomagnesemia

Renal wasting of magnesium, an autosomal recessive trait, occurs as an isolated defect or in association with renal potassium wasting and hypokalemia.[567] Tremor, fasciculations, tetany, and seizures may accompany irritability, apathy, weakness, nausea, and osteochondrosis. All these signs and symptoms resolve with magnesium supplementation of 1 to 2 mEq/kg/day, with additional potassium supplementation in hypokalemic patients.[561] Theoretical anesthetic concerns in these patients would be the potential for interaction between hypomagnesemia and neuronal function, muscular function, and neuromuscular blockade.

Cystic Diseases of the Kidney

The Spectrum of Cystic Diseases

Many diseases may result in renal parenchymal cysts, which in turn may cause varying degrees of renal dysfunction. In some of these diseases the renal lesion may be the most significant; in others, renal involvement is mild and the other systemic manifestations of the illness are by far the most significant, from a

clinical and anesthetic point of view. For example, the medullary cystic dilatations in *medullary sponge kidney* (*precalyceal canalicular ectasia, cystic dilatation of renal collecting tubules*) are the only lesions seen and are associated with only mild renal dysfunction, usually as a result of recurrent pyelonephritis or nephrolithiasis.[570] In contrast, the cystic renal involvement in *Ehlers-Danlos syndrome* and *tuberous sclerosis* may present prior to the other diagnostic stigmata and may cause severe renal disease.[569, 602] Other syndromes, such as *Jeune asphyxiating thoracic dysplasia* or *Zellweger cerebrohepatorenal syndrome*, may occasionally be associated with significant cystic renal disease, but this is usually overshadowed by the other more serious clinical features of the syndromes.[569, 571] The many types of renal parenchymal cysts are shown in Table 7–20, and Table 7–21 lists the various malformation syndromes associated with renal cortical cysts.[569]

Infantile Polycystic Disease

Although termed infantile polycystic disease, this diffuse, bilateral, autosomal recessive illness may be first recognized in adolescence and adulthood. It is characterized by dilation of distal tubules and collecting ducts and takes on several forms which vary in severity and presentation.[569] In the perinatal form the

Table 7–20. CLASSIFICATION OF RENAL PARENCHYMAL CYSTS

Polycystic disease
　Infantile polycystic disease:
　　Polycystic disease of the newborn
　　Polycystic disease of infancy and childhood
　　Congenital hepatic fibrosis
　Adult polycystic disease

Renal cysts in hereditary syndromes
　Diffuse cystic involvement in tuberous sclerosis
　Diffuse cystic involvement in von Hippel–Lindau disease
　Cystic dysplasia in Zellweger cerebrohepatorenal syndrome and Jeune asphyxiating thoracic dysplasia
　Severe cystic involvement in Ehlers-Danlos syndrome
　Cortical microcysts in syndromes of multiple malformation

Renal cortical cysts
　Diffuse glomerular cystic disease
　Juxtamedullary cortical microcysts (Finnish type congenital nephrotic syndrome)
　Solitary and multiple simple cysts
　Segmental and unilateral cystic disease

Renal medullary cysts
　Uremic medullary cystic disease complex:
　　Familial juvenile nephronophthisis
　　Medullary cystic disease
　　Renal-retinal dysplasia
　Medullary sponge kidney

Renal dysplasia
　Cystic dysplasia associated with lower urinary tract obstruction
　Multicystic and aplastic dysplasia
　Hereditary cystic dysplasia
　Focal and segmental cystic dysplasia

From Bernstein J: Polycystic disease. *In* Edelmann CM Jr (Ed.): Pediatric Kidney Disease. Boston, Little, Brown, 1978. Modified from Bernstein J, Gardner KD Jr: Cystic diseases of the kidney and renal dysplasia. *In* Harrison JH, Gittes RF, Perlmutter AD, et al. (Eds.): Campbell's Urology. 4th ed. Philadelphia, W. B. Saunders Co., 1978.

Table 7–21. SYNDROMES OF MULTIPLE MALFORMATION ASSOCIATED WITH RENAL CORTICAL CYSTS

Zellweger cerebrohepatorenal syndrome
Jeune asphyxiating thoracic dysplasia syndrome
Autosomal trisomy syndromes, D and E
Orodigitofacial syndrome
Lissencephaly syndrome
Goldenhar syndrome
Marden-Walker (Schwartz-Jampel) syndrome
Ehlers-Danlos syndrome
Congenital cutis laxa syndrome
Short rib–polydactyly syndrome
DiGeorge syndrome
Noonan syndrome
Turner syndrome
Chromosomal translocation syndromes

From Bernstein J: Polycystic disease. *In* Edelmann CM Jr (Ed.): Pediatric Kidney Disease. Boston, Little, Brown, 1978.

cysts may be enormous and cause oliguria, which may result in oligohydramnios and pulmonary hypoplasia in utero. Abdominal distention may interfere with delivery; if not stillborn, the newborn may suffer from life-threatening renal failure and pulmonary insufficiency.[569, 572] Interstitial pulmonary emphysema and pneumothorax may occur during resuscitative efforts. Malformations other than renal and hepatic cysts are rare and may suggest the presence of a different syndrome.[569] When the disease presents in older children, renal enlargement is less severe and renal insufficiency progresses at a variable rate. Severe systemic hypertension develops in many children and hepatic cysts are usually present, although hepatocellular dysfunction is rare.[573] In a few children systemic and portal hypertension may coexist and result in congestive heart failure, chronic renal failure, and bleeding esophageal varices.[569] As opposed to the oliguria of the neonate, in older children there is typically an impaired tubular ability to concentrate or acidify the urine (renal tubular acidosis).[575]

Infantile polycystic disease is usually progressive and is often fatal in childhood. Medical management is supportive.[565, 574] Appropriate fluid and electrolyte therapy may vary from severe restriction in oliguric neonates to generous salt and water administration in polyuric children. Severe systemic hypertension often requires aggressive medical intervention with its attendant problems, and congestive heart failure may require chronic inotropic support with digitalis. Chronic hemodialysis prolongs survival and allows successful renal transplantation. Portal hypertension may require portacaval shunt in a few children. Anesthetic considerations are determined by the degree and type of renal involvement and resulting systemic manifestations. Congestive heart failure, hepatic involvement, and esophageal variceal bleeding may further influence anesthetic management.

Adult Polycystic Disease in Childhood

A diffuse, bilateral, autosomal dominant disease appearing most frequently in adulthood, adult poly-

cystic disease may present at any age.[572, 576] When it presents in infancy, the disease may be quite severe, perhaps as a result of the presence of two dominant genes (homozygous disease) in these unfortunate infants.[569] It is relatively uncommon in blacks and may rarely occur in association with other hereditary conditions such as *spherocytosis, Peutz-Jeghers syndrome, lobster-claw deformity of the feet, orodigitofacial syndrome,* and *myotonic dystrophy.*[569] In older children and adults the presenting symptom may be flank pain, but in infants palpable flank masses or renal impairment may appear first. Hematuria, proteinuria, and an inability to concentrate the urine precede increasingly severe renal impairment. Renal hemorrhage, lithiasis, and infection complicate the illness and accelerate renal injury. Focal hepatic involvement affects one third of adults with adult polycystic disease; berry aneurysms of the cerebral arteries affect 10 percent and may lead to life-threatening intracranial hemorrhage. Both are infrequent in children.[569] Severe systemic hypertension is common, requiring aggressive therapeutic intervention to prevent accelerated renal deterioration. Secondary congestive heart failure may require digitalization, and renal infection requires prompt recognition and antibiotic therapy. Dialysis prolongs survival in anticipation of renal transplantation. Anesthetic considerations are the same as those for the infantile form, with the exception that the potential presence of cerebral artery aneurysms makes control of blood pressure more critical.

Familial Juvenile Nephronophthisis and Medullary Cystic Disease

Familial juvenile nephronophthisis is an autosomal recessive disorder with onset in childhood, characterized by polyuria and progressive renal failure. *Medullary cystic disease* is an adult-onset, autosomal dominant disease with a urinary concentrating defect and progressive azotemia. Morphologically they are quite similar, which has led to nosological confusion and a variety of descriptions that have been applied to one or the other or both: *cystic disease of the renal medulla, uremic medullary cystic disease, Fanconi nephronophthisis, salt-losing nephritis, uremic sponge kidney,* and *polycystic disease of medullary type.*[579] Variants of familial juvenile nephronophthisis may show ocular, cerebellar, skeletal, and hepatic abnormalities, and the characteristic medullary cystic lesions may be seen with rare syndromes such as *Alström syndrome* (obesity, diabetes mellitus, blindness, and deafness), *Laurence-Moon-Bardet-Biedl syndrome,* and *renal-retinal dysplasia.*[579]

The initial clinical features of familial juvenile nephronophthisis and medullary cystic disease are similar: polydipsia, polyuria, sodium and potassium wasting, azotemia, mild hypertension, anemia out of proportion to the degree of renal failure, and weakness. Both diseases progress inexorably to renal failure over a period of years, culminating in chronic dialysis, transplantation, or death. Treatment is nonspecific and supportive, and anesthetic considerations relate to the individual child's pattern of fluid and electrolyte excretion and degree of renal failure.

Renal Dysplasia, Aplasia, and Hypoplasia

Renal Dysplasia and Aplasia

Renal dysplasia is a condition of abnormal renal development resulting in abnormal nephronic structural organization.[571] It is often associated with obstructive urinary tract malformations, a probable pathogenetic relationship. It may also occur on a hereditary basis and may be associated with varying degrees of structural and functional impairment.

Hereditary cystic dysplasia is a bilateral, diffuse cystic lesion unassociated with urinary tract obstruction. It usually occurs sporadically but may follow an autosomal recessive pattern of occurrence. The degree of renal impairment is variable, but severely affected infants may have suffered from oligohydramnios and may present with life-threatening pulmonary hypoplasia and renal failure. Association with other malformations is common, such as occurs in the *Meckel syndrome*, which consists of cystic renal dysplasia, posterior encephalocele, microcephaly, polydactyly, and cleft lip and palate. In addition to the less significant renal cortical cysts mentioned previously, infants with *Jeune asphyxiating thoracic dysplasia* and *Zellweger cerebrohepatorenal syndrome* may occasionally demonstrate severe cystic renal dysplasia.[571] Infants with *Beckwith-Wiedemann syndrome* (omphalocele, macroglossia, hypoglycemia, and hyperplastic visceromegaly) may demonstrate medullary renal dysplasia, but this is rarely cystic.[571, 580]

Obstructive renal dysplasia, as the name implies, is thought to result from early urinary obstruction causing back pressure and affecting normal renal development.[581, 582] Obstructive renal dysplasia may be associated with any form of congenital urinary tract obstruction and has occurred with *bladder dysfunction due to meningomyelocele, prune belly syndrome, ectopic ureterocele, anterior urethral diverticulum*, and severely obstructive *posterior urethral valves*.[571] Concomitant ureteral reflux may exacerbate the formation of renal dysplasia, and reflux and obstruction may occur asymmetrically, accounting for asymmetrical and unilateral renal dysplasia.[571, 583]

Severe forms of obstructive renal dysplasia are *multicystic* and *aplastic renal dysplasia*, where the involved kidney is severely malformed and nonfunctioning. Both types are associated with ureteropelvic occlusion, which causes the severe dysplasia. Bilateral aplastic or multicystic kidneys are lethal malformations associated with oligohydramnios and stillbirth, or neonatal death from renal failure, pulmonary hypoplasia, or their complications.[571] Unilateral involvement may be silent until recurrent infection, flank pain, or hypertension occur. Because of the difficulty of differentiating the abnormal kidney from one with malignant degeneration, treatment is by surgical removal, which also achieves control of hypertension. The outcome depends on the functional viability of the contralateral kidney and the presence of associated contralateral abnormalities, such as renal or ureteral ectopia and ureteral reflux.

Renal Hypoplasia

Renal hypoplasia, as opposed to dysplasia, is characterized by a diminished number of normally developed nephrons.[584] Most cases are sporadic, but some may occur in association with other malformations. *Unilateral hypoplasia* is a common incidental finding often referred to as a *miniature kidney, doll's kidney,* or *vest pocket kidney*.[571] These small kidneys are prone to infection, lithiasis, and vascular disease causing hypertension.

Segmental hypoplasia (Ask-Upmark kidney) is a form of renal hypoplasia more frequently associated with hypertension due to segmental hypersecretion of renin.[586, 587] Although considered a congenital abnormality by some, infantile vesicoureteral reflux or local vascular injury may account for the segmental renal hypoplasia and scarring.[571] Infection, lithiasis, and severe hypertension, which is difficult to control, are indications for surgical removal of the abnormal segment or whole kidney.

Bilateral renal hypoplasia is an important cause of chronic renal failure in childhood.[571] *Simple bilateral hypoplasia* is rare and is characterized by salt and water wasting, renal tubular acidosis, and refractory hypokalemia.[584] *Oligomeganephronia* is a much more common form of bilateral renal hypoplasia and is characterized by marked hypertrophy of individual nephrons.[585] The cause is unknown, it occurs more frequently in males than females, and cases are sporadic. Clinical manifestations are polyuria, salt wasting, hyperchloremic metabolic acidosis, proteinuria, and slowly progressive azotemia. Hypertension is uncommon. Treatment is supportive and may include dialysis in anticipation of renal transplantation.[571] Anesthetic considerations for all of these lesions are governed by the type and extent of renal impairment.

Systemic Diseases Affecting Renal Parenchyma

As indicated in Tables 7–12, 7–14, 7–15, and 7–17, many systemic diseases may impair renal function and injure the kidney. The renal response to injury in any given disease may be manifested as any combination of interstitial nephritis, glomerulonephritis, the nephrotic syndrome, tubular dysfunction, acute renal failure, and progressive chronic renal failure, depending on the stage of the disease and the extent of renal involvement. For example, extrarenal neoplasms may directly invade renal parenchyma, blood vessels, or ureters; they may cause abnormalities in tubular function resulting in disturbances in excretion of water, sodium, potassium, calcium, and uric acid, or induce membranous glomerulopathy, minimal change nephrotic syndrome, or amyloidosis.[588]

Amyloidosis of the kidney may also result from chronic inflammatory conditions (tuberculosis, osteomyelitis, endocarditis, bronchiectasis, ulcerative colitis, regional ileitis, rheumatoid arthritis), multiple myeloma, and *familial Mediterranean fever*, and it may lead to end-stage renal failure.[589]

Hyperuricemia from chemotherapy of myeloproliferative disorders, genetically abnormal purine metabolism (*Lesch-Nyhan syndrome*), or decreased urate excretion may lead to urolithiasis, urinary obstruction, acute oliguric renal failure as well as renal interstitial inflammation, scarring, and chronic renal failure (*urate nephropathy*).[590] Allopurinol, adequate hydration, and maintenance of an alkaline urine all help prevent intrarenal deposition of urate crystals and should be continued in the perioperative period.

Nephrocalcinosis, nephrolithiasis, and *urolithiasis* leading to obstruction and severe renal impairment may result not only from *Proteus* urinary tract infections, but also from hypercalcemia and hypercalciuria due to thyroid disease, hyperparathyroidism, vitamin D intoxication, fat necrosis, sarcoidosis, and immobilization and idiopathic hypercalcemia.[591] The association of mental retardation, elfin facies, and supravalvular aortic stenosis (*Williams triad*) occurs with *idiopathic hypercalcemia*,[592] in which pulmonary stenosis and seizures have also been observed.

The *lysosomal storage diseases*, recessive hereditary disorders of glycogen, glycosphingolipid, glycoprotein, and mucopolysaccharide metabolism, may all manifest renal involvement. The most dramatic of these is *Fabry disease* (defective alpha-galactosidase A activity), which in addition to cardiac and cerebral vascular disease may cause renal disease presenting as proteinuria, polyuria, tubular dysfunction, and progressive azotemia.[593] Renal transplantation not only treats renal failure but provides genetically normal kidneys with normal alpha-galactosidase A activity to metabolize substrate.[594]

Dysglobulinemia, cryoglobulinemia, and *macroglobulinemia* (including *Waldenström macroglobulinemia*) may all cause renal impairment ranging from focal tubular atrophy to the nephrotic syndrome, to rapidly progressive, diffuse, proliferative glomerulonephritis with hypertension, hematuria, and proteinuria.[595, 596]

Cirrhosis of the liver may be associated with severe and progressive renal failure, know as the *hepatorenal syndrome*. Decreased plasma volume, renal blood flow, and GFR, as well as renal vasoconstriction, have been proposed as pathogenetic mechanisms, but therapeutic measures such as plasma volume expansion, paracentesis, vasodilators, and portacaval anastomosis provide only transient renal improvement.[597-599]

Radiation, drugs, toxins, and heavy metals may all cause renal injury and functional impairment. *Acute lead poisoning* leads characteristically to proximal tubular dysfunction, and occasionally the full-blown *Fanconi syndrome*, while *chronic lead poisoning* has been

associated with the subsequent development of chronic renal failure.[600] *Wilson disease (hepatolenticular degeneration)* is a hereditary disorder of copper metabolism resulting in elevated serum and renal copper levels and aminoaciduria or generalized Fanconi syndrome.[601] Gold remains a useful therapeutic agent in severe *juvenile rheumatoid arthritis* and may cause nephrotoxicity (with proteinuria, hematuria, and tubular dysfunction, and rarely acute tubular necrosis) or a hypersensitivity reaction resulting in the nephrotic syndrome.[600] In addition to amyloidosis and gold therapy, the systemic inflammatory process of *juvenile rheumatoid arthritis* may directly involve the kidney and result in interstitial nephritis, renal papillary necrosis, and focal mesangial proliferative glomerulonephritis.[603] Tubular dysfunction may cause obligatory salt and water loss, hypertension may require aggressive medical therapy, aspirin therapy may cause platelet malfunction, and chronic glucocorticord therapy may require perioperative steroid coverage.

Scleroderma (progressive systemic sclerosis), in addition to myocardial, pericardial, and pulmonary fibrosis, may involve the kidneys in 45 percent of patients, with a mortality of 60 percent.[604, 605] Proteinuria, progressive azotemia, and severe hypertension may all occur. Transplantation has been successful, and subsequent immunosuppression with azathioprine and corticosteroids can improve the systemic manifestations of the disease.[605, 606] *Dermatomyositis (polymyositis)* rarely involves the kidneys, causing focal glomerulosclerosis or membranoproliferative glomerulonephritis and the nephrotic syndrome.[603, 607] Cardiac conduction defects and pulmonary interstitial fibrosis are extrarenal manifestations of concern to the anesthesiologist.[608, 609] Interstitial nephritis, proliferative glomerulonephritis, and membranous glomerulonephropathy have all been reported in children with *mixed connective tissue disease*, and respond well to corticosteroid and immunosuppressive therapy.[610] Although renal disease is reported in only 10 percent of patients, one half of the deaths from mixed connective tissue disease are due to renal failure.[603]

Polyarteritis nodosa (periarteritis nodosa) occurs in an *infantile form* with hematuria, proteinuria, and hypertension, but is rapidly fatal owing to coronary artery involvement and heart failure.[611] The *adult form*, occurring in adolescent males twice as frequently as in females, has an 80 percent incidence of renal involvement with hematuria, proteinuria, hypertension, acute nephritic syndrome, and occasionally acute renal failure. Pulmonary involvement and granulomatous lesions of the upper respiratory tract and ears may precede renal involvement in some types of adult form polyarteritis nodosa (such as *Wegener granulomatosis, allergic granulomatosis, allergic angiitis*, and *the Löffler syndrome*) and may dominate anesthetic considerations.[611] Cyclophosphamide, azathioprine, corticosteroids, and heparin have all been used in different combinations, and have prevented the previously unchecked progression to death from renal failure.[611]

Renal involvement in children with *systemic lupus erythematosus* may occur in up to 80 percent and may present as mesangial, focal or diffuse proliferative, or membranous lupus nephritis.[612] Without adequate therapy the nephrotic syndrome, hypertension, uremia, and progressive renal failure may ensue. Cardiopulmonary and central nervous system involvement are frequent, and must influence anesthetic care. Treatment with corticosteroids, supplemented with immunosuppressive agents, has greatly improved the course and prognosis of childhood systemic lupus erythematosus.[613, 614]

Sickle cell nephropathy may occur with homozygous (SS) disease or heterozygous (AS) sickle cell trait, as well as in sickle cell–thalassemia or SC disease.[615, 616] Polymerization of hemoglobin S and sickling of red blood cells occurs with hypoxemia, hyperosmolarity, acidosis, and increased prostaglandin E_2 levels, all of which may occur in the renal medulla.[616, 617] There are several clinical manifestations of sickle cell nephropathy. Hematuria may be the presenting sign of a sickle cell crisis, but may also occur with sickle trait. It often originates unilaterally from the left kidney.[616, 618] Hyposthenuria resulting from an inability to concentrate the urine is an early and chronic finding, unrelated to changes in GFR or RBF. In the early stage it is reversible by transfusion of normal erythrocytes.[615, 616] The ability to concentrate urine decreases with age, and the large obligate urine output may lead to dehydration, especially if children with sickle cell nephropathy remain NPO without intravenous hydration. A defect of urinary acidification exists in both sickle cell disease and trait, and this, together with the concentrating defect, has led some to describe the functional lesion as a mild form of distal renal tubular acidosis.[615, 616] Membranoproliferative and minimal change glomerulonephritis have been reported in sickle cell patients with the nephrotic syndrome.[616] Renal vein thrombosis also occurs, often in association with the nephrotic syndrome, but whether the primary event is the sickling, thrombosis, or nephrosis is not clear.[619] Pyelonephritis may occur more frequently with sickle cell disease, and unchecked renal infection, as well as an acute vaso-occlusive crisis, may cause renal papillary necrosis and acute renal failure.[616] Renal failure is otherwise rare among children with sickle cell disease, and end-stage renal failure with the need for dialysis or transplantation occurs primarily in adulthood.[620]

Anesthetic care for patients with sickle cell nephropathy requires a recognition of their large obligate urine output. Fluid replacement should err on the generous side, because the ability to produce dilute urine is usually unaffected.[615, 621] Other general principles for anesthesia in patients with sickle cell disease, such as avoidance of hyperosmolarity, dehydration, hypoxia, ischemia, hypothermia, stasis, and extreme anemia, will also help avoid intrarenal sickling and prevent further renal damage.

Renal disease in diabetes mellitus may include a tendency toward bacteriuria, chronic pyelonephritis and renal papillary necrosis, an enhanced susceptibility to contrast media–induced nephropathy, toxin-induced nephropathy and interstitial nephritis, bladder atony and hydronephrosis from diabetic neuropathy, arteriolar nephrosclerosis, and diabetic glomerulosclerosis.[622] *Nodular intercapillary glomerulosclerosis (Kimmelstiel-Wilson nodules)* is a specific lesion present in over 50 percent of patients with diabetes mellitus and is considered pathognomonic of *diabetic nephropathy*.[622, 623] Microvasculopathy affecting the glomerulus (and other microvasculature such as the retina) is a serious threat to longevity in juvenile diabetes mellitus.[622, 623] Proteinuria, once fixed, is an ominous sign, with subsequent decline in GFR by 11 ml per minute each year.[624] Without dialysis or transplantation, survival after the establishment of uremia is usually less than 2 years.[623] Because diabetic nephropathy and glomerulosclerosis are asymptomatic and slowly progressive over 13 to 18 years, it is uncommon for these problems to present prior to adolescence or early adulthood.[622] The initial sign is usually proteinuria, which later progresses to frank nephrotic syndrome and then to relentless renal failure, although nephrotic syndrome may appear in children with diabetes mellitus of recent onset.[625] Hypertension is common and may appear concomitantly with proteinuria. Although the treatment is unproven, tight control of hypertension and serum glucose may slow the progression to renal failure.[623]

Anesthesia for nephrotic diabetics should follow the principles outlined above for nephrotic children, with the understanding that the diabetic may have marginal cardiac reserve and will tolerate intravascular volume changes poorly.[622] One third of each insulin dose is metabolized by the kidney, and as renal function is lost and renal catabolism of exogenous insulin diminishes, juvenile diabetics may suffer hypoglycemic episodes if their insulin is not decreased appropriately.[622] This makes perioperative insulin management more difficult and requires frequent monitoring of serum glucose levels. Finally, with end-stage renal failure treated with hemodialysis in juvenile diabetics, the leading cause of death is myocardial infarction or failure.[626] The anesthetic care of these young adults must address this major potential complication.

Retroperitoneal and Renal Tumors

The systemic manifestations of nonrenal tumors, and their therapy, may induce renal impairment as discussed above. Nonrenal, retroperitoneal tumors may in addition affect renal function by virtue of their location and size. *Neuroblastoma* is the most common retroperitoneal tumor in children, occurring in about 1 in 30,000 children usually before the age of 4. It is more common in females than in males.[628] Over 75 percent secrete catecholamines detectable in the urine, and hypertension may be present. Neuroblastoma may also occur in association with *neurofibromatosis (von Recklinghausen disease)*. Neurofibromas may cause renal artery stenosis and renal hypertension and may be associated with pheochromocytomas, which have many features of importance to the anesthesiologist[629] (see Chapter 12). *Ganglioneuroma* is considered a fully differentiated, benign extreme of neuroblastoma. Levels of catecholamine secretion are lower, and renal impairment is limited to that produced by local pressure effects.[628]

Nephroblastoma (Wilms tumor) is the most common abdominal tumor in children, with a reported incidence from 1 in 100;000 to 1 in 13,500.[627] It is usually diagnosed between 6 months and 5 years of age, and may be bilateral in 8 to 12 percent of cases.[627] Congenital absence of the iris (aniridia), in a familial or a sporadic form, and hemihypertrophy of the body may be associated.[627, 630] Wilms tumor may occur in conjunction with horseshoe kidneys, duplication of the urinary tract, solitary kidney, hypospadias, or with nephritis and male pseudohermaphroditism to form a a distinct syndrome described by Barakat and colleagues.[631] The tumor may extend into the renal vein or inferior vena cava, may cause renovascular distortion and hypertension, and may produce renin with resulting hypertension.[632, 633] An enlarged abdomen or an expanding abdominal mass is the usual presenting symptom, and vomiting, abdominal pain, hematuria, proteinuria, and metastases to para-aortic nodes, liver, and lungs may be present.[627, 634] Mild fever occurs in as many as 30 percent of patients and may accompany hemorrhage into the tumor.[627] It is not a reason to delay surgery. The anemia may be treated either preoperatively or by transfusion during surgery to maintain volume and hemoglobin concentration.[635]

Treatment is by surgical resection, radiation therapy, and chemotherapy. Actinomycin D and vincristine are the most commonly employed chemotherapeutic agents. Vomiting and thrombocytopenia may occur with actinomycin D. Neurotoxicity may accompany vincristine therapy in the form of paresthesias, ptosis, muscular weakness, and rarely convulsions, associated with inappropriate secretion of ADH.[627]

In more advanced stages of the disease cyclophosphamide and adriamycin may be used. Nausea, vomiting, bone marrow suppression and hemorrhagic cystitis may occur with cyclophosphamide. Cardiotoxicity with severe, intractable heart failure may occur when total adriamycin doses exceed 300 mg/m^2.[627] Chest X-ray and electrocardiogram are usually not helpful in detecting early cardiac involvement, but serial echocardiograms may be more useful.[627]

The prognosis in Wilms tumor depends on the age of the child and stage of the disease. Almost 90 percent of children under 2 years of age with an encapsulated tumor and no evidence of spread of disease have no recurrence after 4 years.

Anesthetic considerations for the resection of a Wilms tumor are those of major transabdominal, retroperitoneal surgery in the small child. The large intra-abdominal tumor may predispose the patient to regurgitation on induction. Ventilation may be compromised by the size of the tumor, abdominal retraction, or pulmonary involvement with metastases. Blood loss may be massive. Manipulation of tumor extending into the renal vein and inferior vena cava may require caval cross-clamping and introduces the danger of pulmonary embolism. Large-bore intravenous access must be secured in the upper body.[635] Central venous access via the arms or the subclavian or internal or external jugular veins serves not only as a secure route for transfusion, but also to assess volume status. If a large line is to be placed surgically for postoperative chemotherapy, it is helpful to have this done first, immediately followed by the tumor resection. An arterial line is helpful to monitor respiratory and acid-base status, as well as to provide rapid evaluation of the effects of manipulation and volume changes on blood pressure. The large abdominal exposure may cause significant loss of fluid to the "third space," and great care must be taken to provide adequate replacement to preserve optimal renal function in the remaining kidney, especially in the occasional case in which there is bilateral renal involvement. Baseline preoperative studies provide a guideline for postoperative evaluation of renal function. The large exposure also predisposes to significant heat loss, and all the usual procedures to maintain a normal body temperature are required.

Anesthesiologists may also become involved with Wilms tumor patients for repeated surgery (for example, for venous access for chemotherapy) or for radiation therapy. Particular attention should then be paid to the potential neurological, hematological, immunological, and cardiac impairment caused by chemotherapy (see above).

Sedation for radiation therapy in the uncooperative child may usually be achieved with intramuscular ketamine or rectal brevital, although the latter should probably not be utilized if immunosuppression or mucosal breakdown are present. If venous access is available, intravenous sedation of short duration (as with ketamine, pentothal, or brevital) is also effective.

Congenital mesoblastic nephroma, at times referred to as *neonatal Wilms tumor*, are relatively benign tumors that cause renal impairment because of their location and size. Treatment is by elective nephrectomy at a time when the infant's general condition is stable.[627] These tumors may be so large as to replace the whole kidney, and anesthetic considerations are similar to those cited above.

CONGENITAL ABNORMALITIES OF THE URINARY SYSTEM

Developmental Abnormalities and Associated Anomalies

Many newborns demonstrate anomalies of the urinary tract, and as much as 30 percent of pediatric surgery is dedicated to the correction of these lesions.[635] Some of these infants may also have other congenital anomalies. When these involve the musculoskeletal system, the ears, or facial development they are usually obvious. More subtle, but significant, anomalies may be present in the gastrointestinal, pulmonary, and cardiovascular systems and may escape preoperative detection. An awareness of these associated defects will help in their preoperative detection. Any unexplained cardiovascular or pulmonary response to anesthesia should rekindle the suspicion that other anomalies may coexist.

Cardiovascular malformations (CVM) are variably associated with anomalies of the urinary system and may easily escape detection in the neonatal period.[637] *Horseshoe kidney* may frequently have an associated CVM, with ventricular septal defect (VSD) and endocardial cushion defect being the most common.[637] *Bilateral renal agenesis* is associated with a 75 percent incidence of CVM, while *unilateral renal agenesis* has a 17 percent association, VSD being the most common lesion. Patients with *ectopic kidneys* and *cystic kidneys* have associated CVM in 1 in 7 cases, whereas in *renal dysplasia* the rate of CVM is 1 in 20. Fortunately, the more common congenital urinary malformations requiring surgical intervention, such as *hypospadias, cryptorchidism, urinary duplications, ureteropelvic* and *ureterovesical junction obstructions, exstrophy, urethral valves, genital anomalies,* and *Wilms tumor*, are very rarely associated with CVM.[637, 638]

While the cause for the association of cardiovascular malformations with urinary tract anomalies has not been defined, the etiological relationship between urinary tract anomalies leading to *oligohydramnios and pulmonary maldevelopment* has been established. Fetal urinary production contributes significantly to the production of amniotic fluid, which is essential for normal pulmonary development.[639] Oligohydramnios may also result in fetal compression, causing limb defects and a characteristic *Potter facies.* Severe involvement may lead to the florid *Potter syndrome,* characterized by bilateral renal agenesis (or severe cystic dysplasia) with hypoplastic lungs, the characteristic facies,

skeletal anomalies, and gastrointestinal malformations.[640] The renal agenesis may be primary, or as discussed previously, intrauterine urinary obstruction, if bilateral and severe, may lead to bilateral cystic renal dysplasia.[581, 582] Less severe degrees of obstruction may lead to varying degrees of renal and extrarenal involvement.

If the obstruction is distal, it may lead to the *"prune belly" syndrome (Eagle-Barrett syndrome)* or variations of what has come to be called the *urethral obstruction malformation complex.*[641, 642] Figure 7–15 shows the developmental pathology of the urethral obstruction malformation complex. In addition to pulmonary hypoplasia and deformities due to oligohydramnios, the severely distended bladder is thought to interfere mechanically with the development of surrounding tissues, resulting in other characteristics of the prune belly syndrome: renal dysplasia, abdominal muscular deficiency, excess abdominal skin, cryptorchidism, colonic malrotation, and lower limb deficiency.[642] Figure 7–16 is a picture of an infant with prune belly syndrome, showing his lax abdominal musculature, protuberant abdomen, and small thorax.

The prune belly syndrome occurs in 1 in 40,000 births, with a male to female ratio of 20:1. Interestingly, the females may demonstrate only the abdominal wall involvement.[643] X-linked transmission, association with chromosomal aberration, and sporadic occurrences have all been described, as well as a familial occurrence associated with pulmonic stenosis, mental retardation, and deafness.[644] There is no racial predilection. Survival depends on the severity of the renal and pulmonary involvement, with 20 percent being stillborn or dying within the first month, and 50 percent dying within 2 years.[645] Although the pathogenesis of the prune belly syndrome is still debated, recent reports have confirmed nonspecific distal urinary tract obstruction as an etiology, and in utero ultrasonic diagnosis by 21 weeks' gestation has become possible.[646-648] Furthermore, it has been suggested that early fetal surgical decompression of urinary tract obstruction may prevent the "prune belly" phenotype. Although such intervention at 21 weeks' gestation has resulted in improve-

Figure 7–15. Pathogenesis of the urethral obstruction malformation complex. The pathogenesis of the more severe degrees of this complex is interpreted as the secondary effect of bladder distention on surrounding tissues. (*From* Pagon RA, Smith DW, Shepard TH: Urethral obstruction malformation complex: a cause of abdominal muscle deficiency and the "prune belly." J Pediatr 94:900, 1979.)

Figure 7–16. Prune belly syndrome. (Photograph courtesy of Dr. Babu Koka, The Children's Hospital, Boston.)

ment in the abdominal wall laxity, it did not prevent severe pulmonary and renal involvement.[648] Infants and children with prune belly syndrome come to surgery mainly for genitourinary procedures ranging from cystoscopy to ureteric reconstruction or renal transplantation.

Anesthetic considerations for children with the prune belly syndrome must focus on the compromised renal and pulmonary status.[645, 650, 651] Pulmonary hypoplasia may be complicated by atelectasis, recurrent respiratory infection, and reduced expiratory effort and cough as a result of abdominal muscular deficiency. Preoperative antibiotic treatment of pneumonia and chest physiotherapy have been recommended to optimize the pulmonary status. The use of preoperative sedation has been discouraged for fear of respiratory depression.[649] Rapid-sequence induction with cricoid pressure to avoid regurgitation and gain rapid control of ventilation, as well as routine nasotracheal intubation in anticipation of prolonged postoperative ventilation, have also been suggested.[650, 651] Others have utilized awake intubation or, failing this, have proceeded with a mask induction with assisted ventilation.[645] Controlled intraoperative ventilation with monitoring of airway pressures, tidal volume, end-

tidal P_{CO_2}, transcutaneous hemoglobin saturation, and/or serial blood gases help safeguard the respiratory status. Muscle relaxants are rarely needed, even for extensive intra-abdominal surgery, because of the lax abdominal musculature. Avoiding muscle relaxants eliminates one variable when assessing postoperative hypoventilation. Depending on the surgical procedure, the exposure may be large, predisposing to heat and fluid loss. Preoperative evaluation of renal function will dictate fluid and electrolyte therapy and the possible need for central venous pressure monitoring. Extubation postoperatively is delayed until the patient is vigorous and demonstrates adequate ventilatory exchange as indicated by spirometry and blood gases.[645, 649, 650] Postoperative chest physiotherapy has been recommended.[645]

Obstructive Uropathy

The pathophysiology of acute and chronic obstruction in the developed kidney varies with each individual lesion. The degree and duration of obstruction, the time of onset, and the presence or absence of infection are important factors.[652] Acute ureteral obstruction initially results in an increase in afferent arteriolar blood flow and glomerular capillary pressure to compensate for the rise in tubular pressure.[653] After 24 hours of complete obstruction, however, glomerular capillary pressure and renal blood flow are depressed and GFR is markedly reduced.[653] Parenchymal renal injury may rapidly ensue (see Acute Renal Failure earlier in this chapter).

The pathophysiological changes during partial obstruction (as in *chronic obstructive nephropathy*) differ considerably.[654] Outer cortical nephrons are relatively spared and maintain their GFR, while juxtamedullary nephrons suffer markedly. The ability to concentrate urine may be lost and an obligate urinary flow results. Alterations in renal function due to partial obstruction may remain unchanged for weeks to years.[652]

Recovery of GFR after *complete* obstruction is rapid if the obstruction is relieved within an hour, but otherwise recovery may be delayed or absent.[652] With *partial* obstruction, improvement following relief of obstruction is variable and is related to the presence of hydronephrosis.[652, 654] It is generally felt that the outcome for an individual child with chronic obstructive uropathy is improved with early correction, and in infants with subnormal GFR, intervention within the first year of life appears essential to preserve the capacity to improve glomerular function.[655, 656] Even after early release of partial obstruction, the urinary concentrating capacity may remain diminished.[656] Complications arising from chronic obstruction and urinary stasis include recurrent infection and the tendency to form calculi, both of which may contribute to the progression of renal injury.[657]

Renal Anomalies and Anomalies of the Collecting System and the Lower Urinary Tract

It is because of renal injury, and complications associated with urinary obstruction, that many of the anomalies of the kidney, the collecting system, and the lower urinary tract are significant to the urologist and anesthesiologist.

Renovascular anomalies include renal arterial narrowing due to *fibromuscular dysplasia* or *intrarenal aneurysm* and may result in marked hypertension. Treatment is by segmental or total nephrectomy, percutaneous transluminal angioplasty, or segmental arterial embolization.[124, 658, 659] *Anomalous renal vessels* may become clinically significant because they obstruct ureteral flow.[657, 660] *Supernumary kidneys, malrotation, renal fusion,* and *renal ectopia* (*simple ectopia*, or *crossed ectopia* in which the ureter enters the bladder on the contralateral side) may all be associated with ureteral obstruction. This may be due to bands, aberrant vessels, or tortuous ureteral pathways from kidney to bladder.[661] *Hydronephrosis, ureteral strictures and duplications*, and associated skeletal, central nervous system, cardiovascular, and gastrointestinal tract anomalies may be present.[635] *Fused and ectopic kidneys* may also be more vulnerable to traumatic injury because of their location and fixation.[661]

The ureter may also be the site of developmental anomalies that cause urinary obstruction. The *ureteropelvic junction* is the most common site of supravesical obstruction in children. Such obstruction occurs as a result of intrinsic narrowing or angulation due to aberrant vessels to the lower pole of the kidney or fibrous bands.[657] Obstetric ultrasound may occasionally detect the lesion in utero. Twenty-five percent of such lesions are detected in the first year of life because of a palpable mass, abdominal pain, hematuria, or urinary tract infection. Isosthenuria may occur, but renal insufficiency occurs only late in bilateral obstruction or obstruction of a solitary system.[657] *Ureteral stricture, valves, polyps, retrocaval ureter,* and *idiopathic retroperitoneal fibrosis*[662] may all cause ureteral obstruction.

The second most common site of ureteral obstruction is at the *ureterovesical junction*. The most frequently encountered problem resulting from obstruction at this location is *megaureter*.[657] Although any ureter greater than 1 cm in diameter, regardless of cause, has nonspecifically been called megaureter, *"primary megaureter"* refers to the condition in which the distal ureteral segment is aperistaltic and acts as a functional obstruction.[657] There is a male preponderance, the left side is more frequently involved, and it may be bilateral in 20 percent of children. The usual mode of presentation is with hematuria or urinary tract infection.[663] Treatment is by surgical resection of the aperistaltic segment, tailoring of the dilated ureter, and reimplantation.

Ureteral ectopia, ureteroceles, ureteropelvic and *ureteral* duplications (*complete, partial, or blind-ending*), and *bladder diverticuli* are other developmental anomalies of the urinary collecting system that may cause ureteral obstruction.[657, 661] *Ureteropelvic duplication* is a common anomaly occurring in 1 in 160 individuals, and patients are usually asymptomatic,[635] although obstruction and recurrent infection may occur.

A further major concern in these lesions is *reflux*. *Ureteroureteral reflux* may occur in proximal partial ureteropelvic duplications, but more frequently occurs with *complete ureteral duplications* and *ectopic ureteral implantation*.[661]

Vesicoureteral reflux may occur as a result of these developmental anomalies or secondary to primary incompetence of the functional, interdigitating ureteral–bladder wall valve; elevated intravesical voiding pressures due to bladder malfunction; fixation of the orifice by bladder wall trabeculation; a neurogenic bladder; or even transient, acute inflammation due to infection.[652, 664, 665] The long-term consequences of reflux depend on the cause, severity, age and degree of renal injury at presentation, the presence of infection, the degree of compliance with medical therapy, and probably many other unknown factors.[652, 666, 667] Normal renal function at presentation favors a good prognosis, whereas existing renal impairment represents a poor prognostic sign regardless of medical or surgical intervention.[652]

Because of the heterogeneity of causes and the complexity of factors influencing outcome, controversy persists as to the proper therapeutic approach and the timing of surgery.[664, 665] Large prospective studies are under way to answer these questions.[669] It is clear that even if vesicoureteral reflux is not in itself intrinsically injurious and one half to two thirds of children may outgrow primary vesicoureteral reflux, ascending bacterial infection is severely damaging, especially in younger children.[664] Bilateral vesicoureteral reflux and recurrent infection may cause severe, atrophic parenchymal scarring and renal insufficiency. Unilateral disease may be associated with hypertension and systemic infection, which are risks to long-term well being.[652] Antireflux surgery has been shown to be effective with respect to resolution of reflux and prevention of upper urinary infection.[668, 670] Such surgery obviates the need for long-term antibiotic therapy and repeated radiological investigations. It is clearly indicated for severe reflux, for reflux that is not resolving with age, and for children in families in which compliance with chronic medication and continued medical follow-up is a problem.[652]

Ureteroneocystostomy (ureteral reimplantation) is the usual surgical procedure in primary reflux. A new, relatively long ureteral submucosal tunnel is created and effectively functions as a valve, preventing reflux.[671] Reflux secondary to bladder abnormalities may require urinary diversion.

Anesthetic considerations for surgery for ureteral

obstruction or reflux focus primarily on the type and degree of renal involvement. Hypertension may be present in as many as 25 percent of children with reflux and renal scarring, independent of the degree of azotemia. Antihypertensives may need to be continued perioperatively. Preoperative evaluation should determine whether chronic obstruction has led to a concentrating defect with an obligatory urine output and whether a degree of azotemia exists. Pre- and intraoperative fluid therapy should be managed accordingly. Intraoperative volume assessment may be complicated by the inability to collect and measure urine output because of drainage into the surgical field. An experienced surgeon may be able to estimate the amount of urine flow, or be willing to collect and measure urine in the field; for example, an open ureter may be placed in a sterile glove while not being manipulated. In children with significant renal impairment and/or hypertension, invasive monitoring with an arterial and a central venous pressure catheter will aid in fluid and anesthetic management. All the anesthetic considerations for renal failure discussed previously may need to be observed.

The surgical approach will vary with the procedure and the size of the patient. A lateral decubitus position, flank incision, and retroperitoneal approach may be preferred in older children to avoid bowel manipulation, adhesions, and obstruction. Care must be taken to provide appropriate and adequate padding, and ventilation and blood pressure should be carefully monitored during positioning. Extremes in angulation and tilting may significantly alter pulmonary and cardiovascular dynamics, decrease venous return, and result in hypotension. Smaller infants, and certain procedures, may require a transperitoneal approach. This demands greater abdominal muscular relaxation, and on occasion the avoidance of nitrous oxide to prevent gaseous bowel distention from interfering in the surgical field. A large surgical exposure will predispose to significant heat and fluid loss in small children.

Congenital anomalies of the bladder and urethra such as *duplications, cysts, strictures, polyps, stenoses,* and *valves* may all cause urinary obstruction and stasis. The most significant of these lesions is *posterior urethral valves.* The degree of obstruction is variable, and if minor obstruction is included, it is the most common obstructive anomaly in male children.[672] Severe in utero obstruction may lead to the *urethral obstruction malformation complex* as described above. Male neonates may present with flank masses or a palpable bladder. Hydronephrosis, renal dysplasia, and azotemia may be complicated by acidosis, hyperkalemia, hyponatremia, and sepsis, requiring fluid and electrolyte resuscitation, antibiotic therapy, and emergent urinary drainage.[657] This is usually accomplished with the placement of a small urethral catheter, but may sometimes require a suprapubic vesicostomy or urinary diversion.[657] Older children have less severe obstruction and symptoms

may be limited to urinary hesitancy, frequency, and incontinence. Cystoscopy, voiding cystourethrography, and urodynamic studies will confirm the diagnosis. Transurethral resection is usually possible, but occasionally urethral reconstruction is required.

A *neuropathic bladder* may also cause urinary stasis and obstruction and lead to infection, reflux, and renal parenchymal injury.[673] Myelomeningocele is the most common etiology in children, but neuropathic bladder may also result from diastematomyelia, tethered cord syndrome, sacral agenesis or dysgenesis, spinal tumors, pelvic surgery, trauma, transverse myelitis, and osteomyelitis of the vertebral column.[673] Cystoscopy, voiding cystourethrography, and urodynamic studies are used in the evaluation of the lesion and response to treatment. Aggressive antibiotic therapy, manual expression of the bladder (Credé maneuver), intermittent catheterization, drug therapy, and implantation of artificial sphincters are all designed to prevent the complications of urinary stasis and provide acceptable forms of urinary drainage.[674]

Several pharmacological agents have been employed in an attempt to alter the parasympathetic and sympathetic influence on bladder and urethral sphincter tone. Imipramine, a tricyclic antidepressant that blocks reuptake of norepinephrine in nerve terminals and has prominent anticholinergic effects, increases bladder outlet resistance and decreases bladder contractility. This sometimes leads to continence.[675] Phenoxybenzamine, an alpha-adrenergic blocker, has been used to decrease bladder outlet resistance and allow more complete bladder emptying in children who are able to void voluntarily.[676] On the other hand, ephedrine and phenylpropanolamine have been used as alpha-adrenergic agonists to increase bladder outlet resistance in children on intermittent catheterization programs in whom incontinence has been a problem.[673, 674] Likewise, when incontinence is felt to be due to bladder contraction, anticholinergic agents such as propantheline and oxybutynin have been used to reduce bladder (detrusor muscle) tone. By contrast, bladder contraction has been stimulated with cholinergic agents such as bethanacol and carbachol in cases of transient retention following spinal cord surgery.[673] Finally, diazepam and dantrolene have been used in an attempt to relieve external (voluntary) sphincter spasm,[674, 678] but surgical division by urethrotomy is often required for this problem.[673]

Which drugs are employed in a given child will depend on whether voluntary voiding or catheterization is the goal, whether incontinence is due to increased bladder tone or decreased internal sphincter tone, or whether a large residual urine volume is the principal problem. These drugs have significant interactions with anesthetic, adrenergic, anticholinergic, and neuromuscular blocking and reversal agents commonly employed during anesthesia. In addition, they may interact with antihypertensive medications that the patient may be taking. It is therefore important for the anesthesiologist to determine which, if any, of these drugs the patient is taking, and what interactions might be expected.

Cystoscopy, voiding cystourethrography, and urodynamic studies are important procedures in the urological evaluation of bladder abnormalities. In pediatric practice these studies are usually performed with the patient under anesthesia. Just as the drugs described above may affect bladder and sphincter tone, so also may anesthetics and other drugs commonly employed during anesthesia. As a result, anesthesia for cystoscopy and urodynamic studies must not only address the issues of patient safety but also attempt to provide conditions under which the results of the urodynamic studies are valid. For example, laryngospasm upon urethral instrumentation (the Breuer-Luckhardt reflex) may occur if the depth of anesthesia is inadequate, while a very light anesthetic, almost to the point of awakening, is required to allow voiding to occur for a voiding cystourethrogram.[635] Bladder activity and sphincter tone may be suppressed for up to 10 minutes following the use of thiopental or potent inhalational agents and reliable results during urodynamic measurement requires the use of only nitrous oxide and oxygen.[679] Atropine is commonly used in children to dry secretions, to decrease the potential for laryngospasm, and to counteract bradycardia. Unfortunately, it also relaxes bladder tone and invalidates the results of urodynamic studies.[635] It has been suggested that the risks of regurgitation and laryngospasm, which may accompany the rapid changes required in anesthetic depth, may be diminished if intravenous lidocaine (1 to 1.5 mg/kg repeatable after 5 minutes) is used to smooth out these transitions.[680]

There are many congenital anomalies of the bladder and lower genitourinary tract that do not lead to obstruction and consequent renal involvement but do require surgical intervention. Perhaps the most dramatic of these are the *exstrophic anomalies*, which may range from *epispadias* to complete *cloacal exstrophy*. The cleft may be so large as to extend up the abdomen to the thorax. Associated anomalies are usually genitourinary and gastrointestinal, but may include cleft palate, chromosomal abnormalities, and cardiac malformations.[635]

Bladder exstrophy has an incidence of 1 in 10,000 to 1 in 50,000 live births, with twice as many males affected as females.[681] Exstrophy of the bladder has been reported in twins and siblings, but familial inheritance is rare and sporadic occurrence is the rule.[682] The problems associated with bladder exstrophy include incontinence with subsequent discomfort and social ostracism, squamous metaplasia of bladder mucosa, and a predisposition many years later to malignancy, most commonly adenocarcinoma.[682] Following bladder reconstruction or urinary diversion, the problems of upper urinary tract deterioration, obstruction, formation of calculi, infection, and reflux may lead to renal impairment.[681, 682] Although the timing and

staging of surgical repair remain controversial, several authors suggest that it may be advantageous to perform the surgery on an urgent basis.[681, 682] Early closure may decrease inflammatory changes in the bladder and limit perimuscular fibrosis.[681] Possibly because of the persistent influence of the maternal hormone relaxin, approximation of the pubes may be accomplished without iliac osteotomies in the first day or two of life.[681, 682] After this time it is often necessary to divide the bony pelvic ring to relieve tension at the pubic symphysis. This requires bilateral iliac osteotomies, a major and time-consuming procedure that is done with the patient in the prone position prior to attempted bladder reconstruction and may add significantly to the operative risk.[682] A further advantage to early operative intervention is that if bladder closure can be accomplished prior to bacterial colonization of the gastrointestinal tract, sterility of the urinary system may be more readily preserved.

There are many *anomalies of the urethra and genitalia*, including *malposition, dorsal or ventral duplications*, and *diverticuli*, as well as acquired lesions that are of functional and cosmetic significance.[683-685] The most common of these anomalies is *hypospadias*, which has an incidence of 8 per 1000 male births and varies in severity from the mild coronal variety to the severe penoscrotal type.[683] There is some evidence to suggest that maternal ingestion of synthetic progestins may be a cause of hypospadias,[686] and there have been reports of a familial incidence.[687] Associated anomalies are usually restricted to the lower genitourinary system (hernia, hydrocele, cryptorchidism), but major anomalies of the upper urinary tract may also occur.[685] Although the timing of surgery is still debated, repair may begin by 6 months of age; even with a severe lesion requiring multiple stages, the repair is usually concluded by 4 to 5 years of age.[683, 685]

Almost any form of anesthesia may be used for hypospadias repair, as long as the anesthesiologist takes care to meet the special needs of small infants being anesthetized, such as limitation of heat loss and maintenance of fluid balance. Nitrous oxide plus narcotic anesthesia or light volatile anesthesia may be associated with penile erection, which is bothersome to the surgeon. This is usually easily resolved by deepening the anesthetic with a volatile agent or with intravenous ketamine.[683, 687a, 687b] This problem may also be corrected by the surgeon by manually forcing drainage of the corpora cavernosa and applying a rubber band tourniquet to prevent reinflation. It is important to take note and advise the surgeon of the elapsed tourniquet time in this instance.

Recent anesthetic reports have focused on the use of regional techniques (dorsal penile nerve block versus caudal anesthesia) to provide postoperative analgesia after hypospadias repair or circumcision.[688, 689, 692, 693] Although most of these blocks have been performed at the conclusion of the procedure, some authors have suggested placing caudal blocks immediately after the induction of anesthesia in order to reduce general anesthetic requirements.[690] Spinal anesthesia has been used as the sole anesthetic in high-risk infants for cystoscopy with fulguration of urethral valves and for circumcision.[691] An advantage of caudal and spinal anesthesia is that penile erection is blocked.[683] The techniques of nerve block, caudal, and spinal anesthesia in infants are described in detail elsewhere.[278]

It is important to differentiate penile erection during light anesthesia from pathological *priapism*, as is associated with obstructed venous drainage in *sickle cell anemia, leukemia, trauma*, and *Fabry disease* (a glycosphingolipid storage disease).[683] Regional anesthesia and ketamine are ineffective in these mechanical, obstructive causes and treatment is directed at the underlying illness (oxygenation and hypertransfusion in sickle cell disease, radiation and chemotherapy in leukemia, plasma transfusion in Fabry disease, and surgical drainage in trauma and for other failed therapies).[683, 687a, 687b]

There are many congenital and acquired lesions of the scrotum and testes, some of which require urgent surgical intervention, such as *torsion of the testicle*.[694, 695] *Cryptorchidism* (*undescended testes*) is the most common anomaly, and occurs with an incidence of 1 percent in term infants and much more frequently in prematures, the incidence increasing with decreasing gestational age.[685, 695] The chance of complete spontaneous testicular descent after infancy is small, with the testis suffering degenerative changes proportionate to its delay in reaching the scrotum.[695] Problems associated with cryptorchidism include inguinal hernia, torsion, trauma, malignancy, and infertility.[694, 695] Hormonal treatment to induce descent is only partially successful and is associated with side effects including premature puberty. Orchiopexy is therefore usually performed at an early age in an effort to improve fertility, prevent testicular malignancy (and make it more readily detectable should it occur), and to repair the associated hernia. Anesthesia for orchiopexy includes the same considerations as those for genital and inguinal hernia surgery in infants, and regional techniques for postoperative analgesia (ilioinguinal and iliohypogastric nerve blocks and caudal anesthesia) have been effective.[690] Traction on the testicle and/or peritoneum may induce a marked vagal response in infants, for which anticholinergic blockade with atropine is helpful. On occasion the search for an undescended testicle may extend into an intra-abdominal, retroperitoneal exploration. In this case endotracheal intubation and controlled ventilation may be advisable, and abdominal muscular relaxation may be helpful.

ENDOCRINE FUNCTION AND GENITOURINARY ABNORMALITIES

Renal function and genitourinary development are intimately related to endocrine function. The kidney is not only the target organ for such hormones as aldosterone and antidiuretic hormone but also the endocrine source of renin and erythropoietin and a significant site of metabolism of hormones (for example, gastrin and insulin). The effects of renal injury and failure on some of these interactions have already been discussed.

The *syndrome of inappropriate antidiuretic hormone secretion* (*SIADH*) is an example of a disease state in which normal renal function may lead to a dangerously pathological condition: severe hyponatremia and hypoosmolarity.[696] Excessive secretion of antidiuretic hormone (due to a neurological insult or other causes) promotes tubular reabsorption of water. Although definitive treatment must be directed at the underlying cause of ADH secretion, it may be necessary to impose conditions that make the excessive ADH secretion and the normal renal response appropriate; this is accomplished by severe fluid restriction. Another temporizing solution is to interfere with normal tubular function in order to prevent the detrimental effects of water reabsorption. This may be accomplished by the administration of diuretics, ethanol, or lithium with careful attention to the electrolyte disturbances that may result.[696] In children with convulsions or coma due to hyponatremia, the infusion of hypertonic saline results in transient improvement. (A sodium dose of 6 mEq/kg will transiently raise the serum sodium by 10 mEq/L.[696]) The associated risk is that the hypertonic saline will contribute to the already expanded extracellular volume, inducing circulatory overload.[696] Anesthesia in such children requires careful attention to volume and electrolyte status and therapy.

Adrenogenital syndrome (*congenital adrenal hyperplasia*) is an example of a disease state in which the development of the genitourinary system is affected. Deficiency of adrenal C-21-hydroxylase activity results in virilization of females with occasional severe salt wasting. C-11-hydroxylase deficiency may be associated with severe hypertension.[635, 697] These defects are thought to be autosomal recessive and vary in incidence from 1 in 50,000 live births to 1 in 500 live births among natives of southwestern Alaska.[697] Treatment with exogenous cortisone inhibits ACTH secretion and provides the deficient adrenal end product. This decreases the accumulation of intermediate products of cortisol synthesis that cause virilization, and helps reverse electrolyte abnormalities such as hyponatremia and hyperkalemia.[635, 697] Females will often present for surgical correction of malformed genitalia between 2 and 4 years of age. However, undiagnosed newborn males with dehydration, electrolyte abnormalities, and vomiting may present for surgery with a misdiagnosis of pyloric stenosis or intestinal obstruction.[697] Anesthetic care in these children requires careful preoperative evaluation of their volume and electrolyte status and a continuation of their steroid therapy. The acute stress of surgery or illness may require an increase in their steroid coverage by one and a half times to three times their normal dosage, although excessive administration may lead to sodium retention and hypertension.[680, 697] Since these children are often placed in a extreme lithotomy or knee-to-chest position, endotracheal intubation and controlled ventilation is recommended.[697] Because of the potential for partial recovery from pancuronium neuromuscular blockade following hydrocortisone administration, intraoperative monitoring of neuromuscular blockade is useful.[698, 699]

RENAL AND GENITOURINARY TRAUMA

Blunt or penetrating trauma to the back, abdomen, pelvis, or perineum may result in injury to the kidneys, ureters, bladder, urethra, or genitalia.[700, 701] Up to 7 percent of all childhood injuries may involve the genitourinary system and require urgent surgical intervention.[700] Injury may be obvious, or it may be occult, resulting in retroperitoneal, intrapelvic, or intra-abdominal urinary leakage or bleeding. In up to 40 percent of children, trauma sufficient to cause renal injury is accompanied by cerebral, spinal, bony, pulmonary, abdominal visceral, and vascular trauma which may dictate the initial emergency management.[702] Adequate resuscitation and stabilization should precede radiological investigation, surgical exploration, and operative repair. Complications of renal injury include secondary hemorrhage, persistent urinary extravasation, perinephric abscess, hypertension secondary to segmental ischemia, renal stones, renal scarring, renal atrophy, and renal failure.[700] Anesthetic considerations are those for resuscitation and major trauma, along with the principles of management of patients with impending acute renal failure, as discussed previously.

PSYCHOLOGICAL CONSIDERATIONS

Whether a child suffers from chronic renal failure, requiring frequent medical intervention, or a disfiguring genitourinary malformation, requiring extensive surgical repair, the psychological and social impacts on the child and family are profound.[219] In severe, untreated, or unsuccessfully treated bladder exstrophy, for example, there is a high pubertal incidence of psychiatric problems, including a significant suicide rate.[681] Children made dependent on others by their illness may demonstrate behavior inappropriate to their chronological age, especially in the hospital setting. Additional time, effort, and empathy are required of the anesthesiologist to communicate with the child and his family and to allay anxieties associated with anesthesia and surgery. Time invested preoperatively in gaining a child's understanding and trust is invaluable to the child. It may also be invaluable to the anesthesiologist when soliciting the child's cooperation during difficult venipuncture prior to induction of

anesthesia, or for other unpleasant but necessary interventions.

Supported in part by the Children's Hospital Medical Center Anesthesia Foundation, Inc., Boston, Massachusetts. The author also wishes to acknowledge the advice and support of Milton H. Alper, M.D., Dolly D. Hansen, M.D., Paul R. Hickey, M.D., and Dorothy J. M. Cramolini, R.N.

REFERENCES

1. Berry FA: The Renal System. *In* Gregory GA (Ed.): Pediatric Anesthesia. New York, Churchill Livingstone, 1983, pp 63–128.
2. Spitzer A: Renal physiology and functional development. *In* Edelmann CM Jr (Ed.): Pediatric Kidney Disease. Boston, Little, Brown, 1978, pp 25–128.
3. Bricker NS, Bourgoignie JJ, Licht AA, et al.: Pathophysiology of chronic renal failure. *In* Edelmann CM Jr (Ed.): Pediatric Kidney Disease. Boston, Little, Brown, 1978, pp 205–212.
4. Kuruvila KC, Schrier RW: Chronic renal failure. Int Anesthesiol Clin 22:101, 1984.
5. Easterling RE: Racial factors in the incidence and causation of end stage renal disease. Trans Am Soc Artif Intern Organs 23:28, 1977.
6. Rostand SG, Kirk KA, Rutsky EA, et al.: Racial differences in the incidence of treatment for end stage renal disease. N Engl J Med 306:1276, 1982.
7. Chantler C, Carter JE, Bewick M, et al.: 10 years' experience with regular haemodialysis and renal transplantation. Arch Dis Child 55:435, 1980.
8. Barratt TM, Baillod RA: Chronic renal failure and regular dialysis. *In* Williams DI, Johnston JH (Eds.): Paediatric Urology. London, Butterworth Scientific, 1982, pp 37–47.
9. Schwartz GJ, Feld LG, Langford DJ: A simple estimate of glomerular filtration rate in full term infants during the first year of life. J Pediatr 104:849, 1984.
10. Schwartz GJ, Haycock GB, Edelmann CM Jr, et al.: A simple estimate of glomerular filtration rate in children derived from body length and plasma creatinine. Pediatrics 58:259, 1976.
11. Barratt TM: Renal function. *In* Williams DI, Johnston JH (Eds.): Paediatric Urology. London, Butterworth Scientific, 1982, pp 1–10.
12. Platt R: Structural and functional adaption in renal failure. Br Med J 1:1313, 1372, 1952.
13. Bricker NS: The pathogenesis of the uremic state: the "trade-off" hypothesis. N Engl J Med 286:1093, 1972.
14. Lewy PR, Hurley JK: Chronic renal insufficiency. Pediatr Clin North Am 23:829, 1976.
15. Schrier RW, Regal EM: Influence of aldosterone on sodium, water and potassium metabolism in chronic renal disease. Kidney Int 1:156, 1972.
16. Wilkinson R, Luetcher JA, Dowdy AS, et al.: Studies on the mechanism of sodium excretion in uremia. Clin Sci 42:685, 1972.
17. Carriere S, Wong NLM, Kirks JH: Redistribution of renal blood flow in acute and chronic reduction of renal mass. Kidney Int 3:364, 1973.
18. Kahn T, Mohammad G, Stein RM: Alterations in renal tubular sodium and water reabsorption in chronic renal disease in man. Kidney Int 2:164, 1972.
19. Bourgoignie JJ, Hwang KH, Espinel C, et al.: A natriuretic factor in the serum of patients with chronic uremia. J Clin Invest 51:1514, 1972.

20. Bricker NS, Klahr S, Lubowitz H, et al.: On the biology of sodium excretion: the search for a natriuretic hormone. Yale J Biol Med 48:293, 1975.

21. Fine LG, Bourgoignie JJ, Weber H, et al.: Enhanced end-organ responsiveness of the uremic kidney to the natriuretic factor. Kidney Int 10:364, 1976.

22. Bricker, NS: Sodium homeostasis in chronic renal disease. Kidney Int 21:886, 1982.

23. Bourgoignie JJ, Jacob AI, Sollman L, et al.: Water, electrolyte and acid base abnormalities in chronic renal failure. Semin Nephrol 1:91, 1981.

24. Berl T, Schrier RW: Water metabolism and the hypoosmolar syndromes. In Brenner B, Stein J (Eds.): Chronic Renal Failure. New York, Churchill Livingstone, 1981.

25. Blaufox MD: Systemic arterial hypertension in pediatric practice. Pediatr Clin North Am 18:577, 1971.

26. Kurtzmann NA: Chronic renal failure: metabolic and clinical consequences. Hosp Prac 17:107, 1982.

27. Fine LG, Kaplan M, Bricker NS: Disturbances of salt and water metabolism in chronic renal failure. In Edelmann CM Jr (Ed.): Pediatric Kidney Disease. Boston, Little, Brown, 1978, pp 348–356.

28. Nash MA: Water and solute homeostasis. In Edelmann CM Jr (Ed.): Pediatric Kidney Disease. Boston, Little, Brown, 1978, pp 290–305.

29. Tasker PRW, MacGregor GA, de Wardener HE: Prophylactic use of intravenous saline in patients with chronic renal failure undergoing major surgery. Lancet 2:911, 1974.

30. Trainin EB, Spitzer A: Treatment of acute renal failure. In Edelmann CM Jr (Ed.): Pediatric Kidney Disease. Boston, Little, Brown, 1978, pp 466–474.

31. Bastron RD, Deutsch S: Anesthesia for the functionally anephric patient. In Bastron RD, Deutsch S (Eds.): Anesthesia and the Kidney—The Scientific Basis of Clinical Anesthesia. New York, Grune & Stratton, 1976.

32. Rudolph AM: Disturbances of the cardiovascular system. In Edelmann CM Jr (Ed.): Pediatric Kidney Disease. Boston, Little, Brown, 1978, pp 429–432.

33. Zauder HL: Anesthesia for patients who have terminal renal disease. In Hershey SG (Ed.): Refresher Courses in Anesthesiology. Vol 4, Chapter 14. Park Ridge, IL, American Society of Anesthesiologists, 1976.

34. Koide M, Waud BE: Serum potassium concentrations after succinylcholine in patients with renal failure. Anesthesiology 36:142, 1972.

35. Tammisto T, Leikkonen P, Airaksinen M: The inhibitory effect of D-tubocurarine on the increase of serum creatinine kinase activity produced by intermittent suxamethonium administration during halothane anesthesia. Acta Anaesthesiol Scand 11:333, 1967.

36. Miller RD, Way WL, Hamilton WK, et al.: Succinylcholine-induced hyperkalemia in patients with renal failure. Anesthesiology 36:138, 1972.

37. Walton JD, Farman JV: Suxamethonium, potassium and renal failure. Anaesthesia 28:626, 1973.

38. Roth F, Wüthrich H: The clinical importance of hyperkalemia following suxamethonium administration. Br J Anaesth 41:311, 1969.

39. Powell DR, Miller R: The effect of repeated doses of succinylcholine on serum potassium in patients with renal failure. Anesth Analg 54:746, 1975.

40. Walton JD, Farman JV: Suxamethonium hyperkalaemia in uraemic neuropathy. Anaesthesia 28:666, 1973.

41. Kildeberg P, Engel K, Winter RW: Balance of net acid in growing infants. Acta Paediatr Scand 58:321, 1969.

42. Salcedo JR, Jackson ML, Coleman TN, et al.: Endogenous net acid production in infants, children and adults. Pediatr Res 10:443, 1976.

43. Winters RW, Chan JC, Klenk EL, et al.: Net acid balance in metabolic acidosis. Pediatr Res 5:395, 1971.

44. Lockhart E, Edelmann CM Jr: Acid-base disturbances in renal failure, In Edelmann CM Jr (Ed.): Pediatric Kidney Disease. Boston, Little, Brown, 1978, pp 357–365.

45. de Torrenté A: Acute renal failure. Int Anesthesiol Clin 22:83, 1984.

46. Wrong O, Davies HEF: The excretion of acid in renal disease. Q J Med 28:259, 1959.

47. Schwarz WB, Hall PW, Hays RM, et al.: On the mechanism of acidosis in chronic renal disease. Q J Clin Invest 38:39, 1956.

48. Arruda JAL: Acidosis of renal failure. Semin Nephrol 1:275, 1982.

49. Dubose TD Jr: Acid-base physiology in uremia. Artif Organs 6:363, 1982.

50. Litzow J, Lemann J, Lennon E: The effect of treatment of acidosis on calcium balance in patients with chronic azotemic renal disease. J Clin Invest 46:280, 1967.

51. Avioli LV, Teitelbaum SL: Renal osteodystrophy. In Edelmann CM Jr (Ed.): Pediatric Renal Disease. Boston, Little, Brown, 1978, pp 366–400.

52. Cooke RE, Boyden DG, Haller E: The relationship of acidosis and growth retardation. J Pediatr 57:326, 1960.

53. Burnell S, Villamil M, Vyero B, et al.: Effect in humans of extracellular pH on the relationship between serum potassium concentration and intracellular potassium. J Clin Invest 35:935, 1956.

54. Müller MC: Anesthesia for the patient with renal dysfunction. Int Anesthesiol Clin 22:169, 1984.

55. Goggin MJ, Joekes AM: Gas exchange in renal failure. Dangers of hyperkalemia during anesthesia. Br J Med 2:244, 1971.

56. Norman ME: Vitamin D in bone disease. Pediatr Clin N Am 29:947, 1982.

57. Fine RN, Isaacson AS, Payne V, et al.: Renal osteodystrophy in children: the effect of hemodialysis and renal transplantation. J Pediatr 80:243, 1972.

58. Norman ME, Mazur AT, Borden S, et al.: Early diagnosis of juvenile renal osteodystrophy. J Pediatr 97:226, 1980.

59. Cunningham J, Avioli LV: Systemic acidosis and the bioactivation of vitamin D. In Abstracts of the Fifth Workshop on Vitamin D. Williamsburg, VA, Feb 14–19, 1982.

60. Boischis H, Winterborn MH: Acute renal failure in childhood. Pediatr Ann 3:58, 1974.

61. Ott SM, Coburn JW, Alfrey AC, et al.: The prevalence of bone aluminum deposition in renal osteodystrophy and its relation to the response to calcitriol therapy. N Engl J Med 307:709, 1982.

62. Firor HV, Moore ES, Levitsky LL, et al.: Parathyroidectomy in children with chronic renal failure. J Pediatr Surg 7:565, 1972.

63. McKie BD: Hypocalcaemia and prolonged curarization. Br J Anaesth 41:1091, 1969.

64. Pender JW, Basso LV: Diseases of the endocrine system. In Katz J, Benumof J, Kadis LB (Eds.): Anesthesia and Uncommon Diseases. Philadelphia, W.B. Saunders Co., 1981, pp 155–220.

65. Steele TH, Wen SF, Evenson MA, et al.: The contribution of the chronically diseased kidney to magnesium homeostasis in man. J Lab Clin Med 71:455, 1968.

66. Ferdinandus J, Pederson JA, Whang R: Hypermagnesemia as a cause of refractory hypotension, respiratory depression and coma. Arch Intern Med 141:669, 1981.

67. Ghoneim MM, Long JP: The interaction between magnesium and other neuromuscular blocking agents. Anesthesiology 32:23, 1970.

68. Fried W: Hematologic abnormalities in chronic renal failure. Semin Nephrol 1:176, 1981.

69. Kasanen A, Kalliomaki JL: Correlation of some kidney function tests with hemoglobin in chronic nephropathies. Acta Med Scand 158:213, 1957.

70. O'Brien RT, Pearson HA: Hematologic disturbances in uremia. In Edelmann CM Jr (Ed.): Pediatric Renal Disease. Boston, Little, Brown 1978, pp 401–407.

71. Brown R: Plasma erythropoietin in chronic uremia. Br Med J 2:1036, 1965.

72. Fisher JW, Hatch FE, Roh BL, et al.: Erythropoietin

inhibitors in kidney extracts and plasma from anemic uremic human subjects Blood 31:440, 1968.

73. Radtke HW, Rege AB, LaMarche MB, et al.: Identification of spermine as an inhibitor of erythropoiesis in patients with chronic renal failure. J Clin Invest 67:1623, 1981.

74. Shaw AB: Hemolysis in chronic renal failure. Br Med J 2:213, 1967.

75. Giovannetti S, Balestri PL, Cioni L: Spontaneous in vitro auto-haemolysis of blood from chronic uremic patients. Clin Sci 29:407, 1965.

76. Joske RA, McAlister JM, Prankerd TAJ: Isotope investigations of red cell production and destruction in chronic renal disease. Clin Sci 15:511, 1956.

77. Giovannetti S, Cioni L, Balestri PL, et al.: Evidence that guanidines and some related compounds cause haemolysis in chronic uremia. Clin Sci 34:141, 1968.

78. Shainkin R, Giatt Y, Berlyne G: The presence and toxicity of guanidino-proprionic acid in uremia. Kidney Int 7:S302, 1975.

79. Merrill JP: Uremia. N Engl J Med 282:1014, 1970.

80. Lonergan ET, Semar M, Sterzel RB, et al.: Erythrocyte transketolase activity in dialyzed patients. N Engl J Med 284:1399, 1971.

81. Aherne WA: The "burr" red cell and azotemia. J Clin Pathol 10:252, 1957.

82. Lichtman MA, Miller DR, Abel V, et al.: Erythrocyte glycolysis, 2,3-diphosphoglycerate and adenosine triphosphate concentration in uremic subjects: relationship to extracellular phosphate concentration. J Lab Clin Med 76:267, 1970.

83. Lichtman MA, Murphy MS, Byer BJ, et al.: Hemoglobin affinity for oxygen in chronic renal disease: effect of hemodialysis. Blood 43:417, 1974.

83a. Potter D, Feduska N, Melzer J, et al: Twenty years of renal transplantation in children. Pediatrics 77:465, 1986.

84. Vincenti F, Duca RM, Amend W, et al.: Immunologic factors determining survival of cadaver kidney transplants: effect of HLA serotyping, cytotoxic antibodies and blood transfusions on graft survival. N Engl J Med 299:793, 1978.

85. Opelz G, Terasaki PI: Improvement of kidney graft survival with increased number of transfusions. N Engl Med 299:799, 1978.

86. Eschbach JW, Funk D, Adamson J, et al.: Erythropoiesis in patients with renal failure undergoing chronic dialysis. N Engl J Med 276:653, 1967.

87. Bozzini EE, Devoto FC, Tomio JM: Decreased responsiveness of hematopoietic tissue to erythropoietin in acutely uremic rats. J Lab Clin Med 68:411, 1966.

88. Hoffman GS: Human erythropoiesis following kidney transplantation. Ann NY Acad Sci 149:504, 1968.

89. Miller RD: Complications of massive blood transfusions. Anesthesiology 39:82, 1973.

90. Ellis DE, Stoelting RK: Individual variations in fluroxene, halothane, and methoxyflurane blood-gas partition coefficients and the effect of anemia. Anesthesiology 42:748, 1975.

91. Hampers CL, Blaufox MD, Merrill JP: Anticoagulation rebound after hemodialysis. N Engl J Med 275:776, 1966.

92. Stewart JH: Platelet numbers and life span in acute and chronic renal failure. Thromb Diath Haemorrh 17:532, 1967.

93. Horowitz HI, Stein IM, Cohen BD, et al.: Further studies on the platelet inhibitory effect of guanidinosuccinic acid and its role in uremic bleeding. Am J Med 49:336, 1970.

94. Rabiner SF, Molinas F: The role of phenol and phenolic acids on the thrombocytopathy and defective platelet aggregation of patients with renal failure. Am J Med 49:346, 1970.

95. Eknoyan G, Wacksman SJ, Glueck HI, et al.: Platelet function in renal failure. N Engl J Med 280:667, 1969.

96. Rabiner SF, Hrodek O: Platelet factor 3 in normal subjects and patients with renal failure. J Clin Invest 47:901, 1968.

97. Stewart JH, Castaldi PA: Uremic bleeding: a reversible platelet defect corrected by dialysis. Q J Med 36:409, 1967.

98. Lindsay RM, Moorthy AV, Koens F, et al.: Platelet function in dialyzed and non-dialyzed patients with chronic renal failure. Clin Nephrol 4:52, 1975.

99. Fischback DP, Fogdall RP: Coagulation: The Essentials. Baltimore, William & Wilkins, 1981.

100. Carvalho ACA: Bleeding in uremia—a clinical challenge. N Engl J Med 308:38, 1983.

101. Janson PA, Jubelirer SJ, Weinstein MJ, et al.: Treatment of the bleeding tendency in uremia with cryoprecipitate. N Engl J Med 303:1318, 1980.

102. Watson AJS, Keough JAB: Effect of 1-deamino-8-D-arginine vasopressin on the prolonged bleeding time in chronic renal failure. Nephron 32:49, 1982.

103. Mannucci PM, Remuzzi G, Pusineri F, et al.: Deamino-8-D-arginine vasopressin shortens the bleeding time in uremia. N Engl J Med 308:8, 1983.

104. Deutsch S: Anesthetic management of patients with chronic renal disease. South Med J 68:65, 1975.

105. Linke CL, Merin RG: A regional anesthetic approach for renal transplantation. Anesth Analg 55:69, 1976.

106. Merin RG, Linke CL: Regional anesthesia for renal transplantation. Reg Anaesth 4:13, 1979.

107. Montgomerie JZ, Kalmanson GM, Guze LB: Renal failure and infection. Medicine 47:1, 1968.

108. Kennedy AC, Burton JA, Luke RG, et al.: Factors affecting the prognosis in acute renal failure. Q J Med 42:73, 1973.

109. Kunori T, Fehrman I, Ringdon O, et al.: In vitro characterization of immunological responsiveness of uremic patients. Nephron 26:234, 1980.

110. Soulier JP, Jungers P, Zingraff J: Virus B hepatitis in hemodialysis centers. Adv Nephrol 6:383, 1976.

111. Greenberg HB, Pollard RB, Lutwick LI, et al.: Human leukocyte interferon and hepatitis B virus infection. N Engl J Med 295:517, 1976.

112. du Moulin GC, Hedley-Whyte J: Hospital associated viral infection and the anesthesiologist. Anesthesiology 59:51, 1983.

113. Berry AJ, Isaacson IJ, Hunt D, et al.: The prevalence of hepatitis B viral markers in anesthesia personnel. Anesthesiology 60:6, 1984.

114. Oxman MN: Hepatitis B vaccination of high-risk hospital personnel (editorial views). Anesthesiology 60:1, 1984.

115. Stevens E, Szmuness W, Goodman AI, et al.: Hepatitis B vaccine: immune responses in haemodialysis patients. Lancet 2:1211, 1980.

116. Acosta JH: Hypertension in chronic renal disease. Kidney Int 22:702, 1982.

117. Fergus EB: Infection as a cause and complication of renal disease. J Chron Dis 15:647, 1962.

118. Schoeneman M: Dietary and pharmacologic treatment of chronic renal failure. In Edelmann CM Jr (Ed.): Pediatric Kidney Disease. Boston, Little, Brown 1978, pp 475–486.

119. Guyton AC, Coleman TG, Cowley AW, et al.: Arterial pressure regulation. In Laragh JH (Ed.): Hypertension Manual. New York, Yorke Medical Books, 1974.

120. Kjellstrand CM, Buselmeier TJ: A simple method for anticoagulation during pre- and post-operative hemodialysis, avoiding rebound phenomena. Surgery 72:630, 1972.

121. Laragh JH: Vasoconstriction-volume analysis for understanding and treating hypertension: the use of renin and aldosterone profiles. Am J Med 55:261, 1973.

122. Weidman P, Maxwell MH, Lupu AN: Plasma renin activity and blood pressure in terminal renal failure. N Engl J Med 285:757, 1971.

123. Mulrow PJ, Siegel NJ: Mechanisms in hypertension. In Edelmann CM Jr (Ed.): Pediatric Kidney Disease. Boston, Little, Brown, 1978, pp 325–331.

124. Menster M: Diagnosis and treatment of hypertension in children. Pediatr Clin N Am 29:933, 1982.

125. Versmold HT, Kitterman JA, Phibbs RH, et al.: Aortic

blood pressure during the first 12 hours of life in infants with birth weight 610 to 4,220 grams. Pediatrics 67:607, 1981.

126. de Swiet M, Fayers P, Shinebourne EA: Systolic blood pressure in a population of infants in the first year of life: the Brompton study. Pediatrics 65:1028, 1980.

127. Report of the Task Force on Blood Pressure Control in Children. Pediatrics 59(Suppl):797, 1977.

128. Siegel NJ, Mulrow PJ: The management of hypertension. In Edelmann CM Jr (Ed.): Pediatric Kidney Disease. Boston, Little, Brown, 1978, pp 457–465.

129. Moss AJ, Liebling W, Austin WO, et al.: An evaluation of the flush method for determining blood pressure in infants. Pediatrics 20:53, 1957.

130. Kirkland RT, Kirkland JL: Systolic blood pressure measurements in the newborn infant with the transcutaneous Doppler method. J Pediatr 80:52, 1972.

131. American Heart Association: Recommendations for Human Blood Pressure Determination by Sphygmomanometer. 1981.

132. Pascarelli EF, Bertrand CA: Comparison of blood pressures in the arms and legs. N Engl J Med 270:693, 1964.

133. Whyte RK, Elseed AM, Fraser CB, et al.: Assessment of Doppler ultrasound to measure systolic pressures in infants and young children. Arch Dis Child 50:542, 1975.

134. Koster M, David GK: Reversible severe hypertension due to licorice ingestion. N Engl J Med 278:1381, 1968.

135. Wilkinson R, Scott DF, Uldall PR, et al.: Plasma renin and exchangeable sodium in the hypertension of chronic renal failure: the effect of bilateral nephrectomy. Q J Med 39:377, 1970.

136. Schiff M, Brown RS, Lytton B: The role of bilateral nephrectomy in the treatment of hypertension of chronic renal failure. J Urol 109:152, 1973.

137. Lee JB: Anti-hypertensive activity of the kidney; the reno-medullary prostaglandins. N Engl J Med 277:1073, 1967.

138. Tan SY, Mulrow PJ: Impaired renal prostaglandin E production: a newly identified lesion in hypertensives. Clin Res 25:450A, 1977.

139. Muirhead EE, Germain G, Leach B, et al.: Blood pressure regulation and control. Circ Res (Suppl II) 31:161, 1972.

140. Margolius HS, Horowitz D, Pisano JJ, et al.: Urinary kallikrein excretion in hypertensive man. Circ Res 35:820, 1974.

141. Makker SP, Moorthy B: Rebound hypertension following minoxidil withdrawal. J Pediatr 96:762, 1980.

142. Bruce DL, Croley TF, Lee JS: Pre-operative clonidine withdrawal syndrome. Anesthesiology 51:90, 1979.

143. Maling TJB, Dollery CT: Changes in blood pressure, heart rate and plasma noradrenaline concentration after sudden withdrawal of propranolol. Br Med J 2:366, 1979.

144. Conway J, Lauwers P: Hemodynamic and hypotensive effects of long-term therapy with chlorothiazide. Circulation 21:21, 1960.

145. Repetto HA, Lewy JE, Brando JL, et al.: Furosemide in acute glomerulonephritis. J Pediatr 80:660, 1972.

146. Loggie JMH: Hypertension in children and adolescents. II. Drug therapy. J Pediatr 74:640, 1969.

147. Prys-Roberts C, Meloche R: Management of anesthesia in patients with hypertension or ischemic heart disease. Int Anesthesiol Clin 18:181, 1980.

148. Mohammed S, Hanenson IB, Magenheim HG, et al.: The effects of alpha-methyldopa on renal function in hypertensive patients. Am Heart J 76:21, 1968.

149. Potter DE, Schambelan M, Salvatierra O, et al.: Treatment of high renin hypertension with propranolol in children after renal transplantation. J Pediatr 90:307, 1977.

150. Holland OB, Kaplan NM: Propranolol in the treatment of hypertension. N Engl J Med 294:930, 1976.

151. Koch-Weser J: Drug therapy: hydralazine. N Engl J Med 295:320, 1976.

152. Linas SL, Nies AS: Minoxidil. Ann Intern Med 94:61, 1981.

153. Pennisi AJ, Takahashi M, Bernstein BH, et al.: Minoxidil

therapy in children with severe hypertension. J Pediatr 90:813, 1977.

154. Hansson LM, Hunyor SN: Blood pressure over-shoot due to acute clonidine (Catapres) withdrawal: studies on arterial and urinary catecholamines and suggestions for management of the crisis. Clin Sci Mol Med 45:181s, 1973.

155. Prys-Roberts C: Hemodynamic effects of anesthesia and surgery in renal hypertensive patients receiving large doses of beta-receptor antagonists. Anesthesiology 51(Suppl):122, 1979.

156. Sprague DH: Severe bradycardia after neostigmine in a patient taking propanolol to control paroxysmal atrial tachycardia. Anesthesiology 42:208, 1975.

157. Prys-Roberts C: Adrenergic mechanisms, agonists and antagonist drugs. In Prys-Roberts C (Ed.): The Circulation in Anesthesia. Oxford, Blackwell, 1979.

158. Heel RC, Brogden RN, Speight TM, et al.: Captopril: a review of its pharmacologic properties and therapeutic efficacy. Drugs 20:409, 1980.

159. Friedman A, Chesney RW, Ball D, et al.: Effective use of captopril (angiotensin I–converting enzyme inhibitor) in severe childhood hypertension. J Pediatr 97:664, 1980.

160. McLaine PN, Drummond KN: Intravenous diazoxide for severe hypertension in childhood. J Pediatr 79:829, 1971.

161. Olson DL, Lieberman E: Renal hypertension in children, Pediatr Clin N Am 23:795, 1976.

162. Tinker JH, Michenfelder JD: Sodium nitroprusside: pharmacology, toxicology and therapeutics. Anesthesiology 45:340, 1976.

163. McLain LG: Drugs in the management of hypertensive emergencies in children. Clin Pediatr 15:85, 1976.

164. Davies DW, Greiss L, Kadar D, et al.: Sodium nitroprusside in children; observations on metabolism during normal and abnormal responses. Can Anaesth Soc J 22:553, 1975.

165. Ivankovich AD, Miletich DJ, Tinker JH: Sodium nitroprusside: metabolism and general considerations. Int Anesthesiol Clin 16:1978.

166. Danzig LE: Dynamics of thiocyanate dialysis: the artificial kidney in the therapy of thiocyanate intoxification. N Engl J Med 252:49, 1955.

167. Bedford RF: Increasing halothane concentrations reduce nitroprusside dose requirement. Anesth Analg 57:457, 1978.

168. Tinker JH, Michenfelder JD: Increased resistance to nitroprusside-induced cyanide toxicity in anuric dogs. Anesthesiology 52:40, 1980.

169. Cumming AMM, Davies DL: Intravenous labetalol in hypertensive emergency. Lancet 1:929, 1979.

170. Dillon MJ: Hypertension. In Williams DI, Johnston JH (Eds.): Paediatric Urology. London, Butterworth Scientific, 1982, pp 57–72.

170a. Ferguson RK, Vlasses PH: Hypertensive emergencies and urgencies. JAMA 255:1607, 1986.

171. Agus JC, Frommer JP, Young JB: Cardiac and circulatory abnormalities in chronic renal failure. Semin Nephrol 1:112, 1981.

172. Outwater KM, Treves S, Lang P, et al.: Renal and hemodynamic effects of dopamine in infants following corrective cardiac surgery. Anesthesiology 61:A130, 1984.

173. Kumar S, Lesch M: Pericarditis in renal disease. Prog Cardiovasc Dis 22:357, 1980.

174. Uraemic pericarditis (editorial). Lancet 1:941, 1977.

175. Movin JE, Hollomby D, Gonda A, et al.: Management of uremic pericarditis: a report of 11 patients with cardiac tamponade and review of the literature. Ann Thorac Surg 22:588, 1976.

176. Wray TM, Humphreys J, Perry JM, et al.: Pericardiectomy for treatment of uremic pericarditis. Circulation 50(Suppl 2):268, 1974.

177. Stanley TH, Weidauer HE: Anesthesia for the patient with cardiac tamponade. Anesth Analg 52:110, 1973.

178. Kaplan JA, Bland JW, Dunbar RW: The perioperative management of pericardial tamponade. South Med J 69:417, 1976.

179. Konchigeri HN, Levitsky S: Anesthetic considerations for pericardectomy in uremic pericardial effusion. Anesth Analg 55:378, 1976.

180. Hickey PR, Hansen DD, Cramolini GM: Pulmonary and systemic hemodynamic responses to ketamine in infants with normal and elevated pulmonary vascular resistance. Anesthesiology 61:A438, 1984.

181. Brigham KL, Bernard G: Pulmonary complications of chronic renal failure. Semin Nephrol 1:188, 1981.

182. Martinez WC, Rapin I, Moore CL: Neurologic complications of renal failure. In Edelmann CM Jr (Ed.): Pediatric Kidney Disease. Boston, Little, Brown, 1978, pp 408–420.

183. Alfrey AC: Dialysis encephalopathy syndrome. Ann Rev Med 29:93, 1978.

184. Reese GN, Appel SH: Neurologic complications of renal failure. Semin Nephrol 1:137, 1981.

185. O'Regan S, Matina D, Ducharme G, et al.: Echocardiographic assessment of cardiac function in children with chronic renal failure. Kidney Int 24:S77, 1983.

186. Lock JE, Bass JL, Kulik TJ, et al.: Chronic percutaneous pericardial drainage with modified pigtail catheters in children. Am J Cardiol 53:1179, 1984.

187. Mitschke H, Schmidt P, Kopsa H, et al.: Reversible uremic deafness after successful renal transplantation. N Engl J Med 292:1062, 1975.

188. Jellinek EH, Painter M, Prineas J, et al.: Hypertensive encephalopathy with cortical disorders of vision. Q J Med 33:239, 1964.

189. Maynert EW: Phenobarbital, mephobarbital and metharbital: absorption, distribution and excretion. In Woodbury DM, Penry JK, Schmidt RP (Eds.): Antiepileptic Drugs. New York, Raven Press, 1972.

190. Bennett WM, Singer I, Golper T, et al.: Guidelines for drug therapy in renal failure. Ann Intern Med 86:754, 1977.

191. Woodbury DM, Swinyard E: Diphenylhydantoin: absorption, distribution and excretion. In Woodbury DM, Penry JK, Schmidt RP (Eds.): Antiepileptic Drugs. New York, Raven Press, 1972.

192. Letteri JM, Mellk H, Louis S, et al.: Diphenylhydantoin metabolism in uremia. N Engl J Med 285:648, 1971.

193. Reidenberg MM, Odar-Cederlöf J, Von Bahr ML, et al.: Protein binding of diphenylhydantoin and desmethylimipramine in plasma from patients with poor renal function. N Engl J Med 285:264, 1971.

194. Weir PHC, Chung FF: Anaesthesia for patients with chronic renal disease. Can Anaesth Soc J 31:468, 1984.

195. Arbus GS, Barnor NA, Hsu AC, et al.: Effect of chronic renal failure, dialysis and transplantation on motor nerve conduction velocity in children. Can Med Assoc J 113:517, 1975.

196. Stenzel RB, Semar M, Lonergan ET, et al.: Relationship of nervous tissue transketolase to the neuropathy in chronic uremia. J Clin Invest 50:2295, 1971.

197. Berry AJ, Peterson ML: Hyponatremia after mannitol administration in the presence of renal failure. Anesth Analg (Cleve) 60:165, 1981.

198. Borges HF, Hocks J, Kjellstrand CM: Mannitol intoxification in patients with renal failure. Arch Intern Med 142:63, 1982.

199. Warren SE, Blantz RC: Mannitol. Arch Intern Med 141:493, 1981.

200. Makoff DL, DaSilva JA, Rosenbaum BJ, et al.: Hypertonic expansion: acid base and electrolyte changes. Am J Physiol 218:1201, 1970.

201. Kersh ES, Kronfield SJ, Unger A, et al.: Autonomic insufficiency in uremia as a cause of hemodialysis induced hypotension. N Engl J Med 290:650, 1974.

202. Campese VM, Romoff MS, Levitan D, et al.: Mechanisms of autonomic nervous system dysfunctions in uremia. Kidney Int 20:246, 1981.

203. Mahurkar SD, Dhar SK, Salta R, et al.: Dialysis dementia. Lancet 1:1412, 1973.

204. Alfrey AC, Legendre GR, Kaehny WD: The dialysis encephalopathy syndrome. N Engl J Med 294:184, 1976.

205. McDermott JR, Smith AI, Wark MK, et al.: Brain aluminum concentrations in dialysis encephalopathy. Lancet 1:901, 1978.

206. Zelnic EB, Goyal RK: Gastrointestinal manifestations of chronic renal failure. Semin Nephrol 1:124, 1981.

207. Grodstein G, Harrison A, Roberts C, et al.: Impaired gastric emptying in hemodialysis patients (abstr). Annual Meeting Am Soc Nephrol 182A, 1979.

208. Leiber CS, Lefevre A: Ammonia as a source of gastric hypoacidity in patients with uremia. J Clin Invest 38:1271, 1959.

209. Sullivan SN, Tustanoff E, Slaughter DN, et al.: Hypergastrinemia and gastric acid hypersecretion in uremia. Clin Nephrol 5:25, 1976.

210. Goldstein H, Murphy D, Sokol A, et al.: Gastric acid secretion in patients undergoing chronic dialysis. Arch Intern Med 120:645, 1967.

211. Shepherd AMM, Stewart WK, Wormsley KG: Peptic ulceration in chronic renal failure. Lancet 1:1357, 1973.

212. Black M: Disturbances of the gastrointestinal system. In Edelmann CM Jr (Ed.): Pediatric Kidney Disease. Boston, Little, Brown, 1978, pp 421–428.

213. Manchikanti L, Kraus JW, Edds SP: Cimetidine and related drugs in anesthesia. Anesth Analg 61:595, 1982.

214. Avioli LV: Endocrine disturbances in uremia. In Edelmann CM Jr (Ed.): Pediatric Kidney Disease. Boston, Little, Brown, 1978, pp 442–447.

215. Cohen BD: Disturbances of nitrogen, carbohydrate, and lipid metabolism. In Edelmann CM Jr (Ed.): Pediatric Kidney Disease. Boston, Little, Brown, 1978, pp 432–491.

216. Holliday MA: Growth retardation in children with renal disease. In Edelmann CM Jr (Ed.): Pediatric Kidney Disease. Boston, Little, Brown, 1978, pp 331–341.

217. Emmanouel DS, Lindheimer MD, Katz AI: Endocrine abnormalities in chronic renal failure. Pathogenetic principles and clinical implications. Semin Nephrol 1:151, 1981.

218. Rubenfeld S, Garber AJ: Abnormal carbohydrate metabolism in chronic renal failure. J Clin Invest 62:20, 1978.

219. Korsch BM: Psychological complications of renal disease in childhood. In Edelmann CM Jr (Ed.): Pediatric Kidney Disease. Boston, Little, Brown, 1978, pp 342–347.

220. Anderson RJ: Drug prescribing for patients in renal failure. Hosp Pract 18:145, 1983.

221. Anderson RJ, Schrier RW: Clinical Use of Drugs in Patients with Kidney and Liver Disease. Philadelphia, W.B. Saunders Co., 1981.

222. Bennet WM, Muther RS: Drug metabolism in renal failure. In Brenner B, Stein J (Eds.): Chronic Renal Failure. New York, Churchill Livingstone, 1981, p 287.

223. Wyant GM: The anaesthetist looks at tissue transplantation: three years' experience with kidney transplants. Can Anaesth Soc J 14:255, 1967.

224. Ryan DW: Preoperative serum cholinesterase concentration in chronic renal failure. Br J Anaesth 49:945, 1977.

225. McLeod K, Watson MJ, Rawlins MD: Pharmacokinetics of pancuronium in patients with normal and impaired renal function. Br J Anaesth 48:341, 1976.

226. Miller RD, Sohn YJ, Matteo RS: Enhancement of D-tubocurarine neuromuscular blockage by diuretics in man. Anesthesiology 45:442, 1976.

227. Miller RD: Reversal of muscle relaxants. American Society of Anesthesiologists. ASA Refresher Course Lectures. 32:222, 1981.

228. Brotherton WP, Matteo RS: Pharmacokinetics and pharmacodynamics of metocurine in humans with and without renal failure. Anesthesiology 55:273, 1981.

229. Ghoneim MM, Kramer SE, Bannow R, et al.: Binding of D-tubocurarine to plasma proteins in normal patients with hepatic or renal disease. Anesthesiology 39:410, 1973.

230. Miller RD, Matteo RS, Benet LZ, et al.: The pharmacoki-

netics of D-tubocurarine in man with and without renal failure. J Pharmacol Exp Ther *202*:1, 1977.

231. Cohen EN, Brewer HW, Smith D: The metabolism and elimination of D-tubocurarine-H³. Anesthesiology *28*:309, 1967.

232. Fahey MR, Rupp SM, Fisher DM, et al.: Pharmacokinetics and pharmacodynamics of atracurium in normal and renal failure patients. Anesthesiology *59*:A263, 1983.

233. Hughes R, Chapple DJ: The pharmacology of atracurium: a new competitive neuromuscular blocking agent. Br J Anaesth *53*:31, 1981.

234. Hunter JM, Jones RS, Utting JE: Use of the muscle relaxant atracurium in anephric patients: preliminary communication. J R Soc Med *75*:336, 1982.

235. Brandom BW, Rudd GD, Cook DR: Clinical pharmacology of atracurium in paediatric patients. Br J Anaesth *55*:175, 1983.

236. Goudsouzian NG, Liu LMP, Cote CJ, et al.: Safety and efficacy of atracurium in adolescents and children anesthetized with halothane. Anesthesiology *59*:459, 1983.

237. Brandom BW, Woelfel SK, Cook DR, et al.: Clinical pharmacology of atracurium in infants. Anesth Analg *63*:309, 1984.

238. Nigrovic V, Koechel DA: Atracurium—additional information needed. Anesthesiology *60*:606, 1984.

239. Hennis PJ, Fahey MR, Miller RD, et al.: Pharmacology of laudanosine in dogs. Anesthesiology *61*:A305, 1984.

240. Freeman RB, Sheff MF, Maher JF, et al.: The blood—cerebrospiral fluid barrier in uremia. Ann Intern Med *56*:233, 1962.

241. Upton RA, Nguyen TL, Miller RD, et al.: Renal and biliary elimination of vecuronium (Org NC45) and pancuronium in rats. Anesth Analg *61*:313, 1982.

242. Meistelman C, Lienhart A, Leveque C, et al.: Pharmacology of vecuronium in patients with end stage renal failure. Anesthesiology *59*:293, 1983.

243. Fisher DM, Miller RD: Neuromuscular effects of vecuronium (Org NC45) in infants and children during N_2O, halothane anesthesia. Anesthesiology *58*:519, 1983.

244. Cronnelly R, Stanski DR, Miller RD, et al.: Renal function and the pharmacokinetics of neostigmine in anesthetized man. Anesthesiology *51*:222, 1979.

245. Cronnelly R, Stanksi DR, Miller RD, et al.: Pyridostigmine kinetics with and without renal function. Clin Pharmacol Ther *28*:78, 1980.

246. Everett GB, Allen GD, Kennedy WF, et al.: Renal hemodynamic effects of general anesthesia in outpatients. Anesth Analg *52*:470, 1973.

247. Parsons V, Choudhury AA, Wass JAH, et al.: Renal excretion of fluoride in renal failure and after renal transplantation. Br Med J *1*:128, 1975.

248. Cousins MJ, Mazze RI: Methoxyflurane nephrotoxicity. A study on dose response in man. JAMA *225*:1611, 1973.

249. Cousins MJ, Greenstein LR, Hitt BA, et al.: Metabolism and renal effects of enflurane in man. Anesthesiology *44*:44, 1976.

250. Loehming R, Mazze RI: Possible nephrotoxicity from enflurane in a patient with severe renal disease. Anesthesiology *40*:203, 1974.

251. Harnett MN, Lane W, Bennett WM: Non-oliguric renal failure and enflurane. Ann Intern Med *81*:560, 1974.

252. Eichhorn JH, Hedley-Whyte J, Steinman TI, et al.: Renal failure following enflurane anesthesia. Anesthesiology *45*:557, 1976.

253. Mazze RI, Sievenpiper TS, Stevenson J: Renal effects of enflurane and halothane in patients with abnormal renal function. Anesthesiology *60*:161, 1984.

254. Mazze RI, Cousins MJ, Barr GA: Renal effects and metabolism of isoflurane in man. Anesthesiology *40*:536, 1974.

255. Cousins MJ, Mazze RI, Barr GA, et al.: A comparison of the renal effects of isoflurane and methoxyflurane in Fischer 344 rats. Anesthesiology *38*:557, 1973.

256. Carter R, Heerdt M, Acchiardo S: Fluoride kinetics after enflurane anesthesia in healthy and anephric patients and in patients with poor renal function. Clin Pharmacol Ther *20*:565, 1977.

257. Deutsch S, Bastron RD, Pierce EC, et al.: The effects of anaesthesia with thiopentone, nitrous oxide, narcotics and neuromuscular blocking drugs on renal function in normal man. Br J Anaesth *41*:807, 1969.

258. Philbin DM, Coggins CH: Plasma antidiuretic hormone levels in cardiac surgical patients during morphine and halothane anesthesia. Anesthesiology *49*:95, 1978.

259. Stanley TH, Lathrop GD: Urinary excretion of morphine during and after valvular and coronary artery surgery. Anesthesiology *46*:166, 1977.

260. Don HF, Dieppa RA, Taylor P: Narcotic analgesics in anuric patients. Anesthesiology *42*:745, 1975.

261. Drayes DE: Active drug metabolites and renal failure. Am J Med *62*:486, 1977.

262. Bower S: Plasma protein binding of fentanyl: the effect of hyperlipoproteinaemia and chronic renal failure. J Pharm Pharmacol *34*:102, 1982.

263. Kono K, Philbin DM, Coggins CH, et al.: Renal function and stress response during halothane or fentanyl anesthesia. Anesth Analg *60*:552, 1981.

264. Trudnowski RJ, Mostert JW, Hobika GH, et al.: Neuroleptanalgesia for patients with kidney malfunction. Anesth Analg *50*:679, 1971.

265. Morgan M, Lumley J: Anaesthetic considerations in chronic renal failure. Anaesth Intens Care *3*:218, 1975.

266. Gorman HM, Graythorne NWB: The effect of a new neuroleptic analgesic agent (Innovar) on renal function in man. Acta Anaesthesiol Scand (Suppl 24) *10*:111, 1966.

267. Järnberg PO, Santesson J, Eklund J: Renal function during neuroleptanaesthesia. Acta Anaesthesiol Scand *22*:167, 1978.

268. Mostert JW, Evers JL, Hobika GH, et al.: Circulatory effects of analgesic and neuroleptic drugs in patients with chronic renal failure undergoing maintenance dialysis. Br J Anaesth *42*:501, 1970.

269. Dundee JW, Richards RK: Effect of azotemia upon the action of intravenous barbiturate anesthesia. Anesthesiology *15*:333, 1954.

270. Ghoneim MM, Pandya H: Plasma protein binding of thiopental in patients with impaired renal or hepatic function. Anesthesiology *42*:545, 1975.

271. White PF, Way WL, Trevor AJ: Ketamine—its pharmacology and therapeutic uses. Anesthesiology *56*:119, 1982.

272. Wieber J, Gugler R, Hengstman JH, et al.: Pharmacokinetics of ketamine in man. Anaesthesist *24*:260, 1975.

273. Bevan DR, Budhu R: The effect of ketamine on renal blood flow in greyhounds. Br J Anaesth *47*:634, 1975.

274. Hirasawa H, Yonezawa T: The effects of ketamine and Innovar on the renal cortical and medullary blood flow of the dog. Anaesthesist *24*:349, 1975.

275. Kennedy WF, Sawyer TK, Gerbershagen HU, et al.: Systemic cardiovascular and renal hemodynamic alterations during peridural anesthesia in normal man. Anesthesiology *31*:414, 1969.

276. Kennedy WF, Sawyer TK, Gerbershagen HU, et al.: Simultaneous systemic cardiovascular and renal hemodynamic measurements during high spinal anaesthesia in normal man. Acta Anaesthesiol Scand Suppl *37*:163, 1970.

277. Bromage PR, Gertel M: Brachial plexus anesthesia in chronic renal failure. Anesthesiology *36*:488, 1972.

278. Singler RC: Pediatric regional anesthesia. *In* Gregory GA (Ed.): Pediatric Anesthesia. New York, Churchill Livingstone, 1983, pp 481–518.

279. Strasser K, Abel J, Breuhmann M, et al.: Plasmakonzentration von Etidocain in den erster zwei Stunden nach axillärer Blockade bei Gesunden und bei Patienten mit Niereninsuffizienz. Anaesthesist *30*:14, 1981.

280. Gould DB, Aldrete JA: Bupivacaine cardiotoxicity in a patient with renal failure. Acta Anaesthesiol Scand *27*:18, 1983.

281. Fernando ON: Renal transplantation in children. *In* Williams

DI, Johnston JH (Eds.): Paediatric Urology. London, Butterworth Scientific, 1982, pp 49–56.

282. Mazze RI: Critical care of the patient with acute renal failure. Anesthesiology 47:138, 1977.

283. Slawson KB: Anaesthesia for the patient in renal failure. Br J Anaesth 44:277, 1972.

284. Fine RN, Malekzadeh MH, Pennisi AJ, et al.: Long term results of renal transplantation in children. Pediatrics 61:641, 1978.

285. Ingelfinger JR, Grupe WE, Harmon WE, et al.: Growth acceleration following renal transplantation in children less than 7 years of age. Pediatrics 68:255, 1981.

286. Avner ED, Harmon WE, Grupe WE, et al.: Mortality of chronic hemodialysis and renal transplantation in pediatric end-stage renal disease. Pediatrics 67:412, 1981.

287. Vandam LD, Harrison JH, Murray JE, et al.: Anesthesia aspects of renal homotransplantation in man. Anesthesiology 23:783, 1962.

288. Strunin L: Some aspects of anesthesia for renal homotransplantation. Br J Anaesth 38:662, 1966.

289. Samuel JR, Powell D: Renal transplantation: anaesthetic experience of 100 cases. Anaesthesia 25:165, 1970.

290. Aldrette JH, Daniel W, O'Higgins JW, et al.: Analysis of anesthetic-related morbidity in human recipients of renal homografts. Anesth Analg 50:321, 1971.

291. Levine DS, Virtue RW: Anaesthetic agents and techniques for renal homotransplants. Can Anaesth Soc J 20:259, 1973.

292. Logan DH, Howie HB, Crawford J: Anaesthesia and renal transplantation: 56 cases. Br J Anaesth 46:69, 1974.

293. Strunin L, Davies JM, Filshie JJ: Anesthesia for renal transplantation. Anesthesiol Clin 22:189, 1984.

294. Mauer SM, Howard RJ: Renal transplantation in children. In Edelmann CM Jr (Ed.): Pediatric Kidney Disease. Boston, Little, Brown, 1978, pp 503–530.

295. Mauer SM, Lynch RE: Hemodialysis techniques for infants and children. Pediatr Clin North Am 23:843, 1976.

296. Simmons MA, Levine RL, Lubchenco LO, et al.: Warning: serious sequelae of temporal artery catheterization. J Pediatr 92:284, 1978.

297. Prian GW, Wright GB, Rumack CM, et al.: Apparent cerebral embolization after temporal artery catheterization. J Pediatr 93:115, 1978.

298. Bull MJ, Schreiner RL, Garg BP, et al.: Neurologic complications following temporal artery catheterization. J Pediatr 96:1071, 1980.

299. Downs JB, Rackstein AD, Klein EF Jr, et al.: Hazards of radial artery catheterization. Anesthesiology 38:283, 1973.

300. Miyasaka K, Edmonds JF, Conn AW: Complications of radial artery lines in the paediatric patient. Canad Anaesth Soc J 23:9, 1976.

301. Santiago-Delphin EA, Buselmeier TJ, Simmons RL: Blood gases and pH in patients with artificial arteriovenous fistulas. Kidney Int 1:131, 1972.

302. Hirschman CA, Edelstein G: Intraoperative hyperkalemia and cardiac arrest during renal transplantation in an insulin dependent diabetic patient. Anesthesiology 51:161, 1979.

303. Hirschman CA, Leon D, Edelstein G, et al.: Risk of hyperkalemia in recipients of kidneys preserved with an intra-cellular electrolyte solution. Anesth Analg 59:283, 1980.

304. Ruley EJ, Bock GH: Acute renal failure in infants and children. In Shoemaker WC, Thompson WL, Holbrook PR (Eds.): Society of Critical Care Medicine: Textbook of Critical Care. Philadelphia, W.B. Saunders Co., 1984, pp 604–614.

305. Chesney RW, Kaplan BS, Freedom RM, et al.: Acute renal failure: an important complication of cardiac surgery in infants. J Pediatr 87:381, 1975.

306. Halperin BD, Feeley TW: The effect of anesthesia and surgery on renal function. Int Anesthesiol Clin 22:157, 1984.

307. Byrd L, Sherman RL: Radio-contrast induced acute renal failure: a clinical and pathophysiologic review. Medicine 58:270, 1979.

308. Schreiner SE, Maher JF: Toxic nephropathy. Am J Med 38:409, 1965.

309. Schmidt PJ, Holland PV: Pathogenesis of the acute renal failure associated with incompatible transfusions. Lancet 2:1169, 1967.

310. Rowland LP, Penn AS: Myoglobinuria. Med Clin North Am 56:1233, 1972.

311. Koffler A, Friedler RM, Massry SG: Acute renal failure due to non-traumatic rhabdomyolysis. Ann Intern Med 85:23, 1976.

312. Mattern W, Staab EV: Imaging studies in renal failure: emphasis on selection and sequencing in the clinical setting. CRC Rad Nuc Med 6:459, 1975.

313. Schleigel JV, Lang EK: Computed radionuclide urogram for assessing acute renal failure. AJR 134:129, 1980.

314. Sanders RC, Menon S, Saunders AD: The complementary uses of nuclear medicine and ultrasound in the kidney. J Urol 120:521, 1978.

315. Knochel JP: Rhabdomyolysis and myoglobinuria. Semin Nephrol 1:75, 1981.

316. Nicot GS, Merle LJ, Charmes JP, et al.: Transient glomerular proteinuria, enzymuria and nephrotoxic reaction induced by radiocontrast media. JAMA 252:2432, 1984.

317. Oken DE: Clinical aspects of acute renal failure (vasomotor nephropathy). In Edelmann CM Jr (Ed.): Pediatric Kidney Disease. Boston, Little, Brown, 1978, pp 1108–1122.

318. Ellis D, Gartner JC, Galvis AG: Acute renal failure in infants and children: diagnosis, complications and treatment. Crit Care Med 9:607, 1981.

319. Hodson EM, Kjellstrand CM, Maurer SM: Acute renal failure in infants and children: outcome of 53 patients requiring hemodialysis treatment. J Pediatr 93:756, 1978.

320. Kleinknecht D, Junges P, Chanard J, et al.: Factors influencing immediate prognosis in acute renal failure, with special reference to prophylactic hemodialysis. Adv Nephrol 1:207, 1971.

321. Kennedy AC, Burton JA, Luke RG, et al.: Factors affecting the prognosis of acute renal failure. Q J Med 42:73, 1973.

322. Zech P, Bouletreau R, Moscoutchenko JR, et al.: Infection in acute renal failure. Adv Nephrol 1:231, 1971.

323. Schentag JJ, Cerra FB, Calleri G, et al.: Pharmacokinetic and clinical studies in patients with cimetidine-associated mental confusion. Lancet 1:177, 1979.

324. Counahan R, Cameron JS, Ogg CS, et al.: Presentation, management complications and outcome of acute renal failure in childhood: five years' experience. Br Med J 1:599, 1977.

325. Vertel RM, Knochel JP: Nonoliguric acute renal failure. JAMA 200:118, 1967.

326. Anderson RJ, Linas SL, Berns AS, et al.: Nonoliguric renal failure. N Engl J Med 296:1134, 1977.

327. Shin B, Mackenzie CF, McAslan TC, et al.: Postoperative renal failure in trauma patients. Anesthesiology 51:218, 1979.

328. Clark DA: Times of first void and first stool in 500 newborns. Pediatrics 60:457, 1977.

329. Mathew OP, Jones AJ, James E, et al.: Neonatal renal failure: usefulness of diagnostic indices. Pediatrics 65:57, 1980.

330. Norman ME, Farahnak KA: A prospective study of acute renal failure in the newborn infant. Pediatrics 63:475, 1979.

331. Anand SK, Northway JD, Crussi FG: Acute renal failure in newborn infants. J Pediatr 92:985, 1978.

332. Arant BS Jr: Developmental patterns of renal functional maturation compared in the human neonate. J Pediatr 92:705, 1978.

333. Guignard JP, Torrado A, Da Cunha O, et al.: Glomerular filtration rate in the first three weeks of life. J Pediatr 87:268, 1975.

334. Stonestreet BS, Oh W: Plasma creatinine levels in low birth weight infants during the first three months of life. Pediatrics 61:788, 1978.

335. Sertel H, Scopes J: Rates of creatinine clearance in babies less than one week of age. Arch Dis Child 48:717, 1973.

336. Schwartz GJ, Haycock GB, Spitzer A: Plasma creatinine and urea concentrations in children: normal values for age and sex. J Pediatr 88:828, 1976.

337. Guignard JP, Torrado A, Mazouni SM, et al.: Renal function in respiratory distress syndrome. J Pediatr 88:845, 1976.

338. Chevalier RL, Campbell F, Brembridge AN: Prognostic factors in neonatal acute renal failure. Pediatrics 74:265, 1984.

339. Suki W, Eknoyan G, Rector FC, et al.: Patterns of nephron perfusion in acute and chronic hydronephrosis. J Clin Invest 45:122, 1966.

340. Boichis H, Winterborn MH: Acute renal failure in childhood. Pediatr Ann 3:58, 1974.

341. Sedman AB, Wilkening GN, Warady BA, et al.: Encephalopathy in childhood secondary to aluminum toxicity. J Pediatr 105:836, 1984.

342. Polinsky MS, Gruskin AB: Aluminum toxicity in children with chronic renal failure. J Pediatr 105:758, 1984.

343. Salusky IB, Coburn JW, Paunier L, et al.: Role of aluminum hydroxide in raising serum aluminum levels in children undergoing continuous ambulatory peritoneal dialysis. J Pediatr 105:717, 1984.

344. Espinel CH: The FENa test. Use in the differential diagnosis of acute renal failure. JAMA 236:579, 1976.

345. Miller TR, Anderson RJ, Linas SL, et al.: Urinary diagnostic indices in acute renal failure. A prospective study. Ann Intern Med 89:47, 1978.

346. Gordillo-Paniagua G, Velasquez-Jones L: Acute renal failure. Pediatr Clin North Am 23:817, 1976.

347. Barry KG, Malloy JP: Oliguric renal failure. Evaluation and therapy by the intravenous infusion of mannitol. JAMA 179:510, 1962.

348. Luke RG, Briggs JD, Allison ME, et al.: Factors determining the response to mannitol in acute renal failure. Am J Med Sci 259:168, 1971.

349. Stone AM, Stahl WM: Effect of ethacrynic acid and furosemide on renal function in hypovolemia. Ann Surg 174:1, 1971.

350. Birtch AG, Zakheim RM, Jones LG, et al.: Redistribution of renal blood flow produced by furosemide and ethacrynic acid. Circ Res 21:869, 1967.

351. Lucas CE, Zito JG, Carver KM, et al.: Questionable value of furosemide in preventing renal failure. Surgery 82:314, 1977.

352. Levinsky NG: Pathophysiology of acute renal failure. N Engl J Med 296:1453, 1977.

353. Flamenbaum W: Pathophysiology of acute renal failure. Arch Intern Med 131:191, 1973.

354. Huguenin M, Thiel G, Brunner FP: Mercuric bichloride-induced acute renal failure studied by split drop micropuncture technique in the rat. Nephron 20:147, 1978.

355. Myers BD, Hilberman M, Spence RJ, et al.: Glomerular and tubular function in non-oliguric renal failure. Am J Med 72:642, 1982.

356. Jennings RB, Ganote CE: Mitochondrial structure and function in acute myocardial ischemic injury. Circ Res 38(Suppl 1):80, 1976.

357. Schanne FAX, Kane AB, Young EE, et al.: Calcium dependence of toxic cell death: a final common pathway. Science 206:700, 1979.

358. Siegel NJ, Glazier W, Chandry IH, et al.: Enhanced recovery from acute renal failure by the postischemic infusion of adenine nucleotides and magnesium chloride in rats. Kidney Int 17:338, 1980.

359. Stowe N, Emma J, Magnusson M, et al.: Protective effect of propranolol in the treatment of ischemically damaged canine kidneys prior to transplantation. Surgery 84:265, 1978.

360. Henderson IS, Beattie TJ, Kennedy AC: Dopamine hydrochloride in oliguric states. Lancet 2:827, 1980.

361. Lidner A, Cutler RE, Goodman WG, et al.: Synergism of dopamine plus furosemide in preventing acute renal failure in the dog. Kidney Int 16:158, 1979.

362. Noth RH, McCallum RW, Contino, C, et al.: Tonic dopaminergic suppression of plasma aldosterone. J Clin Endocrinol Metab 51:64, 1980.

363. Chernow B: Hormonal and metabolic considerations in critical care medicine. In Shoemaker WC, Thompson WL, Holbrook PR (Eds.): Society of Critical Care Medicine: Textbook of Critical Care. Philadelphia, W.B. Saunders Co., 1984, pp 646–664.

364. Hilberman M, Maseda J, Stinson EB, et al.: The diuretic properties of dopamine in patients after open-heart operation. Anesthesiology 61:489, 1984.

365. Miller ED Jr: Renal effects of dopamine. Anesthesiology 61:487, 1984.

366. Kebabian JW, Calne DB: Multiple receptors for dopamine. Nature 277:93, 1979.

367. Grodin W, Scantlebury V, Warmington N: Dopaminergic stimulation of renal blood flow and renal function after transplantation. Anesthesiology 61:A129, 1984.

368. Creager MA, Halperin JL, Bernard DB, et al.: Acute regional circulatory and renal hemodynamic effects of converting enzyme inhibition in patients with congestive heart failure. Circulation 61:316, 1980.

369. Dzan VJ, Colvucci WS, Williams GH, et al.: Sustained effectiveness of converting enzyme inhibition in patients with severe congestive failure. N Engl J Med 302:1373, 1980.

370. deTorrenté A, Miller PD, Cronin RE, et al.: Effects of furosemide and acetylcholine in norepinephine-induced acute renal failure. Am J Physiol 235:F131, 1978.

371. Mauk RH, Patak RV, Dadem SZ, et al.: Effect of prostaglandin E administration in a nephrotoxic and a vasoconstrictor model of acute renal failure. Kidney Int 12:122, 1978.

372. Patak RV, Faden SZ, Lifschitz MD, et al.: Study of factors which modify the development of norepinephrine-induced acute renal failure in the dog. Kidney Int 15:227, 1979.

373. Maseda J, Hilberman M, Derry DC, et al.: The renal effects of sodium nitroprusside in post-operative cardiac surgical patients. Anesthesiology 54:284, 1981.

374. Cogan J, Humphreys M, Carlson J, et al.: Renal effects of nitroprusside and hydralazine in patients with congestive heart failure. Circulation 61:316, 1980.

375. Berry KG, Mazze RI, Schwartz FD: Prevention of surgical oliguria and renal hemodynamic suppression by sustained hydration. N Engl J Med 270:1371, 1964.

376. Bush HL, Huse JB, Johnson WC, et al.: Prevention of renal insufficiency after abdominal aortic aneurysm resection by optimal volume loading. Arch Surg 116:1517, 1981.

377. Bidani A, Churchill P, Fleischmann L: Sodium chloride induced protection in nephrotoxic acute renal failure: independence from renin. Kidney Int 16:481, 1979.

378. Kahl FR, Flint JF, Szidon JP: Influence of left atrial distention on renal vasomotor tone. Am J Physiol 226:240, 1974.

379. Mason JM, Ledsome JR: Effects of obstruction of the mitral orifice or distention of the pulmonary vein–atrial junctions on renal and hind-limb vascular resistance in the dog. Circ Res 35:24, 1974.

380. Brosnihan KB, Bravo EL: Graded reductions of atrial pressure and renin release. Am J Physiol 235:H175, 1978.

381. Barry KG, Cohen A, Knochel JP, et al.: Mannitol infusion II. The prevention of acute functional renal failure during resection of an aneurysm of the abdominal aorta. N Engl J Med 264:967, 1961.

382. Flores J, DiBona DR, Beck CH, et al.: The role of cell swelling in ischemic renal damage and the protective effect of hypertonic solute. J Clin Invest 51:118, 1972.

383. Burke TS, Cronin RE, Duchin KL, et al.: Ischemia and tubule obstruction during acute renal failure in dogs. Role of mannitol in protection. Am J Physiol 238:F305, 1980.

384. Eneas JF, Schoenfeld PY, Humphreys MH: The effect of

infusion of mannitol–sodium bicarbonate on the clinical course of myoglobinuria. Arch Intern Med *139*:801, 1979.

385. Morris CR, Alexander EA, Burns SJ, et al.: Restoration and maintenance of glomerular filtration by mannitol during hypoperfusion of the kidney. J Clin Invest *51*:1555, 1972.

386. Stahl WM: Effect of mannitol of the kidney. Changes in intrarenal hemodynamics. N Engl J Med *272*:381, 1965.

387. Barry KG: Post-traumatic renal shutdown in humans: its prevention and treatment by the intravenous infusion of mannitol. Milit Med *128*:224, 1963.

388. Barry KG, Berman AR: Mannitol infusion III. The acute effect of the intravenous infusion of mannitol on blood and plasma volumes. N Engl J Med *264*:1085, 1961.

389. Cantarovich R, Locatelli A, Fernandez JC, et al.: Furosemide in high doses in the treatment of acute renal failure. Postgrad Med J *47*:13, 1971.

390. Epstein M, Schneider NS, Befeler B: Effect of intrarenal furosemide on renal function and intrarenal hemodynamics in acute renal failure. Am J Med *58*:510, 1975.

391. Bailey RR, Natale R, Turnbull DI, et al.: Protective effect of furosemide in acute tubular necrosis and acute renal failure. Clin Sci *45*:1, 1973.

392. Johnston PA, Bernard DB, Levinsky NG: Mechanism of vasodilatory effect of mannitol in the hypoperfused rat kidney: role of renal hormones. Kidney Int *16*:774, 1979.

393. Kleinknecht D, Ganeval D, Gonzalez-Duque LA, et al.: Furosemide in acute oliguric renal failure. A controlled trial. Nephron *17*:51, 1976.

394. Minuth AN, Terrell JB, Suki WN: Acute renal failure: a study of the course and prognosis of 104 patients and of the role of furosemide. Am J Med Sci *271*:317, 1976.

395. Brown CB, Ogg CS, Cameron JS: High dose furosemide in acute renal failure: a controlled trial. Clin Nephrol *15*:90, 1981.

396. Gallagher KL, Jones JK: Furosemide induced ototoxicity. Ann Intern Med *91*:744, 1979.

397. Cooperman LB, Rubin IL: Toxicity of ethacrynic acid and furosemide. Am Heart J *85*:831, 1973.

398. Pillay VKG, Schwartz FD, Aimi K, et al.: Transient and permanent deafness following treatment with ethacrynic acid in renal failure. Lancet *1*:77, 1969.

399. Kelly KJ, Outwater KM, Crone RK: Vasoactive amines in infants and children. Clin Anaesthesiol *2*:427, 1984.

400. Hilberman M: Renal protection. *In* Shoemaker WC, Thompson WL, Holbrook PR (Eds.): Society of Critical Care Medicine: Textbook of Critical Care. Philadelphia, W.B. Saunders Co., 1984, pp 597–604.

401. Lieberman E: Management of acute renal failure in infants and children. Nephron *11*:193, 1973.

402. Abel RM, Beck CH, Abbott WM, et al.: Improved survival from acute renal failure after treatment with intravenous essential L-amino acids and glucose. N Engl J Med *288*:695, 1973.

403. Baek SM, Makabali GG, Bryan-Brown CW, et al.: The influence of parenteral nutrition on the course of acute renal failure. Surg Gynecol Obstet *141*:405, 1975.

404. Abitol CL, Holliday MA: Total parenteral nutrition in anuric children. Clin Nephrol *5*:153, 1976.

405. Giordano C, DeSanto NG, Senatore R: Effects of catabolic stress in acute and chronic renal failure. Am J Clin Nutr *31*:1561, 1978.

406. Blumenkrantz MJ, Kopple JD, Koffler A, et al.: Total parenteral nutrition in the management of acute renal failure. Am J Clin Nutr *31*:1831, 1978.

407. Toback FG, Teergarden DE, Havener LJ: Amino acid–mediated stimulation of renal phospholipid biosynthesis after acute tubular necrosis. Kidney Int *15*:542, 1979.

408. Ellis D, Knappenberger W: Fluid and caloric intake in infants with acute renal failure. Pediatr Res (Abstract) *14*:1017, 1980.

409. Feinstein EI, Blumenkrantz MJ, Healy M, et al.: Clinical and metabolic responses to parenteral nutrition in acute renal failure. Medicine *60*:124, 1981.

410. Conger JD: A controlled evaluation of prophylactic dialysis in post-traumatic acute renal failure. J Trauma *15*:1056, 1975.

411. Kleinknecht D, Jungers P, Chanard J, et al.: Uremic and nonuremic complications in acute renal failure: evaluation of early and frequent dialysis on prognosis. Kidney Int *1*:190, 1972.

412. Parsons FM, Blagg CR, Hobson SM, et al.: Optimum time for dialysis in acute reversible renal failure. Lancet *1*:129, 1961.

413. Esperanca MJ, Collins DL: Peritoneal dialysis efficiency in relation to body weight. J Pediatr Surg *1*:162, 1966.

414. Potter DE: Comparison of peritoneal dialysis and hemodialysis in children. Dial Transplant *7*:800, 1978.

415. Day RE, White RH: Peritoneal dialysis in children. Arch Dis Child *52*:56, 1977.

416. Fine RN: Peritoneal dialysis update. J Pediatr *100*:1, 1982.

417. Vaamonde CA, Michael UF, Metzger RA, et al.: Complications of acute peritoneal dialysis. J Chronic Dis *28*:637, 1975.

418. Soffer O, MacDonnel RC, Finlayson DC, et al.: Intraoperative hemodialysis during cardiopulmonary bypass in chronic renal failure. J Thorac Cardiovasc Surg *77*:789, 1979.

419. Intoni F, Alquati P, Schiavello R, et al.: Ultrafiltration during open heart surgery in chronic renal failure. Scand J Thorac Cardiovasc Surg *15*:217, 1981.

420. Berry AJ: Respiratory support and renal function. Anesthesiology *55*:655, 1981.

421. Priebe HJ, Hedley-White J: Respiratory support and renal function. Int Anesthesiol Clin *22*:203, 1984.

422. Bernstein J, Barnett HL, Edelmann CM Jr.: Glomerular diseases: introduction and classification. *In* Edelmann CM Jr (Ed.): Pediatric Kidney Disease. Boston, Little, Brown, 1978, pp 586–592.

423. Hayslett JP, Siegel NJ, Kashgarian M: Glomerulonephropathy. Adv Intern Med *20*:215, 1975.

424. Hyman LR, Walker PF: Progressive renal failure and nephrotic syndrome in children: a spectrum of glomerulonephropathies. Milit Med *140*:608, 1975.

425. McClusky RT, Klassen J: Immunologically mediated glomerular, tubular and interstitial renal disease. N Engl J Med *288*:564, 1973.

426. Bright R: Cases and observations illustrative of renal disease accompanied by the secretion of albuminous urine. Guy's Hospital Reports *1*:338, 1836.

427. Jordan SC, Lemire JM: Acute glomerulonephritis: diagnosis and treatment. Pediatr Clin North Am *29*:857, 1982.

428. Cochrane CG, Koffler D: Immune complex disease in experimental animals and man. Adv Immunol *16*:185, 1973.

429. Couser WG, Salant DJ: In situ immune complex formation and glomerular injury. Kidney Int *17*:1, 1980.

430. McDonald BM, McEnery PT: Glomerulonephritis in children: clinical and morphologic characteristics and mechanisms of glomerular injury. Pediatr Clin North Am *23*:691, 1976.

431. Jordan SC, Buckingham B, Sakai R, et al.: Studies of immune complex glomerulonephritis mediated by human thyroglobulin. N Engl J Med *304*:1212, 1981.

432. Kaplan BS, Klassen J, Gault MH: Glomerular injury in patients with neoplasia. Ann Rev Med *27*:117, 1976.

433. Barralt TM: Glomerular disease and haematuria. *In* Williams DI, Johnston JH (Eds.): Paediatric Urology. London, Butterworth Scientific, 1982, pp 79–88.

434. George CRP, Clark WF, Cameron JS: The role of platelets in glomerulonephritis. Adv Nephrol *5*:19, 1975.

435. Zimmerman SW, Moorthy AV, Dreher WH, et al.: Prospective trial of warfarin and dipyridamole in patients with membranoproliferative glomerulonephritis. Am J Med *75*:920, 1983.

436. Hayslett JP: Role of platelets in glomerulonephritis. N Engl J Med *310*:1457, 1984.

437. Donadio JV Jr, Anderson CF, Mitchell JC III, et al.: Membranoproliferative glomerulonephritis: a prospective clinical trial of platelet-inhibitor therapy. N Engl J Med *310*:1421, 1984.

438. Lewy JE: Acute post-streptoccocal glomerulonephritis. Pediatr Clin North Am *23*:751, 1976.

439. Dodge WF, Spargo BH, Travis LB: Occurrence of acute glomerulonephritis in sibling contacts of children with sporadic acute glomerulonephritis. Pediatrics *40*:1029, 1967.

440. Kaplan EL, Anthony BF, Chapman SS, et al.: Epidemic acute glomerulonephritis associated with type 49 streptococcal pyoderma. Am J Med *48*:9, 1970.

441. Dodge WF, Spargo BH, Travis LB, et al.: Poststreptococcal glomerulonephritis: a prospective study in children. N Engl J Med *286*:273, 1972.

442. Travis LB: Acute postinfectious glomerulonephritis. *In* Edelmann CM Jr (Ed.): Pediatric Kidney Disease. Boston, Little, Brown, 1978, pp 611–630.

443. McConville JM, West CD, McAdams AJ: Familial and non-familial benign hematuria. J Pediatr *69*:207, 1966.

444. Bernstein J, Kissane JM: Hereditary nephritis. *In* Edelmann CM Jr (Ed.): Pediatric Kidney Disease. Boston, Little, Brown, 1978, pp 571–579.

445. Shaw RF, Kallen RJ: Population genetics of Alport's syndrome: hypothesis of abnormal segregation and the necessary existence of mutation. Nephron *16*:427, 1976.

446. Simila S, Vesa L, Wasz-Hockert O: Hereditary onycho-osteodysplasia (the nail-patella syndrome) with nephrosis-like renal disease in a newborn boy. Pediatrics *46*:61, 1970.

447. Boulton-Jones JM, Sissons JG, Evans DJ, et al.: Renal lesions of subacute infective endocarditis. Br Med J *2*:11, 1974.

448. Dobrin RS, Day NK, Quie PG, et al.: The role of complement, immunoglobulin and bacterial antigen in coagulase-negative staphylococcal shunt nephritis. Am J Med *59*:660, 1975.

449. Meadow SR: Schönlein-Henoch syndrome. *In* Edelmann CM Jr (Ed.): Pediatric Kidney Disease. Boston, Little, Brown, 1978, pp 788–795.

450. Glasgow EF: Renal changes in Henoch-Schönlein purpura. Arch Dis Child *45*:151, 1970.

451. Goldbloom RB, Drummond KN: Anaphylactoid purpura with massive gastrointestinal hemorrhage and glomerulonephritis. Am J Dis Child *116*:97, 1968.

452. Counahan R, Winterborn MH, Meadow SR, et al.: The prognosis of Schönlein-Henoch nephritis. Br Med J *2*:11, 1977.

453. Meadow SR, Glasgow EF, White RHR, et al.: Schönlein-Henoch nephritis. Q J Med *41*:241, 1972.

454. Hurley RM, Drummond KN: Anaphylactoid purpura nephritis: clinopathological correlations. J Pediatr *81*:904, 1972.

455. Lewis EJ: Pulmonary hemorrhage and glomerulonephritis (Goodpasture's syndrome). *In* Edelmann CM Jr (Ed.): Pediatric Kidney Disease. Boston, Little, Brown, 1978, pp 736–744.

456. Proskey AJ, Weatherbee L, Easterling RE, et al.: Goodpasture's syndrome: a report of five cases and review of the literature. Am J Med *48*:162, 1970.

457. Wilson CB, Dixon FJ: Anti–glomerular basement membrane antibody–induced glomerulonephritis. Kidney Int *3*:74, 1973.

458. Beirne GJ, Octaviano GN, Kopp WL, et al.: Immunohistology of the lung in Goodpasture's syndrome. Ann Intern Med *69*:1207, 1968.

459. Lockwood CM, Rees AJ, Pearson TA, et al.: Immunosuppression and plasma exchange in the treatment of Goodpasture's syndrome. Lancet *1*:711, 1976.

460. Maddock RK, Stevens LE, Reetsma K, et al.: Goodpasture's syndrome: cessation of pulmonary hemorrhage after bilateral nephrectomy. Ann Intern Med *67*:1258, 1967.

461. Siegel RR: The basis of pulmonary disease resolution after nephrectomy in Goodpasture's syndrome. Am J Med Sci *259*:201, 1970.

462. Eisinger AJ: Goodpasture's syndrome: failure of nephrectomy to cure pulmonary hemorrhage. Am J Med *55*:565, 1973.

463. Couser WG, Wallace A, Monaco AP, et al.: Successful renal transplantation in patients with circulating antibody to glomerular basement membrane: report of 2 cases. Clin Nephrol *1*:381, 1973.

464. Fong JSC, deChadarevian JP, Kaplan BS: Hemolytic-uremic syndrome: current concepts and management. Pediatr Clin North Am *29*:835, 1982.

465. Gianantonia CA: Hemolytic-uremic syndrome. *In* Edelmann CM Jr (Ed.): Pediatric Kidney Disease. Boston, Little, Brown, 1978, pp 724–735.

466. Upadhyaya K, Barwick K, Fishaut M, et al.: The importance of non-renal involvement in hemolytic-uremic syndrome. Pediatrics *65*:115, 1980.

467. Kaplan BS, Thomson PD, deChadarevian JP: The hemolytic-uremic syndrome. Pediatr Clin North Am *23*:761, 1976.

468. Hellman RM, Jackson DV, Buss DH: Thrombotic thrombocytopenic purpura and hemolytic-uremic syndrome in HLA-identical siblings. Ann Intern Med *93*:283, 1980.

469. Kaplan BS, Drummond KN: The hemolytic uremic syndrome is a syndrome. N Engl J Med *298*:964, 1978.

470. Koster F, Levin J, Walker L, et al.: Hemolytic-uremic syndrome after shigellosis: relation to endotoxemia and circulating immune complexes. N Engl J Med *298*:927, 1978.

471. Katz J, Krawitz S, Sacks PV, et al.: Platelet, erythrocyte and fibrinogen kinetics in the hemolytic-uremic syndrome of infancy. J Pediatr *83*:739, 1973.

472. Remuzzi G, Misiani R, Marchesi D, et al.: Hemolytic uremic syndrome: deficiency of plasma factors regulating prostacyclin activity. Lancet *2*:871, 1978.

473. Ray CG, Portman JN, Stamm SJ, et al.: Hemolytic-uremic syndrome and myocarditis: association with coxsackievirus B infection. Am J Dis Child *122*:418, 1971.

474. Bale JF, Brasher C, Siegler RL: CNS manifestations of the hemolytic-uremic syndrome: relationship to metabolic alterations and prognosis. Am J Dis Child *134*:869, 1980.

475. Rooney JC, Anderson RM, Hopking IH: Clinical and pathological aspects of central nervous system involvement in the haemolytic-uraemic syndrome. Aust Paediatr J *7*:28, 1971.

476. Dolislager D, Tune B: The hemolytic-uremic syndrome. Spectrum of severity and significance of prodrome. Am J Dis Child *132*:55, 1978.

477. O'Regan S, Chesney RW, Mongeau J, et al.: Aspirin and dipyridamole therapy in the hemolytic-uremic syndrome. J Pediatr *97*:473, 1980.

478. Brandt P, Jesperson J, Gregersen G: Post partum haemolytic-uraemic syndrome treated with antithrombin-III. Nephron *27*:15, 1981.

479. Remuzzi G, Misiani R, Marchesi D, et al.: Treatment of the hemolytic-uremic syndrome with plasma. Clin Nephrol *12*:279, 1979.

480. Harden LB, Gluck RS, Salcedo JR: Simultaneous hemodialysis and exchange transfusion in hemolytic uremic syndrome. Clin Pediatr *10*:640, 1980.

481. Denneberg T, Friedberg M, Holmberg L, et al.: Combined plasmapheresis and hemodialysis treatment for severe hemolytic-uremic syndrome following *Campylobacter* colitis. Acta Paediatr Scand *71*:243, 1982.

482. Beattie TJ, Murphy AV, Willoughby MLN, et al.: Plasmapheresis in the haemolytic-uraemic syndrome in children. Br Med J *282*:1667, 1981.

483. Vitacco M, Sanchez-Avalos J, Gianantonio CA: Heparin therapy in the hemolytic-uremic syndrome. J Pediatr *83*:271, 1973.

484. Cerilli CJ, Nelson C, Dorfmann L: Renal homotransplantation in infants and children with the hemolytic-uremic syndrome. Surgery *71*:66, 1972.

485. Howard EJ, Mauer SM, Miller K, et al.: Biopsy proven recurrence of hemolytic uremic syndrome early after kidney transplantation with a favorable outcome. Kidney Int 10:544, 1976.

486. Rance CP, Arbus GS, Balfe JW: Management of the nephrotic syndrome in children. Pediatr Clin North Am 23:735, 1976.

487. McEnery PT, Strife CF: Nephrotic syndrome in childhood: management and treatment in patients with minimal change disease, mesangial proliferation, or focal glomerulosclerosis. Pediatr Clin North Am 89:875, 1982.

488. Barnett HL, Schoeneman M, Bernstein J, et al.: The nephrotic syndrome. In Edelmann CM Jr (Ed.): Pediatric Kidney Disease. Boston, Little, Brown, 1978, pp 679–694.

489. International Study of Kidney Disease in Children: The nephrotic syndrome in children. Prediction of histopathology from clinical and laboratory characteristics at the time of diagnosis. Kidney Int 13:159, 1978.

490. International Study of Kidney Disease in Children: The primary nephrotic syndrome in children. Identification of patients with minimal change nephrotic syndrome from initial response to prednisone. J Pediatr 98:561, 1981.

491. Heymann W, Makker S, Post R: The preponderance of males in the idiopathic nephrotic syndrome. Pediatrics 50:814, 1972.

492. Barnett HL, Schoeneman M, Bernstein J, et al.: Minimal change nephrotic syndrome. In Edelmann CM Jr (Ed.): Pediatric Kidney Disease. Boston, Little, Brown, 1978, pp 695–710.

493. Nash MA: Focal segmental glomerulosclerosis. In Edelmann CM Jr (Ed.): Pediatric Kidney Disease. Boston, Little, Brown, 1978, pp 718–724.

494. International Study of Kidney Disease in Children: Minimal change nephrotic syndrome in children: deaths during the first 5 to 15 year's observation. Pediatrics 73:497, 1984.

495. Futrakul P, Poshyachinda M, Mitrakul C: Focal sclerosing glomerulonephritis: a kinetic evaluation of hemostasis and the effect of anticoagulant therapy: a controlled study. Clin Nephrol 10:180, 1978.

496. Futrakul P: A new therapeutic approach to nephrotic syndrome associated with focal segmental glomerulosclerosis. Int J Pediatr Nephrol 1:18, 1980.

497. White RHR: Membranoproliferative glomerulonephritis. In Edelmann CM Jr (Ed.): Pediatric Kidney Disease. Boston, Little, Brown, 1978, pp 660–678.

498. Habib R, Kleinknecht C, Gübler MC, et al.: Membranous glomerulopathy in children. In Edelmann CM Jr (Ed.): Pediatric Kidney Disease. Boston, Little, Brown, 1978, pp 646–659.

499. Hallman N, Rapola J: Congenital nephrotic syndrome. In Edelmann CM Jr (Ed.): Pediatric Kidney Disease. Boston, Little, Brown, 1978, pp 711–717.

500. Kaplan BS, Bureau MA, Drummond KN: The nephrotic syndrome in the first year of life: is a pathologic classification possible? J Pediatr 85:615, 1974.

501. Bohrer MP, Dean WM, Robertson CR, et al.: Influence of molecular configuration in the glomerular filtration of macromolecules. Kidney Int 14:751, 1978.

502. Chang RLS, Deen WM, Robertson CR, et al.: Permselectivity of the glomerular capillary wall. Restricted transport of polyanions. Kidney Int 8:212, 1975.

503. Rennke HC, Venkatachalam MA: Glomerular permeability: in vivo tracer studies with polyanionic and polycationic ferritins. Kidney Int 11:94, 1977.

504. Cameron JS, Turner DR, Ogg CS, et al.: The long-term prognosis of patients with focal segmental glomerulosclerosis. Clin Nephrol 10:213, 1978.

505. Hulme B, Hardwicke J: Human glomerular permeability to macromolecules in health and disease. Clin Sci 34:515, 1968.

506. Blau EB, Haas DE: Glomerular sialic acid and proteinuria in human renal disease. Lab Invest 28:477, 1973.

507. Carrie BJ, Salyer WR, Myers BD: Minimal change nephropathy: an electrochemical disorder of the glomerular membrane. Am J Med 70:262, 1981.

508. Davison AM, Lambie AT, Verth AH, et al.: Salt-poor albumin in the management of nephrotic syndrome. Br Med J 1:481, 1974.

509. Wilfert CM, Katz SL: Etiology of bacterial sepsis in nephrotic children. Pediatrics 42:841, 1968.

510. Kendall AG, Lohmann RC, Dossetor JB: Nephrotic syndrome—a hypercoaguable state. Arch Intern Med 127:1021, 1971.

511. Lieberman E, Heuser E, Gilchrist GS, et al.: Thrombosis, nephrosis and corticosteroid therapy. J Pediatr 73:320, 1968.

512. Adler AJ, Lundlin AP, Feinroth MV, et al.: Beta-thromboglobulin levels in the nephrotic syndrome. Am J Med 69:551, 1980.

513. Goldbloom RB, Hillman DA, Santulli TV: Arterial thrombosis following femoral venipuncture in edematous nephrotic children. Pediatrics 40:450, 1967.

514. Levin SE, Zamit R, Schmaman A: Thrombosis of the pulmonary arteries and the nephrotic syndrome. Br Med J 1:153, 1967.

515. Egan TJ, Kenny FM, Jarrah A, et al.: Shock as a complication of the nephrotic syndrome. Am J Dis Child 113:364, 1967.

516. Lau SO, Tkachuck JY, Hasegawa DK, et al.: Plasminogen and antithrombin III deficiencies in the childhood nephrotic syndrome associated with plasminogenuria and antithrombinuria. J Pediatr 96:390, 1980.

517. Bang NU, Trygstad CW, Schroeder JE, et al.: Enhanced platelet function in glomerular renal disease. J Lab Clin Med 81:651, 1973.

518. Anderson CF, Jaecks DM, Ballon HS, et al.: Renal handling of creatinine in nephrotic and non-nephrotic patients. Clin Sci 38:555, 1970.

519. McVicar MI, Exeni R, Susin M: Renal glycosuria, an early sign of focal segmental glomerulosclerosis. Pediatr Res 9:376, 1975.

520. Goldstein DA, Haldimann B, Sherman D, et al.: Vitamin D metabolites and calcium metabolism in patients with nephrotic syndrome and normal renal function. J Clin Endocrinol Metab 52:116, 1981.

521. Freedman LR: The interstitial nephritides (interstitial renal inflammation). In Edelmann CM Jr (Ed.): Pediatric Kidney Disease. Boston, Little, Brown, 1978, pp 879–889.

522. Murray T, Goldberg MD: Etiologies of chronic interstitial nephritis. Ann Intern Med 82:453, 1975.

523. Nanra RS, Chirawong P, Kincaid-Smith P: Medullary ischaemia in experimental analgesic nephropathy—the pathogenesis of renal papillary necrosis. Aust NZ J Med 3:580, 1973.

524. Kunin CM: The natural history of recurrent bacteriuria in school-girls. N Engl J Med 282:1443, 1970.

525. Amar AD: Colicotubular backflow with vesico-ureteral reflux. Relation to pyelonephritis. JAMA 213:293, 1970.

526. Hodson CJ: Vesico-ureteric reflux and renal scarring—with and without infection. Kidney Int 5:308, 1974.

527. Winberg J, Bollgren I, Kallenius G, et al.: Clinical pyelonephritis and focal renal scarring. A selected review of pathogenesis, prevention and prognosis. Pediatr Clin North Am 29:801, 1982.

528. Miller T, Phillips S: Pyelonephritis: the relationship between infection, renal scarring, and antimicrobial therapy. Kidney Int 19:654, 1981.

529. Johnston JH: Urinary tract infection: tuberculosis and other specific infections. In Williams DI, Johnston JH (Eds.): Paediatric Urology. London, Butterworth Scientific, 1982, pp 121–127.

530. Kim Y, Michael AF: Infection and nephritis. In Edelmann CM Jr (Ed.): Pediatric Kidney Disease. Boston, Little, Brown, 1978, pp 828–836.

531. Woodroffe AJ, Row PG, Meadows R, et al.: Nephritis in infectious mononucleosis. Q J Med 43:451, 1974.

532. Donckerwolcke RA: Diagnosis and treatment of renal tubular disorders in children. Pediatr Clin North Am 29:895, 1982.

533. Rodriguez Soriano J: Renal tubular acidosis. *In* Edelmann CM Jr (Ed.): Pediatric Kidney Disease. Boston, Little, Brown, 1978, pp 995–1011.

534. Edelmann CM Jr, Rodriguez Soriano J, Boichis H, et al.: Bicarbonate reabsorption and hydrogen ion excretion in normal infants. J Clin Invest 46:1309, 1967.

535. Rodriguez Soriano J, Boichis H, Edelmann CM Jr: Bicarbonate reabsorption and hydrogen ion excretion in children with renal tubular acidosis. J Pediatr 71:802, 1967.

536. Brenes LG, Brenes JN, Hernandez MM: Familial proximal renal tubular acidosis. A distinct clinical entity. Am J Med 63:244, 1977.

537. Sebastian A, McSherry E, Morris RC Jr: Renal potassium wasting in renal tubular acidosis (RTA): its occurrence in types 1 and 2 RTA despite sustained correction of systemic acidosis. J Clin Invest 50:667, 1971.

538. Donckerwolcke RA, van Stekelenburg GJ, Tiddens HA: Therapy of bicarbonate losing renal tubular acidosis. Arch Dis Child 45:774, 1970.

539. Oetliker O, Rossi E: The influence of extracellular fluid volume on the renal bicarbonate threshold: a study of two children with Lowe's syndrome. Pediatr Res 3:140, 1969.

540. Rodriguez Soriano J, Edelmann CM Jr: Renal tubular acidosis. Ann Rev Med 20:263, 1969.

541. McSherry E, Morris RC: Attainment and maintenance of normal stature with alkali therapy in infants and children with classic renal tubular acidosis. J Clin Invest 61:501, 1978.

542. Battle CD, Arruda JAL, Kurkman HA: Hyperkalemic distal renal tubular acidosis associated with obstructive uropathy. N Engl J Med 304:373, 1981.

543. Alon U, Kodroff MB, Broecker BH, et al.: Renal tubular acidosis type 4 in neonatal unilateral kidney diseases. J Pediatr 104:855, 1984.

544. Weinstein SF, Allan DME, Mendoza SA: Hyperkalemia, acidosis and short stature associated with a defect in renal potassium excretion. J Pediatr 85:355, 1974.

545. Brodehl J: The Fanconi syndrome. *In:* Edelmann CM Jr (Ed.): Pediatric Kidney Disease. Boston, Little, Brown, 1978, pp 955–987.

546. Proesmans W, Snoeck L, Sina JKA, et al.: Inhibitors of prostaglandin synthetase as a therapy for cystinosis (abstract). Int J Paediatr Nephrol 2:130, 1981.

547. Dillon MJ, Leonard JV, Buckler JM, et al.: Pseudohypoaldosteronism. Arch Dis Child 55:427, 1980.

548. Joel M, Rosales JK: Fanconi syndrome and anesthesia. Anesthesiology 55:455, 1981.

549. Glorieux FH, Marie PF, Pettifor JM, et al.: Bone response to phosphate salts, ergocalciferol, and calcitriol in hypophosphatemic vitamin-D resistant rickets. N Engl J Med 303:1023, 1980.

550. Rasmussen H, Pechet M, Anast C, et al.: Long-term treatment of familial hypophosphatemic rickets with oral phosphate and 1-alpha-hydroxyvitamin D3. J Pediatr 99:16, 1981.

551. Avoli, LV: Clinical syndromes characterized by disturbances in phosphate transport and excretion. *In* Edelmann CM Jr (Ed.): Pediatric Kidney Disease. Boston, Little, Brown, 1978, pp 1012–1035.

552. Stern P: Nephrogenic defects of urinary concentration. *In* Edelmann CM Jr (Ed.): Pediatric Kidney Disease. Boston, Little, Brown, 1978, pp 987–995.

553. Dousa TP, Valtin H: Cellular actions of vasopressin in the mammalian kidney. Kidney Int 10:46, 1976.

554. Marumo F, Edelman IS: Effects of calcium and prostaglandin E-1 on vasopressin activation of renal adenyl cyclase. J Clin Invest 50:1613, 1971.

555. Jamison RL, Maffly RH: The urinary concentrating mechanism. N Engl J Med 295:1059, 1976.

556. Bennett CM: Urine concentration and dilution in hypokalemic and hypercalcemic dogs. J Clin Invest 49:1447, 1970.

557. Dousa TP: Cellular action of antidiuretic hormone in nephrogenic diabetes insipidus. Mayo Clin Proc 49:188, 1974.

558. Blachar Y, Zadik A, Shemesh M, et al.: The effect of inhibition of prostaglandin synthesis on free water and osmolar clearances in patients with hereditary nephrogenic diabetes insipidus. Int J Pediatr Nephrol 1:48, 1980.

559. Earley LE, Orloff J: The mechanism of antidiuresis associated with the administration of hydrochlorothiazide to patients with vasopressin-resistant diabetes insipidus. J Clin Invest 41:1988, 1962.

560. Spitzer A, Edelmann CM Jr, Goldberg LD, et al.: Short stature, hyperkalemia and acidosis: a defect in renal transport of potassium. Kidney Int 3:251, 1973.

561. Schwartz GJ, Spitzer A: Disorders of renal transport of sodium, potassium and magnesium. *In* Edelmann CM Jr (Ed.): Pediatric Kidney Disease. Boston, Little, Brown, 1978, pp 1079–1093.

562. Bourke E, Delaney V: Bartter's syndrome—a dilemma of cause and effect. Nephron 27:177, 1981.

563. Arant BS, Brackett NC, Young RB, et al.: Case studies of siblings with juxtamedullary hyperplasia and secondary aldosteronism associated with severe azotemia and renal rickets—Bartter's syndrome or disease? Pediatrics 46:344, 1970.

564. Littlewood JM, Lee HR, Medow SR: Treatment of Bartter's syndrome in early childhood with prostaglandin synthetase inhibitors. Arch Dis Child 53:43, 1978.

565. Lechaz G, Arbus GS, Balfe JW, et al.: Effect of ibuprofen on growth in a child with Bartter's syndrome. J Pediatr 95:319, 1979.

566. Abston PA, Priano LL: Bartter's syndrome: anesthetic implications based on pathophysiology and treatment. Anesth Analg 60:764, 1981.

567. Booth BE, Johanson A: Hypomagnesemia due to renal tubular defect in reabsorption of magnesium. J Pediatr 84:350, 1974.

568. Schulman JD, Schneider JA: Cystinosis and the Fanconi syndrome. Pediatr Clin North Am 23:779, 1976.

569. Bernstein J: Polycystic disease. *In* Edelmann CM Jr (Ed.): Pediatric Kidney Disease. Boston, Little, Brown, 1978, pp 557–570.

570. Hayslett JP: Medullary sponge kidney. *In* Edelmann CM Jr (Ed.): Pediatric Kidney Disease. Boston, Little, Brown, 1978, pp 889–893.

571. Bernstein J: Renal hypoplasia and dysplasia. *In* Edelmann CM Jr (Ed.): Pediatric Kidney Disease. Boston, Little, Brown, pp 541–557.

572. Guignard JP: Renal function in the newborn infant. Pediatr Clin North Am 29:777, 1982.

573. Lieberman E, Salinas-Madrigal L, Gwinn JL, et al.: Infantile polycystic disease of the kidneys and liver: clinical, pathological, and radiological correlations and comparison with congenital hepatic fibrosis. Medicine 50:277, 1971.

574. Vuthibhagdee A, Singleton EB: Infantile polycystic disease of the kidney. Am J Dis Child 125:167, 1973.

575. Anand SK, Chan JC, Lieberman E: Polycystic disease and hepatic fibrosis in children. Renal function studies. Am J Dis Child 129:810, 1975.

576. Ross DG, Travers H: Infantile presentation of adult type polycystic kidney disease in a large kindred. J Pediatr 87:760, 1975.

577. Mauer SM, Lynch RE: Hemodialysis techniques for infants and children. Pediatr Clin North Am 23:843, 1976.

578. Guignard JP, Wallimann C, Gautier E: Prevention by verapamil of the hypoxaemia-induced renal vasoconstriction. Kidney Int 20:139, 1981.

579. Bernstein J, Gardner KD Jr: Familial juvenile nephronophthisis—medullary cystic disease. *In* Edelmann CM Jr (Ed.): Pediatric Kidney Disease. Boston, Little, Brown, 1978, pp 580–586.

580. Sotelo-Veila C, Singer DB: Syndrome of hyperplastic fetal visceromegaly and neonatal hypoglycemia (Beckwith's syndrome): a report of seven cases. Pediatrics 46:240, 1970.

581. Beck DA: The effect of intrauterine urinary obstruction upon the development of the fetal kidney. J Urol 105:784, 1971.

582. Bernstein, J: The morphogenesis of renal parenchymal mal-

development (renal dysplasia). Pediatr Clin North Am 18:395, 1971.

583. Cussen JJ: Cystic Kidneys in children with congenital urethral obstruction. J Urol 106:939, 1971.

584. Bernstein J, Meyer R: Some speculations on the nature and significance of developmentally small kidneys (renal hypoplasia). Nephron 1:137, 1964.

585. Carter JE, Lirenman DS: Bilateral renal hypoplasia with oligomeganephronia. Oligomeganephronic renal hypoplasia. Am J Dis Child 120:537, 1970.

586. Royer P, Habib R, Broyer M, et al.: Segmental hypoplasia of the kidney in children. Adv Nephrol 1:145, 1971.

587. Fay R, Winer R, Cohen A, et al.: Segmental renal hypoplasia and hypertension. J Urol 113:561, 1975.

588. Moorthy AV, Zimmerman SW, Burkholder PM: Effects of extra-renal neoplasms on the kidney. In Edelmann CM Jr (Ed.): Pediatric Kidney Disease. Boston, Little, Brown, 1978, pp 811–827.

589. Trainin EB: Renal involvement in amyloidosis. In Edelman CM Jr (Ed.): Pediatric Kidney Disease. Boston, Little, Brown, 1978, pp 799–811.

590. Nyhan WL: Urate nephropathy. In Edelmann CM Jr (Ed.): Pediatric Kidney Disease. Boston, Little, Brown, 1978, pp 894–906.

591. Barratt TM: Urolithiasis: medical aspects. In Williams DI, Johnston JH (Eds.): Paediatric Urology. London, Butterworth Scientific, 1982, pp 351–360.

592. Garcia RE, Friedman WF, Kaback MM, et al.: Idiopathic hypercalcemia and supravalvular aortic stenosis. N Engl J Med 271:117, 1964.

593. Pabico RC, Atanacio BC, McKenna BA, et al.: Renal pathologic lesions and functional alterations in man with Fabry's disease. Am J Med 55:415, 1973.

594. Dresnick RJ, Allen KY, Simmons RL, et al.: Correction of enzymatic deficiencies by renal transplantation: Fabry's disease. Surgery 72:203, 1972.

595. Morel-Maroger L, Basch A, Dannon F, et al.: Pathology of the kidney in Waldenström's macroglobulinemia. N Engl J Med 283:123, 1970.

596. Kaplan NG, Kaplan KC: Monoclonal gammopathy, glomerulonephritis, and the nephrotic syndrome. Arch Intern Med 125:696, 1970.

597. Kew MC, Brunt PW, Varma RR: Renal and intrarenal blood flow in cirrhosis of the liver. Lancet 2:504, 1971.

598. Epstein M, Berk DP, Hollenberg NK, et al.: Renal failure in the patient with cirrhosis: the role of active vasoconstriction. Am J Med 49:175, 1970.

599. Conn HO: A rational approach to the hepatorenal syndrome. Gastroenterology 65:321, 1973.

600. Schwartz GJ, Spitzer A: Metal nephropathy. In Edelmann CM Jr (Ed.): Pediatric Kidney Disease. Boston, Little, Brown, 1978, pp 940–952.

601. Elsas LJ, Hayslett JP, Spargo BH, et al.: Wilson's disease with reversible renal tubular dysfunction: correlation with proximal tubular ultrastructure. Ann Intern Med 75:427, 1971.

602. Stapleton FB, Johnson DL, Kaplan GW, et al.: The cystic renal lesion in tuberous sclerosis. J Pediatr 97:574, 1980.

603. Resnick JS, Michael AF: Renal manifestations in connective tissue disease. In Edelmann CM Jr (Ed.): Pediatric Kidney Disease. Boston, Little, Brown, 1978, pp 768–776.

604. Dabich L, Sullivan DB, Cassidy JT: Scleroderma in the child. J Pediatr 85:770, 1974.

605. Cannon PJ, Hassar M, Case DB, et al.: The relationship of hypertension and renal failure in scleroderma (progressive systemic sclerosis) to structural and functional abnormalities of the renal cortical circulation. Medicine 55:1, 1974.

606. Keane WF, Danielson B, Ray L: Successful renal transplantation in progressive systemic sclerosis. Ann Intern Med 85:199, 1976.

607. Moutsopolous H, Fye KH: Lipoid nephrosis and focal glomerulosclerosis in a patient with polymyositis. Lancet 1:1039, 1975.

608. Singsen B, Goldreyen B, Stanton R, et al.: Childhood polymyositis with cardiac conduction defects. Am J Dis Child 130:72, 1976.

609. Park S, Nyhan WL: Fatal pulmonary involvement in dermatomyositis. Am J Dis Child 129:723, 1975.

610. Singsen BH, Bernstein BH, Kornreich HK, et al.: Mixed connective tissue disease in childhood: a clinical and serologic survey. J Pediatr 90:893, 1977.

611. Meadow R: Polyarteritis nodosa (periarteritis nodosa). In Edelmann CM Jr (Ed.): Pediatric Kidney Disease. Boston, Little, Brown, 1978, pp 796–799.

612. Fish, AJ, Blau EB, Westberg NG, et al.: SLE within the first two decades of life. Am J Med 62:99, 1977.

613. Walravens PA, Chase HP: The prognosis of childhood systemic lupus erythematosis. Am J Dis Child 130:929, 1976.

614. Fish AJ, Vernier RL, Michael AF: Systemic lupus erythematosis. In Edelmann CM Jr (Ed.): Pediatric Kidney Disease. Boston, Little, Brown, 1978, pp 745–767.

615. Alleyene GAO, Statius-Van-Eps LW, Addae SK, et al.: The kidney in sickle cell anemia. Kidney Int 7:731, 1975.

616. Strauss J, McIntosh RM: Sickle cell nephropathy. In Edelmann CM Jr (Ed.): Pediatric Kidney Disease. Boston, Little, Brown, 1978, pp 776–788.

617. Johnson M, Rabinowitz I, Willis AL, et al.: Detection of prostaglandin induction of erythrocyte sickling. Clin Chem 19:23, 1973.

618. Berman LB: Sickle cell nephropathy. JAMA 228:1279, 1974.

619. Strom T, Muehrcke RC, Smith RD: Sickle cell anemia with the nephrotic syndrome and renal vein obstruction. Arch Intern Med 129:104, 1972.

620. Friedman EA, Sreepada TK, Sprung CL, et al.: Uremia in sickle cell anemia treated by maintenance hemodialysis. N Engl J Med 291:431, 1974.

621. Hatch FE, Culbertson JW, Diggs LW: Nature of the renal concentrating defect in sickle cell disease. J Clin Invest 46:336, 1967.

622. Beyer MM: Diabetic nephropathy. Pediatr Clin North Am 31:635, 1984.

623. Knowles HC Jr: Renal disease in juvenile diabetes. In Edelmann CM Jr (Ed.): Pediatric Kidney Disease. Boston, Little, Brown, 1978, pp 806–811.

624. Mogensen CE: Renal function changes in diabetes. Diabetes 25:872, 1976.

625. Urizar RE, Schwartz A, Top F Jr, et al.: The nephrotic syndrome in children with diabetes mellitus of recent onset. N Engl J Med 281:173, 1969.

626. Goldstein DA, Massry SG: Diabetic nephropathy—clinical course and effect of hemodialysis. Nephron 20:286, 1978.

627. Williams DI, Martin J: Renal tumours. In Williams DI, Johnston JH (Eds.): Paediatric Urology. London, Butterworth Scientific, 1982, pp 381–399.

628. Johnston JH: Neuroblastoma, teratoma and other retroperitoneal tumours. In Williams DI, Johnston JH (Eds.): Paediatric Urology. London, Butterworth Scientific, 1982, pp 401–409.

629. Krishna G: Neurofibromatosis, renal hypertension and cardiac dysrhythmias. Anesth Analg 54:542, 1975.

630. Pilling GP: Wilms' tumor in seven children with congenital aniridia. J Pediatr Surg 10:87, 1975.

631. Barakat AY, Papadoulou ZL, Chandra RS: Pseudohermaphroditism, nephron disorder and Wilms' tumor. Pediatrics 54:366, 1974.

632. Sukarochana K, Tolentino W, Kiesewetter WB: Wilms' tumor and hypertension. J Pediatr Surg 7:573, 1972.

633. Spahr J, Demers LM, Shochat SJ: Renin producing Wilms' tumor. J Pediatr Surg 16:32, 1981.

634. Martin J, Rickham PP: Pulmonary metastases in Wilms' tumor. Arch Dis Childhood 45:805, 1970.

635. Stehling LC, Furman EB: Anesthesia for congenital anomalies of the genito-urinary system. In Stehling LC, Zauder HL (Eds.): Anesthetic Implications of Congenital Anomalies in

Children. New York, Appleton-Century-Crofts, 1980, pp 145–165.

636. D'Angio GJ, Beckwith JB, Breslow NE: Wilms' tumor: an update. Cancer 45:1791, 1980.

637. Greenwood RD, Rosenthal A, Nadas AS: Cardiovascular malformations associated with congenital anomalies of the urinary system. Observations in a series of 453 infants and children with urinary malformations. Clin Pediatr 15:1101, 1976.

638. Greenwood RD: Cardiovascular malformations associated with extracardiac anomalies and malformation syndromes: patterns for diagnosis. Clin Pediatr 23:145, 1984.

639. Inselman LS, Mellins RB: Growth and development of the lung. J Pediatr 98:1, 1981.

640. Thomas IT, Smith DW: Oligohydramnios, cause of the nonrenal features of Potter's syndrome, including pulmonary hypoplasia. J Pediatr 84:811, 1974.

641. Pramanik AK, Altshuler G, Light IJ, et al.: Prune-belly syndrome associated with Potter (renal nonfunction) syndrome. Am J Dis Child 131:672, 1977.

642. Pagon RA, Smith DW, Shepard TH: Urethral obstruction malformation complex: a cause of abdominal muscle deficiency and the "prune belly." J Pediatr 94:900, 1974.

643. Belman AB, Kaplan GW: Prune belly syndrome. In Genitourinary Problems in Pediatrics. Philadelphia, W.B. Saunders Co., 1981, pp 254–260.

644. Lockhart JL, Reeve HR, Bredael JJ, et al.: Siblings with prune belly syndrome and associated pulmonic stenosis, mental retardation, and deafness. Urology 14:140, 1979.

645. Chinyanga HM: Cystoscopy and prune-belly syndrome. In Stehling LC (Ed.): Common Problems in Pediatric Anesthesia. Chicago, Year Book Medical Publishers, 1982, pp 77–82.

646. Bovicelli L, Rizzo N, Orsini LF, et al.: Prenatal diagnosis of the prune belly syndrome. Clin Genet 18:79, 1980.

647. Moerman P, Fryns JP, Goddeeris P, et al.: Pathogenesis of the prune-belly syndrome: a functional urethral obstruction caused by prostatic hypoplasia. Pediatrics 73:470, 1984.

648. Nakayama DK, Harrison MR, Chinn DH, et al.: The pathogenesis of prune belly. Am J Dis Child 138:834, 1984.

649. Hannington-Kiff JG: Prune-belly syndrome and general anaesthesia. Br J Anaesth 42:649, 1970.

650. Karamanian A, Kravath B, Nagashima H, et al.: Anaesthetic management of "prune-belly" syndrome: case report. Br J Anaesth 46:897, 1974.

651. Jones AEP, Pelton DA: An index of syndromes and their anaesthetic implications. Can Anaesth Soc J 23:207, 1976.

652. Warshaw BL, Hymes LC, Woodward JR: Long-term outcome of patients with obstructive uropathy. Pediatr Clin North Am 29:815, 1982.

653. Dal Canton A, Corradi A, Stanziale R, et al.: Glomerular hemodynamics before and after release of 24-hour bilateral ureteral obstruction. Kidney Int 17:491, 1980.

654. Wilson DR: Micropuncture study of chronic obstructive nephropathy before and after release of obstruction. Kidney Int 2:119, 1972.

655. Mayor G, Genton N, Torrado A, et al.: Renal function in obstructive nephropathy: long-term effect of reconstructive surgery. Pediatrics 56:740, 1975.

656. McCrory WM, Shibuya M, Leumann E, et al.: Studies of renal function in children with chronic hydronephrosis. Pediatr Clin North Am 18:445, 1971.

657. Belman AB, Kaplan GW: Obstructive uropathy. In Genitourinary Problems in Pediatrics. Philadelphia, W.B. Saunders Co., 1981, pp 92–117.

658. Lorentz WB Jr, Browning MC, D'Souza VJ, et al.: Intrarenal aneurysm of the renal artery in children. Am J Dis Child 138:751, 1984.

659. McCook TA, Mills SR, Kirks DR, et al.: Percutaneous transluminal renal artery angioplasty in a 3 1/2 year old hypertensive girl. J Pediatr 97:958, 1980.

660. Fraley EE: Vascular obstruction of superior infundibulum

661. causing nephralgia: a new syndrome. N Engl J Med 275:1403, 1966.

661. Belman AB, Kaplan GW: Developmental abnormalities of the kidney and urinary collecting system. In Genitourinary Problems in Pediatrics. Philadelphia, W.B. Saunders Co., 1981, pp 225–237.

662. Chan SL, Johnson HW, McLoughlin MG: Idiopathic retroperitoneal fibrosis in children. J Urol 122:103, 1979.

663. Williams DI, Hulme-Moir I: Primary obstructive megaureter. Br J Urol 42:140, 1970.

664. Belman AB: The clinical significance of vesicoureteral reflux. Pediatr Clin North Am 23:707, 1976.

665. Ehrlich RM: Vesicoureteral reflux: a surgeon's perspective. Pediatr Clin North Am 29:827, 1982.

666. Lenaghan D, Whitaker JG, Jensen F, et al.: The natural history of reflux and the long-term effects of reflux on the kidney. J Urol 115:728, 1976.

667. Edwards D, Normand ICS, Prescod N, et al.: Disappearance of vesicoureteral reflux during long-term prophylaxis of urinary tract infection in children. Br Med J 2:285, 1977.

668. Willscher MK, Bauer SB, Zammuto PJ, et al.: Infection of the urinary tract after anti-reflux surgery. J Pediatr 89:743, 1976.

669. Levitt SB, Duckett J, Spitzer A, et al.: Report of the International Reflux Study Committee. Medical versus surgical treatment of primary vesico-ureveral reflux. Pediatrics 67:392, 1981.

670. Lyon RP, Marshall SK, Scott MP: Treatment of vesicoureteral reflux. Urology 16:38, 1980.

671. Belman AB, Kaplan GW: Vesicoureteral reflux. In Genitourinary Problems in Pediatrics. Philadelphia, W.B. Saunders Co., 1981, pp 67–90.

672. Hendren WH: Posterior urethral valves in boys: a broad cliniciai spectrum. J Urology 106:298, 1971.

673. Eckstein HB, Williams DI: The Neuropathic Bladder. In Williams DI, Johnston JH (Eds.): Paediatric Urology. London, Butterworth Scientific, 1982, pp 325–336.

674. Belman AB, Kaplan GW: Neurogenic bladder. In Genitourinary Problems in Pediatrics. Philadelphia, W.B. Saunders Co., 1981, pp 130–147.

675. Cole AT, Fried FA: Favorable experiences with imipramine in the treatment of neurogenic bladder. J Urol 107:44, 1972.

676. Krane RJ, Olsson CA: Phenoxybenzamine in neurogenic bladder dysfunction. I. A theory of micturition. J Urol 110:650, 1973.

677. Diokno AC, Lapides J: Oxybutynin: a new drug with analgesic and anticholinergic properties. J Urol 108:307, 1972.

678. Murdock M, Sax D, Krane RJ: The use of dantrolene sodium in external sphincter spasm. Urology 8:133, 1976.

679. Stehling LC, Patil U, Patil V: Anesthesia for urodynamic studies in children. Anesthesiol Rev 6:13, 1979.

680. Berry FA: Anesthesia for genitourinary surgery. In Gregory GA (Ed.): Pediatric Anesthesia. New York, Churchill Livingstone, 1983, pp 727–771.

681. Belman AB, Kaplan GW: Bladder exstrophy, cloacal exstrophy, and imperforate anus. In Genitourinary Problems in Pediatrics. Philadelphia, W.B. Saunders Co., 1981, pp 238–254.

682. Johnston JH: The exstrophic anomalies. In Williams DI, Johnston JH (Eds.): Paediatric Urology. London, Butterworth Scientific, 1982, pp 299–316.

683. Belman AB, Kaplan GW: Genital abnormalities in the male. In Genitourinary Problems in Pediatrics. Philadelphia, W.B. Saunders Co., 1981, pp 160–198.

684. Williams DI: Male urethral anomalies. In Williams DI, Johnston JH (Eds.): Paediatric Urology. London, Butterworth Scientific, 1982, pp 239–250.

685. Johnston JH: Abnormalities of the penis. In Williams DI, Johnston JH (Eds.): Paediatric Urology. London, Butterworth Scientific, 1982, pp 435–449.

686. Aarskog D: Maternal progestins as a possible cause of hypospadias. N Engl J Med 300:75, 1979.

687. Page LA: Inheritance of uncomplicated hypospadias. Pediatrics 63:788, 1979.

687a. Benzon TH, Leventhal JB, Ovassapian A, et al.: Ketamine treatment of penile erection in the operating room. Anesth Analg 61:457, 1983.

687b. Villalonga A, Beltran, J, Gomar C, et al.: Ketamine for treatment of priapism. Anesth Analg 64:1033, 1986.

688. Kay B: Caudal block for post-operative pain relief in children. Anaesthesia 29:610, 1974.

689. Blaise G, Roy WL: Post-operative pain relief after hypospadias repair in pediatric patients: regional analgesia versus systemic analgesics. Anesthesiology 61:A430, 1984.

690. Hannallah RS, Broadman LM, Belman AB, et al.:Control of post-orchiopexy pain in pediatric outpatients: comparison of two regional techniques. Anesthesiology 61:A429, 1984.

691. Abajian JC, Mellish RWP, Browne AF, et al.: Spinal anesthesia for surgery in the high-risk infant. Anesth Analg 63:359, 1984.

692. Soliman MG, Tremblay NA: Nerve block of the penis for postoperative pain relief in children. Anesth Analg 57:495, 1978.

693. Kirya C, Werthmann MW Jr: Neonatal circumcision and penile dorsal nerve block—a painless procedure. J Pediatr 92:998, 1978.

694. Johnston JH: Abnormalities of the scrotum and the testes. In Williams DI, Johnston JH (Eds.): Paediatric Urology. London, Butterworth Scientific, 1982, pp 451–465.

695. Johnston JH: Acquired lesions of the penis, the scrotum and the testes. In Williams DI, Johnston JH (Eds.): Paediatric Urology. London, Butterworth Scientific, 1982, pp 467–475.

696. Mendoza SA: Syndrome of inappropriate antidiuretic hormone secretion (SIADH). Pediatr Clin North Am 23:681, 1976.

697. Crumrine RS: Adrenogenital syndrome. In Stehling LC (Ed.): Common Problems in Pediatric Anesthesia. Chicago, Year Book Medical Publishers, 1982, pp 119–122.

698. Laflin MJ: Interaction of pancuronium and corticosteroids. Anesthesiology 47:471, 1977.

699. Meyers EF: Partial recovery from pancuronium neuromuscular blockade following hydrocortisone administration. Anesthesiology 46:148, 1977.

700. Belman AB, Kaplan GW: Trauma. In Genitourinary Problems in Pediatrics. Philadelphia, W.B. Saunders Co., 1981, pp 319–329.

701. Johnston JH: Urinary tract injuries. In Williams DI, Johnston JH (Eds.): Paediatric Urology. London, Butterworth Scientific, 1982, pp 369–380.

702. Morse TS, Smith JP, Howard WHR, et al.: Kidney injuries in children. J Urol 98:539, 1967.

8 | DISEASES OF THE GASTROINTESTINAL SYSTEM

DAVID J. STEWARD, M.D.

Disorders of the gastrointestinal system during infancy and childhood are many and varied and may require surgical treatment. In addition, some disorders may be present in patients requiring anesthesia for surgery of an unrelated lesion. Hence, the anesthesiologist must recognize the pathophysiological changes that may accompany pediatric gastrointestinal disease. Some lesions may demand special attention because of their potential to complicate the course of anesthesia. Some diseases that are relatively common in pediatric practice will be discussed because they are not frequently seen by anesthesiologists, but have important anesthetic implications.

DEVELOPMENT OF GASTROINTESTINAL FUNCTION

After birth the infant becomes dependent upon the gastrointestinal tract to provide nutrients, not only to provide for immediate energy requirements but also to sustain a period of rapid growth. The gastrointestinal tract, which has been relatively inactive in utero, must therefore rapidly assume its roles of digestion and absorption.

Intestinal motor activity is evident in the fetus. Swallowing movements begin during the second trimester, and swallowing is an important mechanism in the regulation of amniotic fluid volume. Maternal polyhydramnios frequently accompanies diseases that impair fetal swallowing (for example, esophageal atresia). Gastric emptying and small intestine motor ac-

tivity develop in parallel, and by the time the infant gains the ability to suck, coordinated gastric and small bowel movements are evident.[1] Delayed gastric emptying may accompany respiratory or cardiovascular disease in infants, especially in preterm infants.[2, 3]

Gastric secretions are present during the second trimester of intrauterine life, but are not markedly acidic. The pH of gastric contents at birth is approximately 6, but falls rapidly during the first day of life.[4] Pepsin activity develops during the third trimester, and hence small preterm infants may have limited ability to digest protein.[5]

The digestive enzymes of the pancreas and small bowel appear in a recognized sequence during intrauterine development. This sequence has important implications for the feeding of infants and especially the preterm infant,[6] and formulas should be prepared accordingly.

The ability of the large intestine to conserve water and electrolytes is reduced in infants and this predisposes to the dehydration and electrolyte disturbance that accompanies diarrhea.

COMMON SYMPTOMS OF GASTROINTESTINAL DISEASE

Vomiting and Regurgitation

Vomiting and regurgitation are common in infants up to 1 year of age. Regurgitation is often a result of faulty feeding technique, but if persistent it should suggest the possibility of a gastrointestinal disease. Vomiting in babies may result from many diseases, but is especially common with infections and central nervous system disease. Mechanical obstruction of the digestive tract may result from congenital lesions such as duodenal atresia or congenital hypertrophic pyloric stenosis.

Vomiting in infants, if persistent, results in progressive fluid and electrolyte depletion. The high rate of fluid turnover in infancy dictates that these losses and the accompanying limited intake will rapidly lead to serious dehydration.

Prolonged vomiting leads to several changes in the extracellular fluid.[7] There is a metabolic alkalosis with a varying degree of compensation. Low plasma chloride and potassium concentrations accompany the alkalosis. In addition to these changes in composition, the extracellular fluid may be severely depleted in volume. It is most important that the volume and composition of the extracellular fluid be restored to near normal before induction of general anesthesia in these patients. This will require administration of sodium chloride solution together with appropriate amounts of added potassium chloride when a good urine flow is established. The withholding of oral feeding is also important in the treatment of a child who is vomiting. This decreases the stimulus for gastric secretions and thus decreases fluid and electrolyte losses.

Diarrhea

Diarrhea is a common problem in infancy. The extent of fluid and electrolyte depletion will vary with the etiology of the diarrhea and the extent to which fluid intake is also compromised.[8] The electrolyte content of fluid losses due to diarrhea is lower with viral infections (for example, rotavirus infection) than bacterial infections. Patients with diarrhea also lose potassium in the urine. The net result of diarrhea is dehydration, which may be hypotonic, isotonic, or hypertonic depending upon the extent of electrolyte losses. This dehydration is accompanied by acidosis due to loss of fixed cations and bicarbonate. Hypertonic dehydration is of particular concern, as it may be accompanied by major fluid shifts within the brain and serious neurological complications.

The treatment of dehydration and acidosis due to diarrhea consists of restoration of the intravascular volume, repletion of the remaining fluid and electrolyte deficits, and correction of metabolic acidosis. This treatment may require several days to complete. Hypertonic dehydration and acidosis must be corrected gradually if serious complications are to be avoided.

Malnutrition and Growth Failure

Infants and children with gastrointestinal disease may demonstrate varying degrees of nutritional dep-

rivation. Diseases may cause anorexia, leading to inadequate intake, or may affect absorption of nutrients from the bowel. The normal term infant has a decreased capacity for digestive and absorptive functions, and the preterm infant has an even more limited capacity. Diseases that might affect gastrointestinal function are thus very significant in infancy, and the impact of malnutrition is most obvious at this stage.

The growing infant or child is an anabolic organism and cannot easily cope with starvation and catabolic states.[9] Parenteral nutrition is therefore necessary unless adequate nutrition can be maintained by nasogastric, jejunal, or duodenal feeding.

Malnutrition is common in many underdeveloped countries and may occur in developed countries among poor populations or as a result of diet fads[10] or parental neglect. Serious malnutrition may compromise recovery from a surgical procedure: wound healing is impaired,[11] and the resistance to infection is decreased.[12] The ability of the pediatric patient to survive a critical surgical illness may be severely affected by malnutrition.[13] In North America a population of pediatric surgical patients may include a significant percentage of malnourished children.[14] It has been suggested that a nutritional assessment should be included in the preoperative evaluation of all pediatric surgical patients.[15]

The advent of intravenous hyperalimentation techniques has made it possible to avoid many of the problems of severe nutritional depletion in pediatric surgical patients.

Severe Malnutrition (Kwashiorkor)

Kwashiorkor usually appears soon after weaning and is due to a failure to provide an adequate protein diet. This disease is common in underdeveloped and tropical countries, but cases have occurred in North America.[16] The early clinical signs are of lethargy and irritability. Anorexia, vomiting, and diarrhea are common. Later there is loss of muscle tissue and edema, with increased susceptibility to infection. The edema may conceal a failure of true weight gain. All children with kwashiorkor have a degree of anemia, but this is seldom severe. In late stages of the disease hepatic enlargement with fatty infiltration is common. Mild hypoglycemia may occur secondary to impaired gluconeogenesis. The cardiovascular effects of kwashiorkor range from nonspecific electrocardiographic changes to congestive cardiac failure. Renal function is characterized by reduced renal blood flow, low glomerular filtration rate, and poor tubular function. Hyponatremia is commonly seen as a result of overhydration, and hypokalemia may result from diminished body stores of potassium. Mental changes of apathy, progressing to stupor, coma, and death, occur in the late stages of the disease. The prinicples of treatment of kwashiorkor are supplementation of nonprotein calories and the gradual restoration of an adequate protein intake. An initial high-protein diet may result in liver enlargement, hypoglycemia, and less rapid recovery.

The important considerations for the anesthesiologist in managing children with kwashiorkor are those of reduced plasma protein levels, altered fluid and electrolyte status, reduced muscle mass, and impaired cardiovascular function. Patients with severe disease may be markedly hypovolemic despite overhydration. Drugs that are normally extensively protein-bound in the plasma (for example, barbiturates and muscle relaxants) should be given very cautiously in reduced dosage.

While kwashiorkor demonstrates all the features of malnutrition due to inadequate dietary intake, similar changes may also occur as a result of defective alimentary tract function.

Gastrointestinal Bleeding

Bleeding from the gastrointestinal tract in infants and children may result from many causes. In the neonate the most common cause of upper gastrointestinal bleeding is gastroduodenitis, often as a result of salicylate therapy.[17] Other causes in the newborn include stress ulcers, which may be related to the relatively high gastric acidity in the first few days of life. Neonates with upper gastrointestinal bleeding very rarely require surgery.

Other causes of gastrointestinal bleeding in the infant include hemorrhagic disease of the newborn, for which vitamin K therapy is indicated. In addition, necrotizing enterocolitis (see page 227), midgut volvulus, and infectious diarrhea may cause bleeding. Anal fissure is a very common cause of bleeding in infants under 1 year of age and may require surgical excision.[18] Intussusception results in loss of blood and mucus in feces (red currant jelly stool) and usually occurs in patients under 2 years of age.

In older children vomited blood may have been previously swallowed (for example, during a nosebleed) or may be a result of peptic ulceration, or more rarely esophageal varices. Lower gastrointestinal bleeding may occur from a Meckel diverticulum, intestinal duplication, or polyp. Hemangiomas of the gastrointestinal tract may result in major blood loss and are often associated with cutaneous lesions, as in Osler-Rendu-Weber disease or Klippel-Trenaunay syndrome.

Stress ulceration may be a cause of bleeding in both the neonatal and the pediatric intensive care unit and is particularly common in pediatric burn patients (Curling ulcer) and in association with lesions of the central nervous system (Cushing ulcer). Prophylaxis against stress ulceration is important for all patients at risk. It may consist of cimetidine 2.5 mg/kg every 6 hours,[19] or antacids (for example, Maalox, Gelusil), or a combination of both. Gastric pH should be monitored and maintained at 5 or above. Massive gastric bleeding due to a stress ulcer may require surgical exploration or radiographic embolization.[20] In such patients regurgitation of blood during induction of anesthesia is a major concern. Large-bore intravenous cannulation and a large volume of blood for transfusion must be provided. All blood should be warmed and the coagulation indices regularly monitored during the procedure. Dilutional thrombocytopenia should be anticipated and preparations to obtain platelet concentrates made prior to surgery.

DISEASES OF THE ESOPHAGUS

The esophagus is 3 to 5½ inches in length in the full-term newborn infant and its lumen is 4 to 6 mm in diameter. The development of effective peristaltic waves in the wall of the esophagus normally occurs as the infant acquires a normal sucking pattern. The lower esophageal sphincter is relatively incompetent in infants.[21] The sphincter tone is poor and relaxation is prolonged during swallowing, thus gastroesophageal reflux is common.

Esophageal Atresia

The problems of tracheoesophageal fistula are considered in Chapter 5. When esophageal atresia occurs without a fistulous connection with the trachea, the segment of atretic esophagus is often too long to permit primary anastomosis.[22] The usual management is to perform a gastrostomy for feeding and to attempt to lengthen the upper segment by bougienage. Alternatively, circular myotomies to lengthen the esophageal segments may be performed. Some infants with absence of a long segment of esophagus will require a replacement procedure using a gastric tube or colon interposition. Such a procedure is usually delayed until the child is 1 year of age or more.

Esophageal Duplications

Duplication cysts of the esophagus usually present as an expanding mass originating in the posterior mediastinum. Because of their proximity to the airway, cyanosis and dyspnea may occur together with dysphagia and sometimes vomiting. Cysts that do not communicate with the esophagus contain clear, thick fluid and may grow to a large size. Communicating cysts may contain gastric mucosa and discharge into the esophagus, causing esophagitis and erosion, which may lead to hematemesis. Esophageal duplication may be associated with cervical spine anomalies, including Klippel-Feil syndrome. The treatment of esophageal duplication is by surgical excision. During the operation the anesthesiologist must be alert to the possibility of surgical retraction causing obstruction of the airway and must continuously monitor ventilation.

Gastroesophageal Reflux

A large percentage of infants regurgitate, possibly as a result of poorly coordinated responses to swallowing and a low lower esophageal sphincter (LES) pressure.[23] As the child grows the LES pressure normally increases and regurgitation of stomach contents lessens. Some infants and children, however, have persistent gastroesophageal reflux (GER), which results in serious illness.[24] Many children with GER also have a hiatus hernia, but GER is not an inevitable consequence of hiatus hernia, and serious GER may occur without it.

Older children with GER will complain of symptoms of chest pain and heartburn. Young infants demonstrate regurgitation that is effortless, in contrast to the active vomiting that occurs with pyloric stenosis. Persistent and copious regurgitation results in failure to thrive. The low pH of regurgitated material causes esophagitis, which may lead to bleeding with consequent hematemesis and iron deficiency anemia and eventually may lead to stricture. Gastroesophageal reflux may also lead to pulmonary disease: recurrent aspiration pneumonia and chronic cough and wheezing may be present. GER has also been implicated in neonatal apnea and sudden infant death syndrome.[25]

The medical management of the patient with GER consists of frequent feeding and maintenance of semiupright posture for a period after each feed. Bethanechol may be used to increase the LES pressure and antacids or cimetidine to reduce gastric acidity. Failure of medical therapy to control the serious effects of GER or the presence of a major anatomical abnormality of the gastroesophageal junction are considered to be indications for surgery.

The Nissen fundoplication, which is commonly performed for this condition, consists of encircling the lower esophagus with the fundus of the stomach. The anesthesiologist managing patients for this procedure should be aware of the possibility of reflux and aspiration during induction of anesthesia. Preoperatively cimetidine and antacids should be ordered. A rapid-sequence induction should be performed to secure the airway. During the operation a nasogastric tube is passed before the repair and left in for postoperative management. In patients who are suspected of having associated delayed gastric emptying, a pyloroplasty is also performed. Postoperatively some patients may suffer gastric distention and inability to vomit or burp. This problem may persist for 2 to 3 months after surgery and may require gastric aspiration.[26]

Hiatus Hernia

Hiatus hernia in infants and children is most commonly of the "sliding" type, in which the upper portion of the stomach is drawn into the thoracic cavity by what appears to be a short esophagus. The theory of the "congenital short esophagus" is no longer accepted, but the shortening may be acquired as a result of esophagitis or stricture. Hiatus hernia may be more common in children with cerebral palsy. Sandifer syndrome consists of hiatus hernia and torticollis. The rumination syndrome, characterized by regurgitation of gastric contents into the mouth and subsequent reswallowing after chewing, may occur with hiatus hernia.

Paraesophageal hiatus hernia with a normally situated gastroesophageal junction is much rarer and produces abdominal pain and distention. Surgery is indicated because of the risk of strangulation of the herniated stomach.

Anesthetic management for hiatus hernia should be the same as for gastroesophageal reflux (see above).

Achalasia of the Cardia

Achalasia or cardiospasm may occur in children,[27] but is not usually associated with the voluminous dilation of the esophagus that is seen in adults. There is, however, some dilation of the proximal esophagus and a narrow distal segment. Esophageal motility studies show an absence of peristalsis and a failure of the lower esophageal sphincter to relax on swallowing. Achalasia in childhood produces severe growth retardation, and the extent of pulmonary symptoms due to aspiration is more severe than in adults.[28] The treatment of this condition is by operative myotomy (Heller operation) or by intraesophageal balloon disruption of the constricted cardia. Myotomy is generally preferred in younger children. Gastroesophageal reflux may follow surgery.

The anesthetic management of the patient with achalasia should recognize the possibility of retained food and secretions within the dilated esophagus. A rapid sequence induction following a careful period of fasting is recommended.

Opitz-Frias syndrome (G syndrome, hypospadias-dysphagia syndrome) includes achalasia of the cardia plus craniofacial and genital anomalies.[29] Repeated episodes of pulmonary aspiration occur and may be fatal. Endotracheal intubation may be difficult owing to the craniofacial deformity, and thus a rapid-sequence induction is not possible. It should also be noted that children with this condition have laryngeal hypoplasia[30] and may accept only a very small endotracheal tube.[29] It is recommended that anesthetic management include careful preoperative fasting, preoperative gastric and esophageal aspiration with a nasogastric tube, followed by a careful inhalation induction of anesthesia. A selection of endotracheal tube sizes should be available. By this means the danger of regurgitation and aspiration can be minimized while applying a technique that is appropriate to a patient with a difficult airway problem.

DISEASES OF THE STOMACH AND DUODENUM

Volvulus of the Stomach

Gastric volvulus is a rare condition, usually occurring in the neonatal period, but it may occur throughout childhood. It is due to laxity or absence of the gastric ligaments.[31] The volvulus may be along the axis of the stomach (organoaxial type) or involve the mesentery of that organ (mesenterioaxial type). In either case the disease may progress to gangrene and perforation of the stomach. If there is an associated defect in the diaphragm, the gastric volvulus may be intrathoracic. Acute and subacute or chronic cases are reported.

In acute volvulus the presenting symptoms are persistent regurgitation and vomiting, but respiratory distress may also be prominent.[31] The inability to pass or resistance to advancement of a nasogastric tube is characteristic of the condition. Bleeding may accompany the volvulus as an early symptom.

It is most important that the diagnosis of gastric volvulus be rapidly established. Surgery is urgent to reduce the volvulus and anchor the stomach before ischemic damage occurs. Appropriate fluid resuscitation should be achieved prior to induction of anesthesia, and precautions should be taken to prevent the possibility of regurgitation and aspiration during induction. Awake intubation or a rapid-sequence induction is recommended.

In older children gastric volvulus may present as a chronic recurring disease with episodes of intermittent abdominal pain related to eating.[32]

Rupture of the Stomach

Rupture of the stomach is most common in the neonatal period and is usually iatrogenic, though it may occur spontaneously.[33] The etiology of spontaneous rupture is unknown, but the condition may be related to birth asphyxia, hypoxia, and stress. The usual site of perforation is near the greater curvature on the fundus of the stomach. Males appear to be affected more commonly than females.

The clinical presentation is usually with lassitude, poor feeding, and abdominal distention. In addition the infant may show respiratory distress. Radiological studies demonstrate pneumoperitoneum and absence of the normal gastric air bubble. The infant may progress rapidly to a state of severe shock, and the mortality rate for this condition is high. Prompt, efficient resuscitation and early surgery are required. Nitrous oxide should not be used for general anesthesia in these infants, as there may be considerable free air in the peritoneal cavity. Pneumomediastinum has also been reported in association with acute gastric rupture.[33]

Hypertrophic Pyloric Stenosis

Congenital hypertrophic pyloric stenosis is one of the common gastrointestinal defects of infancy. First-born male patients are most commonly affected, and the incidence is much higher in children of affected parents. The overall incidence may approach 1 in 300 live births, but there are considerable regional variations.

The symptoms usually commence at 2 to 3 weeks of age and consist of bile-free vomiting, which progresses to become a projectile and occurs after every feeding. On examination the infant displays a degree of dehydration that is related to the severity and duration of the symptoms. Visible peristalsis across the left upper quadrant and palpation of a pyloric mass is diagnostic of the disease.[34] Associated anomalies of the renal system may be present in a small percentage of patients.[35] Elevated levels of unconjugated bilirubin may occur in up to 17 percent of patients. This is thought to be due to decreased glucuronyl transferase activity in the liver.[36] Serum bilirubin levels rapidly fall after pyloromyotomy.

Management of the infant with hypertrophic pyloric stenosis must commence with correction of fluid and biochemical derangements. There is never an indication for urgent or emergency surgery.[34] Serum electrolyte determinations will demonstrate a hypochloremic metabolic alkalosis secondary to the loss of chloride and hydrogen ions. Hypokalemia may also be present owing to an intracellular shift of potassium with alkalosis. As the condition of alkalosis persists, potassium may also be lost via the kidneys and severe hypokalemia may result.[37] Optimal preparation of the child with pyloric stenosis for surgery may take several days. Oral feeding should be stopped and a nasogastric tube inserted and connected to gentle suction. Discontinuing oral feeding will decrease secretion of gastric juices and hence decrease electrolyte losses. The management of fluid and electrolyte replacement therapy must be based on the extent of the deficit. In general, the greater the deficit, the greater the role for sodium chloride in replacement fluids. In a patient with only a mild deficit rehydration may be carried out with maintenance fluid and electrolytes. Moderate dehydration requires the use of a solution of 5 percent dextrose with half normal saline infused at 1½ times normal maintenance rates. Severe dehydration requires the rapid infusion of normal saline (20 ml/kg) followed by an infusion of 5 percent dextrose with normal saline at 1½ times maintenance rates. Potassium chloride 3 to 5 mEq/kg/day should be added to these fluids once adequate urine flow is established (1 ml/kg/hour or more). The fluid therapy must be reassessed as the patient's condition improves. Dextrose infusions must be continued until oral feeding is established postoperatively, or serious hypoglycemia may result.[38]

Prior to accepting the patient for general anesthesia the anesthesiologist should check to ensure that the fluid and electrolyte status is fully corrected. There should be no clinical signs of dehydration, a good urine output, and serum electrolytes and acid base values within normal values.

Anesthetic management should commence with passage of a soft gastric tube to empty the stomach. This should be done even if a nasogastric tube has been in place and will often reveal additional stomach fluid content. Lavage of the stomach with normal saline has been recommended, but is not usually necessary. A rapid-sequence induction is recommended to secure the airway. At the end of the operation the infant should be awake and vigorous prior to extubation, which should be performed with the patient in a lateral position.

The patient can usually be fed on the first postoperative day. Postoperative hypoglycemia may occur 2 to 3 hours postoperatively,[38] and respiratory depression in the postoperative period has been described.[39] The child should therefore be in a closely supervised nursing area.

Duodenal Obstruction

Duodenal obstruction may result from an intrinsic block or from extrinsic compression. Intrinsic obstruction may be due to duodenal atresia or stenosis, the latter often due to a web. There is a high incidence of duodenal atresia in Down syndrome. Extrinsic causes of duodenal compression and obstruction include malrotation, Ladd bands, or an annular pancreas.[40]

Infants with duodenal atresia present early in life with bile-stained vomiting and little or no abdominal distention. Duodenal atresia is treated by duodeno-duodenostomy.

Malrotation of the intestines predisposes to midgut volvulus. The infant with this condition commonly presents with abdominal distention, bloody stools, and peritonitis with hypovolemic shock. Such patients require fluid resuscitation prior to urgent laparotomy. Awake intubation or a rapid-sequence induction should be performed because of the danger of regurgitation. If there is doubt about the viability of the bowel, the abdomen may be closed and a "second look" procedure planned for 24 to 48 hours later. In this case the infant may require intensive medical support between operations.

DISEASES OF THE SMALL BOWEL

Meconium Ileus

In this condition the small bowel is blocked by thick, inspissated meconium. This condition is almost always associated with cystic fibrosis, but may very rarely occur as an isolated lesion.[41] The disease is thought to be due to abnormally viscid secretions of

intestinal glands.[42] The infant presents with abdominal distention and a failure to pass meconium. The intestines may be palpable through the abdominal wall, and a radiograph demonstrates a granular appearance of the bowel. A sweat chloride determination will determine the presence of cystic fibrosis. Meconium ileus may be complicated by the presence of ileal atresia, perforation, or meconium peritonitis.

The treatment of uncomplicated meconium ileus may be medical, using a diatrizoate meglumine (Gastrografin) enema.[43] This may be successful in producing disimpaction in up to 50 percent of patients. Other patients require laparotomy, in which case enterostomy and irrigation of the bowel lumen with acetylcysteine solution may be effective. Alternatively, bowel resection may be required. The anesthetic management of these infants must recognize the potential for postoperative pulmonary problems. A rapid-sequence induction or awake intubation should be performed to safeguard the airway. Warmed humidified anesthetic gases should be used and careful aseptic technique used to suction the endotracheal tube.

Postoperative problems to be anticipated in the child with meconium ileus include pneumonia, septicemia, and prolonged bowel dysfunction. Intensive respiratory care and chest physiotherapy must be commenced early, together with appropriate antibiotic therapy for infection.

Intestinal Duplication

This most commonly occurs in the region of the small intestine. The infant presents with abdominal distention, a mass, and possible signs of gastrointestinal bleeding. The diagnosis may be difficult to confirm prior to exploratory surgery. The treatment is excision of the duplicate segment, which may involve resection of adjacent normal bowel.

Neonatal Necrotizing Enterocolitis

Necrotizing enterocolitis (NEC) is a major cause of mortality and morbidity of preterm and small for gestational age (SGA) infants, and is occasionally fatal in term infants as well.[44] The incidence varies considerably between different units, and this may be related to feeding practices or other factors. The mortality rate from NEC may be 30 to 50 percent.[45]

Patients with NEC often have a history of intrauterine fetal distress and/or birth asphyxia.[46] Otherwise, or in addition, a history of respiratory distress syndrome, apnea of prematurity, umbilical artery catheterization, or patent ductus arteriosus may be obtained. The role of all the previously mentioned factors in the etiology of NEC is thought to be due to their potential to reduce the mesenteric flow of oxygenated blood.[47]

The method of feeding and diet may also influence the disease.[48] The presence of a feeding tube and the enteral food may cause mechanical trauma and introduce pathogens or favor their multiplication and colonization. In addition the type of food may promote the growth of specific bacteria. The combination of an ischemic bowel injury and bacterial infection permits endotoxins to pass into the bloodstream. Finally, intestinal perforation or infarction may result.

The epidemiology of the disease and the initial septic manifestations strongly suggest an infective etiology for NEC. Attempts to identify a specific bacterial pathogen for NEC have been unsuccessful, but the fact that the gas present in the bowel wall has a high percentage of hydrogen favors an infective component to the etiology.[49] Cultures from the intestinal contents of affected infants have grown many different organisms, including gas-forming bacilli such as *Clostridium perfringens*. This organism is also, however, a normal bowel inhabitant in healthy infants.[50] It is possible that many organisms that are cultured from NEC patients are not, in fact, the principal pathogen, but are opportunistic colonizers of the diseased bowel. It is suspected that the absence of a "normal" bowel flora might also be an important etiological factor. In summary, the etiology of NEC is thought to involve intestinal ischemia leading to mucosal injury, plus infection and possibly the effect of enteral feeding, in the presence of immature intestinal function.

The clinical signs of NEC include gastric retention of food, thermal instability, and abdominal distention, often with loose, blood-streaked stools. These signs usually appear in the first few days of life and 2 to 3 days after the initiation of feeding. In addition, the infant may appear pale and lethargic and may suffer apnea if not on intermittent positive-pressure ventilation. Later in the disease the infant may show evidence of septic shock and disseminated intravascular coagulation (DIC). Early radiological examination of the abdomen demonstrates distended gas-filled loops of bowel and later the appearance of pneumatosis intestinalis, gas in the wall of the intestine.

The medical treatment of NEC must be initiated promptly. At the first sign of the disease, oral feeding is discontinued and a nasogastric tube is inserted to provide continuous suction. Fluids, electrolytes, and calories must be provided intravenously. Antibiotics effective against gram negative enteric organisms should be administered via the nasogastric tube. Gentamicin and colistin are the most commonly used drugs.[44] The drug selected is given every 4 hours and the nasogastric tube is clamped for 1 hour following each dose. If the disease progresses and signs of sepsis appear, blood cultures are often positive.[51] In such cases patients require systemic antibiotic therapy, and because their humoral immune response is inadequate, they should also receive fresh plasma. Septic shock must be treated by restoration of the intravascular

volume, corticosteroids (hydrocortisone 35 to 50 mg/kg), and inotropic drugs. DIC is common and usually requires exchange transfusion.

The indications for surgical intervention have been a matter of some controversy, but there is some general agreement that bowel perforation evidenced by pneumoperitoneum demands operation.[52, 53] Additional indications include a paracentesis positive for gangrene (0.5 ml or more of fluid that is brown or contains bacteria), abdominal wall erythema, a fixed abdominal mass, or a persistently dilated loop of bowel on serial radiographs.[52]

The successful anesthetic management of the patient with NEC must begin with a thorough preoperative evaluation followed by appropriate therapy to optimize the status of the infant. Many such patients may already be receiving respiratory support, and this must be carefully maintained. Fluid resuscitation is required to correct hypovolemic shock, and fresh blood and platelet concentrates must be administered to restore coagulation mechanisms.

If the infant is not yet intubated, induction of anesthesia and endotracheal intubation should be planned to avoid the possibility of regurgitation and aspiration, as well as to minimize the physiological response to intubation. Awake endotracheal intubation of newborn infants has been demonstrated to result in a large increase in intracranial pressure.[53] In the very sick preterm infant this might well lead to intracranial hemorrhage. Intubation should preferably be facilitated by a relaxant drug and preceded by a very small dose of intravenous barbiturate (for example, thiopentone 2 to 3 mg/kg). Anesthesia should be maintained using fentanyl or low concentrations of isoflurane with a nondepolarizing neuromuscular blocking drug. Appropriate concentrations of oxygen in air should be delivered to maintain an arterial saturation of 90 to 95 percent.[55] Nitrous oxide should not be given, as this may increase the size of gas bubbles in the submucosa and porta hepatis.[56]

Intussusception

An intussusception consists of a segment of bowel that has entered the lumen of the adjacent distal bowel and produced an obstruction. This is the most common cause of obstruction after infancy until the age of 5 years. The obstructing segment of bowel may pass for some distance into the distal bowel and may become ischemic and gangrenous. Viral infection, often with adenovirus, is frequently found in association with intussusception, and enlarged Peyer patches are thought to provide the lead point.

The clinical presentation is usually with sudden onset of abdominal pain, vomiting, and passing blood and mucous in the stool. Frequently a sausage-shaped mass can be palpated in the abdomen. Though most cases are idiopathic, intussusception may also occur secondary to Meckel diverticulum, tumors, suture lines, and duplications and may be associated with cystic fibrosis and Henoch-Schönlein purpura.

The diagnosis of intussusception is confirmed by radiological study of a contrast enema, which may also serve to reduce the intussusception. Indications for laparotomy[57] include signs of peritonitis, obstruction, and failed reduction by enema. Repeated intussusception is also treated surgically after the third episode.

The anesthesiologist must critically analyze the state of hydration of the child prior to operation. It may, however, be necessary to proceed with an emergency laparotomy immediately if the viability of the affected bowel is in doubt. In such a case vigorous fluid resuscitation must accompany the anesthetic. A rapid-sequence induction is indicated to avoid the danger of aspiration.[58] If gangrenous bowel is present, this will require resection. Blood and fluid replacement must be carefully managed during the operation to correct losses.

Meckel Diverticulum and Persistent Omphalomesenteric Duct

The omphalomesenteric duct extends from the embryo into the yolk sac. This duct normally undergoes complete degeneration, but may persist in part, or very rarely in toto. Partial persistence is seen as a Meckel diverticulum or as a cystic remnant in the abdominal wall. Total persistence presents in the newborn as an omphalomesenteric duct, with fecal discharge at the umbilicus. An obliterated, but persistent omphalomesenteric duct may precipitate a volvulus. A persistent omphalomesenteric duct must be surgically excised from the abdominal wall to the bowel.

Meckel diverticulum is the most common remnant to persist and may be present in 2 percent of the population. The diverticulum produces symptoms only if complications occur. These include bleeding, intestinal obstruction, or perforation.[59] The incidence of major complications of Meckel diverticulum is equal to that of appendicitis in infants under 2 years of age. Bleeding from Meckel diverticulum can be very profuse and lead to serious hypovolemic shock. The bleeding originates in ectopic gastric mucosa occurring in the diverticulum. Obstruction may be due to intussusception of the diverticulum or to volvulus around it. Perforation of a Meckel diverticulum is usually at the site of a peptic ulcer in the ectopic gastric mucosa.

The anesthesiologist should carefully assess the fluid status of the child preoperatively. Blood losses may lead to anemia and in some cases to significant hypovolemia. Peritonitis may be present and lead to further fluid deficit. Restoration of an adequate circulating blood volume and hematocrit must precede induction of anesthesia. In all patients with an acute abdomen the airway should be rapidly secured at induction of anesthesia.

MAJOR ABDOMINAL WALL DEFECTS

Omphalocele and Gastroschisis

Omphalocele (or exomphalos) is a congenital herniation of abdominal contents at the umbilicus. The contents are usually covered by a thin membrane that is composed of the fused layers of the amnion and the peritoneum. This membrane may rupture prior to or at birth. The omphalocele, if small, may contain only small bowel. If large it may contain the liver, spleen, stomach, and other abdominal organs. Omphalocele may occur in approximately 1 in 6000 live births, and in 30 percent of cases will be associated with other congenital anomalies. These most commonly affect the gastrointestinal, cardiovascular, genitourinary, or central nervous system.

The Beckwith-Wiedemann syndrome consists of omphalocele, macroglossia, and visceromegaly.[60] Thirty to 50 percent of infants with this syndrome may develop hypoglycemia, which has been demonstrated to be secondary to islet cell hyperplasia and resultant hyperinsulinemia.[61] Hypoglycemia may persist beyond the neonatal period into the first years of life. In addition to hyperinsulinism, patients with this syndrome may show an excessive insulin response to intravenous glucose, resulting in further hypoglycemia. Glucose should therefore be administered by constant infusion (6 to 8 mg/kg/minute) rather than by bolus injection. Blood glucose determinations should be repeated regularly. Infants with Beckwith-Wiedemann syndrome usually lose the tendency to hypoglycemia as they grow older, but in some persistent symptoms may require partial or subtotal pancreatectomy.

Gastroschisis is a full-thickness abdominal wall defect usually situated to the right of a normal umbilical cord. The herniated abdominal contents are not covered by a membrane. Gastroschisis is frequently an isolated lesion with no other congenital defects.

Because omphalocele and gastroschisis pose similar problems and require similar treatment, they are usually considered together.

Infants with major abdominal wall defects may suffer significant heat loss and major fluid shifts into exposed bowel. Intestinal function is often slow to become established, and prolonged periods of intravenous alimentation may be required. The initial treatment of these lesions consists of covering the exposed bowel with sterile moist gauze and a plastic sheet. This will prevent further infection and limit heat and fluid loss from exposed viscera. A nasogastric tube should be inserted to prevent intestinal distention. Warmed intravenous fluids (clear and colloid) should be administered to restore deficits. The volumes of fluid required may be high because of evaporative loss from exposed bowel and third space losses into the intestines.[62] The possibility of Beckwith-Wiedemann syndrome should be recognized and a blood glucose estimation performed if any signs of the syndrome or of clinical hypoglycemia are apparent. An infusion of 10 percent dextrose to provide 6 to 8 mg of dextrose/kg/minute should be commenced and supplemented by administration of balanced salt solution to replace third space losses. The volume administered must be judged by the responses seen in the patient's vital signs.

The optimal surgical management of abdominal wall defects is still the subject of some controversy. Primary closure is favored by some surgeons,[63] whereas others prefer staged closures[64] using a prosthetic sac as a temporary cover for the viscera. If primary closure is planned the patient will usually require continued paralysis and mechanical ventilation into the postoperative period for 24 to 48 hours or more. The proponents of primary closure suggest that this procedure leads to reduced complications of sepsis, sac dehiscence, and prolonged ileus. Primary closure is usually preceded by intraoperative manual stretching of the abdominal wall. The proponents of staged closure suggest that this technique avoids subjecting abdominal viscera to compression and removes the need for prolonged ventilation. In fact, reported results[63, 64] show little difference in overall outcome between the two methods. The overall improvement in survival for infants with abdominal wall defects is considered to be due to improved surgical techniques, the use of intravenous alimentation, and progress in neonatal intensive care.[64] Broad-spectrum antibiotics are usually administered prior to surgery.

Prior to induction of anesthesia the anesthesiologist should ensure that the patient has received optimal fluid replacement. A secure airway should be rapidly established, either by awake intubation or a rapid-sequence induction, since regurgitation and aspiration is a danger. Nitrous oxide should not be used, but air and oxygen provided in proportions to assure optimal PaO_2 or oxygen saturation. Low concentrations of volatile general anesthetic agents and full doses of relaxant drugs should be administered. Ventilation must be carefully controlled and adjusted as required during closure to compensate for increased intra-abdominal pressure. At the end of the procedure, after primary closure a nasotracheal tube is left in place and controlled ventilation is continued.

Prune-Belly Syndrome

This syndrome almost exclusively affects males and consists of congenital absence of abdominal muscles, urinary tract dilation, and undescended testicles. Other congenital defects may occur in association with the syndrome, including malrotation of the gut, pulmonary hypoplasia, cardiac defects, dislocation of the hip, and club feet. Infants are divided into three groups according to the severity of the disease.[65] Group I infants have severe renal and pulmonary defects that are incompatible with survival. Those in group II have

very severe uropathy and will require extensive reconstructive surgery. Infants in group III are healthy as neonates and will require little surgery.

The diagnosis is usually obvious at birth as a result of the lax, wrinkled abdominal wall and bilateral cryptorchidism. Patients in group II have poor renal function and grossly dilated ureters. These infants have disordered micturition and easily acquire renal tract infections. Early high diversion of urine by pyelostomy or ureterostomy is frequently required. Renal function may be significantly impaired.

Group III patients are usually well at birth and demonstrate problems later, usually in association with renal tract infection.

In management of patients with prune-belly syndrome the anesthesiologist must recognize that these patients may have renal failure.[66] They also have a relatively poor cough mechanism owing to absent abdominal muscles and are prone to respiratory infections. Laryngeal atresia has been described in association with prune-belly syndrome.[67] The airway should be rapidly secured with an endotracheal tube, as these patients may regurgitate stomach contents. Muscle relaxants are unnecessary for abdominal surgery, but ventilation should be controlled as spontaneous ventilation may be seriously impaired during anesthesia. Drugs excreted by the kidneys should be avoided. Postoperatively the patient must be carefully managed to detect and treat impending pulmonary complications, which are a potential cause of mortality and morbidity.[68, 69]

NEONATAL CHOLESTATIC JAUNDICE

Defective bile excretion (cholestasis) in the newborn may result from hepatocellular disease or obstruction of the bile ducts.[70] Hepatocellular causes of neonatal cholestasis include infections (hepatitis B, cytomegalovirus, rubella, herpes, and so forth), metabolic diseases, endocrine disease, drug toxicity, and miscellaneous other congenital and acquired defects. Obstruction of the bile ducts may result from atresia, stenosis, or hypoplasia of the ducts or from external compression (as in intestinal duplication). The clinical picture of persistent jaundice, hepatomegaly, pale stools, and dark urine is similar whichever is the etiology. Also similar regardless of etiology are the biochemical features, which will include conjugated bilirubinemia (over 15 percent of total bilirubin), elevated total bilirubin, and elevated alkaline phosphatase and aspartate transaminase levels.

Jaundice is common in the newborn period and indeed is considered physiologic. However, if this jaundice persists for more than 2 weeks, or if conjugated bilirubin levels are found to be elevated, the infant must be urgently investigated. Those infants who have an obstructive component to their cholestasis require early surgical intervention if the best long-term outcome is to be obtained. The problem is to distinguish the infant with extrahepatic biliary obstruction from those with hepatocellular disease.[71] At present there is no single ideal test to diagnose these conditions accurately, and even with multiple studies the diagnosis may be difficult to confirm. Some help in diagnosis may be obtained from the general medical history and the family history. Genetic disorders and metabolic diseases associated with specific syndromes may thus be detected. Ultrasound examination is used to define or exclude mass lesions (for example, choledochal cyst).

Radioisotope scanning using technetium-99m with iminodiacetic acid (99m Tc–IDA) after 5 days of phenobarbital pretreatment is a most valuable test. If the isotope appears in the intestine the bile ducts are patent; however, failure of the isotope to appear is not conclusive evidence of biliary obstruction, as severe hepatocellular disease may also cause this. Percutaneous liver biopsy is therefore required as a complementary test. Fibrosis, bile duct proliferation, and canalicular bile stasis are consistent with a diagnosis of biliary obstruction.[71] The combined use of radioisotope excretion studies and percutaneous liver biopsy should permit identification of 95 percent of cases of extrahepatic biliary atresia.

Biliary Atresia

The extent of obliteration of the bile ducts is very variable. This had led to division of patients into two groups, "surgically correctable" and "noncorrectable." Such a definitive classification is no longer accepted. It is now recognized that obliteration of the biliary system commences in the extrahepatic ducts and spreads to involve the whole system.[72] Intrahepatic ducts are usually patent during the first weeks of life, but progressively become obliterated. The etiology of the disease remains unknown, but viral infection, metabolic abnormalities, and toxic effects of bile acids have been suggested as possible causes. The progressive nature of the disease explains why early surgery is most effective.

The surgical treatment of biliary atresia (Kasai operation) is to resect the extrahepatic bile ducts, including a fibrous mass at the porta hepatis when this is present. The liver at the porta hepatis is dissected to a depth of 2 to 3 mm and a Roux-en-Y jejunal anastomosis to the porta hepatis is performed.[73] There is now general agreement that the earlier the age at operation, the greater is the chance of success.

The anesthetic management of the infant with biliary atresia must include all measures that are normally followed for the sick neonate having major abdominal surgery. In addition, the possibility of preexisting coagulopathy must be recognized, as must the fact that major blood losses may be caused by the surgical procedure. Absence of normal biliary function leads to impaired absorption of fat-soluble vitamins, including vitamin K; hence, prothrombin time may be prolonged. The infant should be treated with intramuscular vitamin K preoperatively, and fresh frozen plasma should be available for the operation. Large-bore intravenous lines should be inserted into the upper limbs or neck for blood replacement during surgery. All blood and intravenous fluids must be warmed. During exploration of the porta hepatis retraction of the liver may restrict flow in the inferior vena cava and cause acute hypotension. The infant must be carefully monitored, therefore, to detect sudden changes in blood pressure. Positioning the patient in a slight Trendelenburg position may facilitate surgery and also optimize venous return via the inferior vena cava. The choice of anesthetic technique may include low concentrations of volatile agents together with a nondepolarizing neuromuscular blocking drug. Halothane has been widely used in infants with biliary atresia without any apparent adverse effects. Curare or atracurium may be used to provide relaxation.

The postoperative course of the infant with biliary atresia may be complicated.[74] Ascending cholangitis is common, particularly for the first few years after operation. Portal hypertension is a frequent sequela and may cause serious bleeding. Fifty to 80 percent of survivors may develop esophageal varices, but only 5 to 10 percent have episodes of bleeding. The use of aspirin in these children may be very dangerous.[71] Recently injection of varices with sclerosing solutions has become the treatment of choice. Malabsorption from lack of bile may lead to poor growth, osteomalacia, and osteoporosis.

Choledochal Cyst

Choledochal cysts are most common in female infants and in Oriental races. The clinical presentation is usually with recurrent pain, fever, and sometimes jaundice and usually the diagnosis is made in children under 10 years of age. In infants jaundice may be the principal sign. Diagnosis is usually confirmed by ultrasound imaging or computed tomography. The "cyst" is most commonly a fusiform dilatation of the common bile duct.[75] If the condition has been undiagnosed until older childhood, the patient may have developed portal hypertension and cirrhosis. The surgical treatment is usually directed at total excision of the bile duct cyst, as there is a high risk of malignancy in remnant cyst wall. The implication of this for the anesthesiologist is that the operation may entail extensive dissection and commensurate blood loss. Large-bore intravenous routes via the upper limbs or neck veins should be established prior to commencement of the operation.

Cholelithiasis

Infants who develop cholelithiasis often have a history of erythroblastosis fetalis, hyperbilirubinemia, parenteral nutrition, or furosemide therapy. The combination of intravenous hyperalimentation with furosemide therapy is particularly likely to result in cholelithiasis. It is thought that furosemide diminishes bile flow and promotes stasis. Older children with gallstones commonly have a history of hemoglobinopathy or cystic fibrosis.

DISEASES OF THE COLON AND RECTUM

Hirschsprung Disease

Hirschsprung disease is a congenital abnormality characterized by an absence of parasympathetic ganglion cells in a portion of the sigmoid colon and rectum.[76] Failure of peristalsis in the affected segment leads to functional obstruction with dilatation and hypertrophy of the proximal colon.[1] There is a family history of the disease in up to 30 percent of patients. Associated conditions include Down syndrome and other forms of mental retardation.

The diagnosis may be made in the neonatal period if the infant does not pass meconium, but is often delayed until the child is several months of age. A history of chronic constipation and abdominal distention is typical. The differential diagnosis is from other causes of chronic constipation, including anal fissure, hypothyroidism, adrenal insufficiency, and other endocrine and nutritional disorders. Confirmation of the diagnosis is by rectal biopsy, which will demonstrate aganglionosis in Hirschsprung disease.

The surgical management of Hirschsprung disease is by means of an initial colostomy, followed by a definitive repair when the child is about 1 year of age. This definitive operation consists of one or other form of a "pull-through" procedure.

Anorectal Anomalies

Agenesis or atresia of the anal canal may affect the entire canal or high, intermediate, or low segments of the canal. Anorectal malformations occur in 1 in 4500 births, with a slight preponderance in males. The more serious types involving a fistula from the colon to the genitourinary tract are also more common in males. In females imperforate anus may be associated with rectovaginal or rectocloacal fistula. Though there are many types of anorectal anomalies,[77] these tend to fall into two main groups based on the location of the blind end of the bowel: the high (supralevator) imperforate anus and the low (translevator) imperforate anus. In either group the rectal pouch may end blindly or communicate via a fistula with an adjacent viscus or the perineal surface.

Sixty percent of patients with anorectal anomalies also have other associated malformations. These most commonly affect the vertebral column (28 percent), the central nervous system (18 percent), the heart (9 percent), and other parts of the gastrointestinal tract (9 percent). Infants with imperforate anus are frequently born prematurely.

The surgical treatment of imperforate anus depends upon the type of anomaly. Low imperforate anus is treated by surgical incision into the pouch. A colostomy is unnecessary, and the outlook for bowel continence is very good. High imperforate anus is more difficult to treat, and the outlook for bowel continence is much less certain. A preliminary colostomy is usually performed and a definitive repair attempted when the infant is 6 to 12 months of age.

Correction of high imperforate anus, especially when this is associated with fistulous connections, requires a major surgical procedure, which may be associated with considerable blood loss. Recently the surgical approach has been by posterior sagittal anorectoplasty.[78] For this procedure the patient is placed in a prone "jackknife" position. An electrostimulator may be used transcutaneously and within the operative wound to map the appropriate anal course by observation of contractions of sphincteric musculature. Though the electrostimulation is primarily direct to the muscle fibers, a clearer response may be seen if neuromuscular blocking drugs are withheld.

CONSIDERATIONS FOR THE ANESTHESIOLOGIST

Assessment of Hydration

It has been stressed that it is most important for the anesthesiologist to accurately assess the degree of dehydration and/or the success of volume replacement when reviewing a patient prior to anesthesia. The fluid and electrolyte status should be determined by consideration of the clinical history, physical examination, and appropriate biochemical studies.[79]

The clinical history will provide some information on the duration of symptoms and the volumes of fluid losses from the gastrointestinal tract. It may also provide valuable information concerning recent weight loss, as each kilogram lost is approximately equal to 1 liter of fluid. Reduction in urine volume is an important sign of dehydration. The older child with dehydration may complain of severe thirst.

The physical examination is most important and can reveal much information concerning fluid status. In the infant, reliable signs of dehydration are a sunken fontanelle and loss of skin turgor. These signs will be evident once a 5 percent weight loss has occurred. More severe dehydration (10 percent weight loss) is accompanied by increased manifestation of these signs plus hypotension, sunken eyes, and loss of ocular tension. Very severe dehydration is accompanied by marked peripheral vasoconstriction, which produces a mottled appearance of the skin. Hyperpyrexia may also occur. A dry tongue may be a sign of dehydration, but may also result from prolonged mouth breathing.

Biochemical studies are essential to confirm the extent of dehydration and to determine the associated electrolyte and acid-base disturbance.

Fluid Therapy for Gastrointestinal Disease

Intravenous therapy to correct dehydration must be planned to progressively restore the existing deficits, while also providing for maintenance fluid plus electrolyte requirements, and the replacement of ongoing losses.

Dehydration due to persistent vomiting requires the replacement of sodium, potassium, chloride, and water.[80] The usual regimen is to replace the estimated deficit with 5 percent dextrose in saline solution. In less severe dehydration 5 percent dextrose in one-third or one-half normal saline is used. Fifty percent of the deficit (estimated from weight loss) may be replaced in the first 24 hours and the remainder in the second 24 hours. Severe disturbances may take longer than 48 hours to correct. In the presence of very severe dehydration due to vomiting, an infusion of normal saline may be required to restore volume rapidly and correct hypotension. As urine output becomes established and increases in volume, potassium chloride should be added to the intravenous infusion at a rate of 3 mEq/kg/24 hours. While replacing deficits, maintenance fluid of 3.5 percent dextrose in 0.3 percent sodium chloride should be infused at a daily rate appropriate for the child. Further losses due to vomiting should be replaced volume-for-volume with isotonic saline.

Dehydration due to persistent diarrhea must be treated according to the proportional losses of water and electrolytes which have occurred. The fluid and electrolyte status will also be influenced by the initial fluid therapy that has been instituted since the onset of diarrhea. The majority of patients will have isonatremic dehydration (serum sodium 130 to 150 mEq/L), but a minority may have hyponatremic dehydration (serum sodium less than 130 mEq/L) or hypernatremic dehydration (serum sodium more than 150 mEq/L). Many patients with diarrhea may be treated with oral carbohydrate and electrolyte solutions, and in all but a few this will maintain and/or restore hydration.[81, 82] Hydration state is monitored by assessing the child's level of activity, body weight, and urine output. If these indicators fail to show improvement, intravenous fluid therapy is required. Infant diarrhea fluid contains approximately 60 mEq/L of sodium, 30 mEg/L of potassium, and 45 mEq/L of chloride. Thus, replacement of fluid deficits with a solution of 5 percent dextrose in water with one-third normal saline plus 20 mEq potassium chloride and 20 mEq of sodium bicarbonate added to each liter is suitable for most infants.[83] Patients with very severe dehydration may

require blood or albumin transfusion to treat persisting hypotension.

Some infants and children may develop hypertonic hypernatremic dehydration with diarrhea, especially if high-solute feedings are initially used as therapy. The treatment of hypertonic dehydration consists of administration of more fluid than solute to restore hydration. This treatment must, however, be applied over an extended period (48 to 72 hours). Too rapid administration of hypotonic solutions may result in movement of excessive fluid to the intracellular compartment and the possibility of seizures. A replacement fluid containing approximately 50 mEq/L of sodium is commonly used.

Hyponatremic dehydration is treated by administration of isotonic solutions over a period of a few days. Added sodium may be administered, but hypertonic saline is unnecessary unless frank signs of water intoxication (for example, convulsions) are present. Hypotonic solutions must be avoided for patients with hyponatremic dehydration, as they may cause further hyponatremia.

In the assessment of the patient who has been treated for dehydration from any cause, the anesthesiologist should look for evidence of signs of good replacement of deficits. The most important indicators are a normal flat fontanelle, well-filled veins, normal skin turgor, a good urine output, and a normal sensorium. Biochemical indices should be within normal limits.

Intravenous Alimentation

Total parenteral nutrition (TPN) has become refined as a technique to the point where nutrition can be maintained despite very severe gastrointestinal disease. Principal gastrointestinal indications for the use of TPN in pediatric patients are short bowel syndrome, intractable diarrhea, and conditions in which normal bowel function is compromised for a prolonged period (such as following omphalocele repair). TPN may also be used for infants with respiratory distress syndrome, sepsis, and other medical conditions, to maintain nutrition during intensive medical therapy.

Short bowel syndrome following massive intestinal resection was associated with a high incidence of morbidity and mortality prior to the introduction of TPN. A length of small bowel of not less than 30 cm was considered essential for survival.[84] Since the advent of TPN, a length of less than 15 cm is compatible with survival.[85] Many infants who are supported with TPN for short bowel syndrome will ultimately develop adequate bowel function.[86]

Solutions for TPN contain amino acids, glucose, electrolytes and trace metals, lipids and carnitine, biotin, vitamins, and iron. They may be delivered by a peripheral intravenous route, but are usually delivered via a central venous line.[87] A two-line system is used to mix lipid and amino acid solutions close to the infusion site. Each patient must be stabilized on a regimen that will provide energy requirements, electrolyte replacements, and other essentials suitable to his or her individual needs. The process of stabilization on TPN may require 2 to 3 days, during which frequent blood and urine glucose estimations must be performed. Once the child is stable, glucose and electrolyte levels are monitored every second or third day.

The most common complication of TPN is sepsis. The central line may become infected by improper handling, but more often becomes secondarily infected by organisms entering elsewhere.[88] Thus, every child on TPN should be managed with meticulous attention to asepsis in all invasive maneuvers (endotracheal intubation, vascular cannulation, and so forth).

Whenever possible, if a child on TPN presents for anesthesia, the TPN line should be left totally undisturbed. Injections should not be made into the line, and the line should not be used as a central venous pressure monitor. Obviously, there will be exceptions to these principles when desperately sick infants require care but have limited routes for venous access. Some drugs are compatible with intravenous hyperalimentation amino acid solutions.[89] These include many antibiotics, cimetidine, furosemide, heparin, hydrocortisone, and phenobarbital. Drugs that are not compatible with TPN solutions include pentobarbital and thiopental, diazepam, morphine, sodium bicarbonate, and digoxin. Since the lipid solutions are unstable with most drugs, these must be temporarily discontinued if any drugs are infused via a TPN solution line.

Management of the Pediatric "Full Stomach" Patient

Many patients with gastrointestinal disease may present to the anesthesiologist the challenge of providing safe anesthesia in the presence of the risk of regurgitation and aspiration of stomach contents. There are some special considerations for infants and children that should be recognized by the anesthesiologist when meeting this problem.

If time permits, pretreatment of the patient with drugs may reduce the volume and acidity of the gastric contents. Glycopyrrolate has been demonstrated to be the most effective of the anticholinergic drugs in reducing acid secretions.[90] It should be given in a dose of 0.01 mg/kg IM at least 30 minutes prior to induction of anesthesia. Cimetidine has also been shown to reduce gastric acidity in pediatric patients.[91] It should be given in an oral dose of 7.5 mg/kg 1 to 3 hours before anesthesia.[91] Sodium citrate may be administered to increase the pH of the stomach contents. Metoclopramide is a dopamine antagonist that has central antiemetic properties and also promotes gastric emptying into the small bowel.[92] Metoclopramide increases the tone of the lower esophageal sphincter.[93] It should be given in a dose of 0.1 to 0.2 mg/kg

intravenously 30 minutes prior to induction of anesthesia. Anticholinergic drugs interfere with the action of metoclopramide and should be withheld until induction of anesthesia is commenced.

Awake intubation has been advocated for the management of infants with a potentially full stomach. This is a relatively simple procedure to perform in the neonate and has been considered a very safe approach. The airway protective reflexes are intact up to the moment of intubation. In addition, if intubation fails for any reason, the infant will maintain his airway and continue to ventilate spontaneously. More recently, however, there are concerns that the physiological response to awake intubation, and particularly any associated increase in cerebral intravascular pressure, might predispose some preterm infants to intracranial hemorrhage. It is recognized that the stressed preterm infant has impaired autoregulation of cerebral blood flow;[94] cerebral blood flow is related directly to mean arterial blood pressure. A surge in mean arterial pressure, such as might accompany intubation, will be directly transmitted to fine cerebral vessels. Thus, it might be concluded that the stressed preterm infant should be as carefully managed during intubation as is the adult with an intracranial aneurysm. Awake intubation of preterm infants is still widely practiced, both in the operating room and in the neonatal intensive care unit. This approach should be reviewed, especially in the sick, hypoxic, preterm infant. Induction of anesthesia with a small dose of barbiturate (such as thiopental, 2 to 3 mg/kg), fentanyl (20 to 30 μg/kg), neuromuscular blockade, and the administration of lidocaine IV (1 mg/kg) all may diminish the increase in blood pressure associated with intubation. When practical, a suitable combination of these methods should be applied before intubation. Awake intubation of the term neonate may still be the method of choice in some situations, such as in the presence of a tracheoesophageal fistula.

Awake intubation has not been widely practiced in older children. They become very upset and vigorously oppose efforts to intubate them awake, unless they are moribund. Such older patients will require another technique to rapidly establish a safe airway. For many years an inhalation induction of anesthesia with the child in a lateral position was advocated as an acceptable technique for the full-stomach patient. More recently most authorities would suggest that the pediatric patient should be managed similarly to the adult, with a rapid-sequence induction and cricoid pressure.

A rapid-sequence induction in infants and children must be undertaken with some considerations similar to those in adults. Hypovolemia should be first corrected, the drugs should be rapidly injected after a period of preoxygenation, and cricoid pressure should be initiated as soon as sleep intervenes. A suitable endotracheal tube should be inserted as soon as adequate relaxation is present. Some considerations are different in infants and young children. Little is to be gained by elevation of the head of the table; the vertical height gained is insufficient to significantly diminish the risk of passive regurgitation.[95] Succinylcholine does not increase intragastric pressure in young patients,[96] (under 10 years); therefore, pretreatment with a nondepolarizing relaxant is unnecessary.

Cuffed endotracheal tubes are not routinely used for infants and small children, because the added bulk of the cuff limits the internal diameter of the tube. Despite this, there are few reports of significant aspiration once the endotracheal tube is in place. This might be a problem if large volumes of fluid regurgitate into the pharynx due to surgical manipulation.[97] If such a situation is anticipated, a large gastric tube should be inserted and connected to continuous suction, and in older children a cuffed endotracheal tube should be inserted.

The risk of regurgitation and aspiration during emergence from anesthesia must be recognized. All patients with a potentially full stomach should be allowed to awaken completely prior to extubation, which should be performed with the patient in a lateral position.

The foregoing recommendations for the management of the "full stomach" patient must, of course, be modified if other disease is present. A standard "crash induction" is not recommended in a hypovolemic patient or in one with an airway abnormality that may render intubation difficult. Ketamine is a useful induction agent for the patient who cannot be fully volume-restored prior to induction. Following preoxygenation, 2 to 4 mg/kg of ketamine with 0.02 mg/kg of atropine IV and 1 to 2 mg/kg of succinylcholine IV may be used for a rapid-sequence induction. Cricoid pressure should be applied as soon as the patient loses consciousness.

The patient with a possible full stomach who also has an abnormality of the airway presents special problems. A crash induction is unsafe if any doubt exists as to the ease of laryngoscopy and intubation. Awake direct laryngoscopy in such a patient is unlikely to be successful and will be very distressing for the patient. Awake flexible laryngoscopy may be practical, but many pediatric patients would find this distressing also.

If possible the child with a difficult airway should be prepared by appropriate fasting, continuous gastric aspiration, and administration of cimetidine, glycopyrrolate, and sodium citrate. Anesthesia should then be induced by inhalation of halothane and oxygen, and the anesthetic level should be rapidly deepened while spontaneous ventilation is maintained.

When the patient is deeply anesthetized laryngoscopy (direct or flexible) may be attempted and intubation performed if possible. Lidocaine, 2 mg/kg administered IV 2 to 3 minutes prior to attempts at laryngoscopy, will minimize the risk of coughing or breath holding.

When surgery is completed, the child with a difficult airway should be allowed to awaken completely and placed in a lateral position before extubation.

REFERENCES

1. Milla PJ: Development of intestinal structure and function. *In* Tanner MS, Stocks RJ (Eds): Neonatal Gastroenterology: Contemporary Issues. Newcastle on Tyne, Intercept Ltd., 1984, p 6.
2. Cavell B: Gastric emptying in preterm infants. Acta Paediatr Scand 68:725, 1979.
3. Cavell B: Gastric emptying in infants with congenital heart disease. Acta Paediatr Scand 70:517, 1981.
4. Ebers DW, Smith DI, Gibbs GE: Gastric acidity on the first day of life. Pediatrics 18:800, 1956.
5. Werner B: Peptic and tryptic capacity of the digestive tract of newborns. Acta Paediatr Scand 35(Suppl 70):1, 1948.
6. Lebenthal E, Lee PC, Heitlinger LA: Impact of development of the gastrointestinal tract on infant feeding. J Pediatr 102:1, 1983.
7. Winters R.W. The Body Fluids in Pediatrics. Boston, Little, Brown, 1973, pp 412–413.
8. Chandra M: Dehydration and acidosis. *In* Lifshitz F (Ed.): Common Pediatric Disorders, New York, Marcel Dekker Inc., 1984, p 106.
9. Barltrop D, Wharton BA, Arneil GC, et al.: Nutrition and nutritional disorders. *In* Forfar JO, Arneil GC (Eds.): Textbook of Pediatrics. 3rd ed. New York, Churchill-Livingstone, 1984.
10. Shull MW, Reed RB, Valadian I, et al.: Veolocities of growth in vegetarian preschool children. Pediatrics 60:410, 1977.
11. Mullen JL, Gertner MH, Buzby G, et al.: Implications of malnutrition in the surgical patient. Arch Surg 114:121, 1979.
12. Katz M, Stiehm ER: Host defense in malnutrition. Pediatrics 59:490, 1977.
13. Pollace MM, Wiley JS, Yeh TS, et al.: Effect of nutritional depletion on physiologic stability (abstr). Crit Care Med 10:205, 1982.
14. Merritt RJ, Suskind RM: Nutritional survey of hospitalized pediatric patients. Am J Clin Nutr 32:1320, 1979.
15. Cooper A, Jakobowski D, Spiker J, et al.: Nutritional assessment; an integral part of the preoperative pediatric surgical evaluation. J Pediatr Surg 16:554, 1981.
16. Berlin CM Jr, Tinker DE: Kwashiorkor in a child in central Pennsylvania. A seven year follow-up. Am J Dis Child 136:822, 1982.
17. Stevenson RJ: Gastrointestinal bleeding in children. Surg Clin North Am 65:1455, 1985.
18. Raffensperger JG, Luck SR: Gastrointestinal bleeding in children. Surg Clin North Am 56:413, 1976.
19. Chhattriwalla Y, Colon AR, Scanlon JW: The use of cimetidine in the newborn. Pediatrics 65:301, 1980.
20. Morden RS, Schullinger JN, Mollitt DL, et al.: Operative management of stress ulcers in children. Ann Surg 196:18, 1982.
21. Strawczinski H, Beck I, McKenna R, et al.: The behavior of the lower esophageal sphincter in infants and its relationship to gastroesophageal regurgitation. J. Pediatr 64:17, 1964.
22. Vaage S, Levorstad F, Efskind L: Congenital atresia of the esophagus. Scand J Thorac Cardiovasc Surg 9:68, 1975.
23. Moroz SP, Espinza J, Cumming WA, et al.: Lower esophageal sphincter function in children with and without gastroesophageal reflux. Gastroenterology 71:236, 1976.
24. Euler AR, Ament ME: Gastroesophageal reflux in children: clinical manifestations, diagnosis, pathophysiology and therapy. Pediatr Ann 5:678, 1976.
25. Walsh, JK, Farrell MK, Keenan WJ, et al.: Gastroesophageal reflux in infants: relation to apnea. J. Pediatr 99:196, 1981.

26. Nissen R. The treatment of hiatal hernia and esophageal reflux by fundoplication. *In* Nyhus LM, Harkins HN (Eds.): Hernia. Philadelphia, J.B. Lippincott Co., 1964, p 488.
27. Payne W, Ellis F, Olson AM: Treatment of cardiospasm (achalasia of the esophagus) in children. Surgery 50:731, 1961.
28. Azizkhan RG, Tapper D, Eraklis A: Achalasia in childhood: a 20 year experience. J Pediatr Surg 15:452, 1980.
29. Bolsin SN, Gillbe C: Opitz-Frias syndrome: a case with potentially hazardous anaesthetic implications. Anaesthesia 40:1189, 1985.
30. Little JR, Opitz JM: The G syndrome. Am J Dis Child 121:505, 1971.
31. Idowu J, Aitken DR, Georgeson KE: Gastric volvulus in the newborn. Arch Surg 115:1046, 1980.
32. Asch MJ, Sherman NJ: Gastric volvulus in children: report of two cases. J Pediatr Surg 12:1059, 1977.
33. Rosser SB, Clark CH, Elechi EN: Spontaneous neonatal gastric perforation. J Pediatr Surg 17:390, 1982.
34. Stevenson RJ: Non-neonatal intestinal obstruction in children. Surg Clin North Am 65:1224, 1985.
35. Atwell JD, Levick P: Congenital hypertrophic pyloric stenosis and associated anomalies in the genitourinary tract. J Pediatr Surg 16:1029, 1981.
36. Wooley MM, Felsher BF, Asch MJ, et al.: Jaundice, hypertrophic pyloric stenosis and glucuronyl transferase. J Pediatr Surg 9:359, 1974.
37. Winters RW: Metabolic alkalosis of pyloric stenosis. *In* Winters RW (Ed.): The Body Fluids in Pediatrics. Boston, Little, Brown, 1973, p 402.
38. Shumake LB: Post-operative hypoglycemia in congenital hypertrophic pyloric stenosis. South Med J 68:223, 1975.
39. Daly AM, Conn AW: Anaesthesia for pyloromyotomy: a review. Canad Anaesth Soc J 16:316, 1969.
40. Ghory MJ, Sheldon CA: Newborn surgical emergencies of the gastrointestinal tract. Surg Clin North Am 65:1083, 1985.
41. Rickham PP, Boeckmann CR: Neonatal meconium obstruction in the absence of mucoviscidosis. Am J Surg 106:173, 1965.
42. Kalayoglu M, Sieber WK, Rodman JB, et al.: Meconium ileus: a critical review of treatment and eventual prognosis. J Pediatr Surg 6:290, 1971.
43. Mabogunje OE, Wang CI, Mahour GH: Improved survival of neonates with meconium ileus. Arch Surg 117:37, 1982.
44. Brown EG, Sweet AY: Neonatal necrotizing enterocolitis. Pediatr Clin North Am 29:1149, 1982.
45. Sweet AY: Epidemiology. *In* Brown EG, Sweet AY (Eds.): Neonatal Necrotizing Enterocolitis. New York, Grune and Stratton, 1980, p 13.
46. Brady P, Garite T, German JC: Fetal heart rate patterns in infants in whom necrotizing enterocolitis develops. Arch Surg 115:1050, 1980.
47. Touloukian RJ: Etiologic role of the circulation. *In* Brown EG, Sweet AY (Eds.): Neonatal Necrotizing Enterocolitis. New York, Grune and Stratton, 1980, p 41.
48. Goldman HI: Feeding and necrotizing enterocolitis. Am J Dis Child 134:553, 1980.
49. Engel RR, Vernig ML, Hunt CE, et al.: Origin of gas in necrotizing enterocolitis. Pediatr Res 7:292, 1973.
50. Holdman LV, Moore WEC: Anaerobic Laboratory Manual. Blacksburg, VA, Virginia Polytechnic Institute, 1972.
51. Kleigman RM: Neonatal necrotizing enterocolitis: implications for an infectious disease. Pediatr Clin North Am 26:327, 1979.
52. Rowe MI, Marchildon MB: Surgical management. *In* Brown EG, Sweet AY (Eds.): Neonatal Necrotizing Enterocolitis. New York, Grune and Stratton, 1980, p 167.
53. Kosloske A, Papile LA, Burstein J: Indications for operation in acute necrotizing enterocolitis of the neonate. J Pediatr Surg 87:532, 1980.
54. Raju, TNK, Vidyasagar D, Torres C, et al.: Intracranial pressure during intubation and anesthesia in infants. J. Pediatr 96:860, 1980.
55. Deckhart R, Steward DJ: Noninvasive arterial hemoglobin oxygen saturation versus transcutaneous oxygen tension monitoring in the preterm infant. Crit Care Med 12:935, 1984.
56. Dierdorf SF, Krisna G: Anesthetic management of neonatal surgical emergencies. Anesth Analg 60:204, 1981.
57. Rosenkrantz JG, Cox JA, Silverman FN, et al.: Intussusception in the 1970's: indications for operation. J Pediatr Surg 12:367, 1977.
58. Evrard M: Anesthesia problems in the infant with acute intestinal intussusception. Anesth Analg (Paris), 30:1085, 1973.
59. Meguid M, Canty T, Eraklis AJ: Complications of Meckel's diverticulum in infants. Surg Gynecol Obst 139:541, 1974.
60. Filippi G, McKusick VA: The Beckwith-Wiedemann syndrome. Medicine 49:279, 1970.
61. Schiff D, Colle E, Wells D, et al.: Metabolic aspects of the Beckwith-Wiedemann syndrome. J. Pediatr 82:258, 1973.
62. Philippart AI, Cantry TG, Filler RM: Acute fluid volume requirements in infants with anterior abdominal wall defects. J Pediatr Surg 7:553, 1972.
63. Canty TG, Collins DL: Primary fascial closure in infants with gastroschisis and omphalocele: a superior approach. J Pediatr Surg 8:707, 1983.
64. Schwartz MZ, Tyson KRT, Milliorn K, et al.: Staged reduction using a Silastic sac is the treatment of choice for large congenital abdominal wall defects. J Pediatr Surg 18:713, 1983.
65. Woodhouse CRJ, Ransley PG, Innes-Williams D: Prune belly syndrome—report of 47 cases. Arch Dis Child 57:856, 1982.
66. Hannington-Kiff JG: Prune belly syndrome and general anaesthesia: case report. Br J Anaesth 42:649, 1970.
67. Lyon AJ: Congenital atresia of the larynx in association with prune belly syndrome. J Army Med Crops 129:118, 1983.
68. Hendren WH: Prune belly syndrome. *In* Devine C, Stecker JF (Eds.): Urology in Practice. Boston, Little, Brown, 1978, p 361.
69. Chinyanga HM: Cystoscopy and prune belly syndrome. *In* Stehling LC (Ed.): Common Problems in Pediatric Anesthesia. Chicago, Year Book Medical, 1982, p 77.
70. Johnston DI: Neonatal cholestatic jaundice. *In* Tanner MS, Stocks RJ (Eds.): Neonatal Gastroenterology: Contemporary Issues. Newcastle on Tyne, Intercept Ltd., 1984, pp 139–153.
71. Altman RP, Stolar CJH: Pediatric hepatobiliary disease. Surg Clin North Am 65:1245, 1985.
72. Howard ER: Extrahepatic biliary atresia: a review of current management. Br J Surg 70:193, 1983.
73. deVries PA, Cox KL: Surgical treatment of congenital and neonatal biliary obstruction. Surg Clin North Am 61:987, 1981.
74. Barkin RM, Lilly JR: Biliary atresia and the Kasai operation: continuing care. J. Pediatr 96:1015, 1980.
75. Todani T, Watanabe Y, Narusue M, et al.: Congenital bile duct cysts. Am J Surg 134:263, 1977.
76. Martin LW, Torres AM: Hirschsprung's disease. Surg Clin North Am 65:1171, 1985.
77. deVries PA, Cox KL: Anorectal anomalies. Surg Clin North Am 65:1139, 1985.
78. deVries PA, Pena A: Posterior sagittal anorectoplasty. J Pediatr Surg 17:638, 1982.
79. Vaughan VC, McKay RJ, Behrman RE (Eds.): Nelson Textbook of Pediatrics. 11th ed. Philadelphia, W.B. Saunders Co., 1979, pp 290–291.
80. McGeowin M: Clinical Management of Electrolyte Disorders. Boston, Martinus Nijhoff, 1983, p 90.
81. Santosham M, Daum RS, Diuman L, et al.: Oral rehydration therapy of infantile diarrhea. A controlled study of well nourished children hospitalized in the United States and Panama. N Engl J Med 306:1070, 1982.
82. Hamilton JR: Treatment of acute diarrhea. Pediatr Clin North Am 32:419, 1985.
83. Collins RD: Illustrated Manual of Fluid and Electrolytes. 2nd ed. Philadelphia, J.B. Lippincott Co., 1983, p 107.

84. Wilmore DW: Factors correlating with a successful outcome following extensive intestinal resection in infants. J. Pediatr *80*:88, 1972.

85. Klish WJ, Putman TC: The short gut. Am J Dis Child *135*:1056, 1981.

86. Heird WC, Winters RW: Total parenteral nutrition: the state of the art. J. Pediatr *86*:2, 1975.

87. Zlotkin SH, Stallings VA, Pencharz PB: Total parenteral nutrition in children. Pediatr Clin North Am *32*:381, 1985.

88. Miller RC, Grogan JB: Incidence and source of contamination of intravenous nutritional infusion systems. J Pediatr Surg *8*:195, 1973.

89. Farago S: Compatibility of antibiotics and other drugs in total parenteral nutrition solutions. Can J Hosp Pharm *36*:43, 1983.

90. Salem MR, Wong AY, Mani M, et al.: Premedicant drugs and gastric juice pH and volume in pediatric patients. Anesthesiology *44*:216, 1976.

91. Goudsouzian NG, Cote CJ, Liu LMP, et al.: The dose response effect of oral cimetidine on gastric pH and volume in children. Anesthesiology *55*:533, 1981.

92. Albibi R, McCallum RW. Metoclopramide: pharmacology and clinical application. Ann Intern Med *98*:86, 1983.

93. Stanciu C, Bennett JR: Metoclopramide in gastro-esophageal reflux. Gut *14*:275, 1973.

94. Lou HC, Lassen NA, Friis-Hansen B: Impaired autoregulation of cerebral blood flow in the distressed newborn infant. J. Pediatr *94*:118, 1979.

95. Salem MR, Wong AY, Fizzotti GF: Efficacy of cricoid pressure in preventing aspiration of gastric contents in paediatric patients. Br J Anaesth *44*:401, 1972.

96. Salem MR, Wong AY, Lin YH: The effect of suxamethonium on intra-gastric pressure in infants and children. Br J Anaesth *44*:166, 1972.

97. Roy WL: Intraoperative aspiration in a paediatric patient. Canad Anaesth Soc J *32*:639, 1985.

9 || PEDIATRIC HEAD AND NECK SYNDROMES

C. F. WARD, M.D.

Several decades have passed since the discovery of the vaccine and the conquest of polio. The organization that once devoted itself to polio alone now largely concerns itself with birth defects and has recruited a medical ally, the dysmorphologist, who possesses special knowledge concerning anatomical associations and the probabilities of recurrence of malformations. The specialist and the organization have both tremendously expanded the understanding of human malformation, as well as presenting another etiological concept of abnormal anatomy, that of in utero growth restraint leading to *deformation*. Much of what follows is based on this foundation, provided over the past 30 years.

This particular chapter is the first of three constrained by anatomy and morphology. Wherever possible, the author has attempted to remain within the assigned boundaries; however, it is important to realize that numerous other diseases and syndromes have craniofacial presentation that may be of anesthetic significance and will not be so easily restricted. For example, Table 9–1 presents a compilation of the many syndromes associated with micrognathia. By no means will all such issues be dealt with here, and investigation of other publications may well be necessary to thoroughly understand some pathology, especially that resulting from chromosome abnormalities or trauma.

The question of nomenclature is prominent in any discussion of birth defects. Descriptions applied in this chapter are those found in the *Birth Defects Compendium* with additional titles or descriptions added as thought appropriate to assist in historical correlation.

EMBRYOLOGY

Typically, those engaged in the practice of anesthesia possess a dominant interest in physiology and pharmacology, with a near aversion to anatomy, except as it pertains directly to the clinical situation. This aversion usually becomes withdrawal when embryology is mentioned; however, tracing the origin of head and neck anatomy is worthwhile because of the understanding such pursuit lends to what *may be*. Many an operating room visit planned for the child with unusual craniofacial appearance is an aggressive examination with the child under anesthesia, occasionally followed by removal or rearrangement of malpositioned or malproportioned parts. Those who schedule such visits usually know well the anatomical possibilities. As the surface area in question encompasses the brain and the airway, both of which are of interest to anesthetists, it seems prudent to briefly review development as an aid to foreseeing what these possibilities may be.

The Skull

The upper portion of the cranial vault develops from mesenchyma that undergoes membranous ossification. This part of the skull consists of flat bones that join edge-to-edge to form sutures, or form fontanelles where more than two bones meet. The two frontal bones oppose at the mid-forehead, forming the metopic suture. The frontal bones oppose the parietal bones bilaterally, creating the coronal suture, and the anterior fontanelle results from both matched bone pairs joining in the midline. The two parietal bones oppose to form the sagittal suture, and posteriorly contact the occipital bone to form the lambdoid suture. At the junction of these three bones, the posterior fontanelle is formed.

The base of the skull is formed from separate cartilage that create the base of the occipital bone, the sphenoid, the ethmoid, and the petrous bone, along with portions of the temporal bone. Where the base of the skull, consisting primarily of the squamous

Table 9–1. SYNDROMES ASSOCIATED WITH MICROGNATHIA

Abnormality, Primary Name	Associated Names, Descriptions
Syndromes Caused by Known Chromosome Abnormality	
4 p −	Wolf
5 p −	Cri du chat
13 trisomy	
14 q proximal partial trisomy	
11 q −	
11 q partial trisomy	
18 q −	
18 p −	
18 trisomy	Edwards
21 monosomy	
Syndromes Caused by Other Than Known Chromosome Abnormality	
Acrocephalopolysyndactyly	
Acrocephalosyndactyly	
Arthro-ophthalmopathy	Stickler
Auditory canal atresia	
C	
Campomelic dysphasia	
Cerebrocostomandibular	
Cerebrohepatorenal	Bowen or Zellweger
Cerebro-oculofacioskeletal	COFS
Chrondrodystrophic myotonia	
Cleft palate	
Craniofacial dysostosis with diaphyseal hyperplasia	
Craniofacial dyssynostosis	
Deafness and ear pits	
Dubowitz	
Ear, absent tragus	
Fetal trimethadione	
Frontometaphyseal dysplasia	
G	Opitz-Frias
Gingival fibromatosis, Cowden type	
Hanhart	
Hemifacial microsomia	
Laryngomalacia	
Lissencephaly	
Mandibulofacial dysostosis	
Marden-Walker	
Meckel	
Megalocornea—mental retardation	
Mesomelic dysplasia, Langer type	
Noonan	
Nose, posterior atresia	Choanal atresia
Oculoauriculovertebral dysplasia	Goldenhar
Oculomandibulofacial dysplasia	Hallermann-Streiff
Opitz-Kaveggia FG	
Osteodysplasty	Melnick-Needles
Pierre Robin	
Progeria	Hutchinson-Gilford
Pyle disease	
Seckel	
Smith-Lemli-Opitz	
Thrombocytopenia with absent radius	TAR
Thymic agenesis	DiGeorge
Trichorhinophalangeal, type II	Langer-Giedion
Turner	
Williams	

p − Nomenclature indicates partial or total absence of chromosome short arm.

q − Nomenclature indicates partial or total absence of chromosome long arm.

temporal bone, opposes the parietal bone, the squamous suture is created; where these two bones meet the frontal bone and occipital bone, the anterolateral and posterolateral fontanelles are, respectively, formed.

The face develops from two origins. Upper midline structures develop primarily from the frontal prominence, while lateral and middle facial anatomy additionally trace their origin to the branchial or pharyngeal arches. The arches are originally bars of mesenchymal tissue, separated from one another by the branchial or pharyngeal clefts. Both of these structures develop coincidentally with the foregut, or pharyngeal, pouches. Each of these three structures will be described in turn. It is well worthwhile remembering the various arch components, especially the first, for developmental abnormalities involving a visible portion of an arch may also affect other less prominent anatomy.

The first branchial arch gives origin to the maxilla, the mandible, the zygoma, and a portion of the temporal bone. A small portion of this arch also contributes the incus and malleus. The muscles of mastication, the mylohyoid, the tensor tympani, tensor palatini, and anterior belly of the digastric also originate here. Each arch has its own cranial nerve component, in this case the trigeminal nerve.

The second arch gives rise to the stapes, the styloid process of the temporal bone, the stylohyoid ligament and the lesser horn, and a portion of the body of the hyoid bone. The muscles are the stapedius, stylohyoid, posterior belly of the digastric, the auricular, and all the facial expression muscles. The nerve supply is from the facial nerve.

The third arch gives rise to the remainder of the hyoid, while the lone muscle derived from this structure is the stylopharyngeal, with innervation from the glossopharyngeal nerve.

The fourth arch provides the laryngeal cartilage, along with the pharyngeal constrictors, the levator palatini, and the cricothyroid muscles, with innervation from the fourth arch nerve, the superior laryngeal branch of the vagus. The sixth arch provides the intrinsic laryngeal muscles with nerve supply from the recurrent branch of the vagus.

The first pharyngeal pouch creates the eustachian tube and middle ear, the second pouch forms the tonsillar fossa, and the third pouch creates the thymus and a portion of the parathyroid. The fourth pouch contributes the rest of the parathyroids, while the fifth pouch develops into the portion of the thyroid gland that secretes calcitonin.

Of the clefts, only the first, between the first and second arches, forms a definitive structure—the external ear. However, if the second arch does not grow caudally over the third and fourth arches, as it normally should, the second, third, and fourth clefts can remain in contact with skin surface, forming branchial fistulas anywhere between the inferior border of the mandible and the clavicle, anterior to the sternocleidomastoid muscle. The tongue surface, although originating primarily from first arch structures, also receives major contributions from the second, third, and fourth arches, as evidenced by its changing sensory nerve supply. To complicate matters still further, the bulk of the tongue probably originates from occipital somites, thus accounting for the hypoglossal nerve innervation of the tongue musculature.

The thyroid gland originates as a cell proliferation at the foramen cecum in the tongue, then migrates, anterior to the gut, caudad to its eventual location anterior to the larynx. During this transition, the gland remains connected to the tongue via the thyroglossal duct, which eventually disappears. Should this not occur, it is worth recalling the migration, for although 75 percent of thyroglossal cysts are near the hyoid, they may be found anywhere along the track from the foramen cecum.

The mid-face is created by a very complex lateral-to-medial transition of first arch structures, along with evolution of the frontal prominence. The first arch contributions begin as maxillary, medial nasal, and lateral nasal swellings. During their midline fusion process, these structures create the intermaxillary segment. If one considers the upper jaw as an arch, this segment is the keystone. It comprises the philtrum of the lip, a jaw segment with the four incisor teeth, and a triangular component, called the primary palate, the vertex of which is the incisive foramen. This foramen marks the demarcation point between a cleft lip and a cleft (secondary) palate. The majority of the definitive palate arises from the maxillary swellings and grows medially to a midline fusion, also giving rise to the uvula. Returning to the arch analogy, it becomes easier to comprehend the location of the usual cleft lip, along the off-midline border of the "keystone" intermaxillary segment, and equally well, the midline location of the isolated cleft palate.

GENERAL ASSESSMENT

Prior to discussion of specific pathology, and immediately after discussion of embryology, I draw to the reader's attention that there is a separate chapter (Chapter 4) that concerns itself with central nervous system disease. This is quite appropriate, and it is equally so to note that despite the close proximity of the face, skull, and brain, they are not subject to a uniform pathological discussion. That lovely children may develop debilitating brain disease seems intellectually acceptable. Slightly more awkward, however, is the fact that an infant with near-monstrous appearance may, for the moment at least, be intellectually normal and quite able to survive. One must overlook the overall appearance of the package and instead consider the contents. A physician's initial expression of dismay when first viewing a child with a cloverleaf skull or facial burn may be witnessed by the parents and

accidentally destroy all chance to establish confidence with them. The goal, then, must be to evaluate such children strictly as a physician without contamination from personal aesthetic values. To do otherwise does all concerned a terrible disservice.

CONGENITAL CRANIOFACIAL DEFORMITIES

The *Birth Defects Compendium* provides an encyclopedic approach to development gone awry and provides descriptions of over 1000 birth defects. Numerous tables in the volume list anatomical areas involved by these defects; the face alone receives nearly 300 such citations, with mention of the facial segments and skull proper receiving about an equal number. Obviously, many of these tables involve duplicate listings of the same syndrome. Nevertheless, a discussion of congenital craniofacial deformities must cover a panoply of anatomy, roughly divided into three areas: (1) chromosome defects; (2) syndromes named for the original author(s) involved; and (3) syndromes named to describe the anatomical defect. A failure to recognize members of category 1 or 2 has always seemed somewhat understandable to the author, for many are exceedingly rare and complex; furthermore, disease descriptions involving proper names are somewhat passé. The third category is rather more embarrassing, for specific anatomical information is available in the names; unfortunately, the words are alien to the rest of medicine and seem altogether more appropriate to a description of long-deceased reptiles. Therefore, the following is a guide to the terms involved in this subject.

A *synostosis* is a union between adjacent bones. A *dysostosis* refers to a defect in ossification. A cranial suture dysostosis refers in a nonspecific way to a primary defect in suture formation. *Craniosynostosis* refers to a premature closure of a skull suture. Harken back to the description of embryology and it becomes apparent that the resultant anatomy will be highly dependent on which suture is involved. Keep clearly in mind that brain growth is the driving force behind cranial expansion; if one dimension is eliminated, growth may well be diverted to the others.

Closure of the sagittal suture prevents lateral skull growth. This results in an elongated skull, referred to as *scaphocephaly* (scapho—boat-shaped) or *dolichoscaphocephaly* (dolicho—long, narrow). Closure of the coronal suture prevents anterior-posterior skull growth. This results in a widened skull, referred to as *brachycephaly* (brachy—broadened) or *acrobrachycephaly* (acro—extreme). If both the sagittal and coronal sutures close, skull growth is impeded in two dimensions, resulting in vertical growth. The result is *turricephaly* (turri—tower), *oxycephaly* (oxy—pointed), or *oxyturricephaly*. An unusual varient of multiple suture closure results in vertical and inferolateral expansion, referred to as *Kleeblattschädel* or more simply as a *cloverleaf* dysostosis. Premature closure of the metopic suture creates the very visible *trigonocephaly* (trigono—triangular), characterized by a mid-forehead "keel." Finally, an asymmetrical suture closure may create a tilted cranium, referred to as *plagiocephaly* (plagio—slanting). Reduced symmetrical cranial size is *microcephaly*, usually due to deficient brain growth, while nonspecific symmetrical skull enlargement is *macrocephaly*, which may be due to causes *other* than hydrocephalus, to which it is often reflexly attributed.

The Craniosynostoses

Given these terms, logic would dictate a unified classification scheme, probably based primarily on suture involvement and resultant cranial vault shape. However, even if the specific pathology of each defect were known (they are not), this classification model would be valid only if syndrome anatomy proved relatively constant (it does not). Each leading text rearranges some or all of these defects, based on the particular author's viewpoint. This sort of internecine activity is useful in an evolutionary sense, but it makes the occasional reader's task a good bit more difficult. To those interested in a previously diagnosed specific syndrome, much of this is superfluous. Consequently, what follows is a consensus compilation of craniosynostosis syndromes, listed in alphabetical order, with an inclusion of anatomy that either generally occurs with the syndrome or has special relevance to anesthesia. Particular note should be taken of what is *not* included here—anesthesia for craniofacial reconstructive surgery. The strides made by Gilles, Obwegeser, Converse, Munro, and especially Tessier in remodeling the entire cephalad portion of a deformed human are absolutely astounding. In these aggressive techniques, only the brain and attendant cranial-nerve-supplied organs are sacrosanct; everything else is movable and/or removable. However, the most liberal estimate of centers required to perform this surgery is 1 per 20 million population. Assuming, then, that the author is in one such hospital, a discussion of anesthesia for this radical surgery would be directed to 11 other centers in the United States, in turn attending to about 1200 to 1500 patients per year requiring plastic repair. Therefore, rather than simply being presented with a rearrangement of published phrases, the interested reader is directed to obtain and thoroughly read original articles, in some detail. In such reading it should be particularly noted that major postoperative neurological sequelae and intraoperative demise are almost invariably mentioned, usually in groups consisting of only 15 to 20 patients. In this context, the fact that the trachea can be extubated because the entire mid-face advances 3 cm seems almost insignificant. It is, therefore, the author's opinion that surgery *on* a patient with a craniosynostosis is reasonable when and wherever otherwise indicated. However, surgery

for the craniosynostosis is a much different matter and literally requires a cast of thousands, of which the anesthetist is but one. Following a perusal of the literature, patient referral for definitive repair will usually appear eminently more reasonable.

The Acrocephalo(poly)syndactylies

This group of deformities includes Apert syndrome, Carpenter syndrome, Pfeiffer syndrome, and Saethre-Chotzen syndrome.

In addition to the above list, the following syndromes are listed for the sake of completeness, although often only one report of each is present in the literature: Herrmann-Opitz type, Sakati syndrome, Summitt type, and Waardenburg type (not Waardenburg syndrome). Because of their extraordinary rarity, these will not be discussed further.

Apert Syndrome (Fig. 9–1)

In 1906, Apert first noted a syndrome of acrobrachycephaly with syndactyly or webbing between the fingers and toes (usually second to fifth). This particular combination is in general referred to as acrocephalopolysyndactyly; Apert described but one variation. This syndrome is thought to occur about 1 in 160,000 live births, is transmitted as autosomal dominant with a male:female ratio of 1:1, and is rarely linked with advanced paternal age. Mental retardation is common and life span should be normal.

Clinical Features. Craniosynostosis is of a variable degree, primarily affecting the coronal suture, associated with sphenoethmoidomaxillary hypoplasia. The characteristic appearance is of turribrachycephaly with a wide, high forehead, marked in infancy by a supraorbital ridge. As the mid-face is hypoplastic, the mandible is relatively prominent. There is hypertelorism, proptosis, downward slanting palpebral fissures, and generally a small nasal bridge. Hydrocephalus, with several presentations, has been variably reported. The symmetrical limb defect creates a fusiform mass that generally contains the second, third, and fourth digits at a minimum. Slightly less than one third of these patients will also have a cleft palate. Later in life, there is progressive skeletal involvement, which has been reported to involve the cervical spine.

Pfeiffer Syndrome (Fig. 9–2)

A recent addition to the category acrocephalopolysyndactyly was made in 1964 when Pfeiffer described eight members of one family with what is now "his" syndrome. Owing to the recentness of the report, statements concerning incidence are unwarranted. The male:female ratio is probably 1:1, and transmission is autosomal dominant with complete penetrance and variable expressivity. Intelligence is usually unaffected and life span should be normal, although the latter statement has only 2 decades of support at this writing.

Figure 9–1. Apert syndrome. (Reproduced by permission from Cohen MM Jr: Dysmorphic syndromes with craniofacial manifestations. *In* Stewart RE, Prescott GH [Eds.]: Oral Facial Genetics. St. Louis, 1976, The C.V. Mosby Co.)

Clinical Features. The skull is towering and wide, with "syndactyly" usually presenting in the form of unusually broad thumbs and great toes. The maxilla is hypoplastic, as is the nasal bridge, leading to relative prognathism. There may also be hypertelorism, downward slanting palpebral fissures, proptosis, and strabismus. Malocclusion and submucous cleft palate, along with low-set ears, have been associated also.

Saethre-Chotzen Syndrome (Fig. 9–3)

Saethre, in a 1931 report of three patients, followed in 1932 by Chotzen with a further three patients,

described another variant of acrocephalopolysyndactyly. The incidence of this syndrome is uncertain, with the male:female ratio probably 1:1. Transmission is autosomal dominant with a high degree of penetrance and variable expressivity. Intelligence is frequently normal and life span is presumed unaffected. Some experts contend this is a frequently misdiagnosed syndrome, either being labeled as a mild normal variant or as another of the acrocephalopolysyndactylies.

Clinical Features. The skull is usually wide and towering, with a flat forehead and low anterior hairline. Frequently the involvement is asymmetrical, causing plagiocephaly. The nasal bridge is small, while the mandible is prominent. Hypertelorism, strabismus, lacrimal duct defects, high-arched palate, and low-set ears have also been associated. Mild conductive hearing loss is common. The limb malformations are generally minimal, presenting as webbing between the second and third fingers and/or clinodactyly (medially or laterally "bent" fingers).

Carpenter Syndrome (Fig. 9–4)

In this case, history has been kind, for Carpenter's description of this syndrome in 1909 was not placed into perspective until Temtamy's observations in 1966, yet the original name remained somehow associated. This is a variant of acrocephalopolysyndactyly, of rare but uncertain incidence, transmitted in an autosomal recessive manner. The male:female ratio is probably 1:1. Mental retardation is severe. Life span is adversely affected by the occurrence of congenital heart disease; as of 1978, the oldest known patient was 25 years old.

Clinical Features. The skull is widened and towering, often to an extreme degree. This is thought to be due to premature closure of all cranial sutures, with the coronal being last to fuse. Occasionally, this

Figure 9–2. Pfeiffer syndrome. (Reproduced by permission from Goodman RM, Gorlin RJ: Atlas of the Face in Genetic Disorders. 2nd ed. St. Louis, 1977, The C.V. Mosby Co.)

Figure 9–3. Saethre-Chotzen syndrome. (From Cohen MM Jr: An etiologic and nosologic overview of craniosynostosis syndromes. *In* Bergsma D [Ed.]: Malformation Syndromes. New York, American Elsevier Publishing Co., Inc., for the National Foundation—March of Dimes, BD: OAS XI(2):137–189, 1975.)

produces a cloverleaf skull. The eyes are wide-spread and "downthrust," with a flat nasal bridge and hypoplastic mandible. The patient is often short, with a particularly short neck; weight is commonly above average. Omphalocele and atrial ventricular septal defect, pulmonary stenosis, and tetralogy of Fallot have been associated. The upper limbs are often short with webbing between the third and fourth digits. There

may be associated minor lower extremity defects as well.

Crouzon Syndrome (Fig. 9–5)

Crouzon reported, in 1912, the association of a widened towering skull with proptosis, maxillary hy-

Figure 9–4. Carpenter syndrome. (From Cohen MM Jr: An etiologic and nosologic overview of craniosynostosis syndromes. *In* Bergsma D [Ed.]: Malformation Syndromes. New York, American Elsevier Publishing Co., Inc., for the National Foundation—March of Dimes, BD:OAS XI(2):137–189, 1975.)

Figure 9–5. Crouzon syndrome. (Reproduced by permission from Cohen MM Jr: Dysmorphic syndromes with craniofacial manifestations. *In* Stewart RE, Prescott GH [Eds.]: Oral Facial Genetics. St. Louis, 1976, The C.V. Mosby Co.)

poplasia, and a beaked nose. This initial report, in both a mother and her son, is the first description of craniofacial dysostosis; subsequent descriptions have variously added and subtracted features, largely owing to the variability of the syndrome. Transmission is autosomal dominant with complete penetrance and highly variable expressivity. This latter characteristic makes statements concerning incidence somewhat suspect; additionally, about 25 percent of reported cases seem to represent fresh mutations. Life span should be normal, while mental capacity may be highly dependent on the interaction between suture closure and brain growth. Generally, intelligence is normal. The male:female ratio is 1:1.

In 1963, Stanesco reported a syndrome, found in seven members of one family, that may be a variant of Crouzon syndrome. The seven patients all presented with craniofacial features found in Crouzon syndrome, plus diaphyseal hyperplasia and small stature. Referred to as Stanesco dysostosis, or craniofacial dysostosis with diaphyseal hyperplasia, this syndrome is transmitted as autosomal dominant with nearly complete expression. The incidence is unknown.

Clinical Features. In distinction from many other forms of craniosynostosis, suture closure generally begins well after birth in Crouzon syndrome, usually becoming complete by age 2 or so. Commonly the involved sutures are the coronal and sagittal, occasionally with inclusion of the lambdoidal as well. Because of this variability, no characteristic cranial shape can be described. Brachycephaly, scaphocephaly, trigonocephaly, and even the cloverleaf skull have been reported. Hypertelorism and exophthalmos are fairly constant features, as are strabismus and nystagmus. The maxillae are hypoplastic, creating the appearance

of prognathism. The palate is often high-arched, short, and occasionally cleft, and malocclusion is common. Increased intracranial pressure may be associated with Crouzon syndrome, although this is not the norm.

Craniofacial Dyssynostosis

This syndrome was reported by Neuhauser in 1976. It is transmitted as autosomal recessive, although there is some thought that this syndrome has several different possible etiologies. The male:female ratio is 1:1 and the incidence is unknown. The majority of children are mentally retarded, perhaps secondary to elevated intracranial pressure.

Clinical Features. The skull may be long or wide and towering with occipital prominence, usually secondary to lambdoid and posterior sagittal suture closure. There may also be facial and/or cranial asymmetry. Macrocephaly and microcephaly have both been reported. The face is characterized by hypoplastic supraorbital ridges, short maxillae, and micrognathia. Ocular signs include strabismus and nystagmus. EEG recordings are often abnormal and seizures may be associated. Hydrocephalus is common, and almost all patients are of short stature. Associated congenital heart disease has been reported as well.

Craniocarpotarsal Dysplasia (Whistling Face or Freeman-Sheldon Syndrome) (Fig. 9–6)

This extraordinarily rare disorder was first reported by Freeman and Sheldon in 1938. It is transmitted as an autosomal dominant, is of unknown incidence, and

Figure 9-6. Freeman-Sheldon syndrome. (Reproduced by permission from Goodman RM, Gorlin RJ: Atlas of the Face in Genetic Disorders. 2nd ed. St. Louis, 1977, The C.V. Mosby Co.)

presents a male:female ratio of 1:1. Intelligence and life span should both be normal.

Clinical Features. The face is flat, stiff, and mask-like. The eyes are sunken; hypertelorism, strabismus, and blepharophimosis are common. The central segment of the cheeks bulge as though the patient were whistling, apparently secondary to a facial muscle defect. The mouth is frequently strikingly small and the lips pursed, often with a V-shaped fibrous tissue band at the mid-chin. Bilateral talipes equinovarus is associated, causing delay in ambulation.

Anesthetic Considerations

The unusual appearance of many children with congenital craniofacial abnormalities, in conjunction with an impressive syndrome title, can at times become the definitive statement about the patient's health. Unfortunately, when this occurs, the anesthetist is left with numerous unanswered questions about the current status of the life-support system for this strange craniofacial complex. Not only is it necessary to temporarily overlook the obvious, it is also necessary to question about the usual—children with Crouzon disease still get upper respiratory infections, for example. Only after the questions about associated defects and other diseases have been answered can the more obvious anesthetic problems of these children be addressed.

The mental and neurological status of the child must be assessed early in the planning of anesthetic treatment, based on how well the patient has met developmental milestones and current evaluations. The more severe the deformity, the more thoroughly the chart should be reviewed, if for no other reason than to facilitate the rapid development of the parents'

confidence during the interview. As well, this information allows for a thoughtful approach to premedication and induction plans. For the infant, general activity and muscle tone are primary, with lesser attention paid to intellectual progression, as it little affects initial drug selection. The older child should be premedicated based on physical status and developmental age. As a general rule all children, and perhaps these especially, look with disfavor on injection; this suggests use of oral premedicants, given 60 to 90 minutes prior to transport to the operating room.

Intracranial pressure (ICP) obviously influences the premedication and induction sequence significantly. In this group of patients, as only about one third will have normal ICP, it is probably safest to depend only on "certain" statements and discard usual assumptions. "Certain" statements are those that clearly note the presence or absence of raised ICP based on examination, while much less "certain" is the child with an unusual cranium about whom nothing has been said regarding ICP. Furthermore, beyond documented elevated ICP there is the consideration of intracranial compliance. The safe administration of drugs that cause rises in $Paco_2$ and/or cerebral blood volume depends in large measure on the assumption that the cranial vault is not only fairly accommodative, but uniformly so. A child with turricephaly may have marginally sufficient total intracranial volume to tolerate 1.3 MAC N_2O/O_2/halothane with spontaneous ventilation, yet lack the necessary room in one or more dimensions. In essence, while blood and CSF can follow the path of least resistance, the brain may not. In one series of patients with craniosynostosis, 14 percent of children with single suture involvement were found to have elevated ICP. Given this uncertainty, the most reasonable course seems to be to select premedication associated with lesser degrees of respiratory depression—for example, chloral hydrate instead of morphine—and administer more potent drugs only under personal control at induction. Finally, if drugs known to raise $Paco_2$ and/or cerebral blood volume are selected, thought must be given to emergence and the postoperative period; no matter how efficacious, hyperventilation eventually must cease, and spontaneous ventilation must resume.

Although, as stated earlier, many strange-appearing children are intellectually normal, the complete picture is that many are not. As a part of this, the ability of one mentally retarded child to defeat the efforts of a half dozen supposedly bright adults concerning elimination of preoperative oral intake is living testimony to the motivational power of hunger. In the author's experience, the probability of a full stomach rises in the environmental progression: concerned, bright parents→hospital→unconcerned, less-intelligent parents→custodial nursing facility. This situation is magnified by the number of hours awake and starved, strongly suggesting a rapid transition from A.M. awakening to the operating room.

Laboratory assessment should include hematocrit and urinalysis at the minimum, along with liver function tests for patients received from chronic institutional care. Chest x-ray and ECG are usually not needed unless indicated by the history or physical exam.

Adding up the features noted thus far presents a variably retarded child with a potential for an unusual airway, full stomach, and raised ICP. As with most such complex situations there is no "right" answer. However, one approach is oral chloral hydrate premedication, rectal barbiturates (if needed), N_2O/O_2 with spontaneous mask ventilation and controlled mask hyperventilation (with cricoid pressure) as indicated, and then halothane, until the patient is intubated and IV access is established. At this point, the stomach should be decompressed and relaxants and/or narcotic employed as desired. If the stomach proves relatively empty, the patient can be extubated at operation's end while still anesthetized, switching to mask ventilation to decrease anesthetic depth. If the stomach proves full, ventilation must continue via the endotracheal tube until drug effects are eliminated, dissipated, or reversed, at which time the patient is extubated awake.

The problem of pain control in a patient with potentially raised ICP requires caution in the use of narcotics; preferably, small incremental doses should be given IV rather than a larger dose IM. In situations where applicable, the use of regional analgesia may also provide a reasonable alternative in these patients, although narcotics may still be required for the child with defects of mentation, hearing, or vision. In conjunction with this, those responsible for care of this strange-appearing child must be given a very clear understanding of the patient's preoperative neurological status, developmental age, and any defects in sensory reception or speech. Parental visitation in the recovery room is very much a matter of local policy, but in many cases a visit by the child's mother may be more helpful as well as safer than morphine.

ACQUIRED CRANIOFACIAL DEFORMITIES

Trauma

Infants and children are highly exposed to head and neck trauma, suffering damage from falls and motor vehicle accidents like their parents, while at risk for birth injury, dog bites, and child abuse in a way their elders are not. The injuries children suffer are modified favorably by very rapid healing and highly elastic bones that are difficult to actually fracture. Unfortunately, these injuries are adversely affected by derangement of suture lines, osseous development, and tooth eruption along with an increased ease of airway obstruction from hemorrhage or aspiration. All this is without consideration of the devastating psychological impact on a child of suddenly becoming unattractive or blind

and then facing, perhaps, several attempts at surgical reconstruction.

Any attempt to consider pediatric trauma restricted along anatomical boundaries immediately runs afoul of a child's construction and the forces of physics. Children have relatively larger heads, weaker necks, and thinner and more flexible bones; the patient's smaller size makes it likely that more than the skull will be injured and that mass-velocity relationships will transfer tremendous amounts of kinetic energy to the patient. As a consequence, blunt thoracoabdominal injuries and head injuries are more likely to be coincident in children than in adults. The evaluation of this combination is very difficult and must be performed in a logical manner, without any regard to the initial training and orientation of the physician responsible. For those working in trauma centers, this is already accomplished. For those anesthetists working elsewhere, a frequently discovered principle is that each specialist perceives a human to be a mobile life support system for an organ system of interest. Neurosurgery excepted, adherence to this concept has the potential for great misadventure. Any child who presents with upper body trauma must first have established the basics of CPR. An airway must be established (while accounting for deciduous teeth), respiration assured, and circulation confirmed. Any bleeding must be stopped, followed by a rapid evaluation of the central nervous system, skull, and cervical spine. The actual incidence of spinal cord injury, with or without fracture, is low in children below age 13. The clinical evaluation is made more difficult because the majority of cases of pediatric cord trauma do *not* have associated fractures.

Next, cardiothoracic and abdominal evaluation should proceed in conjunction with a bladder catheter, and, if indicated, an intravenous pyelogram. Moving peripherally, long bone and other fractures are evaluated and soft tissue injuries dealt with. In this sequence, the head and neck are at the periphery if the CNS is considered independently. The patient who is cardiovascularly stable should be nursed head up (not reverse Trendelenburg), with the chin midline to decrease ICP and swelling. The only significance afforded to the head and neck during the first critical moments should be because: (1) blood loss from scalp and facial lacerations, even though now no longer active, may have been substantial; and (2) any evidence of a major midface fracture, although not found commonly in children, is a relative contraindication to the blind nasal passage of anything, nasogastric tubes included, lest the skull be entered.

Following this evaluation, there is often pressure to operate on the child to close lacerations and/or stabilize facial fractures. This is usually motivated by a desire to obtain a quick return to normal appearance, coupled with the knowledge that the face will rapidly swell and fractures become "sticky," making subsequent work difficult. However, before this occurs the anesthetist must ensure that the patient is stable from a neurological and cardiopulmonary standpoint. If a major cerebral concussion was sustained, the neurosurgeon must be made aware that no neurological examination will be possible for several hours during the operation. On occasion, this may prompt the insertion of a device to monitor ICP as, and while, the patient is anesthetized. Any evidence of blunt trauma to the body absolutely demands a recent postresuscitation hematocrit measurement and chest x-ray—hours-old data are insufficient. Additionally, if anterior thoracic trauma is suspected, an ECG should be obtained. The anesthetist should ensure that blood is available as needed. Finally, intravenous access must be well established and hydration accomplished, not only to insure hemodynamic stability but to allow for rapid drug administration when required.

The patient should be brought to the operating room with analgesic premedication as tolerated by CNS status. The induction process is often a matter of selecting the drugs less contraindicated by the injuries; for example, ketamine offers hemodynamic stability and analgesia, but adversely affects ICP. Whatever sequence is selected, several points are worth mentioning:

1. Suction capability must be redundant and assured—the stomach is full.

2. Mask oxygenation preinduction should be complete, timed by clock and not by guess.

3. Oral intubation is generally best, at least initially.

4. Laryngoscopy must be visually analyzed from start to finish, as loose teeth, aspiration, hemorrhage, or airway disruption may be so diagnosed.

5. The incidence of oxygenation defects after major trauma, from aspiration, pulmonary contusion, pneumothorax or hemothorax, and so forth is so high as to suggest use of >90 percent O_2 until blood gases are sampled.

A fair amount of information will be presented after induction, and requires interpretation. The response to positive-pressure ventilation often unmasks occult hypovolemia; crystalloid infusion to correct this will lower a marginal hematocrit level yet further. As well, this same ventilation may rapidly enlarge an undiagnosed pneumothorax, requiring constant reassessment of symmetrical chest movement for at least 10 to 15 minutes after intubation. For the patient brought very suddenly to operation, hypothermia is a major concern. Later in the hospital course, patients with maxillofacial trauma often develop fever, not infrequently intraoperatively.

During the major portion of the operation, the anesthetist should add to his or her usual duties the continuing reevaluation of the acute patient. Despite the heroic image associated with liver trauma, slow blood loss can occur from these injuries and this can be diagnosed intraoperatively by increased fluid requirements, falling hematocrit, and enlarging abdomen. If some aspects of a case do not make sense,

questions should be verbalized, as the pattern may be recognizable to others.

Finally, special vigilance is reserved for the airway itself. Tube malfunction, circuit disconnections, and surgical transgression of the airway can all occur, occasionally presenting as unusual one-way partial obstructions to gas exchange that are difficult to diagnose.

At the end of surgery, a full stomach and a generally swollen face are indications for leaving the patient intubated. The frequent use of intermaxillary fixation usually requires an intraoperative transition to a nasal tube, or, when the nasal complex or meninges were involved, even a tracheostomy. The latter, fortunately, eliminates the temptation to remove the tube prematurely; no matter how easy nasal intubation was initially, it will not be so straightforward to reinsert the tube in an awake patient. When the time seems eventually appropriate for extubation, any question should be assessed via direct visualization of the upper airway with a fiberoptic device. Any mechanical difficulty in tube removal requires an AP and lateral skull x-ray to rule out transfixation by wires or pins.

The patient should be nursed semi-sitting in the recovery room, supplied with humidified air/oxygen, and pain should be very carefully controlled with small incremental doses of narcotics (morphine 0.025 mg/kg). Not infrequently, these patients will have one nostril filled with nasogastric tube, while the mouth is wired shut and filled with swollen tongue. One somewhat edematous nostril leaves little margin for error in gas exchange; if respiratory difficulty ensues, a nasal airway should be gently inserted before the oral wires are hurriedly cut. This airway can be in the form of a shortened endotracheal tube that can be easily connected to an oxygen source and used to buy time to reevaluate the situation.

Burns

Burn injuries account for over 3000 deaths per year in children below age 15 years, with three times this number being disabled. Thermal and electrical burns are the second most common cause of death from age 1 to 4 years, and the third most common cause between ages 5 and 14 years. The majority of childhood burns, fortunately, are not serious and do not require inpatient therapy. Such burns are due to scalds, usually affecting the lower body, from a bathtub, or the upper body, from spilled liquids. The child is otherwise subjected to burns for the same reason as the parent, substituting curiosity for stupidity where matches and flammable liquids are concerned.

The general tendency in the care of these patients has been to refer patients with burns over a large surface area, those with more complicated burn injuries, or younger burned children to centers specializing in their care. This is appropriate management in intellectual isolation, but reality is the chance that any combination of child plus uncontrolled heat can create a critical mass demanding initial, or very late stage, anesthetic care wherever the child happens to be. This can be for anything from life-saving intubation and establishment of vascular access, to anesthesia for scar revision. The elaborate detail required to describe this full spectrum requires, and has recently received, a chapter unto itself (Ward, 1984). The following is a consolidation of pertinent facts that represents the *minimum* data base for caring for a child with damage to a portion of his or her largest organ, where the center of the injury area is occupied by multiple special senses and access to the respiratory tract.

Anesthetic Management

The preanesthetic assessment of a burned child is truly an emotionally difficult task. Even with substantial experience in an adult burn population, everyone who in any way cares for children must steel themselves for the sight of an infant or small child suffering the pain and disfigurement of a head and neck burn. As a part of this, the anesthetist must also prepare for a preanesthetic interview with parents, who often seem to possess a terribly short attention span and who oscillate between twin pillars of rage and guilt. In general, the majority of these children will have been healthy prior to the thermal insult, thus easing the interview, but the incidence of associated diseases is still high enough to deserve the usual questions. Additionally, there is a significant probability of other associated trauma compounding the burn, for which major allowances must be made in management.

Beyond the medical history of the child who *was*, obtained from the parents, there is the medical history of the child who *is*, obtained from the current chart. Preeminent in this review must be the evaluation of pulmonary function, for facial burns are often associated with significant airway damage. The awareness of everyone caring for burn patients that the upper airway may be injured is very high, and while criteria may vary from unit to unit, a request by an experienced burn surgeon to intubate a child, on admission or preoperatively, should be very seriously considered—nearly taken as mandatory, in fact. While true lung burn, steam inhalation excepted, is rare, upper airway burns are common; furthermore, the rate of edema formation after a major burn can be absolutely astounding. A straightforward, apparently unnecessary, intubation can become critical and impossible in 4 hours as normally mobile anatomy becomes swollen and woodlike. While the section on the difficult airway (see page 264) covers the appropriate strategy, an extra concern for the burn patient is tube fixation. When the face is freshly burned, adhesive tape is not useful. Later, during reconstruction, such tape may injure new grafts. The swelling that ensues after resuscitation will actually enlarge the head, so any form of circumcranial tube restraint may need to be acutely readjusted

to remain nonconstrictive. A very interesting technique to stabilize a nasal tube, reported by Galvis, is to split the tube longitudinally down to the nostril and tie umbilical tape to the resultant ends. One other answer to this is a back-and-forth suture in the nasal membranous septum, tied around the tube. While this is not the place to discuss the issue, a nasal tube seems more secure than an oral tube in these patients and is recommended as the final airway. However, their use requires an index of suspicion for otitis media and sinus infection whenever an unexplained fever occurs. Lastly, whatever tube is selected must have an airway leak, if uncuffed; if cuffed, it must be minimally inflated. Previously damaged tracheal cartilage cannot tolerate further insult.

There is a reasonable possibility that a child with burns of the head and neck, oral electrical injury excepted, will also have burns of the remainder of the upper body. These, in turn, may require escharotomy, and if anesthesia is requested for this, the anesthetist must remember to inquire about inhalation injury and carbon monoxide poisoning. The former demands anesthetic gas heat and humidification, along with arterial gas sampling; the latter suggests >90 percent O_2 if more than 10 percent carboxyhemoglobin is measured.

During the preoperative visit for these patients, obtaining excessive detail about ongoing care is nearly impossible. The airway and ventilation data must include: (1) tube size, depth of insertion (external and internal measure), leak/cuff pressure, and ease of suctioning; (2) ventilator settings with matched blood gases; and (3) chest x-ray and endoscopic evaluation of airway insult. The intake and output data must also include not just quantity, but how administered, as venous access can be very difficult. Monitoring must be noted; usually easy questions such as "where to place ECG pads" often evolve awkward answers. Drug therapy must be recorded and then reflected upon. The chronic pain and analgesic therapy these patients receive requires a readjustment in thinking, lest the anesthetist discover the selected preoperative intravenous dose of morphine is 50 percent *less* than the patient's usual increment. The author's preference is to order analgesic premedication alone, with little else, for patients in the acute phase of a burn, unless ventilation is mechanically controlled. Once the chronic phase begins, usual individual premedication practice for patients subjected to multiple painful procedures should be followed. Beware the perfectly calm child; an emotional decompensation in the operating room can be expected if he or she is treated as if the inside matched the outside.

Burned children resemble prematures in their vulnerability to cold. The operating room should be warm and draft-free when these patients arrive. A heating blanket should be on the bed, with an initial temperature set at 37°C, to be then decreased to 30 to 32°C for a prolonged case or for any situation in which the patient essentially sits semi-upright on the blanket. Although difficult to quantify exactly, the time-related potential for thermal injury to weight-bearing surfaces only requires consideration of how well the anesthetist would enjoy sitting absolutely immobile on a 37°C surface for several hours to prompt moderation in temperature settings. A heated gas humidifier is strongly recommended for all but short, late-stage reconstruction. Prolonged ventilation with cool dry gas is not appropriate therapy for an already insulted airway. The drugs selected for the anesthetic are usual in name, but not in quantity. Morphine, thiopental, and nondepolarizing relaxants should all be at least available in larger quantities. Succinylcholine should be eliminated from use in all but chronic, fully covered burns—and probably even from those, as it is potentially harmful and rarely essential. For larger surface area burns, $CaCl_2$ is very useful to have readily at hand, in a dilution such that 5 mg/kg is easy to administer as treatment for unexplained cardiovascular depression.

Monitoring again needs consideration, with an automatic blood pressure cuff or Doppler monitor nearby if the legs alone are available and an arterial catheter is not desired. Fluids should be passed through a warmer, most especially if the venous catheter tip is central. Additionally, if this is the case, flow must be evaluated early on—fluid in a 6-inch, 18-gauge central catheter flows less than half as well as in the usual 18-gauge peripheral catheter.

During induction and maintenance the anesthetist must attend to the airway problems (see page 264) while striving to stay up with fluid and thermal caloric losses. Keep very clearly in mind just how stressed these patients already are and that the skin preparation is noxious and actually begins the operation. The anesthetic should require large quantities of busy preparation, but should be designed to run on automatic pilot during the case. The author favors moderate muscle paralysis, 50 percent N_2O/O_2, low-dose volatile vapor, and morphine 0.2 to 0.5 mg/kg, all with controlled ventilation. The task then becomes vernier adjustment of anesthesia, monitoring, and intake and output control—the latter to maintain perfusion and urine output at 0.5 to 1 ml/kg/hr.

Deliberate induction of hypotension may have a place in head and neck burn surgery, provided the patient, anesthetist, monitoring, and vascular access all coincide. The entire subject is much too broad to deal with here, except for three caveats: (1) hypotension should never be a last-minute addition to the anesthetic; (2) hypovolemia and high MAC-multiple inhalation anesthesia is a terrible combination that devastates the cardiac index, and it should not be employed; and (3) positioning and anesthesia should be flawless before hypotensive pharmacology is employed.

Once the débridement has finished and grafts have been placed, the wound must be covered and the patient awakened. If the wound extends onto the chest and circumferential dressings are to be applied, it becomes all easy to impede thoracic wall and upper abdominal respiratory movement during this process. Five to 10 cm of positive end-expiratory pressure at this stage, carried through until the patient is awake and breathing well, will assist in maintaining functional residual capacity and oxygenation. Extubation, if indicated, should usually be a thoughtful process in a comfortable patient, perhaps an hour or so postoperatively, unless the surgery was minor. Striving for rapid extubation without analgesia has almost no place in the care of such chronically tormented children. In the recovery room, the anesthetic record should be reviewed thoroughly for detail. Whether the immediately preceding anesthesic was perfect or not, it represents a significant data point in the child's history and can be invaluable to those that follow. The paradigm of senseless morbidity is the same error on the same patient—occasionally by the same anesthetist. These children are much too ill for repetitive first order approximations at optimum anesthesia.

DEFORMITIES OF THE EXTERNAL EAR

The auricle serves as a gathering device. By design, it is a gathering device for sound energy, but when deformed, it becomes, by default, a gathering device for attention. Many of the adjectives applied to the deformed external ear, excepting complete agenesis, are subjective and involve terms descriptive of size and location. As such, barring interference with hearing, such defects would appear to be of concern to the patient and his or her surgeon solely because of cosmetic considerations. However, review briefly the embryology, and the possibilities for associated defects looms large. The external ear originates from the first pharyngeal, or branchial, cleft; the first pharyngeal pouch opposes the cleft and creates the eustachian tube and middle ear. The ossicles develop from the first and second branchial arch, and the entire apparatus rests along the base of the skull near the temporal bone. Potentially, then, an event affecting the external ear could equally well disrupt development in the near vicinity. In addition to malformations related by embryological continuity, external ear defects may also serve as a marker for more significant generalized abnormalities. There are therefore two general categories in which external ear defects may be placed. The first, primary ear defects, is presented in Table 9–2, along with a listing of associations, genetics, incidence, intelligence and life span predictions, and appropriate clinical features. The second category, in Table 9–3, is that of external ear abnormalities generally found in specific syndromes, although the described abnormality is by no means the primary diagnosis. Some, such as skin tags associated with Goldenhar syndrome, are visually obvious. Others,

Table 9–2. PRIMARY EXTERNAL EAR DEFECTS AND ASSOCIATIONS

Defect	Associated	Genetics	Incidence	Intelligence/ Life Span	Clinical Features
Absent tragus	Agnathia	?	?	Normal/Normal	Absent tragus
AV fistula	—	?	?	Normal/Normal	Enlarged pink or blue pulsatile auricle
Cupped ear	Pierre Robin	Autosomal dominant	?	Normal/Normal	Pinna cupped forward, ear projects laterally, usually bilateral
Ectopic pinna	Middle ear malformation	?	?	Normal/Normal	Pinna located without relation to ear canal
Echondrosis	—	Autosomal dominant	?	Normal/Normal	Cartilaginous lump on posteromedial pinna
Absent lobe	Bird-headed dwarfism	?	?	Normal/Normal	Absent ear lobe
Lobe pit	—	Autosomal dominant	?	Normal/Normal	Incomplete pit, or hole, in ear lobe
Attached lobes	—	?	High in Germany	Normal/Normal	Lower portion of ear attached to skull without free-hanging lobes
Hypertrophic lobes	Malformed incus	Autosomal dominant	?	Normal/Normal	Fibrotic large ear lobes, conductive hearing loss
Long, narrow, posteriorly rotated ears	Rubinstein-Taybi syndrome, osteogenesis imperfecta	?	?	Normal/Normal	Elongated ear, rotated backwards on skull more than 10%
Lop ear	Trisomy 21, conductive hearing loss	Autosomal dominant	1:5000	Normal/Normal	Large concha, protruding ear, floppy helix
Low-set ears	Multiple syndromes	?	?	Retardation/ Normal or reduced	Helix below line from outer canthus to occipital protuberance
Mozart ear	—	?	?	Normal/Normal	Bulging superior aspect of pinna
Ear pits	Branchial fistulas, cleft palate, spina bifida, imperforate anus, renal defects	Autosomal dominant	2:1000	Normal/Normal	Frequently draining tracts on/near helix
Prominent anthelix	Multiple syndromes and chromosome defects	?	?	Variable/Variable	Prominent anthelix, poorly formed helix
Small ear with folded-down helix	Trisomy 21, conductive hearing loss	?	?	Normal/Normal	Small ear; poorly developed, folded helix

Table 9–3. SECONDARY EXTERNAL EAR DEFECTS AND ASSOCIATIONS

Defect	Association	Defect	Association
Cauliflower ear	Diastrophic dwarfism	Large ear(s) *Continued*	Osteodysplasty
Crumpled ear	Contractural arachnodactyly		Bilateral renal agenesis
	Microtia-atresia		Trichorhinophalangeal syndrome, type II
Cup ear	Syndrome with conductive deafness	Small ear(s)	Auditory canal atresia
	Fetal trimethadione		Auriculo-osteodysplasia
Folded ear	Cranio-oculodental syndrome		C syndrome
	Syndrome with conductive deafness		Chromosome 13 trisomy syndrome
Lop ears	Anus-hand-ear syndrome		Chromosome 21 trisomy syndrome
	Chromosome 18 p− syndrome		Cranio-oculodental syndrome
	Deafness and ear pits		Craniosynostosis−radial aplasia syndrome
Preauricular fistula	Deafness and ear pits		Deafness and ear pits
	Mandibulofacial dysostosis		Hemifacial microsomia
	Oculoauriculovertebral dysplasia (Goldenhar)		Hypertelorism, microtia, facial clefting and conductive deafness
Preauricular pit	Chromosome 4 p− syndrome		Microtia-atresia
	Deafness and ear pits		Renal, genital, and middle ear anomalies
	Lip pits	Dysplastic ear(s)	Acrocephalopolysyndactyly(ies)
Preauricular tag	Chromosome 5 p− syndrome		C syndrome
	Deafness and ear pits		Cervico-oculoacoustic syndrome
	Lateral facial clefts		Chromosome 18 trisomy syndrome
	Hemifacial microsomia		Chromosome 4 p− trisomy syndrome
	Iris coloboma and anal atresia syndrome		Pierre Robin syndrome
	Limbal dermoid		Craniofacial dysostosis
	Mandibulofacial dysostosis		Craniosynostosis−radial aplasia syndrome
	Marden-Walker syndrome		Lateral facial cleft
	Microtia-atresia		Fetal warfarin syndrome
	Oculoauriculovertebral dysplasia (Goldenhar)		Limb-oto-cardiac syndrome
Large ear(s)	Auditory canal atresia		Lissencephaly syndrome
	Cerebro-oculofacial syndrome (COFS)		Mandibulofacial dysostosis
	Chromosome 8 trisomy syndrome		Median clefts of lip, mandible, and tongue
	Chromosome 18 p− syndrome		Prader-Willi syndrome
	Chromosome 13 q− syndrome		Short rib−polydactyly syndrome, Majewski type
	Chromosome 21 monosomy syndrome		Thymic agenesis
	Deafness, peripheral pulmonary stenosis, and brachytelephalangy		
	Ear AV fistula		
	Leprechaunism		
	Macrotia		

such as the association of peripheral pulmonary stenosis with large ears, are far from apparent, but nonetheless significant.

The preoperative assessment may find significant systemic disease, but this is not usually the case. What may be discovered instead is a 6-year-old who knows he or she is going to have an operation because he or she looks funny. For those unable to relate to this, the Walt Disney movie "Dumbo" is recommended. Premedication should be ordered accordingly. Otherwise, these diagnoses rarely demand special measures.

Anesthetic Management

Access to both ears is generally crucial during reparative surgery, not only for the obvious reason that defects may be bilateral, but because symmetry is so important to appearance. As a consequence, the surgeon may well request that both ears be visible and that 270° access to the head be afforded. If the former alone is desired, an endotracheal tube in line with the patient's longitudinal axis will suffice. This can be either an oral precurved tube (see Cleft Lip and Palate on page 252) or a nasal tube, again precurved if possible. If free 270° availability is needed, then the oral tube is best, leading to an anesthesia circuit that also follows the longitudinal axis. The eventual arrangement of the operating table is generally turned 90 to 180° from the traditional orientation, influenced by preference and the possible intent to take a skin graft for the ear repair.

The patient should be placed slightly head up (20°) to prevent bleeding, with little fear of air emboli unless bone is to be entered. Not infrequently, lidocaine with epinephrine is injected along the incision line for hemostasis, markedly decreasing the anesthetic requirements—until the surgeon moves to an unanesthetized area or turns the head (for epinephrine dose limits with halothane, see page 254). This situation, except for a more favorable position for ventilation, is akin to that found in a cleft palate repair. The anesthetist must watch the airway move 4 feet away and then disappear beneath drapes, all the while maintaining the patient's spontaneous ventilation prompted by minimal stimulus. Muscle paralysis is one answer to this quandary, while another is controlled ventilation alone. In either case, the troublesome period is the start of surgery, when anesthetic concentration is rising; the author generally employs controlled ventilation early on, changing to spontaneous ventilation, if possible, as the case progresses. Whatever the solution arrived at, a probably unacceptable combination is high inspired concentrations of volatile anesthetic, spontaneous ventilation, and minimal or absent surgical stimulation. The hypoventilation and myocardial depression associated with this combination can be literally deadly.

A prominent exception to this low anesthetic requirement is the harvesting of costal cartilage, usually from the eighth, ninth, and tenth ribs. Not only does this necessitate a second incision, but the area in question can never be fully immobilized to decrease pain. Additionally, this raises the possibility of pneumothorax with the attendant concerns of N_2O use thereafter.

Strangely, given the preceding warnings about diminished anesthetic requirements, small doses of narcotics (morphine 0.025 mg/kg) may be required in the recovery room for children who have undergone bilateral repairs, as they awaken functionally deaf from surgical dressings. Obviously, the requirement for analgesia will be substantially greater for the child from whom costal cartilage was harvested for the auricular repair, unless regional anesthesia is utilized prior to emergence to provide postoperative pain relief. A chest x-ray examination in the recovery room is probably worthwhile to ensure the absence of pneumothorax.

CLEFT LIP AND PALATE

This topic would seem relatively straightforward, requiring brief mention of several combinations and variations on two central themes. The realization that this anatomy has an entire medical journal devoted to it, and that the abnormality occurs in association with over 150 syndromes (accounting, however, for less than 10 percent of clefts), exclusive of the Pierre Robin anomalad, points out the spectrum of the malformations. A good bit of this interest is due to a combination of two features: (1) surgically reparable defects in appearance and speech, and (2) frequency. Cleft lip and palate occur at a rate of about 1.5 per 1000 live births, with isolated cleft lip, or cleft palate, occurring about one third as often. Complicating these statements, however, is the realization that while cleft lip is almost invariably reported by birth certificate, cleft palate often is not; indeed, estimates of under-reporting are as high as 60 percent. The left:right:bilateral relationship is about 6:3:1. There is a male excess in cleft lip and palate, with a female excess in isolated

cleft palate. Intelligence and life span should both be normal, although an estimated 10 to 20 percent of infants do not survive the first year of life, usually owing to associated other defects, especially congenital heart disease.

Clinical Features

Much of the distinction between cleft lip and cleft palate is based on an arcane landmark, the incisive foramen, and a missing word—secondary. Cleft *lip* usually refers to a pre–incisive foramen defect that may be anything from a minor incomplete skin cleft to a complete interruption of skin, gum, alveolar ridge, and primary palate. Cleft *palate* actually refers to a cleft secondary post–incisive foramen palate. Bilateral cleft lip usually involves both primary and secondary palate, but may involve only the primary. As a consequence of all this, the diagnosis of cleft lip may refer to a highly variable spectrum of defects, while cleft palate may not be apparent in any way until the patient's mouth is opened. Indeed, some forms of palate defects may not be obvious even then. In addition to the cosmetic defects, however, cleft lip may present major impediments to the development of normal dentition, while cleft palate may cause velopharyngeal incompetence with resultant hypernasality of speech. Cleft palate may also present feeding problems in infancy, as the normal separation between food and air is absent, creating a nonphysiologic mixing chamber in the nasopharynx. Not infrequently, this is associated with chronic rhinorrhea that must be distinguished preoperatively from infection.

Beyond the familiar clefts of the lip and palate, there is also a range of much rarer midline, median, and lateral facial clefts. These occur in an incidence of 1 to 4 percent of all clefts. Several classification schemes have been proposed to make sense of these unusual defects, with none being totally satisfactory. Their rarity and variability defy general statements, although in all such cases, a thorough search should be made for other associated abnormalities. A number of these rarer defects would seem to pose significant difficulties to airway management by mask; intubation does not appear so formidable, as almost all these malformations affect only the mid-face.

Although clefts of the lip and palate appear to be in anatomical continuity, it seems fairly clear that isolated cleft palate is somewhat unique. While the incidence of simultaneously occurring additional abnormalities varies from series to series, isolated cleft palate almost invariably has twice the percentage of such associations when compared with isolated cleft lip or cleft lip with cleft palate. The most common non–syndrome related abnormalities found in association with any of these clefts are umbilical hernia, clubfoot, and limb and ear deformities; the most common syndromes are Klippel-Feil and the Pierre Robin anomalad. The incidence of congenital heart disease is fairly low in surgical series; however, this is because a large number of infants younger than 6 months with severe cardiac malformations are too ill, or have not survived, to enter such series. Among such infants, 66 percent have severe heart disease, while less than 2 percent of infants older than 6 months do so. There is also an increased incidence of cervical spine abnormalities in cleft palate patients, although these generally do not become symptomatic in children.

Anesthetic Management

Repair of an isolated cleft lip will usually take place between the ages of 3 months and 6 months, while repair of cleft secondary palate is delayed until age 12 months or more so that growth can occur and ease the technical problems of the procedure. Preoperative assessment is typical for a child of this age, modified by the presence of additional defects. Intraoperative blood transfusion can be anticipated very rarely for lip repairs, uncommonly for palate repairs, and occasionally for pharyngoplasty. For any of these procedures, the patient should be brought to the operating room unpremedicated, excepting atropine 0.01 to 0.02 mg/kg, given 30 minutes or less prior to, or coincident with, induction. The operating room should be warm (25°C) and draft-free, with a heating blanket (37°C) placed on the table. Induction is usually uneventful, utilizing N_2O/O_2/halothane and spontaneous ventilation, although a large palate defect may require placement of an oral airway fairly early on. Laryngoscopy in a patient with a cleft lip is generally straightforward, but a cleft palate has the capability to trap and immobilize a straight blade, occasionally in a subtle fashion that befuddles an endoscopist unaware of the possibility. Should this occur, the anesthetist must first recognize the lateral immobility of the laryngoscope for what it is (this requires some thought, for the problem area is not always in direct view) and then consider inserting a gauze pack or dental roll in the cleft prior to the next attempt to visualize the vocal cords. Some anesthetists feel that specific laryngoscope blades such as the Robertshaw or Oxford infant blades (Fig. 9–7), are especially useful in this setting.

The endotracheal tube itself is chosen for internal diameter (ID), according to age; in children older than 12 months, this can be determined by using the formula:

$$\frac{16 + \text{age in years}}{4} = \text{ID in mm}$$

While some prefer a straight tube with a curved 15-mm connector, most anesthetists now select a precurved tube for lip and/or palate surgery. Insertion of such a precurved tube is somewhat easier with a stylet, and use of a stylet is recommended. To achieve a cosmetic repair, symmetry is essential, so the tube should exit the mouth in the midline without facial distortion from either the tube itself or the securing tape. As this tape will disappear beneath the surgical drapes, the use of a cutaneous adhesive, such as

Figure 9–7. Blades for laryngoscopy. *A,* Robertshaw blade. *B,* Oxford infant blade. *C,* Seward blade. (Courtesy of Penlon USA, Division of Bear Medical Systems, Inc., Riverside, CA.)

benzoin, is recommended to ensure adherence. It may be necessary to suture the tube to the lower gum in some circumstances.

Adhesive tape for precurved tube stabilization should be applied in two layers. The first layer crosses the straight external tube extension parallel to the lower lip and fixes the tube laterally. However, if narrow tape is used for this purpose (most often the case), the tube can still pivot or rotate. Consequently, a second piece of tape should be placed further distal on the tube extension, with divided ends extending to the face over the right and left mandibular rami. This layer effectively restricts longitudinal and axial motion. Following tube fixation, stomach decompression with an in-and-out orogastric tube is recommended. After this step, bilateral chest ventilation should be assured with the patient in essentially the position required for the surgery. For a cleft lip, this is fairly neutral, but for a cleft palate, moderately extreme cervical extension is required. Next, a pharyngeal pack of moistened ribbon gauze is inserted for cleft lip repairs; cleft palate surgery requires a tongue gag, and this cannot be placed correctly if the pack is in place. Once the gag has been inserted into a cleft palate patient, the surgeon can insert a pharyngeal pack, if it does not interfere with the surgical anatomy. Following gag and pack insertion, ventilation should be reassessed, as tube compression may have occurred. If a pack is used, consider writing the word "pack" on a piece of tape applied to the anesthesia machine or the patient's forehead, as a reminder at the end of surgery. Sterile ointment should be placed in both eyes; the application of tape to close the eyelids is according to surgical preference. If not already placed, secondary monitors (temperature, ECG, BP) should be applied and intravenous access established. The latter should be selected for cleft palate patients with the distinct possibility that blood transfusion might be required, especially if a pharyngeal flap is planned.

The patient can now be positioned for surgery. The top of the infant's skull should be as near the head of the table as possible. For the cleft lip patient, this is generally sufficient, but the cleft palate patient frequently requires exaggerated neck hyperextension with a 15° Trendelenburg tilt that, following 90 to 180° table rotation, nearly places the patient's head in the surgeon's lap. In either situation, a low metal screen can sometimes be mounted on the table with the horizontal bar a few cm over the patient's abdomen, serving to support the surgical drapes free of the infant's thorax.

Following positioning and surgical preparation, the drapes are applied. If the patient's temperature has not fallen below 36°C, external heating devices should be turned off at this point, as hyperthermia is easily achieved when all but 5 percent or so of the patient's surface area is covered. If the temperature has fallen substantially, warming should continue until 36°C is reached. In any case, the room can now be cooled, as the patient is environmentally isolated.

Occasionally in cleft lip repair, and always in cleft palate repair, lidocaine with epinephrine is injected early on. The volume is small, to prevent anatomical distortion, but nevertheless raises the recurrent question of "How much epinephrine is allowed?" In general, children seem less susceptible to dysrhythmias than adults, although the reasons for this are not clear. The most specific and aggressive recommendations are those of Karl and associates, who suggest a maximum epinephrine dose of 10 µg/kg through a wide range of end-tidal halothane concentrations—in *normocarbic children*. This should be placed in the context of a 1-year-old infant, covered in layers of surgical drapes, positioned head down and breathing through a convoluted, long, high-resistance tube. The decision to utilize a spontaneous or controlled ventilation technique involves a number of considerations, but the obstacles to adequate spontaneous alveolar ventilation, for the cleft palate patient to a major degree, and the cleft lip patient somewhat less, are substantial. Clearly, if a dysrhythmia does occur following epinephrine injection, one available option is to assure normocarbia via controlled ventilation. A further consideration following this injection of local anesthesia is the elimination of some, or all, of the surgical stimulus to the patient. Failure to adjust inspired anesthetic concentration in response to this can lead to a relative overdose.

At the conclusion of the procedure, extubation should occur only when the patient is fully awake. Any other decision raises the specter of postextubation

airway problems in which oral and nasal airways, and perhaps even masks, threaten the surgical repair. Many anesthetists make it a practice to remove any pharyngeal packs under direct vision while the patient is still anesthetized, to ensure an airway free of blood at the time of tube removal.

To prevent the infant from disrupting the repair, patient arm restraints are utilized; these may interfere with the function of upper extremity intravenous infusions as well as requiring blood pressure to be measured in the legs rather than the arms. Before the patient is left in the recovery room, the anesthetist must ensure that the flow of intravenous infusions can be maintained and that blood pressure can be monitored.

Pain therapy in the infant is a matter of some discussion. Options available vary from mother's comfort and oral intake to small doses of narcotics. If the parents are prepared for the postoperative appearance of their infant, their presence may be quite beneficial. If narcotics are felt needed, a suggested increment is morphine 0.025 mg/kg intravenously repeated no more frequently than every 10 minutes, to a total dose not to exceed 0.1 mg/kg. The author's habit is to write no repeat orders for any patient after pharyngoplasty, but instead to reevaluate personally from time to time, as these patients are at some risk postoperatively from airway obstruction.

If possible, these infants should be nursed slightly head up in the postoperative period to decrease edema formation. A variety of so-called infant seats can be employed to accomplish this.

BRANCHIAL ARCH DEFECTS

The clarity of this embryologically based title belies the facts, or at least the facts as different specialists perceive them. For example, one dysmorphology text presents a syndrome of high-arched palate, beak nose, micrognathia, zygomatic hypoplasia, antimongoloid palpebral fissures, broad thumbs, and broad great toes—the Rubinstein-Taybi syndrome—as one of the most important first arch syndromes. Another similar text places this syndrome in a separate classification, while a plastic surgery text doesn't mention the syndrome at all. At the outset, then, there appears to be not only confusion about what belongs in this classification but also whether, indeed, more than one syndrome "qualifies." The *Birth Defects Compendium* applies this primary title of first (and second) branchial arch syndrome to hemi(cranio)facial microsomia. The following discussion follows this convention.

Hemifacial Microsomia (Fig. 9–8)

Also known as otomandibular dysostosis, this syndrome was apparently described as early as 2000 B.C. By 1845, it was recognized that the structures involved

Figure 9–8. Hemifacial microsomia. (Reproduced by permission from Cohen MM Jr: Dysmorphic syndromes with craniofacial manifestations *In* Stewart RE, Prescott GH [Eds.]: Oral Facial Genetics. St. Louis, 1976, The C.V. Mosby Co.)

were primarily derived from the first and second branchial arches, including the intervening first cleft. Providing a reasonable estimate of incidence is made difficult by yet another disagreement over terminology—in this case, whether or not this syndrome can cause *bilateral* deformity. However, as the supposed incidence of bilateral disease is only about 10 to 12 percent, it has little impact on an estimated incidence of 1 in 4000 to 6000 live births. As will be apparent from the description of the unilateral version, a bilateral presentation seems barely distinguishable from the Treacher Collins syndrome, except possibly by genetics. The male:female ratio has been variably reported at 1:1 or 2:1. The etiology is unknown. The patient's intelligence and life span should not generally be affected.

Clinical Features. The minimal diagnostic criteria are unilateral ear abnormalities and unilateral hypoplasia of the mandibular condyle and ramus. The ear abnormalities may vary from absence of the external ear to mild prominence of the auricle. Mandibular hypoplasia may virtually eliminate the ramus, causing the body of the mandible to curve up and join the condyle. The chin is generally deviated toward the affected side. Malocclusion and late tooth eruption occur frequently. The muscles of mastication, especially the lateral pterygoid, are impaired in some of these patients. This can limit the patient's ability to move the mandible, either forward or laterally, and when the mandible is externally depressed, the unaffected side may nearly dislocate downward and laterally, while the affected condyle barely moves. Abnormalities of the eye and eyelid have been reported, including deviated palpebral fissure and choroid coloboma, along with strabismus. Pulmonary hypoplasia on the affected side has been noted as well. Agenesis

of a portion of the facial nerve is the most common CNS defect noted, but any cranial nerve can be affected. Hearing loss on the affected side may obviously be associated; usually this is of a conductive type and is due to the canal abnormalities.

Oculoauriculovertebral Dysplasia (Goldenhar Syndrome) (Fig. 9–9)

In 1952, Goldenhar described in detail a syndrome of preauricular appendages and fistulas, associated with mandibulofacial dysostosis. Since that time, slightly

Figure 9–9. Goldenhar syndrome. (Reproduced by permission from Goodman RM, Gorlin RJ: Atlas of the Face in Genetic Disorders. 2nd ed. St. Louis, 1977, The C.V. Mosby Co.)

more than 110 cases have been reported, extending the clinical presentation widely. The incidence is uncertain, as are the genetics. The male:female ratio is 1:1; life span and intelligence are both usually normal. This syndrome is currently thought to be a variation of the first (and second) branchial arch syndrome.

Clinical Features. There is no universally accepted constellation of features. Eye abnormalities include epibulbar dermoids, extraocular muscle defects, and coloboma. Auricular defects include external ear abnormalities, skin tags, and hearing loss. Rather more interesting from the anesthetist's view is micrognathia, unilateral mandibular hypoplasia, and cleft palate, in association with a 40 percent incidence of vertebral abnormalities and a 35 percent incidence of congenital heart disease. The former association frequently involves the upper neck, with vertebral fusion and odontoid elongation being noteworthy. The cardiac defects include septal defects and tetralogy of Fallot.

Increasingly, the term facioauriculovertebral anomalad has been applied to both this and hemifacial microsomia owing to increasing clinical experience that suggests a continuum rather than a separation.

Mandibulofacial Dysostosis (Berry Syndrome; Treacher Collins Syndrome; Franceschetti-Zwahlen-Klein Syndrome)

Simply based on the number of names involved, the struggle involved in classifying this constellation of defects can be easily surmised. Berry, an ophthalmologist, reported several family members with lower lid coloboma, and Treacher Collins subsequently reported an 8-year-old child who also had malar hypoplasia. Finally, Franceschetti and colleagues pointed out the associated ear and mandibular deformities and emphasized that the minimal manifestation of the syndrome may only be downward-slanting palpebral fissures and lid coloboma. As well, these latter authors subdivided the syndrome into five categories: complete, incomplete, unilateral, abortive, and atypical. The so-called unilateral form is probably actually hemi(cranio)facial microsomia and will not be further considered here. The incidence is approximately 1 in 8000 to 10,000 live births, and over 200 cases have been reported. The syndrome is transmitted as autosomal dominant with high penetrance and highly variable expressivity.

Patients with this syndrome do not generally suffer intellectual impairment, except as a function of hearing loss. However, those patients with pronounced facial maldevelopment in conjunction with such hearing loss may suffer enormously from being perceived as retarded. The prognosis for a normal life span is excellent, provided the patient survives infancy. Unfortunately, a number of children suffer fatal respiratory complications during the first few months of life.

Clinical Features. The complete form includes downward-slanting palpebral fissures, notching or coloboma of the lower eyelid, hypoplasia of facial bones (especially the zygoma and mandible), malformation of the ear (external, middle, and occasionally inner), macrostomia with high palate and abnormal dentition, blind fistulas between the ear and the angle of the mouth, and patchy projections of hair from the sideburns onto the cheeks. Very commonly, the palate may be cleft, as well. As a matter of interest, Tessier, in presenting a new classification of craniofacial clefts in 1973, felt that the entire syndrome could be explained by a combination of three different clefts (numbers 6, 7, and 8 in his system). While a decade is insufficient time to establish this concept, it may provide an attractive unification of the syndrome presentations.

The incomplete form usually presents with lesser degree of deformity, frequently with associated deafness. This presentation is probably the original Treacher Collins syndrome. The abortive form involves only the eyes, while the atypical type consists of defects, partly typical and partly quite unusual, such as microphthalmos and temporomandibular joint dysfunction. The inclusion of cases into this category is often subject to debate.

The incomplete form, or Treacher Collins syndrome (Fig. 9–10), has received a rather large amount of attention considering its rarity. Externally, many children with Treacher Collins syndrome somewhat resemble those with Pierre Robin anomalad, suggesting upper airway obstruction from similar causes—glossoptosis and micrognathia. However, several investigators have examined children with Treacher Collins syndrome in some detail and have discovered a slightly more complex situation. Utilizing multiview video-

Figure 9–10. Treacher Collins syndrome. (Reproduced by permission from Goodman RM, Gorlin RJ: Atlas of the Face in Genetic Disorders. 2nd ed. St. Louis, 1977, The C.V. Mosby Co.)

fluoroscopy and fiberoptic nasopharyngoscopy, patients with Treacher Collins syndrome were compared with normal controls and with a group of patients with isolated cleft palate. It was clearly demonstrated that every patient with Treacher Collins syndrome had pronounced narrowing of the pharynx in the lateral dimension, usually at the tongue base. This was associated with some anteroposterior narrowing as well, markedly reducing the cross-sectional area of the airway at a point well above the larynx. To put this finding into perspective, the mean pharyngeal width reported for controls was 32 mm, while patients with the Treacher Collins syndrome were reported to have a mean width of 14 mm—including one 11-year-old with a lateral measurement of only 5 mm. To worsen the situation, the correlation between the visible penetrance of the syndrome and pharyngeal hypoplasia was adjudged poor, so that predicting an excessively narrow airway from the patient's appearance was improbable. Interestingly, despite the fact that 80 percent of the patients in this report with Treacher Collins syndrome also had cleft palates, those patients with isolated cleft palate possessed increased lateral pharyngeal dimensions—mean width 36 mm—emphasizing that similar features do not create identical situations. However, it is worth considering the implications of cleft palate and Treacher Collins syndrome, for if such a patient speaks with a nasal quality, the traditional approach might be to correct velopharyngeal incompetence with a pharyngoplasty. In at least one reported Treacher Collins patient, this produced a subsequent sleep apnea syndrome; this demonstrates that despite the multifactorial requirements currently thought necessary to develop sleep apnea, a major contribution from any one sector can precipitate the syndrome. (For further considerations, see the following discussion of Pierre Robin Anomalad, and Chronic Airway Obstruction, page 263.)

Two questions are immediately generated from this progression. First, does this pharyngeal hypoplasia occur in the other forms of mandibulofacial dysostosis? Second, how many other syndromes primarily manifested in maldevelopment of the first and second branchial arch might involve airway constriction? At the moment, both await further data.

Pierre Robin Anomalad (Fig. 9–11)

Micrognathia and glossoptosis (tongue falling backward), often in association with a cleft palate, compose this assemblage, which is more correctly called an anomalad, or group of anomalies. It was undoubtedly known prior to Pierre Robin's 1923 paper, but he does deserve credit for drawing attention to the clinical significance of the association. (In further writings Robin developed the significance of this combination to the point he felt that it was present in 60 percent of children and caused, among other things, flat feet.) The anomalad may occur in isolation in about 1 in

Figure 9–11. Pierre Robin anomalad. (Reproduced by permission from Goodman RM, Gorlin RJ: Atlas of the Face in Genetic Disorders. 2nd ed. St. Louis, 1977, The C.V. Mosby Co.)

30,000 live births or as a part of other syndromes, especially the campomelic syndrome, the cerebrocostomandibular syndrome, the persistent left superior vena cava syndrome, and Stickler syndrome. The etiology is uncertain, although intrauterine malposition and pressure are frequently mentioned. While this initially seems a simplistic explanation, alternatives are not clearly available, as the structures involved develop at different times and from different sources. The male:female distribution is 1:1. The patient's intelligence and life span are normal, except in cases involving significant airway compromise and associated other defects. Unfortunately, 60 percent of patients have such other defects, largely accounting for the associated mortality of 20 to 25 percent.

Clinical Features. The essential features of the anomalad are micrognathia and glossoptosis. Cleft palate is almost an invariable addition; the defect is usually U-shaped, thought secondary to tongue interference with palatal fusion. Twenty-five percent of cases are associated with known syndromes, while 36 percent of patients have other defects, most frequently cardiac, not associated with identified syndromes.

These infants can present major problems almost immediately after delivery. It is actually difficult to imagine upper airway anatomy more vexing than in this anomalad. In pronounced cases, the nasopharynx will fill with tongue (via the cleft palate) whenever the baby is supine, causing total airway occlusion, with the generation of negative respiratory pressures of up to 60 mmHg serving only to aggravate the posterior tongue displacement. The baby may frequently try to maintain its airway by constant struggling and crying, only to suffer obstruction very abruptly when exhausted. Prodigious amounts of nursing attention, prone positioning, and extraordinary care in feeding may buy time during which the tongue-mandible relationship may improve or, alternatively, time in which the infant improves tongue musculature control.

When traditional medical means have been inadequate, traditional surgical measures have usually been employed. Such measures include suturing the tongue anteriorly in one of several methods (including permanent glossopexy) or passing a Kirschner wire anterior to the mandibular angles and transfixing the tongue.

Two unusual other management techniques have recently been employed with these babies. One is to nurse the baby prone with the skull suspended by a traction cap. The other concept, very comfortable to anesthetists, is to use an 8- to 9-cm long, 3- to 3.5-mm I.D. endotracheal tube as a nasopharyngeal airway. This latter technique has been evaluated in some detail, and with appropriate nursing care it appears to have substantial merit.

Chronic upper airway obstruction represents a constant threat to these unfortunate infants in two ways. First, prolonged hypoventilation and marginal oxygenation may cause pulmonary artery hypertension and cor pulmonale. This clinical situation has been associated with an increased incidence of pulmonary edema, which was originally thought to be due to changes in central blood volume and intrapleural pressure but, in view of current research on right-left ventricular interaction, may also be partly due to interventricular septal shift secondary to chronic right ventricular overload. Associated with this cardiopul-monary dysfunction may well be failure to thrive subsequent to feeding difficulties and to a two- to threefold increase in the work of breathing. The second threat is abrupt respiratory failure, superimposed on chronic disease, due to exhaustion, aspiration, or infection, all of which are common.

With time, usually a few months, infants with this anomalad generally, but not always, "improve" such that the airway is less perilous. However, cleft palate repair involving the use of a pharyngeal flap may recreate the neonatal situation of airway compromise. This particular sequence has recently been implicated in the postoperative demise of a child.

The preceding discussion sets the basis for considerations of elective tracheostomy in these children, with full recognition that decannulation may require months. While this may be viewed as somewhat archaic in this advanced age of oral and nasal plastics, note well the duration and severity of the pathology before rejecting a permanent artificial airway. As will be discussed on page 264, supraglottic intubation of a child with a severe form of this syndrome may simply prove impossible, leaving no other option.

Oculomandibulofacial Syndrome (Hallermann-Streiff) (Fig. 9–12)

As is often the case, history has been unkind, for this syndrome was probably first described by C. Audry in 1893. Hallermann and Streiff, independently, further clarified the components of the syndrome and pointed out the ophthalmological aspects, thus gaining lasting recognition. Although this syndrome has constant manifestations that extend well beyond the head and neck, it is included in discussion here because the anatomical description seems to warrant it.

This syndrome is very rare, with somewhat more

Figure 9–12. Hallermann-Streiff syndrome. (Reproduced by permission from Cohen MM Jr: Dysmorphic syndromes with craniofacial manifestations. *In* Stewart RE, Prescott GH [Eds.]: Oral Facial Genetics. St. Louis, 1976, The C.V. Mosby Co.)

than 50 cases in the literature. The male:female ratio is 1:1, with the mode of genetic transmission unknown. In theory, life span should be normal, but the impact of lower facial malformation has led to death in childhood, usually directly linked to recurrent respiratory infections and feeding problems. Intelligence should be normal, although the effect on development of strange facies, possibly diminished hearing, and probably decreased vision may be profound.

Clinical Features. Proportionate dwarfism is almost invariably present, along with diminished scalp and body hair. The skull is often wide, occasionally with macrocephaly and lambdoid suture dehiscence, although microcephaly has also been reported. Ophthalmological defects include microphthalmia, downward-slanting palpebral fissures, blue sclerae, congenital cataracts (which, strangely, may spontaneously resorb), nystagmus, strabismus, and decreased visual acuity. The face usually appears small, with a narrow beaked nose, that generates an impression of a "birdlike" face. Malar bone hypoplasia may be present, while micrognathia and mandibular hypoplasia are almost invariably so. Interestingly, the entire temporomandibular joint may be displaced up to 2 cm forward. The palate has a high arch, while dentition is disturbed, allowing for severe malocclusion, absent teeth, extra teeth, and persistent deciduous teeth. Deafness is occasionally noted, as are general skeletal problems such as lordosis, scoliosis, and spina bifida. The scalp veins are often noted to be prominent, generally secondary to cutaneous atrophy, not to hydrocephalus.

Anesthetic Management

In general, hemifacial microsomia, oculoauriculovertebral dysplasia, mandibulofacial dysostosis, Pierre Robin anomalad, and oculomandibulofacial syndrome all present to the anesthetist the dual challenge of the difficult airway and difficult intubation, compounded by other assorted systemic defects. The airway constraints are very real and, despite the progression described in the section on Management of the Difficult Pediatric Airway and Intubation (see page 264), can defeat a very skilled anesthetist on any given day.

Hemifacial microsomia, strictly speaking, is unilateral and the unaffected side may represent a point of attack, especially for lateral laryngoscope insertion. The three-dimensional asymmetry can be expected to make fitting a mask very difficult.

Oculoauriculovertebral dysplasia poses the very tough combination of cervical spine abnormalities, including odontoid elongation, with micrognathia. Not only can this serve to make mask fit and intubation difficult, the possibility of actual cord trauma exists. Compounded with congenital heart disease, especially a tetralogy, this can set the stage for disaster. Airway management is often extremely difficult in affected children, and the capability to add tracheostomy rap-

idly to the scheduled procedure is a must. The concept of a continuum of facioauriculovertebral anomalad suggests that the anesthetic considerations applying to the entire continuum should be kept in mind in managing patients with oculoauriculovertebral dysplasia or hemifacial microsomia.

Mandibulofacial dysostosis is highly variable in appearance and difficulty. The detailed description of Treacher Collins syndrome should probably be assumed to apply to all variations until proved otherwise. The very narrow posterior upper airway should be kept in mind during laryngoscopy, as distortion of this plane, at this location, could adversely affect blade mobility and tube passage.

Pierre Robin anomalad is the best known of these very difficult airways. Difficulty here is related to a large palate defect, other systemic abnormalities, and micrognathia. These infants, too, may require tracheostomy because intubation cannot be accomplished by the outlined measures. However, with Pierre Robin anomalad and all these syndromes, it is worth considering a request for help from the best pediatric fiberoptic endoscopist available if personal expertise is not up to the task.

Oculomandibulofacial syndrome presents a risk for obstructive sleep apnea and a difficult airway with difficult intubation. The occasional displacement of the temporomandibular joint is difficult to assess, as it might possibly diminish problems. By no means, however, should this be counted on, as clinical experience is minimal. The isolated case report of anesthesia for a patient with this syndrome commented on micrognathia, fragile teeth, and temporomandibular joint restrictions, along with diminished nostril size, as potential problems. In point of fact, the actual management of this case involved awake direct laryngoscopy and oral intubation without much difficulty. The patient was, however, an adult; management would probably have been more difficult for a child.

All of the children should be carefully assessed postoperatively and extubated awake. Near-prone positioning may help the patient to sustain a natural airway, and humidified oxygen should be supplied after extubation. Serious thought should be given to staffing patterns in the recovery room. If continuous one-on-one coverage with an experienced nurse who is comfortable with children is not the plan, then the plan must be rearranged or the anesthetist must stay close at hand. To have one of these patients get into difficulty in the immediate postoperative period, after all the anxiety and effort in the operating room, is truly to snatch defeat from the jaws of victory.

BRANCHIAL CYSTS AND FISTULAS

Despite the brief and seemingly straightforward opening discussion of branchial cleft embryology, uniform agreement as to the true origin of these cysts and fistulas has yet to be achieved. The most generally accepted theory is that presented in the initial review of embryology, and for discussion purposes, this will be accepted here. From the management standpoint, however, it is worthwhile to note that some authors feel the cysts are of a different origin than the fistulas and will therefore refer to these lesions as cervical cysts instead. By themselves, neither cysts nor fistulas generally impact on the patient's life span, intelligence, or well being. A rare exception to this is a case of malignant degeneration in a cyst or fistula late in life.

Clinical Features

These lesions may present at any age, are more common in males, and are generally unilateral. Cysts outnumber fistulas about three to one. A confusing entity in this area is the very common preauricular sinus, which may be associated with other defects but generally exists independently. This type of sinus presents as a dimple anterior to the tragus and usually ends in a blind pouch against the superior conchal fossa. Unless inflamed, such a sinus usually requires little medical attention.

A first branchial cleft cyst or fistula is found entirely above the hyoid bone, communicates with the external auditory canal, and can be easily confused with a parotid tumor. The primary significance of these lesions, like parotid tumors, is their proximity to the facial nerve. A more common sinus or fistula originates from the second branchial cleft. They may appear externally anywhere along the anterior border of the lower two thirds of the sternocleidomastoid muscle, generally most often at the junction of the lower and middle third. About 50 percent of these particular cleft defects will have a fistula with origins in the tonsillar fossa, traversing between the internal and external carotid arteries and presenting at the skin. The third branchial cleft opens externally at about the same location as the second, but presents internally at the pyriform sinus after traveling down the sheath of the common carotid, deep to the internal carotid artery. Cysts or fistulas of the fourth cleft are theoretically possible but are reported rarely; they should pass from upper esophagus to mediastinum.

Anesthetic Management

The symptoms presented by these cysts or fistulas are generally only cosmetic, although the possibility of infection and prior attempts at removal may certainly be part of the patient's history. Preoperative assessment and preparation are unremarkable for this diagnosis.

The patient will eventually be positioned with the neck extended and the head rotated away from the lesion. There exists some possibility that intraoral manipulation will be required, suggesting a contralateral nasal tube as a final airway. If a nasal tube is chosen, the precurved variety provides for a low profile as well as minimizing dead space. Recommendations

for passing a nasal tube are found in the section on the Difficult Pediatric Airway (see pages 266 and 267). During the actual procedure, the patient should be positioned slightly (20°) head up (not, however, in the reverse Trendelenburg position) to decrease bleeding. Overaggressiveness in elevating the head also raises the possibility of air emboli; this should be avoided unless the position is felt to be so beneficial that all the measures associated with a sitting craniotomy are also taken. For procedures on first cleft defects, the proximity of the facial nerve suggests minimal use of long-acting relaxants, particularly if a nerve stimulator is included on the sterile field. Defects of the lower clefts involve dissection around the carotid artery with the attendant problem of bradycardia; after hypoxia has been eliminated as a cause, such heart rate changes may require atropine therapy.

Following an excision of a first cleft lesion, extubation can usually be performed immediately. Procedures for second and third cleft defects may involve substantially more paratracheal dissection, with the possibility of attendant cervical swelling, and this suggests awake extubation. In either case, the patient should be nursed semi-sitting in the postoperative period to minimize swelling.

CYSTIC HYGROMA

Adolph Wernher published a monograph in 1843 concerning one variety of what is today called a lymphangioma. Wernher described the gross pathology of these lesions; pointed out that while they are common in the neck, they may occur elsewhere (as in the abdomen); and applied the clinically established but nonspecific term cystic hygroma. It remained for a number of pathologists to establish the lymphatic origin of these lesions, and even today there is controversy concerning their true nature. The current leading hypothesis is that cystic hygromas are the result of congenital dysplasia of lymphatics, although the possibility still exists that hamartoma or true neoplasm may be a more applicable classification.

Lymphangioma may be classified into one of three general categories: (1) simplex, made up of small lymphatics, usually confined to skin or mucous membranes; (2) cavernous, made up of larger lymphatics, with deep diffuse extension; and (3) cystic, or cystic hygroma, involving multilobular, multilocular collections of small cysts filled with clear, yellow-tinged or bloody fluid. None of these presentations are considered common.

Clinical Features

Cystic hygroma most often occurs in the neck (60 to 70 percent), generally in the posterior triangle, although occasionally a cyst will communicate beneath the clavicle with a hygroma in the axilla, the next most common location (20 percent). Less frequently, a hygroma will appear in the anterior triangle, generally high up, and will then be associated with intraoral lymphangiomas. This presentation is the one most often associated with airway compromise, occasionally compounded by mediastinal extension of the hygroma. This latter possibility strongly suggests radiological evaluation of the chest in all infants with a diagnosis of cystic hygroma.

The usual history of these lesions is presentation at birth or shortly thereafter, often with subsequent alarmingly rapid enlargement. Infection is certainly possible, while spontaneous regression is doubtful. Simple incision and drainage leads to chronic fluid loss, while decompression of the cyst, or cysts, pre- or intraoperatively has been described as a major impediment to complete cure—being then, in turn, partly responsible for the 10 to 25 percent recurrence rate of hygromas. The word "recurrence" requires some elaboration, for on occasion these cysts have refilled, with either clear fluid or blood, in periods of only a few days.

Anesthetic Management

First and foremost, it is necessary for the anesthetist to have a clear picture of the limits of the disease. In general, these lesions are tolerated amazingly well by the infants, but any history vaguely suggestive of respiratory problems, feeding difficulties, or even cough should be pursued to discover possible intraoral or mediastinal disease. The presence of cysts in the visible oral cavity may warn of extension into the supraglottic area, while mediastinal compression may require endotracheal tube insertion to, or perhaps beyond, the carina. While such preoperative assessment must be thorough, it should not be tardy, for the possibility that the cysts will enlarge is quite real, thus making a known difficult situation into an unknown worse one.

The patient should be brought to the operating room unpremedicated except for atropine, given 30 minutes or less prior to, or coincident with, induction. For a neonate, an awake intubation with continuous oxygen insufflation may be preferred. For the older infant, a spontaneous ventilation N_2O/O_2/halothane mask induction allows for gradual assumption of the airway and upon demonstration of bilateral chest expansion without gastric distention during a positive-pressure breath, the anesthetist has total airway control—as yet, however, without assurance of intubation. Even at this stage, it is best to maintain spontaneous ventilation until the trachea has been intubated, as despite preoperative assessment the supraglottic airway may possess unsuspected abnormalities, such as epiglottic cysts. In general, these structures can be avoided under direct vision, given the time available with adequate oxygenation and anesthesia. If the intubation is prolonged, it may be worthwhile to insufflate the anesthetic mixture via a nasopharyngeal catheter or airway, provided it does not also serve to anesthetize the endoscopist. (See also the section on the Difficult Airway and Intubation, page 264).

After the trachea has been intubated orally, some thought may be given to substituting a nasal tube, especially if the lesion extends into the mouth. To change the tube is very much the decision of the anesthetist, and no further steps should be taken if the maneuver is thought excessively difficult. In either case, bilateral ventilation must be reconfirmed once the baby is finally positioned for surgery.

Taking advantage of halothane-induced cutaneous vein prominence, it is highly desirable to insert at least one, preferably two, substantial intravenous catheter(s) early on, not only to offset the dehydration/inhalation combination, but in anticipation of the occasionally substantial blood and fluid losses that occur in the resection of these cysts. An intra-arterial catheter is suggested if the cyst is large, and *strongly* suggested if the lesion extends into the mediastinum. Central venous pressure monitoring is desirable; unfortunately, the most direct access to the right atrium, via the jugular veins, may be impossible. For all but the most limited lesions, an indwelling bladder catheter connected to calibrated drainage is indicated.

Following tracheal intubation, spontaneous or controlled ventilation techniques may be employed, as indicated. The anesthetist's task then becomes fluid and thermal energy replacement in the face of steady substantial losses of both. Clearly identifying what type of fluid is being lost may be rather difficult, emphasizing the value of intermittent blood sampling.

The possibility of surgically induced bradycardia should be considered whenever the dissection nears branches of the vagus nerve or the carotid sinus. However, bradycardia remains foremost a warning of hypoxia in infants, despite the anatomy. Only after this cause is eliminated should atropine be employed.

Postoperative airway management is largely dictated by the procedure. For removal of an isolated small cyst, extubation is straightforward. In general, however, the possibility of oropharyngeal edema suggests a cautious delay in extubation. Indeed, if the situation so warrants, elective tracheostomy may even be indicated at the time of the excision, rather than delaying 2 weeks and performing the operation under less optimal conditions.

The patient should spend a short stay in an intensive care unit following most such operations. If the endotracheal tube, nasal or oral, is left in place, position should be confirmed by chest x-ray. Provisions for humidified air/oxygen should be made, and all those responsible for postoperative care should be informed of fluid therapy, the potential for swelling, and possible nerve dysfunction (such as vocal cord weakness) from surgery. As well, the connection between massive swelling and hypovolemia should be gently emphasized lest intravascular volume slowly translocate, without replacement, into the neck.

THYROGLOSSAL DUCT CYST

This is the most common case of a midline neck mass in a child. The two other fairly common causes are dermoid cysts and midline cervical clefts, both of which are simply and easily locally excised. As was reviewed in the discussion of embryology, thyroglossal duct cyst represents a somewhat more complex situation.

Clinical Features

The thyroid gland originates as a cellular rest at the foramen cecum in the tongue and migrates in the anterior midline of the neck to its permanent location by the eighth week of development. In the usual situation, the thyroglossal duct is obliterated by the tenth week, but should this not occur, a neck mass may present anywhere along the path followed by the gland. In fact, over 75 percent of these cysts present in close proximity to the hyoid bone. Early excision is recommended before infection or occasional malignant degeneration occurs. The majority of these cysts appear after the second birthday, with 50 percent being identified by age 10.

The removal of the cyst requires dissection of the tract to the foramen cecum. Rather than widely opening the anterior neck, the surgeon should employ a series of stepladder-style incisions until digital pressure, applied intraorally over the foramen cecum, brings the tongue nearer the skin incision, such that the entire tract can be removed flush with the tongue epithelium.

Anesthetic Management

The symptoms presented by these cysts are generally only cosmetic, occasionally compounded by external drainage and rarely by infection. Thyroid function is not involved. Preoperative assessment and preparation are unremarkable for this diagnosis. Very rarely, fluid can be expressed from the cyst into the mouth, but neither the frequency nor quantity recommend special airway precautions.

The patient will eventually be placed in position essentially like that for tracheostomy. The surgical field can be expected to include the mouth, as intraoral digital pressure assists the dissection. The patient can be intubated orally, although it seems more reasonable to progress from an oral tube, the insertion of which confirms correct tracheal fit, to a nasal tube, thus removing the airway from the surgical field. If a nasal tube is chosen, the precurved variety provides for a low profile as well as minimizing dead space. A pharyngeal pack is rarely indicated, as the operation never truly enters the oral cavity. During the actual procedure, the patient should be positioned slightly (20°) head up to decrease bleeding. Overaggressiveness in elevating the head raises the possibility of air embolism; this should be avoided unless the position is felt to be so beneficial that all the measures associated with a sitting craniotomy are also taken.

Following a straightforward excision in an older child, the tube can be removed and the patient then awakened. A more difficult procedure, or operation on a smaller infant, suggests awake extubation. In either case, the patient should be nursed semi-sitting in the postoperative period to minimize swelling.

SALIVARY GLAND TUMORS

This topic generally brings to mind tumors of the parotid gland, or radical extirpative surgery for oropharyngeal cancer—all in adults. Salivary gland tumors constitute about 3 percent of all tumors, with only about 0.3 to 1.3 percent of this 3 percent found below patient age of 16. Unfortunately, when such tumors are found in children, the majority are malignant. The anatomical possibilities include the paired glands—parotid, submandibular, and sublingual—or any of the 400 to 800 individual glands found in the oropharynx; however, 75 percent will be located in the parotid gland. In those circumstances in which the other paired glands are involved, the incidence of malignancy may be as high as 70 percent. As with most cases of malignant disease, the etiology is unknown, although a history of head and neck radiation has been estimated to increase the incidence ninefold. The majority of patients should be cured by surgery.

Clinical Features

The usual clinical presentation is of a 1- to 2-cm firm and slowly enlarging mass, often in the parotid gland, brought to a physician's attention when the patient is about 1 year of age. The facial nerve is rarely involved, and the child does not otherwise appear to have cancer. Airway compromise is extraordinarily uncommon in the usual case; occasionally a ranula, a cyst of the sublingual gland duct, may present some minor difficulty.

Surgical approach to the parotid is via an incision anterior to the auricle, to the submandibular gland via an incision parallel to the horizontal ramus of the mandible beneath the floor of the mouth, and to the sublingual gland intraorally. In general, the largest element of concern is preserving vital structures while removing the entire tumor, as recurrences can be more aggressive. The most prominent such vital structure is the facial nerve as it divides and weaves its way through the parotid gland, in one of multiple patterns. On occasion, despite the importance of the facial nerve, it or one of its branches must be sacrificed; in such a situation, immediate repair, either by direct anastomosis or free nerve grafting, is recommended. The nerve is rather sensitive to trauma, and facial muscle weakness after nerve manipulation is not uncommon.

Anesthetic Management

The symptoms presented by these lesions are usually cosmetic, although terribly magnified by the fear of malignancy. The airway is rarely involved. Therefore, preoperative assessment and preparation for these tumors are unremarkable.

The patient will be placed in moderate cervical extension with the head possibly rotated away from the lesion. An oral tube will usually suffice, although a nasal tube can certainly be used. A pharyngeal pack is not indicated. A lesion in the parotid suggests that long-acting neuromuscular block be avoided.

Following surgery, the tube can usually be removed in a straightforward manner, although dissection in the floor of the mouth may favor extubation awake. In either case, the patient should be nursed semi-sitting in the postoperative period to minimize swelling.

CHRONIC UPPER AIRWAY OBSTRUCTION AND SLEEP APNEA

Examination of one of any number of current anesthesia textbooks could lead to the assumption that the trachea is separated from the environment by an uninteresting and amorphous area simply referred to as "the upper airway." This construct is not unique to anesthesiology, for until recently, this anatomy was also largely ignored by respiratory physiologists and clinicians in other specialties. In the mid-1960's, the key feature of the "pickwickian" syndrome was recognized to be oropharyngeal occlusion that occurred only during sleep. About 10 years later, Remmers presented a concept of airway occlusion during sleep that emphasized the role of oropharyngeal inspiratory muscle activity. Following these prominent advances, a number of studies have increased general knowledge of this unknown territory between the teeth and trachea. Some of these studies, in attempting to answer why the airway closes during sleep in some patients, have posed an even more fundamental question: Why does the airway stay open in anyone during sleep? Initially, this research was directed toward a seemingly small adult population, but as has proved true in other newly described entities, the actual scope and size of the population affected by upper airway obstruction was soon found to be substantially greater than expected.

The current understanding of sleep apnea generally includes two categories: *central*, or arrhythmic, apnea characterized by absent gas flow and lack of respiratory effort, and *obstructive* apnea, characterized by absent gas flow despite respiratory effort. Given that most patients with this problem do not have obstruction when awake, the majority of obstructive types must have some defect in central drive to airway musculature, leading to a third group aptly called *mixed* apnea. Perfectly normal people may experience, usually on a nonrecurring basis, short (10- to 20-second) episodes of apnea during sleep. It has been suggested that those with sleep apnea syndromes demonstrate repetitive (20 per hour) episodes, each greater than 10 seconds in duration. The exact pathology responsible for these

syndromes, and there may be multiple causes, is unclear, but theories include the following:

1. A small airway that requires greater inspiratory pressure than a normal-sized airway, and that passively closes as tone is reduced in sleep.

2. A small airway that requires active dilator muscle activity to remain patent—inspiratory pressure is normal.

3. A normal airway with excessive loss of muscle tone (predominantly the genioglossus).

4. A normal airway, including muscle tone, with abnormal respiratory control/feedback.

The usual symptoms are snoring, enuresis, sleepwalking, daytime sleepiness, morning headaches, personality changes, dyspnea with exercise intolerance, and insomnia. However, failure to thrive in infants has also been attributed to this syndrome.

The pediatric literature initially approached chronic obstruction from the perspective of mechanical high-grade occlusion from "visible" sources, such as hypertrophied adenoids and tonsils or severe micrognathia. This situation was often the source for case reports of chronic hypercapnia and hypoxemia with subsequent right ventricular dysfunction from pulmonary artery hypertension. Beyond this presentation, there was a suggested possible association with sudden infant death syndrome that is still unclear. However, the parallel adult and pediatric approaches to upper airway disorders have become more nearly coincident recently and a number of authors have suggested a continuum in age and presentation, extending from infants with Pierre Robin anomalad to sixth-decade males (it is a male-preponderant population) with severe snoring.

Although the emphasis in pediatric patients was originally on airway obstruction with subsequent right heart disease, a connection to adult sleep apnea research was made in a report of postoperative sleep obstruction in a patient with Treacher Collins syndrome. Admittedly, the pharyngeal hypoplasia associated with Treacher Collins syndrome would seem to present an unusual mechanical restriction in the airway, but even so, there must be some additional component responsible for sleep obstruction since few of these patients are in distress while awake. Studies of non–syndrome-related sleep apnea patients have also suggested combinations of reduced airway cross-sectional area in conjunction with some deficiency in respiratory drive during natural sleep. In general, this deficiency is best described as a respiratory dysrhythmia, or failure of rhythm control, but there is also an element of decreased responsiveness to CO_2. Furthermore, during sleep, the breathing of increased oxygen concentration will improve saturation at the cost of prolongation of apnea duration. Clearly, a patient with a natural unresponsiveness to CO_2, failure of respiratory rhythm control, reduced cross-sectional area of the airway, and a tendency to retain CO_2 when administered oxygen requires strict attention to airway management and respiratory monitoring in the postanesthetic recovery period. Unfortunately, the only visible clue available to identify these patients, other than morbid obesity, comes from the work of Coccagna and associates, who noted that a "birdlike facies" with micrognathia was highly suggestive of sleep apnea. For the moment, the anesthetist must remain aware of the syndrome, in its several presentations, and be advised to question the patient, or parents, about sleeping problems or snoring whenever obesity or facial anatomy suggests the syndrome. If responses to this line of questioning support the diagnosis, premedication should be ordered cautiously. (As an example of the risks involved, consider the case of a 4-year-old child with sleep apnea who succumbed following ingestion of a usual dose of cough syrup, containing promethazine and codeine, ostensibly due to the effect of these two drugs on deficient respiratory drive.) The postoperative management of sleep apnea patients may be benefited by the application of nasal continuous positive airway pressure, which seems to offer great promise for amelioration of symptoms during normal unmedicated sleep. However, this technique has not yet been tested in sedated patients.

MANAGEMENT OF THE DIFFICULT PEDIATRIC AIRWAY AND INTUBATION

Achieving control of a patient's airway is the anesthetist's forté and primary task. Without expertise in this area, the rendering of a person unconscious with respiratory depressant drugs becomes unacceptably hazardous. A first consideration of this crucial subject might therefore place "intubation" into the larger category of "airway" management; on further thought and clinical experience, it is clear that difficulty with management of the nonintubated airway is not always associated with difficulty in intubation. Laryngotracheomalacia is one example of such a situation. Furthermore, given reasonable assurance that the airway is manageable, most anesthetists face the difficult elective intubation as a challenge, armed with numerous techniques, publications, and mechanical devices. The difficult airway, on the other hand, is an altogether undesirable addition to any anesthetic, for which the publications and devices have much less to offer. Indeed, many authors seem to feel that their principal task, and a major contribution, is to forewarn the anesthetist of a difficult airway and trust to experience thereafter. The following is an approach to the recognition and management of the difficult airway, and then to its less threatening associate, the difficult intubation. This is necessitated by the fact that a number of head and neck syndromes present both problems in rapid succession.

Preoperative assessment begins the management of the difficult airway and/or difficult intubation, for first the problem must be recognized. Every anesthetist has memories of dealing with such challenges, but the clearest recall is always demonstrated for the unsuspected difficulty or the uncertain situation in which

someone thought all would be well and pressed on, only to be completely defeated in a few short minutes. It is interesting to reflect for a moment on the concept of a "difficult airway," as perceived by an anesthetist, for often at the time this description is applied, the patient appears completely unperturbed by this problem. The trouble, therefore, is that resulting from the combination of anesthetic-induced muscle relaxation and respiratory depression plus preexisting anatomy. Consider an extreme example of a difficult airway, the Pierre Robin anomalad. Micrognathia is a hallmark here, along with a tongue that "falls backward." White and Kander examined the difficult intubation in adults and found that the most significant anatomical measurement associated with difficulty in laryngeal visualization was the depth (or vertical height) of the mandible as measured from the alveolar ridge at the third molar to the lower border of the mandible. They felt that this anatomy, especially if it was combined with a relatively short mandible, placed soft tissue more posteriorly into the oropharynx and hindered intubation. When this line of reasoning is applied to the aforementioned child with Pierre Robin anomalad, the similarity is striking. Practically every illustration drawn to describe a child with micrognathia and glossoptosis portrays a condensed mass of soft tissue, including the tongue, in the posterior oropharynx. In essence, the compression of soft tissue into a space defined by a mandible relatively deficient in length seems to pose a spectrum of problems, varying in severity from functional intrusion into the airway, patient awake, to functional intrusion, patient anesthetized, to the least threatening situation, that of interference only with laryngeal visualization. This continuum was also recently suggested, somewhat obliquely, in study of airway stability in micrognathic infants. In general, the transition through this panoply appears to be part of normal growth, which allows for relative airway enlargement beyond critical lower limits, perhaps in conjunction with improvement in oropharyngeal muscle tone and control. That this airway improvement should occur is probably due to the impact of fluid flow being inversely proportioned to the fourth or fifth power of the length of the radius, and is analogous to the enormous declines in flow resistance associated with the smallest endotracheal tubes as they increase internal diameter by 0.5-mm increments.

Another approach to the difficult airway was offered by Nichol and Zuck, who looked at a frequent preanesthetic exercise, that of asking a patient to tip his or her head back as far as possible, from the view of determining what actually restricts his movement. The authors noted that the atlanto-occipital distance largely defines these limits, and attempts to forcefully continue extension after atlanto-occipital contact apply leverage to the cervical spine posteriorly, producing an anterior bowing of the vertebral column, thereby lifting the larynx further anteriorly out of view. This relationship was examined in adults and children only but, despite the anatomical differences in infants, is interesting in view of the strong clinical dictum not to extend an infant's head beyond neutral for laryngoscopy. It is certainly easy to suspect that the very prominent occiput of an infant may restrict this axis of motion. Unfortunately, while this is intriguing, the clinical recommendation must remain simply to continue the current practice of evaluating head extension preoperatively, as cervical spine x-rays on every patient are impractical. Furthermore, functional demonstration is probably more valuable than static measurement. There are, however, a limited number of congenital abnormalities of the cervical spine that may adversely affect ease of laryngoscopy, or spinal cord function, during neck hyperextension. These may require further radiological evaluation; they are listed in Table 9–4.

Consequent to this and previous evaluations, the patient's appearance, and the range of motion at the temporomandibular and atlanto-occipital joints, must be examined in detail. The child's face must be seen in three dimensions, so a full lateral view must be obtained. This will reveal defects in proportion, such as small jaw or malar hypoplasia. The former's significance should now be clear; the latter may create an almost flat face that cannot be well matched to a traditional semi-rigid Rendell-Baker mask, but instead requires a more adult-style small mask with a moldable pneumatic cushion. The anterior gliding movement of the temporomandibular joint can be evaluated by asking the child to oppose the upper and lower incisors, while a request to open the mouth wide is the best test of that axis of movement.

From the perspective of the endoscopist, the atlanto-occipital and temporomandibular joints seem to represent the only available sites of motion that can possibly assist in the task of "straightening" the upper airway into alignment with the trachea. However, the larynx is one end of a movable conduit and, as such, can itself be repositioned to assist in visualization. In circumstances where full displacement of both skeletal sites is inadequate to visualize the larynx, manual pressure posteriorly and/or laterally over the thyroid cartilage will often bring at least some recognizable anatomy into view. As intubation under direct vision requires both of the endoscopist's hands to be occupied, an assistant can stand to the patient's right and provide this extra degree of movement on command from the anesthetist. As well, the assistant can insert one of any number of atraumatic surgical retractors (Green loop, vein, Army-Navy, small Richardson) into the right corner of the mouth, laterally and superiorly displacing the entire orifice such that substantially more "working room" is available for intubation. Decreasing the soft tissue obstruction caused by the ipsilateral cheek can often ease actual tube passage to a striking degree. Yet another role for the assistant can be to "elevate" the larynx into view by tongue withdrawal with forceps, as described by Miyabe and colleagues.

In dealing with a subject as vexing as this, any absolute statement is suspect. However, a strong recommendation to preserve spontaneous ventilation comes reasonably close to being such an absolute. Even following a successful induction, maintaining the option offered by a breathing patient will occasionally rescue the situation from an unanticipated last-moment obstacle—as well as serving to prevent the reduction in the anesthetist's coronary artery flow associated with the sudden appreciation of the obstacle.

Accepting this concept, premedication should be selected to assist, rather than impair, the induction process. Consequently, drugs such as barbiturates, benzodiazepines, or chloral hydrate are suggested as examples of suitable choices instead of narcotics, which are more prone to decrease minute ventilation. Although atropine is usually given primarily to block

Table 9–4. CONGENITAL ABNORMALITIES OF THE CERVICAL SPINE AND ASSOCIATIONS

Abnormalities	Association	Symptom Onset
Basilar impression (for platybasia)	Atlanto-occipital fusion, atlas hypoplasia, abnormal odontoid, Klippel-Feil syndrome, skeletal dysplasias, bifid post-atlas arch	Uncommon until 2nd, 3rd decade
Congenital atlantoaxial instability	Congenital scoliosis, Down syndrome, bone dysplasia, spondyloepiphyseal dysplasia, osteogenesis imperfecta, neurofibromatosis	Usually by 2nd decade; childhood presentation; generalized weakness
Atlanto-occipital fusion	Jaw anomalies, cleft palate, ear deformities, cervical rib, urinary tract anomalies	Usually in 3rd, 4th decade
Odontoid hypoplasia/aplasia or os odontoideum	Down syndrome, Klippel-Feil syndrome, skeletal dysplasias, spondyloepiphyseal dysplasia	Variable; frequently diagnosed after episode of significant trauma
Congenital laxity of transverse atlantal ligament	Down syndrome (20%)	Variable; recommend C1-C2 articulation be evaluated in all Down prior to general anesthesia
Klippel-Feil syndrome (congenital synostosis of cervical vertebrae)	Scoliosis, renal abnormalities, Sprengel deformity, deafness, synkinesia, congenital heart disease	Symptoms uncommon

the cardiac response to vagal stimulation, in this situation atropine can also be given by mouth, primarily to decrease secretions. As all of these sedating compounds, except the newer benzodiazepines, are long-acting in effective doses, their use must be based on both the preoperative and postoperative situations—chloral hydrate 50 mg/kg is not well suited to early same-day discharge. Another consideration for the difficult airway is that of gastric contents. Although it is far from universal practice, the author administers cimetidine 10 mg/kg, every 6 hours, beginning the night prior to surgery, to selected patients anticipated to have problems with a difficult airway. Implementation of this step requires knowledge of the drug interactions associated with cimetidine, but the seemingly greater margin of safety suggests this as a worthwhile step.

Finally, the method of anesthetic induction seems crucial to success, as spontaneous ventilation and oxygenation must both be preserved. Undoubtedly, a "proper" dose of ketamine or barbiturate can be selected, such that apnea does not occur, but the consequences of misjudgment must be recognized. The author's preference is to administer oxygen alone for several minutes, followed by halothane, increased by 0.25 percent every three breaths, until 4 to 5 percent inspired concentration is reached. On occasion, this may have to be accomplished with the patient semi-sitting, at least initially, to prevent abrupt obstruction while the patient is still awake. A useful adjunct to this sequence is an intravenous infusion, established several hours preoperatively such that the child does not develop a fluid deficit. A full right atrium assists the smooth leisurely establishment of inhalation anesthesia remarkably well—especially if the patient must be positioned head up during the induction.

Initial operating room management of the airway usually centers on the interface between the anesthesia mask and the patient's face. All anesthesia masks roughly create a funnel with a small peripheral invagination for the chin and a larger one for the nose. A lateral facial view of a child with Pierre Robin anomalad, as an example, shows that the usual plane created by the maxilla and mandible does not exist, thereby creating a break in the mask-to-face seal over the mandible. One answer to this might be a custom mask, while another and more practical answer might be to "build up" the mandible artificially with gauze until contact is obtained. While either may help achieve a mask fit, ensuring oxygen and anesthetic delivery to the face, the basic pathology remains unaffected and the airway may still be obstructed.

Therefore, in distinction to usual practice, the airway must first be established prior to general anesthesia. Consequently, assuming mask positive pressure alone appears insufficient, the nasopharynx or oropharynx should be topically anesthetized (lidocaine 4 mg/kg, cocaine 3 mg/kg, tetracaine 1 mg/kg) and the appropriate device inserted. When a nasal airway is used, the lubricant should be only that, not a concentrated anesthetic preparation, as drug administration will be neither recognized nor controlled. Furthermore, some topical anesthetic preparations dry into stalactites and can potentially cause airway obstruction. If a shortened endotracheal tube is used as a nasal airway, ready connection with an anesthetic apparatus will be facilitated via the 15-mm connector.

Complications to the above are epistaxis, emesis, and failure to establish an airway. Epistaxis is rarely a problem with infants; for the older child, topical application of 0.125 percent phenylephrine or 0.025 percent oxymetazoline will effectively vasoconstrict the mucosa. When applied first, this step should also theoretically decrease absorption of local anesthetic. The older child also is at risk of having a cylindrical biopsy of hypertrophied adenoids taken during nasal tube insertion. This can be avoided by first passing a small soft catheter through the tube, then (through the nostril) into and (via the mouth) back out of the oropharynx. The tube is then passed into the oropharynx via the nose while gentle tension is maintained on the catheter, thus directing the tube anteriorly away from the adenoids; once the tip passes these tissues, the catheter is removed and the tube is placed in final position in a conventional manner. Obviously, this step generally requires an anesthetized patient.

Emesis, like epistaxis, does not seem to be a major problem with infants. For the older child, topical anesthesia to the oropharynx will usually limit this. Failure to establish an airway is generally due to the variation of Murphy's Law that predicts the device selected will be too large or too small. An excessively large oral airway has the potential to aggravate the obstruction by occluding or compressing the larynx, while an airway that is too small simply fails to displace the tongue from the posterior pharyngeal wall. An oversized nasal tube either will not pass the nostril or after insertion extends into the esophagus and worsens the entire situation. To avoid this, an external estimate of length should be made before the nasal airway is inserted. In any case, if the situation does not improve following airway insertion, the tube should be removed immediately and the approach to intubation should be reassessed.

All of the preceding serves to establish a passage for gas exchange and possibly even for mask positive-pressure ventilation. This may prove adequate for some surgery, but more likely what it serves to do is provide a calm, well-oxygenated patient for intubation attempts or possibly tracheostomy. However, one exception to this progression to endotracheal intubation is provided by the use of a supraglottic nasal endotracheal tube, or nasal airway with an added 15-mm connector, as a final method to administer anesthesia. With sufficient patience to achieve adequate depth, even assisted ventilation can be provided in this way. Obviously, this situation is not as desirable as a properly fitting translaryngeal endotracheal tube, but it is superior to a tracheostomy for a revision of a syndactyly repair. If this method is eventually selected, a high degree of vigilance is required to detect gastric distention; if that is suspected, a 10- to 14-gauge catheter must be quickly passed via the mouth into the stomach. As this is such a distinct possibility, the presence of any form of esophageal pathology that makes gastric intubation hazardous poses a relative contraindication to this nasopharyngeal technique, at least if positive airway pressure is to be employed.

If endotracheal intubation is indicated, the tube will generally be inserted via the mouth, at least initially. For the overwhelming majority of patients, this is a straightforward task. The variety of laryngoscope blades commercially available stands in mute testimony to the exceptions. The occasional pediatric anesthetist may be acquainted with numerous adult blades, but perhaps only one, frequently the Miller, for children. (It is enlightening to compare the currently available Miller blade with the original; from this, one can speculate that the first version may well have been the best.) Often other blades are useful for the difficult intubation, and it is worthwhile having a selection at hand for this situation. In the United States, the following are generally available: (1) Miller, (2) Wisconsin, (3) Wis-Foregger, (4) Wis-Hipple, (5) Alberts, (6) Michaels, (7) Flagg, (8) Guedel, (9) Bennet, (10) Seward, (11) Robertshaw, and (12) Oxford Infant. When the patient's anatomy allows the usual right-sided oral laryngoscope insertion, followed by lateral movement to the midline, the author has found the Seward or Robertshaw blade (see Fig. 9–7) useful. For those situations in which the blade must be passed via, and remain in, the far right lateral aspect of the mouth, the smaller cross-sectional area of the Miller blade seems best. The limited view of the glottis afforded by this lateral approach may require removal of the 15-mm connector from the tube to prevent loss of view of the larynx during intubation. A very interesting variation of this technique utilizes a pediatric Jackson anterior commissure laryngoscope to visualize the larynx, followed by tube insertion over an optical stylet, through the laryngoscope. The tube is then fixed in position with long alligator forceps while the stylet and laryngoscope are withdrawn and the 15-mm connector is inserted into the tube. In this, or any situation in which the connector has been left off during insertion, the tube must be left long enough to grasp and the connector initially firmly preinserted to facilitate subsequent reinsertion after intubation. Not infrequently during these maneuvers, the tube becomes slippery; the silent struggle to control 1 cm of lubricated plastic of 4 mm ID tube well enough to insert a connector, without extubating the child, is amusing only to the uninitiated.

In any of the techniques involving difficult laryngoscopy, two additional general measures must be attended to: someone must observe and care for the patient, and oxygen, usually with anesthetic, must be provided. The answer to the former is to obtain assistance. The latter is satisfied by insufflation, intermittently via the laryngoscope, or preferably continuously via a nasopharyngeal catheter or airway. Finally, the child's fragile teeth must be protected, either by a commercial dental guard or by cotton gauze.

An alternative to conventional laryngoscopy is the use of a fiberoptic bronchoscope, as a flexible stylet, as a visualization device when the bronchoscope is too large to pass through the tube, or as the first step of a guide wire—cardiac catheter—endotracheal tube sequence. Expertise with the device comes with practice, most easily acquired in adult patients first. The difficult small airway is most certainly not the place to launch a new skill.

The Hopkins telescope can be used as a rigid optical stylet in certain cases, either as previously described, or as part of a more conventional laryngoscopy-bronchoscopy technique.

A large number of devices have been used as nonoptical guides to direct tube passage into the larynx in instances when only the most posterior aspect of the larynx could be visualized. Any malleable object thin enough to pass through a tube and long enough to be manageable while intubating can be, and probably has been, used. An interesting commercially produced variation allows for variable flexion of the guide tip; this device has recently become available in a size that will accommodate tubes as small as 4.5 mm ID, at a cost about that of a laryngoscope blade.

If laryngoscopy and oral intubation prove impossible, blind nasal intubation is usually the next option. The endotracheal tube is passed with the same consideration as when used an an airway, except it is cut somewhat longer. This method is much less hurried in a patient spontaneously breathing an anesthetic mixture via an airway in the other nostril, although occasionally the airway may need to be withdrawn slightly to prevent interference with the advancing tube. Alternatively, the anesthesia circuit may be connected directly to the endotracheal tube being passed, although this removes the audible cues to intubation. Atraumatic insertion can be facilitated by heating the tube, in a warmer or in fluids, to a temperature of 40 to 50°C. Berry recently reported an impressive 96 percent success rate for blind nasal intubation aided by an 8- or 14-gauge pliable stylet, formed to desired shape and inserted into the endotracheal tube *after* the tube tip was in the oropharynx. Interested readers should consult the original, very specific, reference. Great care must be taken with these blind techniques in children, as the larynx may be easily traumatized by intubation attempts. A recent report of arytenoid dislocation in a child, caused by vigorous coughing, emphasizes the fragility of these periglottic structures.

It is possible, during a difficult nasal intubation, to tunnel the tube submucosally, generally via a tear near the sphenoid prominence. Once this tissue plane has been entered, it is surprisingly easy to advance the tube, although obviously never successfully into the airway. Consequently, whenever a tube appears to have passed from the nasopharynx into the oropharynx, without accompanying audible evidence of respiration emanating from the tube, it is worthwhile to inspect the oropharynx visually and confirm the proper plane of advance.

On occasion following a successful oral intubation, a transition to a nasal tube is planned. One device that facilitates this exchange under direct vision is an Aillon tube forceps, which can nicely redirect an anterior tube tip down the tracheal axis, thereby eliminating the "hang-up" so often encountered with a nasal tube.

An interesting technique, now largely forgotten, may prove useful when visual and traditional blind methods fail. Well described by Hudon, this method is perhaps most appropriately titled tactile intubation. This technique involves guiding the tube through the glottis with fingers inserted into the oral cavity, after ensuring adequate anesthesia and with the mouth held open with a gag. The initial route of intubation, oral or nasal, appears immaterial in this technique; Hudon actually seemed to feel this represented a preferred means of intubation. This approach can be useful in difficult situations, provided some prior practice is obtained in straightforward cases. The original article should be read in some detail by those interested, as it is extremely thorough.

A useful addition to a stylet is a light source at the tip, creating a device referred to as a "lightwand." This provides optical assistance to an otherwise blind technique, by allowing visualization of light source entry into the cervical trachea via transillumination of the thyroid cartilage. This adaptation is most often described as an adjunct to Hudon's technique, but recently was suggested as a means to confirm endotracheal tube tip location in the cervical trachea. However, as always, there must be some negative component to this addition; in this case, it was loss of the light bulb into a bronchus.

If intubation from above proves initially impossible, a reasonable next step would be to establish a reliable mechanical path into the airway from below. This technique was initially made popular with a large bore needle–epidural catheter–retrograde oral tube sequence across the cricothyroid membrane, but has recently been reported as a modified Seldinger technique, utilizing a 20-gauge needle and a 0.021-inch guide wire. When this technique is employed, the wire should be passed into the endotracheal tube via the Murphy side hole rather than the larger end hole, to allow insertion of an additional 1 cm or so of tube into the larynx before wire withdrawal. Obviously, this technique also demands a fairly still patient during needle insertion to prevent internal laryngeal injury.

Should none of these techniques prove effective, two options remain: tracheostomy and other. Tracheostomy seems quite attractive at first, but often proves less so when the entire picture of small child, movement, possible supine airway obstruction, and unfavorable anatomy becomes clearer. In essence, the very problems initially confronting the anesthetist are still there, compounded by surgical access requirements. It is important to remember that tracheostomy is still surgery, and there are good reasons why surgery without general anesthesia is rarely scheduled for children. This is most especially true if the child is mentally retarded and/or has a hearing or vision defect.

"Other" refers to the innovation required when all else fails. For example, while most extremity procedures are performed while patients are supine, it may be possible to obtain reasonable operating conditions with the patient in a lateral or semi-prone position that more favors the natural airway. Perhaps the most extreme example of how useful position may be is a report of blind nasal intubation in the prone position, employed in an infant with Pierre Robin anomalad, for whom all other techniques had failed. Additionally, local or regional anesthesia may play a role, providing *very* strict attention to protection from overdose is maintained, as convulsion or cardiac depression without airway control seems a highly undesirable situation. Finally, alternative methods of analgesia or relative immobility, such as a continuous ketamine infusion, may alone, or in conjunction with the previous variations, allow successful surgery. This infusion technique has often been useful for the burned child with severe cervical flexion contractures, for whom other techniques would have been quite difficult. For any of these approaches it is critical that the team members be made aware of the anesthetist's concerns and management plan, for proceeding with an operation without any reasonable possibility of providing general endotracheal anesthesia, even if required, is a major departure from usual practice. A hasty discussion about the situation after a request for muscle paralysis is untimely and seems poorly designed for good future working relations.

The author gratefully acknowledges the excellent editorial assistance and typing of this chapter by Ms. Allyn Charney.

REFERENCES

Embryology

Wilson DB: Embryonic development of the head and neck. Part 2. The branchial region. Head Neck Surg 2:59, 1979.

Wilson DB: Embryonic development of the head and neck. Part 3. The face. Head Neck Surg 2:145, 1979.

Congenital Craniofacial Deformities

Apert E: De l'Acrocephalosyndactylie. Bull Soc Med 23:1310, 1906.

Bergsma D: Birth Defects Compendium. New York, Alan R. Liss, 1979.

Carpenter G: Two sisters showing malformations of the skull and other congenital abnormalities. Rep Soc Study Dis Child Lond 1:110, 1901.

Chotzen F: Eine eigenartige familiare Entwicklungsstorung. (Akrocephalosyndaktylie, Dysostosis craniofacialis und Hypertelorismus.) Monatsschr Kinderheilkd 55:97, 1932.

Cohen MM: Dysmorphic syndromes with craniofacial manifestations. In Steward R, Prescott G (Eds.): Oral Facial Genetics. St. Louis, C. V. Mosby Co., 1976.

Converse JQ, Wood-Smith D, McCarthy JG: Report of a series of 50 craniofacial operations. Plast Reconstr Surg 55:283, 1975.

Crouzon O: Dysostose cranio-faciale hereditaire. Bull Mem Soc Med Hop (Paris) 33:545, 1912.

Davies DW, Munro IR: The anesthetic management and intraoperative care of patients undergoing major facial osteotomies. Plast Reconstr Surg 55:50, 1975.

Dyken P, Miller M: Facial Features of Neurologic Syndromes. St. Louis, C.V. Mosby Co., 1980.

Gorlin RJ: Developmental anomalies of the face and oral structures. In Gorlin RJ, Goldman HM (Eds.): Thoma's Oral Pathology. 6th ed. St. Louis, C.V. Mosby Co., 1970.

Handler SD, Beaugard ME, Whitaker LA, et al.: Airway management in the repair of craniofacial defects. Cleft Palate J 16:16, 1978.

Marchac D: Discussion: Early surgery for craniofacial synostosis: an 8-year experience. Plast Reconstr Surg 73:531, 1984.

McCarthy JG, Epstein F, Sadove M, et al.: Early surgery for craniofacial synostosis: an 8-year experience. Plast Reconstr Surg 73:521, 1984.

Pfeiffer RA: Dominant erbliche Akrocephalosyndaktylie. Z Kinderheilkd 90:301, 1964.

Powazek M, Billmeier GJ: Assessment of intellectual development after surgery for craniofacial dysostosis. Am J Dis Child 133:151, 1979.

Renier D, Sainte-Rose C, Marchac D, et al.: Intracranial pressure in craniostenosis. J Neurosurg 57:370, 1982.

Saethre H: Ein Beitrag zum Turmschadelproblem. (Pathogenese, Erblichkeit und Symptomatologie.) Dtsch Z Nervenheilkd 117:533, 1931.

Shillito J, Matson DD: Craniosynostosis: a review of 519 surgical patients. Pediatrics 41:829, 1968.

Smith DW: Recognizable Patterns of Human Malformation. 2nd ed. Philadelphia, W.B. Saunders Co., 1976.

Stanesco V, Maximilian C, Poenaru S, et al.: Syndrome hereditaire dominant reunissant une dysostose cranio-faciale de type particulier, une insuffisance de croissance d'aspect chondrodystrophique et un epaississement massif de la corticale des os longs. Rev Fr Endocrinol 4:219, 1963.

Temtamy SA: Carpenter's syndrome: acrocephalopolysyndactyly, an autosomal recessive syndrome. J Pediatr 69:111, 1966.

Tessier P: Anatomical classification of facial, cranio-facial and latero-facial clefts. J Maxillofac Surg 4:69, 1976.

Acquired Craniofacial Deformities: Trauma

Converse JM: Facial injuries in children. In Mustarde JC (Ed.): Plastic Surgery in Infancy and Childhood. Edinburgh, Churchill Livingstone, 1979.

Karlson TA: The incidence of facial injuries from dog bites. JAMA 251:3265, 1984.

Luce EA, Tubb T, Moore A: Review of 1,000 major facial fractures and associated injuries. Plast Reconstr Surg 63:26, 1979.

Palmer J, Rees M: Dog bites of the face: a 15 year review. Br J Plast Surg 36:315, 1983.

Sayers M: Craniocerebral trauma. In Touloubian R (Ed.): Pediatric Trauma. New York, John Wiley, 1978.

Venes J, Collins W: Spinal cord injury. In Touloubian R (Ed.): Pediatric Trauma. New York, John Wiley, 1978.

Wiseman NE, Chochinov H, Fraser V: Major dog attack injuries in children. J Pediatric Surg 18:533, 1983.

Acquired Craniofacial Deformities: Burns

Galvis AG, Mestad PH: Modified endotracheal tube for airway management of children with facial burns. Anesth Analg 60:116, 1981.

Molinaro JR: The social fate of children disfigured by burns. Am J Psychiatry 135:979, 1978.

Ward CF: Anesthesia for head and neck burn surgery. In Wachtel T, Frank D (Eds.): Burns of the Head and Neck. Philadelphia, W.B. Saunders Co., 1984, pp 34–55.

Ward CF, Alfery DD, Saidman LJ, et al.: Deliberate hypotension in head and neck surgery. Head Neck Surg 2:185, 1980.

Deformities of the External Ear

Bergsma D: Birth Defects Compendium. New York, Alan R. Liss, 1979.

Edgerton M: Auricular deformities. In Ravitch M, Welch K, Benson C, et al. (Eds.): Pediatric Surgery. 3rd ed. Chicago, Year Book, 1979.

Posivillo D: The pathogenesis of the first and second branchial arch syndromes. Oral Surg 35:302, 1973.

Tanzer R, Bellucci R, Converse J, et al.: Deformities of the auricle. In Converse JM (Ed.): Reconstructive Plastic Surgery. Vol. 3. 2nd ed. Philadelphia, W.B. Saunders Co., 1977.

Cleft Lip and Palate

Bethmann W, Hockstein H: Anesthesiological experiences in 4,000 operations on infants and children for cleft lip and palate. Plast Reconstr Surg 41:129, 1968.

Cohen MM: Syndromes with cleft lip and cleft palate. Cleft Palate J 15:306, 1978.

Conway H, Bromberg B, Hochn R, et al.: Causes of mortality in patients with cleft lip and cleft palate. Plast Reconstr Surg 37:51, 1966.

Fraser GR, Cahran JS: Cleft lip and palate: seasonal incidence of birth weight, birth rank, sex, and site, associated malformations and parental age. Arch Dis Child 36:420, 1961.

Furnas DW, Allison GR: Circummandibular or nasomaxillary suture with pullout loop for secure placement of endotracheal tube. Am J Surg 139:887, 1980.

Gorlin RJ, Cervenba J, Pruzansky S: Facial clefting and its syndromes. Birth Defects 7:3, 1971.

Karl HW, Swedlow DB, Lee KW, et al.: Epinephrine-halothane interactions in children. Anesthesiology 58:142, 1983.

Maue-Dickson W, Dickson DR: Anatomy and physiology related to cleft palate: current research and clinical implications. Plast Reconstr Surg 65:83, 1980.

McClelland RM, Patterson TJ: The preoperative, anesthetic and postoperative management of cleft lip and palate. Plast Reconstr Surg 29:642, 1962.

Morgan GA, Steward DJ: A pre-formed paediatric orotracheal tube design based on anatomical measurements. Can Anaesth Soc J 29:9, 1982.

Morgan GA, Steward DJ: Linear airway dimensions in children: including those with cleft palate. Can Anaesth Soc J 29:1, 1982.

Salanitre E, Rackow H: Changing trends in the anesthetic management of the child with cleft lip–palate malformation. Anesthesiology 23:610, 1962.

Shah CV, Pruzansky S, Morris W: Cardiac malformations with facial clefts. Am J Dis Child 119:238, 1970.

Wall MA: Infant endotracheal tube resistance: effects of changing length, diameter, and gas density. Crit Care Med 8:38, 1980.

Whalen JS, Conn AW: Improved technics in anesthetic management for repair of cleft lips and palates. Anesth Analg 46:355, 1978.

Zook EG, Salmon JH: Anomalies of the cervical spine in the cleft palate patient. Plast Reconstr Surg 60:96, 1977.

Branchial Arch Defects

Audry C: Variete d'alopecie congenitale; alopecie suturale. Ann Dermat et Syph (Ser 3) 4:899, 1893.

Berry GA: Note on a congenital defect (coloboma) of the lower lid. Ophthal Hosp Rep 12:255, 1888.

Braver RD: Congenital cysts and tumors of the neck. In Converse

JM (Ed.): Reconstructive Plastic Surgery. Vol. 5. 2nd ed. Philadelphia, W.B. Saunders Co., 1977.

Burge D, Middleton A: Persistent pharyngeal pouch in the neonate. J Ped Surg 18:230, 1983.

Carey J, Fineman R, Ziter F: The Robin sequence as a consequence of malformation, dysplasia and neuromuscular syndromes. J Pediatr 101:858, 1982.

Collins S: The pathogenesis of the Treacher Collins syndrome. Br J Oral Surg 13:1, 1975.

Deane SA, Telander R: Surgery for thyroglossal duct and branchial cleft anomalies. Am J Surg 136:348, 1978.

Dennison WM: The Pierre Robin syndrome. Pediatrics 36:336, 1965.

Feingold M, Baum J: Goldenhar's syndrome. Am J Dis Child 132:136, 1978.

Fletcher M, Blum S, Blanchard C: Pierre Robin syndrome: pathophysiology of obstructive episodes. Laryngoscope 79:547, 1969.

Franceschetti A, Klein D: Mandibulo-faciale dysostosis; a new hereditary syndrome. Acta Ophthalmol 27:143, 1949.

Franceschetti A, Zwahlen P: Un syndrome nouveau, la dysostose mandibulofaciale. Bull Schweiz Akad Med Wissensch 1:60, 1944.

Freeman MK, Manners JM: Cor pulmonale and the Pierre Robin anomaly. Anaesthesia 35:282, 1980.

Goldenhar M: Associations malformatives de l'oeil et de l'oreille, en particular le syndrome et dermoide epibulbaire-appendices auriculaires-fistula auris congenita et ses relations avec le dysostose mandibulo-faciale. J Genet Humaine 1:243, 1952.

Grabb WC: The first and second branchial arch syndrome. Plast Reconstr Surg 36:485, 1965.

Hallerman W: Vogelgesicht und Cataracta congenita. Klin Monatsbl Augenheilkd 113:315, 1948.

Hanson JW, Smith DW: U-shaped palatal defect in the Robin anomalad: developmental and clinical relevance. Pediatrics 87:30, 1975.

Heaf DP, Helms PJ, Dinwiddie R, et al.: Nasopharyngeal airways in Pierre Robin syndrome. J Pediatr 100:698, 1982.

Henzel J, Pories W, DeWeese M: Etiology of lateral cervical cysts. Surg Gynecol Obstet 125:87, 1967.

Jackson P, Whitaker LA, Randall P: Airway hazards associated with pharyngeal flaps in patients who have the Pierre Robin syndrome. Plast Reconstr Surg 58:184, 1976.

Jeresaty RM, Huszar RJ, Basu S: Pierre Robin syndrome. Cause of respiratory obstruction, cor pulmonale, and pulmonary edema. Am J Dis Child 117:710, 1969.

Johnson G, Todd D: Cor pulmonale in severe Pierre Robin syndrome. Pediatrics 65:152, 1980.

Luke MJ, Mehrizi A, Folger GM, et al.: Chronic nasopharyngeal obstruction as a cause of cardiomegaly, cor pulmonale, and pulmonary edema. Pediatrics 37:762, 1966.

Mallory SB, Paradise JL: Glossoptosis revisited: on the development and resolution of airway obstruction in the Pierre Robin syndrome. Pediatrics 64:946, 1979.

Olsen KD, Maragos N, Weiland L: First branchial cleft anomalies. Laryngoscope 90:423, 1980.

Pearl W: Congenital heart disease in the Pierre Robin syndrome. Pediatr Cardiol 2:307, 1982.

Posivillo D: The pathogenesis of the first and second branchial arch syndromes. Oral Surg 35:302, 1973.

Ravidson R, Stoops CM: Anesthetic management of a patient with Hallermann-Streiff syndrome. Anesth Analg 53:254, 1979.

Roa NL, Moss KS: Treacher-Collins syndrome with sleep apnea: anesthetic considerations. Anesthesiology 60:71, 1984.

Robin P: Backward lowering of the root of the tongue causing respiratory disturbances. Bull Acad Nat Med 89:37, 1923.

Robin P: De la physiologique de la tetee au sein et de la forme que doit avoir tetine dur bibeion. Bull Soc Pediat Paris 27:55, 1929.

Ross ED: Treacher Collins syndrome. Anaesthesia 18:350, 1963.

Shprintzen RJ, Croft C, Berkman MD, et al.: Pharyngeal hypoplasia in Treacher Collins syndrome. Arch Otolaryngol 105:127, 1979.

Sklar GS, King BD: Endotracheal intubation and Treacher-Collins syndrome. Anesthesiology 44:247, 1976.

Stehling L: Goldenhar syndrome and airway management. Am J Dis Child 132:818, 1978.

Stern LM, Fonkalsrud EW, Hassakis P, et al.: Management of Pierre Robin syndrome in infancy by prolonged nasoesophageal intubation. Am J Dis Child 124:78, 1972.

Streiff EB: Dysmorphie mandibulofaciale et alterations oculaire. Ophthalmologica 120:79, 1950.

Thomson A: A description of congenital malformation of the auricle and external meatus of both sides in three persons. Proc Roy Soc Edinburgh 1:443, 1845.

Treacher Collins E: Case with symmetrical congenital notches in the outer part of each lower lid and defective development of the malar bones. Trans Ophthal Soc UK 20:190, 1900.

Weissman C, Damask MC, Yang J: Noncardiogenic pulmonary edema following laryngeal obstruction. Anesthesiology 60:163, 1984.

Williams AJ, Williams MA, Walker CA, et al.: The Robin anomalad (Pierre Robin syndrome)—a follow up study. Arch Dis Child 56:663, 1981.

Cystic Hygroma

Barrand KG, Freeman NV: Massive infiltrating cystic hygroma of the neck in infancy. Arch Dis Child 48:523, 1973.

Bill AH, Sumner DS: A unified concept of lymphangioma and cystic hygroma. Surg Gynecol Obstet 120:79, 1965.

Braver RD: Congenital cysts and tumors of the neck. In Converse JM (Ed.): Reconstructive Plastic Surgery. Vol. 5. 2nd ed. Philadelphia, W.B. Saunders Co., 1977.

Evans P: Intubation problem in a case of cystic hygroma complicated by a laryngotracheal haemangioma. Anaesthesia 36:696, 1981.

Grosfeld J, Weber T, Vane D: One-stage resection for massive cervicomediastinal hygroma. Surgery 92:693, 1982.

Lindsay WK: The neck. In Mustarde JC (Ed.): Plastic Surgery in Infancy and Childhood. 2nd ed. New York, Churchill Livingstone, 1979.

Ninh TN, Ninh TA: Cystic hygroma: a report of 126 cases. J Pediatr Surg 9:191, 1974.

Pounds L: Neck masses of congenital origin. Pediatr Clin North Am 28:841, 1981.

Weller RM: Anaesthesia for cystic hygroma in a neonate. Anaesthesia 29:588, 1974.

Wernher A: Die angeborenen Zysten-Hygrome und die ihnen verwandten Geschwulste in anatomischer, diagnostischer und therapeutischer Beziehung. Giessen, G.F. Heyer, 1843, p 76.

Wilson RD, Putnam L, Phillips MT, et al.: Anesthetic problems in surgery for varying levels of respiratory obstruction in infants and children. Anesth Analg 53:878, 1974.

Zitelli B: Neck masses in children. Pediatr Clin North Am 28:813, 1981.

Thyroglossal Duct Cyst

Braver RD: Congenital cysts and tumors of the neck. In Converse JM (Ed.): Reconstructive Plastic Surgery. Vol. 5. 2nd ed. Philadelphia, W.B. Saunders Co., 1977.

Brereton RJ, Symonds R: Thyroglossal cysts in children. Br J Surg 65:507, 1978.

Deane SA, Telander R: Surgery for thyroglossal duct and branchial cleft anomalies. Am J Surg 136:348, 1978.

Pounds L: Neck masses of congenital origin. Pediatr Clin North Am 28:841, 1981.

Zitelli B: Neck masses in children. Pediatr Clin North Am 28:813, 1981.

Salivary Gland Tumors

Attie JN: Tumors of major and minor salivary glands: clinical and pathologic features. Curr Probl Surg 18:65, 1981.

Bianchi A, Cudmore RE: Salivary gland tumors in children. J Pediatr Surg 13:519, 1978.

Krolls SD, Tradahl JN, Boyers RC: Salivary gland lesions in children. Cancer 40:459, 1972.

Schuller DE, McCabe BF: The firm salivary mass in children. Laryngoscope 87:1891, 1977.

Tipton JB: Carcinoma of a minor salivary gland in an 18 month old child: case report. Plast Reconstr Surg 62:790, 1978.

Chronic Upper Airway Obstruction and Sleep Apnea

Brouilette RT, Fernbach SK, Hunt CE: Obstructive sleep apnea in infants and children. J Pediatr 100:31, 1982.

Cherniack NS: Sleep apnea and its causes. J Clin Invest 73:1501, 1984.

Coccagna G, Cirignotta F, Lugaresi E: Sleep Apnea Syndromes. New York, Alan R. Liss, 1978.

Coccagna G, di Donata G, Verucchi P, et al.: Hypersomnia with periodic apnea in acquired micrognathia. Arch Neurol 33:769, 1976.

Conway WA, Bower GC, Barnes ME: Hypersomnolence and intermittent upper airway obstruction. JAMA 237:2740, 1977.

Felman A, Loughlin G, Leftridge C: Upper airway obstruction during sleep in children. Am J Roentgenol 133:213, 1979.

Gastaut H, Tassinari CA, Duron B: Polygraphic study of the episodic diurnal and nocturnal (hypnic and respiratory) manifestations of the Pickwick syndrome. Brain Res 2:167, 1966.

Kravath RE, Pollak CP, Borowiecki B, et al.: Obstructive sleep apnea and death associated with surgical correction of velopharyngeal incompetence. J Pediatr 96:645, 1980.

Littner M, Young E, McGinty D, et al.: Awake abnormalities of control of breathing and of the upper airway. Chest 86:573, 1984.

Mealer WR, Fisher JC: Cor pulmonale and facio-auriculo-vertebral sequence. Cleft Palate J 21:100, 1984.

Remmers JE, de Groot WJ, Sauerland EK, et al.: Pathogenesis of airway occlusion during sleep. J Appl Physiol 44:931, 1978.

Remmers JE, Sterling JA, Thoratinsson B, et al.: Nasal airway positive pressure in patients with occlusive sleep apnea. Methods and feasibility. Am Rev Respir Dis 130:1152, 1984.

Roberts JL, Reed WR, Mathew OP, et al.: Assessment of pharyngeal airway stability in normal and micrognathic infants. J Appl Physiol 58:290, 1985.

Rowland TW, Nordstrom LG, Bean MS, et al.: Chronic upper airway obstruction and pulmonary hypertension in Down's syndrome. Am J Dis Child 135:1050, 1981.

Sullivan CE, Berthon-Jones M, Issa FG, et al.: Reversal of obstructive sleep apnoea by continuous positive airway pressure applied through the nares. Lancet 1:862, 1981.

Weinberg S, Kravath R, Phillips L, et al.: Episodic complete airway obstruction in children with undiagnosed obstructive sleep apnea. Anesthesiology 60:356, 1984.

Management of the Difficult Pediatric Airway and Intubation

Alfery DD, Ward CF, Harwood IR, et al.: Airway management for a neonate with congenital fusion of the jaws. Anesthesiology 51:340, 1979.

Borland LM, Swan DM, Leff S: Difficult pediatric endotracheal intubation: a new approach to the retrograde technique. Anesthesiology 55:577, 1981.

Bourke D, Levesque PR: Modification of retrograde guide for endotracheal intubation. Anesth Analg 53:1013, 1974.

Brown AC, Sataloff T: Special anesthetic techniques in head and neck surgery. Otolaryngol Clin North Am 14:587, 1981.

Burtner DD, Goodman M: Anesthetic and operative management of potential upper airway obstruction: Arch Otolaryngol 104:657, 1978.

Chatterji S, Gupta NR, Mishra TR: Valvular glottic obstruction following extubation. Anaesthesia 39:246, 1984.

Fan LL, Flynn JW: Laryngoscopy in neonates and infants: experience with the flexible fiberoptic bronchoscope. Laryngoscope 91:451, 1981.

Handler SD, Keon TP: Difficult laryngoscopy/intubation: the child with mandibular hypoplasia. Ann Otol Rhinol Laryngol 92:401, 1983.

Hemmer D, Lee T, Wright BD: Intubation of a child with a cervical spine injury with the aid of a fiberoptic bronchoscope. Anaesth Intens Care 10:163, 1982.

Hensinger RN, MacEwen GD: Congenital anomalies of the spine. In Rothman RH, Simeone FA (Eds.): The Spine. Philadelphia, W.B. Saunders Co., 1982.

Hudon F: Intubation without laryngoscopy. Anesthesiology 6:476, 1945.

Katz RL, Berci G: The optical stylet—a new intubation technique for adults and children with specific reference to teaching. Anesthesiology 51:251, 1979.

Manchibanti L, Kraus J, Edds S: Cimetidine and related drugs in anesthesia. Anesth Analg 61:595, 1982.

Miller RA: A new laryngoscope. Anesthesiology 2:317, 1941.

Miyabe M, Dohi S, Homma E: Tracheal intubation in an infant with Treacher-Collins syndrome—pulling out the tongue by a forceps. Anesthesiology 62:213, 1985.

Nichol HC, Zuck D: Difficult laryngoscopy—the "anterior" larynx and the atlanto-occipital gap. Br J Anaesth 55:141, 1983.

Populaire C, Lundi JN, Pinaud M: Elective tracheal intubation in the prone position for a neonate with Pierre Robin syndrome. Anesthesiology 62:214, 1985.

Salem MR, Mathrubhutham M, Bennet EJ: Difficult intubation. N Engl J Med 295:879, 1976.

Seraj MA, Yousif M, Channa AB: Anaesthetic management of congenital fusion of the jaws in a neonate. Anaesthesia 39:695, 1984.

Stiles CM: A flexible fiberoptic bronchoscope for endotracheal intubation of infants. Anesth Analg 53:1017, 1974.

Stone DJ, Stirt JA, Kaplan MJ, et al.: A complication of lightwand-guided nasotracheal intubation. Anesthesiology 61:780, 1984.

Watson CB, Clapham M: Transillumination for correct tube positioning: use of a new fiberoptic endotracheal tube. Anesthesiology 60:253, 1984.

White A, Kander PL: Anatomical factors in difficult direct laryngoscopy. Br J Anaesth 47:468, 1975.

10 || OPHTHALMOLOGICAL DISEASES

NANCY KNUTSEN FRANCE, M.D.

Congenital Cataracts
Effects of Anesthetic Drugs and
   Techniques on Intraocular Pressure
Penetrating Trauma of the Globe

Glaucoma
Retinoblastoma
Retinopathy of Prematurity
Retinal Detachment

Anesthetic considerations specific to pediatric eye surgery are the same for both normal children and those with syndromes of congenital abnormalities. For example, maintaining stable intraocular pressure (see the sections on Congenital Cataracts, Penetrating Trauma, and Glaucoma later in this chapter) and an awareness of the potential for eliciting the oculocardiac reflex (see the section on Retinoblastoma) are important concerns for the anesthesiologist with *all* pediatric patients.

Frequently, however, children with uncommon diseases and congenital abnormalities have a disproportionate number of ophthalmic lesions requiring surgery. In formulating a preoperative anesthetic plan for such children, the anesthesiologist must be aware of any associated systemic abnormalities apart from the eye lesion. Table 10–1, designed to provide a handy reference for the anesthesiologist, outlines ocular lesions associated with pediatric syndromes and the manifestations of these syndromes, including associated systemic disorders, and highlights the major anesthesia concerns. It is beyond the scope of this table to elaborate on details of anesthesia for multisystem anomalies, although a few are listed. One frequent problem is upper airway deformity leading to a difficult or impossible intubation, especially in cases of craniofacial anomalies. In such cases, topical anesthesia followed by an awake intubation, either blind or with the aid of a small-diameter fiberoptic bronchoscope, is often required.

The purpose of this chapter is to inform the anesthesiologist of the surgical approach and anesthetic concerns related to the relatively uncommon pediatric ocular lesions. The more common lesions such as strabismus or lacrimal duct probe are amply described elsewhere.

CONGENITAL CATARACTS

Clouding of the crystalline lens of the eye is termed a cataract. Congenital cataracts of sufficient size or density severely limit retinal stimulation and restrict development of vision. Cataracts never regress; therefore, early identification and treatment is necessary.[1]

The most effective treatment of bilateral complete congenital cataracts is surgical removal as early in life as possible. A unilateral complete congenital cataract also should be removed in the neonatal period to prevent severe deprivation amblyopia and a poor visual outcome. These conditions are likely to develop when surgery is delayed beyond 6 months of age.[1, 2]

Approximately 50 percent of congenital cataracts are idiopathic. The remainder are associated with various pediatric syndromes including inborn errors of metabolism, chromosomal disorders, intrauterine infections, trauma that ruptures the lens capsule, or drugs (for example, corticosteroids)[1–3] (see Table 10–1). At least 30 percent of children with congenital cataracts have an associated nonocular anomaly of another organ system;[1] cardiac anomalies, as commonly occur in the congenital rubella syndrome and Down syndrome, are of particular concern to the anesthesiologist.

Lenses that become malpositioned owing to dislocation or subluxation, as seen in Marfan syndrome and homocystinuria (80 percent and 100 percent of patients, respectively) require similar surgical removal[1] (Table 10–2).

Anterior chamber aspiration of the lens is performed using an operating microscope and a mechanical suction–cutting instrument. An optimal surgical field requires an immobile, maximally dilated pupil for observation of the red reflex to assure complete removal of lens material.[2]

A gravity infusion of 1:200,000 epinephrine in saline via a small needle inserted into the anterior chamber will immediately induce dilatation of the iris and intense vasoconstriction, which presumably also delays absorption of intraocular epinephrine. Simultaneous with the epinephrine infusion, a second motorized cutting needle is placed in the anterior chamber for aspiration of its contents along with a considerable volume of the epinephrine-saline solution.[2] The total volume of epinephrine infusion required varies considerably from patient to patient and depends on the duration of the procedure and on fluid losses from needle sites in the anterior chamber.

The arrhythmogenic potential of systemically absorbed epinephrine in the child receiving a potent inhalation anesthetic is a very real concern to the anesthesiologist. Compared with adults, children ap-

272

Text continued on page 278

Table 10–1. OCULAR SURGICAL LESIONS IN PEDIATRIC SYNDROMES

Disorder	Inheritance	Defect	Surgical Lesions	Manifestations	Anesthesia Concerns
Chromosomal Aberrations					
Numerical Abnormalities					
Trisomy 13 (Patau syndrome)	Sporadic; rarely inherited as translocation	Trisomy of chromosome 13	Cataracts, glaucoma, retinal detachment	Cleft lip/palate; digital abnormalities; CHD; arhinencephaly; MR; hypotonia; low-set ears; deafness; high infant mortality (18% survive first year); surgical therapy probably not indicated	
Trisomy 18 (Edwards syndrome)	Sporadic; rarely inherited as translocation	Trisomy of chromosome 18	Cataracts, glaucoma, ptosis	MR; microcephaly; digital, central venous, and renal abnormalities; rocker-bottom feet; apneic spells; micrognathia; majority die before 1 year	Difficult intubation; CHD precautions; caution with renally excreted drugs
Trisomy 21 (Down syndrome)	Sporadic; 5% familial translocation	Trisomy of chromosome 21	Cataracts, strabismus	Mental and physical retardation; hypotonia; chronic infections; partial upper airway obstruction during sleep; characteristic facies; atlanto-occipital instability or dislocation; CHD: endocardial cushion defect, ventricular septal defect, PDA, tetralogy of Fallot, ± pulmonary vascular disease	Standard doses of atropine; heavy sedation pre- or postop likely to accentuate airway obstruction and hypoventilation; cannulation may be difficult owing to hypoplastic peripheral vessels; small subglottic area—choose endotracheal tube that allows air leak with ventilation; gentle manipulation of cervical spine during laryngoscopy; blood pressure significantly lower than normal; ketamine, inhalation agents satisfactory; CHD precautions
"Cat eye" syndrome		Extra acrocentric chromosome	Cataracts	Imperforate anus; variable renal, central venous, and digital anomalies; micrognathia; MR; iris resembles the cat's vertical pupil	Difficult intubation
Cornelia de Lange syndrome	Unknown	Small % chromosomal aberrations	Ptosis, strabismus	Short stature; MR; microcephaly; hirsutism and bushy eyebrows; weak cry; malformed hands and feet	
Fanconi syndrome with pancytopenia	Autosomal recessive	High % of chromated breaks and unusual chromosomal alignments	Strabismus, ptosis	Microcephaly and short stature; MR; pigmentation of skin; absence of radii and thumbs; pancytopenia; leukemia frequently occurs	Severe anemia, leukopenia—Rx with blood transfusions and androgenic steroids
Prader-Willi syndrome	Unknown	Occasional chromosome 15 abnormalities	Strabismus	Uncontrollable hyperphagia; small, obese stature; MR; hypotonia; cryptorchidism; ± diabetes	Monitor for hypoglycemia—Rx glucose infusion; extreme obesity may impair ventilation postop.
Structural Abnormalities					
Deletion 4p− (Wolf-Hirschorn syndrome)	Sporadic or may be familial	Deletion (4p−)	Strabismus, cataracts	MR; seizures; cleft lip/palate; deformed nose; hydrocephalus	
Deletion 5p− (Cri-du-chat)	Sporadic, may be familial	Deletion (5p−)	Cataracts, strabismus	Cat-like cry secondary to abnormal larynx; cleft lip/palate; microcephaly; micrognathia; ± CHD; hypotonia; MR	Airway stridor due to laryngomalacia; difficult intubation; CHD precautions
Deletion 11p−	Sporadic or familial translocation	Deletion (11p−)	Glaucoma, cataracts	Aniridia; MR; genitourinary anomalies; associated with Wilms tumor	± Hypertension—Rx with hydralazine and propranolol; avoid ketamine
Deletion 13q−	Sporadic or familial translocation	Deletion (13q−)	Cataract, retinoblastoma, strabismus, ptosis	Microcephaly; micrognathia; MR; hypospadias	Avoid ketamine
Deletion 18p−	Sporadic, occasional familial translocation	Deletion (18p−)	Ptosis, strabismus	Microcephaly; MR; webbed neck; immunoglobulin abnormalities; diabetes; thyroiditis; severe form has cyclopia	
Deletion 18q−	Sporadic, occasional familial translocation	Deletion (18q−)	Cataracts	Microcephaly; midface hypoplasia; carp-like mouth; deafness; abnormalities of hands and feet	
Sex Chromosomes					
Turner syndrome (Monosomy X)	Sporadic	XO (80% have 45 chromosomes, a single X, no sex chromatin) XO/XX mosaics	Strabismus, ptosis, cataracts	Sexual infantilism; short stature; webbed neck; small mandible; cubitus valgus; coarctation of aorta; dissecting aneurysm of aorta; autoimmune disease (diabetes and thyroiditis); recurrent ear infections	± Hypertension secondary to coarctation of aorta; avoid ketamine
Klinefelter syndrome	Sporadic	XXY XXXY XXXXY XXYY XYY (for chromatin positive)	Strabismus, retinal detachment, dislocation of lens	± MR; scoliosis; microcephaly; CHD; gynecomastia; prognathism; tall stature; aggressive or bizarre behavior; hypogenitalism; increasing X chromosomes associated with mental and physical impairment	

Table continued on following page

Table 10–1. OCULAR SURGICAL LESIONS IN PEDIATRIC SYNDROMES *Continued*

Disorder	Inheritance	Defect	Surgical Lesions	Manifestations	Anesthesia Concerns
Defects of Lipid Metabolism					
Familial Hypolipoproteinemia					
Bassen-Kornzweig syndrome (Abetalipoproteinemia)	Autosomal recessive	Absent betalipoprotein	Retinal abnormalities, strabismus, ptosis	Spinocerebellar degeneration with ataxia; steatorrhea; acanthocytes; vitamin A deficiency	
Tangier disease (Analphalipoproteinemia)	Autosomal recessive	Deficiency of high-density lipoprotein	Corneal haziness	Accumulation of cholesterol esters in RE system (large orange tonsils, hepatosplenomegaly); peripheral neuropathy and muscle wasting; anemia and thrombocytopenia; premature coronary disease; decreased plasma cholesterol and phospholipids	Check hemoglobin and platelets
Lipoidoses					
Gaucher disease I, II, III	Autosomal recessive	Defect in glucocerebrosidase; ceramide glucosidase accumulates	Corneal opacities, strabismus	Hepatosplenomegaly; hypersplenism and abnormal bruising; elevated serum acid phosphatase; bone pain, joint swelling, and fractures; chronic lung disease secondary to aspiration; spasticity; tremors; failure to thrive; progressive dementia	Anemia and coagulation disorders second to platelet deficiency
Fabry disease (angiokeratoma corporis diffusum)	X-linked recessive	Deficiency of ceramide trihexosidase	Corneal dystrophy, cataracts	Lipid deposition in blood causes painful extremities and dark purple maculopapular eruption; edema of legs and face; hypertension; progressive renal failure; myocardial ischemia and premature death in adult	Cardiac and renal function compromised
Gangliosidoses					
Tay-Sachs disease (GM2 type I) (infantile cerebromacular degeneration)	Autosomal recessive	Deficiency of hexosaminidase A	Optic atrophy, blindness	Begins 6–12 mos.—death by 3 years; dementia; hypotonia; hyperacusis; visceromegaly; spastic paralysis; seizures	Neurological deficit leads to respiratory disability
Refsum syndrome (heredopathia atactica polyneuritiformis)	Autosomal recessive	Deficiency of phytanic acid alpha-hydroxylase	Optic nerve atrophy, cataracts, glaucoma	Peripheral polyneuropathy; ichthyosis; limb weakness; nerve deafness; cerebellar ataxia; ECG changes and premature death in adulthood	
Familial cerebrotendinous xanthomatosis	Autosomal recessive	Increased serum cholestanol	Cataracts	Cerebellar ataxia; enlargement of tendons	
Defects of Amino Acid Metabolism					
Albinism 1. Oculocutaneous 2. Ocular	1. Autosomal recessive 2. X-linked	Defect in converting tyrosine to melanin	Strabismus	Hypopigmentation; increased susceptibility to skin neoplasia	
Cystinosis (Fanconi syndrome with renal tubular defects)	Autosomal recessive	Enzyme defect unknown	Corneal transplant (benign or adult form)	Deposition of cystine in RE system, renal tubular cells, and cornea; small stature; aminoaciduria; renal tubular acidosis; hypophosphatemic rickets; nephrotic syndrome and renal failure (benign form, kidneys spared)	Monitor acid-base and electrolytes Caution when using renally excreted drugs
Homocystinuria	Autosomal recessive	Deficiency of cystathionine B synthase	Dislocated lens, secondary glaucoma, strabismus, retinal detachment	MR; seizures; marfanoid habitus; osteoporosis; thromboembolic episodes secondary to platelet adhesiveness	Preop correction of platelet function; maintain hydration and peripheral perfusion
Alkaptonuria and ochronosis	Autosomal recessive	Deficiency of homogentisic acid oxidase	Scleral pigmentation	Renal calculi; osteoarthritis; valvular heart disease and atherosclerosis; black urine on standing secondary to homogentisic acid	Cardiac and renal precautions
Hyperlysinemia	Autosomal recessive	Deficiency of lysine ketoglutarate reductase	Subluxation of lens, strabismus	Lax ligaments; hypotonic muscles; seizures; hyperlysinemia and lysinuria	
Defects of Carbohydrate Metabolism					
Galactosemia	Autosomal recessive	1. Deficiency of galactose-1-phosphate uridyl transferase	Cataracts	Galactosemia and galactosuria; hepatosplenomegaly; hepatic failure and jaundice; MR; vomiting and failure to thrive; Rx eliminate galactose from diet	

Table continued on opposite page

Table 10–1. OCULAR SURGICAL LESIONS IN PEDIATRIC SYNDROMES *Continued*

Disorder	Inheritance	Defect	Surgical Lesions	Manifestations	Anesthesia Concerns
Defects of Carbohydrate Metabolism *Continued*					
		2. Deficiency of galacto-kinase	Cataracts	More benign; galactosuria and galactosemia; Rx eliminate galactose from diet	
Mucopolysaccharidoses (Types I–VII)	All autosomal recessive except Hunter syndrome, which is X-linked recessive	Defects in lysosomal acid hydrolases	Cloudy cornea, retinal changes, glaucoma	Variable changes depending on type—coarse facies, short neck, hepatosplenomegaly, dwarfism, stiff joints, cardiac involvement, respiratory disability	Upper airway obstruction Difficult intubation
Hurler syndrome (gargoylism)	Autosomal recessive	Deficiency of L-iduronidase	Cloudy cornea, ptosis, strabismus, glaucoma	Deposition of acid mucopolysaccharide in every system of body; MR; large head; short neck; coarse features; dwarfism; kyphoscoliosis; hepatosplenomegaly; myocardial and valvular infiltration cause angina, myocardial infarction, CHF; respiratory difficulties: infections, abnormal tracheobronchial cartilages, large tongue, infiltration of lymphoid tissue of larynx and lungs; most die by 10 years of age	Upper airway obstruction; difficult intubation; CHF; arrhythmias, postop respiratory difficulties
Glycogen storage disease (Von Gierke disease) unknown (hepatorenal glycogenosis type I)		Deficiency of glucose-6-phosphatase	Macular lesions	Hepatosplenomegaly; renal hyperplasia; poor muscular development; macroglossia; hypoglycemia; lactic acidosis; hyperlipemia; dwarfism; bleeding diathesis with thrombocytosis	Dehydration and acidosis—monitor acid base; fasting blood glucose very low—maintain at physiologic levels
Glucose-6-phosphate dehydrogenase (G-6-PD) deficiency (Favism)	X-linked recessive	Deficiency of glucose-6-phosphate dehydrogenase	Cataracts, vitreous hemorrhage	Fava bean, sulfonamides, antimalarials, and phenacetin induce an acute hemolytic anemia	
Defects of Metal Metabolism					
Wilson disease (hepatolenticular degeneration)	Autosomal recessive	Deficiency of serum ceruloplasmin	Kayser-Fleischer rings of cornea; "sunflower" cataracts	Copper accumulation in liver, brain, kidney, and cornea; degeneration of lenticular nucleus and basal ganglia; hepatic cirrhosis and jaundice; malabsorption syndrome; renal tubular damage and aminoaciduria	Treatment with penicillamine (copper chelator which lowers body content of copper); anemia; anesthetic compatible with hepatic and renal failure
CNS Disorders					
Marinesco-Sjögren syndrome	Autosomal recessive		Cataracts, strabismus	Oligophrenia and spinocerebellar ataxia; MR	
Sjögren syndrome	Autosomal recessive		Cataracts	Oligophrenia	
Meckel syndrome	Autosomal recessive		Cataracts	Occipital encephalocele; polycystic kidneys; polydactyly; CHD; abnormal genitalia	
Musculoskeletal Disease					
Chondrodysplasia punctata	Autosomal recessive and autosomal dominant	Bone dysplasia	Cataracts	Bone dysplasia; joint contractures; calcification of tracheal cartilages; recessive form lethal in 1st year of life	
Myotonic dystrophy (Steinert disease)	Autosomal dominant	Muscle defect	Ptosis, cataracts, strabismus	Myotonia with muscle atrophy and weakness; conduction defects and arrhythmias; impaired ventilation, frequent aspiration and pneumonia; hypogonadism	Can induce myotonia with succinylcholine, neostigmine, halothane; jaw easily dislocated; sensitive to respiratory depressants—anticipate postop pulmonary problems; regional or local anesthesia preferred
Albright hereditary osteodystrophy	Autosomal dominant	Skeletal dysplasia	Cataracts	Skeletal dysplasia; obesity; MR; intracranial and subcutaneous calcifications; neuromuscular problems and seizures	
1. Pseudohypoparathyroidism (PH) 2. Pseudo-pseudohypoparathyroidism (PPH)				1. Hypocalcemic 2. Normocalcemia	Hypocalcemia with possible cardiac conduction defects, neuromuscular problems; avoid relaxants
Stickler syndrome (progressive arthro-ophthalmomyopathy)	Autosomal dominant		Cataracts, retinal detachment, glaucoma	Tall; joint laxity with arthritis; cleft palate; kyphoscoliosis; deafness; micrognathia; flat facies	Difficult intubation
Robert syndrome	Autosomal recessive		Cataracts	Tetraphocomelia; cleft lip/palate	

Table continued on following page

Table 10–1. OCULAR SURGICAL LESIONS IN PEDIATRIC SYNDROMES *Continued*

Disorder	Inheritance	Defect	Surgical Lesions	Manifestations	Anesthesia Concerns
Musculoskeletal Diseases *Continued*					
Marfan syndrome	Autosomal dominant	Connective tissue degeneration of the elastic lamellae	Subluxation of lens, glaucoma, retinal detachment, strabismus	Arachnodactyly; hyperextensibility; hypotonia; scoliosis; hernias; aortic aneurysm; aortic valve insufficiency; mitral valve prolapse	± Propranolol therapy
Weill-Marchesani syndrome	Autosomal recessive	Connective tissue disorder	Dislocation of lens, secondary to glaucoma	Brachydactyly; short stature; stiff immobile joints; ± cardiac anomalies	
Ehlers-Danlos syndrome (7 forms)	Autosomal dominant Also recessive Also X-linked	Connective tissue disorder; deficiency of protocollagen lysyl hydroxylase	Subluxation of lens, keratoconus, glaucoma, retinal detachment	Hyperextensibility of joints and skin; easy bruisability; wide nasal bridge; gastrointestinal bleeding; kyphoscoliosis; dissecting aortic aneurysm; mitral valve prolapse; conduction defects; hernias	Avoid trauma to skin, eyes, joints; difficult to maintain IV routes; adequate vascular access; risk of excessive bleeding; potential for spontaneous pneumothorax
Bird-headed dwarfism (Seckel syndrome)	Autosomal recessive		Strabismus	Microcephaly; prominent nose; intrauterine growth retardation; short stature; MR	
Klippel-Feil syndrome	Autosomal dominant, ? autosomal recessive		Strabismus	Congenital fusion of cervical vertebrae, especially synostosis of atlas and axis; short neck, immobile, often torticollis; spastic paraplegia; deafness; ± MR	Difficult intubation
Mieten syndrome	Autosomal recessive		Strabismus	MR; small stature; short forearms, dislocation of radius with flexion contracture elbow	
Spondyloepiphyseal dysplasia, congenital (pseudoachondroplasia)	Autosomal dominant		Retinal detachment, cataracts	Short trunk and limbs; deformity of sternum, hands and feet; skeletal abnormalities of vertebral column and hips; deafness	
Thrombocytopenia—absent radius syndrome	Autosomal recessive		Strabismus	Thrombocytopenia, ± eosinophilia; absence or hypoplasia of radius; ± CHD; 35% die in 1st year of life of intracranial hemorrhage	Platelet transfusion pre- and intraop
Renal Diseases					
Lowe syndrome (Oculocerebrorenal syndrome)	X-linked recessive		Cataracts, glaucoma, strabismus	MR; hypotonia; renal tubular dysfunction with hyperchloremic acidosis; aminoaciduria; osteoporosis; renal rickets; seizures	Rx large doses Vit D, Ca, Na supplements; monitor acid base, electrolytes, calcium; caution with renally excreted drugs
Alport syndrome (hereditary nephritis with deafness and ocular abnormalities)	X-linked recessive or ? Autosomal dominant		Cataracts, retinal detachment	Sensorineural deafness; glomerulopathy and chronic renal failure	Caution with renally excreted drugs
Cerebrohepatorenal syndrome (Zellweger syndrome)	Autosomal recessive		Glaucoma, cataracts	Mental and growth retardation; flat facies; hepatomegaly; polycystic kidneys and albuminuria; hypotonia; PDA; hypospadias; calcific deposits in long bones; death in early infancy	Rx hypoprothrombinemia; caution with renally excreted drugs
Hartnup disease	Autosomal recessive	Defect in transport of tryptophan by intestinal mucosa and renal tubules	Strabismus	Aminoaciduria; photosensitive skin and pellagra-like skin rash; ataxia; mental deterioration; excess urinary indole excretion; Rx with nicotinamide and high-protein diets	
Dermatological Disorders					
Cockayne syndrome	Autosomal recessive		Cataracts	Dwarfism with prognathism; MR; deafness; thick skull bones; hepatosplenomegaly; photosensitive dermatitis; premature senility	
Rothmund-Thomson syndrome (poikiloderma atrophicans vasculare)	Autosomal recessive		Cataracts	Atrophic telangiectatic dermatosis; sparse hair; defective dentition; congenital bone defects; hypogenitalism	
Bloch-Sulzberger syndrome (incontinentia pigmenti)	X-linked dominant (lethal in male)	Mesenchymal and ectodermal defect	Cataracts, strabismus	Generalized ectodermal dysplasia; bullous eruptions; hyperpigmentation; hypoplasia of dentition; MR; skeletal abnormalities; microcephaly; ± cardiac abnormalities	

Table continued on opposite page

Table 10–1. OCULAR SURGICAL LESIONS IN PEDIATRIC SYNDROMES *Continued*

Disorder	Inheritance	Defect	Surgical Lesions	Manifestations	Anesthesia Concerns
Dermatological Disorders *Continued*					
Goltz syndrome (focal dermal hypoplasia)	Unknown	Mesenchymal and ectodermal defect	Strabismus	Areas of hypoplasia and altered pigmentation of skin; dystrophic nails; enamel hypoplasia; syndactyly; multiple papillomas of mucous membranes and skin; occurs mainly in females	Airway may contain papillomas
Histiocytic dermatoarthritis	Autosomal dominant		Glaucoma, cataracts	Histiocytic nodules on face, hands, feet; seronegative arthritis; bony resorption of hands, wrists	
Ataxia-telangiectasia (Louis-Bar syndrome)	Autosomal recessive	Probable thymus dysfunction	Strabismus	Cutaneous telangiectasia of ears, cheeks, antecubital space; cerebellar ataxia; deficiency of IgA; lymphoreticular malignancy; recurrent sinopulmonary infections (bronchiectasis); anemia; MR	Correct anemia; anesthesia for chronic lung disease; reverse isolation techniques
Ichthyosis					
Ichthyosis vulgaris	Autosomal dominant	Abnormal stratum corneum	Cataracts	Skin changes appear after 3 mos. of life (mildest form); dryness; keratosis pilaris, increased markings on palmar and plantar skin	
Congenital ichthyosis (harlequin fetus)	Autosomal recessive	Abnormal stratum corneum	Cataracts	Hyperkeratosis with thick scaly skin and hyperhidrosis (lethal in neonatal period)	
Ichthyosis and cataracts	Autosomal recessive	Abnormal stratum corneum	Cataracts	Same as congenital ichthyosis	
Oculocerebral syndrome with keratosis follicularis and aminoaciduria	X-linked		Cataracts, glaucoma	Keratosis follicularis; aminoaciduria; alopecia; MR	
Hamartoses (Abnormal Mixtures of Normal Tissues)					
Sturge-Weber syndrome (encephalotrigeminal angiomatosis)	Unknown		Glaucoma when hemangioma involves lid or conjunctiva	Flat facial hemangioma (usually unilateral), 5th cranial nerve distribution; meningeal hemangiomas; seizures; paresis; mental deficiency, cerebral calcifications	Angioma may involve airway
Klippel-Trenaunay-Weber (giant hemangioma with localized hypertrophy or gigantism)	Unknown		Glaucoma when hemangioma involves lid or conjunctiva	Similar to Sturge-Weber syndrome, except hemangioma also affects body and limbs with hypertrophy of one or more limbs; varicose veins	
Von Recklinghausen syndrome (neurofibromatosis)	Autosomal dominant		Glaucoma	Multiple neurofibromas in skin and meninges; café-au-lait spots; skeletal defects; scoliosis; neurological symptoms with involvement of cranial or spinal nerve roots	Hypertension may indicate pheochromocytoma
Oculodermal melanocytosis (nevus of Ota)	Sporadic		Glaucoma	Unilateral ocular melanocytosis; increased pigmentation of lids and periorbital skin	
Basal cell nevus (carcinoma) syndrome	Autosomal dominant		Glaucoma, strabismus, cataracts	Multiple cutaneous nevoid basal cell carcinomas; cysts of mandible; scoliosis; intracranial calcifications; mental deficiency	
Craniofacial Malformations					
Hallermann-Streiff syndrome (oculomandibulo) or François syndrome	Autosomal dominant or sporadic		Cataracts, strabismus	Dyscephaly; mandibular and malar hypoplasia; small mouth; faulty dentition; atrophy of skin and hypotrichosis; dwarf stature; limitation of mouth opening secondary to maldevelopment of temporomandibular joint	
Rubinstein-Taybi syndrome	Unknown ? recessive	Unknown ? small Chromosomal abnormality	Cataracts, glaucoma, ptosis, strabismus	Broad thumbs and toes; beaked nose; MR; antimongoloid slant of eyelids; very short stature; may have vertebral, cardiac, renal abnormalities	Cardiac (pulmonary stenosis) and renal compromise
Smith-Lemli-Opitz syndrome	Autosomal recessive		Ptosis, cataracts, strabismus	Microcephaly; micrognathia; hypotonia; pyloric stenosis; MR; hypospadias and cryptorchidism; syndactyly	Difficult intubation

Table continued on following page

Table 10–1. OCULAR SURGICAL LESIONS IN PEDIATRIC SYNDROMES *Continued*

Disorder	Inheritance	Defect	Surgical Lesions	Manifestations	Anesthesia Concerns
Craniofacial Malformations *Continued*					
Marshall syndrome (? synonymous with Stickler syndrome)	Autosomal dominant		Cataracts	Saddle nose; sensorineural deafness	
Cerebro-oculo-facial–skeletal (COFS) syndrome	Autosomal recessive	Degenerative disorder	Cataracts, blepharophimosis	Hypotonia; microcephaly; micrognathia; flexion contractures; death common in first few years of life	
Möbius syndrome	Autosomal dominant	Cranial nerve palsy VI and VII, bilateral	Strabismus, ptosis	Deafness; muscular weakness of tongue, neck, and chest; immobility (palsy) of face; difficulty chewing and swallowing	
Crouzon disease (craniofacial dysostosis) (Apert syndrome is a manifestation of greater expressivity and penetrance)	Autosomal dominant	Defect unknown	Cataracts, strabismus, tarsorrhaphy	Craniofacial dysostosis; deafness; beaked nose; hypoplastic maxilla; hypertelorism and proptosis; soft palate against posterior pharyngeal wall, mouth breathing necessary; syndactyly associated with Apert syndrome	Difficult intubation; upper airway obstruction
Pierre Robin syndrome	? Autosomal dominant	1st and 2nd arch syndrome	Cataracts, glaucoma, retinal detachment, strabismus	Micrognathia with glossoptosis and cleft palate; upper airway obstruction and swallowing difficulties	Upper airway obstruction; difficult intubation
Goldenhar syndrome (oculoauriculovertebral syndrome)	Sporadic	Anomalies of development of 1st and 2nd branchial arches	Glaucoma, cataracts, strabismus	Bulbar dermoids or lipodermoids; ± cleft lip/palate; ± CHD; deafness; malar and manidibular hypoplasia; malformed low-set ear; hypoplasia of cervical vertebrae; condition usually unilateral	Difficult intubation
Oculodento-digital syndrome	Unknown		Glaucoma	Hypoplastic tooth enamel; abnormal digits; ± cleft lip/palate; deafness; hip dislocation	
Rieger syndrome	Autosomal dominant		Glaucoma	Hypodontia; malar hypoplasia; myotonic dystrophy; MR; hypertelorism	
Axenfeld syndrome and Peter anomaly			Glaucoma	Similar to Rieger syndrome, probably represents a different manifestation of same dysgenetic defect	
Miscellaneous Disorders					
Kartagener syndrome	Autosomal recessive		Cataract	Dextrocardia; bronchiectasis and sinusitis; dysfunctional cilia; heart block; male sterility	Anesthesia for chronic pulmonary disease
Laurence-Moon syndrome	Autosomal recessive		Strabismus	Hypogenitalism; MR; spastic paraplegia; ± CHD and renal abnormalities; retinitis pigmentosa	Precautions if cardiac or renal abnormalities present
Werner syndrome	Autosomal recessive		Cataracts	Retinitis pigmentosa; arrest of growth at puberty; ± MR scleroderma-like changes; premature graying, alopecia; arteriosclerosis; hypogonadism; diabetes	Manage as for atherosclerotic heart disease and diabetes
Hypercalcemia (Williams syndrome)	Unknown		Strabismus	Elfin facies; supravalvular aortic stenosis; hypercalcemia in infancy, dental abnormalities	Monitor serum calcium; avoid cardiac depressants if fixed cardiac output, left ventricular failure and myocardial ischemia, cardiac surgery; correction must precede eye surgery

CHD = congenital heart disease; MR = mental retardation; PDA = patent ductus arteriosus; RE = reticuloendothelial; CHF = congestive heart failure.
Data from references 96 to 103.

pear to have a higher threshold to and lower incidence of dysrhythmias induced by exogenous epinephrine during halothane anesthesia.[5–9] However, studies determining the upper limit of subcutaneously injected epinephrine compatible with halothane cannot necessarily be applied to the absorption of intraocular epinephrine. Measurements of systemic epinephrine levels in children have not been reported during this infusion technique, and there are no reports of adverse dysrhythmias with intraocular epinephrine infusion under anesthesia.[10, 11] Nevertheless, caution is war-

ranted and halothane may be avoided in favor of less arrythmogenic agents, such as isoflurane, ethrane, or a narcotic-relaxant combination.[5]

EFFECTS OF ANESTHETIC DRUGS AND TECHNIQUES ON INTRAOCULAR PRESSURE

Maintaining a near-normal intraocular pressure (IOP) throughout surgery is essential to prevent loss of vitreous or intraocular contents associated with elevated IOP in the surgically opened eye. IOP is determined by the balance between aqueous humor formation and drainage in the anterior segment of the eye. The most important determinant of IOP is the systemic central venous pressure; it is reflected in the periocular venous system, which receives both blood and aqueous humor drainage from the eye. A sudden explosive Valsalva maneuver or cough immediately raises the central venous pressure, retards drainage of aqueous humor into the venous plexus, increases the intraocular blood volume, and markedly elevates the intraocular pressure.[12] An adequate depth of anesthesia until the last suture has closed the open wound is the best protection against such an unfortunate occurrence. If necessary, a nondepolarizing muscle relaxant can be used to immobilize the patient. If the child unexpectedly moves in response to surgical stimulation, immediate and rapid administration of thiopental will quiet the patient. In this instance, succinylcholine should be avoided as it will acutely raise the IOP owing to its unique effect of tonic contracture of the extraocular muscles.[13]

All of the central nervous system depressants in the anesthesiologist's armamentarium tend to decrease intraocular pressure and are, therefore, all acceptable agents in intraocular surgery.[14-19] Similarly the nondepolarizing muscle relaxants, atropine premedication, alteration in arterial blood pressure, and modest variations in P_{CO_2} have minimal or no effect on IPO.[13, 18, 20-23] Studies of ketamine effects on the normal eye have shown conflicting results of either elevated or unchanged IOP; it should be used cautiously if at all in the open eye.[24-27]

Succinylcholine, although contraindicated when the eye is surgically open, may be used during the early induction and intubation period. The transiently increased IOP returns to baseline within 5 minutes of intravenous succinylcholine, presumably by autoregulation with increased outflow of aqueous humor; however, the tonic contracture of the extraocular muscles persists for up to 15 to 20 minutes.[13] In theory, the continued contracture and pull of the extraocular muscles on the sclera may cause the ocular contents to be expelled upon incision into the globe. In practice, however, succinylcholine has been widely used to facilitate laryngoscopy without documented increased hazard during cataract surgery.

Many of the patients presenting for congenital cataract aspiration are infants—term or premature—in the first few days of life. An effective and safe anesthetic technique for the neonate includes fentanyl (5 μg/kg) and pancuronium (0.06 mg/kg) or atracurium (0.4 mg/kg), titrated and reversed with the aid of ulnar nerve stimulation. The potential for hyperoxia-induced retinopathy of prematurity dictates maintenance of an arterial oxygen tension less than 100 torr in the premature; monitoring transcutaneous oxygen tension or hemoglobin saturation is very helpful in determining safe concentrations of nitrous oxide and oxygen to be administered.[28-33]

Avoiding prolonged periods of high inspired oxygen in the full-term neonate is recommended because of variations in retinal maturation until 44 weeks postconceptional age.[34]

Postoperatively, it is desirable to have a quiet, drowsy patient and to again minimize large swings in venous pressure and IOP. The very young infant who has received a narcotic-balanced combination of anesthetics will continue to have residual sedation in the recovery room, but the older infant or child who

Table 10–2. ECTOPIA LENTIS REQUIRING SURGICAL REMOVAL

	Abnormalities of Eye	Abnormalities of Skeleton	Abnormalities of Central Venous System	Therapy
Marfan syndrome	Lens subluxated or dislocated (also glaucoma, retinal detachment, strabismus)	Arachnodactyly; tall, slender build; kyphosis; scoliosis; chest deformities; muscles flaccid with joint hyperextensibility	Aneurysm of ascending aorta; aortic or mitral regurgitation; mitral valve prolapse	Propranolol (? retard aortic dilation) Antibiotic prophylaxis (Not necessary for eye surgery, for intubation)
Homocystinuria	Lens dislocated (also glaucoma, retinal detachment, strabismus)	Marfanoid habitus; osteoporosis	Thromboembolic lesions	Pyridoxine (vitamin B_6)
			Deficiency of cystathionine-beta-synthase	Dipyridamole (anti-platelet utilization)
			Homocystine irritates vascular endothelium and induces platelet consumption and thrombosis	Surgery when platelet function within normal limits Anesthesia: adequate hydration and peripheral blood flow; hypoglycemia second to hyperinsulinemia requires monitoring serum glucose

received inhalation anesthetics may require additional postoperative sedation with diazepam (0.1 to 0.2 mg/kg) or droperidol (0.075 to 0.1 mg/kg).

PENETRATING TRAUMA OF THE GLOBE

Perforating wounds of the eye are common in children and vary from small punctures to extensive lacerations complicated by prolapse of intraocular contents. Apart from mechanical damage at the time of injury, the subsequent risk of intraocular infection and the potential for development of sympathetic ophthalmia involving the contralateral eye are very real hazards.[42]

Early wound closure and removal of any foreign body present the anesthesiologist with the dual challenge of maintaining a stable IOP to prevent further ocular damage and inducing anesthesia in the small child with a full stomach.

IOP can best be maintained within a normal range by preventing elevated central venous pressure due to breath-holding, crying, struggling, and vomiting, and by avoiding drug-induced IOP changes following administration of succinylcholine or ketamine.

A safe, rapid induction technique designed to minimize IOP elevation includes preoxygenation of a well-sedated child and gentle mask placement to prevent extrinsic pressure on the globe; thiopental, 5 to 7 mg/kg intravenously; a nondepolarizing muscle relaxant of intermediate-acting duration such as pancuronium,* 0.15 mg/kg, or atracurium, 0.4 mg/kg; cricoid pressure, which will allow gentle positive-pressure ventilation, minimizing gastric inflation and passive regurgitation; intravenous lidocaine, 1 mg/kg, to blunt the stimulation of intubation and its adverse effect on IOP; and laryngoscopy as soon as the child is fully paralyzed as indicated by a peripheral nerve stimulator.[43-47]

However, the small, frightened, uncooperative child may do considerable additional damage to his open eye injury by excessive crying or struggling during attempts to place an intravenous catheter. Flexibility and an alternate induction technique are necessary for this situation. A rectal barbiturate in the presence of the parents or a gentle mask induction followed by cricoid pressure and intravenous catheter placement as soon as the child is asleep is acceptable; the remainder of induction is as previously described.[48, 49]

Efforts to avoid a succinylcholine-induced rise in IOP with a small, nonparalyzing dose of a nondepolarizing muscle relaxant have met with inconsistent success.[50-54] It is, therefore, more advantageous to use a nondepolarizing drug such as atracurium, 0.4 mg/kg, achieving full paralysis within 2 minutes to facilitate intubation.[55]

*In practice the relaxant drug can be given immediately *before* the thiopental to further hasten good intubating conditions.

At the conclusion of wound closure, the stomach should be aspirated and the trachea extubated when the child is awake with full return of airway reflexes. Again, intravenous lidocaine, 1 to 2 mg/kg, will diminish vigorous coughing on the endotracheal tube while the child is awaiting an awake extubation.[56]

GLAUCOMA

In infants and children glaucoma, an elevated IOP which produces damage to ocular structures or function, is caused either by maldevelopment of the eye (developmental glaucoma) or, secondarily, by other ocular diseases such as neoplasm or trauma.[57] In addition, many syndromes and anomalies may have associated glaucoma (see Table 10–1).

Congenital glaucoma occurs at or shortly after birth; 75 percent of the cases are bilateral. The cardinal signs in the infant are enlarged and cloudy cornea due to edema, tearing, photophobia, and blepharospasm. Under 3 years of age the eye is quite elastic and will enlarge as a result of increased IOP; this is termed buphthalmos or ox eye.[57, 58] Glaucomatous cupping of the optic disc appears early in infants with increased IOP and may also disappear rapidly after the IOP is controlled.[58]

Congenital glaucoma occurs because of impaired outflow; surgical therapies such as goniotomy, trabeculotomy, and trabeculectomy are designed to open a route for aqueous flow into Schlemm's canal, normalizing IOP. Cases that fail to respond to such surgery may require cyclocryotherapy. This technique involves freezing (to −60 to −80°C) the aqueous-producing portion of the ciliary body; the lesions are extremely painful postoperatively, and patients require generous narcotic analgesia.

The infant suspected of having congenital glaucoma requires a general anesthetic for an examination and IOP measurement. Preparations should be made to follow the examination with a surgical procedure if the diagnosis is confirmed. A sleep dose of rectal methohexital plus a topical ocular anesthetic is often sufficient for the initial exam.[49]

All general anesthetics and central nervous system depressants tend to lower IOP (with the exception of ketamine) and are also acceptable. One simply needs to be aware of the modest lowering or slight elevation (ketamine) of IOP from the baseline levels in the unanesthetized eye when evaluating the measured pressure.[59, 60] Fortunately, the diagnosis of congenital glaucoma is not based solely on the numerical IOP reading, but also on the unmistakable ocular signs of glaucoma (corneal edema, tears in Descemet's membrane, cupping of the optic nerve).[58]

Succinylcholine and intubation, both causes of acute IOP elevation, should be avoided before the IOP reading, but may be used in preparation for the subsequent operative procedure.[46]

Infants with glaucoma should be examined periodically with repeat IOP measurements under general anesthesia. In order to evaluate the success of therapy, the drugs must be continued up to the time of anesthesia and consideration given to the potential systemic side effects (Table 10–3).

RETINOBLASTOMA

Retinoblastoma is an intraocular tumor that occurs in 1 per 20,000 live births and accounts for 1 percent of all cancer-related deaths in children.[70] The tumor is either inherited in an autosomal dominant gene, as a chromosomal abnormality with a partial deletion of the long arm of chromosome 13 (13 q), or as a sporadic mutation.[71, 72] One third of retinoblastoma cases are bilateral. The tumor is very aggressive and may extend along the optic nerve to the brain and metastasize to skull, long bones, lung, and lymph nodes. The affected child may present clinically with a white pupil, strabismus, a red painful eye, glaucoma, or poor vision.[70, 71] An urgent examination with the patient under anesthesia is required to determine the extent of the disease. Enucleation and irradiation are the primary modes of therapy and, depending on the tumor staging, secondary treatment may also include chemotherapy, photocoagulation, and cryotherapy. The remaining eye should be examined periodically for tumor and treatment as necessary.

The potential to elicit the oculocardiac reflex (a trigeminovagal arc) is fairly high during the manipulation of enucleation through traction on the extraocular muscles and during digital pressure deep within the empty orbit. Vigorous (as opposed to gentle) surgical handling of the extraocular muscles will both increase the frequency and severity of the oculocardiac reflex, as will hypercapnia.[73] The incidence of the oculocardiac reflex can be minimized by atropine (0.04 mg/kg p.o.; 0.02 to 0.03 mg/kg IM; 0.01 to 0.02 mg/kg IV) either preoperatively or during the induction period.[74–78]

The most common manifestation of the oculocardiac reflex is a sinus bradycardia, but multiple varieties of dysrhythmias may occur including junctional rhythm, periods of sinus arrest, and extrasystoles. No treatment is necessary for modest decreases in heart rate; however, the anesthesiologist should observe the ECG and blood pressure closely and wait for vagal escape or fatigue of the reflex.[73, 79]

Should the oculocardiac reflex decrease the heart rate to less than 100 beats per minute in small infants, less than 80 beats per minute in young children, or less than 60 beats per minute in older children, the surgeon should promptly discontinue traction or stimulation of the globe. The rate can be expected to return to baseline, and (particularly when hypotension has accompanied the relative bradycardia) small intravenous increments of atropine 0.01 mg/kg should be given before resumption of surgical traction.[74]

On the rarer occurrence of ventricular dysrhythmias, increments of lidocaine, 1 to 2 mg/kg IV, may return the rhythm to a normal sinus pattern. These dysrhythmias are more difficult to treat and frequently are abolished only at the conclusion of surgery and ocular traction.

Table 10–3. DRUG THERAPY FOR GLAUCOMA

Drug	Action	Potential Systemic Effects
Pilocarpine topical (1–4%)	Short-acting parasympathomimetic Pupillary constriction and ciliary muscle contraction Facilitates outflow of aqueous humor	
Epinephrine topical (0.25–2%)	Decreases aqueous humor production Increases facility of outflow	Sympathomimetic reactions
Timolol maleate topical (0.25–0.5%)[61–64]	Nonselective adrenergic blocking agent Decrease aqueous humor production	Bradycardia, bronchospasm, and aggravation of preexisting asthma
Echothiophate iodide (0.03–0.25%) (Phospholine iodide)[65–69]	Long-acting anticholinesterase miotic Decreases resistance to outflow of aqueous humor	Decrease in plasma (pseudo) cholinesterase activity for 4–6 weeks after discontinuing drug Prolonged neuromuscular block of succinylcholine and ester-linked local anesthetics Avoid succinylcholine or titrate small doses and monitor peripheral nerve stimulator Fresh frozen plasma will increase plasma cholinesterase (but value of this is questionable)
Acetazolamide (Diamox)	Carbonic anhydrase inhibitor Decreases aqueous humor production Used in combination with a miotic and/or epinephrine	Dehydration, GI disturbances, hypokalemia, metabolic acidosis
Osmotic agents	Rapid increase in plasma osmolarity Fluid shifts from eye to circulation, shrinking vitreous	Hyperglycemia (or glycosuria) Disorientation, seizures

Frequently, infants and children with retinoblastoma require daily radiation therapy for many weeks. The children need to be motionless for a short time (about 10 minutes) during radiotherapy and ideally should return to normal activity and eating within a few hours. Satisfactory anesthetic agents and techniques include rectal (25 mg/kg) or intramuscular (10 mg/kg) methohexital, intravenous or intramuscular ketamine combined with atropine, or a brief period of an inhalational agent.[80–83] Ketamine is usually quite satisfactory as long as the anesthesiologist is mindful of its potential to produce tachyphylaxis and the need for increasing dosage over time.[84] An indwelling catheter may be placed (with the patient under intramuscular ketamine) and securely taped, and patency can be maintained by flushing with heparinized (50 μg/ml) saline solution four times a day.[85] This can simplify daily intravenous administration of the anesthesiologist's drug of choice without the trauma of multiple injections or the unpredictability of rectal absorption. Recommendations for care of the indwelling cannula include a 5-day (Monday through Friday) period of use, removal during the weekend, and reinsertion each Monday for the following week of treatment.[85]

RETINOPATHY OF PREMATURITY

The continuing problem of retinopathy of prematurity (ROP) has long been a concern of neonatologists and ophthalmologists. Increasingly, anesthesiologists too are sharing this concern, as the very young premature infant requires a general anesthetic and oxygen administration for cardiovascular, gastrointestinal, or central nervous system surgery.[28–31]

ROP acutely presents as a vascular retinopathy at the developing edge of the eye and evolves to a cicatricial form in which scar tissue places the retina under traction, causing detachment and loss of vision.[31]

Each year in the United States, about 2000 neonates incur some degree of permanent ROP and a quarter of these are affected by blindness. It is well known that the incidence of ROP is inversely related to birthweight, although one third of healthy premature infants who received high concentrations of oxygen (for example, FIO_2 0.5 for 28 days) developed cicatricial ROP, according to data from the 1950's. However, we do not know the incidence of ROP in the tiny sick premature population receiving only moderate concentrations of oxygen for short periods of time, such as during the course of a general anesthetic.[31]

Logistical risk analysis considering surgery (requiring use of anesthetic gases) as a risk variable demonstrated that surgery does not contribute to the risk of ROP in small prematures as compared with those who did not require surgery.[31]

Arbitrarily, anesthesiologists regulate the FIO_2 of oxygen–nitrous oxide or oxygen-air mixtures to maintain PaO_2 at less than 100 torr as monitored by intra-arterial blood sampling or by a transcutaneous sensor, both of which must sample the oxygen tension above the level of the ductus arteriosus. Any condition, such as systemic hypotension or the pulmonary hypertension syndrome, that places the infant's circulation in the fetal pattern of right-to-left shunting at the ductus level requires assessment of the oxygen tension in the ascending aorta as an indication of oxygen concentration perfusing the eye.[28, 32, 33]

But the old dogma that stresses oxygen as the sole culprit responsible for inducing ROP is being challenged by the recognition that it is a multifactorial disease.[30, 86] The continued high incidence of ROP among very-low-birth-weight infants in spite of frequent monitoring of oxygen use, the reports of ROP in premature infants who have received little or no oxygen, the occurrence of ROP in premature infants with cyanotic congenital heart disease, and its rare occurrence in full-term neonates all suggest causes other than oxygen-induced vasoconstriction.

In infants smaller than 1250 gm there is a significant correlation of ROP with apnea requiring mask and bag ventilation without an increase in oxygen concentration, prolonged parenteral nutrition, a greater number of blood transfusions, and episodes of hypoxemia (PaO_2 less than 40 torr), hypercarbia, and hypocarbia.[87] Specifically, episodes of hypocarbia with $PaCO_2$ less than 25 torr and an arterial pH above 7.55 were often associated with ROP. It appears that the retinal vasculature may also be responsive to this deficit, and the anesthetic plan should include monitoring to avoid severe hyperventilation.[87]

Thirty years after the initial observation that vitamin E supplements were associated with a reduced incidence of ROP, therapy with prophylactic intramuscular and oral vitamin E is again showing promise in protecting the preterm infant against severe ROP. Vitamin E is an andogenous antioxidant that protects against free radical damage (plasma levels are severely depressed in the premature), and supplementation to adult physiologic levels is nontoxic.[88, 89] The drug must be initiated on the first day of life and maintained continuously until the retinal vasculature matures.

The maturation of the retinal vasculature shows considerable variation until 44 weeks postconception, suggesting that excessively long periods of high oxygen concentration should be minimized throughout the neonatal period.[34]

Caution is necessary when an infant who was born prematurely requires eye or nonocular surgery early in life. Those younger than 41 to 46 weeks conceptual age with a history of idiopathic apnea are predisposed to postoperative life-threatening apneic episodes.[90] Nonessential surgery in preterm infants should be delayed until 44 weeks conceptual age or later. When surgery is necessary, these infants must be monitored for apnea for 18 hours postoperatively, and the means to ventilate the infant mechanically should be kept at hand.[91]

RETINAL DETACHMENT

A retinal detachment occurs when subretinal fluid causes a separation of the outer layers of the sensory retina away from the retinal pigment epithelial layer.[92, 93] Retinal detachments in the pediatric age group are classified as rhegmatogenous, traction, or exudative.

Rhegmatogenous retinal detachments in children are most frequently a sequela of trauma, usually contusion of the globe, and to a lesser extent of myopia, aphakia, and retinopathy of prematurity. Breaks through all of the inner areas of the retina allow vitreous fluid to enter the subretinal space, dissecting it off the retina. Classic scleral buckling procedures are successful in reattaching this type of detachment in most cases.[92]

The traction detachment is a complication seen with retinopathy of prematurity, diabetes, and sickle retinopathy and occurs when vitreoretinal traction separates the retinal pigment epithelium from the retina. Scleral buckling, scleral resection, or vitrectomy may be indicated in cases of traction detachment that extend into the macular or foveal area.[92]

Exudative retinal detachments follow accumulation of subretinal fluid without evidence of retinal break and can be seen with retinoblastoma, choroidal hemangioma or melanoma, angiomatosis retinae, and severe renal disease.[92]

Reattachment of the retina to the pigment epithelium is managed with scleral buckling surgery consisting of a combination of techniques.[93] First, cryotherapy or laser therapy may be used to produce a chorioretinal scar, sealing the retinal break. The second part of the surgical procedure consists of physical indentation of the sclera by a variety of buckling materials to bring the retinal tear closer to the pigment epithelium. Third, reattachment may be facilitated by external drainage of the subretinal fluid. In more complicated cases, vitrectomy surgery using a suction-cutting instrument may be combined with scleral buckling.

In addition, an intraoperative technique of internal tamponade by air injected into the vitreous may help hold the retina in place; the air remains in the eye for 6 to 10 days until resorbed.[93] Use of this technique is of special concern as regards the concurrent use of nitrous oxide. Because nitrous oxide rapidly diffuses into the air-containing space, the volume of gas increases two- to threefold and is responsible for an associated significant increase in intraocular pressure.[94, 95] Compromised retinal circulation poses a potential risk to the eye as a consequence of elevated intraocular pressure.[94] Conversely, when nitrous oxide is discontinued at the conclusion of surgery, the sudden washout of nitrous oxide and shrinkage of the gas bubble (causing a lower than original IOP) may also be detrimental to the surgical outcome.[94, 95]

This potential problem can be avoided by discontinuing nitrous oxide 15 minutes before the air is injected into the vitreous so that there will be little change in bubble size. An inhalation agent and 100 percent oxygen can be used for the balance of the procedure without affecting intravitreal gas dynamics.[95]

Any combination of induction and inhalation anesthetic agents is acceptable for retinal detachment procedures, applying the basic principles of anesthetic care for pediatric ophthalmic surgery as previously discussed. Regard for the potential to elicit the oculocardiac reflex with traction on the globe, especially during placement of the scleral buckle, is also an important consideration.

REFERENCES

1. O'Neill JF, Bateman JB: The lens and pediatric cataracts. In Metz HS, Rosenbaum AL (Eds.): Pediatric Ophthalmology. New York, Medical Examination Publishing Co., 1982, pp 235–261.
2. France TD, Baker JD, Rogers GL, et al.: Diagnosis and treatment of cataracts in children. American Academy of Ophthalmology, 1980, Instruction Section, Course 58.
3. Kohn BA: The differential diagnosis of cataracts in infancy and childhood. Am J Dis Child 130:184, 1976.
4. Cross HE, Jensen AD: Ocular manifestations in the Marfan syndrome and homocystinuria. Am J Ophthalmol 75:405, 1973.
5. Johnston RR, Eger EI, Wilson C: A comparative interaction of epinephrine with enflurane, isoflurane, and halothane in man. Anesth Analg 55:709, 1976.
6. Rao CC, Dierdorf SF, Wolfe TM, et al.: Effect of age on epinephrine-induced arrhythmias during halothane anaesthesia in pigs. Can Anaesth Soc J 31:20, 1984.
7. Karl HW, Swedlow DB, Lee KW, et al.: Epinephrine-halothane interactions in children. Anesthesiology 58:142, 1983.
8. Ueda W, Hirakawa M, Mae O: Appraisal of epinephrine administration to patients under halothane anesthesia for closure of cleft palate. Anesthesiology 58:574, 1983.
9. Pepple J: Epinephrine-halothane interaction in children versus adults. Anesthesiology 60:76, 1984.
10. Smith RB: Intra-ocular adrenaline and halothane anaesthesia. Br J Anaesth 43:1200, 1971.
11. Smith RB, Douglas H, Petruscak J, et al.: Safety of intraocular adrenaline with halothane anaesthesia. Br J Anaesth 44:1314, 1972.
12. MacDiarmid IR, Holloway KB: Factors affecting intraocular pressure. Proc R Soc Med 69:601, 1976.
13. France NK, France TD, Woodburn JD, et al.: Succinylcholine alteration of the forced duction test. Ophthalmology 87:1282, 1980.
14. Kornblueth W, Aladjemoff L, Magora F, et al.: Influence of general anesthesia on intraocular pressure in man. AMA Arch Ophthalmol 61:84, 1959.
15. Joshi C, Bruce DL: Thiopental and succinylcholine: action on intraocular pressure. Anesth Analg 54:471, 1975.
16. Famewo CE, Odugbesan CO, Osuntokun OO: Effect of etomidate on intra-ocular pressure. Can Anaesth Soc J 24:712, 1977.
17. Runciman JC, Bowen-Wright RM, Welsh NH, et al.: Intraocular pressure changes during halothane and enflurane anaesthesia. Br J Anaesth 50:371, 1978.
18. Ausinsch B, Graves SA, Munson ES, et al.: Intraocular pressures in children during isoflurane and halothane anesthesia. Anesthesiology 42:167, 1975.
19. Presbitero JV, Ruiz RS, Rigor B, et al.: Intraocular pressure during enflurane and neurolept anesthesia in adult patients undergoing ophthalmic surgery. Anesth Analg 59:50, 1980.

20. Litwiller RW, DiFazio CA, Rushia EL: Pancuronium and intraocular pressure. Anesthesiology 42:750, 1975.
21. Cunningham AJ, Kelly CP, Farmer J, et al.: The effect of metocurine and metocurine-pancuronium combination on intraocular pressure. Can Anaesth Soc J 29:617, 1982.
22. Balamoutsos NG, Tsakona H, Kanakoudes PS, et al.: Alcuronium and intraocular pressure. Anesth Analg 62:521, 1983.
23. Schwartz H, de Roetth A, Papper EM: Preanesthetic use of atropine and scopolamine in patients with glaucoma. JAMA 165:144, 1957.
24. Corssen G, Joy JE: A new parenteral anesthetic—CI-581: its effect on intraocular pressure. J Pediatr Ophthal 4:20, 1967.
25. Yoshikawa K, Murai Y: The effect of ketamine on intraocular pressure in children. Anesth Analg 50:199, 1971.
26. Peuler M, Glass DD, Arens JF: Ketamine and intraocular pressure. Anesthesiology 43:575, 1975.
27. Ausinsch B, Rayburn RL, Munson ES, et al.: Ketamine and intraocular pressure in children. Anesth Analg 55:773, 1976.
28. Phibbs RH: Oxygen therapy: a continuing hazard of the premature infant. Anesthesiology 47:486, 1977.
29. Betts EK, Downes JJ, Schaffer DB, et al.: Retrolental fibroplasia and oxygen administration during general anesthesia. Anesthesiology 47:518, 1977.
30. Merritt JC, Sprague DH, Merritt WE, et al.: Retrolental fibroplasia: a multifactorial disease. Anesth Anal 60:109, 1981.
31. Flynn JT: Oxygen and retrolental fibroplasia: update and challenge. Anesthesiology 60:397, 1984.
32. Horbar JD, Clark JT, Lucey JF: The newborn oxygram: automated processing of transcutaneous oxygen data. Pediatrics 66:848, 1980.
33. Lucey JF: Transcutaneous diagnosis in the high-risk neonate. Hosp Pract 16:108, 1981.
34. Quinn GE, Betts EK, Diamond GR, et al.: Neonatal age (human) at retinal maturation. ASA Abstracts, Anesthesiology 55:A326, 1981.
35. Pyeritz RE, McKusick VA: The Marfan syndrome: diagnosis and management. N Engl J Med 300:772, 1979.
36. Boucek RJ, Noble NL, Gunja-Smith Z, et al.: The Marfan syndrome: a deficiency in chemically stable collagen cross-links. N Engl J Med 305:988, 1981.
37. Harker LA, Slichter SJ, Scott CR, et al.: Homocystinemia: vascular injury and arterial thrombosis. N Engl J Med 291:537, 1974.
38. Brown BR, Walson PD, Taussig LM: Congenital metabolic diseases of pediatric patients: anesthetic implications. Anesthesiology 43:197, 1975.
39. Crooke JW, Towers JF, Taylor WH: Management of patients with homocystinuria requiring surgery under general anaesthesia. Br J Anaesth 43:96, 1971.
40. McGoldrick KE: Anesthetic management of homocystinuria. Anes Rev 8:42, 1981.
41. Parris WC, Quimby CW: Anesthetic considerations for the patient with homocystinuria. Anesth Analg 61:708, 1982.
42. Hicks E: Ocular trauma. In Metz HS, Rosenbaum AL (Eds.): Pediatric Ophthalmology. New York, Medical Examination Publishing Co., 1982, pp 25–47.
43. Salem MR, Wong AY, Fizzotti GF: Efficacy of cricoid pressure in preventing aspiration of gastric contents in paediatric patients. Br J Anesth 44:401, 1972.
44. Salem MR, Wong AY, Mani M, et al.: Efficacy of cricoid pressure in preventing gastric inflation during bag-mask ventilation in pediatric patients. Anesthesiology 40:96, 1971.
45. Brown EM, Krishnaprasad D, Smiler BG: Pancuronium for rapid induction technique for tracheal intubation. Can Anaesth Soc J 26:489, 1979.
46. Donlon JV: Anesthesia factors affecting intraocular pressure. Succinylcholine and endotracheal intubation. Anesth Rev 8:13, 1981.

47. Stoelting RK: Circulatory changes during direct laryngoscopy and tracheal intubation: influence of duration of laryngoscopy with or without prior lidocaine. Anesthesiology 47:381, 1977.
48. Smith RM: Choice of inhalation agents. In Anesthesia for Infants and Children. St. Louis, C. V. Mosby Co., 1980, pp 109–127.
49. Goresky GV, Steward DJ: Rectal methohexitone for induction of anaesthesia in children. Can Anaesth Soc J 26:213, 1979.
50. Borman B, Babinski M, Bunegin L, et al.: Succinylcholine: intraocular and intracranial pressure. ASA Abstracts, Anesthesiology 51:S272, 1979.
51. Miller RD, Way WL, Hickey RF: Inhibition of succinylcholine-induced increased intraocular pressure by non-depolarizing muscle relaxants. Anesthesiology 29:123, 1968.
52. Bowen DJ, McGrand JC, Palmer RJ: Intraocular pressures after suxamethonium and endotracheal intubation in patients pretreated with pancuronium. Br J Anaesth 48:1201, 1976.
53. McLeskey CH, Pavlin EG, Hornbein TF: Effectiveness of pancuronium in blocking succinylcholine induced elevation of intraocular pressure. ASA Annual Meeting—Abstracts of Scientific Papers, 1977, pp 319–320.
54. Meyers EF, Krupin T, Johnson M, et al.: Failure of nondepolarizing neuromuscular blockers to inhibit succinylcholine-induced increased intraocular pressure, a controlled study. Anesthesiology 48:149, 1978.
55. Goudsouzian NG, Liu LM, Cote CJ, et al.: Safety and efficacy of atracurium in adolescents and children anesthetized with halothane. Anesthesiology 59:459, 1983.
56. Baraka A: Intravenous lidocaine controls extubation laryngospasm in children. Anesth Analg 57:506, 1978.
57. Hoskins HD: Pediatric glaucomas. In Metz HS, Rosenbaum AL (Eds.): Pediatric Ophthalmology. New York, Medical Examination Publishing Co., 1982, pp 262–302.
58. Kolker AE, Hetherington J: Congenital glaucoma. In Kolker AE, Hetherington J (Eds.): Diagnosis and Therapy of the Glaucomas. St. Louis, C.V. Mosby Co., 1976, pp 276–321.
59. Adams AK: Ketamine in paediatric ophthalmic practice. (Letter.) Anaesthesia 28:212, 1973.
60. Duncalf D: Anesthesia and intraocular pressure. Bull NY Acad Med 51:374, 1975.
61. Kim JW, Smith PH: Timolol-induced bradycardia. Anesth Analg 59:301, 1980.
62. Schoene RB, Martin TR, Charan NB, et al.: Timolol-induced bronchospasm in asthmatic bronchitis. JAMA 245:1460, 1981.
63. Samuels SI, Maze M: Beta-receptor blockade following the use of eye drops. Anesthesiology 52:369, 1980.
64. Williams T, Ginther WH: Hazard of ophthalmic timolol. (Letter.) N Engl J Med 306:1485, 1982.
65. Eilderton TE, Farmati O, Zsigmond EK: Reduction in plasma cholinesterase levels after prolonged administration of echothiophate iodide eyedrops. Can Anaesth Soc J 15:291, 1968.
66. Ellis PP, Esterdahl M: Echothiophate iodide therapy in children. Arch Ophthalmol 77:598, 1967.
67. Pantuck EJ: Echothiopate iodide eye drops and prolonged response to suxamethonium. Br J Anaesth 38:406, 1966.
68. Donati F, Bevan DR: Controlled succinylcholine infusion in a patient receiving echothiophate eye drops. Can Anaesth Soc J 28:488, 1981.
69. Brodsky JB, Campos FA: Chloroprocaine analgesia in a patient receiving echothiophate iodide eye drops. Anesthesiology 48:288, 1978.
70. Rosenbaum AL, Bremer DL: Ocular tumors in children. In Metz HS, Rosenbaum AL: Pediatric Ophthalmology. New York, Medical Examination Publishing Co., 1982, pp 391–403.
71. Bensinger RE, Mills M: Retinoblastoma: diagnosis and treatment. Res Staff Phys 46–49, 1982.

72. Weichselbaum RR, Zakov ZN, Albert DM, et al.: New findings in the chromosome 13 long-arm deletion syndrome and retinoblastoma. Ophthalmology 86:1191, 1979.

73. Blanc VF, Hardy JF, Milot J, et al.: The oculocardiac reflex: a graphic and statistical analysis in infants and children. Can Anaesth Soc J 30:360, 1983.

74. Meyers EF, Tomeldan SA: Glycopyrrolate compared with atropine in prevention of the oculocardiac reflex during eye-muscle surgery. Anesthesiology 51:350, 1979.

75. Steward DJ: Anticholinergic premedication for infants and children. Can Anaesth Soc J 30:325, 1983.

76. Mayhew JF: Are anticholinergics needed in strabismus surgery? Anesth Rev 11:24, 1984.

77. Joseph MC, Vale RJ: Premedication with atropine by mouth. Lancet 2:1060, 1960.

78. Brzustowicz RM, Nelson DA, Betts EK, et al.: Efficacy of oral premedication for pediatric outpatient surgery. Anesthesiology 60:475, 1984.

79. Moonie GT, Rees DL, Elton D: The oculocardiac reflex during strabismus surgery. Can Anaesth Soc J 11:621, 1964.

80. Amberg HL, Gordon G: Low-dose intramuscular ketamine for pediatric radiotherapy: a case report. Anesth Analg 55:92, 1976.

81. Cronin MM, Bousfield JD, Hewett EB, et al.: Ketamine anaesthesia for radiotherapy in small children. Anaesthesia 27:135, 1972.

82. Samuels SI, Lim F, Maze A: Failure to produce satisfactory operating conditions following large doses of ketamine hydrochloride. Anesth Rev 5:23, 1978.

83. Smith HS: Anaesthesia for radiotherapy. (Letter.) Can Anaesth Soc J 31:236, 1984.

84. Byer DE, Gould AB: Development of tolerance to ketamine in an infant undergoing repeated anesthesia. Anesthesiology 54:255, 1981.

85. Rodarte A: Heparin-lock for repeated anesthesia in pediatric radiation therapy. Anesthesiology 56:316, 1982.

86. McGoldrick KE: Factors influencing development of retrolental fibroplasia. (Letter.) Anesth Analg 60:539, 1981.

87. Shohat M, Reisner SH, Krikler R, et al.: Retinopathy of prematurity: incidence and risk factors. Pediatrics 72:159, 1983.

88. Hittner HM, Speer ME, Rudolph AJ, et al.: Retrolental fibroplasia and vitamin E in the preterm infant—comparison of oral versus intramuscular:oral administration. Pediatrics 73:238, 1984.

89. Hittner HM, Kretzer FL, Rudolph AJ: Prevention and management of retrolental fibroplasia. Hosp Pract 19:85, 1984.

90. Liu LM, Cote CJ, Goudsouzian NG, et al.: Life-threatening apnea in infants recovering from anesthesia. Anesthesiology 59:506, 1983.

91. Gregory GA, Steward DJ: Life-threatening perioperative apnea in the ex-"premie." (Editorial.) Anesthesiology 59:495, 1983.

92. Hammer, ME: Pediatric diseases of the retina. In Metz HS, Rosenbaum AL (Eds.): Pediatric Ophthalmology. New York, Medical Examination Publishing Co., 1982, pp 331–373.

93. Marcus DF, Bovino JA: Retinal detachment. JAMA, 247:873, 1982.

94. Smith B, Carl B, Linn JG, et al.: Effect of nitrous oxide on air in vitreous. Am J Ophthalmol 78:314, 1974.

95. Stinson TW, Donlon JV: Interaction of intraocular SF_6 and air with nitrous oxide. ASA Abstracts, Anesthesiology, 51:S16, 1978.

General References for Table 10–1

96. Harley RD (Ed.): Pediatric Ophthalmology. 2nd ed. Philadelphia, W.B. Saunders Co., 1983.

97. Metz HS, Rosenbaum AL (Eds.): Pediatric Ophthalmology. New York, Medical Examination Publishing Co., 1982.

98. Behrman RE, Vaughan VC III (Eds.): Nelson Textbook of Pediatrics. 12th ed. Philadelphia, W.B. Saunders Co., 1983.

99. Gregory GA: Pediatric Anesthesia. New York, Churchill Livingstone, 1983.

100. Steward DJ: Manual of Pediatric Anesthesia. New York, Churchill Livingstone, 1979.

101. Stehling LC: Common Problems in Pediatric Anesthesia. Chicago, Year Book Medical Publishers, 1982.

102. Stehling LC, Zauder HL (Eds.): Anesthetic Implications of Congenital Anomalies in Children, New York, Appleton-Century-Crofts, 1980.

103. Kobel M, Creighton RE, Steward DJ: Anaesthetic considerations in Down's syndrome: experience with 100 patients and a review of the literature. Can Anaesth Soc J 29:593, 1982.

11 | OTOLARYNGOLOGICAL DISEASES

JAMES D. MORRISON, M.D.

No area of surgery demands closer cooperation between surgeon and anesthetist than does that of the upper airway. A cooperative approach to airway control demands the operator and anesthetist be aware of each other's problems and intentions, and this in turn requires each to have a competent understanding of the diseases and lesions with which they are dealing. The anesthetist, in his role of resuscitator, also requires the ability to recognize and appropriately treat respiratory obstruction, particularly in neonates and infants. Not only is it important to know when tracheostomy is required, it is also necessary to know when it, and its associated morbidity, can safely be avoided. An informed anesthetist can also perform a valuable diagnostic role, in that he is often the first physician to examine the larynx in cases of respiratory obstruction.

The diseases discussed in this chapter are uncommon, and perhaps for most practitioners many of them will remain textbook descriptions of lesions they will never see at first hand. A few are trivial but most are serious and life-threatening, some devastatingly so. Almost all, however, by their intimate involvement with the airway have the potential for rapid progression to ventilatory problems of frightening proportions. These problems can be greatly compounded by medical, particularly anesthetic, mismanagement. The diseases and conditions included do not form a comprehensive catalogue of all the conditions affecting the upper airway, but they do form a representative sample of the main groups.

NOSE AND NASOPHARYNX

Choanal Atresia

Lack of continuity of the air passages between the nasal cavity and the nasopharynx is a rare congenital defect, and varies from partial unilateral obstruction to complete bilateral atresia. The defect is usually due to obstruction by a bony plate, but in 10 percent the obstruction lies more posteriorly and is membranous rather than bony. This difference, although interesting on embryological grounds, has little practical bearing on diagnosis or treatment. Unilateral choanal atresia is of much lesser importance, as significant respiratory obstruction is unlikely; patients with such an atresia may go undetected for many years, eventually presenting with symptoms of unilateral nasal obstruction such as chronic discharge or reduced olfactory sensation.

Congenital Bilateral Choanal Atresia

Babies born with complete bilateral atresia are at grave risk of sudden death from asphyxia, because the newborn breathes only through the nose, mouth breathing being a learned rather than spontaneous activity in humans.[1] Bilateral choanal atresia therefore usually presents as an acute respiratory crisis soon after birth. This may take the form of spontaneous asphyxial episodes associated with signs of upper respiratory obstruction, or occasionally as asphyxial episodes during sucking. The respiratory obstruction is spontaneously relieved during crying, as this breaks the seal between tongue and palate and permits mouth breathing.

The diagnosis is confirmed by immediate response to appropriate emergency treatment, which is to insert a tongue depressor or an oropharyngeal airway into the mouth to break the seal between tongue and palate and thus allow mouth breathing. The diagnosis is further confirmed by the inability to pass a soft catheter through the nose into the pharynx. If doubt remains, the diagnosis can be finalized by contrast radiological studies or posterior rhinoscopy.[1]

Management

First aid management is simple: use a tongue depressor or oropharyngeal airway to allow mouth

286

breathing. Such measures are only makeshift, however, and do not permit feeding the infant. Although puncture of the atretic area at the time of diagnosis was suggested as long ago as the middle of the nineteenth century,[2] this treatment fell into disuse because of the invariable restenosis. Instead, conservative management during the first year of life followed by definitive repair in the older infant has become the more or less universal treatment.

Effective conservative management followed the demonstration by Hough[3] that an orogastric tube would not only maintain an oral airway and hence effective mouth breathing, but would also provide a route by which the infant could be fed. (Inability to breath through the nose makes sucking impossible.) This management, although very effective, requires prolonged close observation in a hospital, as babies may be slow to learn spontaneous mouth breathing. Until this skill has been acquired, the orogastric tube must be kept in place.

The alternative "conservative" treatment, which has largely been superseded, is tracheostomy.[1, 2] This allows effective respiratory exchange but is not without its own problems of morbidity and even mortality in this age group.

Definitive Surgical Correction

Traditionally corrective surgery for bilateral choanal atresia is performed when the patient is about 1 year of age. Access to the posterior part of the nose is not easy, and various operations have been tried. The choanae may be approached through the nose, through the septum, through the antrum, or, most commonly, through the palate.[4] None of these operations is entirely satisfactory, and there is a high recurrence rate of the atresia. Plastic surgery is often required later to repair and reconstruct the secondary defects produced by the effects of the surgery on normal facial bone growth. The transpalatine technique is perhaps the simplest, giving good access to the atretic area,[5] but has the disadvantage of interfering with subsequent transmaxillary growth. This may be corrected later by definitive palatal repair and orthodontic treatment.[6] Similarly, the transseptal approach necessitates later plastic reconstruction of the nose. The transnasal operation avoids this growth disturbance but gives poorer access to the atresia, and operations done by this route suffer a higher relapse rate.[5]

Recently, attention has again become focused on primary endonasal puncture in the neonatal period, despite the earlier poor results of this type of operation. This is because the addition of stenting tubes to maintain postoperative patency of the choanae has dramatically reduced the restenosis rate. This offers a fairly simple operation with good initial results that allows the infant to feed and breath normally and often entirely obviates the need for later surgery.[1, 2]

Operation. The infant is anesthetized and orally intubated, and then a nasopharyngoscope is inserted through the mouth into the pharynx, and under direct vision a metal bougie is passed through the nose to puncture the atretic plate or membrane. In the neonate, unlike the older infant, there is usually no difficulty in perforating the atresia. The procedure is repeated on the other side and a double-barrelled stent is inserted. This is made from a polyvinyl chloride endotracheal tube folded and partially cut through to give patency to both sides. It is inserted into the nostrils from the nasopharynx and secured in place by suturing the two ends together in front of the nasal columella. The tube must fit loosely to avoid pressure against the posterior nasal septum and possible interference with growth. The stent is left in place for 3 months. After its removal weekly dilation of the choanae may be required to prevent constriction by scar tissue. If more frequent dilations are necessary, the stent is reintroduced and left in place for a further period. Postoperatively, the patient usually establishes normal feeding and breathing patterns within a few days and does not require prolonged hospitalization.[1, 2] In older infants operation is much more difficult, because of the growth of the atresia into a substantial bony obstruction requiring destructive surgical dissection and also because of difficulty of instrumental access to the atretic area. Use of the operating microscope is usually necessary.

Anesthetic Management

Neonates. Endonasal puncture of the atresia in the neonate presents several problems for the anesthetist. There are the general problems of neonatal anesthesia related to immaturity and size, thermoregulation and fluid and electrolyte balance, and the additional problems of operating within the airway. Access to the patient is limited if an operating microscope is used. Postoperatively the presence of foreign bodies within the nose may cause problems.

If it is desired to induce anesthesia before intubation, care must be taken to ensure a good oral airway at all times before successful intubation. Tracheal intubation is probably better performed with the patient awake. An oral RAE* or similar tube should be used and brought down over the chin and secured so as to neither impede operation nor be at risk of accidental displacement or disconnection by the operator. Following intubation, anesthesia may be continued using assisted or controlled ventilation with halothane, or halothane and a muscle relaxant. Other agents can be substituted, but narcotic-based techniques should be used with caution to avoid postoperative respiratory depression. A reliable intravenous cannula should be placed, and minimum monitoring must include precordial auscultation with a stethoscope, blood pressure and temperature measurements, and electrocardiograph. Blood loss is not usually significant during endonasal puncture in the neonatal period. Before

---

*RAE tube, National Catheter Corp.

extubation at the end of operation, the anesthetist must ensure that the new nasal airway is clear and that the stents are secure and will not themselves be liable to cause obstruction. Postoperatively the nasal tubes must be kept clear by frequent suctioning using small soft catheters.

Older Infants. For the reasons mentioned above, definitive surgery in older infants is a much more major undertaking than neonatal endonasal puncture. The operation is usually prolonged and there is likely to be substantial blood loss requiring replacement.

Anesthetic management is similar to that outlined above for the neonate. Limited access to the patient while the microscope is in use necessitates careful attention to securing of the tracheal tube and monitors. Particular attention to measurement and replacement of blood loss is required.

Nasopharyngeal Tumors

The majority of tumors of the nose in children are benign. Some can nonetheless be life-threatening owing to respiratory obstruction, potential for serious bleeding, or aggressive local expansion. They may also cause considerable interference with normal growth of the face.[7]

Angiofibroma

Juvenile nasal angiofibroma is a benign tumor with an aggressive local growth pattern that renders it a dangerous disease for the patient.[8] It occurs predominantly in males, usually at about the age of adolescence, but occasionally in older patients.[9] These tumors are deep-seated, arising from the vault of posterior wall of the nasopharynx. Their growth is accompanied by considerable erosion of surrounding tissues, and the tumor may extend into the cranium through the base of the skull or the orbit. The usual presentation is with episodic epistaxis, and the presence of a tumor is confirmed by x-ray. These tumors are very vascular, and because of the inaccessible position bleeding can be difficult to control. For this reason it is usual to avoid biopsy. Diagnosis depends on definition of the extent of the tumor by computed tomography, and determination of its major vascular components (which are usually derived from the internal maxillary artery) by carotid angiography.

Surgical removal of these tumors usually involves a staged procedure. The first requirement is to reduce the vascularity, and this may be done by selective embolization of the feeder vessels under radiological control at the time of carotid angiography[10] or by ligation of the feeders if accessible. Following successful devascularization, a transpalatal approach is used to expose the body of the tumor. Dissection is often difficult, and bleeding may still be troublesome in spite of devascularization. Incomplete removal may necessitate repeated operation. Those tumors that have extended into the cranium or orbit are particularly difficult to treat surgically and are more often treated by radiotherapy.

The special problems of anesthetic management for surgery of nasal angiofibromas are preexisting nasal obstruction, possible anemia due to persistent epistaxis, and the possibility of considerable, sometimes massive, bleeding during dissection. Because of the staged nature of surgical management, the patient is likely to have a series of investigations or operations requiring repeated general anesthetics in a relatively short time. Preoperative assessment should pay particular attention to the degree of nasal obstruction and the possible need for preoperative blood transfusion. During induction of anesthesia early insertion of an oral airway will compensate for nasal obstruction. The trachea should be intubated orally using a cuffed RAE or similar tube, and a pharyngeal pack should be inserted. The tube must be secured very carefully because of lack of access to it once the operation is under way. A reliable, large-bore intravenous cannula is essential in case rapid blood infusion becomes necessary. Maintenance of anesthesia can be by any suitable method, but generally a relaxant technique with controlled ventilation is preferred, particularly if controlled hypotension is used. This can be of great help to the surgeon by making dissection much easier. If sodium nitroprusside is used to induce hypotension, monitoring should include means to assess blood loss, including central venous pressure and direct intra-arterial blood pressure measurement. Postoperatively, there may be residual nasal obstruction, and continuing oozing from the operation site. The tracheal tube should therefore be left in place until the patient is fully awake.

Other Nasal Tumors in Children

Teratomas, dermoids, nasal encephaloceles, and gliomas may occur due to abnormal embryological protrusion of intracranial contents into the nose. All may present as congenital nasal masses[11] and, if large, cause airway obstruction. In neonates nasal airway obstruction is tantamount to complete airway obstruction because of obligatory nasal breathing, but the airway may readily be restored by insertion of an oropharyngeal airway. Proper treatment depends on accurate diagnosis and delineation of the extent of the tumor by radiography and computed tomography. Particular search must be made for any intracranial component; surgery should not be undertaken until these investigations are complete, as these lesions are often more extensive than at first anticipated. Nasal tumors with intracranial extensions or connections should not be approached intranasally but rather by frontal craniotomy.[11] Purely intranasal tumors are approached through a midline or lateral rhinotomy. Anesthetic management is similar to that for nasal angiofibroma except insofar as bleeding is unlikely to be a major problem, and deliberate hypotension will rarely be required.

Malignant Tumors of the Nose and Nasopharynx

Malignant tumors of the nose and nasopharynx are exceedingly rare in childhood, and are usually treated by radiation rather than surgery.

Nasopharyngeal Mucocele

Nasal polyps are rare in children but do occur in association with cystic fibrosis.[12] Such polyps inevitably lead to obstruction of the nasal airway and chronic nasal infection. Surgical removal is necessary, and anesthetic management is complicated not only by the local obstruction due to the polyps but also by the patient's chronic respiratory disease. Such patients may have reduced pulmonary function, chronic hypoxia, cor pulmonale, and bronchiectasis with copious purulent sputum. They must be carefully prepared for operation, with every effort made to reduce the volume of retained secretions by physiotherapy, postural drainage, and bronchodilators, along with antibiotics to control the infection. Anesthetic management should take into account the local obstruction caused by the lesion, its propensity to bleed during removal, and the special requirements of the chronic respiratory disease. Preoperatively it is usual to avoid all sedative and anticholinergic drugs, because of effects on ventilation and on the viscosity of secretions respectively. Preoxygenation, intravenous induction, and oral intubation followed by oxygen and halothane anesthesia with controlled ventilation is a suitable technique that ensures control of the airway and allows optimum ventilation with reduced airway reactivity. Humidified gases should be used for ventilation. Throughout the operation, the tracheal tube should be aspirated frequently but gently, using a soft catheter. Profuse bleeding may occur during polypectomy in these circumstances, and blood transfusion may be required. At the end of operation, the tracheal tube may be removed early unless there is persisting nasal obstruction (for example, by packing) or persisting bleeding. In this case the tube must remain in place until the patient is fully awake. It is important to recommence active chest treatment as soon as possible in the postoperative period, preferably in the recovery room. The preoperative regimen of physiotherapy, postural drainage, bronchodilators, and antibiotics should be continued.

MOUTH AND PHARYNX

Congenital Conditions Requiring Surgery

Ranulas

Ranulas are simple, thin-walled cysts with a characteristic bluish appearance. They occur in the floor of the mouth, and are formed by myxomatous degeneration of the salivary glands. Ranulas occur in all age groups, including infants and older children. They may burst and drain spontaneously but invariably recur. Although uncomfortable, they rarely, if ever, cause obstruction. The only reliable way to avoid recurrence is total excision of the cyst, but this is often technically difficult because of the very thin wall. Marsupialization, with high probability of recurrence, may be the best that can be offered. Dissection is made easier by partial removal of the contents of the cyst, but unfortunately the contents are usually too viscid to allow easy aspiration. Ranulas are therefore frustrating for surgeon and patient alike, but cause little morbidity and are of no danger to the patient except insofar as multiple operations are likely to be required for their eventual elimination. General endotracheal anesthesia via a nasal tube with packing off of the pharynx as for any other straightforward intraoral operation will give satisfactory operating conditions. Blood loss is usually minimal.

Ankyloglossia (Tongue Tie)

Primary tethering of the tongue in infants and children is caused by shortening of the lingual frenulum. Secondary ankyloglossia, such as that which occurs in carcinoma of the tongue or following damage to the glossopharyngeal nerve, is exceedingly rare in childhood.

Tongue tie is difficult to evaluate in terms of functional impairment of speech, and it is doubtful if there is ever serious interference with sucking in infancy. Difficulty in clearing the buccal sulcus with the tongue is the main indication for surgery. For these reasons there is no particular urgency to perform release of tongue tie. If release is thought to be indicated, it can be safely postponed until the child is about a year old without affecting normal development of speech.

Although lingual frenulectomy is a simple operation, there is danger of bleeding, and such bleeding may be difficult for the surgeon to control in less than ideal operating conditions. For this reason these patients should be treated as for any intraoral operation, that is, given general anesthesia with nasotracheal intubation and pharyngeal packing.

Pharyngeal Infections of Surgical Importance

Although it is generally thought that serious infective complications of tonsillitis are less common than a generation or two ago, and that the severity of such abscesses has been reduced since the availability of specific antibiotic therapy, this may not be entirely true. There is some evidence that the incidence of extratonsillar abscess is rising again, and this increase may be related to the generally decreased rate of tonsillectomy.[13] Nonetheless, early antibiotic treatment of pyogenic extratonsillar pharyngeal infection usually prevents progression to frank abscess formation and the necessity for surgical drainage. This is fortunate, because a large pharyngeal abscess is a life-threatening condition. Not only does the airway be come obstructed by the pharyngeal swelling but there is the added risk of sudden aggravation of this obstruction by rupture of the abscess, flooding the pharynx with pus and possibly allowing aspiration of infected material into the trachea. Rupture occurring during induction of anesthesia, when the patient's protective reflexes are obtunded and before the airway has been secured and adequately sealed off from the pharynx, is particularly dangerous, and general anesthesia in these circumstances can be hazardous in the extreme.[14]

Peritonsillar Abscess (Quinsy)

Peritonsillar abscess forms by the spread of infection beyond the tonsillar capsule, most usually into the soft palate in the region of the superior pole of the tonsil. In most cases, peritonsillar abscess affects one side only but in a few patients, less than 10 percent, bilateral abscesses may occur. Older children and young adults account for most cases, and rather more males are affected than females.[15, 17] The most commonly cultured organisms are streptococci, including beta-hemolytic streptococci, but pneumococci, enterococci, and, occasionally, Haemophilus species are also seen. Since many of these patients have been treated with antibiotics, a proportion of the abscesses prove to be sterile on culture.[13, 18]

The usual presentation is of a patient who complains of severe sore throat, with trismus and difficulty in swallowing, and signs of systemic toxicity. The voice is often affected, speech becoming difficult and muffled. If there is marked swelling of the pharynx, there may also be signs of respiratory obstruction. Most patients who present with signs of early peritonsillar infection may be managed successfully by conservative treatment with antibiotics—usually penicillin—and do not proceed to abscess formation. Such patients should have elective tonsillectomy as soon as possible after this episode because the chance of recurrence remains high in spite of apparently complete resolution.[15, 16] Alternatively these patients, and those with small peritonsillar abscesses, can be treated by immediate tonsillectomy, ("tonsillectomy a chaud"). However, some perfer to treat the patient for a day or so with antibiotics and intravenous fluids before proceeding to surgery.[3, 19] At operation the tonsil on the unaffected side is removed first, and under no circumstances is adenoidectomy carried out at the same time. Bleeding on the affected side is usually greater than in most tonsillectomies but is readily controlled by the usual means and has not proved a serious problem.[13] The results of immediate tonsillectomy are encouraging, as judged by duration of hospitalization. They are as good as, if not better than, those of conservative treatment alone, and there is the added benefit for the patient of not requiring later interval tonsillectomy.

Patients with obvious pointing large abscesses are not suitable for tonsillectomy a chaud and require incision and drainage into the pharynx. Because of the hazard of aspiration this should be done, if at all possible, in the fully awake patient, with neither general anesthesia nor deep sedation.[17] Unfortunately this is not usually possible in children, and general anesthesia will be required.

Management of General Anesthesia in Patients with Peritonsillar Abscess. The special problems of anesthesia in these circumstances are:

1. The likelihood of aggravating preexisting respiratory obstruction during induction and loss of consciousness.

2. Trismus may not resolve even with muscle relaxation, thus making laryngoscopy and intubation difficult or impossible.

3. Pharyngeal swelling and distortion of normal anatomy add to the difficulty of intubation.

4. The abscess may rupture at any time during induction or laryngoscopy and flood the pharynx with pus. This causes immediate respiratory obstruction and allows aspiration of infected material into the lungs, also adding greatly to the immediate difficulty of intubation.

5. Patients with large abscesses may be severely ill, pyrexial, toxic, and dehydrated.

A seriously toxic and dehydrated patient must be prepared for operation by rehydration with intravenous fluids, antibiotic therapy, and measures to lower his temperature. The most difficult problem for the anesthetist then remains management of the airway. If, after examination of the patient's mouth and pharynx, the anesthetist has any doubt that the patient can be intubated successfully, the safer course is to perform a preliminary tracheostomy with the patient under local anesthesia. General anesthesia can then be induced after the airway has been secured. However, most instances of peritonsillar infection are not so florid, and it is reasonable to proceed to induction of general anesthesia in those patients in whom it has been possible to inspect the throat preoperatively, there is no significant respiratory obstruction, and the abscess is still intact. In these circumstances, preoxygenation followed by a rapid-sequence intravenous induction and intubation (avoiding positive-pressure ventilation of the patient before intubation if at all possible) is a suitable technique.

If, on the other hand, preoperative examination of the patient shows a degree of trismus sufficient to make opening of the mouth difficult, or if there has been any suggestion of respiratory obstruction due to the pharyngeal swelling, then it becomes imperative to maintain spontaneous ventilation until absolutely sure that intubation can be achieved. Anesthesia should be induced in these circumstances with oxygen and halothane, and the patient should be allowed to become sufficiently deeply anesthetised, provided adequate ventilation is maintained, to allow laryngoscopy. If the glottis can be easily seen and there is no apparent hindrance to intubation, the trachea may be intubated directly. Alternatively, to avoid coughing and straining and possible abscess rupture, an assistant can give succinylcholine intravenously while the anesthetist maintains direct vision of the glottis and proceeds to intubate when the cords are fully relaxed. The prolonged period of oxygen breathing during induction usually allows 1 or 2 minutes of apnea without leading to hypoxia, and most often it is unnecessary to ventilate the patient artificially before intubation.

Once the airway has been secured by intubation, the hazards are greatly reduced and anesthesia can be continued in any appropriate way. The area of incision is hyperemic, and considerable bleeding is common and may be difficult to control; particular attention should be paid to adequate blood replacement. At the end of operation the patient should be turned on his side and allowed to regain consciousness before extubation.

Occasionally a similar clinical picture is seen in infectious mononucleosis, in which marked involvement of the lymphoid tissue of the nasopharynx can cause gross enlargement of the tonsils and respiratory obstruction sometimes severe enough to be fatal.[20] If there is no response to conservative treatment, tonsillectomy will become urgently required. However, because of the friability and hyperemia of the tonsillar and other lymphoid tissue in the nose and pharynx, along with the possibility of secondary pyogenic bacterial infection, the problems and hazards of attempting induction of general anesthesia are the same as those in peritonsillar abscess. Where there is any doubt about the ease of intubation, preinduction tracheostomy offers much greater safety for the patient.[21]

Retropharyngeal Abscess

There are two distinct types of retropharyngeal abscess. The first, which is related to acute pyogenic infection and abscess formation in the lymphatic tissue that lies between the prevertebral fascia and posterior pharyngeal wall in children, occurs as a direct extension of infection from the tonsil, nose, or middle ear. The clinical features are severe sore throat, respiratory obstruction due to forward dislocation of the posterior pharyngeal wall, and marked general toxicity. Retropharyngeal abscess of this type presents the same threat to the patient's airway as does quinsy, for if it ruptures it does so into the pharynx itself. The treatment is similar to that described for peritonsillar abscess. Drainage, if required, has of necessity to be into the pharynx because of the abscess's position relative to the prevertebral fascia.

The other form of retropharyngeal abscess occurs behind the prevertebral fascia, usually because of extension from osteomyelitis of a vertebral body, and is more usually chronic than acute. Because of the barrier presented by the prevertebral fascia these abscesses do not tend to point into the pharynx and the appropriate drainage route is to the exterior of the neck. This may be readily accomplished through a skin incision made behind the sternomastoid. Induction of general anesthesia in these circumstances is much safer and simpler than in other forms of pharyngeal abscess because of the lesser degree of obstruction of the pharynx by swelling and the prevention of pharyngeal soiling by the intact prevertebral fascia.

Ludwig Angina

This is a severe pyogenic (usually streptococcal) cellulitis of the submandibular and sublingual region associated with inflammatory edema of the mouth and tongue. Edema develops rapidly, and the tongue swells and is pushed forward through the open mouth and upward against the palate. Cellulitis spreads into the neck below the deep cervical fascia, and respiratory obstruction may occur with great rapidity. Intubation of the trachea is usually impossible, and should respiratory obstruction become severe there is no option but to perform emergency tracheostomy with the patient under local anesthesia alone. General anesthesia is fraught with danger of provoking complete respiratory obstruction, and must be avoided. If an abscess forms, which is unusual, it should be incised and drained externally through a submental cervical incision. Indeed, even in the absence of a defined abscess, if edema and swelling of the neck do not subside rapidly following institution of antibiotic therapy, a similar incision may still be indicated to decompress the closed fascial space beneath the mylohyoid muscle and reduce the potential for airway obstruction. This incision should be made with the patient under local anesthesia alone, and is left open until the swelling subsides.

TONGUE

Macroglossia

Macroglossia is a loosely applied term covering many disparate conditions. The tongue may be truly enlarged, owing for example to hypertrophy of its own tissues or to invasion by tumor, or there may be merely apparent enlargement secondary to a relative diminution in the size of the oral cavity, such as occurs in Down syndrome. To avoid confusion, the term "macroglossia" should be reserved to those conditions in which there is chronic, usually painless, enlargement of the tongue, and the term "acute parenchymatous glossitis" used to describe those conditions in which the tongue enlarges acutely and rapidly, for example as a result of inflammatory edema. The various causes of chronically enlarged tongue in childhood are summarized in Table 11–1.

The definition of macroglossia is confused, however, and has been extended by some to include all cases in which the tongue is incapable of being withdrawn behind the anterior teeth (or gums). Others have limited its application to only those instances in which obstructive symptoms occur. Because of this problem of definition estimates of the incidence of macroglossia

Table 11–1. CLASSIFICATION OF MACROGLOSSIA IN CHILDHOOD

Category	Type	Remarks
Congenital	Idiopathic hyperplasia	If unilateral, often associated with other somatic anomalies
	Relative	Associated with Down syndrome, cretinism, glycogen storage diseases
Secondary	Cystic tumors	Lymphangioma (cystic hygroma)
		Lingual thyroid
		Dermoid cyst
	Solid tumors	Neurofibroma
		Rhabdomyoma
		Fibrolipoma
		Carcinoma
		Sarcoma

in the population are equally confusing. Primary macroglossia has been described as being "common,"[22] "uncommon,"[23] and "rare."[24]

Symptoms associated with macroglossia vary with the degree of enlargement of the tongue relative to the mouth. These vary from minor effects on development of speech and dentition to profound obstruction of both respiration and swallowing. Speech cannot, of course, be evaluated in infancy, but in older children secondary macroglossia causes interference with speech related not only to the overall degree of enlargement of the tongue but also to the exact site, particularly in smaller lesions. Minor degrees of obstruction cause little noticeable effect apart from excess salivation, but more pronounced obstruction causes dysphagia. Almost all patients with primary or secondary macroglossia of any significant degree have difficulty in swallowing, often being able to manage only liquids. In gross enlargements of the tongue the anterior part becomes permanently exteriorized, the surface is dry and fissured, and ulceration is common. Respiratory obstruction is a feature of the grosser forms of macroglossia and occurs particularly in those instances in which the pathology involves not only the tongue, but also the floor of the mouth and the tissues of the neck (for example, lymphangioma).

Some Specific Causes of Enlarged Tongue

Primary Macroglossia. This is a benign condition, and operation to reduce the size of the tongue is usually required only if there are major obstructive effects. Some recommend that reduction glossoplasty should be carried out in most cases to prevent later dental malocclusion,[24] and claim that if such surgery is performed in infancy the need for orthodontic treatment and speech therapy later in childhood is greatly reduced.[23] Operations directed to prevention of speech impairment alone should be postponed until the age of 3 years, after which further spontaneous improvement in articulation is unlikely to occur and the degree of speech deficit can be accurately assessed.

Lymphangioma. Cystic hygroma usually occurs in infancy; most cases presenting soon after birth and 95 percent of all cases are seen before the age of 2 years.[25] It most commonly occurs in the posterior triangle of the neck, but more rarely may arise in the anterior triangle close to the mandible. In this latter group the tumor usually extends into the floor of the mouth and the base of the tongue. Cystic hygroma involving the tongue is much rarer than other forms of cervical lymphangioma but causes severe pharyngeal obstruction, and the patient usually presents with acute respiratory obstruction at birth. The histological appearance of cystic hygroma is that of a multilocular, endothelium-lined, thin-walled tumor that arises from lymphatic vessels but often contains areas of more solid lymphoid tissue and a large number of thin-walled blood vessels. It is not malignant but it infiltrates tissues, making dissection difficult and often necessitating multiple operations for its eradication. The tumor is prone to sudden enlargement, sometimes due to contained hemorrhage or infection, but more often for no apparent reason.

Lingual Thyroid. Thyroid tissue may occur in the tongue in the form of a complete ectopic thyroid gland as a result of failure to complete proper "descent" during development of the thyroid from the thyroglossal duct. In other cases in which there is a normally situated thyroid gland, accessory thyroids may occur along the tract of the thyroglossal duct and presumably represent ectopic "rests" of thyroid tissue.[26] Lingual thyroid of any variety is rare; it is more common in females, and usually occurs in the region of the foramen cecum, or between it and the epiglottis in the posterior third of the tongue. Symptoms depend on the size of the ectopic gland, and small lingual thyroids may remain symptomless and undetected. In other patients presenting features are dysphagia and dyspnea, and occasionally bleeding. Once suspected, the diagnosis can be confirmed by radionuclide scanning.

Treatment largely depends on the degree of symptoms; if the patient is asymptomatic there may be no indication for any treatment at all. It must, however, be borne in mind that some 5 percent of all lingual thyroids may eventually undergo malignant transformation.[22] If the patient is symptomatic, thyroid supplementation therapy usually results in reduction in the size of the gland, often to the point of rendering the patient asymptomatic. Alternatively, the ectopic thyroid tissue may be excised, in which case the patient will often require thyroid replacement therapy. To avoid the need for lifelong replacement therapy, the excised thyroid tissue may be implanted elsewhere in the body.[27, 28]

Cysts of the Tongue. Solitary cysts of a variety of pathological types occur in the tongue, including salivary, dermoid, and epidermoid growths. Symptoms are dependent on size and site, and most cysts will require operation. Simple salivary cysts can usually be effectively cured by marsupialization, but most other cysts require definitive removal.

Other Tumors of the Tongue. Apart from lymphangioma, other diffuse neoplastic tumors including hemangioma, fibromatosis, and fibrolipomatous dysplasia are also rare causes of macroglossia. Smaller, discrete simple tumors of the tongue have also been reported occasionally.[29, 30] Malignant tumors of the tongue are exceedingly rare in childhood, but lingual carcinoma[31] and rhabdomyosarcoma[32] have been known to occur. Treatment of malignant tumors of the tongue in children is similar to that in adults, including radiation and aggressive surgery, possibly with hemimandibulectomy and radical cervical node dissection.

Surgery for Macroglossia

When surgery of the tongue is required, the operation should be designed not only to remove the bulk of the tumor or cyst but also to preserve as far as possible function and appearance. This means that attention must be given to the shape and mobility of the tongue as well as size, and that preservation of speech and taste should also be ensured if at all possible. Various operations have been devised to fulfill these goals.[22] Among the least damaging partial glossectomies are those that are limited to the anterior and superficial two thirds of the tongue and avoid the lingual and hypoglossal nerves. Operations on the posterior part of the tongue may damage these nerves, as well as the glossopharyngeal nerve.

Anesthesia for Tongue Surgery

The special problems that may be encountered by the anesthetist during operations on the tongue are related to:
1. The degree of pharyngeal obstruction. Severe macroglossia will cause marked obstruction of the airway, although if the enlargement is confined to the anterior part of the tongue, obstruction in the oropharynx may be bypassed by the nasal airways. Thus, even in the absence of obvious respiratory obstruction there may be sufficient intraoral obstruction to make laryngoscopy and intubation difficult. Lesions that involve not only the tongue but also the floor of the mouth are particularly likely to cause difficulty during laryngoscopy and intubation.
2. The need to secure the airway and isolate it from the surgical field.
3. Intraoperative bleeding, which may be considerable and require extensive replacement therapy.
4. Acute postoperative edema and swelling, which may cause severe, albeit temporary, pharyngeal and respiratory obstruction. This is particularly likely if the operation involves the posterior third of the tongue. Swelling of the anterior two thirds is usually well tolerated by patients who have unobstructed nasal airways. (Postoperative airway obstruction due to an acutely enlarged tongue is not limited to patients with an already existing tongue lesion but has also been reported as occurring secondarily to venous obstruction of the tongue during anesthesia in the sitting position.[33])

In the preoperative assessment of patients requiring glossectomy particular attention should therefore be paid to signs and symptoms of respiratory obstruction, and even in patients without clinical evidence of significant obstruction a careful examination of the pharynx and neck should be made for the degree of soft tissue enlargement. The nasal airways should also be checked for patency.

Intraoperative Management

Patients in Whom There Is No Respiratory Obstruction. Laryngoscopy and intubation in this group, although occasionally difficult, is rarely impossible. Nevertheless, if there are any doubts, after preoperative examination of the patient, that intubation will be other than straightforward, it is wise to avoid intravenous agents or muscle relaxants until the airway has been secured. Awake laryngoscopy and intubation may be possible in some of these patients, particularly infants; otherwise a gentle inhalational induction to a deep plane of anesthesia sufficient to allow intubation is the technique of choice (as described earlier in the section on Peritonsillar Abscess). If the tongue lesion is placed anteriorly and there are no indications of potential difficulty in intubation, any technique of induction that might otherwise be used will be suitable.

Nasotracheal intubation is the route of choice. It offers the advantage of removing the tube as far as possible from the surgical field, allows better fixation, and is more suitable for retention in the immediate postoperative period. Pharyngeal packing to protect against tracheobronchial soiling is necessary. Monitoring and maintenance of anesthesia are as for any other common pharyngeal operations, with particular attention to accurate estimation of blood loss and replacement of blood volume depletion when indicated.

At the end of operation, it is important to assess the possible degree of postoperative respiratory obstruction that may occur secondary to edema and swelling. This is particularly likely to cause trouble if the operation has involved the posterior part of the tongue or if the patient has preexisting nasal obstruction. If there is any indication that there may be some postoperative obstruction of this nature, then the airway must be secured and maintained by artificial means until postoperative edema and swelling have subsided. This may be achieved either by maintaining nasotracheal intubation for 1 or 2 days postoperatively, or by elective tracheostomy. It is much easier to anticipate problems and provide for them than to have to cope with an acute episode of severe respiratory obstruction occurring perhaps hours after operation.

Patients in Whom There Is Preexisting Respiratory Obstruction. These are usually infants with cystic hygromas involving the anterior tongue, and the usual presentation is of acute respiratory distress at birth.[22] (It must be emphasized that only a very small proportion of infants with cystic hygromas fall into this group.[34]) The primary objective is to achieve and maintain an adequate airway. Although intubation may be difficult, there is little alternative, as these tumors often infiltrate the floor of the mouth and the neck, making tracheostomy technically very difficult (and unlikely to be successful if required to be done urgently for resuscitation). Every effort should therefore be directed to intubating the trachea as the initial resuscitative measure. (In the newborn infant this should be performed without anesthesia.) A selection of laryngoscope blades, endotracheal tubes, and stylets should be prepared, and skilled assistants should be available. In some instances it may be possible to establish the airway only by using a bronchoscope, and in this case a tracheostomy should be performed with the bronchoscope in place. Once the airway is secured by intubation, the immediate emergency is over and time can be taken to complete resuscitation and assessment of the child. Because of the difficulty in dissection of these tumors and their unpredictable behavior in terms of acute size changes, long-term tracheostomy is usually required for airway management. Many other patients may require tracheostomy for the immediate perioperative period. As stressed above, tracheostomy in these patients is difficult and should be carried out as a planned procedure in an already intubated patient. Once a satisfactory airway has been secured, further management is as described above for nonobstructed patients, except that in this group it is absolutely mandatory to maintain the artificial airway well into the postoperative period.

Patients with lesser degrees of respiratory obstruction will not require immediate respiratory resuscitation, but must be considered as candidates for complete respiratory obstruction during induction of anesthesia and be treated accordingly. The techniques that may be most safely used are awake intubation; intubation following gentle inhalational induction alone; or, occasionally in those patients whose lesions do not involve the neck, primary tracheostomy using infiltration anesthesia alone.

ACUTE OBSTRUCTIVE INFECTIONS OF THE UPPER AIRWAY

Any lesion producing partial obstruction of the larynx or trachea causes characteristic noisy breathing (stridor),[35] but in previously healthy children stridor of acute onset is almost always attributable to laryngitis, epiglottitis, or laryngotracheal foreign body.[36] Much rarer causes include trauma, smoke inhalation, and external compression of the trachea. The classification and descriptions of acute infections has until recently been the subject of much confusion, but it is now generally accepted that there are two broad categories of illness responsible for infectious stridor in children (Table 11–2). On the one hand is viral laryngotracheobronchitis, commonly called croup, of rather slower onset and usually running a benign course over a few days, and on the other is bacterial infection

Table 11–2. SOME FEATURES OF ACUTE EPIGLOTTITIS AND LARYNGOTRACHEOBRONCHITIS

	Acute Epiglottitis	Laryngotracheo- bronchitis
Incidence	Rare (<5%)*	Common (>80%)*
Age	Mostly 2–6 yrs.; sometimes older	6–36 months
Onset	Sudden: <24 hours	Gradual: usually preceded by 2–3 days of upper respiratory tract symptoms
Clinical features		
1. Stridor	Yes, but may decrease as respiratory obstruction worsens	Yes
2. Cough	No	Yes
3. Voice	Usually does not speak	Hoarse
4. Posture	Sits upright, head forward	
5. Drooling	Yes	No
X-ray	Swollen epiglottis	Narrow subglottis
Laryngoscopy	Erythema and edema of epiglottis and periglottic tissues	Normal glottis
Etiology	Bacterial: *Haemophilus influenzae* group b	Viral: Parainfluenzal, influenzal
Treatment	Intubation Antibiotics Rehydration	Humidification Racemic epinephrine Steroids Intubation (rare)
Course	24–48 hours	3–6 days

*Refers to proportion of children with stridor requiring hospital admission.

of the epiglottis and surrounding tissues, characterized by sudden onset and rapid progression to potentially lethal respiratory obstruction within hours. Although there is a characteristically different clinical picture in typical cases of laryngotracheobronchitis and acute epiglottitis, in many patients initial diagnosis may be difficult, and it may be quite impossible to distinguish one from the other.[36–38] A small proportion of patients with laryngotracheobronchitis also proceed to severe respiratory obstruction requiring similar airway intervention to that used in managing acute epiglottitis, and for this reason every instance of sudden onset of stridor in a child must be considered potentially lethal and treated accordingly.[36]

Acute Epiglottitis (Supraglottitis)

This is a potentially fatal bacterial infection of the larynx, with dangerously rapid onset, affecting primarily the epiglottis, aryepiglottic folds, arytenoid cartilages, and surrounding tissues. Inflammatory swelling and edema of the involved tissues not only produces the characteristic swollen cherry-red epiglottis but encroaches on the airway and can produce severe, or indeed complete, respiratory obstruction. Variations from this classic pattern of tissue involvement can occur. There have been reports of isolated involvement of paraepiglottic tissues with minimal swelling of the epiglottis itself, with, however, typical respiratory obstructive symptoms.[39, 40]

Acute epiglottitis most commonly occurs in children between the ages of 2 and 8 years;[41] most cases occurring in preschool children,[42] but it has also been known to occur in infants[43] and in adults.[44] It may occur at any time of the year. Most series show a definitive decline during the summer months,[42, 45] although others report no such seasonal predilection.[40, 46] There may be a slightly higher incidence in males.[47]

This disease has a high mortality, entirely related to respiratory obstruction, but if the respiratory obstruction is adequately treated the infection generally resolves quickly and the patient recovers fully. In spite of this, unnecessary deaths still occur, even in patients who arrive at the hospital before the onset of respiratory failure.[47] This should not happen and usually is the consequence of inappropriate diagnostic or therapeutic efforts.[47, 48]

Bacteriology

Most cases of acute epiglottitis are due to infection by Group B *Haemophilus influenzae*,[45] but occasionally other organisms, notably pyogenic staphylococci and beta-hemolytic streptococci,[41] have been responsible. The infecting organism is more readily identified from blood cultures than from direct swabs from the larynx. A higher positive rate is obtained when blood cultures are taken after instrumentation of the larynx, but even so, about half of such cultures will be sterile.[41] Serum counterimmunoelectrophoresis may also be useful in determining the bacteriological etiology.[49]

H. influenzae is generally sensitive to ampicillin, but in the past few years an increasing incidence of infections due to beta-lactamase–producing strains resistant to ampicillin have been reported. For this reason some authorities now recommend starting treatment with both ampicillin and chloramphenicol, later modifying the antibiotic according to the results of sensitivity tests from the blood cultures.[42] A few instances of chloramphenicol resistant *H. influenzae* have also been reported,[50] and in these cases the cephalosporin cefamandole may be substituted.

Clinical Picture

Acute epiglottitis is typically described as sudden onset of sore throat, dysphagia, and shortness of breath progressing rapidly to inspiratory stridor in a previously well child. The total time span from onset of first symptoms to severe respiratory distress is usually only 6 to 12 hours. In other cases, however, the patients are found to have a history of feeling unwell, with fever, sore throat, or a "cold" for 24 hours or more before the onset of stridor. The child appears toxic with pyrexia, tachycardia, and tachypnea, and prefers to sit up, leaning forward with the chin pushed out and the neck hyperextended. Drooling of saliva

occurs because of dysphagia. The symptoms are exacerbated by lying down. There is no cough, and the child usually makes little effort to speak. As respiratory obstruction worsens, hypercapnia and hypoxia cause further distress, and the onset of cyanosis or obvious air hunger signals impending respiratory arrest. Even when respiratory distress does not appear to be particularly severe, sudden complete respiratory obstruction and arrest may be caused at any time by laryngospasm. Stress, anxiety, and crying can all contribute to an increased oxygen requirement and exacerbation of symptoms.[47]

Diagnosis

The diagnosis of acute epiglottitis is essentially clinical and is made by history and examination. Laboratory studies play only a retrospective role in establishing precise bacteriology. The important differential diagnoses in acute epiglottitis are viral laryngotracheobronchitis (Table 11–2) and inhaled foreign body. Laryngotracheobronchitis and acute epiglottitis are usually described as being quite different in history, pathology, presentation, and course. Airway intervention is rarely required in laryngotracheobronchitis, most cases being mild and responding quickly to humidification. However, more severe cases of laryngotracheobronchitis may show a similar sudden deterioration in ventilatory status to acute epiglottitis, often due to increasing respiratory obstruction caused by laryngeal edema or secondary bacterial laryngitis, or simply by retention of tenacious secretions. In individual cases, therefore, diagnosis may be difficult.[36, 37] This is of limited practical importance, as the treatment of severe respiratory obstruction is similar no matter the precise cause. It is essential to proceed with airway management rather than to delay intervention to allow more diagnostic efforts while the patient's condition rapidly deteriorates.[51] Laryngeal foreign body is usually diagnosed by history of sudden onset of stridor after choking, eating, or playing with small objects, the lack of systemic toxicity, and radiography.[35]

Although diagnosis of epiglottitis can be confirmed by direct inspection of the throat, the extent of examination compatible with safety remains controversial. Most authorities continue to advise against any effort to examine the patient's throat before definitive airway management is available, lest such examination provoke respiratory arrest and turn a serious situation into a crisis. Others suggest that direct laryngeal inspection is not so dangerous as formerly stated[40] and that gentle inspection of the larynx, using a well-lubricated curved laryngoscope blade of the Macintosh pattern, is often well tolerated by these patients; however, advocates of this approach still advise that such examination should take place only in situations in which the apparatus and expertise to secure an artificial airway immediately are present.[43] Visualization of a hyperemic edematous epiglottis or swollen aryepiglottic folds confirms the diagnosis. Occasionally the swollen epiglottis may even be ulcerated.

If the patient's condition warrants it, x-ray of the neck not only helps to differentiate acute epiglottitis from laryngotracheobronchitis but also is useful in the exclusion of laryngotracheal foreign body.[35, 36] The lateral view is particularly useful and in acute epiglottitis typically shows swelling and rounding of the epiglottis and distention of the hypopharynx.

Blood studies are of no immediate diagnostic value and may be positively dangerous if they lead to crying and laryngospasm or to temporizing by the medical staff. Such studies are better left undone until the airway has been secured. Arterial blood gas levels are of no predictive value in assessing the need for airway intervention.

Treatment

The management of patients with severe stridor has been, and remains to some extent, the subject of controversy,[40] but the consensus is toward immediate admission to an intensive care unit. As soon as possible laryngoscopy should be performed with the patient anesthetized, and the airway should be secured by tracheal intubation. Specific etiological diagnosis is made on the basis of blood culture, and specific treatment with antibiotics and rehydration is then instituted. To avoid possible delays in treatment, many centers have established protocols to be followed in cases of suspected acute epiglottitis. The following account of management of patients with suspected acute epiglottitis is that followed in the author's hospital.

When the hospital is notified that a patient with suspected acute epiglottitis is being sent in, the anesthesia and intensive care unit staffs are alerted to ensure the presence of an anesthetist in the emergency room when the patient arrives, and to allow arrangements to be made for probable admission to the intensive care unit and availability of an operating room. In some centers, management of these cases is undertaken by the otorhinolaryngology service, in which case an ENT surgeon would be called in addition to the anesthetist.

On arrival, the patient is subject to the very minimum of examination or interference, and can generally be immediately categorized into one of three groups by simple inspection:

1. If he is in gross respiratory distress or moribund, immediate resuscitation must be attempted; hence the need for skilled airway management to be available from the moment of admission. If an artificial airway is not instantly available it is often possible to ventilate by face mask and positive pressure,[52] but if respiratory obstruction cannot be overcome quickly, cricothyroidotomy should be performed. Following successful resuscitation and securing of the airway, the patient should be transferred to the intensive care unit and specific treatment of the epiglottitis should be contin-

ued along the lines suggested below. Every effort should also be made to minimize the detrimental effects of tissue hypoperfusion and hypoxia that will have occurred during the period of cardiac arrest, particularly with respect to control of cerebral edema and prevention of any increase in cerebral oxygen demand. Use of anticonvulsants, artificial ventilation, and neuromuscular blockade is well established in these circumstances, while therapy with corticosteroids, barbiturate coma, and/or hypothermia is more controversial.[52a]

2. If the patient has obvious stridor with air hunger, as evidenced by use of accessory muscles of respiration, he is not examined or x-rayed, but is allowed to remain sitting up and is transferred at once to the intensive care unit or operating room for immediate endoscopy and intubation. The only therapeutic endeavor allowed is oxygen (preferably humidified) by face mask. Examination of the throat is avoided for fear of provoking profound respiratory obstruction and with the knowledge that little will be gained by such examination, as the patient will almost certainly require an artificial airway irrespective of the findings. For similar reasons, x-rays are contraindicated in these circumstances. Routine blood work should be postponed not only because drawing blood will cause an unnecessary delay in getting on with more definitive treatment but also, and more importantly, because increasing the patient's distress will increase oxygen demand and hence put him further at risk.

3. The third group of patients are those in whom although there is stridor there is no obvious respiratory distress. It is important to distinguish those who are in the early stages of epiglottitis or possibly severe laryngotracheobronchitis and who are likely to progress to severe respiratory obstruction from those with mild laryngotracheobronchitis who will require little treatment apart from humidification and possibly racemic epinephrine. In this group a lateral neck radiograph can be invaluable in showing incipient obstruction.[53] However, the patient must be accompanied at all times by a physician with the capability and necessary equipment to establish an emergency artificial airway. Patients in whom radiological signs of epiglottic swelling are seen are intubated and admitted to the intensive care unit. If there are no x-ray changes but stridor persists even without respiratory distress, the patient is admitted to the intensive care unit but treated for laryngotracheobronchitis with frequent reassessment. If at any time respiratory obstruction worsens to the point of producing distress, the patient proceeds to laryngoscopy and intubation. If, however, stridor lessens, then the patient is assumed to have resolving laryngotracheobronchitis and is transferred out of intensive care to a general pediatric ward.

Laryngoscopy and Intubation. Before the patient arrives in the operating room, all necessary airway equipment should have been prepared. This should include a range of tracheal tubes, rigid bronchoscopes, and a tracheostomy set. On arrival, the patient should be disturbed as little as possible and allowed to remain in the sitting position while a gentle inhalational induction of anesthesia, using halothane in oxygen, is started. As induction proceeds, a little positive pressure applied via the reservoir bag often improves ventilation noticeably. So long as the patient does not become cyanosed, anesthesia should be continued in this manner until the patient is in a fairly deep plane of surgical anesthesia. The time required to achieve this state provides an opportunity to establish an intravenous infusion, administer atropine, and apply the usual monitors (EKG, blood pressure cuff, and so forth), none of which is done while the child is still fully awake lest it increase his or her apprehension and stress. When the child is adequately anesthetised, and this will probably take at least 15 minutes, laryngoscopy is performed, note is taken of the appearance of the epiglottis and surrounding tissues, and an oral tracheal tube is passed, without the aid of muscle relaxants. Generally there is no great difficulty in doing this, although a smaller than normal tube may be required. If the laryngeal opening cannot be seen because of swelling, external pressure on the chest usually allows its identification by the expulsion of air bubbles into the pharynx. If a tube cannot be passed, a small bronchoscope should be used to secure the airway. If total respiratory obstruction occurs with inability to achieve any airway through the mouth, an attempt should be made to ventilate the patient by facemask and positive pressure. If adequate ventilation cannot be achieved promptly, a cricothyroidotomy should be performed.

Once the airway is established, anesthesia is continued in the same way, blood cultures and glottic bacteriology swabs are taken, and the oral tracheal tube is changed to a nasal tracheal tube, which is then carefully secured. Once blood cultures have been obtained, intravenous antibiotic therapy is started with ampicillin and chloramphenicol. The patient is allowed to waken and is returned to the intensive care unit, where treatment is continued with antibiotics and intravenous fluids. Most patients tolerate the nasotracheal tube well, but some may require sedation. Spontaneous ventilation using humidified air or oxygen-enriched air via a T-piece is usually all that is required. Accidental displacement of the tube at this stage is not usually followed by immediate total airway obstruction, probably because of the "stenting" effect reducing the degree of glottic edema. Nonetheless all patients with epiglottitis must be kept in an intensive care unit, and all routine care for an intubated patient is given. In circumstances in which a nursing unit skilled in the care of patients with nasotracheal tubes is not available, it is probably safer to proceed to elective tracheostomy once oral intubation has been achieved.

Bacterial epiglottitis usually resolves very quickly, within 24 to 48 hours, but viral laryngotracheobronchitis takes rather longer. The average duration of nasotracheal intubation is about 36 hours in acute epiglottitis, but there is considerable individual variation,[54] so it is not possible to set an arbitrary time for extubation. Evidence of improvement includes resolution of the pyrexia and development of an air leak around the tracheal tube. These events are usually a better guide to the time to extubate than repeated laryngoscopies under general anesthesia because the appearance of the larynx under these circumstances does not correlate well with the patient's ability to maintain an adequate airway without help.[47] The safety and freedom from complications of short-term nasotracheal intubation in acute epiglottitis has been established. This is not the case for the longer-term intubation occasionally required in the treatment of laryngotracheobronchitis, particularly in children less than 1 year old, in whom the incidence of postintubation subglottic stenosis is high.[55] Complications of acute epiglottitis include cervical lymphadenitis, pneumonia, otitis media,[56] and very rarely meningitis.

Role of Steroids. The use of expectant corticosteroid therapy to reduce inflammation and edema is becoming more common;[41] although doubt remains about whether this has any advantageous effect on the rate of resolution of the edema over that of conventional treatment,[47] it may have a useful role in reducing postintubation subglottic edema. By far the most controversial aspect of steroid therapy in acute epiglottitis is reliance on steroids to reduce edema to the extent of deliberately avoiding the necessity for intubation or tracheostomy.[52] This approach has received little support and has indeed been specifically condemned for management of childhood epiglottitis.[57]

Diphtheria

Although this formerly dreaded infectious disease has largely disappeared from the developed world since the adoption of active immunization, it has not been eradicated, as evidenced by continuing sporadic outbreaks.[58, 59] In recent years such outbreaks have generally occurred in subjects who were debilitated[60] or lacking in immunity for other reasons,[61] but they serve to remind that danger of epidemics of diphtheria may be expected to recur should immunization policies be allowed to lapse. There is some evidence that such policies are no longer being so actively pursued as formerly.[62, 63] Furthermore, because diphtheria can be spread by asymptomatic carriers, travelers and immigrants from regions in which there has not been universal active immunization may be expected to be constantly reintroducing the infection. Hence it is important to maintain a high level of active immunity in the population at large.[59]

Diphtheria occurs predominantly in temperate zones, and epidemics tend to be more common in winter but may occur at any time of the year. In the absence of active immunization, this is very much a disease of childhood. It rarely occurs before 6 months of age, due to transplacental transfer of maternal antibody, but thereafter the incidence increases to a maximum at about 5 to 7 years of age and becomes comparatively rare after age 10. Girls are rather more commonly affected than boys, but there is a higher mortality in boys because of the more frequent involvement of the larynx. Recent outbreaks in immunized communities, however, have predominantly involved older patients and largely reflected individual immunity deficiencies (due for example to avoidance of active immunization for religious reasons.)[58] In nonimmunized communities the disease still predominantly affects children.[61]

The infecting organism, *Corynebacterium diphtheriae*, is usually transmitted by droplet infection, and although the bacteria remain largely confined to the site of infection, widespread and devastating systemic effects are produced by its powerful exotoxin. The virulence and toxigenicity of the organism vary widely and independently of morphological differences.[64]

The incubation period is short, usually 2 to 5 days, although it can be as short as 24 hours or as long as 8 days. Mortality rates of 10 to 30 percent were not uncommon in epidemics occurring before immunization became widely adopted. The onset is insidious; the patient feels unwell, may complain of a sore throat, and has a low-grade fever. Inspection of the throat at this stage may show no more than a redness of the pharynx due to hyperemia. However, within a day whitish spots appear on the tonsils, rapidly enlarging and growing together so that by the second day the typical leathery pseudomembrane may be seen. This pseudomembrane consists of necrotic tissue, exudate, and blood, varies in color from dirty white to near black, and has sharply defined margins. It can be removed only with difficulty and leaves a raw and bleeding surface. Apart from the local effects of membranous pharyngitis, toxic systemic effects may occur at any time. Organs particularly vulnerable to the exotoxin are the heart, in which disturbances of conduction and contractility occur, and the peripheral nervous system, particularly the cranial nerves. Clinical evidence of myocardial involvement is seen in about half of all patients with diphtheria and histological evidence in almost all patients who die from the disease, while peripheral nerve palsies occur in about one fifth of all patients. Both local and systemic symptoms usually begin to subside after about 5 days, but even after apparently complete local resolution late cardiac and/or neurological complications may occur. However, in patients who survive there are usually no permanent neurological or cardiac impairments. Death may occur at any time, and is most commonly due to either respiratory obstruction or myocardial failure.

Membranous pharyngitis is not pathognomonic of diphtheria, and important differential diagnoses include infections with other *Corynebacterium* species, for example *C. haemolyticum*,[65] infectious mononucleosis, streptococcal pharyngitis, candidiasis, and Vincent infection, although in these instances the membrane tends to be more easily removed and does not leave a bleeding surface. A similar but nonbacterial membranous pharyngitis can be caused by oral ingestion of the herbicide paraquat.[66]

When diphtheria is suspected, efforts must be made to confirm the diagnosis bacteriologically. Swabs should be taken before antibiotics are given. In general, direct staining of pharyngeal smears is unreliable and cultures of pharyngeal swabs, which also allow testing for virulence, are required. These investigations, however, take a considerable time to complete and treatment cannot be allowed to await the results. Isolation of beta-hemolytic streptococcus does not preclude a diagnosis of diphtheria, as the streptococcus often appears as a secondary invader.

Variations of Diphtheria

Malignant or "bull-neck" diphtheria is a particularly severe form in which the disease follows an accelerated course, progressing to involve the entire pharynx with marked swelling and necrosis of tissues along with cervical lymphadenitis and cellulitis. Toxemia is marked and mortality is high.

Other manifestations of diphtheria occur depending on the site of infection, and include:

1. Nasal diphtheria, in which the infection is limited to the anterior nares, is usually unassociated with constitutional symptoms, and may take a long time to resolve without specific treatment. Affected patients are carriers and are a great danger to the community.

2. Laryngeal diphtheria. In most patients involvement of the larynx is by direct spread from the pharynx, but in a few the larynx is the site of primary infection. The disease presents with hoarseness and loss of voice. Patients with laryngeal diphtheria are at particular risk from respiratory obstruction, and the mortality is high.

3. Cutaneous diphtheria is largely confined to tropical climates, and occurs when otherwise insignificant skin wounds are invaded by *C. diphtheriae*, leading to chronic ulceration, membrane formation, and secondary toxic complications.

Treatment

The mainstays of treatment are specific antitoxin, antibiotics, relief of respiratory obstruction, prolonged bed rest, isolation, and public health measures to prevent spread. Antitoxin neutralizes circulating toxin but has no effect on toxin already taken up by tissues and so should be given early, on suspicion of diphtheria, and with full precautions against sensitivity to horse serum. Penicillin and erythromycin suppress the growth of *C. diphtheriae* and should be given along with antitoxin. The risk of respiratory obstruction is always present when there is pharyngeal membrane formation of moderate degree, and increases should the membrane spread to the glottis, larynx, and trachea. Even in the recovery period sudden death may still occur by laryngeal obstruction due to loosened membrane being aspirated from the pharynx or coughed up from the trachea.

Formerly tracheostomy was reserved for severe diphtheritic respiratory obstruction and was frequently performed in circumstances of great urgency. It would seem that with modern facilities elective tracheostomy should be performed early in patients with any form of membranous pharyngitis, even before the onset of respiratory symptoms. Indications for tracheostomy in these circumstances would include (1) stridor, (2) membrane extending beyond the tonsils to encroach on the periglottic tissues, and (3) any other evidence of laryngeal involvement. If tracheostomy is delayed until evidence of respiratory obstruction or failure becomes apparent it may be too late.[58, 67] Emergency intubation of such patients is likely to be difficult due to involvement of periglottic tissues and difficulty in clearing away the obstructing membrane. Should complete respiratory obstruction occur in patients with diphtheria it would probably be better to proceed directly to cricothyroidotomy rather than to attempt intubation.

Because of the high incidence of toxic myocarditis, general anesthesia is probably better avoided in these patients and tracheostomy should be carried out using local infiltration anesthesia without prior intubation.

Bed rest is important, and should continue for 2 or 3 weeks after local manifestations have resolved, until the usual period in which toxic myocarditis may occur has passed.

Prognosis

The outcome in diphtheria not only is dependent on the virulence of the particular strain of *C. diphtheriae* involved and the degree of immunity possessed by the patient but also is related to the age of the patient, the location and extent of the membrane, and the promptness of diagnosis and the institution of specific antitoxin and antibiotic treatment. Older patients tend to do better than younger, probably because older persons have bigger laryngeal airways and are therefore relatively more tolerant of partial occlusion. Spread of the membrane from the pharynx into the larynx and trachea is associated with a higher mortality. Mortality is greatly reduced if the antitoxin is given early.

LARYNX

The immediate threat to the child presented by anatomical defects or diseases of the larynx is that of respiratory obstruction. Congenital malformations and lesions involving the larynx are uncommon, and when they do occur they usually cause respiratory symptoms

Table 11–3. SOME COMMON AND UNCOMMON CAUSES, OF LARYNGEAL OBSTRUCTION IN CHILDREN

Congenital	Within the larynx	Laryngomalacia
		Congenital subglottic stenosis
		Laryngeal web
		Laryngotracheoesophageal cleft
		Congenital laryngeal paralysis
		Laryngeal tumors
		1. Hemangioma
		2. Lymphangioma
		3. Saccular cyst
		4. Laryngocele
	Extralaryngeal	Congenital macroglossia
		Cervical tumors (lymphangioma)
Acquired	Infections	Laryngotracheobronchitis
		Acute epiglottitis
		Diphtheria
		Infectious mononucleosis
		Pharyngeal abscesses
	Trauma	Inhaled foreign body
		Laryngeal edema
		Postintubation
		Chemical
		Thermal
		Acquired subglottic stenosis
		Cervical trauma
		Open
		Closed
	Neoplasms	Juvenile laryngeal papillomatosis
		Extrinsic tumors of tongue and neck

at birth or shortly thereafter. Acquired diseases involving the larynx and causing respiratory difficulty occur commonly in older children, and are responsible for the general syndrome of croup. Some of the causes, common and uncommon, of laryngeal obstruction in children are shown in Table 11–3.

Congenital Laryngeal Anomalies

Stridor, that is, noisy breathing, is the cardinal symptom of laryngeal obstruction but is not a complete diagnosis in itself and may have many different causes.[35, 68] High-pitched inspiratory stridor is suggestive of obstruction at the glottic or supraglottic level, while the addition of an expiratory component suggests a level below that of the glottis. Expiratory wheeze alone suggests that there is no laryngeal obstruction, but is associated with obstruction in the bronchi. The quality of the cry may give further evidence of the site of the lesion. Most laryngeal lesions are associated with a weak or absent cry, even in patients with little or no demonstrable respiratory obstruction. A hoarse cry is suggestive of a lesion at the level of the glottis. The presence of stridor does not necessarily mean that respiratory distress will inevitably develop, but stridor along with signs of respiratory distress is an indication that airway support will probably be necessary, and adds urgency to the need for a definitive diagnosis. Signs of increasing respiratory distress in infants are increased respiratory rate, flaring of the alae nasi, sternal indrawing, decreased breath sounds, head retraction, tachycardia, restlessness, and cyanosis. Overflow of saliva and aspiration pneumonia will also occur where there is interference with normal laryngeal protective functions.

The assessment of an infant with stridor requires considerable care because of the myriad causes of respiratory problems in this age group. In the presence of stridor in an infant with respiratory distress it cannot be assumed that the cause of the respiratory distress is necessarily laryngeal obstruction. Nor should the absence of respiratory distress in an infant with stridor be assumed to mean that the infant is in no danger. In such patients otherwise trivial events such as minor upper respiratory infections can provoke profound respiratory obstruction.[69] For these reasons it is necessary to take every effort to make a correct anatomical diagnosis and to assess the degree of respiratory obstruction accurately. A careful history and physical examination will go a long way to exclude other common causes of respiratory distress, for example, congenital heart disease. Where a laryngeal lesion is present, particular attention to the quality of the stridor, the effect of posture change on the degree of stridor, and the quality of the cry will often make possible a fairly accurate diagnosis of the type of laryngeal lesion to be made. Particular care should be taken to palpate the neck for evidence of cervical lesion (for example, cyst or tumor) that may cause laryngeal obstruction either by compression or by invasion of the larynx. Further help in diagnosis may be obtained from inspiratory and expiratory lateral cervical radiographs. Definitive diagnosis is made by endoscopy, but in general it is better to postpone laryngoscopy until the child has been fully examined and x-rays have been obtained. However, if the patient is already in respiratory distress, laryngoscopy must be undertaken urgently, with a high probability that the patient will require an artificial airway.

Laryngomalacia

Laryngomalacia is the most common form of congenital laryngeal obstruction; 75 percent of all infants with stridor are found to have this disease.[70] The laryngeal cartilages are abnormally soft and flaccid, so that during inspiration the supraglottic tissues, lacking intrinsic rigidity, tend to fold in toward the glottis, causing partial obstruction and accounting for the characteristic inspiratory noise. Babies born with this condition usually have stridor from birth, although it may be intermittent and tends to disappear during periods of rest and to be exaggerated during crying. The stridor is usually most marked when the infant is lying on his back.[68] Respiratory distress is rare in laryngomalacia. On lateral x-ray of the neck there is a characteristic anterior and downward displacement of the aryepiglottic folds during inspiration. The diagnosis is confirmed by laryngoscopy performed with the patient awake, which reveals a small glottis with a long, narrow epiglottis and floppy aryepiglottic folds that can be seen to fold in toward the glottis during inspiration. Occasionally they also vibrate during inspiration, imparting a "fluttering" quality to the stridor. During expiration, the epiglottis and aryepiglottic folds are blown back out of the way and no longer offer any resistance to air flow. Thus in laryngomalacia the supraglottic tissues act rather like a one-way valve, and these characteristic appearances have suggested the alternative name of "inspiratory laryngeal collapse" for this entity.[68]

Laryngomalacia almost always runs a benign course, and symptoms tend to disappear with growth, usually by about 18 months of age. Treatment is rarely required, and there are no long-term sequelae. However, in a very small proportion of cases severe respiratory obstruction does occur, and in these patients airway support is necessary, generally entailing long-term tracheostomy. In those patients in whom the epiglottis is primarily responsible for the obstruction, lasting relief can sometimes be obtained by suturing the epiglottis to the base of the tongue.[71]

The etiology of laryngomalacia is unknown, and although various nutritional and other factors have been suggested, its natural history indicates that it can best be considered a relative immaturity of the cartilages representing no more than a slowing of normal development.

Another and very much rarer form of congenital laryngeal cartilage dystrophy is complete absence of the epiglottis. In this condition there is no direct respiratory obstruction, but inadequate protection of the glottis during swallowing leads to choking and persistent aspiration pneumonia.

Laryngeal Web

Obstruction of the larynx by membranous webs or partial fusion of the cords is a very rare cause of stridor in infants, occurring in less than 5 percent of those studied by Holinger and Brown.[70] The most common form of web occurs at the level of the cords, and may consist of a thin membrane lying across the cords, a thick web, or partial fusion joining the cords firmly together. The supraglottic web, which is the least common of the laryngeal webs, is a partial fusion of the false cords. In extreme cases there is failure of cannulation, that is, total fusion or atresia of the larynx. Laryngeal atresia is, of course, incompatible with life unless recognized quickly at birth, but a few cases have been reported in which immediate tracheostomy or forceful bronchoscopy has been successful in resuscitation of infants with this anomaly. It is likely that laryngeal atresia is the cause of occasional stillbirths in which the respiratory obstruction has gone unrecognized. Even after routine autopsy (in which the larynx is often only superficially examined), laryngeal atresia may be missed, so that the true incidence may be greater than usually reported.[72]

Laryngeal webs produce symptoms of respiratory obstruction proportional to the degree of narrowing, which may vary from mild to extreme. Definitive diagnosis is made by laryngoscopy. In general, the treatment of severe degrees of laryngeal web remains unsatisfactory,[73] and the outcome of treatment is related more to the type and thickness of the web rather than to the particular form of treatment chosen. Simple membranous webs may require little more than endoscopic division with scissors to restore laryngeal patency. Thicker webs can be treated in the same way but tend to recur, making repeated endoscopic dilatations imperative. If a satisfactory airway cannot be obtained in this way, there is no alternative but to proceed to tracheostomy. In such cases eventual open operation by laryngofissure with insertion of a prosthetic keel implant will be required. Although this operation usually restores an adequate laryngeal airway, good phonation is often difficult to achieve. Alternative endoscopic operations for reconstruction of the larynx and insertion of Silastic keels, avoiding the need for laryngofissure, have been described.[74]

Congenital Subglottis Stenosis

Soft tissue thickening of the larynx, usually most marked 2 to 3 mm below the level of the true cords, may cause stridor from birth, or the onset of symptoms may be delayed for up to 6 months.[75] This anomaly has a particular association with other congenital defects, notably Down syndrome. Infants with mild degrees of congenital subglottic stenosis may be asymptomatic but are at increased risk of developing laryngeal obstruction secondary to upper airway infection or edema. They occasionally present first because of recurrent episodes of laryngotracheobronchitis. Congenital subglottic stenosis is rare (about 6 percent of all congenital laryngeal anomalies) but is of relative importance because it accounts for the majority of tracheostomies required in the first year of life.[72] Diagnosis is confirmed by endoscopy, and treatment depends on the severity of obstruction. If the condition is mild, little may be required apart fom careful observation, while more severe cases may require repeated dilatations.[76, 77] In the most severe cases, tracheostomy[68] or anterior cricoid split with temporary stenting intubation[78, 79] will be necessary. The degree of stenosis gradually lessens with growth, and eventual restoration of a normal patency of the larynx usually takes place without serious sequelae.[80] However, infants who have required prolonged tracheostomy may not be so fortunate, as the tracheostomy itself may produce chronic and sometimes intractable secondary acquired subglottic stenosis. In these cases reconstructive surgery of the larynx may be necessary.[80, 81]

Laryngotracheoesophageal Cleft

This is a very rare family of conditions in which there is incomplete separation of the larynx from the esophagus. The degree of malformation varies from simple absence of the interarytenoid muscle, producing only mild symptoms, to complete fusion of the larynx, trachea, and esophagus into one tube in the most severe form.[82] Between these extremes intermediate degrees of cleft are represented by failure of posterior fusion of the cricoid and possibly the first one or two tracheal cartilages.

The infant presents with a clinical picture similar to that of tracheoesophageal fistula (which itself can coexist in the same patient). The most prominent features are profuse pharyngeal secretions, aspiration pneumonia, and choking and respiratory distress provoked by attempts at feeding. Stridor may or may not be present. Apart from a separate tracheoesophageal fistula, which is found in about 20 percent of these patients, a wide variety of congenital anomalies of other organs, often extensive and severe, occur in association with laryngotracheoesophageal cleft. The endoscopic appearances are confusing and difficult to interpret, and frequently fail to produce the diagnosis. The disease is best confirmed by probing the posterior wall of the larynx during endoscopy, when parting of the mucosal folds may not only reveal the cleft but also allow its extent to be determined. It is probable that because of the difficulty in making this diagnosis the true incidence is consistently underestimated.

Tracheostomy to secure the airway is comparatively ineffective, except in very minor degress of cleft, because of the propensity for the tracheostomy tube to find its way through the defect and into the esophagus. A better approach to the immediate airway problem is to maintain endotracheal intubation and proceed to early reconstructive surgery.[83, 84] In some cases the cleft can be repaired intraluminally using the suspension laryngoscope and simply suturing the mucosal defect, but if this is not possible, or if such a repair persistently breaks down, then correction by open operation will be required. Open operation is usually attempted through a lateral pharyngotomy incision, the larynx being reconstructed over the tracheal tube, which remains in place as a stent. A gastrostomy is maintained during the period of healing. Such reconstructions are technically very difficult and are prone to breakdown or later development of secondary laryngeal stenosis or esophageal stricture or both.[68]

Laryngoceles and Congenital Laryngeal Cysts

Epithelium-lined, simple cystic tumors of the larynx are rare causes of respiratory obstruction in children and may occur in one of two forms: laryngocele or congenital laryngeal cyst.[85] A laryngocele is an abnormal development of the saccular appendage of the laryngeal ventricle and communicates freely with the lumen of the larynx. This free communication accounts for the most remarkable feature of the laryngocele, that is, the great variation in size that can take place rapidly with changes in intralaryngeal pressure. On the other hand congenital laryngeal cysts, or saccular cysts, although also arising from the saccular appendage, do not communicate with the laryngeal cavity and are fluid-filled.

Laryngeal symptoms are proportional to the degree of respiratory obstruction. Investigation is largely by radiology and endoscopy, but frequently may be difficult and require repeated examination before a firm diagnosis can be established. Laryngoscopy may sometimes provoke a sudden increase in size, due to bleeding or edema formation, and cause severe respiratory obstruction. Such obstruction can, however, usually be relieved by endoscopic aspiration of the cyst. Reduction of the volume of the cyst in this way will relieve the symptoms temporarily. Recurrence is the rule after aspiration, however, and a more effective treatment is to unroof the cyst and strip its lining epithelium as far as possible. This can be done through the laryngoscope, but again recurrence rates are high and multiple operations may be required.[86, 87] A more satisfactory approach might be to allow some months for the infant to grow, maintaining security of the airway by tracheostomy, and then proceed to open neck operation.[68]

Other congenital cystic swellings in the neck, for example cystic hygroma, may also cause laryngeal obstruction, either by external compression of the larynx or by extension into it.

Congenital Laryngeal Paralysis

Paralysis of the vocal cords secondary to central or peripheral nervous system disorder, which is the second most common cause of congenital laryngeal obstruction,[68] arises from a variety of primary causes. Congenital laryngeal paralysis is often associated with gross anomalies in other systems, particularly the central nervous system. It can be apparent at birth or, when it is due to expanding lesions elsewhere, there may be considerable delay in the onset of symptoms. In one series the average age at onset of symptoms was 38 days.[88] Among the central causes of laryngeal paralysis are intracerebral hemorrhage, cerebral agenesis, myelomeningocele with Arnold-Chiari malformation, and hydrocephalus.[89, 90] Peripheral motor nerves may be damaged by birth trauma or by involvement in malformations or congenital lesions in the mediastinum and neck.[88] Damage to the recurrent laryngeal nerve may also occur during operations to relieve other congenital anomalies, for example during thoracotomy for repair of heart and esophageal defects. In many cases a definite cause cannot be identified and the paralysis is often temporary. Half of all patients with unilateral congenital cord paralysis eventually recover fully. Similarly, a rather smaller proportion, about a third, of patients with bilateral paralysis show a good recovery.[88]

Symptoms are proportional to the severity of obstruction and the degree of laryngeal incompetence to protect the airway. The infant presents with varying degrees of stridor, respiratory distress, dysphagia, and aspiration pneumonia. Dysphonia is uncommon. Diagnosis is confirmed by awake laryngoscopy with careful observation of cord motility.[91]

Unilateral paralysis, which is usually due to a peripheral lesion, is more common than bilateral, and the left side is more often affected than the right, presumably because the longer course of the recurrent laryngeal nerve on the left exposes it to greater risk of damage. Unilateral lesions are often associated with quite severe feeding problems, marked by coughing and choking. Accompanying stridor may be markedly dependent on position, lessening or even disappearing when the infant is lying on the affected side. Bilateral paralysis is usually indicative of a central nervous system lesion; respiratory obstructive symptoms are more obvious and of greater degree than in unilateral paralysis.

The need for treatment is determined by the degree of obstruction. In some cases of isolated unilateral paralysis no treatment is required. Good phonation can develop by compensation by the normal cord, even without recovery on the affected side. However, tracheostomy is required if there are persistent problems of respiratory obstruction or continuing aspiration. Arytenoidectomy to remove the obstructive component should be delayed for several years to allow for spontaneous recovery. Alternatively, the use of innervated muscle pedicle grafts to restore function has been explored.[92]

Congenital Hemangioma

Laryngeal and subglottic hemangiomas commonly occur in association with similar cutaneous lesions,[93] and should be suspected in any child with a strawberry nevus in the head region who develops stridor. Girls are affected twice as frequently as boys. Phonation is not usually affected, as the tumor usually lies below the cords, leaving them uninvolved. Obstructive symptoms generally appear before 6 months of age, usually first as stridor during crying, but tending to worsen during the growth of the tumor. The diagnosis should be suspected in any baby with a history of fluctuating respiratory obstruction but normal cry. Diagnosis is confirmed by radiography of the airway, possibly helped by contrast radiography of the esophagus, and endoscopy. However, endoscopic diagnosis is not always easy, because the overlying mucosa is normal and the angioma empties as pressure is applied so that inspection may show only an apparently normal larynx. Thus the diagnosis may be missed, particularly in those patients without the clue of concomitant skin nevi. Growth of the tumor is usually limited, and most laryngeal hemangiomas tend to regress. Many patients become asymptomatic by the age of 2 years. However, it is difficult to predict the behavior of any individual tumor, and repeated endoscopy is usually required to follow the progression of the disease. Spontaneous bleeding from these tumors is not a problem, nor does bleeding usually occur during diagnostic laryngoscopy or tracheal intubation.[94]

Because of the natural history of the disease tending to spontaneous regression, treatment should be conservative and limited to those patients in whom the degree of obstruction makes relief imperative. Tracheostomy should be avoided if at all possible for fear of seeding the tumor into the trachea. Repeated partial endoscopic resection, using the carbon dioxide laser or cryoprobe rather than sharp dissection to minimize bleeding, along with systemic steroids is the treatment of choice.[71, 95] In the past radiation therapy has been used, but there is considerable doubt about its therapeutic efficacy.[93] It also has the unfortunate sequelae of permanent scarring and chronic laryngeal obstruction and dysfunction, and also has been implicated in the etiology of thyroid cancer.[96] In a very small minority of patients the tumor continues to grow in spite of all therapeutic endeavors, and in such patients there may be no alternative to eventual laryngofissure and surgical excision.[97]

Laryngeal Tumors

Simple squamous papillomas, though rare, are the most common of the laryngeal tumors.

Juvenile Papillomatosis

Multiple papillomas (juvenile laryngeal papillomatosis) are most common in children 5 to 15 years of age and usually present as hoarseness. These tumors, although benign, are aggressive in growth and local spread.[98, 99] They tend to recur frequently and rapidly, and may spread throughout the larynx, pharynx, and trachea and occasionally even into the lung tissue itself. In spite of this aggressive behavior they rarely, if ever, become malignant. Nevertheless, their presence within the laryngotracheal tract presents a serious threat of respiratory obstruction, and resulting mortality rates in excess of 10 percent have been reported fairly recently.[99] The natural history of juvenile laryngeal papillomatosis is erratic and unpredictable. Prolonged periods of quiescence can be followed by a sudden outburst of activity, and initially good results from local therapy may not be maintained. Evaluation of differing treatment modalities is particularly difficult, and long-term follow-up is required even after apparently complete regression.[100] Fortunately, in most patients the papillomatosis tends to regress and finally disappear around the time of puberty.

It has long been suspected that these papillomas are of viral origin, and an association between neonatal papillomas and maternal genital warts has been noted.[101] There is increasing evidence for existence of a human papilloma virus.[100, 102]

The usual treatment is repeated surgical removal during endoscopy, using sharp dissection, cryotherapy, or laser dissection. If the papillomatous mass becomes very big, respiratory obstruction may necessitate tracheostomy, but this brings the added danger of papillomas seeding to the tracheostomy. Less morbidity and reduced mortality can be achieved by aggressive surgical treatment with careful atraumatic dissection using the microscope and suspension laryngoscope, repeated regularly before the development of respiratory symptoms. Additional benefits have been obtained from the adjuvant use of podophyllum[99] and from interferon therapy.[103] Apart from avoidance of respiratory obstruction, it is probable that regular endoscopic excision of the papillomas will help to preserve vocal quality.

In spite of undoubted advances in endoscopic surgery, the treatment of juvenile laryngeal papillomatosis remains frustrating, and achieves little more than control of the growth of the tumors until, in most cases, spontaneous regression takes place.

Vocal Cord Nodules

Vocal cord nodules, which are fairly common in adults as "singer's nodes," are less common in childhood, in which they are possibly better described as "screamer's nodes." The usual presentation is of hoarseness in a child with a history of voice abuse.[71] These nodules are harmless and are treated conservatively in the first instance with voice rest and speech therapy. Very occasionally persistent nodules require surgical removal.

Postintubation granulomas are similar in most respects to singer's nodes, but do not tend to resolve spontaneously and generally require surgical removal.

Malignant Tumors of the Larynx

Malignancy arising in the larynx in childhood is exceedingly rare, as is involvement of the larynx in malignancy arising is other tissues of the neck.[7]

Acquired Structural Defects of the Larynx

Acquired Subglottic Stenosis

By far the most common cause of acquired subglottic stenosis at any age is prolonged endotracheal intubation.[104] The premature infant with respiratory distress syndrome is particularly at risk,[105, 106] and better survival rates for such infants have been paralleled by an increased incidence of postintubation subglottic stenosis. Much less frequently, subglottic stenosis occurs as a complication of tracheostomy, particularly a high tracheostomy, direct laryngeal trauma, or respiratory burns.

Most acquired stenoses are at the level of the cricoid cartilage. The stenosis may be apparent at the time of attempted extubation, but more usually there is a variable length of time between extubation and development of symptoms of respiratory obstruction. The patient presents later with recurrent lower respiratory tract infections, stridor, and hoarseness.[75] In contrast to congenital subglottic stenosis, the acquired variety does not tend to resolve and is much more difficult to manage.[75] The need for treatment is likely to be prolonged over years rather than months. Almost all patients with acquired subglottic stenosis (unless treated by immediate reconstructive surgery) will require tracheostomy, compared with fewer than 50 percent of those with congenital subglottic stenosis. Thus, there is a higher degree of associated morbidity and mortality. Mortality rates in infants with acquired subglottic stenosis and long-term tracheostomy have been reported to be as much as 24 percent.[107]

The treatment of acquired subglottic stenosis is difficult, and many different methods have been explored. In general, the initial approach is a conservative one, similar to the management of congenital subglottic stenosis: tracheostomy to maintain the airway while the patient undergoes repeated endoscopic dilatations. The aim each time is to achieve sufficient stretching to increase the airway diameter while simultaneously avoiding any degree of trauma sufficient to cause more scarring and hence the possibility of increased stenosis.

Endoscopic resection using a urethral resectoscope[108] or laser dissection of scar tissue[109] has in some cases decreased the need for repeated dilatations and made management easier, but these approaches are not applicable to all patterns of stenosis.

With conservative treatment it can be difficult to know when decannulation of the trachea will be tolerated, and indeed restoration of the tracheostomy may be required weeks, or even months, after apparently successful decannulation.[76] If the stenosis persists in spite of prolonged dilatation, surgical reconstruction of the larynx offers the only hope of avoiding a permanent tracheostomy. Among the operations that have been described for this are laryngofissure with grafting, open laryngotracheoplasty, and vertical incision of the cricoid cartilage with insertion of a cartilage graft to maintain a wider lumen.[76] These operations do not remove the need for prolonged tracheostomy and are therefore burdened by all the complications of tracheostomy. This fact, along with the relatively poor results of conservative treatment of acquired subglottic stenosis, has encouraged attempts at immediate surgical correction of acquired stenoses with avoidance of tracheostomy if possible.[110]

In the anterior cricoid split operation,[78, 111] the cricoid cartilage and upper trachea are exposed in the neck and a vertical midline incision is made through the cricoid cartilage and mucosa, down to the endotracheal tube, and extended downward through the first two tracheal rings. No effort is made to close the incision by grafting or other means. The endotracheal tube is left in place as a stent, and every effort is made to minimize further laryngeal trauma, including in some instances keeping the patient paralyzed and artificially ventilated.[111] The endotracheal tube can usually be removed after 7 to 10 days.

Posttraumatic laryngeal stenosis that occurs in association with blunt cervical trauma can be among the most difficult of all to treat, particularly in small children. Excision of the scarred area and medium- to long-term use of a prosthetic stent may be required.[112, 113]

Acquired Laryngeal Paralysis

The distinction between congenital and acquired vocal cord paralysis is entirely artificial, acquired laryngeal paralysis being in all aspects similar to congenital laryngeal paralysis. The investigation and treatment are the same. Causes of acquired vocal cord paralysis in children include surgical trauma (particularly associated with mediastinal operations and thyroid surgery), blunt trauma to the neck, and compression by cervical tumors. Laryngeal paralysis is usually unilateral and may be asymptomatic or present as hoarseness. The diagnosis is confirmed by awake indirect endoscopic examination, which reveals an immobile cord fixed in an intermediate position.

Anesthetic Considerations in Laryngoscopy

Of all therapeutic interventions requiring general anesthesia in infants and children, few have greater potential than laryngoscopy for producing danger for the patient, urgent problems for the anesthetist, and considerable difficulty for the operator. Disaster can strike with rapidity if respiratory obstruction occurs, and in this circumstance tragedy can be averted only by rapid action. This requires a clear understanding of what is happening and immediate implementation of predetermined plans to deal with complications.

The particular problems associated with laryngoscopy include:

1. The airway has to be shared between operator and anesthetist, who must ensure constant control of the airway, which is vital to the patient's safety.

2. Adequate alveolar ventilation must be maintained, despite upper airway pathology further embarrassed by the presence of surgical instruments.

3. During the operation blood and debris must be removed to prevent aspiration into the lower respiratory tract.

4. Laryngoscopy and surgery are made difficult or impossible if there is any movement. Reflex coughing, bucking, or laryngospasm must be suppressed.

5. Sophisticated instruments and operative techniques (for example, the carbon dioxide laser) add further constraints to anesthetic management.

6. Speedy recovery of protective reflexes at the end of operation is essential.

7. Severe respiratory obstruction may arise in the postoperative period owing to laryngeal edema.

The sometimes apparently conflicting requirements can be met only by cooperation and understanding between anesthetist and surgeon, and require that each be fully cognizant of the other's problems. Many different anesthetic techniques have been described for laryngoscopy but none is ideal in all respects. Choice of technique of anesthetic management will depend on the nature of the disease and the planned operative procedure. Precise details will have to be matched to the individual patient. However, certain general principles apply and are discussed in the following paragraphs.

Diagnostic Laryngoscopy in Neonates

The usual indication for laryngoscopy is the presence of stridor, and proper endoscopic examination requires evaluation of vocal cord movements as well as inspection of laryngeal anatomy. This requires observation of the glottis during normal inspiration and expiration and during phonation or crying. For these reasons, and because newborns often tolerate awake laryngoscopy surprisingly well, general anesthesia is not used. However, because there is always danger of provoking respiratory arrest or obstruction, the examination should take place in a fully equipped operating room, with the assistance of an anesthetist to monitor the baby. The anesthetist should be prepared to intubate and ventilate the patient should respiratory problems arise, or to induce anesthesia should tracheostomy or other operation become indicated.

Although general anesthesia is not often required, these patients should be given atropine, 0.1 mg/10 kg with a minimum of 0.1 mg, prior to the examination. Reflex bradycardia commonly occurs from stimulation of the larynx, and reduction of salivation contributes to the ease of endoscopy. During neonatal laryngoscopy the tip of the blade should be placed in the vallecula; if the blade is inserted on the epiglottis it not infrequently fixes the right cord, and this could be misinterpreted as right-sided vocal paralysis.

Diagnostic Direct Laryngoscopy in Older Infants and Children

Older infants and children will not readily tolerate awake laryngoscopy, and general anesthesia is required. In order to allow the endoscopist unimpeded view of the glottis it is preferable to avoid intubation, and this is most readily accommodated by using volatile anesthesia agents and having the patient maintain spontaneous ventilation throughout the examination. Sedative premedications should be avoided in patients with obstructive respiratory symptoms, but atropine should be given for the reasons outlined above. Anesthesia is induced with oxygen, nitrous oxide, and halothane. When the patient is deeply anesthetized the glottic area is sprayed with lidocaine (maximum dose 4 mg/kg). After a further few minutes of oxygen and halothane the facemask is removed and endoscopy can take place. With the facemask removed the level of anesthesia begins to lighten but usually there is sufficient time to allow adequate examination of the laryngeal anatomy. Maintaining the endoscope in place as the level of anesthesia lightens also allows movement of the cords to be observed. During laryngoscopy oxygen and halothane can be delivered to the pharynx by catheter. Throughout the procedure the patient must be monitored fully and carefully. At any sign of respiratory inadequacy the laryngoscope should be removed, the airway secured by intubation or by rigid bronchoscope, and the patient ventilated. Again, if the endoscopy shows the need for immediate tracheostomy or other operative intervention, the patient should be intubated and anesthesia continued according to the requirements of the particular operation involved.

Most pediatric laryngologists prefer rigid endoscopes for diagnostic investigation of the upper airway in infants and children. However, some authors have reported the transnasal use of small flexible fiberoptic bronchoscopes and claim excellent visualization of the supraglottic, glottic, and subglottic structures.[114]

Anesthesia for Suspension Microlaryngoscopy

Suspension laryngoscopy with the use of the microscope is commonly used for both diagnostic and operative purposes. Preoperative sedative drugs should be avoided in patients with preexisting respiratory obstruction, who should be given atropine alone. Endotracheal tubes and a rigid bronchoscope of appropriate size should be available and the patient must be fully monitored to allow immediate detection of ventilatory inadequacy. Good conditions for general diagnostic and operative laryngoscopy are obtained by maintenance of spontaneous ventilation using inhalational agents,[115] allowing the minimum of competition between surgeon and anesthetist for access to the airway, along with retention of normal laryngeal function, which greatly eases the interpretation of any apparently abnormal appearances and movements of the airway structures. Other advantages claimed for this technique include excellent surgical access,[116] a quiet unreactive glottis,[116–118] reduced postoperative coughing and edema,[116] and a history of safety in use.[118, 119]

Following induction with nitrous oxide, oxygen, and halothane, the glottis is sprayed with lidocaine in appropriate dosage, and a small endotracheal tube or catheter[117, 120] is passed through the cords. Anesthesia is continued by insufflation of oxygen and halothane,[116] a constant check being made to ensure the tube does not become obstructed by surgical manipulation. An alternative method of insufflation is to use a side channel incorporated in the laryngoscope blade.[115] If intubation is used it is important that the size of the tube be such that it does not impede the surgeon's access to the particular area of the larynx in which he is interested. The addition of a continuous intravenous infusion of procaine during manipulation of the larynx has been claimed to enhance operating conditions by reducing laryngeal reactivity during operation, and to decrease the incidence of postoperative laryngospasm and stridor.[121]

Following operative interventions in the larynx, edema is likely and may produce significantly increased obstruction. Postoperative laryngeal edema may not be entirely avoidable, but it can be reduced by maintaining a meticulous and gentle approach to laryngeal manipulations and dissection. Its effects can be minimized in the immediate postoperative period by routine administration of humidified gases by mask or tent.

Many alternative techniques for ventilation of the lungs during operative laryngoscopy have been described, and the relative merits of each remains a matter of some controversy. Among these are the jet Venturi system, which has the advantages of offering an unobstructed view of the larynx and enabling good alveolar ventilation in a paralyzed but unintubated patient. Its disadvantage is the potential for producing very high airway pressures, with the risk of mediastinal emphysema and tension pneumothorax, particularly in the presence of laryngeal obstruction and if the tip of the injector is in the trachea rather than in the laryngoscope.[122-124] The risk of barotrauma is increased in the smaller-diameter airways of children. For this reason jet ventilation is generally considered unsuitable for use in children,[117, 118, 125] although, because of the absolute immobility of the cords ensured in the paralyzed patient, some still believe that it remains the technique of choice for laser surgery even in smaller children.[126]

More recently high-frequency ventilation using a small-bore catheter within the trachea has been suggested as a safer technique than jet ventilation,[127, 128] because it provides the same advantages of good surgical access and reliable alveolar ventilation without the risk of barotrauma. Its usefulness in children remains unexplored. Intubation of the trachea using a relatively small-bore cuffed tube to allow controlled ventilation and muscle paralysis during laryngoscopy has been used in adults,[129, 130] but is not a suitable technique for small children because of the relative sizes of tube and trachea.

Carbon Dioxide Laser. Use of the laser adds further special considerations for the anesthetist. The laser beam, which is invisible, is reflected by metal surfaces but will be absorbed by biological tissues and other substances, where its energy is dissipated as heat. All operating room personnel should be guarded from the risk of corneal and retinal burns by wearing protective goggles, and the patient's eyes should be protected by taping the eyelids closed and covering with moist pads. The risk of random reflection can be greatly reduced by ensuring that all metal surfaces are matte black. Rubber or plastic tracheal tubes are liable to

ignite if struck directly by the laser beam[131-133] and must be protected by wrapping in aluminum foil tape or in wet muslin that is itself kept constantly wet by repeated applications of saline lest it, too, catch fire. Ignition of the endotracheal tube demands immediate action; all gases should be discontinued and the tube should be removed immediately.

Laryngeal Trauma

Injuries to the neck may involve the larynx or the cervical trachea, or both. Unfortunately children are not immune to such accidents, although serious injury to the laryngotracheal airway in the neck is uncommon. Open injuries of the neck are usually the result of road traffic accidents and are most commonly caused by laceration of the neck by broken glass. Other forms of open wound of the neck, such as suicidal cut throat or gunshot wounds, are met in older age groups. The larynx is less at risk in this type of injury than is the cervical trachea, being relatively well protected by the laryngeal cartilages. The larynx can also be severely damaged by compression against the cervical spine, even in the absence of any external evidence of injury to the neck. In many ways this is more dangerous than an open neck injury, for it is easy to overlook closed injury, since the symptoms and signs may be confusing and often do not correspond well with the degree of disruption of the airway.[134, 135] Such laryngeal fractures may be caused by sharp blows on the front of the neck as might be sustained by running against a taut rope or wire or falling against the edge of a table or across the handlebar of a bicycle.

Tracheal damage in these circumstances usually takes the form of longitudinal tears, but laryngeal damage can involve complete anatomical disruption with dislocation of the arytenoid cartilages and disruption of the cricoarytenoid joint so that the arytenoid itself may obstruct the glottis. Obstruction by such injuries will be further aggravated by the associated bleeding, swelling, and edema formation.

In large open wounds, involvement of the larynx or trachea may be obvious on inspection, but subcutaneous emphysema, dyspnea, hoarseness, coughing, and hemoptysis are all signs of airway involvement, and the onset of respiratory distress with stridor or cyanosis is evidence of critical respiratory obstruction. Voice change after a blow on the neck almost always signifies laryngeal damage. Anterior cervical emphysema can quickly produce a dangerous vicious circle in which increasing respiratory obstruction causes increased respiratory effort and further increases the air leak, which in turn increases the emphysema. Positive-pressure ventilation, struggling, and coughing will also increase the degree of emphysema. There is no constant relationship between the degree of injury and the degree of emphysema.

Isolated damage to the airway is unlikely in cervical

injuries owing to the concentration of vital structures within the neck. Associated injuries that may add to the difficulties of managing these patients include gross hemorrhage, arterial and/or venous, with the possibility of cerebral ischemia if the carotid vessels are involved or compressed; air embolism through torn cervical veins; hemopneumothorax where penetrating neck wounds involve the dome of the pleura; and cervical spine injury.

Surgical Management

Injuries to the larynx and trachea are usually fairly simple to repair. Tracheal injuries require little more than suturing. Even quite complex laryngeal fractures are reconstructed by wiring; good potential for recovery of function exists if they are treated early.[136, 137] In general, a tracheostomy is performed below the level of the injury and the airleak is closed with reconstruction of the airway. If possible the use of a stent is avoided. The tracheostomy is maintained until healing is complete. However, the surgery of cervical trauma is rarely limited to the airway. There are likely to be associated injuries to the blood vessels, pharynx, and esophagus,[138, 139] and such injuries must be sought and treated at the same time that the airway is repaired. Esophageal tears, in particular, cause a marked increase in morbidity and mortality if missed.

Initial Airway Management

Emergency resuscitation of patients with cervical wounds who develop respiratory distress presents an urgent problem of restoration of an airway. Unfortunately, it also presents the danger that therapy will further aggravate the degree of injury and respiratory obstruction.[140] In very rare cases, a transected cervical trachea may be seen in the wound, and the distal segment can then be intubated directly. In other circumstances in which there is suspicion of laryngotracheal injury, attempts at intubation may produce further disruption of anatomy, or the tube, apparently passed safely through the glottis, may in fact leave the airway through the tear, creating a false passage and total respiratory obstruction. For this reason it is better to secure the airway by bronchoscopy[11] if this is possible, or, in those cases with gross disruption of anatomy, to proceed to immediate tracheostomy or cricothyroidotomy.[142]

Anesthetic Management

Most patients with cervical injury who survive and arrive at the hospital do not develop respiratory distress so quickly as to require resuscitation as just described, but most will require early surgical exploration.[139, 143] The particular problems facing the anesthetist in these circumstances include:

1. The general problems of induction of anesthesia in the injured patient, especially those related to hypovolemia and the full stomach.

2. The risk of laryngotracheal damage causing sudden respiratory obstruction during induction.

3. Difficulty in laryngoscopy and intubation because of distortion of the normal anatomy by injury and swelling.

4. The presence of blood and debris (including foreign bodies) in the pharynx, adding further difficulty in laryngoscopy along with the risk of aspiration.

5. Associated injuries, particularly of the cervical spine.

6. The risk of venous air embolism in open cervical wounds.

7. Distant injuries (for example, ruptured spleen) resulting from the same accident.

Awake intubation is preferable if at all possible, but the use of heavy sedation to permit "awake" intubation should be avoided lest undue depression of the patient provoke respiratory obstruction. However, small doses of narcotics, given intravenously, can be of great help in suppressing the continual coughing that is often a feature in these cases. Slow, gentle insertion of the laryngoscope with careful topical anesthesia of the glottis (unless there is risk of aspiration before the tracheal tube is passed) and constant reassurance of the patient will often allow successful awake oral intubation.[144, 145] Primary nasotracheal intubation is to be avoided not only because of its increased difficulty but also because attempts at passing a tube through the nose may make matters worse by provoking nasopharyngeal bleeding.

If awake intubation is not possible, the alternatives are to perform tracheostomy with use of local anesthesia, or to postpone intubation until after induction of anesthesia. Although the patient must be assumed to have a full stomach, it is probably unwise to attempt to aspirate stomach contents through a gastric tube for fear that the tube will aggravate the injury. Similarly, cricoid pressure must not be used over a damaged larynx; quite apart from aggravating the damage, this maneuver is likely to cause complete respiratory obstruction if the intrinsic anatomical integrity of the larynx has been lost. Use of intravenous induction agents or muscle relaxants before the airway has been secured is contraindicated in all patients in whom there is risk of total respiratory obstruction. The preferred technique is gentle inhalational induction with halothane and oxygen (nitrous oxide should be avoided in the presence of surgical emphysema) and maintenance of spontaneous ventilation until the patient will tolerate laryngoscopy and intubation. Intravenous lidocaine, 1.5 mg/kg prior to laryngoscopy, can be used to help prevent coughing. A rigid bronchoscope must be available in case there is difficulty in passing or positioning the tracheal tube. If ventilation is adequate, it may be advantageous to postpone intubation until after the larynx and trachea have been exposed and the extent of the damage has been assessed. Intubation can then be done with certainty that the tube has been properly placed in relation to the damaged airway. Once the airway is secure, anesthesia can be continued in any appropriate way, but positive-pressure ventilation should not be used so long as there is any doubt about the extent of the laryngotracheal damage. Positive-pressure ventilation is safe only when the damaged region has been isolated by the use of a cuffed endotracheal or endobronchial tube.

REFERENCES

1. Winther LK: Congenital choanal atresia. Arch Otolaryngol 104:72, 1978.
2. Lantz HJ, Birck HG: Surgical correction of choanal atresia in the neonate. Laryngoscope 91:1629, 1981.
3. Hough JVD: The mechanism of asphyxia in bilateral choanal atresia. South Med J 48:588, 1955.
4. Stoksted P, Greisen O, House L: A survey of the diagnosis and treatment of congenital choanal atresia. Int Rhinol 10:3, 1972.
5. Freng A: Surgical treatment of congenital choanal atresia. Ann Otol Rhinol Laryngol 87:346, 1978.
6. Hengerer AS, Strome M: Choanal atresia: a new embryologic theory and its influence on surgical management. Laryngoscope 922:913, 1982.
7. Snow JB: Neoplasms of the head and neck in children. Adv Otorhinolaryng 23:115, 1978.
8. Sessions RB, Zarin DP, Bryan N: Juvenile nasopharyngeal angiofibroma. Am J Dis Child 135:535, 1981.
9. Zakzouk SM, Elgarem A, Hafiz MA: An unusual case of nasopharyngeal angiofibroma. Ear Nose Throat J 58:351, 1979.
10. Biller HF, Sessions DG, Ogura JH: Angiofibroma: a treatment approach. Laryngoscope 84:695, 1974.
11. Bradley PJ, Singh SD: Congenital nasal masses: diagnosis and treatment. Clin Otolaryngol 72:87, 1982.
12. Moller NE, Thomsen J: Mucocele of the paranasal sinuses in cystic fibrosis. J Laryngol Otol 92:1025, 1978.
13. Richardson KA, Birck H: Peritonsillar abscess in the pediatric population. Otolaryngol Head Neck Surg 89:907, 1981.
14. Majumdar B, Stevens RW, Obara LG: Retropharyngeal abscess following tracheal intubation. Anaesthesia 37:67, 1982.
15. Beeden AG, Evans JNG: Quinsy tonsillectomy—a further report. J Laryngol Otol 84:443, 1970.
16. Bonding P: Tonsillectomy a chaud. J Laryngol Otol 87:1171, 1973.
17. Tucker R: Peritonsillar abscess—a retrospective study of medical treatment. J Laryngol Otol 96:639, 1982.
18. Muller SP: Peritonsillar abscess: a prospective study of pathogens, treatment, and morbidity. Ear Nose Throat 57:439, 1978.
19. Yung AK, Cantrell RW: Quinsy tonsillectomy. Laryngoscope 86:1714, 1976.
20. Wolfe JA, Rowe LD: Upper airway obstruction in infectious mononucleosis. Ann Otol Rhinol Laryngol 89:430, 1980.
21. Catling SJ, Asbury AJ, Latif M: Airway obstruction in infectious mononucleosis. Anaesthesia 39:699, 1984.
22. Velcek FT, Klotz DH, Hill CH, et al.: Tongue lesions in children. J Pediatr Surg 14:238, 1979.
23. Gupta OP: Congenital macroglossia. Arch Otolaryngol 93:378, 1971.
24. Shafer AD: Primary macroglossia. Clin Pediatr 7:357, 1968.
25. MacDonald DJF: Cystic hygroma. An anaesthetic and surgical problem. Anaesthesia 21:66, 1966.
26. Katz AD, Zager WJ: The lingual thyroid. Arch Surg 102:582, 1971.
27. Danis RK: An alternative to management of lingual thyroid: excision with implantation. J Pediatr Surg 8:869, 1973.
28. Wertz ML: Management of undescended lingual and sublingual thyroid glands. Laryngoscope 84:507, 1974.
29. Solomon MP, Tolete-Velcek F: Lingual rhabdomyoma (adult variant) in a child. J Pediatr Surg 14:91, 1979.
30. Das S, Sengupta P, Chatterjee SK, et al.: Oncocytoma of tongue in a child. J Pediatr Surg 11:113, 1976.
31. Pichler AG, Williams JR, Moore JA: Carcinoma of the tongue in childhood and adolescence. Arch Otolaryngol 95:178, 1972.
32. Rao TV, Satyanaryana CV: Rhabdomyosarcoma. Indian J Pediatr 44:377, 1977.
33. McAllister RC: Macroglossia—a positional complication. Anesthesiology 40:199, 1974.
34. Ninh TN, Ninh TX: Cystic hygroma in children: a report of 126 cases. J Pediatr Surg 9:191, 1974.
35. Maze A, Bloch E: Stridor in pediatric patients. Anesthesiology 50:132, 1979.
36. Valman HB: Stridor. Br Med J 283:294, 1981.
37. Rowlandson P: Stridor. Br Med J 283:863, 1981.
38. Couriel J: Acute stridor in preschool child. Br Med J 288:1162, 1984.
39. Tucker JA: Obstruction of the major pediatric airway. Otolaryngol Clin North Am 12:329, 1979.
40. Fried MP: Controversies in the management of supraglottitis and croup. Pediatr Clin North Am 26:931, 1979.
41. Rowe LD: Advances and controversies in the management of supraglottitis and laryngotracheobronchitis. Am J Otolaryngol 1:235, 1980.
42. Schultz RL, Morrison WV: Short-term intubation in children with acute epiglottitis. South Med J 75:158, 1982.
43. Diaz JH, Lockhart CH: Early diagnosis and airway management of acute epiglottitis in children. South Med J 75:399, 1982.
44. Bishop MJ: Epiglottitis in the adult. Anesthesiology 55:701, 1981.
45. Briggs WH, Althenau MM: Acute epiglottitis in children. Otolaryngol Head Neck Surg 88:665, 1980.
46. Cohen SR, Chai J: Epiglottitis: twenty year study with tracheotomy. Ann Otol Rhinol Laryngol 87:461, 1978.
47. Welch DB, Price DG: Acute epiglottitis and severe croup. Experience in two English regions. Anaesthesia 38:754, 1983.
48. Marjolis CZ, Ingram DL, Meyer JH: Routine tracheotomy in Hemophilus influenzae type b epiglottitis. J Pediatr 81:1150, 1972.
49. Smith EWP, Ingram DL: Counterimmunoelectrophoresis in Hemophilus influenzae type b epiglottitis and pericarditis. J Pediatr 86:571, 1975.
50. Philpott-Howard J, Williams JD: Increase in antibiotic resistance in Haemophilus influenzae in the United Kingdom since 1977: report of study group. Br Med J 284:1597, 1982.
51. Schuller DE, Birck HG: The safety of intubation in croup and epiglottitis: an eight year follow up. Laryngoscope 85:33, 1975.
52. Glicklich M, Cohen RD, Jona JZ: Steroids and bag and mask ventilation in the treatment of acute epiglottitis. J Pediatr Surg 14:247, 1979.
52a. Grenrik A, Safar P: Brain Failure and Resuscitation. New York, Churchill Livingstone, 1981, pp 155–184.
53. Rapkin RH: The diagnosis of epiglottitis: simplicity and reliability of radiographs of the neck in the differential diagnosis of the croup syndrome. J Pediatr 80:96, 1972.
54. Rothstein P, Lister G: Epiglottitis—duration of intubation and fever. Anesth Analg 62:785, 1983.
55. Zulliger JJ, Schuller DE, Beach TP, et al.: Assessment of intubation in croup and epiglottitis. Ann Otol Rhinol Laryngol 91:403, 1982.
56. Molteni RA: Epiglottitis: incidence of extra-epiglottic infection. Pediatrics 58:526, 1976.
57. Hawkins DB: Corticosteroids in the management of laryngotracheobronchitis. Otolaryngol Head Neck Surg 88:207, 1980.

58. Dobie RA, Tobey TN: Clinical features of diphtheria in the respiratory tract. JAMA 242:2197, 1979.

59. Hodes HL: Diphtheria. Pediatr Clin North Am 26:445, 1979.

60. Heath CW, Zusman J: An outbreak of diphtheria among skid row men. N Engl J Med 267:809, 1962.

61. Brooks GF, Bennett JV, Feldman RA: Diphtheria in the United States, 1959–1970. J Infect Dis 129:172, 1974.

62. McDaniel DB, Patton EW, Mather JA: Immunization activities of private-practice physicians: a record audit. Pediatrics 56:504, 1975.

63. Nelson LA, Peri BA, Rieger CHL, et al.: Immunity to diphtheria in an urban population. Pediatrics 61:703, 1978.

64. Pappenheimer AM, Gil DM: Diphtheria. Recent studies have clarified the molecular mechanisms involved in its pathogenesis. Science 182:353, 1973.

65. Green SL, LaPeter KS: Pseudodiphtheritic membranous pharyngitis caused by Corynebacterium hemolyticum. JAMA 245:2330, 1981.

66. Stephens DS, Walker DH, Schaffner W, et al.: Pseudodiphtheria: prominent pharyngeal membrane associated with fatal paraquat ingestion. Ann Intern Med 94:202, 1981.

67. Naiditch MJ, Bower AG: Diphtheria: a study of 1,433 cases observed during a ten year period at the Los Angeles County Hospital. Am J Med 17:229, 1954.

68. Cotton RT, Richardson MA: Congenital laryngeal anomalies. Otolaryngol Clin North Am 14:203, 1981.

69. Kahn A, Baran D, Spehl M, et al.: Congenital stridor in infancy. Clin Pediatr 16:19, 1977.

70. Holinger PH, Brown WT: Congenital webs, cysts, laryngoceles and other anomalies of the larynx. Ann Otol Rhinol Laryngol 76:744, 1967.

71. Fearon B: Laryngeal surgery in the pediatric patient. Ann Otol Rhinol Laryngol (Suppl) 89:146, 1980.

72. Cundy RL, Bergstrom LB: Congenital subglottic stenosis. J Pediatr 82:282, 1973.

73. Benjamin B: Congenital laryngeal webs. Ann Otol Rhinol Laryngol 92:317, 1983.

74. Hardingham M, Walshe-Waring GP: The treatment of a congenital laryngeal web. J Laryngol Otol 89:273, 1975.

75. Holinger PH, Kutnick SL, Schild JA, et al.: Subglottic stenosis in infants and children. Ann Otol 85:591, 1976.

76. Fearon B, Crysdale WS, Bird R: Subglottic stenosis of the larynx in the infant and child. Ann Otol 87:645, 1978.

77. Kotton B: The treatment of subglottic stenosis in children by prolonged dilatation. Laryngoscope 89:1983, 1979.

78. Cotton RT, Seid AB: Management of the extubation problem in the premature child. Anterior cricoid split as an alternative to tracheotomy. Ann Otol 89:508, 1980.

79. Fearon B, Cotton R: Surgical correction of subglottic stenosis of the larynx. Ann Otol 81:508, 1972.

80. Fearon B: Management of subglottic stenosis of the larynx in infants and children. Adv Otorhinolaryngol 23:97, 1978.

81. Evans JNG, Todd GB: Laryngotracheoplasty. J Laryngol Otol 88:689, 1974.

82. Armitage EN: Laryngotracheo-oesophageal cleft. A report of three cases. Anaesthesia 39:706, 1984.

83. Yamashita M, Chinyanga HM, Steward DJ: Posterior laryngeal cleft—anaesthetic experiences. Can Anaesth Soc J 26:502, 1979.

84. Kingston HGG, Harrison MW, Smith JD: Laryngotracheoesophageal cleft—a problem of airway management. Anesth Analg 62:1041, 1983.

85. Donegan JO, Strife JL, Seid AB, et al: Internal laryngocele and saccular cysts in children. Ann Otol 89:409, 1980.

86. Van DeWater FW: Laryngeal cysts: their surgical management. Laryngoscope 83:1185, 1973.

87. Holinger LD, Barnes DR, Smid LJ: Laryngocele and saccular cysts. Ann Otol Rhinol Laryngol 87:675, 1978.

88. Cohen SR, Geller KA, Birns JW, et al.: Laryngeal paralysis in children. A long term retrospective study. Ann Otol Rhinol Laryngol 91:417, 1982.

89. Bluestone CD, Delerme AN, Samuelson GH: Airway obstruction due to vocal cord paralysis in infants with hydrocephalus and meningomyelocele. Ann Otol 81:778, 1972.

90. Holinger PC, Holinger LD, Reichert TJ, et al.: Respiratory obstruction and apnea in infants with bilateral abductor vocal cord paralysis, meningomyelocele, hydrocephalus, and Arnold-Chiari malformation. J Pediatr 92:368, 1978.

91. Dedo HH: The paralysed larynx: an electromyographic study in dogs and humans. Laryngoscope 80:1455, 1970.

92. Tucker HM: Human laryngeal reinnervation. Laryngoscope 86:769, 1976.

93. Leikensohn JR, Benton C, Cotton R: Subglottic hemangioma. J Otolaryngol 5:487, 1976.

94. Lee MH, Ramanathan S, Chalon J, et al.: Subglottic hemangioma. Anesthesiology 45:459, 1976.

95. Cohen SR, Wang C-I: Steroid treatment of hemangioma of the head and neck in children. Ann Otol 81:584, 1972.

96. Saenger GL, Silverman FM: Neoplasia following therapeutic irradiation for benign conditions in childhood. Radiology 74:889, 1960.

97. Calcaterra TC: An evaluation of the treatment of subglottic hemangioma. Laryngoscope 78:1956, 1968.

98. Cohen S, Seltzer S, Geller K, et al.: Papilloma of the larynx and tracheobronchial tree in children. Ann Otol Rhinol Laryngol 89:497, 1980.

99. Dedo HH, Jackler RJ: Laryngeal papilloma: results of treatment with the CO_2 laser and podophyllum. Ann Otol Rhinol Laryngol 91:425, 1982.

100. Szpunar J: Juvenile laryngeal papillomatosis. Otolaryngol Clin North Am 10:67, 1977.

101. Strong MS, Vaughn CW, Healy GB, et al.: Recurrent respiratory papillomatosis—management with the CO_2 laser. Ann Otol Rhinol Laryngol 85:508, 1976.

102. Lancaster WD, Jenson AB: Evidence for papillomavirus genus-specific antigens and DNA in laryngeal papillomas. Intervirology 15:204, 1981.

103. Haglund S, Lundquist, PG, Cantell K, et al.: Interferon therapy in juvenile laryngeal papillomatosis. Arch Otolaryngol 107:327, 1981.

104. Hawkins DB: Glottic and subglottic stenosis from endotracheal intubation. Laryngoscope 87:339, 1977.

105. Ratner I, Whitfield J: Acquired subglottic stenosis in the very low birth weight infant. Am J Dis Chil 137:40, 1983.

106. Papsidero MJ, Pashley NRT: Acquired stenosis of the upper airway in neonates. Ann Otol 89:152, 1980.

107. Fearon B, Cotton R: Surgical correction of subglottic stenosis of the larynx in infants and chidren. Ann Otol 83:428, 1974.

108. Downing TP, Johnston DG: Excision of subglottic stenosis with the urethral resectoscope. J Pediatr Surg 14:252, 1979.

109. Holinger LD: Treatment of severe subglottic stenosis without tracheotomy: a preliminary report. Ann Otol Rhinol Laryngol 91:407, 1982.

110. Cotton R: Management of subglottic stenosis in infancy and childhood. Ann Otol 87:649, 1978.

111. Frankel LR, Anas NG, Perkin RM, et al.: Use of anterior cricoid split operation in infants with acquired subglottic stenosis. Crit Care Med 12:395, 1984.

112. Grahne B: Operative treatment of severe chronic traumatic laryngeal stenosis in infants up to three years old. Acta Otolaryngol 72:134, 1971.

113. Schuller DE: Long term stenting for laryngotracheal stenosis. Ann Otol 89:515, 1980.

114. Vauthy P, Reddy R: Acute upper airway obstruction in infants and children. Evaluation by the fiberoptic bronchoscope. Ann Otol 89:417, 1980.

115. Kennedy MG, Chinyanga HM, Steward DJ: Anaesthetic experience using a standard technique for laryngeal surgery in infants and children. Can Anaesth Soc J 28:561, 1981.

116. Hadaway EG, Page J, Shortridge RT: Anaesthesia for microsurgery of the larynx. (Letter.) Ann R Coll Surg 64:279, 1982.

117. Steward DJ, Fearon B: Anaesthesia for laryngoscopy. Br J Anaesth 53:320, 1981.

118. Steward DJ, Fearon B: Laryngeal microsurgery. Br Anaesth 54:364, 1982.
119. Talmage EA: Endotracheal tube is not necessary for laryngeal microsurgery. Anesthesiology 55:332, 1981.
120. Young, PN, Robinson JM: Anaesthesia for microsurgery for the larynx. Ann R Coll Surg 65:135, 1983.
121. Lawson LW, Rogers D, Seifen A, et al.: Intravenous procaine as a supplement to general anaesthesia for carbon dioxide laser resection of laryngeal papillomas in children. Anesth Analg 58:492, 1979.
122. Vivori E: Anaesthesia for laryngoscopy. Br J Anaesth 52:638, 1980.
123. Oliverio R, Ruder CB, Fermon B, et al.: Pneumothorax due to ball valve obstruction during jet ventilation. Anesthesiology 51:255, 1979.
124. Tate N: Excessive airway pressure during anaesthesia. Anaesthesia 34:212, 1979.
125. Norton ML, Strong MS, Snow JC, et al.: Endotracheal intubation and Venturi (jet) ventilation for laser microsurgery of the larynx. Ann Otol 85:656, 1976.
126. Oliverio RM, Ruder CB, Abramson AL: Jet ventilation for laryngeal microsurgery. Br J Anaesth 53:1010, 1981.
127. Borg U, Eriksson I, Sjostrand U: High frequency positive pressure ventilation (HFPPV): a review based upon its use during bronchoscopy and for laryngoscopy and microlaryngeal surgery under general anaesthesia. Anesth Analg 59:594, 1980.
128. Smith RB: Ventilation at high respiratory frequencies. Anaesthesia 37:1011, 1982.
129. Coplans MP: A cuffed nasotracheal tube for microlaryngeal surgery. Anesthesia 31:430, 1976.
130. Keen RI, Kotak PK, Ramsden RT: Anaesthesia for microsurgery of the larynx. Ann R Coll Surg 64:112, 1982.
131. Rita L, Seleny F: Endotracheal tube ignition during laryngeal surgery with resectoscope. Anesthesiology 56:60, 1982.
132. Wainwright AC, Moody RA, Carruth JAS: Anaesthetic safety with the carbon dioxide laser. Anaesthesia 36:411, 1981.
133. Cozine K, Rosenbaum LM, Askanazi J, et al.: Laser-induced endotracheal tube fire. Anesthesiology 55:583, 1981.
134. Holinger PH, Schild J: Pharyngeal, laryngeal and tracheal injuries in the pediatric age group. Ann Otol 81:538, 1972.
135. Thomas RJS: Rupture of the cervical trachea. Med J Aust 1:415, 1972.
136. Olson NR Surgical treatment of acute blunt laryngeal injuries. Ann Otol 87:716, 1978.
137. Schaefer SD: Primary management of laryngeal trauma. Ann Otol Rhinol Laryngol 81:399, 1982.
138. Defore WW, Mattox KL, Hansen HA, et al.: Surgical management of penetrating injuries of the esophagus. Am J Surg 134:734, 1977.
139. Pate JW, Casini M: Penetrating wounds of the neck: explore or not? Am Surg 46:38, 1980.
140. Sirkir D, Clarke MM: Rupture of the cervical trachea following a road traffic accident. Br J Anaesth 45:909, 1973.
141. Donchin V, Vered IY: Blunt trauma to the trachea. Br J Anaesth 48:1113, 1976.
142. Boyd AD, Romita MC, Conlan AA, et al.: Clinical evaluation of cricothyroidotomy. Surg Gynecol Obstet 149:365, 1979.
143. Grover FL, Ellestad C, Arom KV, et al.: Diagnosis and management of major tracheobronchial injuries. Ann Thorac Surg 28:384, 1978.
144. Duncan JAT: A case of severely cut throat. Br J Anaesth 47:1327, 1975.
145. Sims J, Giesecke AH: Airway management. Clin Anesth 11:71, 1976.

DISEASES OF THE ENDOCRINE SYSTEM

12

THOMAS P. KEON, M. D. ● *JOSEPHINE J. TEMPLETON, M. D.*

Abnormalities of endocrine function may be the primary indication for a surgical procedure or may be present in patients who require surgery for unrelated diseases. An understanding of the pathophysiology of diseases of the endocrine glands is essential for optimal anesthetic management of these patients. This chapter will review normal endocrine physiology and diagnostic studies, pathology, and current management of endocrine diseases in the pediatric patient. Anesthetic considerations including preoperative assessment, operative management, and postoperative care will be discussed with emphasis on the infant, child, or adolescent. Inevitably, for some disorders, the majority of the data that are available have been taken from studies in adult patients.

PITUITARY GLAND

The pituitary, a complex endocrine gland located in the sella turcica at the base of the brain, is connected to the hypothalamus by the pituitary stalk, which is composed of glandular, vascular, and neural elements. The anterior pituitary (adenohypophysis) develops from an outgrowth of the buccal mucosa called Rathke's pouch and is connected to the hypothalamus by a complex portal vascular system that provides hypothalamic control of pituitary function. The posterior pituitary (neurohypophysis) is composed of the terminal endings of neurons that originate in the hypothalamus.

Normal Pituitary Function

Anterior Pituitary (Adenohypophysis)

Hormones secreted by the anterior pituitary gland include adrenocorticotropic hormone (ACTH), thy-roid-stimulating hormone (TSH), growth hormone (GH), prolactin (PRL), luteinizing hormone (LH), follicle-stimulating hormone (FSH), and melanocyte-stimulating hormone (MSH). The regulation of hormone secretion from the anterior pituitary is controlled by hypothalamic neurohormonal substances (releasing and inhibiting hormones) produced in the neurons of the tuber cinereum, particularly within the median eminence.[1] These hypothalamic hormones are secreted intermittently in response to decreasing levels of circulating end-organ hormones or to neural stimuli, and are transported by the venous system of the pituitary stalk to the sinusoidal capillaries of the anterior lobe of the pituitary gland.

The median eminence, which forms the base of the hypothalamus and third ventricle, appears to be the common pathway for humoral and neural control of the anterior pituitary. The identification in the median eminence of nerve endings containing dopamine, nor-epinephrine, and serotonin that arise from neurons in the hypothalamus suggests that the secretion of hypothalamic releasing hormones and consequently pituitary hormones is controlled by secretion of biogenic aminergic neurons. In addition, target organ products such as estrogen, testosterone, thyroid, and adrenal hormones can exert feedback at either the hypothalamic or the pituitary level (Fig. 12–1).

Posterior Pituitary (Neurohypophysis)

The supraoptic and paraventricular nuclei of the hypothalamus synthesize the posterior pituitary hormones vasopressin (antidiuretic hormone; ADH) and oxytocin. These hormones are attached to specific carrier proteins, neurophysins, and are transported along the pituitary stalk in secretory granules. The stimulus for the release of these hormones arises in the hypothalamus.

The primary functions of antidiuretic hormone are regulation of plasma osmolality and maintenance of

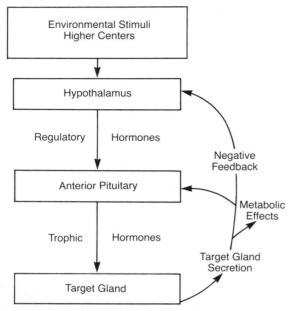

Figure 12–1. The endocrine system. Hormonal control by feedback mechanisms.

extracellular fluid volume. ADH secretion, hence extracellular fluid osmolality, is regulated by osmoreceptors in the region of the supraoptic nuclei and blood volume receptors located in the left atrium and pulmonary veins. The most potent stimulus to ADH secretion is hypotension due to blood loss. The release of ADH produces peripheral vasoconstriction in addition to conservation of water by the kidneys. ADH acts on the distal tubules, collecting tubules, and a portion of the loops of Henle to make them permeable to water such that most of the water in the urine is reabsorbed. In the absence of ADH these structures are almost impermeable to water.[2] Conservation of free water as a result of the release of antidiuretic hormone also results in a decrease in urinary output. Painful stimulation due to trauma or surgery and positive airway pressure are additional factors that result in the release of antidiuretic hormone and conservation of free water.[3] Disorders of posterior pituitary function are manifested as either diabetes insipidus or inappropriate (excessive) antidiuretic hormone secretion. The physiological role of oxytocin is to stimulate contraction of the uterus, and to promote milk secretion by the mammary glands.

The endocrine disorders associated with tumors in the pituitary hypothalamic area result from interference of pituitary function by the tumor. The clinical manifestations of endocrine abnormalities vary with the age of the patient as well as the type of lesion. Tumors involving the pituitary-hypothalamic area usually result in deficiency of pituitary trophic hormones and less commonly in excessive secretion. In children, the tumors most frequently associated with endocrine dys-

function are craniopharyngiomas, gliomas of the optic nerve and optic chiasm, hypothalamic gliomas, hamartomas, and pineal tumors. Pituitary adenomas, more common in adults, are rarely encountered in the first two decades of life.

Hypopituitarism

The most common demonstrable cause of panhypopituitarism in children is compression of the pituitary gland by a craniopharyngioma. Hypothalamic tumors, tuberculosis, sarcoidosis, toxoplasmosis, and aneurysms are less common causes. In more than half of children with hypopituitarism the cause is not known[4] and there is no demonstrable lesion of the pituitary or hypothalamus. Panhypopituitarism may also follow head injury, radiation therapy, or surgical hypophysectomy and is manifested as multiple endocrine gland dysfunction. Deficiency of growth hormone in childhood results in dwarfism, but when it occurs in adults it does not produce symptoms. Treatment of panhypopituitarism is with specific hormone replacement, which may include gonadotropins, cortisol, and thyroxine. The administration of a mineralocorticoid is usually unnecessary because aldosterone release continues in the usual fashion.[5]

Craniopharyngioma

This tumor accounts for approximately 10 percent of all intracranial tumors in patients under 14 years of age.[6] Peak incidence occurs at age 7 years, with males more frequently affected than females. The lesion is benign and usually well encapsulated, and its size may vary from that of an olive to that of an orange. In the majority of cases it extends above the sella, indenting the hypothalamus and stretching the optic chiasm.

The characteristic triad of clinical features includes growth failure, increased intracranial pressure, and visual loss. Tumors presenting in childhood frequently produce hydrocephalus and symptoms of increased intracranial pressure, which may obscure the endocrine abnormalities. However, multiple endocrine abnormalities may be manifested by short stature, hypothyroidism, diabetes insipidus, lack or arrest of sexual development, obesity, and less commonly hypoadrenalism. Skull x-rays may reveal suprasellar calcifications, and a computed tomography scan revealing a calcified suprasellar tumor is virtually pathognomonic.

Surgical removal of the tumor is the treatment of choice. Radiation therapy is prescribed for tumors that cannot be removed completely.[7] Deficiencies of adrenocorticotropic hormone and antidiuretic hormone may exist prior to surgery or develop following extirpation of the tumor.

Hypothalamic Tumors

Tumors growing in the region of the hypothalamus, optic nerves, and optic chiasm may be associated with specific endocrine and metabolic abnormalities. The diencephalic syndrome, with a peak incidence in the first 6 months of age, is manifested by extreme emaciation, hyperkinesis, vomiting, inappropriate euphoria, nystagmus, and pallor without anemia.[8] Endocrine abnormalities include growth hormone deficiency and lack of diurnal variation in plasma cortisol levels.

Precocious puberty may be associated with tumors in the floor of the third ventricle, the posterior hypothalamus, and the tuber cinereum, often in the median eminence. Boys are more commonly affected, and clinical features include all the signs of puberty associated with gonadal maturation. The mechanism by which these tumors produce sexual precocity is unclear. Pressure from the tumor may result in increased secretion of gonadotropin-releasing hormone by interference with inhibitory neural stimuli.

Pituitary Tumors

Pituitary adenomas are uncommon in children and represent only 1 percent of all intracranial tumors. The endocrine abnormalities associated with pituitary tumors result from lack of secretion due to compression of the normal gland, impairment by the tumor of the hypophyseal-portal circulation, or excessive production of pituitary hormones. The diagnosis is suggested by the presence of endocrine abnormalities and visual field defects and confirmed by abnormalities of the sella turcica seen on x-ray. In prepubertal children the earliest clinical findings are decreased linear growth and delayed development of secondary sex characteristics. Hypothyroidism and hypoadrenalism may occur later.

Diabetes Insipidus

Central diabetes insipidus results from diminished or absent ADH synthesis or release. If not present before pituitary surgery, diabetes insipidus usually becomes manifest 6 to 12 hours after surgery, as a result of direct hypothalamic injury or ischemia, stalk edema, or high pituitary stalk transection. In some of these patients diabetes insipidus lasts only 24 to 36 hours, after which urine output decreases and urinary specific gravity increases, suggesting normal ADH activity. However, in the majority recovery lasts for only 3 to 5 days, following which permanent diabetes insipidus develops. Transient recovery of ADH function is thought to result from lysis of surgically damaged cells containing ADH.

Urinary volume and specific gravity and serum electrolytes should be monitored in the intraoperative and postoperative periods. The urine volume may be as high as 10 to 20 ml/kg/hr, with osmolality usually between 50 and 150 mOsm/L. Specific gravity will be between 1.001 and 1.005, and a urine to serum osmolality ratio of less than 1:1 indicates a negative water balance. The differential diagnosis includes diuresis from mannitol, glucose, or excessive crystalloid fluid administration.

Diabetes insipidus will result in dehydration and hypernatremia if fluid and electrolyte balance is not carefully monitored. Vasopressin (Pitressin) administered subcutaneously at 6- to 8-hour intervals, or as a nasal spray, will control the symptoms of ADH deficiency. After the fifth postoperative day when the patient has demonstrated a normal thirst mechanism and no longer requires intravenous fluids, a longer-acting form of vasopressin (Pitressin tannate in oil) can be administered intramuscularly every 48 hours. Alternately, a synthetic analogue of arginine vasopressin (1-deamino-8D-arginine vasopressin, DDAVP) which lacks the pressor activity of Pitressin can be administered intranasally twice daily and appears to be an effective therapy for diabetes insipidus.[9]

Hyperpituitarism

Gigantism

Gigantism is rare in early childhood but is usually recognized during adolescence when clinical features of both acromegaly and gigantism are present.[11] It is due to excessive secretion of growth hormone associated with an eosinophilic or chromophobic pituitary adenoma. Clinical features in children include increased growth velocity, excessive height, and enlargement of hands and feet without associated virilization. The diagnosis is confirmed by measuring an increased basal growth hormone concentration and the presence of sellar abnormalities. Lack of suppression or a paradoxical increase in growth hormone levels during hyperglycemia is characteristic. Glucose intolerance and hyperinsulinemia are commonly found.[12]

Acromegaly

Excessive growth hormone secretion following puberty results in acromegaly. Clinical manifestations result from a general overgrowth of skeletal, soft, and connective tissues. Facial features are coarse and the mandible increases in thickness and length. Excessive enlargement of the tongue and epiglottis may contribute to upper airway obstruction, and intubation may be difficult.[13] Stridor or a history of dyspnea suggests involvement of the larynx, and subglottic narrowing of the trachea may be present.[14] Peripheral neuropathies occur because of trapping of nerves by skeletal, connective, and soft tissue overgrowth.

Cushing Disease

This condition is the result of excessive secretion of adrenocorticotropic hormone (ACTH). The characteristic clinical features in children consist of obesity, stunted growth, retarded bone age, and osteoporosis. Bilateral hyperplasia of the adrenal glands is found, although a pituitary adenoma may not be evident. A high incidence of pituitary microadenomas has been documented at surgery in patients with Cushing disease even when sellar changes were not detected on routine skull films.[15] The diagnosis is confirmed by demonstrating elevated plasma ACTH and cortisol levels, absence of diurnal variation, and failure of dexamethasone to suppress serum cortisol and urinary 17-hydroxycorticosteroids. Cushing disease and syndrome are thoroughly discussed in the section on adrenal diseases later in this chapter.

Syndrome of Inappropriate Antidiuretic Hormone Secretion (SIADH)

This condition exists in patients when excessive quantities of ADH are produced in the absence of a physiological stimulus. It is found in association with a variety of illnesses including brain diseases of inflammatory, neoplastic, vascular, and traumatic origin, pulmonary disease, and malignancies of the larynx, duodenum, and pancreas. Clinical features include hyponatremia, decreased serum osmolality, reduced urine output, and urine with a high osmolality. Acute reductions in serum sodium can lead to seizures. Diagnosis is based on evidence that the urine osmolality is unusually high when related to the markedly decreased osmolality of the plasma. Patients with SIADH usually do not show signs of impaired renal, adrenal, or hepatic function. Peripheral edema and arterial hypertension are not present. Hyponatremia occurs because of decreased free water clearance as well as excessive natriuresis, which even in conjunction with a high sodium input generally leads to a negative sodium balance. Treatment is initiated by restriction of fluid intake, which may be sufficient for asymptomatic patients. Demeclocycline (DMC), lithium, furosemide, and hypertonic saline may be necessary in selected patients unresponsive to fluid restriction.[16]

Other Pituitary Hormone–Secreting Tumors

Pituitary tumors that secrete thyrotropin (TSH), prolactin (PRL), and the gonadotropins luteinizing hormone (LH) and follicle-stimulating hormone (FSH) have not been reported in children. However pituitary adenoma may result from long-standing hypothyroidism and hypogonadism, suggesting that early diagnosis and treatment of hormonal deficiencies with continuous replacement therapy may be important in the prevention of some pituitary tumors.[17]

Anesthetic Management

Preoperative Assessment

Preoperative evaluation of patients with pituitary dysfunction requires a familiarity with normal anterior and posterior pituitary physiology. Panhypopituitarism is more common with nonfunctioning tumors than with hormone-producing tumors. In the former, diagnosis is usually delayed until the growth of the tumor disrupts normal pituitary function. The important anesthetic considerations are assessment and management of the endocrine dysfunctions as well as

management of intracranial hypertension or reduced intracranial compliance. Adrenocortical, thyroid, and antidiuretic hormone dysfunction are the three principal endocrine problems that must be evaluated. Accurate radioimmunoassay methods are presently available for all hormones, but traditional laboratory tests are still frequently utilized.

Adrenocortical hormone activity must be maintained when pituitary-adrenocortical function has been or will be disrupted. The normal secretory rate of cortisol in children is 12 mg/m^2/day, and a maximal adrenal cortisol production rate of 270 mg/1.73m^2/day has been reported.[18] Cortisol measurements in adults under conditions of major stress have revealed maximal cortisol production of 250 to 300 mg/day. Intramuscular hydrocortisone hemisuccinate in a dosage of 100 mg every 6 hours in adults produces plasma corticosteroid values that compare favorably with levels observed in normal adult patients undergoing surgery.[19] Commercial steroid preparations have variable absorption rates. The hemisuccinate and phosphate ester conjugates are water soluble and readily absorbed parenterally, and hence are useful for infusions during surgical procedures. The acetate and diacetate forms are relatively insoluble in water and are absorbed slowly over days to weeks when given intramuscularly. Different coverage protocols have been recommended but the administration of 2 mg/kg of hydrocortisone every 6 hours should exceed the maximal cortisol production of a normal adrenal gland and hence is appropriate for major surgical procedures.

Thyroid function, as measured by blood levels of TSH, triiodothyronine (T_3), and thyroxine (T_4) as well as clinical signs, should be determined. Hypothyroidism must be corrected with appropriate amounts of thyroxine. The patient may require up to 2 weeks to achieve a euthyroid state. Patients with normal preoperative thyroid function who undergo hypophysectomy usually will not need thyroid replacement therapy for a few weeks following surgery (see the section on the Thyroid Gland later in this chapter).

Diabetes insipidus is rarely present preoperatively but commonly occurs in the immediate postoperative period. Urine output, serum sodium, serum osmolality, and urine osmolality are necessary for diagnosis and must be monitored frequently. Therapy has been discussed previously.

Hypophysectomy causes minimal alterations in carbohydrate metabolism in nondiabetic patients. However, in patients with diabetes mellitus the postoperative requirements for insulin are markedly reduced. Usually about one third of the preoperative dose of insulin will be required postoperatively. Sex hormone and mineralocorticoid hormone replacement are not necessary in the immediate postoperative period but may be required on a long-term basis.[20]

Signs of raised intracranial pressure must be sought in children with brain tumors. Headache, vomiting, papilledema, tense fontanelle in infants, and alteration of consciousness are indicative of increased intracranial pressure. Preoperative treatment with corticosteroids, fluid restriction, and diuretics usually results in temporary improvement.

Premedication with central nervous system depressants should not be given to patients with reduced intracranial compliance or signs of increased intracranial pressure. Preoperative anticholinergics are useful to reduce oral secretions and permit secure fixation of the endotracheal tube. Corticosteroid coverage should begin in the preoperative period.

Operative Management

The three surgical approaches that have been utilized are stereotactic, transsphenoidal, and frontal craniotomy. The transsphenoidal operation involves incision through the nasal septum and vomer to the sphenoid or through an incision in the maxilla. A frontal craniotomy necessitates retraction and elevation of the frontal lobe. When evidence exists of extension of the tumor into the cavernous sinuses, an increased risk of air embolism and excessive blood loss must be anticipated.[21, 22]

A neuroanesthesia induction sequence of intravenous thiopental (4 to 6 mg/kg) and pancuronium (0.12 mg/kg) with hyperventilation prior to endotracheal intubation should be utilized. If considered necessary, cricoid pressure can be maintained during the period of mask ventilation to prevent passive regurgitation of gastric contents. Intravenous fentanyl (12 to 15 μg/kg) and lidocaine (1.5 mg/kg) are administered prior to tracheal intubation to attenuate cardiovascular and intracranial pressure changes associated with laryngoscopy and insertion of the endotracheal tube. The eyes should be protected with sterile lubricant and taped closed. The endotracheal tube tip should be placed at mid-trachea and firmly secured with meticulous care.

Monitors should include esophageal stethoscope, blood pressure cuff, temperature probe, and electrocardiogram. An intra-arterial catheter allows continuous monitoring of the arterial pressure and provides for regular sampling for hematocrit, electrolytes, blood gases, and osmolality. Continuous end-tidal CO_2 monitoring permits constant control of arterial carbon dioxide tension, is a sensitive monitor for air embolism, and reduces the number of arterial gas samples that must be obtained. If the patient is in the sitting position or there is an increased likelihood of air embolism, a central venous catheter should be placed through the internal jugular or femoral vein. The precordial Doppler device should be applied for sensitive diagnosis of venous air embolism. A urinary catheter is essential if diuretics are given and for accurate measurement of hourly urine output. Neuromuscular blockade should be monitored with a nerve stimulator to ensure continuous paralysis.

Maintenance of anesthesia is continued with nitrous oxide (70 percent) and oxygen (30 percent), with isoflurane (0.5 to 1.2 percent) added as needed. The arterial carbon dioxide tension is maintained at 25 to 30 torr and mannitol or furosemide is administered when clinical swelling of the brain is observed. Intravenous fluids consisting of 5 percent dextrose and 0.45 normal saline are restricted to maintenance amounts and the fasting deficit is not replaced. Preoperative volume status, intraoperative blood loss, and urine output must be considered in determining intraoperative fluid management.

Nasogastric tubes should not be inserted in patients with pituitary tumors. Large tumors may erode the sella and the sphenoid sinus and permit direct intracranial penetration of tubes or catheters with potentially serious complications.

Patients operated upon in the sitting position are prone to venous air embolism. Therapy for this complication includes lowering the head, flooding the operative field with saline, discontinuation of nitrous oxide, application of bilateral jugular pressure, and aspiration of air through a previously placed right atrial catheter.[23]

At the termination of surgery discontinuation of the anesthetic agents usually results in prompt recovery of consciousness. Intravenous lidocaine (1 to 2 mg/kg IV) may be utilized to prevent coughing on the tracheal tube. A regular and adequate respiratory pattern, normal neuromuscular function, and spontaneous eye opening are satisfactory criteria for extubation.

Postoperative Management

Vigilant, comprehensive monitoring must be continued in the postoperative period. The following complications or problems should be anticipated:

1. **Diabetes Insipidus.** The most significant complication is diabetes insipidus. Urine output, serum sodium and osmolality, and urine osmolality must be measured frequently. If the urine output exceeds 3 ml/kg/hr, hypernatremia is present, urine osmolality is decreased, and the urine to serum osmolality ratio is less than 1:1, vasopressin should be administered. Diabetes insipidus occurs in approximately 20 per cent of patients and may subside in a few days.[24] Therapy includes replacement of urine losses with a hypotonic solution, replacement of potassium, and subcutaneous Pitressin tannate or nasal insufflation of DDAVP. Administration of glucose solutions must be carefully monitored because hyperglycemia may contribute to the diuresis. Preoperative prophylactic therapy with Pitressin is not advised because excessive fluid retention with volume overload could result and diabetes insipidus occurs in a minority of patients. Diabetes insipidus occurs with greater frequency following a transfrontal craniotomy than with the transsphenoidal approach.

2. **Hormone Deficiency.** Adrenocortical hormone therapy at maximum stress dosage (8 mg/kg/day) should be continued for 48 hours before reduction to maintenance levels is begun. Unless thyroxine was required preoperatively, this hormone can be started

in 1 to 2 weeks. Testosterone (in males), estrogen and progesterone (in females), and mineralocorticoid are usually begun a few weeks following surgery.

3. Reduced Insulin Requirement. Insulin-dependent diabetics develop a drastically reduced insulin requirement. Urine and blood sugar determinations must be done frequently, and the daily insulin dose is often only one third of the preoperative dose.

4. Hyperthermia. Hypothalamic temperature-regulating mechanisms may be disrupted, and temperature should be monitored continuously. Symptomatic therapy is indicated to maintain normathermia.

5. Seizures. Postoperative seizures may occur and phenytoin medication may be given as a prophylactic measure.

6. Cerebrospinal Fluid Leak. Following transsphenoidal hypophysectomy, cerebrospinal fluid leak is an infrequent complication. Therapy includes antibiotic administration to prevent meningitis and may require surgical reexploration.

THYROID GLAND

Thyroid hormone influences many physiological processes but is particularly important in the maintenance of body temperature, cardiovascular activity, gastrointestinal motility, and reflex neurological function. During fetal life and in the first 2 years it is essential for normal growth and development of the central nervous system and the skeletal system. Thyroid hormones play a role in the biological processes of essentially every organ system.

Normal Thyroid Function

Thyroxine (tetraiodothyronine, T_4) and triiodothyronine (T_3) are the active thyroid gland hormones that influence cells to alter the rate of biochemical reactions. Approximately one third of T_3 comes from thyroid gland secretion, whereas two thirds is the result of peripheral tissue deiodination of T_4.[25] T_3 is approximately four to five times as active as T_4 in bioassays. Circulating T_4 and T_3 are more than 99 percent bound to serum proteins, especially thyroxine-binding globulin and prealbumin.[26] Only the free thyroid hormone is biologically active, and therefore the ratio of free hormone to bound hormone, rather than the total serum concentration, will determine the level of metabolic activity.

The major regulator of thyroid hormone production is thyroid-stimulating hormone (TSH), which is secreted from the anterior pituitary. A closed feedback loop functions to control the production of thyroid hormones (Fig. 12–2). The negative feedback produced by circulating T_4 or T_3 on the production of TSH has the dominant effect. TSH release is also affected by thyrotropin-releasing hormone (TRH), which is produced in the hypothalamus and transported to the

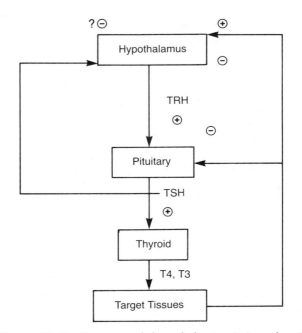

Figure 12–2. Concept of hypothalamic-pituitary-thyroid axis. The closed feedback loop controls the production of thyroid hormones. ⊕ stimulation of gland; ⊖ inhibition of gland.

anterior pituitary by the hypophyseal portal venous system. Hence thyroid gland dysfunction can reflect disease processes involving the hypothalamus, the anterior pituitary, or the thyroid gland itself.

The biosynthesis of thyroid hormone can be divided into four steps: (1) iodide trapping by the gland, (2) oxidation and iodination of tyrosine, (3) coupling of iodotyrosines and hormone storage as part of thyroglobulin, and (4) proteolysis with release of T_3 and T_4. Various drugs are administered to alter thyroid function and may act at different stages of thyroid hormone production. Thiocyanate and perchlorate both inhibit iodine trapping by the gland. Propylthiouracil and methimazole inhibit the oxidation of inorganic iodide and formation of monoiodotyrosine and diiodotyrosine. The proteolytic step necessary for the release of active hormone is stimulated by thyroid-releasing hormone and inhibited by the administration of iodides or lithium.[27]

The mechanism of action of thyroid hormone at the cellular level is complex, with multiple mechanisms rather than a solitary mode of action. Effects occur on the plasma membrane and the mitochondrial inner membrane with activation of mitochondrial energy metabolism. The activation of mitochondrial energy metabolism probably accounts for increased oxygen consumption seen within a few hours of injection of T_3.[28]

Development of Thyroid Function

The embryonic thyroid gland is evident in the first month of fetal life as an invagination of the endoderm of the foregut. The first evidence of thyroid activity is the synthesis of thyroglobulin as early as the eighth fetal week.[29] By the twelfth week colloid formation is apparent histologically and fetal pituitary TSH secretion occurs. The fetal hypothalamic-pituitary-thyroid axis is functional by 20 weeks and develops free of maternal influence. Neither thyroid-stimulating hormone (TSH), thyroxine (T_4), nor triiodothyronine (T_3) cross the placental barrier to any significant degree.[30] Thus, the fetal pituitary-thyroid axis functions independently of the maternal axis, and maternal thyroid hormones do not protect against congenital hypothyroidism.

Premature infants delivered prior to maturation of the hypothalamic-pituitary-thyroid system respond to extrauterine life with qualitatively similar but quantitatively decreased changes in serum TSH and iodothyronine concentrations. The TSH response to birth is reduced and, although a subsequent increase in T_4 concentration occurs, T_4 levels remain below those seen in full-term infants throughout the first few weeks of life.[31] Thyroid hormone levels are highest in infancy, gradually decline throughout childhood, and reach adult levels at about the age of 15 years.

Thyroid Function Tests

Tests of thyroid function include (1) quantitation of thyroid hormone levels in blood, (2) measurement of iodine turnover in the thyroid gland, (3) assessment of peripheral effects of thyroid hormone, and (4) tests of the hypothalamic-pituitary-thyroid axis.

Serum Thyroxine and Triiodothyronine

Most of the T_4 and T_3 circulating in the blood is bound to various thyroid-binding proteins. The bound forms of the hormone are inactive, and only the small proportion of circulating free hormone is active at the tissue level. Radioimmunoassay levels of T_4 and T_3 measure both the bound and free moieties. Drugs or conditions that alter the level of thyroid-binding proteins can cause major changes in the levels of total serum T_4 or T_3 and therefore do not reflect a thyroid abnormality or an excess of free hormones at the tissue level. A list of the more common conditions and medications altering total T_4 and T_3 are given in Table 12–1. Correction of the total T_4 or T_3 levels for thyroid-binding protein abnormalities has been achieved by combining them with the direct measurement of thyroid-binding protein levels or, more commonly, with the T_3 resin uptake test.

Triiodothyronine Resin Uptake

This test measures the unsaturated binding sites available to bind radioactive T_3. In situations where the level of binding proteins is normal but the patient's serum T_4 or T_3 levels are high (hyperthyroidism) or low (hypothyroidism), the T_3 resin uptake (T_3RU) is similarily raised or lowered. However, elevation or

Table 12–1. FACTORS AFFECTING THYROID BINDING PROTEINS

Increase
High total T_4 + low T_3RU
Estrogens
Pregnancy
Methadone
Liver disease
Porphyria
Decrease
Low total T_4 + high T_3RU
Androgens
Anabolic steroids
Asparaginase
Steroids
Phenytoin—competes with T_4 for binding
Salicylates—compete with T_4 for binding
Severe liver disease
Severe illness

lowering of blood levels of thyroid binding proteins alters the T_3RU inversely to serum T_4 or T_3. Thus, in most cases, multiplying the T_4 or T_3 with the T_3RU corrects for thyroid-binding protein abnormalities. This is the basis of the free thyroxine index (FTI) test reported by some laboratories.

Free Thyroxine

New techniques have been developed to measure free T_4 and free T_3 in the serum, and these tests will soon replace the combination of measurements of the total serum T_4 or T_3 level with the T_3RU or measurement of thyroid-binding proteins.

Radioactive Iodine Uptake (RAIU)

This test measures the uptake of radioactive iodine by the thyroid gland in a given period of time. The uptake of isotopes by the thyroid gland is influenced by the iodine content of the body. Although elevations of iodine-131 uptake usually indicate hyperthyroidism and decreases usually indicate hypothyroidism, iodine deficiency or excess can give similar results. An alternative test measures uptake of radioactive technetium.

Thyroid-Stimulating Hormone

The measurement of serum TSH has become an essential tool in the diagnosis of primary and secondary hypothyroidism. Primary hypothyroidism will result in a low level of serum T_4 and an elevated serum TSH.

Thyroid Scanning

Various isotopes of iodine can be used, but the most common scanning material is technetium-99, which gives off lower doses of radiation than the standard iodine-131. Isotope scanning gives an outline picture of the thyroid tissue including its size, shape, and location. In addition scanning can outline areas of decreased function (cold) or increased function (hot) in a gland. It cannot distinguish the malignant from the nonmalignant nor, in the case of a cold area, whether it is solid or cystic.

Additional Tests

Ultrasonography of the thyroid gland permits reliable discrimination between cystic and solid nodules. Computed tomography (CT) may be used to complement the other structural investigations of the thyroid gland. Xerography is an x-ray technique that is useful in determining the degree of tracheal or esophageal compression from a large goiter or nodule. The detection of thyroid antibodies (antithyroglobulin and antimicrosomal) are important in the diagnosis of Hashimoto thyroiditis.

Hypothyroidism

Hypothyroidism results from deficient production of thyroid hormone and is among the most common of the endocrine disorders of childhood. Hypothyroidism in children may be congenital or acquired; however, when symptoms appear after a period of apparently normal thyroid function, a disorder may appear "acquired" but result from a congenital defect in which the manifestation of the deficiency is delayed. In the pediatric age group, approximately one third of patients with hypothyroidism present in infancy (less than 1 year of age), and two thirds during childhood.

Goiter

A goiter is an enlargement of the thyroid gland. Goiter may be congenital, acquired, endemic, or sporadic. A patient with an enlarged thyroid gland may have normal function of the gland (euthyroidism), thyroid deficiency (hypothyroidism), or overproduction of hormones (hyperthyroidism). A large goiter may be seen rarely in an infant born to a mother who has received thionamide medication or iodide for hyperthroidism. Both these goitrogens cross the placenta to the fetal side and inhibit fetal thyroid hormone production. The resultant fetal TSH secretion and thyroid gland hypertrophy may produce life-threatening airway obstruction.

Congenital Hypothyroidism

The estimated frequency of congenital hypothyroidism is between 1 in 4000 and 1 in 7000 live births.[29] An unexplained 2:1 ratio of affected females to affected males exists with this disorder. Developmental defects of the thyroid gland are the most common causes of congenital hypothyroidism and are referred to as thyroid dysgenesis. Other causes include maternal goitrogen ingestion or radioactive iodine treatment, iodine deficiency (endemic goiter), autoimmune thyroiditis, and hypopituitarism.

The term cretinism is often used synonymously with congenital hypothyroidism but is best applied to infants with neurological sequelae of congenital hypothyroidism.

Acquired Hypothyroidism

The incidence of acquired hypothyroidism is difficult to estimate, but it is approximately twice as common as congenital hypothyroidism. Causes include chronic lymphocytic thyroiditis, previous thyroidectomy or iodine-131 treatment, infiltrative diseases (cystinosis, histiocytosis X), sick euthyroid syndrome, and hypopituitarism.

Manifestations of Hypothyroidism

At birth signs of hypothyroidism are usually absent or so nonspecific that the diagnosis is missed. Because irreversible damage to the central nervous system may take place before clinical manifestations suggest the diagnosis, screening programs have been developed to detect the disorder in newborns by laboratory testing before signs become clinically manifest.

It is uncommon for infants to present with a palpable goiter. Classical features of congenital hypothyroidism include a puffy face; wide fontanelles and sutures; flattened nasal bridge with pseudohypertelorism; a large protruding tongue with an open mouth; a hoarse cry; a protuberant abdomen with an umbilical hernia; cold, mottled, or jaundiced skin; and sluggish reflexes. The risk of mental retardation appears to exist when hypothyroidism is present in a child under 2 years of age.

Hypothyroidism in childhood or adolescence may be insidious in onset, and the most common sign is a decrease in growth velocity. Clinical features include lethargy, cold intolerance, bradycardia, low pulse pressure, myxedema, delayed dentition, goiter, precocious sexual development, and a dull, placid expression. Myxedema coma is rare in children and is characterized by extreme lethargy, severe hypothermia, respiratory depression, hyponatremia, and congestive heart failure.

Laboratory Diagnosis

The biochemical hallmarks of primary hypothyroidism are a low serum T_4, normal or low serum T_3 resin uptake, and an elevated TSH. The elevated TSH is the most sensitive test for primary hypothyroidism. Serum cholesterol is elevated in hypothyroidism in childhood (not in infants), but this is not a diagnostic finding. The development of programs for screening newborns is an important advance in the diagnosis of congenital hypothyroidism. Most of the programs perform an initial T_4 on a filter paper blood sample obtained at a few days of life; if this is low, a TSH assay is performed on the same filter paper specimen.

Treatment

Untreated congenital hypothyroidism will have devastating effects on the growth and development of a child. Synthetic sodium levothyroxine is administered in a dose of 5 to 6 µg/kg in the first year of life, then

4 μg/kg after age 2 years and 3 to 4 μg/kg in late childhood and adolescence.[32]

In the infant one will observe an increase in activity, an improvement in skin color and temperature, reversal of other signs of hypothyroidism, plus normal growth and skeletal advancement. Serum T_4, T_3 resin uptake, and TSH should be monitored. Serum TSH that is in the normal range appears to be the best biochemical indicator of adequate therapy. If hypothyroidism develops after age 2 years, there does not appear to be a risk of permanent intellectual impairment, and all changes should be reversible with treatment.

Anesthetic Management

Preoperative Assessment. The degree of dysfunction in hypothyroidism may range from subclinical to overt with myxedema coma. Hypothyroidism should be corrected prior to a planned surgical procedure. At least 2 weeks are usually necessary to render a patient euthyroid. Treatment must begin slowly in patients with underlying myxedematous heart disease because of rare reports of sudden deaths in infants after 2 to 3 weeks of treatment.[29] Both serum T_4 and TSH will be normal in adequately treated patients.

Depending on the degree of physiological derangement, any or all of the following problems should be anticipated.

1. Sensitivity to Depressant Drugs. Cardiovascular and respiratory depression occur more readily with sedative, narcotic, or anesthetic agents.[33] Narcotics, including fentanyl and morphine, may be associated with prolonged recovery from anesthesia.[34] The increased sensitivity of hypothyroid patients to morphine may in part be related to decreased hepatic metabolism.[35]

2. Hypodynamic Cardiovascular Function. Cardiac output may decrease as much as 40 percent owing to reductions in both stroke volume and heart rate. Peripheral vascular resistance is increased with narrowing of the pulse pressure. Myocardial depression may be partly due to myxedematous infiltration but also reflects impaired cellular metabolism resulting from deficient thyroid hormone activity.[36] Baroreceptor dysfunction has been demonstrated and may contribute to the hypotension that occurs with anesthetic agents.[37]

3. Impaired Respiratory Function. The normal ventilatory response to hypoxia and hypercarbia are impaired in overt hypothyroidism.[38] Depressant anesthetic drugs and hypothermia may further impair this function, necessitating postoperative ventilation.

4. Decreased Intravascular Volume. Intravascular volume may be reduced 10 to 24 percent below normal values. Chronic peripheral vasoconstriction is present. Use of drugs or anesthetic agents that cause vasodilation will lead to marked hypotension.[36]

5. Hypothermia. Basal metabolic rate may be reduced to 55 percent of normal because of a decrease in the activity of mitochondrial enzymes and a general slowing of substrate oxidation. This results in an inability to increase core temperature which renders these patients susceptible to intraoperative and postoperative hypothermia. In infants such hypothermia is associated with apnea, bradycardia, and hypotension.

6. Adrenal Insufficiency. There is an increased incidence of adrenocortical insufficiency in patients with hypothyroidism, and the adrenocorticotropic hormone (ACTH) response to stress is impaired. Patients with severe hypothyroidism should receive daily steroid coverage during any acute stress.[39]

7. Hyponatremia. Inappropriate secretion of ADH as well as changes in renal function may also be of consequence in drug elimination.

8. Anemia. Anemia is often present and is refractory to treatment with hematinics.

9. Hypoglycemia. Intravenous dextrose solutions are necessary to prevent hypoglycemia from prolonged fasting.

10. Delayed Gastric Emptying Time. Emptying of the stomach is delayed and precautions to prevent gastric regurgitation and pulmonary aspiration are necessary.

Premedication. Sedative premedication should be avoided in hypothyroid patients who are symptomatic. Anticholinergics can be administered intravenously prior to the induction of anesthesia. Patients taking thyroid replacement therapy should continue the usual dose regimen in the perioperative period. Full stress response doses of hydrocortisone (2 mg/kg every 6 hours) should be given if concomitant pituitary disease exists or if associated adrenal insufficiency is suspected.

Operative Management. Regional nerve blocks offer a major advantage for some procedures but frequently are not accepted and may be unsatisfactory in the pediatric patient. The dose of any local anesthetic agent used should be minimal to avoid toxicity secondary to impaired rates of metabolism of these drugs.

Induction. Because of increased sensitivity to all anesthetic agents the induction agent must be administered in small increments with continuous monitoring of the cardiovascular system. Excessive peripheral vasodilation or myocardial depression may precipitate cardiovascular collapse. Inhalation agents must be titrated slowly. Ketamine may offer advantages in these functionally hypovolemic patients by stimulating increased sympathetic activity. Thiopental must be used cautiously in small doses to avoid excessive myocardial depression.[40] Endotracheal intubation is recommended both for airway protection and for controlled ventilation. Respiratory dysfunction should be expected.

Maintenance. Balanced anesthesia with nitrous oxide in oxygen and small amounts of fentanyl and diazepam with a muscle relaxant have been used successfully.[34] Muscle relaxation utilizing pancuronium is advantageous because of the drug's sympathomimetic effects. Curare may induce vasodilatation and hypotension. Potent inhalational agents must be used cautiously because of the known reduced myocardial reserve of these patients.

Animal studies indicate that the level of thyroid activity has minimal effect on anesthetic requirements or MAC.[41] The increased sensitivity of hypothyroid patients to anesthetic agents may represent secondary effects. Decreases in cardiac output shorten induction time with inhalation agents. This combined with a decreased intravascular volume and altered baroreceptor function may readily produce hypotension in the hypothyroid patient. In addition, reduced hepatic drug metabolism and renal drug excretion can prolong elimination of drugs and delay recovery from anesthesia.[36]

Patients undergoing major surgical procedures with significant blood loss require continuous arterial monitoring of blood pressure. Central venous pressure should also be measured because of a contracted blood volume and the need to maintain an adequate but not excessive intravascular volume. Intraoperative fluids must contain dextrose to prevent hypoglycemia. Administration of sodium-containing solutions and monitoring of serum electrolyte levels will prevent serious hyponatremia.

Aggressive practices must be used to prevent hypothermia. The temperature of the operating suite should be maintained at 25°C or above. An overhead radiant heater, warming mattress, heated humidified inspired gases, warmed irrigation solutions, and a blood warmer have proved effective. Reduction of the patient's temperature reduces anesthetic requirements for volatile drugs as well as slowing the hepatic biotransformation and renal elimination of injected drugs.

Postoperative Management. The vigilance of the operative period must be continued postoperatively. Emergence from anesthesia may be delayed with a prolonged obtunded period. Continued respiratory and cardiovascular monitoring is essential until the effects of the anesthetic drugs have dissipated. Normal body temperature should be restored and maintained. Hypothermia will contribute to incomplete reversal of neuromuscular blockers, respiratory depression, and bradycardia. Corticosteroid therapy must continue and thyroid maintenance is reinstituted.

Hyperthyroidism

Hyperthyroidism results from excessive secretion of thyroid hormone. The most common causes in children are congenital (transient neonatal) hyperthyroidism and Graves disease. Rare causes of hyperthyroidism observed in children include toxic uninodular goiter (Plummer disease), hyperfunctioning thyroid carcinoma, thyrotoxicosis factitia, and acute suppurative thyroiditis. Hyperthyroidism is a frequent concomitant

of McCune-Albright syndrome (precocious puberty with polyostotic fibrous dysplasia and abnormal pigmentation). Graves disease is often associated with other autoimmune disorders such as pernicious anemia, idiopathic adrenal insufficiency, myasthenia gravis, and disseminated lupus erythematosus.

Congenital Hyperthyroidism

Transient neonatal hyperthyroidism is considered to result from the transplacental transfer of thyroid-stimulating immunoglobulins from the mother, but the thyroid function status of the mother does not seem to play a role in the transmission of the disease. The hyperthyroid state is short-lived because of the half-life of maternal immunoglobulins (up to 3 months). Frequently long-acting thyroid stimulator (LATS) can be demonstrated in both infant and mother when the mother has a history of active or recently active Graves disease.[42]

Affected infants are frequently premature and the majority will have a goiter. Sex predominance is not found. Hypermetabolic signs may be severe with tachycardia, respiratory distress, and congestive heart failure. Accelerated bone maturation with premature craniosynostosis may be present. When the mother has been taking antithyroid medication all symptoms in the infant may be suppressed until a week after birth owing to the effect of maternal antithyroid medication.

Graves Disease

This is the most common cause of juvenile thyrotoxicosis, with the peak incidence occurring during adolescence. The disease is four to five times more common in females than in males.[43] There is substantial evidence that immune factors are important in the pathogenesis, and immunoglobulins, such as long-acting thyroid stimulator, can be identified.[44] In general, the disease is less debilitating and not as fulminant in children as in adults. Thyroid storm and apathetic hyperthyroidism rarely occur in children.[42]

Manifestations of Hyperthyroidism

The onset of the disease is usually gradual with nervousness, increased sweating, heat intolerance, increased appetite, and palpitations. Physical findings include thyroid enlargement (goiter), eye prominence and exophthalmos, tremor, tachycardia, hypertension, and a wide pulse pressure. Skeletal muscle weakness is frequently present.

The hyperdynamic cardiovascular system is characterized by tachycardia, increased cardiac output, and low peripheral resistance. Though this is a sympathetic-type response, serum catecholamines are not elevated, suggesting that adrenergic receptors may be sensitized by thyroid hormone. Nevertheless, there is no direct evidence that cardiovascular responsiveness to exogenous catecholamines is altered by increased or decreased activity of the thyroid gland. Persistent excessive release of thyroid gland hormones may produce an increase in the number of beta-adrenergic receptors.[5]

Laboratory Diagnosis

Serum T_4 and T_3 levels are usually elevated. Elevation of T_3 with normal T_4 (T_3 toxicosis) is frequently described in adults but it is rare in children. However, at the time of presentation of the disease the T_3 level is usually markedly elevated, making it the best single screening test for hyperthyroidism. Levels of thyroid hormone are higher in children, and an erroneous diagnosis of hyperthyroidism can be made if age-adjusted normal values are not used.[45] T_3 resin uptake will help distinguish abnormally elevated values associated with excess thyroid-binding globulin. Radioactive iodide uptake testing may be utilized, and the detection of immunoglobulins is useful in confirming the diagnosis.

Treatment

Initial treatment of congenital hyperthyroidism attempts to control the excessive cardiovascular stimulation. Propranolol, 1 to 2 mg/kg/day in three divided doses, is administered. In addition, hypersecretion of the thyroid gland is suppressed using propylthiouracil 5 to 10 mg/kg/day and saturated solution of potassium iodide one drop every 8 hours. Symptomatic improvement occurs in 1 or 2 weeks, whereas laboratory abnormalities may not return to normal until 4 to 6 weeks after initiation of therapy.

Radioactive iodide therapy in children may be associated with genetic damage, thyroid cancer induced by the radiation, and development of hypothyroidism. Surgical treatment necessitates that the patient be well controlled with medical therapy prior to the operation. Generally the indications for treatment by radioactive iodides or surgery are a drug reaction or noncompliance. Medical therapy is the treatment of choice for children, and remission occurs in one third of patients in 2 to 3 years.[45]

Thyroid Storm

Thyroid storm or acute uncompensated thyrotoxicosis is extremely rare in children. In adults, it most commonly occurs 6 to 18 hours postoperatively and is manifested by hyperthermia, tachyarrhythmias, hypotension, and coma. Thyrotoxic storm is a clinical diagnosis and may mimic malignant hyperthermia.[46]

Treatment of thyroid storm must be aggressive with both specific and supportive therapy. Hyperthermia may require ice packs, a cooling blanket, and cold crystalloid solutions. Glucose-containing solutions and balanced salt solutions are necessary to maintain intravascular volume. Propranolol intravenously is titrated to reduce the peripheral effects of thyroid gland hormones on the cardiovascular system. Propylthiouracil 5 to 10 mg/kg inhibits the synthesis of thyroid gland hormone. Sodium iodide can be administered following the thiouracil; the iodide will inhibit the release of active hormone from the gland. Hydrocortisone, 2 mg/kg every 6 hours, has been reported to increase survival, although documented adrenal insufficiency among patients in thyroid storm is rare.[47]

Anesthetic Management

Preoperative Assessment. Patients should be pharmacologically euthyroid prior to a planned surgical procedure. Six to 8 weeks of thiouracil therapy is usually necessary, and Lugol's iodine solution is started 1 week prior to surgery to decrease vascularity and hyperplasia of the overactive gland. Propranolol is administered to reduce the heart rate to a normal range and should be continued on the day of surgery. The euthyroid state is substantiated by improvement of clinical symptoms, a normal resting pulse, and normal laboratory findings. A large goiter should be evaluated with lateral neck x-rays, xeroradiography, or computed tomography scans to determine the length and extent of tracheal compression.

Premedication. A calm, sedated patient is the goal. Pentobarbital, 4 mg/kg, provides effective sedation with the advantage that barbiturates suppress thyroid gland function. Anticholinergics have been avoided because they interfere with the sweating mechanism and normal heat regulation. Chronically administered antithyroid drugs and beta-adrenergic blockers should be administered on the morning of surgery.

Operative Management. Patients with large goiters or signs of upper airway obstruction should be managed with techniques appropriate for children with upper airway obstruction. The airway must be secured awake or an inhalation induction is used with the maintenance of spontaneous ventilation until a satisfactory airway has been established. A firm armored endotracheal tube should be placed beyond the area of obstruction if tracheal compression has been demonstrated.

Induction. Thiopental is preferred because the thiourea structure lends antithyroid activity to this agent. Inhalational inductions are prolonged in patients with an increased cardiac output because additional time is required to increase the alveolar concentration of inhaled agent. In contrast to a common clinical impression, an increased anesthetic requirement has not been demonstrated in well-controlled animal studies.[41] Airway instrumentation and stimulation should be avoided until a deep level of anesthesia has been achieved. Prominent eyes will demand meticulous care with the instillation of lubricant and careful protective covering.

Muscle relaxants with the least cardiovascular effects (atracurium and vecuronium) are recommended. Continuous monitoring of neuromuscular blockade will permit assessment of the degree of coexisting muscle weakness that may be present.

Maintenance. Anesthetic agents that stimulate the sympathoadrenal axis or have sympathomimetic effects should be avoided (ether, cycloproprane, ketamine, pancuronium). Because of accelerated drug biotransformation in hyperthyroidism, drugs exhibiting a significant degree of biotransformation to toxic products are potentially more hazardous. An animal model made hyperthyroid by pretreatment with triiodothyronine resulted in hepatotoxicity associated with halothane anesthesia, which did not occur with enflurane anesthesia.[48] Isoflurane, which does not undergo significant biotransformation and does not sensitize the myocardium to catecholamines, appears to be a good choice for the maintenance of anesthesia.

Controlled mechanical ventilation will prevent hypercapnia with consequent sympathetic activity. Carotid sinus stimulation resulting from surgical manipulations can produce profound bradycardia. Continuous electrocardiographic and esophageal stethoscope monitoring will permit immediate detection. Treatment consists of stopping the stimulation as well as administering atropine intravenously. Venous air embolism is rare but is possible because of head elevation and large neck veins.

Continuous intraoperative and postoperative monitoring is essential to detect increased thyroid activity and thyroid storm. Temperature elevation, tachycardia and cardiovascular instability are indications for invasive monitoring and institution of the steps outlined previously to treat thyroid storm.

Postoperative Management. A number of postoperative complications may occur and therefore continuous postoperative monitoring is essential. Problems include airway obstruction, hypoparathyroidism, thyroid storm, and thoracic air dissection.[49]

Upper airway obstruction may occur owing to mucosal edema (postintubation croup), tracheomalacia, vocal cord paralysis, or compression by hematoma. Postintubation croup can be managed with humidified air and/or oxygen and racemic epinephrine inhalation. Bilateral recurrent laryngeal nerve injury secondary to surgical trauma results in obstruction due to unopposed adduction of the vocal cords and closure of the glottic aperture. This unusual complication necessitates reintubation followed by tracheotomy. Unilateral recurrent nerve injury often is not noticed because of compensatory overadduction of the uninvolved cord. Tracheal collapse due to preexisting chondromalacia of the tracheal rings may necessitate intubation for a period of time postoperatively. Postoperative hematoma in the neck may obstruct the trachea and requires the prompt removal of the dressing and opening of the surgical incision.

Hypoparathyroidism may occur because of inadvertent surgical removal of the parathyroid glands. Signs of hypocalcemia commonly do not develop for 24 to 72 hours but may become manifest immediately in the recovery room. Below-normal serum ionized calcium is diagnostic. Signs of tetany, including spasm of the laryngeal muscles, will diminish with the intravenous administration of calcium.

Thyroid storm is rare in children but in adults occurs most commonly 6 to 18 hours postoperatively. Supportive and specific therapy for thyroid storm was discussed earlier.

Subcutaneous emphysema, pneumothorax, and pneumomediastinum may occur with the surgical dissection of extensive thyroid tumors. A postoperative chest film should be reviewed for these complications.

Thyroiditis

Chronic Lymphocytic Thyroiditis

Also known as Hashimoto thyroiditis, this disease is the most common thyroid disorder in children and adolescents. The overall incidence in children is 1 percent, with a 4:1 to 8:1 female predominance. It is the most common cause of nontoxic goiter, and thyroid enlargement occurs in 90 percent of cases.[50]

Clinical features may include signs of hypothyroidism or hyperthyroidism. The usual course is either uneventful recovery or slow progression to hypothyroidism. Thyroid hormone supplementation in replacement doses is indicated when laboratory tests confirm hypothyroidism.

The disease is caused by an autoimmune process, and antibodies to thyroglobulin or thyroid microsomes can be demonstrated. It is commonly seen in Down syndrome (Trisomy 21), and in sex chromosome abnormalities such as Turner and Klinefelter syndromes, and is associated with diabetes mellitus, Addison disease, congenital rubella, and toxoplasmosis.[51] Corticosteroids in pharmacologic doses may have some temporary effect in reducing goiter size and increasing the serum T_4 level but do not change the long-term outlook.

Anesthetic considerations will be determined by the functional status of the thyroid gland and have been outlined previously.

Thyroid Tumors

Thyroid tumors in children are uncommon. The important benign lesions are thyroiditis, thyroid adenoma, thyroid cysts, and ectopic thyroids. A solitary and nonfunctioning ("cold") nodule in the thyroid gland will be malignant in 10 to 30 percent of patients, with the greatest incidence occurring in patients less than 20 years of age. Common features of thyroid carcinoma in children include abnormal cervical lymph nodes, metastatic lesions, abnormal hardness of the nodule, and a history of radiation to the head and neck.[52]

Medullary thyroid gland carcinoma characteristically produces large amounts of calcitonin, but hypocalcemia does not occur despite an excess of calcitonin in the circulation. Multiple endocrine adenomatosis (MEA) comprises a group of endocrine disorders that can occur by autosomal dominant genetic transmission. Sipple syndrome (MEA II) consists of medullary carcinoma of the thyroid, pheochromocytoma, and parathyroid hyperplasia. The important anesthetic considerations for medullary carcinoma of the thyroid are the presence or absence of these syndromes.

ADRENAL GLAND

The adrenal gland consists of two distinct endocrine systems. The cortical system is responsible for the synthesis of glucocorticoid, mineralocorticoid, and androgenic hormones, and the medullary system synthesizes the endogenous catecholamines dopamine, norephinephrine, and epinephrine.

Adrenal Cortex

The cortex is divided into three functional zones, each responsible for the synthesis of a specific group of hormones. The glucocorticoids are synthesized in the middle zona fasciculata and are so named for their ability to conserve glucose at the expense of other substrates. The mineralocorticoids, synthesized in the zona glomerulosa, are important in salt and water balance.

Cortisol, the major glucocorticoid synthesized by the adrenal cortex, affects the metabolism of most tissues (Fig. 12–3). Cortisol exerts a catabolic effect, resulting in a degradation of protein into amino acids with subsequent formation of glucose. In addition, cortisol inhibits utilization of glucose by the cells, an effect that is in direct opposition to the action of insulin. Thus hyperglycemia, which is present in syndromes of hypercorticism, is in part a reflection of both gluconeogenesis and decreased peripheral utilization of glucose. In the liver cortisol has a prominent anabolic effect, which results in an increase of protein and glycogen synthesis.

In the medulla cortisol must be present to facilitate the conversion of norepinephrine to epinephrine. As a result hypertension is a common feature in syndromes of hypercorticism. The anti-inflammatory activity of cortisol with its ability to stabilize cell membranes is used at advantage in treating conditions of hypersensitivity.

The mean cortisol production rate in children is approximately 12 mg/m²/day. Plasma levels range from 7 to 18 μg/100 ml in the early morning hours, with lower plasma concentrations of 2 to 9 μg/100 ml occurring at midnight, thereby establishing a diurnal variation. Adrenocorticotropic hormone (ACTH), synthesized in the pituitary, controls the secretion of

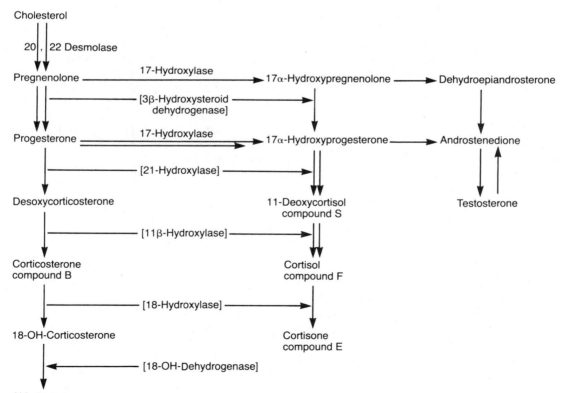

Figure 12–3. Synthesis of hydrocortisone. Double arrows indicate principal pathway of steroid synthesis. Single arrows indicate alternate pathways. Brackets denote enzymatic defects leading to virilizing adrenal hyperplasia.

cortisol by a negative feedback mechanism. A diurnal variation in the secretion of ACTH is used to advantage during steroid therapy. Exogenous steroids administered in the early morning hours when cortisol levels are already high and ACTH secretion is low will cause less suppression of the pituitary-adrenal axis.

Aldosterone is the principal mineralocorticoid; others, including desoxycortisone and corticosterone, are secreted in small quantities. The synthesis and secretion of aldosterone is regulated by the renin-angiotensin system and the serum concentration of potassium (Fig. 12–3). Renin is a proteolytic enzyme released from the juxtaglomerular cells of the kidney in response to hypovolemia, hypotension, or hyponatremia. In the presence of the angiotensin converting enzyme secreted by the lung, angiotensin I is converted to angiotensin II, which acts primarily on the adrenal cortex to secrete aldosterone. The kidney responds to aldosterone by increasing sodium reabsorption and increasing potassium excretion.

Dehydroepiandrosterone, androstenedione, and testosterone are androgenic hormones synthesized in the adrenal cortex (Fig. 12–3). The androgenic properties of these hormones are most conspicuous under pathological conditions such as congenital adrenal hyperplasia. These hormones are metabolized in the liver and are excreted by the kidney in the form of 17-ketosteroids. In the female, urinary measurement of 17-ketosteroids can be accepted as an index of their production; whereas, in the male, only two thirds of the urinary 17-ketosteroids are of adrenal cortical origin. The remaining one third are produced by the testicle. Prior to 8 to 10 years of age, the urinary excretion of these hormones is small, but there is a constant increase throughout adolescence until adult levels are reached.

Laboratory Tests of Adrenal Function

Metapyrone Test. Metapyrone inhibits the conversion of 11-deoxycortisol to cortisol. 11-Deoxycortisol, or compound S, is physiologically inert and therefore cannot suppress ACTH output by the pituitary. The absence of cortisol causes the pituitary to increase the secretion of ACTH. Thus the adrenal gland is stimulated to increase production of 11-deoxycortisol. A normal pituitary ACTH secretion and a normal adrenal responsiveness are indicated by a sharp increase in compound S or 11-deoxycortisol following the administration of metapyrone. If the measured level of 11-deoxycortisol in plasma, after metapyrone is injected, is greater than 7 μg/100 ml it can be concluded that the subject has a normal pituitary adrenal axis. The metapyrone test remains the best method for demonstrating cortisol deficiency with a normal pituitary-adrenal responsiveness.

ACTH or Cortrosyn Stimulation Test. The ACTH or cosyntropin (Cortrosyn) stimulation test is used to establish whether the abnormality of the pituitary-adrenal axis is located in the pituitary, hypothalamus, or adrenal glands. The test is carried out by administering 250 μg of Cortrosyn intravenously. Serum cortisol levels are then measured 1 hour after injection. A normal test is one in which there is a baseline cortisol level of at least 5 μg/100 ml, an increment between baseline and stimulated level greater than 7 μg/100 ml, and a stimulated cortisol level of greater than 18 μg/100 ml.

Dexamethasone Suppression Test. The dexamethasone suppression test is the most useful method for screening hypercorticism. This test is carried out by administering 1 mg of dexamethasone in older children (10 years and older) and 0.5 mg in younger children at 11:00 P.M. and then measuring the plasma cortisol levels the next day at 8:00 A.M. prior to ingestion of food. In the normal individual the cortisol level should be below 5 μg/100 ml. It is also useful to determine whether a diurnal variation of cortisol levels is present. In the normal individual, after 6:00 P.M. the serum cortisol level is less than 75 percent of the 8:00 A.M. level.

Adrenal Insufficiency

The syndrome of adrenal insufficiency (Addison disease) results from a deficient production of cortisol and aldosterone attributed to congenital and acquired lesions of the hypothalamus, pituitary, and adrenal cortex. As originally described by Addison, the syndrome occurred in patients whose adrenals were destroyed by tuberculosis. Today the most important cause of adrenal insufficiency is an autoimmune phenomenon, which may coexist with other autoimmune diseases such as chronic lymphocytic thyroiditis, hypoparathyroidism, diabetes mellitus, pernicious anemia, and hypopituitarism.[53, 54] Bilateral adrenal hemorrhage in those individuals who survive the acute episode results in adrenal insufficiency. It is interesting to note that in the newborn bilateral adrenal hemorrhage and subsequent calcification does not result in adrenal insufficiency.

Clinical Manifestations. The symptoms and clinical manifestations are secondary to glucocorticoid and mineralocorticoid insufficiency. The age of onset and the severity of symptoms will depend on the specific etiology involved. In chronic adrenal insufficiency the outstanding features are progressive weakness and hyperpigmentation. Pigmentation is more obvious over the extensor surfaces of knees and elbows, giving the appearance of dirty skin. The weakness present in these patients is due in part to glucocorticoid insufficiency with hypoglycemia, anorexia, and muscular weakness. If aldosterone insufficiency is also present, dehydration with hyponatremia and hyperkalemia secondary to urinary salt losses will coexist with anemia, hypotension, and a small cardiac silhouette on chest x-ray. The increase in pigmentation seen in these patients is a result of high levels of ACTH and unopposed melanophore-stimulating hormone (MSH) as a result of cortisol insufficiency.

If adrenal insufficiency is not recognized, an adrenal crisis may supervene in which the patient suddenly becomes cyanotic with a weak and rapid pulse and cold extremities. Hypotension is present with rapid and labored respirations. If therapy is not immediate and aggressive, death ensues. In patients with inadequately treated adrenal insufficiency adrenal crises can be precipitated by trauma, infection, excessive fatigue, or drugs such as morphine, barbiturates, thyroid hormone, laxative, or insulin.

Characteristic laboratory findings are decreased serum sodium concentration with increased serum concentration of potassium. Urinary electrolytes mirror serum findings with increased excretion of sodium and chloride and a decrease in urinary potassium. Hypoglycemia may be present or become manifest with prolonged fasting. Anemia is generally present and circulating levels of eosinophils are often increased in number. Roentgenographic examination of the chest will reveal a small, narrow heart.

Treatment. Administration of glucocorticoids and mineralocorticoids forms the basis for the treatment of adrenal insufficiency. To treat adrenal insufficiency adequately, it is sufficient to replace normal production of cortisol. In general, daily administration of cortisol 12 to 15 mg/m^2 is considered adequate replacement. In times of illness or stress the dosage is increased by 50 to 100 percent. Fludrocortisone (Florinef), an oral mineralocorticoid, is administered in a dosage of 0.05 to 0.1 mg irrespective of age or weight. This dose is adjusted to maintain normal serum levels of sodium and potassium without producing hypertension. In times of crisis when the patient is unable to ingest oral medications, the mineralocorticoid is given by intramuscular injection.

In the acute situation, hypoglycemia and sodium loss are treated by the intravenous administration of 5 to 10 percent glucose in isotonic saline, at a rate of 100 to 120 ml/kg for the first 24 hours. Twenty to 25 percent of the total replacement is administered in the first 2 hours. Fluid therapy after the initial 24 hours will depend on the status of the child and assessment of continuing losses. A water-soluble form of hydrocortisone such as hydrocortisone hemisuccinate, initial dose of 2 mg/kg, is administered and followed by an infusion at 0.6 mg/kg/hr until symptoms subside. In this manner high levels of cortisol can be achieved instantaneously. Invasive monitoring with an arterial cannula, central venous pressure line, and urinary catheter should be instituted early and continued until cardiovascular stability is attained. Intramuscular injections of cortisone acetate (2 mg/kg) are given daily for a few days to provide a sustained and prolonged cortisol level. These doses can then be reduced progressively over 24 hours if progress is satisfactory. A salt-retaining hormone in the form of intramuscular deoxycorticosterone (DOCA) in doses of 1 to 3 mg is added daily to maintain electrolyte balance. This therapy is administered for 48 hours. If oral intake is satisfactory, the intravenous fluids are discontinued and cortisol can be given orally at 0.5 mg/kg in three divided doses. DOCA is administered daily and continued throughout the period of treatment.

Once the acute episode is under control, the patients will require chronic replacement therapy with cortisol and aldosterone deficiency. The intramuscular administration of DOCA is replaced by the oral administration of fluorohydrocortisone in doses of 0.05 mg to 0.1 mg daily regardless of age. Appropriate dosage of fluorohydrocortisone is regarded as that at which electrolyte balance can be maintained without signs of hypertension.[55]

Anesthetic Management. The anesthetic management of the child with documented adrenal insufficiency must include the provision for exogenous corticosteroids. Preoperative assessment should particularly focus on the adequacy of corticosteroid supplementation (refer to the section of The Steroid-Treated Patient later in this chapter). However, the selection of anesthetic agents is not influenced by the presence of treated hypocorticism. Plasma cortisol concentrations predictably increase during surgery, but the rise is in response to surgical stimulus rather than the anesthetic agent.[56] In the literature there are frequent suggestions that unexplained intraoperative hypotension and even death reflect undiagnosed adrenal insufficiency, but there is no supportive evidence for this etiology.[57]

Should emergency surgery become necessary in a situation of untreated or partially treated hypoadrenocorticism, the patient is regarded as one with impending acute adrenal insufficiency and is therefore treated aggressively with fluids, glucocorticoids, and a mineralocorticoid.

Corticosteroids should be administered well above the physiologic dose of 12 mg/m^2/day: the preparation of choice is cortisone succinate, which provides an immediate serum level. The administration of 2 mg/kg of hydrocortisone every 6 hours is appropriate for most surgical procedures. Anesthetic agents must be titrated because patients with adrenal insufficiency are sensitive to the myocardial depression induced by potent anesthetic agents. Muscle relaxants must be titrated to produce the desired effect in view of the skeletal muscle weakness. The response to relaxant drugs is monitored by a peripheral nerve stimulator. Invasive monitoring of arterial blood pressure and cardiac filling pressures may be indicated for major procedures. Serum concentrations of electrolytes and blood glucose must be evaluated frequently in the perioperative period. Glucocorticoid and mineralocorticoid supplementation must be continued in the postoperative period.

Congenital Adrenal Hyperplasia

Congenital adrenal hyperplasia is characterized by ambiguous genitalia, severe salt-losing crises, virilization, and in rare cases hypertension. It is inherited as

Table 12–2. CONGENITAL ADRENAL HYPERPLASIA

Enzymatic Defect	Urine		Plasma		Electrolyte Abnormality	Symptoms	Treatment
21-Hydroxylase, salt-losing	↑ ↑ ↓	Pregnanetriol 17-Ketosteroids Aldosterone	↑ ↑ ↑ ↓	17-Hydroxyprogesterone Dehydroepiandrosterone Renin Aldosterone	↓ Na ↑ K	Virilization Muscle weakness Dehydration	DOCA + cortisol for acute crisis Fluorohydrocortisone + cortisone for maintenance therapy
21-Hydroxylase, non–salt-losing	↑ ↑	Pregnanetriol 17-Ketosteroids	↑ ↑ ↑ ↑	17-Hydroxyprogesterone Dehydroepiandrosterone Renin Aldosterone	Normal	Virilization	Cortisone
11-Hydroxylase	↑ →	Tetrahydro-S Pregnanetriol	↑ →↓ →↓	Compound S Renin Aldosterone	↑ NA ↓ K	Incomplete virilization Hypertension	Cortisone
17-Hydroxylase	↓	17-Ketosteroids	↑ ↑ ↑	Progesterone Corticosterone 11-Deoxycorticosterone	Normal		
3-β-Dehydrogenase, salt-losing	↑	17-Ketosteroids	↑	Pregnenolone	↓ Na ↑ K	Dehydration	DOCA + cortisol for acute crisis Fluorohydrocortisone + cortisone for maintenance therapy

an autosomal recessive gene. The primary defect of congenital adrenal hyperplasia is failure to synthesize cortisol with consequent lack of suppression of ACTH. Increased ACTH secretion from the anterior pituitary will lead to increased production of adrenal androgen hormones. There are several forms of congenital adrenal hyperplasia, the most common of which is 21-hydroxylase deficiency (Table 12–2). This enzymatic defect leads to failure of conversion of 17-hydroxyprogesterone to 11-deoxycortisol (compound S) and accumulation of 17-hydroxyprogesterone in the serum. In both females and males the cardinal feature of the disease is virilization. In females this is manifested by ambiguous external genitalia. If the disease is not treated, virilization will be progressive with premature growth of pubic and axillary hair and progressive growth of the penis or clitoris. Muscles are well developed and ossification is well advanced for chronological age. Initially growth will be accelerated, but because of early epiphyseal closure with untreated adrenal hyperplasia individuals will be short in stature. Salt-losing crises occur in about half of all patients with 21-hydroxylase deficiency as a result of a concomitant aldosterone deficiency. In those patients who do not have salt-wasting crises, there is actually an increase in aldosterone production in time of stress. Salt loss is aggravated by the presence of two metabolic intermediates, 17-hydroxyprogesterone and progesterone, both of which antagonize the action of aldosterone on the renal tubule. In the newborn with ambiguous genitalia, the possibility of congenital adrenal hyperplasia exists and the infant should be monitored for signs of salt loss. These signs include poor feeding, vomiting, lethargy, and shock. Serum sodium concentration is below normal and serum potassium is abnormally high. The electrocardiogram may show sharply peaked T waves and shortening of the S-T segment, consistent

with hyperkalemia. Urea nitrogen and creatinine are increased secondary to prerenal diversion of the circulation.

An increase in the plasma concentration of 17-hydroxyprogesterone establishes the diagnosis. Serum concentrations of 200 ng/100 ml are considered normal in the first month of life, after which there is a gradual decrease to 100 ng/100 ml until puberty. In patients with 21-hydroxylase deficiency these levels are 20- to 500-fold above normal.

Treatment. There are three essential components to treating salt-losing crises: intravenous fluids containing sodium, mineralocorticoids (deoxycorticosterone), and cortisol. If the infant is moribund, initial treatment is begun with the intravenous infusion of normal saline at 20 ml/kg administered over a short period of time. With improvement of the circulatory status, treatment is then continued as for acute adrenal insufficiency crises.

In the patient receiving fludrocortisone (Florinef) blood pressure is measured frequently, since hypertension is an early sign of overdosage. Fludrocortisone is administered in a dosage of 0.05 to 1 mg orally; the requirements do not seem to increase with age, although the reasons for this are unclear. The dosage of cortisol to maintain adequate bone maturation, growth and steroid levels is normally two and one-half to three times the normal secretory rate of cortisol. The average dose of cortisol for patients with congenital adrenal hyperplasia is in the range of 30 to 36 mg/m²/day or 1 to 1.5 mg/kg/day. Two thirds of the dose is administered in the evening hours, when the major surge of ACTH occurs, and one third in the morning hours.

In salt losers discontinuation of mineralocorticoids at any time carries the risk of acute adrenal insufficiency. These children will need close observation should infection develop and in preparation for surgery. In these situations their requirements for corticosteroids and mineralocorticoids will be increased.

Anesthetic Management. The preoperative assessment of this patient must include evaluation of the state of hydration, serum electrolytes, urea nitrogen, blood glucose, and acid-base status. Glucocorticoids and mineralocorticoids are continued in the usual doses up to the time of surgery. Blood pressure measurement is important to evaluate the adequacy of mineralocorticoid replacement. On the day of surgery the usual therapeutic cortisone dose is increased by 50 to 100 percent. Thus a child receiving a daily morning dose of 8 mg of cortisone should have the dose increased to 12 mg administered by intravenous injection. The initial dose should be followed by a continuous infusion of 0.4 mg/kg/hr throughout the period of surgery or given as individual doses of 1.5 to 2 mg/kg at 6-hour intervals. Intramuscular DOCA should be administered in dosages of 1 to 3 mg daily and continued until the patient is able to resume oral medication. The use of invasive monitoring in these patients must be decided based on the severity of the surgical procedure and physical status of the patient. Electrolytes, blood glucose, and acid-base status must be evaluated frequently during the surgical procedure. Any anesthetic agent, whether volatile or intravenous, may be used in these patients. One agent does not seem to have any advantage over another. Postoperatively these patients must be observed closely for signs of adrenal insufficiency.

The Steroid-Treated Patient

Cortisone, when administered, must be converted to cortisol to become biologically active. This conversion occurs even in the absence of adrenals.[5] Similarly prednisolone, a synthetic steroid, must be converted to prednisone to become biologically active. In managing patients on corticosteroid therapy it is important to distinguish between plasma and biological half-life of the steroid preparations (Table 12–3). The biological half life appears to be manifested well after the glucocorticoid has left the circulation and is reflected in the duration of the hypothalamic pituitary-adrenal (HPA) suppression. It is also known that the duration of the HPA suppression approximates the duration of the anti-inflammatory activity of the glucocorticoid when this is given orally. By examining the HPA suppression it has been possible to estimate the duration of the therapeutic effects of cortisol and its analogues.

Important factors in determining the degree of HPA suppression are not only the potency and the tissue half-life of the glucocorticoid but also the dosage, the time of day, and the total duration of steroid therapy. The peak activity of the pituitary-adrenal interaction occurs in the early morning hours, with high levels of plasma cortisol being measured at approximately 8:00 A.M. The resultant feedback maximally suppresses further ACTH release. If exogenous steroids are administered at this time, there will be minimal suppressive effect on the pituitary-adrenal axis.[58]

It is generally accepted that significant HPA suppression occurs after 10 days of high-dose corticosteroid therapy and may be detected as early as 5 days. The recovery time from HPA suppression is not as definite and can be as long as 12 months after only 2 weeks of supraphysiologic doses of steroids (Table 12–4).

In the recovery phase ACTH levels increase before the adrenal cortex is capable of responding to ACTH. However, without evaluation of the axis, it is difficult to draw conclusions regarding recovery of the HPA axis. Preoperative evaluation of the pituitary-adrenal axis, as suggested by Symreng and colleagues, would provide a more intelligent approach to coverage of the corticosteroid-treated patient.[59] However, since evaluation of the HPA axis is often difficult and impractical, it is wise to administer steroid supplementation to patients who will experience medical or surgical stress within 1 year of cessation of corticosteroid therapy.

Knowledge of the absorption rates of commercial steroid preparations is important in preparing these patients for surgery. For example, the hemisuccinates and phosphate preparations are water soluble and therefore are readily absorbed when administered par-

Table 12–3. DIFFERENCES IN STEROID PREPARATIONS

	Biological Half-Life (hr)	Plasma Half-Life (min)	Glucocorticoid Potency	Equivalent Glucocorticoid (mg)	Mineralocorticoid Activity
Short-Acting					
Cortisol	8–12	90	1	20	2+
Cortisone	24–36	30	0.8	25	2+
Prednisone	24–36	30	4	5	1+
Prednisolone	12–36	200	4	4	1+
Methylprednisolone	12–36	200	5	4	0
Intermediate-Acting					
Triamcinolone	12–36	200	5	4	0
Long-Acting					
Bethamethasone	36–54	300	25	0.60	0
Dexamethasone	36–54	300	30	0.75	0

Table 12-4. RECOVERY OF HYPOTHALAMIC-PITUITARY-ADRENAL FUNCTION AFTER WITHDRAWAL OF STEROIDS

Recovery Time (mo)	Plasma 17-Hydroxycorticoid Values	Plasma ACTH Values	Adrenal Response to Exogenous ACTH	Response to Metyrapone
1	Low	Low	Low	Low
2–5	Low	High	Low	Low
6–9	Normal	Normal	Low	Low
> 9	Normal	Normal	Normal	Normal

enterally. These preparations are useful in acute situations as well as for prolonged infusions. The acetate and diacetate forms are insoluble in water, and when given intramuscularly are absorbed slowly over a period of days or weeks and can be used parenterally for short-term continuous therapy in place of oral steroids. The pivalates and hexacetonide are long-acting and are absorbed over weeks or months.

The preoperative coverage of the corticosteroid-treated pediatric patient is based on adult protocols. We know that the adrenal cortex of the normal adult under perioperative conditions is able to secrete 116 to 185 mg of cortisol daily.[60] During periods of maximum stress, the adult is able to secrete 200 to 500 mg daily. Good correlation also seems to exist between the response of the adrenal gland and the severity and duration of surgical stress. In one study the mean maximal plasma cortisol level during the major surgery was 47 μg/100 ml (range, 22 to 75 μg/100 ml) and values remained above 26 μg/100 ml for a maximum of 72 hours. The mean maximal cortisol level during minor surgery was 28 μg/100 ml (range, 10 to 44 μg/100 ml).[61]

In the child hydrocortisone hemisuccinate, 2 mg/kg, is administered every 6 hours on the day of surgery. For major surgery this therapy is continued for the next 3 days and either discontinued abruptly or tapered over the next 5 days. For minor surgery, such as a herniorrhaphy, 24-hour coverage with 2 mg/kg of hydrocortisone hemisuccinate every 6 hours is sufficient protection, whereas for short procedures as esophagoscopy a single injection of 2 mg/kg of hydrocortisone hemisuccinate on the day of surgery is sufficient.[62]

Hypercorticism

Cushing syndrome is characterized by chronic excessive production of glucocorticoid hormones. In 1932, Harvey Cushing described bilateral adrenal hyperplasia secondary to basophilic adenomas. This form of the syndrome, bilateral adrenal hyperplasia caused by excessive production of ACTH, became known as Cushing disease and is distinguished from other forms of the syndrome. Cushing disease was formerly thought rare but is now being detected with increasing frequency. The initiating factor appears to be a hypothalamic disturbance giving rise to pituitary tumors. However, enlargement of the sella turcica in children is extremely rare. Characteristic of the syndrome is

increased secretion of corticotropin, with loss of the circadian rhythm and resistance to suppression by the dexamethasone test.

Excessive production of biologically active ACTH by nonendocrine tumors such as thymoma, bronchogenic carcinoma, islet tumor of the pancreas, neuroblastoma, and ganglioneuroblastoma will give rise to a symptom complex known as ectopic Cushing syndrome. More commonly in children, a clinical pattern identical to Cushing syndrome results from prolonged exogenous administration of glucocorticoids.

In infants with adrenal involvement the lesion is usually a functioning tumor, frequently a malignant cortical carcinoma. These patients present with increased production of androgens, estrogens, and aldosterone, giving a mixed picture of hypercorticism.

Clinical Features. A moon facies and centripetal fat distribution with thin extremities and truncal obesity are the most outstanding features. Growth retardation is a useful sign to distinguish this syndrome from exogenous obesity, which is usually characterized by excessive growth. Osteoporosis is present with delayed epiphyseal maturation due to decreased matrix formation and impaired calcium reabsorption. Hypertension occurs as a result of increased catecholamine secretion with salt and fluid retention. Hyperglycemia or frank diabetes mellitus results from inhibition of peripheral utilization of glucose and concomitant gluconeogenesis. Hypokalemic alkalosis may be present, although this is more commonly seen in the ectopic ACTH syndrome. The lympholytic and immunosuppressive effects of glucocorticoids make these patients more susceptible to infections. Glucocorticoids also have a negative effect on wound healing, which is only in part reversed by vitamin A.[63]

Diagnosis. Demonstration of increased plasma and urine concentrations of cortisol forms the basis of the diagnosis of hypercorticism. Dexamethasone will suppress production of cortisol in the normal patient but not in the patient with hypercorticism; testing for cortisol production after administration of dexamethasone is the most useful method for screening patients for hypercorticism. An elevated plasma level of adrenocorticotropic hormone suggests the presence of a pituitary gland tumor or an ectopic hormone-producing tumor. A very high level of ACTH is highly suggestive of an ectopic tumor. Carcinoma of the adrenal cortex, which produces an excess of glucocorticoids, is likely to secrete an excess of androgens, leading to increased urinary excretion of 17-ketosteroids and sometimes to signs of virilization.

Preoperative Evaluation. Special preoperative considerations in children with hypercorticism are directed toward the establishment of the diagnosis, the indication for surgery, and the specific hormonal abnormalities present. In cases of glucocorticoid excess emphasis is placed on regulating hyperglycemia and hypertension, ensuring that the intravascular volume is adequate and that electrolyte concentrations are normal. Evaluation of acid-base disturbances is particularly important in cases of ectopic ACTH production, in which hypokalemic alkalosis may be marked. Radiographs of the skeletal system should be reviewed for evidence of osteoporosis and presence of subclinical pathological fractures. This is important in terms of subsequent positioning of the patient.

In addition to the evaluation of the specific medical conditions of the patient, specific considerations are directed to the particular surgery contemplated.

There is no reason to alter the preoperative medication schedule, since hypercorticism does not influence drug metabolism. Holaday and associates report decreased morphine metabolism in patients following bilateral adrenalectomy.[64]

Anesthetic Management. Surgical stress will predictably increase the release of cortisol from the adrenal cortex. It does not seem likely, however, that these patients would be affected differently from normal patients. Halothane, ethrane, isoflurance, or a nitrous oxide–narcotic relaxant technique can be chosen according to the personal preference of the anesthetist. Mechanical ventilation of the lungs is suggested in view of the muscle weakness that frequently accompanies hypercorticism. Muscle relaxant doses may need to be reduced, especially if hypokalemia coexists. The need for invasive monitoring is dependent on the type of surgery and the physical status of the patient. For adrenalectomy, the size, vascularity, and location of the tumor must be considered. Once the secreting tumor is removed the patient should receive supplemental exogenous intravenous glucocorticoids, (as discussed previously in the section on Adrenal Insufficiency). Supplementation is required by patients undergoing unilateral as well as bilateral adrenalectomy, since the contralateral adrenal may be quiescent as a result of low levels of ACTH. Postoperatively, the glucocorticoid may be tapered to a maintenance therapy level.

Primary Aldosteronism

Primary aldosteronism usually occurs in the third decade of life and is rare in children. It is generally attributable to a functional adrenal tumor. In children hyperaldosteronism has been associated more commonly with adrenal hyperplasia. However, demonstration of a low renin serum level should suggest a primary adrenal defect.

Clinical Manifestations. The clinical symptoms are due to excess production of mineralocorticoids, which results in hypertension. Other symptoms include polydipsia, polyuria, nocturia, paresthesias, visual disturbance, intermittent paralysis, tetany, fatigue, muscle weakness, and discomfort. The severe growth retardation and muscle weakness that may occur are probably a result of potassium depletion. The urine is alkaline or neutral, and the kidneys lose their ability to concentrate. The serum pH carbon dioxide content, and sodium concentration are all elevated, and serum potassium and chloride levels are decreased. Tetany may occur in spite of a normal serum calcium. Urinary excretion of 17-ketosteroids and 17-hydroxycorticosteroids is within normal limits, but urinary excretion of aldosterone is increased.

Primary aldosteronism must be differentiated from secondary hyperaldosteronism, in which there is an increased secretion of aldosterone secondary to low body sodium and excessive accumulation of potassium and/or dehydration. Secondary hyperaldosteronism is present in congestive cardiac failure, cirrhosis of the liver, and the nephrotic syndrome. The most important diagnostic clue is the level of serum renin, which is high in secondary hyperaldosteronism but low in primary aldosteronism, in which the renin-angiotensin system is suppressed.

Diagnosis. A serum potassium of less than 3.5 mEq/L in a patient with hypertension suggests hyperaldosteronism. The diagnosis is confirmed by the demonstration of an increased plasma concentration of aldosterone and elevated urinary potassium. Measurement of plasma renin activity allows differentiation between primary hyperaldosteronism with low activity and secondary hyperaldosteronism with increased secretion. The patient's drug history should be considered in interpreting laboratory values (Table 12–5).

Anesthetic Management. The preoperative evaluation of the patient with hyperaldosteronism must be directed toward assessment of the electrolyte status, correction of hypertension, and hypokalemia. The anesthetic management is simplified if hypokalemia is corrected preoperatively, since hyperventilation can further decrease the serum concentration of potassium.

Either intravenous or inhaled anesthetic agents are acceptable choices; however, the choice of ethrane may be questionable if a nephropathy exists preoperatively. Invasive monitoring of arterial blood pressure and central venous pressure is suggested for adequate eval-

Table 12–5. DRUGS THAT ALTER PLASMA RENIN ACTIVITY

Increased Activity	Decreased Activity
Thiazide diuretics	Propranolol
Nitroprusside	Alpha-methyldopa
Hydralazine	Clonidine
Chlorpromazine	
Thyroxine	

uation of intravascular volume as well as of the response to intravenous fluids. Unexpected hypotension in response to vasodilating anesthetic agents and positive-pressure ventilation may be the result of aggressive preoperative preparation to reduce the excess intravascular volume. Acid-base status and serum electrolytes must be monitored frequently during the perioperative period. Supplementation with exogenous cortisol is not indicated in the case of a solitary adenoma. However, when multiple adenomas are to be excised with bilateral mobilization of the adrenal gland, transient hypocorticism may develop and the need for exogenous cortisol exists. In this situation a continuous infusion of cortisone hemisuccinate should be administered to attain immediate high serum levels.

Adrenal Medulla

The adrenal medulla is composed of chromaffin tissue derived from the neural crest. By its capability to synthesize epinephrine and norepinephrine, the medulla becomes an integral part of the sympathetic nervous system (Fig. 12–4). With the exception of the sweat glands and the pilomotor nerves, norepinephrine forms the neurotransmitter for the postganglionic fibers of the sympathetic nervous system. Epinephrine is produced entirely in the medulla from methylation of norepinephrine by the action of the enzyme phenylethanolamine transferase. The presence of cortisol is essential for this reaction to take place. This synergistic action of cortisol partly explains the hypertension that occurs in syndromes of hypercorticism.

The half-life of catecholamines is short because deactivation occurs rapidly by means of enzymatic degradation (catechol-O-methyltransferase) or conjugation (with sulfate or glucuronide). The secretion of catecholamines is under the direct control of the nervous system. Factors such as mental stress, hypoxia, and acidemia favor the release of epinephrine. In addition, histamine can stimulate the release of epinephrine from the adrenal medulla. This explains why the administration of D-tubocurarine, which releases histamine, can produce a rise in blood pressure when used in a patient with pheochromocytoma.

Knowledge of the pharmacology of catecholamines is important in understanding the clinical and anesthetic implications of catecholamine-secreting tumors. Alquist's classification of catecholamines as possessing alpha- or beta-adrenergic activity was artificially based on chemical and pharmacological differences.[65] Under this classification, norepinephrine was described as possessing alpha-adrenergic activity and producing systemic vasoconstriction with reflex bradycardia. However, as a neurotransmitter of the sympathetic nervous system, norepinephrine has direct cardiac effects or beta activity. The beta activity of norepinephrine will become evident in the presence of an agent such as phentolamine, which will block the alpha receptors.

Epinephrine is considered to possess both alpha and beta activity. The peripheral vascular effects of epinephrine vary in different vascular beds and with different drug concentrations. In the arterioles of skeletal muscle where both alpha and beta receptors are present, vasodilatation occurs at low concentration of epinephrine. By contrast, in the presence of high concentration of epinephrine, the alpha effects predominate and vasoconstriction occurs. The vessels of the skin and mucous membranes will respond almost always with vasoconstriction. The effect of epinephrine on the heart is similar to that of norepinephrine. The major difference between norepinephrine and epinephrine is their effect on body metabolism. An injection of exogenous epinephrine is associated with a sharp increase in oxygen consumption. Insulin secretion is inhibited by epinephrine, while blood levels of glucose, lactate, and glycerol are increased.

Dopamine is now generally accepted as a neurotransmitter with specific receptors in certain organs such as

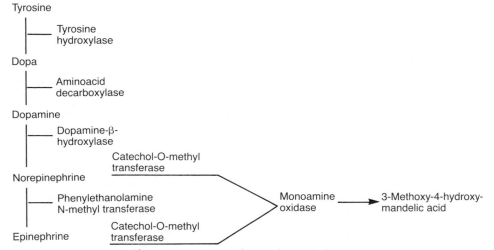

Figure 12–4. Biosynthesis of catecholamines.

the kidney.[66] At low concentrations the beta-adrenergic activity of dopamine is evident, whereas at higher concentrations the alpha effects predominate. Dopamine is often the major catecholamine secreted by a neuroblastoma.

Neuroblastoma

Neuroblastoma is a malignant solid tumor of childhood that arises from the adrenal medulla or paravertebral ganglia. As a tumor derived from the neural crest, a neuroblastoma may occur in the mediastinum or abdomen or invade the spinal canal, where it can cause compression of the spinal cord. A neuroblastoma will generally reach a large size before clinical symptoms become evident. Common sites of metastases include bone marrow, liver, and brain. Radiological studies, including intravenous urograms, computed tomography, and radionuclide scans, are used together with bone marrow and spinal tap to establish the diagnosis. If there is evidence of cord compression, myelography is performed immediately in preparation for emergency decompression.

The diagnosis of neuroblastoma is established by measurement of urinary catecholamines and their metabolites. Abnormally high levels of dopamine, homovanillic acid, norepinephrine, normetanephrine, vanillylmandelic acid, and other metabolites are found in the urine of most patients with neuroblastoma. Radioisotope studies and tumor analysis show that there is increased catabolism of catecholamines with release of metabolically inactive compounds. Thus hypertension secondary to catecholamine secretion is not always present.

Anesthetic Management. The size and location of the tumor, extent of the disease, biological effects of the tumor, symptoms related to the presence of the tumor, and the extent of chemotherapy are important factors for the anesthetic management of the child with neuroblastoma.

A large number of children may have metastases present at the time of diagnosis. Since neuroblastomas frequently metastasize to the liver, lymph nodes, bone marrow, and skeleton, the preoperative evaluation should include x-ray views of the abdomen and chest, intravenous pyelography, and a skeletal survey. Serum electrolytes and urea nitrogen should be measured, particularly in the patient who presents with vomiting and diarrhea, which may result from vasoactive peptide secretion by some neuroblastomas.

Blood loss equal to the patient's blood volume during the resection of a neuroblastoma is not uncommon. Third space fluid sequestration secondary to the generous exposure needed for the resection should be replaced by lactated Ringer's solution at 8 to 10 ml/kg/hr.

In the young child the size of the tumor may cause symptoms of intestinal obstruction and, particularly in the infant, respiratory failure may be present. Where spinal compression is suspected and an emergency myelogram required, the induction of anesthesia may be further complicated by the presence of a full stomach.

Intravenous catheters must be placed in the upper extremities so that infusion of fluids occurs independently of the status of the inferior vena cava. Urine output should be measured by means of a urinary catheter. In thoracic tumors as in large abdominal tumors, a pulse oximeter in addition to measurement of arterial blood gas levels is useful to detect sudden changes in arterial oxygenation. The use of invasive arterial monitoring is necessary to measure changes in blood pressure. A large catheter in a central vein should be used to measure cardiac filling pressure and to administer added volume and resuscitation drugs. Heat losses are common in these patients, and precautions to avoid hypothermia should be taken.

Anesthesia may be induced with thiopental or by the use of an inhalation agent, preferably enflurane or isoflurane. If signs of intestinal obstruction are present, a rapid-sequence induction is preferred. Isoflurane and enflurane, with their ability to protect the myocardium from catecholamine stimulation and control blood pressure, remain the anesthetic agents of choice. Atracurium and vecuronium are similarly chosen for their minimal cardiovascular effects, and pancuronium has been used in the past without difficulty. Hypertension may be present, and alpha-adrenergic blocking agents such as nitroprusside and phentolamine should be available.

Since most children with neuroblastoma have normal pulmonary function, extubation of the trachea is usually possible at the completion of the surgical procedure. The postoperative care of these patients requires close monitoring of the fluid status as measured by arterial and central venous pressure and urine output. If the cardiovascular or respiratory system is not stable, or losses of blood and fluid have been substantial, these patients should be admitted to the intensive care unit for more attentive supervision.

Pheochromocytoma

Pheochromocytoma is a catecholamine-secreting tumor that originates from chromaffin cells. It is most commonly found in the adrenal medulla but may be found wherever chromaffin tissue is present. Extraadrenal tumors are usually located in the abdomen along the sympathetic chain, although they have been described in the neck and in the mediastinum. In the bladder they may arise from sympathetic ganglia present in the wall. Pheochromocytoma is a rare tumor in the pediatric population and occurs more commonly at puberty. Over 95 percent of the tumors arise in the abdominal cavity, including approximately 90 percent in the adrenal medulla, with a predilection for the right side. A malignant pheochromocytoma is rare in children. Bilateral or multiple tumors may occur. A pheochromocytoma may occur as part of multiple

Table 12–6. MULTIPLE ENDOCRINE ADENOMATOSIS

	Organ	Disorder
Werner syndrome	Pituitary	Hypoglycemia
(Type I)	Parathyroid	Hypercalcemia
	Pancreas	Peptic ulcer
Sipple syndrome	Thyroid	Medullary carcinoma
(Type II)	Parathyroid	Hyperplasia
	Adrenal medulla	Pheochromocytoma
(Type III)	Nervous system	Multiple neuromas
	Thyroid	Medullary carcinoma
	Adrenal medulla	Pheochromocytoma

endocrine adenomatosis (Table 12–6) in association with pituitary and/or parathyroid gland adenoma.[67]

Clinical Manifestations. The symptoms of pheochromocytoma are the result of the physiological and pharmacological effects of an increased plasma concentration of norepinephrine and epinephrine. Headache, nausea, and vomiting are common findings in the child with hypertension due to a pheochromocytoma. Arterial blood pressure may reach levels of over 250 mmHg systolic with concomitant elevated diastolic pressure. The child often appears pale, weak, and anxious and has cool extremities. Abdominal pain, polydipsia, and polyuria are also common findings.[68] Hypertensive encephalopathy may occur and may be confused with intracranial neoplasm.

Diagnosis. The importance of diagnosing a pheochromocytoma before anesthesia and surgery cannot be overemphasized. Pheochromocytoma can be totally quiescent when the tumor is not actively secreting catecholamines but suddenly cause a stormy hypertensive crisis as catecholamines are rapidly secreted into the circulation. Cardiomyopathy is rare in children but more common in the adult patient. Small tumors are more likely to produce the classic intermittent type of hypertension with normotension between crises. Apparently small tumors release active metabolites, including normetanephrine and metanephrine. Sustained hypertension is more common in children and is a feature of large tumors, which predominantly secrete norepinephrine. The catecholamine composition of the tumor will regulate the type and severity of hypertensive crises even to the extent that a hypotensive crisis may occur in dopamine-epinephrine mixed tumors. Measurement of urinary catecholamines or their metabolites provides a useful screening method, but diagnosis is difficult owing to the high percentage of false positives. Measurement of plasma catecholamines reliably establishes the presence of a pheochromocytoma even in those cases in which normotension exists.[70]

Preoperative Preparation. The child should be admitted several days before surgery, at which time any additional laboratory tests and preparation may be conducted. Although not common in the pediatric age group, active myocarditis was found in 15 of 26 patients with pheochromocytoma in a study reported by the Mayo Clinic.[71] James reported that the coronary arteries of one patient with pheochromocytoma had platelet aggregates, supporting the role of catecholamines in platelet aggregation.[72]

The preoperative preparation of the patient with pheochromocytoma should include measurement of serum electrolytes, creatinine, and fasting blood glucose levels and, if indicated, a glucose tolerance test. Cardiac evaluation with an electrocardiogram and an echocardiogram should be performed to exclude cardiomyopathy. The blood volume in patients with pheochromocytoma is contracted. A falling hematocrit in response to alpha-adrenergic blocking drugs is generally an indication of restoration of blood volume. The abnormal function of other endocrine glands should be screened by reviewing the history and by laboratory evaluation.

Preoperative localization of the tumor can be achieved by the use of computed tomography. Arteriography will establish the vascular connections of the tumor, which are important for surgical resection. General anesthesia for arteriography should be conducted with the same precautions as are taken for anesthesia for resection of the tumor. Radiocontrast materials may cause histamine release when injected during the vascular study, and this may cause the tumor to secrete catecholamines. Formerly used pharmacological provocative tests with agents such as histamine, glucagon, and phentolamine are rarely used because of their associated risks. Venous samples from different locations in the vena cava can often supplement radiological evaluation.[73]

Phenoxybenzamine given orally in increasing doses several days to weeks prior to surgery is the drug of choice for the preoperative preparation of the patient with pheochromocytoma. Phenoxybenzamine, a long-acting alpha blocking drug, acts by strongly binding with the receptor so that it cannot be displaced by circulating catecholamines. Thus, excessive vasoconstriction is prevented in spite of variable surges of catecholamines that can occur during manipulation of the tumor,[74] and the preoperative intravascular volume is partly restored.

Cardiac arrhythmias and tachycardia are very rare in the pediatric patient with pheochromocytoma. If supraventricular arrhythmias should occur, control can be attained by the use of a beta blocker such as propranolol. Beta blockade should not be instituted in the absence of alpha-adrenergic block.[75] There is at least a theoretical concern that a heart depressed by beta blockade could not maintain an adequate cardiac output in the face of unopposed alpha-mediated vasoconstriction. Beta blockade is not generally required in children with pheochromocytoma.

An additional approach to the preparation of the child with pheochromocytoma is the use of alpha-methyltyrosine, which interferes with the hydroxylation of tyrosine and thereby inhibits the further production of catecholamines. This mode of therapy has been used with some success in children.[75]

Anesthetic Management. Patients with pheochromocytoma require adequate preoperative medication to minimize anxiety-induced catecholamine release. Oral diazepam, 0.1 mg/kg, approximately 90 minutes before induction of anesthesia followed by morphine sulfate, 0.1 mg/kg, and glycopyrrolate, 0.01 mg/kg, 1 hour before produces reliable sedation. Glycopyrrolate is the preferred anticholinergic because of its minimal effects on heart rate, whereas scopolamine may produce behavioral dysfunction in some children. The use of morphine with the release of histamine has been questioned in patients with pheochromocytoma, but hypertensive crises have not been reported in well-blocked patients.

Anesthesia is induced by the intravenous administration of thiopental or diazepam or by inhalation of isoflurance or enflurane. Thiopental releases histamine and might cause a hypertensive response, although this has never been reported in children. Enflurane and isoflurane are selected because they do not sensitize the myocardium to the dysrhythmic effects of catecholamines and they are able to reduce the activity of the sympathetic nervous system. In contrast, halothane increases myocardial sensitivity to catecholamines. Intubation is facilitated by the use of a nondepolarizing muscle relaxant, such as atracurium, metacurine, or vecuronium, that produces minimal cardiovascular effects. The histamine release produced by D-tubocurarine and the vagolytic effects of pancuronium and gallamine make these drugs unattractive in the patient with pheochromocytoma.[76] Succinylcholine has been used in patients with pheochromocytoma without adverse effects, but there is concern that fasciculations may cause release of catecholamines. Clinical experience, however, has not supported this theory.

Intubation of the trachea should be performed only after establishment of adequate depth of anesthesia and muscle relaxation as determined by a nerve stimulator. To further minimize increases in blood pressure, the administration of intravenous lidocaine, 1 to 2 mg/kg 1 minute before intubation, is quite effective. Nitroprusside, 1 to 4 µg/kg/min, or phentolamine, 30 to 60 µg/kg, is effective for treating acute rises in blood pressure.

Maintenance of anesthesia can be accomplished with enflurane or isoflurane and nitrous oxide.[77-79] The delivered concentration of these agents is adjusted in response to blood pressure changes. Nitrous oxide narcotic combinations do not suppress sympathetic activity; in addition, should hypotension occur, the reduction in depth of anesthesia is not as easily attainable when intravenous agents are used. Droperidol may provoke hypertension by interfering with the uptake of norepinephrine into the postganglionic sympathetic nerve endings or may stimulate the release of catecholamines directly into the tumor.[80]

Continuous infusions of nitroprusside or phentol-amine are necessary if hypertension should occur in the presence of adequate anesthesia.[81] Trimetaphan is not recommended because of histamine release and frequent occurrence of tachyphylaxis. The potential rapidity and magnitude of blood pressure changes requires continuous intra-arterial pressure measurements. An intra-arterial catheter is introduced after the induction of anesthesia. During induction of anesthesia arterial blood pressure can be reliably measured by means of a Doppler flowmeter. The use of a pulmonary artery catheter, which permits determination of cardiac output, left heart function, and vascular resistance, has generally been limited to patients in whom there is evidence of myocardial dysfunction. In children, a central venous pressure catheter is used as an alternative with the understanding that left ventricular dysfunction may not be appreciated by this method.

Serial measurement of arterial blood gases, electrolytes, blood glucose concentration, urine output, and body temperature is required to follow rapid changes in these parameters. Blood glucose is followed closely, since hypoglycemia may occur when catecholamine secretion decreases following the removal of the tumor.[82] Serial electrocardiograms should also be taken. Also with tumor removal rapid blood and fluid infusions are usually required to combat hypotension, even if apparently full alpha blockade was established preoperatively.

Reversal of the neuromuscular blockade at the completion of the procedure is accomplished by the use of anticholinesterase and anticholinergic agents. There is no evidence to suggest that this combination should be avoided.

Postoperatively invasive monitoring should be continued until cardiovascular stability has been established. Generally the arterial blood pressure will return to normal within 24 to 48 hours after surgery; failure to do so is an indication that residual catecholamine tumor is still present.[83] While the blood pressure will return to normal levels, the plasma concentration of catecholamines will not for at least 7 to 10 days after excision of the pheochromocytoma.

PARATHYROID GLANDS

The parathyroid glands, located behind the upper and lower poles of the thyroid, synthesize a polypeptide known as parathyroid hormone (PTH). Secretion of PTH into the circulation depends on the serum calcium concentration and indirectly on the serum concentration of phosphorus and magnesium. Thus an increased concentration of calcium will inhibit the secretion of PTH, whereas a decreased concentration of calcium will stimulate secretion of parathyroid hormone. An increase in serum concentration of phosphorus will cause a decrease in serum concentration of calcium to maintain the calcium-times-phosphorus product constant. The resulting decrease in calcium concentration will further stimulate the parathyroids to secrete PTH. Magnesium impairs secretion of PTH as well as decreasing the peripheral response to PTH.

The function of PTH is to maintain a normal serum concentration of calcium by promoting the absorption of calcium from three main sites: the kidney, the intestinal tract, and the skeletal system. In the kidney PTH promotes the conversion of 25-hydroxycalciferol (vitamin D_3) to 1,25-dihydroxycalciferol, the active metabolite. Vitamin D increases tubular reabsorption of calcium while it enhances renal excretion of phosphorus. In renal disease in which phosphorus clearance is decreased, accumulation of phosphate in the circulation will result in a decrease in the serum concentration of calcium and stimulation of the parathyroid gland to secrete PTH.

Similarly, the effect of PTH on the gastrointestinal tract is to induce the synthesis of vitamin D, which in turn enhances calcium absorption. On the skeletal system PTH releases calcium by its activity on the osteoclastic cells. Evidence of this activity is seen in cystic areas in bone which may be the cause of pathological fractures.

Calcium exists in the body in two main forms: an inactive protein-bound fraction and an active ionized fraction. Several factors will alter the distribution between these two fractions and must be considered in interpreting serum calcium levels (Table 12–7). A fall in total protein concentration of 0.8 mg will decrease serum calcium by 1 mg/100 ml. Unless other conditions such as alkalosis exist, this decrease may not be accompanied by symptoms of hypocalcemia since it occurs only in the protein-bound fraction and not in the ionized fraction. Similarly, an increase in total protein may increase the total serum calcium but not the ionized fraction, and symptoms of hypocalcemia may exist.[84]

The ionized calcium fraction regulates the permeability of cell membranes to sodium and potassium. Thus, calcium becomes important in the excitation of skeletal and cardiac muscle. As the serum concentration of ionized calcium increases, the permeability of the cell membrane to sodium and potassium decreases. The effect will be a spontaneous slowing of the cardiac rhythm with an increase in the ventricular arrhythmogenicity, decreases in muscular excitability, and disturbances in mentation. In contrast, when the ionized calcium level is decreased, membrane permeability to sodium and potassium increases, thereby increasing muscle and nervous tissue excitability.

Finally, calcitonin produced by the C cells of the thyroid and thymus glands is important in maintaining serum calcium equilibrium by directly opposing the actions of PTH. Secretion of calcitonin decreases the serum calcium concentration.

Hyperparathyroidism

The recognition of hyperparathyroidism has increased in recent years for several reasons: routine evaluation of serum calcium levels, increased survival of patients undergoing renal dialysis who may need a parathyroidectomy to control bone and metastatic calcification; increased awareness of hyperparathyroidism as an etiology of renal stones; fluoridation of drinking water, which decreases calcium and magnesium content with subsequent stimulation of the parathyroid glands, and iatrogenic factors such as the use of steroids and diuretics.

Hyperparathyroidism can be classified into a primary or idiopathic form, a secondary form, and pseudohyperparathyroidism.

Primary Hyperparathyroidism

Primary hyperparathyroidism is the result of malregulated hypersecretion of the parathyroid gland. Although considered more common in the adult, hyperparathyroidism is now recognized increasingly frequently in children as a result of improved methods of diagnosis. Hyperparathyroidism may be the result of generalized hyperplasia, a benign adenoma, or carcinoma of the parathyroid gland. It also may exist in association with other endocrine disorders as in multiple endocrine adenomatosis. In childhood, a parathyroid adenoma is the more common etiology.

The clinical manifestations of hyperparathyroidism are secondary to hypercalcemia and can be grouped according to the major bodily systems they affect (Table 12–8). In the newborn, primary hyperparathyroidism presents with hypotonia, poor feeding, weight loss, dehydration, anemia, and respiratory distress from a poorly developed rib cage.

Diagnosis. The presence of an elevated ionized serum calcium concentration is diagnostic of primary hyperparathyroidism. The serum chloride is also elevated. This reflects increased renal excretion of bicarbonate producing a mild metabolic acidosis. Serum concentration of phosphate is decreased with increased urinary excretion of phosphate. As the disease pro-

Table 12–7. SERUM CALCIUM CONCENTRATION IN VARIOUS CONDITIONS

Increased	Decreased
Milk alkali syndrome	Malabsorption syndrome
Hyperparathyroidism	Hypoparathyroidism
Vitamin A and D excess	Subtotal parathyroidectomy
Idiopathic hypercalcemia of infants	Neonatal tetany
Adrenocortical deficiency	Excessive fluoride intake
PTH-like neoplasms	
Acidosis increases ionized fraction	Alkalosis increases protein fraction
Sarcoidosis	
Immobilization	
Thiazide diuretics	
Acute renal failure	

From Nimmagadda U, Salem MR, Ivankovich AD: Anesthesia and parathyroid disease. Semin Anesth 3:175, 1984.

Table 12–8. CLINICAL MANIFESTATIONS OF HYPERCALCEMIA

Nervous system	Psychosis
	Somnolence
	Hypesthesia
Cardiac	Hypertension
	Short Q-T interval
	Prolonged P-R interval
Gastrointestinal	Abdominal pain
	Peptic ulcer
	Pancreatitis
	Vomiting
Renal	Polyuria
	Lithiasis
	Decreased GFR
Neuromuscular	Muscle weakness
Articular	Calcifications
Ocular	Band keratopathy
	Conjunctivitis
Hematopoietic	Anemia

gresses, renal dysfunction is reflected by elevation of serum creatinine. Finding of an increased serum concentration of parathyroid hormone establishes the diagnosis of hyperparathyroidism.

Secondary Hyperparathyroidism

Secondary hyperparathyroidism results from a compensatory increase in the secretion of parathyroid hormone in response to hypocalcemia, hyperphosphatemia, or hypomagnesemia produced by other disease processes. A common cause is renal disease, which impairs the elimination of phosphorus and the synthesis of vitamin D. Gastrointestinal diseases that impair calcium absorption will result in hypocalcemia. After renal transplantation transient hypercalcemia may exist as a result of the inability of a hyperactive parathyroid to adapt to the normal renal handling of calcium, phosphorus, and vitamin D. In time the parathyroid function will generally return to normal.

Pseudohyperparathyroidism

Sometimes called ectopic hyperparathyroidism, pseudohyperparathyroidism results from the increased secretion of parathyroid hormone or of a substance with similar endocrine properties from tissues other than the parathyroid glands. More commonly this is caused by carcinoma of the lung, breast, pancreas, kidney, or lymphoid tissues.

Secondary Hypercalcemia

Hypercalcemia may be present in association with conditions not related to the parathyroid gland. Certain tumors can be the cause of hypercalcemia, as occurs with carcinoma of the lung, hepatoma, fibrosarcoma, renal cancer, leukemia, pheochromocytoma, and bone metastases.[83, 85-87] Ectopic parathyroid tissue may also produce hypercalcemia. Hypercalcemia in these conditions is related to the secretion of PTH, similar hormone production of prostaglandin (PGE_2) with

osteoclastic activity, or tumor-produced osteoclastic stimulating factor.

Hypercalcemia can result from vitamin D intoxication when doses above 400 units are ingested daily or from vitamin A overdosage as a result of food faddism or treatment for acne.

Thiazide therapy potentiates the hypercalcemic effect of PTH.[88] Milk alkali syndrome similarly can be an important cause of hypercalcemia in patients using large quantities of milk and alkali for peptic ulcer disease.

Immobilization for fractures, burns, or other causes can lead to a rise in serum calcium, which is seen beginning on the fourth day and reaches a peak in 6 days.[89] Total calcium levels may reach 18 mg/100 ml. Nephrocalcinosis, hypertension, and hypertensive encephalopathy occur in addition to other more typical signs. Thyrotoxicosis and decreased glucocorticoid secretion have been associated with elevated calcium levels as well.[90]

Benign familial hypercalcemia is inherited as an autosomal dominant trait and presents as mild hypercalcemia with serum calcium levels generally under 12 mg/100 ml and without apparent ill effects.

In infants fat necrosis can lead to calcium levels as high as 19 mg/100 ml. Fat necrosis occurs in traumatic vaginal deliveries, especially of large infants. Areas subjected to greatest pressure, including shoulders, upper arms, back, and outer thighs, can form necrotic lesions. Hypercalcemia develops after a week or several weeks, suggesting gradual mobilization of calcium to extracellular space from the existing necrotic areas.

Idiopathic hypercalcemia of infancy is thought to be part of a syndrome consisting of mental retardation, elfin facies, and supravalvular aortic stenosis. Clinically, failure to thrive, vomiting, constipation, hypotonia, and nephrocalcinosis may be present.

Treatment

The treatment of hyperparathyroidism is directed toward the lowering of the serum concentration of calcium by decreasing bone resorption and increasing urinary calcium excretion. The intravenous infusion of normal saline alone can decrease calcium levels by 2 to 3 mg/100 ml. Loop diuretics such as furosemide are used to promote urinary calcium loss. This mode of therapy results in the loss of large quantities of electrolytes in the urine; therefore, close monitoring of the cardiovascular and electrolyte status is necessary. Electrocardiography is important to monitor changes in Q-T intervals and occurrence of arrhythmias.[91]

Mitramycin as an inhibitor of RNA synthesis when administered in a dose of 25 μg/kg will block osteoclastic activity induced by parathyroid hormone. A rapid reduction in the serum concentration of calcium occurs within 12 to 36 hours.[92, 93] Mitramycin has a tendency to produce rebound hypercalcemia after an initial decrease, thereby decreasing its effectiveness.

Calcitonin causes no toxicity and can be administered intravenously and intramuscularly in doses of 8 units per kg every 6 hours. Dialysis is used when renal failure is present. By the use of a low-calcium dialysate approximately 300 mg/hr can be removed. Ethylenediaminetetraacetic acid is a chelating agent that binds calcium but has a substantial nephrotoxicity. Prosphate is administered orally to avoid causing symptoms of hyperphosphatemia.

Specific therapy of hypercalcemia is aimed at treating the cause of hyperparathyroidism. In patients with diffuse hyperplasia, familial hyperplasia, multiple endocrine adenomatosis syndrome, or several adenomas a subtotal parathyroidectomy is performed to lessen the incidence of postoperative hypocalcemia.

A particular group of patients are the hyperparathyroid patients with a serum calcium level above 15 mg/100 ml. These patients are seriously ill with a condition referred to as hypercalcemic crisis, which if not treated promptly can lead to coma and even death. If scheduled for emergency surgery these patients are lethargic and are dehydrated with electrolyte imbalance from vomiting and polyuria. Hypertension is a common finding.

Preoperative Evaluation. The preoperative evaluation of the hyperparathyroid patient includes a careful history and physical examination with particular emphasis on the cardiovascular, renal, and gastrointestinal systems. Blood pressure and electrolytes should be carefully noted. Several authors have described ECG changes in hyperparathyroidism. These include a prolonged P-R interval and a rate-corrected, Q-T interval that is inversely proportional to the serum calcium level up to 16 mg/100 ml. Above this level T waves are prolonged and rounded and the Q-T interval becomes disproportionately long. Although tachycardia is often mentioned, Bronsky found no change in cardiac heart rate in 35 patients with hypercalcemia.[94]

The patient should be well hydrated, the serum calcium should be decreased to an acceptable level, and other electrolyte abnormalities should be corrected before parathyroidectomy is attempted. The bones are very fragile in these patients, who must be handled very gently to avoid pathological fractures.

Anesthetic Management. Anesthesia can be induced by means of intravenous thiopental or the use of an inhalational agent. Before or soon after the induction of anesthesia a large-bore intravenous tube should be inserted. Alterations in heart rate with severe bradycardia may occur if the carotid sinus is stimulated during mobilization of the parathyroid glands. A precordial stethoscope is used to monitor cardiac rhythm and ventilation. The use of an esophageal stethoscope is felt by some surgeons to interfere with neck dissection and to cause laryngeal edema.[95] There is experimental and clinical evidence that nasogastric tubes left in place for prolonged periods of time give rise to laryngeal edema,[96] but there is as yet no definite evidence that the same occurs with short-term placement of the esophageal stethoscope.

Urine output should be monitored by means of a Foley catheter. This is particularly important in cases of acute hypercalcemic crises to diagnose renal shutdown. Temperature monitoring is necessary, especially in the young child, in whom heat loss may be a cause of acidosis and increased serum calcium concentration. Lidocaine, 1 to 2 mg/kg, intravenously or by spray 1 minute before intubation, is useful to suppress laryngeal reflexes. The airway may then be secured by a well-positioned endotracheal tube allowing for air leak below 30 cm of H_2O as suggested by Lee.[97] A supine position with slight elevation of the head and moderate extension of the neck will provide good surgical conditions, increase venous drainage, and decrease bleeding.

In patients with hypercalcemic crises ketamine may be useful in avoiding precipitous falls in blood pressure. Arterial and venous hypertension is to be avoided, and slight hypotension may be useful in providing a bloodless surgical field. Mild respiratory alkalosis will reduce ionized calcium levels in the blood. Hyperventilation must be used carefully in the patient with hypercalcemic crises, in whom alkalosis may cause calcium to precipitate with further damage to the kidney. The action of calcium on the cell membrane may alter the effect of muscle relaxants; in general, this is a problem only in hypercalcemic crises, and in this case the dose of muscle relaxants should be decreased.

Blood loss generally is not significant. Possible exploration of the mediastinum must be considered whenever surgery on the parathyroid glands is undertaken. At the end of the surgical procedure when vital signs are stable, intravenous lidocaine, 1 to 2 mg/kg, is administered to suppress laryngeal reflexes, and the trachea is extubated.

Postoperative Management. During the early postoperative period the patient must be observed in a high-surveillance area. The patient's head is maintained in a 30° elevation and humidified oxygen is administered. The immediate postoperative complications may lead to airway obstruction. These include hematoma with airway obstruction, bilateral recurrent laryngeal nerve injury, and laryngeal edema.

Bilateral vocal cord paralysis in the postoperative period is a result of bilateral recurrent laryngeal nerve injury.[98] The vocal cords appear flaccid and paralyzed in an intermediate position; the airway may or may not be compromised. Bilateral vocal cord paralysis is suspected in patients with stridor and cyanosis shortly after extubation. If the stridor is mild and laryngeal edema is suspected, treatment with humidified oxygen is warranted. Racemic epinephrine in normal saline administered by nebulizer is useful for airway edema causing obstruction.

Muscular hyperexcitability with muscle cramps, paresthesias, and cardiac irregularities with prolongation of the Q-T interval may be present in milder forms of hypocalcemia. The more serious forms are manifested by tetany. Symptoms may appear 3 or 4 days after surgery and may persist for 3 to 6 months until the remaining parathyroid tissue is able to produce an adequate amount of parathyroid hormone. Treatment for symptomatic hypocalcemia is administration of calcium gluconate, 30 mg/kg, or calcium chloride, 10 mg/kg, through a central catheter. Calcium should be administered with ECG monitoring.

A rare complication is injury to the cervical sympathetic trunk leading to a Horner syndrome. Other complications may involve damage to the phrenic nerve, transection of the spinal accessory nerve, and damage to the right lymphatic duct.

Hypoparathyroidism

In the pediatric age group there are two classic forms of hypoparathyroidism: primary or idiopathic hypoparathyroidism, in which there is decreased production of parathyroid hormone, and pseudohypoparathyroidism, in which there is an increase of parathyroid hormone production with deficient end-organ responsiveness.

Pseudohypoparathyroidism is an inherited disorder in which the release of parathyroid hormone is intact. The children are typically short in stature with round faces, short thick necks, and short metacarpals. Mental retardation is a prominent feature. Pseudopseudoparathyroidism is characterized by similar findings but there is an inadequate secretion of parathyroid hormone.

More commonly, hypoparathyroidism results from the inadvertent removal of parathyroid glands during thyroid surgery or during subtotal parathyroidectomy, when the function of the residual parathyroid is decreased.[99]

Deficiency of parathyroid hormone decreases serum and urinary phosphorus excretion, resulting in an elevated serum phosphorus level with a decreased calcium level.

Clinical Manifestations

Signs and symptoms of hypoparathyroidism are a reflection of the serum concentration of calcium. The severity of the symptoms depends on the rapidity of the reduction in serum calcium concentration. Acute hypocalcemia, such as that which occurs when parathyroids are inadvertently removed, manifests itself with perioral paresthesias, restlessness, and neuromuscular irritability. A positive Chvostek or Trousseau sign is confirmatory of neuromuscular irritability. In the nonverbal child, inspiratory stridor may be the first sign of hypocalcemia.

A chronic reduction in serum concentration of calcium is associated with fatigue and skeletal muscle cramps. The common cause of chronic hypocalcemia is chronic renal failure. Prolonged P-R interval with unchanged QRS complex frequently provides electrocardiographic evidence of hypocalcemia. Cardiac rhythm remains normal.

Diagnosis

Diagnosis of hypoparathyroidism is based on a reduced serum calcium concentration. Urinary excretion of calcium and phosphorus is decreased. A decrease in urinary excretion of cyclic adenosine monophosphate is an indication of low serum concentration of parathyroid hormone. Diagnosis of pseudohypoparathyroidism is made on the basis of the presence of hyperphosphatemia.

Treatment

Treatment of acute hypocalcemia is with intravenous infusion doses of calcium gluconate 10 percent (0.45 mEq/ml) 30 mg/kg or calcium chloride 10 percent (1.36 mEq/ml) 10 mg/kg until signs of neuromuscular irritability, particularly cardiac irritability, disappear. Calcium is administered with the use of electrocardiography to monitor cardiac rhythm until a serum level of 4 mEq/100 ml is reached.

Hypocalcemia from chronic hypoparathyroidism is treated by the administration of oral calcium and vitamin D. Thiazide diuretics cause sodium depletion without calcium excretion. This tends to increase serum calcium concentration and can be used as an alternative mode of therapy.

Anesthetic Management. Elective surgical procedures in patients with hypoparathyroidism should be postponed until appropriate therapy to raise the serum concentration of calcium can be administered. If the procedure cannot be postponed, intravenous calcium therapy is administered with continuous ECG monitoring.

If emergency surgery is to be performed, the anesthetic management is designed to prevent further decreases in the serum concentration of calcium. Respiratory or metabolic alkalosis, which can occur with hyperventilation or after the infusion of bicarbonate for the treatment of a metabolic acidosis, can cause a decrease in the serum ionized calcium concentration. Administration of whole blood with a citrate preservative does not reduce serum calcium concentrations appreciably since the body can mobilize calcium rapidly from its stores. However, the rapid administration of citrated whole blood (1 ml/kg/min) or plasma may cause hypocalcemia, particularly in patients with cirrhosis, in whom a decreased metabolism of citrate may occur.

Arterial blood gases must be monitored frequently during anesthesia with particular regard to pH, serum protein level, and ionized calcium concentration. Muscle relaxants should be administered with the use of a nerve stimulator, but the choice of anesthetic agents should be dictated by the needs of the particular patient and the preference of the anesthesiologist.

Hypocalcemia in the Newborn

The anesthetic management of the newborn infant during the first week of life can be further complicated by the presence of hypocalcemia and hyperphosphatemia. Three groups of infants are particularly prone to neonatal hypocalcemia. These are: premature infants, infants of diabetic mothers, and infants with birth asphyxia.

Hypocalcemia in the neonate is thought to be related to several factors: renal immaturity, direct action of phosphate on calcium deposition and/or resorption, and a relative hypoparathyroidism. The newborn kidney excretes phosphate less efficiently as a result of its low glomerular filtration rate. To increase urinary phosphate excretion the neonate must increase the serum concentration of phosphate. The high serum phosphorus concentration inhibits calcium resorption in order to maintain a normal calcium-times-phosphorus product. In addition, the newborn kidney is relatively refractory to parathyroid hormone, with the result that phosphate excretion is further decreased. Connelly and Crawford found that the newborn responded to exogenous parathyroid hormone on the first day of life with an increase in serum phosphate concentration, but the renal phosphaturic response was minimal.[100] By the third day, the renal response was adequate to lower the serum phosphorus level. An increase in urinary cyclic AMP excretion during the first 3 days of life is associated with an increase in phosphate excretion and phosphate clearance. At the end of the second week of life, the renal response to parathyroid hormone is similar to that of the adult.[98, 101] Thus, the hypoparathyroidism that exists in the newborn is transient, lasting a few days, and calcium serum concentration should return to normal after the first week of life. The term newborn infant is capable of maintaining a normal serum calcium concentration, probably by parathyroid bone calcium mobilization.[102]

The decrease in parathyroid function is a prominent factor in premature infants and infants of diabetic mothers,[103, 104] whereas increased production of calcitonin may play a role in the hypocalcemia seen in the infant with birth asphyxia.

GONADS

Testis

In the male, testosterone is the principal hormone secreted by the testis. Testosterone is responsible for the development of secondary sex characteristics and spermatogenesis in the adult. Dysfunction of the testis is reflected by Klinefelter syndrome, which is characterized by the presence of two X chromosomes and one Y chromosome. Plasma concentration of testosterone is reduced and the testes are small. Diagnosis is made by the demonstration of clumps of Barr bodies in mucosal cells. The syndrome does not pose anesthetic problems.

Ovary

The principal hormones produced by the ovary are estrogen and progesterone. Dysfunction of hormonal secretion includes gonadal dysgenesis and polycystic ovary.

Gonadal Dysgenesis

Gonadal dysgenesis, or Turner syndrome, is due to absence of the second X chromosome, giving a chromosome pattern of XO. These patients generally are of short stature, are mildly obese, and have a webbed neck that may present problems at intubation. Their anesthetic management may be further complicated by the presence of coarctation of the aorta and pectus excavatum.

Polycystic Ovary

Polycystic ovary syndrome (Stein-Leventhal syndrome) is characterized by an increased production of androgens with associated findings of primary amenorrhea, hirsutism, and muscularity. Height is usually normal and congenital anomalies are unlikely. The patients do not present particular anesthetic problems.

PANCREAS

The pancreas contains two types of secreting glands: acinar tissue responsible for exocrine secretion, and islet cells (islands of Langerhans) responsible for endocrine secretion. This section is not concerned with disorders of the exocrine pancreas. Islet cells secrete insulin (beta cells) and glucagon (alpha cells). Hypofunction of these cells results in diabetes mellitus, and hyperactivity results in hypoglycemia.

Diabetes Mellitus

Diabetes mellitus is the most common endocrine disease in childhood. It results from an absolute or functional deficiency of insulin, which leads to an impairment of glucose transport, a decrease in the storage and synthesis of lipid, and a decrease in the synthesis of protein. These metabolic abnormalities produce long-term effects through changes in small and large vessels resulting in retinopathy, nephropathy, neuropathy, ischemic heart disease, and large vessel obstruction. The accumulated clinical, experimental, and biochemical evidence links the development of complications from diabetes to the degree of control of the metabolic disturbances found in diabetes. Hence, the pediatrician's aim is to maintain as near normal metabolism as is compatible with the well-being of each individual child.

Diabetes mellitus has an overall prevalence of 1.89 per 1000 school-age children and affects some 100,000 persons under the age of 20 in the United States.[105] Males and females appear to be equally affected, and there is no correlation to socioeconomic status. Prevalence rates in the United States are similar to those reported in England and Sweden.[106]

The Diabetes Branch of the National Institutes of Health (NIH) recommends dividing patients with diabetes mellitus into two principal types: type I, the insulin-dependent group (IDDM) and type II, the non–insulin-dependent group (NIDDM). Diabetes in children is of the insulin-dependent variety previously called juvenile diabetes mellitus. However, insulin-dependent diabetes may present in adulthood, and hence the term juvenile diabetes mellitus should be abandoned. Type I diabetes is characterized by insulin deficiency, intermittent ketoacidosis, and association with other autoimmune diseases. Type II diabetes is characterized by normal or high plasma insulin levels, absence of ketoacidosis, a strong hereditary pattern, and onset in the third and fourth decades of life or later.

Pathogenesis

The cause of pancreatic beta-cell failure in IDDM may be an autoimmune destruction of pancreatic islets in predisposed individuals. Type I diabetes is known to be associated with disorders such as Addison disease and Hashimoto thyroiditis, in which autoimmune disturbances are known to be pathogenic.[108]

Circulating antibodies directed against the surface components of islet cells have been demonstrated and are not the insulin antibodies found universally in insulin-treated diabetic patients. Environmental triggering factors such as a viral infection may initiate the immune response in susceptible individuals.

Although insulin deficiency is the primary defect, secondary hormonal changes also contribute to metabolic abnormalities. Levels of growth hormone, catecholamines, and cortisol are elevated in decompensated diabetes and are restored to normal with adequate insulin therapy.[105] The important metabolic effects of insulin include the transfer of glucose across the cell membrane into the cell, the formation of glycogen, the conversion and storage of glucose as fatty acids in adipose tissue, and the passage of potassium into cells with glucose. Insulin deficiency results in hyperglycemia secondary to glycogenolysis; gluconeogenesis and decreased peripheral glucose utilization; and lipolysis in fat tissue, which increases free fatty acids and conversion of free fatty acids to ketone bodies (acetoacetic acid and betahydroxybutyric acid). Acetone formed from acetoacetic acid is responsible for the characteristic fruity odor of the breath.

Epinephrine produces hyperglycemia by stimulating liver glycogenolysis, decreasing glucose uptake by muscle, and directly inhibiting pancreatic insulin release. The glucocorticoids exert their diabetogenic action by increasing hepatic gluconeogenesis from proteins, decreasing glucose uptake by adipose tissue, and stimulating the formation of an ill-defined circulating insulin antagonist.

Clinical Features

Initially, children usually present with a history of polyuria, polydipsia, polyphagia, and weight loss. An insidious onset with lethargy, weakness, and weight loss is also quite common. A minority of children (10 to 20 percent) present with frank diabetic ketoacidosis manifested by hyperglycemia, ketonemia, vomiting, dehydration, obtundation, air hunger, acetone breath, glucosuria, and ketonuria.

Abdominal pain with leukocytosis that mimics appendicitis is common in children with ketoacidosis and may be associated with an elevated serum amylase level that does not necessarily indicate the existence of pancreatitis. Hyperglycemia with blood glucose exceeding 300 mg/100 ml must be demonstrated for this diagnosis to be made. With the administration of fluid and electrolyte therapy and insulin replacement, the abdominal pain resolves after several hours.

Renal glycosuria either as an isolated finding or as part of the Fanconi syndrome in a child with vomiting and starvation ketosis may mimic the urinary findings of ketoacidosis (glycosuria and ketonuria). Blood glucose levels are normal, however, and insulin therapy is not indicated.

The average total daily dose of insulin in children when replacement is necessary is on the order of 0.5 to 1.0 units per kg. With a single daily dose regimen, two thirds of the total dose is intermediate acting insulin (NPH, lente) and the remainder is fast-acting regular insulin, given 30 minutes before breakfast. Adjustments in the dose are made depending on the pattern of blood glucose or urine glucose. Each increase should be approximately 10 percent and subsequent changes should be made at 2- to 3-day intervals depending on response. Twice daily injections may also be utilized, with two thirds given before breakfast and one third before the evening meal; each injection consists of intermediate- and short-acting insulin in the proportion of 2:1 or 3:1. For infants and children less than 5 years old twice daily injections result in smoother control of blood glucose and fewer episodes of hypoglycemia.

Nearly all patients can be demonstrated to have antibodies to insulin after several months of insulin therapy. Rarely, children with antibodies develop true insulin resistance characterized by an insulin requirement in excess of 2 units per kg per day. A change to a preparation of pure beef or pure pork insulin usually resolves the problem; if it does not, a course of steroids may be necessary.[105]

Following initial stabilization when insulin requirements are quite high, there is in many children a progressive reduction in insulin requirements to daily doses of 0.3 unit per kg or less. The duration of this honeymoon phase is variable, lasting a few months or as long as 1 to 2 years.

Hypoglycemic reactions occur in all diabetic children sometime during the course of their disease. The signs of hypoglycemia develop suddenly over a few minutes, whereas signs of diabetic ketoacidosis develop over hours or days. Symptoms and signs of hypoglycemia include trembling, shaking, sweating, apprehension, tachycardia, mood changes, mental confusion, seizures, and coma. When the child is cooperative a drink with sugar or candy should be taken. Glucagon, 0.5 to 1 mg intramuscularly, is useful when the patient is losing consciousness or vomiting.

Hypoglycemic episodes that alternate with hyperglycemia, ketosis, glycosuria, and ketonuria should suggest the diagnosis of the Somogyi phenomenon.[110] This syndrome has been described as "hypoglycemia begetting hyperglycemia," and is believed to be caused by excessive insulin and the counterregulation of its hypoglycemic effects by hyperglycemic hormones. The occurrence of "brittle" diabetes with daily insulin doses of more than 2 units per kg suggests that the phenomenon is present and the insulin dose should be reduced. The Somogyi phenomenon is the most common cause of instability or brittleness.

Diabetic Ketoacidosis

Criteria for diagnosis include hyperglycemia (glucose greater than 300 mg/100 ml), ketonemia (ketones strongly positive at greater than 1:2 dilution of serum), acidosis (pH less than 7.30), glycosuria, and ketonuria. Clinical findings include dehydration, hyperventilation, obtundation, and a strong odor of acetone on the breath. A few other conditions with ketoacidosis, such as starvation, organic acidemias, and ingestion of ethanol or salicylates, have to be considered and excluded. Precipitating factors include stress such as trauma, infections, vomiting, and psychological disturbances.

Insulin deficiency results in a pattern of starvation and catabolism with gluconeogenesis, ketogenesis, and enhanced lipolysis. Overproduction of ketones and glucose result in their accumulation in the blood and urine. Hyperglycemia increases serum osmolality, with a shift of water from the intracellular space producing intracellular dehydration. Excessive diuresis results in a net loss of water greater than that of electrolytes and a decrease in the intravascular fluid volume. In the presence of acidosis potassium leaves the cells and, although serum potassium may be high, total body stores are depleted. Metabolic acidosis occurs mainly because of the buildup of organic acids. Dehydration and impairment in renal acidification also contribute to acidosis. Severe systemic acidosis may cause hypotension and impair myocardial function. Hyperosmolality and brain cell dehydration are the main causes of obtundation. In the treated patient, further obtundation may occur, with a rapid lowering of blood glucose to 250 mg/100 ml and below. A shift of water from the extracellular fluid to the relatively hyperosmolar brain cells causes cerebral edema.[111]

The treatment of diabetic ketoacidosis consists of fluid and electrolyte replacement, insulin administration, and frequent laboratory and clinical monitoring.

The child differs little from the adult in basic pathophysiological disturbances and clinical features. However, in children there is a greater need for precision in the quantity, composition, and rate of fluid and electrolyte therapy, as well as in insulin dosage. A flow chart should include fluid intake and output, weight, vital signs, blood glucose, electrolytes, bicarbonate, and pH. These parameters should be monitored at intervals of 2 to 4 hours. Hourly blood glucose readings should be made during the first 6 to 10 hours.

A fluid and electrolyte deficit of 10 percent or more is present in moderate to severe diabetic ketoacidosis. This deficit of 100 ml/kg of fluid should be replaced over 24 hours in addition to the normal maintenance requirements. Normal saline solution (20 ml/kg) should be given in the first hour. Half the deficit should be replaced in the first 8 hours. When the serum glucose declines below 300 mg/100 ml, 5 percent glucose and 0.45 normal saline solution should replace the normal saline solution. Potassium should be added to the solution in the absence of hyperkalemia, provided that renal function is intact. Therapy results in a shift of potassium back to the intracellular compartment and may result in hypokalemia if potassium supplementation is inadequate. The administration of potassium phosphate will also replace phosphate, which can be significantly depleted in acidosis. Provision of phosphate promotes the formation of 2,3-diphosphoglycerate (2,3-DPG), which shifts the oxygen dissociation curve to the right, releasing oxygen to tissues and resulting in correction of acidosis.[112]

Metabolic acidosis usually corrects spontaneously with the administration of fluids, electrolytes, and insulin owing to the interruption of ketogenesis, the metabolism of ketones to bicarbonate, and the generation of bicarbonate by the distal renal tubule. Bicarbonate administration may be deleterious because alkalosis shifts the oxygen dissociation curve to the left, accelerates entry of potassium into the intracellular space, and may lead to worsening in cerebral acidosis. Hence bicarbonate is not administered unless the pH is below 7.2.

A regimen of constant infusion of small doses of insulin is simple to follow and permits close monitoring of the relationship of dose to effect.[114] Initially 0.1 unit per kg of regular insulin is administered by bolus intravenously. This is followed by the administration of 0.1 unit per kg per hour intravenously by constant infusion. 50 units of regular insulin in 250 ml of isotonic saline yields 0.2 unit of insulin per ml of solution. A few milliliters are run through the tubing and discarded to saturate the insulin-binding sites in the tubing. The rate of insulin infusion can be modified to produce a decrease of 75 to 100 mg/100 ml/hr in blood glucose concentration. When the blood glucose concentration reaches 250 to 300 mg/100 ml, 5 percent glucose should be added to the intravenous solutions. The infusion is discontinued when control has been achieved and regular insulin can be given subcutaneously every 6 to 8 hours. Intermediate-acting insulin is usually begun within 24 to 36 hours after commencing therapy, but 3 to 5 days is the usual time required to stabilize the insulin dose.

Preoperative Assessment

General Principles. The majority (85 to 90 percent) of adult patients with diabetes in the United States have type II, non–insulin-dependent diabetes and are treated with diet and the oral hypoglycemic agents (tolbutamide, tolazamide, chlorpropamide, acetohexamide). Some of these agents have hypoglycemic effects for 24 to 36 hours, which may result in hypoglycemic episodes in fasting patients. A review of the perioperative management of adult diabetics has recently been published.[115]

Diabetic patients in the pediatric age group virtually all have type I, insulin-dependent diabetes. In children a careful history must be obtained with respect to age of onset, types and dose of insulin, dietary habits, and frequency of hypoglycemic or ketotic episodes. The perioperative management of children is best accomplished with the help of the patient's pediatrician or endocrinologist. Their familiarity and knowledge of the patient will be useful in formulating a mutually acceptable management plan. There are advantages to "same day" surgery for patients with stable, well-controlled diabetes undergoing relatively minor surgical procedures. However, those with unstable or brittle diabetes may need hospitalization for a few days prior to surgery for stabilization and optimal preparation.

Associated Conditions. The complications of diabetes, including microangiopathy of the kidneys, coronary artery disease, hypertension, retinopathy, and peripheral neuropathies, are rarely observed in children. The "functional age" of a diabetic is estimated to equal the sum of the patient's chronological age and the number of years following onset of the disease. Hence a prematurely senile vascular system may be present in youthful-appearing patients. Autonomic neuropathy affects cardiovascular reflexes and may impair the catecholamine response to hypoglycemia.[116] Gastric emptying may be delayed on the same basis. In children delayed puberty and a reduction of height are the major sequelae. The designation Schmidt syndrome is applied to the association of insulin-dependent diabetes, chronic lymphocytic thyroiditis, pernicious anemia, and vitiligo.[108]

Laboratory Studies. Frequent preoperative determinations of blood glucose and ketones will be necessary for unstable patients. Urinary sugar and ketone levels are optimally recorded before each meal and at bedtime. Monitoring of serum electrolytes, creatinine, and blood urea nitrogen values may also be indicated. Associated physiological disturbances that require surgical intervention demand more extensive investigation in some patients.

Premedication

Anxiety, trauma, and stress associated with illness and surgery result in sympathetic discharge and neuroendocrine changes termed the stress response. Reduction of anxiety and the establishment of rapport with the diabetic child during the preoperative visit will prove beneficial. Premedication with barbiturates, diazepam, narcotics, and anticholinergics do not have a significant effect on glucose metabolism and should be administered in the usual doses. Solid food is withheld for 12 hours and clear fluids are permitted 6 to 8 hours prior to induction of anesthesia. The surgical procedure should be scheduled for the early morning to avoid a prolonged period of fasting. The plan for insulin administration and glucose infusion should be individualized for each patient after consultation with the child's pediatrician or endocrinologist.

Operative Management

The primary goals of management are the avoidance of hypoglycemia and excessive hyperglycemia with ketosis. Ketosis and protein breakdown can be prevented by the administration of dextrose and insulin. Many plans have been described for the management of diabetic patients undergoing surgery, but no particular perioperative regimen has been shown to be superior to others.[117, 118] An infusion of 5 percent dextrose and 0.45 normal saline solution should be started prior to 8 A.M. on the day of surgery and continued at a calculated maintenance rate until oral intake is reinstituted. The method of insulin administration will depend on the individual patient's needs and the preference of the anesthesiologist and pediatrician.

One method is to give one half of the usual intermediate-acting insulin dose in the morning following the initiation of the dextrose infusion. Blood glucose determinations prior to induction and at 2-hour intervals permits further therapy to maintain plasma glucose between 100 and 250 mg/100 ml. Regular insulin, 0.1 mg/kg, can be given intravenously when the plasma level approaches 250 mg/100 ml. However, the administration of the partial dose of insulin in the morning has been associated with hypoglycemia, and an intravenous bolus of regular insulin may not reach the peak effect for 3 hours.[117, 119] Another alternative to the preoperative administration of a portion of the normal daily dose of insulin is the continuous intravenous infusion of a low dose of regular insulin during the procedure. A constant infusion of 5 percent dextrose is maintained and the rate of insulin infusion is adjusted to maintain blood glucose levels between 100 and 200 mg/100 ml.[118] New electronic techniques for monitoring and infusing insulin and glucose are being tested, and these automated devices may someday improve on current practices.

The effects of anesthetic drugs on blood glucose concentration and insulin release are clinically insignificant to the total management of anesthesia in the diabetic patient. Hyperglycemia occurs with surgery and is probably due to increases in cortisol, growth hormone, and sympathetic stimulation.[120] No particular anesthetic agents are specifically beneficial for diabetes, nor are any of the agents contraindicated. The management of fluid and electrolytes should be indicated by a continuous infusion of dextrose.

Postoperative Management

A blood glucose determination should be done in the recovery room and a plan formulated in conjunction with the surgeon and pediatrician for subsequent management. Walts and associates were impressed at finding a large number of adult patients who had postoperative plasma glucose values greater than 400 mg/100 ml.[116] They attributed the hyperglycemia to poorly monitored dextrose infusion rates and infrequently monitored plasma glucose values. Children will need monitoring every 4 to 6 hours until they are able to resume their normal oral intake.

Hyperinsulinism

Hyperinsulinism is the most common cause of persistent hypoglycemia in the first year of life. At this age, hypoglycemia is often severe and intractable; if it is not treated effectively, irreversible brain damage is likely to result. Hyperinsulinism may result from a number of pancreatic abnormalities termed "islet-cell dysmaturation syndrome." The pathology of islet-cell dysmaturation syndrome ranges from microadenomas and islet-cell adenomas to islet-cell dysplasia and nesidioblastosis. At the present time no way has been found to predict the nature of the lesion responsible for hyperinsulinism in infants and children preoperatively. In infants under 1 year of age, diffuse pancreatic involvement appears to be as likely as a localized resectable lesion.[121] In the older child an islet-cell adenoma is likely and surgery is indicated. A trial of medical therapy with diazoxide (10 to 20 mg/kg/day) is indicated in infants because diffuse lesions are frequently present and subtotal pancreatectomy has not necessarily been curative.

Anesthetic Management

During the preoperative evaluation a plan is formulated that will continue the current medical management and avoid hypoglycemia during the operative procedure. The patient must be transported to the surgical suite without disruption of the intravenous glucose or medical therapy including diazoxide and hydrocortisone. An arterial catheter or central venous line should be inserted that will permit frequent monitoring of blood glucose concentration. The anesthetic technique and selection of agents will have minimal influence on intraoperative blood glucose levels. Smooth stable anesthesia with adequate depth will attenuate the stress response to the surgical procedure. Blood glucose determinations should be made

every 15 minutes with Dextrostix and laboratory samples sent every 30 minutes for confirmation. Transient falls in blood glucose may occur with manipulation of the tumor. Complete removal of an insulinoma may produce a rise in blood sugar within 30 minutes, but this is not reliable evidence that an adenoma has been removed.

Postoperatively, frequent monitoring of blood glucose should continue for early detection of persistent hypoglycemia or hyperglycemia. Diabetes mellitus may develop when minimal pancreatic tissue is left behind. Children who continue to exhibit hypoglycemia resistant to diazoxide will need reexploration with an extended subtotal pancreatectomy.

REFERENCES

1. Blackwell RE, Guillemin R: Hypothalamic control of adenohypophysial secretions. Ann Rev Physiol 35:357, 1973.
2. Hays RM: Antidiuretic hormone. N Engl J Med 295:659, 1976.
3. Philbin DM, Coggins CH: Plasma antidiuretic hormone levels in cardiac surgical patients during morphine and halothane anesthesia. Anesthesiology 49:95, 1978.
4. Behrman RE, Vaughan VC III (Eds.): Nelson Textbook of Pediatrics. Philadelphia, W.B. Saunders Co., 1983, p 1435.
5. Tasch MD: Endocrine diseases. In Stoelting RK, Dierdorf SF (Eds.): Anesthesia and Co-Existing Disease. New York, Churchill Livingstone, 1983.
6. Banna M, Hoare RD, Stanley P, et al.: Craniopharyngioma in children. J Pediat 83:781, 1973.
7. Hoffman HJ, Hendrick EB, Humphreys, RP, et al.: Management of craniopharyngioma in children. J Neurosurg 47:218, 1977.
8. Burr IM, Slonim AE, Danish RK, et al.: Diencephalic syndrome revisited. J Pediatr 88:439, 1976.
9. Becker DJ, Foley TP: 1-Deamino-8-D-arginine vasopressin in the treatment of central diabetes insipidus in childhood. J Pediatr 92:1011, 1978.
10. Matjasko J: Perioperative management of patients with pituitary tumors. Semin Anesth 3:155, 1984.
11. Costin G, Fefferman RA, Kogut MD: Hypothalamic gigantism. J Pediatr 83:419, 1973.
12. Nelson JC, Kollar DJ, Lewis JE: Growth hormone secretion in pituitary disease. Arch Intern Med 133:459, 1974.
13. Southwick JP, Katz J: Unusual airway difficulty in the acromegalic patient — indication for tracheotomy. Anesthesiology 51:72, 1979.
14. Hassan SZ, Matz G, Lawrence AM, et al.: Laryngeal stenosis in acromegaly. Anesth Analg 55:57, 1976.
15. Tyrrell JB, Brooks RM, Fitzgerald PA, et al.: Cushing's disease—selective trans-sphenoidal resection of pituitary microadenomas. N Engl J Med 298:753, 1978.
16. Finsterer U, Beyer A, Jensen R, et al.: The syndrome of inappropriate secretion of antidiuretic hormone (SIADH) — treatment with lithium. Intens Care Med 8:223, 1982.
17. Samaan NA, Osborne BM, MacKay G, et al.: Endocrine and morphologic studies of pituitary adenomas secondary to primary hypothyroidism. J Clin Endocrinol Metab 45:903, 1977.
18. Kenny FM, Preeyasombat C, Migeon CJ: Cortisol production rate in normal infants, children and adults. J Pediat 37:34, 1966.
19. Plumpton FS, Besser GM, Cole PV: Corticosteroid treatment and surgery. I. Investigation of the indications for steroid cover. II. The management of steroid cover. Anesthesia 24:3, 1969.

20. Raven MB, Feinberg G: Anesthetic management of hypophysectomy. NY State J Med 24:776, 1968.
21. Newfield P, Albin M, Chestnut JS, et al.: Air embolism during transsphenoidal pituitary operations. Neurosurgery 2:39, 1978.
22. Messick JM, Laws ER, Abboud CV: Anesthesia for transsphenoidal surgery of the hypophyseal region. Anesth Analg 57:206, 1978.
23. Munson ES: Effect of nitrous oxide on the pulmonary circulation during venous air embolism. Anesth Analg 50:785, 1971.
24. Shucart WA, Jackson I: Management of diabetes insipidus in neurosurgical patients. J Neurosurg 44:65, 1976.
25. Surks MI, Schadlow AR, Stock JM: Determination of iodothyronine absorption and conversion of L-thyroxine (T4) to L-triiodothyronine (T3) using turnover rate techniques. J Clin Invest 52:805, 1973.
26. Inglar SH, Woebar KA: The thyroid gland. In Williams RH (Ed.): Textbook of Endocrinology. Philadelphia, W.B. Saunders Co., 1981, pp 117–247.
27. Gilman AG, Murad F: Thyroid and antithyroid drugs. In Goodman LS, Gilman A (Eds.): The Pharmacological Basis of Therapeutics. New York, Macmillan, 1980, pp 1397–1419.
28. Sterling K: Thyroid hormone action at the cell level. N Engl J Med 300:117, 1979.
29. La Franchi SH: Hypothyroidism. Pediatr Clin North Am 26:33, 1979.
30. Fisher DA, Drissault JH, Sach J, et al.: Ontogenesis of hypothalamic-pituitary-thyroid function and metabolism in man, sheep, and rat. Recent Prog Hormone Res 33:59, 1977.
31. Fisher DA, Klein AH: Thyroid development and disorders of thyroid function in the newborn. N Engl J Med 304:702, 1981.
32. Rezvani I, DiGeorge AM: Reassessment of the daily dose of oral thyroxine for replacement therapy in hypothyroid children. J Pediatr 90:291, 1977.
33. White VA, Kumagai LF: Preoperative endocrine and metabolic considerations. Med Clin North Am 63:1321, 1979.
34. Kim JM, Hackman L: Anesthesia for untreated hypothyroidism: report of three cases. Anesth Analg 56:299, 1977.
35. Kato R, Takanaka A, Takahashi A: Effect of thyroid hormone on the substrate interaction with p450 in the oxidation of drugs by liver microsomes. J Biochem 68:613, 1970.
36. Murkin JM: Anesthesia and hypothyroidism: a review of thyroxine physiology, pharmacology and anesthetic implications. Anesth Analg 61:371, 1982.
37. McBrien DJ, Hindle W: Myxoedema and heart failure. Lancet 1:1066, 1963.
38. Zwillich CW, Pierson DJ, Hofeldt FD, et al.: Ventilatory control in myxedema and hypothyroidism. N Engl J Med 292:662, 1975.
39. James ML: Endocrine disease and anesthesia. Anesthesia 25:232, 1970.
40. Abbott TR: Anesthesia in untreated myxoedema: report of two cases. Br J Anaesth 39:510, 1967.
41. Badad AA, Eger EI: The effects of hyperthyroidism and hypothyroidism on halothane and oxygen requirements in dogs. Anesthesiology 29:1087, 1968.
42. Lee WN: Thyroiditis, Hyperthyroidism, and Tumors. Pediatr Clin North Am 26:53, 1979.
43. Barnes HV, Blizzard RM: Antithyroid drug therapy for toxic diffuse goiter (Graves' disease): thirty years experience in children and adolescents. J Pediatr 91:313, 1977.
44. Brown J, Solomon DH, Beall GN, et al.: Autoimmune thyroid diseases, Graves' and Hashimoto's. Ann Intern Med 88:379, 1978.
45. Fisher DA, Sack J, Oddie TH, et al.: Serum T4, TBG, T3 uptake, T3, reverse T3, and TSH concentrations in children 1 to 15 years of age. J Clin Endocrinol Metab 45:191, 1977.
46. Peters KR, Nance P, Wingard DW: Malignant hyperthyroidism or malignant hyperthermia? Anesth Analg 60:613, 1981.
47. Mackin JF, Canary JJ, Pittman CS: Thyroid storm and its management. New Engl J Med 291:1396, 1974.
48. Wood M, Berman ML, Harbeson RD, et al.: Halothane induced hepatic necrosis in triiodothyronine pretreated rats. Anesthesiology 52:470, 1980.
49. Caldarelli DD, Holinger LD: Complications and sequelae of thyroid surgery. Otolaryngol Clin North Am 13:85, 1980.
50. Rallison ML, Dobyns BM, Kealing FR, et al.: Occurrence and natural history of chronic lymphocytic thyroiditis in childhood. J Pediatr 86:675, 1975.
51. Fisher DA, Oddie TH, Johnson DE, et al.: The diagnosis of Hashimoto's thyroiditis. J Clin Endocrinol Metab 40:795, 1975.
52. Fisher DA: Thyroid nodules in childhood and their management. J Pediatr 89:866, 1976.
53. Knowlton AI: Addison's disease: a review of its clinical course and management. In Christy NR (Ed.): The Human Adrenal Cortex. New York, Harper and Row, 1971, pp 329–358.
54. Blizzard RN, Solomon IL: Autoimmune disorders of endocrine glands. J Pediatr 63:1021, 1963.
55. Kaplan SA: Disorders of the adrenal cortex. Pediatr Clin North Am 26:70, 1979.
56. Oyama T: Endocrine response to general anesthesia and surgery. In Endocrinology and the Anesthetist. Monographs in Anesthesiology. Vol. 11. Amsterdam, Elsevier, 1983.
57. Knudsen L, Christiansen LA, Lorentzen JE: Hypotension during and after operation in glucocorticord-treated patients. Br J Anaesth 53:295, 1981.
58. Axelrod L: Glucocorticoid therapy. Medicine 55:39, 1976.
59. Symreng T, Karlberg BE, Kågedal B, et al.: Physiological cortisol substitution of long-term steroid-treated patients undergoing major surgery. Br J Anaesth 53:949, 1981.
60. Roizen M: Semin Anesth 3:000, 1984.
61. Plumpton FS, Besser GM, Cole PV: Corticosteroid treatment and surgery. 1. An investigation of the indication for steroid cover. 2. The management of steroid cover. Anaesthesia 24:3, 1969.
62. Kehelet H: A rational approach to dosage and preparation of parental glucocorticoid substitution therapy during surgical procedures. Acta Anaesth Scand 19:260, 1975.
63. Ehrlich HP, Hunt TP: Effects of cortisone and vitamin A on wound healing. Ann Surg 167:324, 1968.
64. Holaday JW, Law P-Y, Loh HH, et al.: Adrenal steroids indirectly modulate morphine and beta-endorphin effects. J Pharmacol Exp Ther 208:176, 1979.
65. Alguist RP: Studies on the adrenotropic receptors. Am J Physiol 153:586, 1948.
66. Goldberg LI: Cardiovascular and renal actions of dopamine: potential clinical applications. Pharmacol Rev 24:1, 1972.
67. Vorhees ML: Disorders of the adrenal medulla and multiple endocrine adenomotoses. Pediatr Clin North Am 26:209, 1979.
68. Melicow NM: One hundred cases of pheochromocytoma at the Columbia Medical Center. Cancer 40:1987, 1977.
69. Iversen LL: Uptake of circulating catecholamines into tissues. In Blasko H, Sayers G, Smith AD (Eds.): Handbook of Physiology, Section 7. Endocrinology. Vol. 6: Adrenal. Washington, DC, American Physiological Society, 1975, pp 713–722.
70. Bravo EL, Tarazi RC, Ray WG, et al.: Circulatory and urinary catecholamines in pheochromocytoma. N Engl J Med 301:682, 1978.
71. Van Vliet PD, Burchell HB, Titus JL: Focal myocarditis associated with pheochromocytoma. N Engl J Med 274:1102, 1966.
72. James TN: On the cause of sudden death in pheochromocytoma. Circulation 54:348, 1976.

73. Davies RA, Patt NL, Sole MJ: Localization of pheochromocytoma by selective venous catheterization and assay of plasma catecholamines. Can Med Assoc J 120:539, 1979.

74. Maddern PJ, McGrew I, Oh T: Pheochromocytoma: aspects and management. Anaesth Intens Care 4:156, 1976.

75. Robinson RG, DeQualtro V, Grushkin CM, et al.: Childhood pheochromocytoma: treatment with alpha methyl tyrosine for resistant hypertension. J Pediatr 91:143, 1977.

76. Jones RB, Hill AB: Severe hypertension associated with pancuronium in a patient with pheochromocytoma. Can Anaesth Soc J 28:394, 1981.

77. Desmonts JM, le Houelleur J, Remond P, et al.: Anaesthetic management of patients with phaeochromocytoma. A review of 102 cases. Br J Anaesth 49:991, 1977.

78. Suzukawa M, Michaels IAL, Ruzbarsky J, et al.: Use of isoflurane during resection of pheochromocytoma. Anesth Analg 62:100, 1983.

79. Janeczko GF, Ivankovich AD, Glisson SN, et al.: Enflurane anesthesia for surgical removal for pheochromocytoma. Anesth Analg 56:62, 1977.

80. Bittar DA: Innovar induced hypertensive crises in patients with pheochromocytoma. Anesthesiology 50:366, 1979.

81. Csanky-Treels JC, Lawick van Pabst WP, Brands JW, et al.: Effects of sodium nitroprusside during the excision of pheochromocytoma. Anesthesia 31:60, 1976.

82. Martin R., St. Pierre B, Molinar OR, et al.: Pheochromocytoma and postoperative hypoglycemia. Canad Anaesth Soc J 26:260, 1979.

83. Knill-Jonens RP, Buckle RM, Parsons V, et al.: Hypercalcemia and increased parathyroid hormone activity in primary hepatoma. N Engl J Med 282:704, 1970.

84. Melian FC, Hastings AB: Clinical estimation and significance of calcium ion concentration in blood. Am J Med Sci 189:601, 1935.

85. Stein RC: Hypercalcemia in leukemia. J Pediatr 89:1029, 1976.

86. Swinton NW: Hypercalcemia and familial pheochromocytoma correction after adrenalectomy. Ann Intern Med 76:455, 1972.

87. Stapleton FB, Lukert BP, Linshaw MA: Treatment of hypercalcemia associated with osseous metastases. J Pediatr 89:1029, 1976.

88. Porter RH, Cox BG: Treatment of hypoparathyroid patients with chlorothiazide. N Engl J Med 198:577, 1978.

89. Heath H III, Earle JM: Serum ionized calcium during bed rest in fracture patients on normal man. Metabolism 21:633, 1972.

90. Rude RK, Oldham SB, Singer FR, et al.: Treatment of thyrotoxic hypercalcemia with propranolol. N Engl J Med 294:431, 1976.

91. Heath DA: Emergency management of disorders of calcium and magnesium. Clin Edocrinol Metab 9:487, 1980.

92. Nimmagadda U, Salem MR, Ivankovich AD: Anesthesia and parathyroid disease. Semin Anesthesia 3:175, 1984.

93. Schweitzer VG, Thompson NW, Harness JK, et al.: Management of severe hypercalcemia caused by primary hyperparathyroidism. Arch Surg 113:373, 1978.

94. Bronsky D, Dubin A, et al: Calcium and the electrocardiogram. Electrocardiographic manifestations of hyperparathyroidism and of marked hypercalcemia from various etiologies. Am J Cardiol 7:833, 1961.

95. Paloyan E, Lawrence AM: Hyperparathyroidism. New York, Grune and Stratton, 1973, p 180.

96. Friedman H, Baun H: Laryngeal injuries secondary to nasogastric tubes. Ann Otol Rhinol Laryngol 90:469, 1981.

97. Lee KW, Dugal RM, Templeton JJ, et al.: Tracheal gas leak and intraoperative tracheal aspiration in children. Anesth Analg 64:185, 1985.

98. McCrory WW, Forman CW, McNamara H, et al.: Renal excretion of inorganic phosphate in newborn infants. J Clin Invest 31:357, 1952.

99. Waldster SS: Medical complications of thyroid surgery. Otolaryngol Clin North Am 13:99, 1980.

100. Connelly JP, Crawford JD: Studies of neonatal hyperphosphatemia. Pediatrics 30:425, 1962.

101. Linarelli LG: Newborn urinary cyclic AMP and developmental renal responsiveness to parathyroid hormone. Pediatrics 50:14, 1972.

102. David L, Anast C: Calcium metabolism in newborn infants. J Clin Invest 54:187, 1974.

103. Tsang RC, Chen IW, Friedman MA, et al.: Neonatal parathyroid function: role of gestational age and postnatal age. J Pediatr 83:728, 1973.

104. Tsang RC, Chen IW, Friedman MA, et al.: Parathyroid function in infants of diabetic mothers. J Pediatr 86:399, 1975.

105. Sperling MA: Diabetes mellitus. Pediatr Clin North Am 26:149, 1979.

106. Calnan M, Peckham CS: Incidence of insulin dependent diabetes in the first 16 years of life. Lancet 1:589, 1977.

107. Cahill GF Jr, McDevitt HO: Insulin dependent diabetes mellitus: the initial lesion. N Engl J Med 304:1454, 1981.

108. MacCuish AC, Irvine WJ: Autoimmunological aspects of diabetes mellitus. Clin Endocrinol Metab 4:435, 1975.

109. Valerio D: Acute diabetic abdomen in childhood. Lancet 1:66, 1976.

110. Bloom ME, Mintz DH, Field JB: Insulin induced posthypoglycemic hyperglycemia as a cause of "brittle" diabetes: clinical clues and therapeutic implications. Am J Med 47:891, 1969.

111. Duck SC, Weldon VV, Pagliara AJ: Cerebral edema complicating therapy for diabetic ketoacidosis. Diabetes 25:111, 1976.

112. Alberti KG, Hockaday TD.: Diabetic coma: a reappraisal after five years. Clin Endocrinol Metab 6:421, 1977.

113. Kaye R: Diabetic ketoacidosis—the bicarbonate controversy. J Pediatr 87:156, 1975.

114. Edwards GA, Kohaut EC, Wehring B: Effectiveness of low-dose continuous intravenous insulin infusion in diabetic ketoacidosis. A prospective comparative study. J Pediatr 91:701, 1977.

115. Roizen MF: Endocrine abnormalities and anesthesia: implications for the anesthesiologist. American Society of Anesthesiologists Refresher Courses, No. 12. Philadelphia, J.B. Lippincott Co., 1984.

116. Loughran PG, Giesecke AH: Diabetes mellitus: anesthetic considerations. Semin Anesth 3:207, 1984.

117. Walts LF, Miller J, Davidson MB, et al.: Perioperative management of diabetes mellitus. Anesthesiology 55:104, 1981.

118. Meyer EJ, Lorenzi M, Bohannon WV, et al.: Diabetic management by insulin infusion during major surgery. Am J Surg 137:323, 1979.

119. Fletcher J, Langman MJS, Kellock TD: Effect of surgery on blood sugar levels in diabetes mellitus. Lancet 2:52, 1965.

120. Clarke RSJ: Anesthesia and carbohydrate metabolism. Br J Anaesth 45:237, 1973.

121. Gauderer M, Stanley CA, Baker L, et al.: Pancreatic adenomas in infants and children: current surgical management. J Pediatr Surg 13:591, 1978.

GENETIC METABOLIC DISEASES | 13

LINDA C. STEHLING, M.D.

The history of human biochemical genetics began when Sir Archibald Garrod initiated studies of patients with alkaptonuria at the turn of the century. He developed the concept that certain diseases arise because of a deficiency of enzymes that govern specific metabolic steps.[1] It is now possible, using the map of the human genome, to locate the pathological region of deoxyribonucleic acid (DNA) responsible for many disorders of metabolism. For example, the mutation that causes Tay-Sachs disease is located on chromosome 15 and that for Gaucher disease is on chromosome 1.[2]

The terminology used to describe many of the disorders is confusing and often misleading. Eponyms, acronyms, biochemical defects, physical features, and the names of patients are used singly or in combination. It is impossible to become familiar with even the more common disorders, necessitating access to appropriate reference sources.[1, 3–10] The classification of some of the diseases also varies from text to text. Gaucher disease, for example, is listed alternately as a lysosomal disorder and as a lipid disorder.

GENETIC SCREENING

The first laws mandating screening of newborns were intended to detect phenylketonuria (PKU). Now it is estimated that at least 90 percent of infants born in the United States are screened, as are those in several other countries. The diseases for which screening is performed vary, but PKU and hypothyroidism are the most common.[11, 12] The blood specimen is collected on filter paper and mailed to a central facility. At the reference laboratory small discs of the filter paper are placed on agar gels containing bacteria and growth media. The amount of bacterial growth around the dics is proportional to the concentration of the metabolite in the blood. This type of bacterial assay is suitable for several inborn errors of metabolism including PKU, galactosemia, homocystinuria, and maple syrup urine disease. Radioimmunoassay for thyroxine (T_4) and thyroid-stimulating hormone (TSH) are the usual screening tests for hypothyroidism. Transient abnormalities of no clinical significance are frequently detected. The majority of infants with mild to moderately abnormal test results do not, in fact, have a metabolic disorder.[11] However, any positive or questionable results must be confirmed by further examination because the adverse effects of many disorders can be prevented with early therapy.

There are several tests employed when inborn errors of metabolism are suspected. Some disorders can be identified by accumulated or missing metabolites in urine. Diagnosis of enzymatic defects can be made by direct assay of blood or tissue. Liver biopsy is necessary in some children. Although percutaneous biopsy using local anesthesia is usual in adults, it is dangerous in children because they cannot be expected to cooperate. General anesthesia is therefore recommended for percutaneous biopsy and is mandatory for open liver biopsy. Electrophoresis and cell culture studies are employed for identification of protein variants. Skin fibroblasts are usually used for the latter studies because skin is the most accessible tissue.

345

Special screening programs are indicated in certain high-risk populations. For example, the frequency of the carrier state for Tay-Sachs disease is 1 in 30 to 60 in American Jews of northeastern European ancestry—approximately ten times greater than in the general population.[1] Both identification of the carrier state and antenatal diagnosis are possible.

Antenatal diagnosis of many inborn errors of metabolism is possible through amniocentesis (Table 13–1). Direct examination of the amniotic fluid is of some value, but assay of specific enzymes in cultured fetal cells is necessary for diagnosis of most disorders. Experience with chorionic biopsy, a minor procedure that can be performed earlier in pregnancy than amniocentesis, is limited.

TREATMENT OF METABOLIC DISEASES

Treatment of genetic metabolic disorders depends upon definitive diagnosis and understanding of the

Table 13–1. INBORN ERRORS OF METABOLISM FOR WHICH PRENATAL DIAGNOSIS IS FEASIBLE

Disorders of Carbohydrate Metabolism
Glycogen storage diseases types II, III, and IV
Galactosemia
Galactokinase deficiency
Pyruvate decarboxylase deficiency
Disorders of Amino Acid Metabolism
Argininosuccinic aciduria
Citrullinemia
Homocystinuria
Maple syrup urine disease
Methylmalonic aciduria
Isovaleric acidemia
Ketotic hyperglycemia
Disorders of Lipoprotein and Lipid Metabolism
Homozygous familial hypercholesterolemia
Refsum syndrome
Disorders of Lysosomal Enzymes
Mucopolysaccharidosis, type I (Hurler syndrome)
Mucopolysaccharidosis, type II (Hunter syndrome)
Mucopolysaccharidosis, type III (Sanfilippo syndrome)
Mucopolysaccharidosis, type VI (Maroteaux-Lamy syndrome)
Mucopolysaccharidosis, type VII (beta-glucuronidase deficiency)
I-cell disease
Lysosomal acid phosphatase deficiency
Wolman syndrome
Cholesteryl ester storage disease
Fabry disease
Gaucher disease
Krabbe disease (globoid cell leukodystrophy)
Metachromatic leukodystrophy
Niemann-Pick disease
Tay-Sachs disease
Sandhoff disease
Generalized gangliosidosis
Juvenile gangliosidosis
Fucosidosis
Mannosidosis
Farber disease (lipogranulomatosis)

Modified from Stanbury JB, Wyngaarden JB, Fredrickson DS, et al.: The Metabolic Basis of Inherited Disease. 5th ed. New York, McGraw-Hill, 1983, p 31.

Table 13–2. EXAMPLES OF TREATABLE INBORN ERRORS OF METABOLISM

Method of Treatment	Disorder
Dietary restriction of substrate	
Phenylalanine	Phenylketonuria
Galactose	Galactosemia
Replacement of deficient end product	
Uridine	Orotic aciduria
Depletion of storage substance	
Cystine removal by D-penicillamine	Cystinuria
Amplification of enzyme activity	
Pryidoxine (vitamin B_6)	Homocystinuria
Organ transplantation	
Kidney	Fabry disease
Palliative surgery	
Portacaval shunt	von Gierke disease

pathophysiology of the diseases (Table 13–2). However, no specific treatment is available for the majority of the disorders to be discussed.

ANESTHETIC IMPLICATIONS

Unfortunately, the anesthesiologist cannot predict which child scheduled for a hernia repair or eye examination under anesthesia has a congenital metabolic disorder of major anesthetic significance. Thus, some familiarity with the more common disorders and knowledge of available resources is essential.

Emphasis is placed on those disorders with specific anesthetic implications. Many of the disorders that are discussed are rare and will never be encountered by most anesthesiologists. Some diseases that are extremely rare have been omitted.

Unless otherwise specified, the mode of inheritance of the disorders discussed is presumed to be autosomal recessive. The prevalence is indicated for disorders for which estimates are available.

DISORDERS OF CARBOHYDRATE METABOLISM (Table 13–3)

Glycogen Storage Diseases (Table 13–4)

Type I (Von Gierke Disease)

Children with type I glycogen storage disease are deficient in glucose-6-phosphatase, the enzyme that causes release of glucose from glucose-6-phosphate. Glucose-6-phosphate does not, however, accumulate. Some enters the Embden-Meyerhof pathway resulting in lactic acid accumulation; it is also shunted into the pentose phosphate pathway, leading to uric acid accumulation. Pyruvate, triglycerides, phosphates, and cholesterol are also elevated. Glycogen accumulation in the liver results in massive hepatomegaly, usually evident at birth. The large liver may preclude palpation of the kidneys, which are also enlarged. Liver function

Table 13–3. DISORDERS OF CARBOHYDRATE METABOLISM

Disorder	Prevalence	Clinical Features	Anesthetic Implications
Galactosemia	1:65,000	Cataracts, vomiting, jaundice, hepatomegaly, cirrhosis, hypoglycemia, failure to thrive, mental retardation	Hypoglycemia
Galactokinase deficiency	1:40,000 to 1:100,000	Cataracts	None
Benign fructosuria	1:130,000	1+ test for reducing substances in urine, negative for glucose	Confusion with diabetes
Hereditary fructose intolerance	1:20,000 Swiss	Hypoglycemia, vomiting, jaundice, hepatosplenomegaly, failure to thrive	Dehydration, hypoglycemia, acidosis, hypokalemia
Fructose-1,6-diphosphatase deficiency	Rare	Hypoglycemia, hypotonia, acidosis, hepatomegaly	Dehydration, acidosis, hypoglycemia
Pentosuria	1:2500 Ashkenazi Jews	Benign; 1+ test for reducing substances in urine, negative for glucose	Confusion with diabetes
Glycogen storage diseases—see Table 13–4			

tests are normal, however. Splenomegaly is rare. The patients are of short stature with poorly developed musculature. Hypoglycemia is severe and may result in convulsions. Paradoxically, blood glucose levels may be as low as 10 mg/100 ml without clinical symptoms.

A Fanconi-like syndrome characterized by aminoaciduria, glycosuria, and phosphaturia is seen in these patients. A bleeding diathesis is common. Clotting studies are usually normal, but the bleeding time is commonly prolonged, indicating platelet dysfunction. Despite the severe metabolic derangements and multisystem disease, many patients live to adulthood. Mental retardation is not a feature of the disease. Diagnosis is made by assaying glucose-6-phosphatase in liver tissue, usually obtained by open liver biopsy. Portacaval shunts have been performed in a few patients with encouraging results.

If the history suggests easy bruising or other evidence of coagulopathy, a bleeding time determination should be performed preoperatively. If it is abnormal, a hematologist should be consulted.

The primary perioperative problem is avoidance of hypoglycemia. The child should receive glucose-containing solutions and the blood sugar should be measured frequently. A rapid-sequence induction is indicated because of the increased intra-abdominal pressure caused by the enlarged liver. None of the halogenated anesthetic agents currently in use are contraindicated. Renal function is not ordinarily impaired to a degree that warrants omission of muscle relaxants that depend on renal excretion. Monitoring of arterial blood gases to detect metabolic acidosis is recommended during long procedures.[13] Sodium bicarbonate therapy is rarely required.

Table 13–4. GLYCOGEN STORAGE DISEASES

Disorder		Prevalence	Clinical Features	Anesthetic Implications
Type I	von Gierke disease	1:100,000 to 1:200,000	Hypoglycemia, hepatomegaly, short stature, lactic acidosis, hyperlipidemia, bleeding diathesis, nephropathy, hyperuricemia	Increased intra-abdominal pressure, hypoglycemia, bleeding, acidosis
Type II	Pompe disease	1:100,000 to 1:200,000	Hypotonia, hepatomegaly, cardiomegaly, macroglossia, recurrent pneumonia	Airway difficulties, congestive heart failure, pulmonary disease
Type III	Cori disease	1:100,000 to 1:200,000	Hepatomegaly, splenomegaly, cardiomegaly, hypoglycemia, seizures, muscle wasting, growth retardation	Hypoglycemia, myopathy
Type IV	Andersen disease	1:500,000	Hepatosplenomegaly, failure to thrive, cirrhosis	Muscle weakness, hypoglycemia
Type V	McArdle disease	1:500,000	Muscle cramps, myoglobinuria	Muscle damage secondary to tourniquet, myoglobinuria or hyperkalemia with depolarizing relaxants, confusion with malignant hyperthermia
Type VI	Hers disease	1:200,000	Hepatomegaly	Hypoglycemia
Type VII	Tauri disease	1:500,000	Muscle cramps, myoglobinuria	Confusion with malignant hyperthermia

Type II (Pompe Disease)

In this disorder, acid maltase, the lysosomal enzyme that cleaves small oligosaccharides and the outer branches of glycogen into glucose, is absent, resulting in accumulation of glycogen in lysosomes. All tissues are involved, but muscle is the most severely affected. Hypotonia and muscle weakness are evident, although the muscle mass appears normal. Cardiomegaly is usually severe. In the most common variant, the infantile form of the disease, symptoms appear before 6 months of age and death occurs within the first year. Pneumonia and congestive heart failure occur in virtually all patients. The liver is normal in size or moderately enlarged. There are no abnormalities of glucose metabolism, and lactate, uric acid, and lipid levels are normal.

In the juvenile form of the disease, symptoms occur in early childhood and the disease progresses more slowly. Muscle weakness and hypotonia are pronounced, but cardiac disease is absent. Death due to respiratory failure usually occurs by the mid to late teens. There are a few reported cases in which onset of the disease occurred in adulthood and progressed slowly. In all patients histological examination of muscle tissue reveals an increase in glycogen. Diagnosis is confirmed by demonstration of acid maltase deficiency in leukocytes, liver, or muscle tissue. There is no treatment available.

Narcotics should be administered with caution because of their respiratory depressant effects. A preoperative chest x-ray examination is mandatory and an electrocardiogram desirable. Macroglossia may cause difficulty with airway maintenance and endotracheal intubation. Following all but the most minor procedures, children should be observed in a special care unit. Mechanical ventilation may be required. None of the volatile anesthetic agents or muscle relaxants are contraindicated.

Type III (Cori Disease)

Amylo-1,6-glucosidase (debranching enzyme) deficiency in liver and muscle causes deposition of glycogen in these tissues because only the outer chains of glycogen can be broken down. The patients resemble those with Von Gierke disease, but the clinical course is milder. The hepatomegaly is not as severe and may resolve at puberty, and splenomegaly and muscle wasting are common. Hypoglycemia, acidosis, and hyperuricemia occur. Although cardiomegaly may be evident, signs and symptoms of heart disease are not prominent features of the disease. The diagnosis is made by enzyme analysis of liver or muscle tissue. Many patients live to adulthood, despite the fact that there is no therapy. Anesthetic management is influenced by the severity of the disease. The principles outlined for type I and II disease apply.

Type IV (Branching Enzyme Deficiency)

Branching enzyme deficiency or amylopectinosis is characterized by progressive liver deterioration. Progressive hepatosplenomegaly, muscle weakness, and failure to thrive develop when the child is a few months old. Death due to cirrhosis usually occurs by 2 years of age. Although the abnormal glycogen is deposited in muscle as well as liver, cardiomyopathy does not occur. Mild fasting hypoglycemia is common. Diagnosis is confirmed by assay of branching enzyme in leukocytes or cultured skin fibroblasts. There is no treatment.

Type V (McArdle Disease)

Children with this deficiency of muscle phosphorylase are usually asymptomatic. Adolescents and adults complain of easy fatigability, severe muscle cramps, and inability to perform vigorous exercise. Muscle wasting is evident in older patients. Exercise tolerance is limited because rapid glycogenolysis cannot occur owing to the myophosphorylase deficiency. Liver phosphorylase is normal. Cardiac disease is not a feature of the disorder. A few cases of acute renal failure secondary to myoglobinuria associated with excessive exercise have been reported.[14] A venous blood sample drawn from an extremity that has been vigorously exercised will not have an elevated lactate level. Biochemical analysis of muscle tissue reveals absence of phosphorylase activity. The only therapy is avoidance of strenuous exercise.

A history of severe muscle cramping and myoglobinuria, which occurs in one half to two thirds of these patients, is suggestive of malignant hyperthermia. However, there is no association between the two disorders. Theoretically, malignant hyperthermia is unlikely because of the patient's limited ability to generate a hypermetabolic state.[15]

A glucose-containing solution should be infused to serve as an energy source. Succinylcholine should be avoided in older patients, because of the risk of myoglobinuria and renal failure. Succinylcholine may also induce hyperkalemia in patients with muscle wasting. Should myoglobinuria occur, forced diuresis with mannitol and furosemide is indicated. The absence of acidosis should readily differentiate myoglobinuria due to McArdle disease from that produced by malignant hyperthermia.

Intravenous regional anesthesia (Bier block) should not be used because muscle ischemia can, at least theoretically, lead to muscle atrophy.[16] If the success of a surgical procedure on the extremity depends upon provision of a bloodless field, use of a tourniquet is justified.

Type VI (Hers Disease)

Patients with hepatic phosphorylase complex deficiency usually have only mild hepatomegaly secondary to glycogen accumulation. Mild fasting hypoglycemia occurs in some patients and should be considered when NPO orders are written. Acidosis is not a feature of the disease. Anesthesiologists must also be aware that life-threatening hypoglycemia may be precipitated by illness in these patients.

Type VII (Tauri Disease)

The conversion of glucose to pyruvate does not proceed normally if there is a deficiency of muscle phosphofructokinase. Muscles are unable to utilize glucose for energy, and lactate does not accumulate during exercise. Children are usually asymptomatic. Vigorous exercise produces muscle cramps and myoglobinuria in adults. There is no therapy other than avoidance of strenuous activity. Although the disease is much less severe than McArdle disease, the same anesthetic considerations may apply.

Type VIII Disease

The enzyme deficiency responsible for this extremely rare disorder has not yet been demonstrated. Progressive brain degeneration and hepatomegaly are the clinical features of the few patients with this presumptive diagnosis.

Types IX and X Disease

These disorders are due to deficient hepatic enzymes and are less well described. A case of hyperthermia and ketoacidosis during anesthesia has been described in a child thought to have type IX disease.[17]

Disorders of Galactose Metabolism

Both disorders caused by deficiency of the enzymes that metabolize galactose result in cataracts; together they are responsible for approximately 4 percent of cataracts seen in children under 1 year of age. As galactose accumulates, it diffuses into the lens of the eye and is converted to galactitol, which cannot diffuse out of the lens. Osmotic overhydration and swelling occur and the lens fibers are eventually destroyed.

Classic Galactosemia

"Classic" galactosemia is due to deficiency of galactose-1-phosphate uridyl transferase. Failure to thrive is often the presenting symptom. Vomiting, dehydration, hypoglycemia, jaundice, hepatomegaly, and cirrhosis occur. Diagnosis is made by enzyme assay of liver tissue, red or white cells, or cultured fibroblasts. Elimination of galactose from the diet is essential and is accomplished by avoiding milk products. Cataracts and cirrhosis regress if not advanced at the time of diagnosis and initiation of dietary restrictions. Mental retardation, which occurs in varying degrees, is not reversible.

Galactokinase Deficiency

The only pathology in children with galactosemia due to galactokinase deficiency is cataracts.

Disorders of Fructose Metabolism

Benign Fructosuria

Fructokinase deficiency does not produce any pathology beyond the inability to metabolize ingested fructose. The disorder may be confused with diabetes mellitus because fructose is excreted in the urine. Urine examination will be positive with Clinitest and negative with Clinistix, revealing that the reducing substance is not glucose. Chromatography is necessary for definitive diagnosis.

Hereditary Fructose Intolerance

Infants who lack hepatic fructose-1-phosphate aldolase are asymptomatic until they ingest fructose or the disaccharide sucrose. Vomiting, hypoglycemia, and failure to thrive rapidly ensue. Apneic episodes, seizures, coma, and brain damage may result from the hypoglycemia. Hepatosplenomegaly, coagulopathy, and renal tubular defects also occur. Albuminuria and excessive loss of potassium result in hypoproteinemia and hypokalemia. Acidosis occurs because of excessive renal bicarbonate excretion and enhanced conversion of fructose to lactate. Chromatographic analysis of urine and a fructose tolerance test are useful diagnostic tools, but measurement of hepatic fructose-1-phosphate aldolase is required for confirmation. Exchange transfusion has been employed in critically ill children; however, omission of fructose, sucrose, and sorbitol from the diet is all that is required for remission of symptoms and resumption of normal growth in most children.

Deficiency of Fructose-1,6-Diphosphatase

Symptoms of fructose-1,6-diphosphatase deficiency are initiated by introduction of fructose-containing foods in the diet. Children are free of symptoms as long as they ingest only human milk. Hypoglycemia is the usual presentation with hyperventilation the most common symptom in the newborn. Hypotonia, hepatomegaly, and metabolic acidosis may also occur. The latter is due to accumulation of lactate and ketone bodies. The disease is exacerbated by infection or prolonged fasting. Diagnosis is made through enzyme assay using leukocytes or hepatic tissue. Death may result from severe metabolic derangement. Therapy consists of dietary restriction of fructose and sucrose and results in regression of hepatomegaly.

Since hypoglycemia occurs with prolonged fasting, especially during periods of fever, it is important to minimize the time children with the latter two disorders are kept NPO prior to surgery. The anesthesiologist must also remember not to order fruit juice or other foods containing fructose for oral hydration. Use of invert sugar, which contains fructose and glucose, is also contraindicated. Intravenous solutions containing glucose should be administered freely.

All surgical procedures except those for life-threatening conditions must be deferred in children who are severely acidotic or hypokalemic. Intermittent sampling of blood for glucose and blood gas determinations is indicated during major surgery to ensure that hypoglycemia and acidosis are not present.[18]

Pentosuria

Essential benign pentosuria, which occurs almost exclusively in Jewish populations, is only of clinical significance when confused with diabetes mellitus. Affected patients cannot degrade L-xylulose derived from glucuronic acid. The urine shows a 1+ reaction for reducing substances but is negative for glucose. Blood sugar is normal. The pentose reacts with Clinitest but not with glucose oxidase test papers such as Testape or Clinistix dipsticks.

DISORDERS OF AMINO ACID METABOLISM

Phenylketonuria

The most common of the amino acid disorders, phenylketonuria (PKU), results from a deficiency of phenylalanine hydroxylase, which normally is found primarily in the liver. The reported incidence varies from 1 in 11,000 to 1 in 15,000. Lack of the enzyme leads to accumulation of phenylalanine and classic, or type I, hyperphenylalaninemia. Lesser enzyme deficiencies result in milder forms of the disorder. Discussion will be limited to type I disease.

The most significant consequence is progressive mental retardation, which first becomes manifest in mid-infancy. Accumulation of phenylalanine or its metabolites interferes with brain maturation and myelination. Less than 2 percent of untreated children have an IQ above 70; in most it is under 20. However, with scrupulous dietary management, mental development should proceed normally. The children are usually hyperactive and aggressive. Occasionally the disorder is confused with autism. At least one fourth have seizures.

Untreated children have hypopigmentation of the skin, hair, and irises. A mousey or musty order, due to accumulation of phenylacetic acid, is characteristic. Eczema is common. An increased incidence of pyloric stenosis has been reported in these patients.

Levels of phenylalanine are normal at birth. With institution of protein intake, the level rises rapidly and by 4 to 5 days of age is at least ten times normal. In order to prevent the sequelae of high levels of phen-

ylalanine, dietary restriction must be instituted very early. Accordingly, screening of newborns for PKU is mandatory in most of the United States. It is of interest that mass screening programs have identified an unexpectedly large number of patients with hyperphenylalaninemia who do not have PKU.

There are no unique anesthetic considerations for children with PKU. In fact, it should not be seen in children born in countries with neonatal screening programs. Affected children with seizures should be maintained on anticonvulsant medication in the perioperative period. If eczema is present, careful handling and positioning are indicated to prevent further damage to the skin, including omitting adhesive tape to secure the intravenous cannulae and endotracheal tube. Although it has been stated that children with PKU are very sensitive to narcotics and central nervous system depressants,[8] no documentation for this statement is provided and it does not seem intuitively obvious that such should be the case.

Transient Neonatal Tyrosinemia

Hypertyrosinemia occurs in many newborns, especially prematures. Although the levels of tyrosine may be very high, the liver and kidneys are not affected. Aside from transient lethargy, there are no clinical findings. The tyrosine levels decrease to normal within a few weeks, and no treatment is required. Data regarding the merits of vitamin C supplementation, reduction of dietary protein, and breast feeding are contradictory.

Tyrosinemia

Type I

There are two forms of tyrosinemia due, at least in part, to a deficiency of para-hydroxyphenylpyruvic acid oxidase. Large quantities of tyrosine, para-hydroxyphenylpyruvic acid (P-HPPA), and their lactic and acetic acid derivatives are found in the patient's urine. Both tyrosine and methionine are elevated in the plasma. There is an acute infantile form of the disorder in which vomiting, diarrhea, failure to thrive, hepatosplenomegaly, and jaundice occur within the first few months. A renal tubular defect causes acidosis, aminoaciduria, and polyuria. Rickets may result from phosphaturia. Glucosuria leads to hypoglycemia. Rapid deterioration in liver function occurs and most children with this form of the disorder die within the first year.

The second form of the disease has a later onset and a more chronic course. The majority of children with this variant die within the first decade of life. Liver function progressively deteriorates and hypertension is common, probably secondary to enhanced catecholamine synthesis from tyrosine. Elevated concentrations of most of the amino acids are found in both blood and urine, but tyrosine and methionine predominate. Dietary restriction of tyrosine and phenylalanine is the primary therapy. Vitamin D is used to prevent or treat rickets. The disease is rare but the incidence is much greater in French Canadians than in the general population.

Modifications of anesthetic technique may be required, depending upon the degree of hepatic and renal disease. Chronic anemia is common; however, transfusion is not indicated unless the hematocrit is very low or acute blood loss has occurred. Hypoglycemia should be avoided by minimizing the NPO period and infusing a glucose solution. The presence of liver or renal disease does not contraindicate use of the halogenated anesthetic agents. Renal excretion of muscle relaxants is not affected unless renal damage is severe. In such cases, use of a relaxant such as atracurium, which does not depend upon renal excretion, is preferable.

Type II (Richner-Hanhart Syndrome)

A rare disease, type II or Oregon tyrosinemia is due to a deficiency of hepatic tyrosine aminotransferase. Keratosis of the soles and palms and corneal erosions and plaques are usually evident within the first few months of life. The severity of the skin and ocular lesions is related to the degree of tyrosine deposition. There are no hepatic or renal abnormalities. Treatment is dietary restriction as in type I tyrosinemia.

Alkaptonuria

Alkaptonuria is the disorder that led to elucidation of the concept of inborn errors of metabolism by Garrod in 1902. It is a rare disease in which homogentisic acid, an intermediary product in the metabolism of phenylalanine and tyrosine, cannot be further metabolized, leading to pigmentation of the connective tissue (ochronosis). Progressive degenerative arthropathy and spondylitis occur in adults, but symptoms are not present in children. The relationship between the metabolic defect and the clinical syndrome has not been explained. Theoretically, dietary restriction should be beneficial if patients can be identified early. There are no special anesthetic considerations in children, and those appropriate for adults with other types of arthritis apply to those with alkaptonuria.

Maple Syrup Urine Disease

There are five clinical phenotypes of maple syrup urine disease. Only the classic type, which has an incidence of approximately 1 in 600,000, will be discussed since other variants are even more rare and less severe. The first step in degradation of the three branched-chain amino acids leucine, isoleucine, and valine involves transamination to the corresponding ketoacids. The next step is mediated by two or three different ketoacid decarboxylases. In the absence of the decarboxylases, ketoacids accumulate. Both the amino acids and the ketoacids are readily detected in the urine. Enzyme assay of fibroblasts is used to confirm the diagnosis. Prenatal diagnosis is possible through study of cultured amniotic cells. Routine screening of newborns is performed in a manner similar to that for PKU.

Poor feeding, vomiting, and a high-pitched cry are noted within the first week or two. The typical maple syrup or burnt sugar odor of the urine may be the first clue to the diagnosis. Hypotonicity or hypertonicity may be prominent features. It is not unusual for the two to alternate initially. Seizures, loss of deep tendon reflexes, stupor, and coma ensue. Severe hypoglycemia and ketoacidosis occur. Death usually occurs within weeks to months in untreated babies.

Treatment must be initiated within the first week to 10 days to prevent central nervous system damage and physical and mental retardation. Although exchange transfusion has been used, peritoneal dialysis is the preferred method for clearing accumulated amnio acids and ketoacids. Dialysis may also be required during life-threatening illness. Infection or trauma may be fatal because of catabolism of protein stores. Dietary treatment is difficult, but possible. A few aggressively treated patients have survived into childhood both physically and mentally normal.

The primary anesthetic consideration in children who are well controlled and require elective surgery is prevention of hypoglycemia and acidosis.[19] The period of dietary restriction pre- and postoperatively should be minimized and a glucose solution providing 125 to 150 kcal/kg/day administered intravenously throughout the perioperative period. If the surgical procedure is prolonged or complex, blood sugar and arterial blood gas determinations should be made intermittently. The child who is in a catabolic state as a result of an infectious process or trauma may require dialysis prior to surgery.

Homocystinuria

Accumulation of homocystine leads to homocystinuria, which has a prevalence of 1 in 200,000 to 1 in 300,000. Deficiency of hepatic cystathionine synthase causes elevated plasma and urinary levels of both methionine and homocystine, with other amino acids less commonly detected in the urine. Cystathionine synthase is dependent on vitamin B_6 (pyridoxine). At least two different enzyme mutations can result in the syndrome, as evidenced by the fact that some patients respond to treatment with vitamin B_6 and others do not.

Afflicted children usually have fair skin and light-colored, brittle hair as well as growth abnormalities.

Malar flushing, livedo reticularis, and formation of telangiectasia are common. Dislocation of the ocular lens usually occurs within the first few years and may lead to myopia, glaucoma, and retinal detachment. Hepatomegaly is not unusual, but liver function studies are normal. Bony abnormalities include osteoporosis, pectus excavatum or carinatum, kyphosis, scoliosis, and arachnodactyly. Some patients have a Marfan-like habitus. Growth retardation has also been reported. Many children have a "Charlie Chaplin" type of gait. About half are moderately retarded.

By far the most serious manifestation of the disease is arterial and venous thrombosis. Although the exact mechanism of the thrombotic diathesis is not defined, both abnormalities of the arterial walls and hypercoagulability appear to contribute. The latter is probably due to increased platelet adhesiveness. Vascular occlusion may occur as early as the first decade, and is common in older children. Death results from vascular thrombosis by the mid-twenties in half of the patients.

Administration of vitamin B_6 is beneficial in approximately half of the patients. Dietary restriction is practiced in those unresponsive to vitamin B_6.

Although spontaneous thrombosis of the cerebral, pulmonary, renal, mesenteric, and coronary arteries occurs, it is more common in the perioperative period. Any preexisting neurological deficit must be carefully documented. A preoperative electrocardiogram should be obtained in all patients. Although the effectiveness of prophylactic salicylates is unknown, they are employed. If spinal or epidural anesthesia is considered in a patient on aspirin therapy, a coagulation study should be performed. If the bleeding time is abnormal, another technique should be chosen or the aspirin discontinued (and bleeding time rechecked) because of the potential for epidural hematoma formation. Intraoperative administration of dextran has been recommended to decrease platelet adhesiveness.[20]

Invasive radiographic studies requiring intravenous administration of contrast media are especially hazardous because the dye induces an osmotic diuresis, which may lead to dehydration and increased blood viscosity. It is imperative that intravenous fluid administration equal or exceed urinary loss. Hypothermia also increases viscosity and predisposes to thrombosis.

During lengthy operative procedures, it is critical that the patient be positioned in a manner that minimizes venous stasis. Wrapping the extremities with Ace bandages and elevating the foot of the operating table are recommended.

Albinism

Albinism describes a heterogeneous group of disorders of melanin metabolism found in many animal species. However, clinical use of the term should be restricted to congenital hypomelanosis limited to the eye or involving the eye and integument in patients who also have nystagmus, photophobia, and decreased visual acuity. There are ten distinct forms of oculocutaneous albinism, which can be distinguished on the basis of clinical, biochemical, and genetic characteristics. Nine are inherited as autosomal recessive traits; one is autosomal dominant. Two forms are of interest to the anesthesiologist: the Hermansky-Pudlak syndrome and the Chédiak-Higashi syndrome.

The hallmark of the Hermansky-Pudlak syndrome is a bleeding diathesis due to morphological, chemical, and functional platelet defects. In addition, there is accumulation of a ceroid-like material in the reticuloendothelial system, lung, and oral and intestinal mucosa. Restrictive lung disease, ulcerative colitis, and occasionally renal dysfunction are seen in older patients. The basic metabolic defect is unknown but is presumed to be an enzyme alteration. It affects 1 in 5000 Puerto Ricans and approximately 1 in 60,000 Caucasians.

Patients should be questioned about easy bruisability and excess bleeding associated with minor trauma. If the bleeding time is abnormal, platelet aggregation studies and consultation with a hematologist regarding use of cryoprecipitate or other hemotherapy in the perioperative period are indicated.

The Chédiak-Higashi syndrome is a rare, usually fatal disease. The pathognomonic feature is the presence of peroxidase-positive lysosomal granules in granulocytes of the peripheral blood. Giant granules can also be identified in Schwann cells and other tissues. Repeated infections, usually due to gram positive staphylococci or streptococci, occur. Those who survive the infections often develop a terminal lymphoreticular malignancy characterized by progressive anemia, thrombocytopenia and neutropenia, mediastinal and hilar lymphadenopathy, and hepatosplenomegaly. Bruising, gastrointestinal bleeding, and prolonged bleeding times are usually evident in the accelerated phase of the disease.

Both cranial and peripheral nerves are involved in the progressive neuropathy evident by 5 to 6 years of age. Muscle weakness, an abnormal gait, diffusely abnormal EEG, and sensory deficits are characteristic. The use of succinylcholine is avoided in children with Chédiak-Higashi syndrome because of the potential for inducing hyperkalemia.

Cystinuria

Cystine is the least soluble of the amino acids in urine. A defect in cellular transport of cystine and the dibasic amino acids ornithine, lysine, and arginine in the proximal renal tube leads to cystinuria, which is the cause of approximately 5 percent of renal calculi in children. Cystinuria is one of the most prevalent inherited disorders with an overall incidence of approximately 1 in 7000. Newborn screening programs have demonstrated an incidence of 1 in 2000 in

England, 1 in 4000 in Australia, and 1 in 15,000 in the United States. Treatment consists of a high fluid intake and therapy with D-penicillamine, which reacts with urinary cystine to form a compound 50 times more soluble than cystine, thus reducing the incidence of renal calculi. The value of attempting to alter urinary pH is questionable.

It is essential that patients with this disorder receive adequate fluid therapy in the perioperative period, especially at night when urine is more concentrated. Accordingly, an IV should be started prior to surgery and continued until the patient can resume oral intake. Pancytopenia and proteinuria are side effects of penicillamine therapy that can be detected by preoperative blood count and urinalysis.

Hartnup Disease

The prevalence of Hartnup disease may be as high as 1 in 18,000, although many patients with the disorder are asymptomatic. Most of the manifestations are secondary to defective intestinal absorption of the essential amino acid tryptophan, a major source of nicotinamide. The resulting niacin deficiency leads to a pellagra-like syndrome. An intermittent red, scaly rash appears following exposure to sunlight. Attacks of cerebellar ataxia, emotional instability, and frank psychoses are common and may follow infection, stress, poor nutrition, or sulfonamide therapy.

If patients with Hartnup disease require anesthesia during an acute episode, special care must be taken to protect involved skin. Adhesive tape should not be used to secure IV cannulae or the endotracheal tube. No metabolic derangements are associated with the disease.

Hypophosphatasia

There appear to be three types of hypophosphatasia: infantile, childhood, and adult. The precise biochemical defect is unknown. The overall incidence is approximately 1 in 100,000. Perinatal or neonatal death is common. Premature cranial synostosis, hypercalcemia, failure to thrive, and several bony defects occur.

The childhood form becomes evident between 6 months and 2 years of age. It is characterized by premature shedding of deciduous teeth and increased susceptibility to infection. Skeletal manifestations may be absent or mild rickets evident. Patients with the adult form may have spontaneous fractures or be entirely asymptomatic.

Surgical decompression is required in infants with increased intracranial pressure due to craniosynostosis. The usual precautions apply, including avoidance of drugs such as ketamine that increase intracranial pressure. The major intraoperative concern is blood loss. Adequate blood must be crossmatched preoperatively and reliable infusion routes established.

Other Amino Acid Disorders

There are numerous disorders of amino acid metabolism that do not lead to clinical sequelae. Others, though clinically significant, are extremely rare. The anesthesiologist who enounters a child with any of these disorders should refer to specialized texts devoted to metabolic disorders and consult with the child's pediatrician.

Generalized Aminoaciduria

Enhanced excretion of all of the amino acids normally found in the urine, loosely termed generalized aminoaciduria, can result from a number of disease states, including several genetically transmitted metabolic disorders. The amino acid losses per se are usually not of sufficient magnitude to cause deleterious clinical effects. However, dysfunction of the proximal renal tubules also results in poor absorption of water, organic acids, sugars, bicarbonate, sodium, potassium, phosphate, and uric acid. The Fanconi syndrome is characterized by increased renal clearance of these substances plus childhood rickets.

Disturbance of fluid and electrolyte homeostasis are of variable severity. Of these, dehydration, acidosis, and hypokalemia are significant to the anesthesiologist. These children should have an IV started the night prior to surgery. It is preferable that surgery be scheduled in the morning to minimize the period of fasting. During long procedures and those associated with significant volume shifts and metabolic derangements, electrolytes, glucose, and blood gases should be determined frequently.

DISORDERS OF LIPID AND LIPOPROTEIN METABOLISM

Familial Hyperlipoproteinemia

Approximately half of the children found on routine screening to have high serum cholesterol levels have elevated low density lipoprotein levels. Among the other causes of high cholesterol levels are diabetes, nephrotic syndrome, systemic lupus erythematosus, pancreatitis, and hypothyroidism. It is essential that the differential diagnosis be established because of the marked variations in therapeutic implications and prognosis. There are five recognized types of familial hyperlipoproteinemia, two of which present during childhood and are associated with significant morbidity and mortality.

Type I

Type I familial lipoproteinemia is a rare disorder usually detected late in the first decade of life. Severe abdominal pain is the most common presenting symptom. In addition to recurrent pancreatitis, cutaneous xanthomatosis and hepatosplenomegaly characterize the disease. The skin lesions usually appear abruptly when the triglyceride levels are very high and resolve over the ensuing weeks.

The disorder is due to a deficiency of the lipolytic enzyme lipoprotein lipase, which is responsible for hydrolysis and removal of chylomicrons and triglycerides from the blood. The enzyme is released into the blood by heparin and can be assayed either in plasma following heparin administration or directly in biopsied adipose tissue. Serum levels of chylomicrons, cholesterol, and trigylcerides are very high and the severity of symptoms correlates with the degree of chylomicronemia. Strict dietary restriction is essential.

Premature atherosclerosis is not a feature of the disease. However, pancreatitis may be life-threatening. Children may be subjected to laparotomy if pancreatitis is confused with other intra-abdominal disease, for example, appendicitis. Major fluid deficits may be present owing to third space sequestration in the presence of pancreatitis. Use of central venous and urinary catheters facilitates fluid management.

Type II

Familial hypercholesterolemia, type II A and B hyperlipoproteinemia, is transmitted through a single autosomal dominant gene. The heterozygous state may be as frequent as 1 in 500; the incidence of homozygosity is only about 1 in 1,000,000. Homozygotes have severe disease which is manifest early in childhood. Heterozygotes may exhibit only the biochemical anomaly in lipid metabolism or clinical signs of the disease. Hypercholesterolemia occurs in both variants. Low density lipoproteins are increased in type IIA, but triglycerides are normal. In addition to low density lipoproteins, very low density lipoproteins and triglycerides are elevated in patients with type IIB disease. The definitive diagnosis is made by measuring low density lipoprotein receptor function in cultured skin fibroblasts.

Generalized atherosclerosis with severe coronary artery involvement usually leads to death prior to age 20. Xanthomas are evident by age 4 years in homozygotes and may even be present at birth. Arcus corneae develop in the first decade.

Management of heterozygotes includes dietary restriction and therapy with cholestyramine or colestipol exchange resins, which bind cholesterol and increase its excretion via the intestine. Clofibrate lowers serum triglyceride and very low density lipoproteins, but not cholesterol. Nicotinic acid may be added to enhance the effect of the ion exchange resins. Neither dietary modification nor medical therapy is beneficial in homozygotes. Chronic plasmapheresis has been successfully tried in some patients to lower cholesterol levels. Portacaval shunts and ileal bypasses have been performed in a limited number of patients with disappointing results.

The anesthesiologist must presume that children with the homozygous form of the disease have coronary artery disease. In addition to an electrocardiogram, the preoperative workup should include consultation with a pediatric cardiologist. Placement of a Swan-Ganz catheter and arterial cannula is recommended prior to anesthesia for major operative procedures. Blood loss during portacaval shunts may be significant, necessitating careful measurement of blood loss and administration of appropriate component therapy.

DISORDERS OF LYSOSOMAL ENZYMES

Lysosomal enzyme deficiencies result in accumulation of mucopolysaccharides, glycoproteins, and sphingolipids, singly or in combination (Table 13–5). The skeleton, central nervous system, and viscera are affected. Although deposition of the stored material begins prior to birth, the onset of clinical manifestations can be delayed several years. The mucopolysaccharidoses are the largest subgroup of disorders of

Table 13–5. DISORDERS OF LYSOSOMAL ENZYMES

Disorder	Prevalence
Mucopolysaccharidosis, type I	
Hurler syndrome	1:100,000
Scheie syndrome	1:500,000
Hurler-Scheie syndrome	1:100,000
Mucopolysaccharidosis, type II (Hunter syndrome)	1:150,000
Mucopolysaccharidosis, type III (Sanfilippo syndrome)	1:24,000
Mucopolysaccharidosis, type IV (Morquio syndrome)	1:100,000
Mucopolysaccharidosis, type VI (Maroteaux-Lamy syndrome)	1:100,000
Mucopolysaccharidosis, type VII (Sly syndrome)	Rare
Mucolipidosis I	Rare
Mucolipidosis II (I-cell disease)	Rare
Mucolipidosis III (pseudo-Hurler polydystrophy)	Rare
Mannosidosis	Rare
Sialidosis	Rare
Aspartylglycosaminuria	Rare
Fucosidosis	Rare
Acid lipase deficiency (Wolman disease and cholesteryl ester storage disease)	Rare
Ceramidase deficiency (Farber disease)	Rare
Niemann-Pick disease	1:25,000 US Jews
Gaucher disease, type I	1:2000 US Jews
type II, type III	Rare
Galactosylceramide lipidosis (Krabbe disease)	1:50,000 Swedes
Metachromatic leukodystrophy	1:100,000
Multiple sulfatase deficiency	Rare
Alpha-galactosidase A deficiency (Fabry disease)	1:40,000
GM_1 gangliosidosis	Rare
Tay-Sachs disease	1:3000 US Jews

Modified from Stanbury JB, Wyngaarden JB, Fredrickson DS, et al.: The Metabolic Basis of Inherited Disease. 5th ed. New York, McGraw-Hill, 1983, pp 47–50.

lysosomal storage and are also associated with the most significant anesthetic problems.

Mucopolysaccharidoses

Deficiency of the lysosomal enzymes involved in the degradation of dermatan sulfate, heparan sulfate, and keratan sulfate leads to accumulation and increased urinary excretion of partially degraded mucopolysaccharides. The clinical features of the disorders are similar and, although mucopolysacchariduria is readily detected by employing spot tests, enzyme assay of leukocytes or cultured fibroblasts is often necessary for definitive diagnosis.

Type I

There are three different forms of alpha-L-iduronidase deficiency, which can be distinguished on the basis of age of onset and clinical course. The first of these, the Hurler syndrome, is the prototype for all the mucopolysaccharidoses. Children with the Hurler syndrome appear normal in infancy. However, toward the end of the first year they are noted to be unusually large with proportionately large heads. Dwarfing and increased head size become evident by 2 to 3 years of age. Coarse facies are a prominent characteristic of the disorder. Macroglossia and patulous lips are accentuated, since the children are usually mouth breathers because the nose is obstructed by secretions and the adenoids and tonsils are large. The gums are hyperplastic and the teeth abnormally shaped and widely spaced. The neck is short and thick. Narrowing of the laryngeal inlet and tracheobronchial tree may occur as a result of deposition of the mucopolysaccharides.[21] Progressive clouding of the cornea occurs and some children also develop glaucoma. Hydrocephalus may occur secondary to thickening of the meninges. The skin is thickened and there is generalized hirsutism. The abdomen is protuberant, and the liver and spleen are enlarged. Umbilical and inguinal hernias are frequently seen. Joint mobility is decreased, flexion contractures and thoracolumbar kyphosis usually occur, and the hands are often clawlike. Sensorineural deafness is frequent. Severe coronary artery disease and valvular disease occur in young children.[22, 23] Cardiomyopathy also results from deposition of mucopolysaccharides in the myocardium. Severe mental retardation is a consistent feature of the disorder. Death from cardiac failure usually occurs in the first decade. Restrictive lung disease due to thoracic cage abnormality is compounded by recurrent pulmonary infection.

Children with Scheie syndrome are, as a rule, less severely affected than those with the Hurler syndrome. Coarseness of the facial features, corneal clouding, glaucoma, retinal degeneration, deafness, and aortic valvular disease are common. Sleep apnea severe enough to require tracheotomy has been reported.[24] Intelligence and life span are usually normal. Patients may present for aortic valve replacement, carpal tunnel release, or ophthalmological procedures.

Hurler-Scheie disease is an intermediate phenotype. Patients are short, have joint involvement, and are usually of moderate intelligence. Valvular lesions are usually more severe than in children with Scheie disease. Micrognathia is a consistent feature. Death usually occurs by the second decade.

There are multiple causes of the significant morbidity and mortality associated with operative procedures in these children. In addition to myocardial ischemia and valvular heart disease, most have chronic pulmonary disease. It is difficult to determine the optimal time for elective surgery because the children usually have chronic otitis media and nasal stuffiness, which must be differentiated from an acute infectious process.

Cervical spine x-rays should be obtained preoperatively because odontoid hypoplasia and atlantoaxial subluxation, although more common in other forms of mucopolysaccharidosis, have been reported.[25] In addition, the diameter of the trachea can be assessed although this is better defined with a CT scan. A chest x-ray examination is indicated to determine the degree of pulmonary disease and cardiomegaly. A preoperative electrocardiogram should be obtained.

Unless the child has narrow-angle glaucoma, an antisialagogue should be administered preoperatively. Sedatives should be used only in small doses or avoided altogether because of the potential for airway obstruction. Administration of an antacid such as sodium citrate or an H_2 antagonist such as cimetidine is recommended in children with gross hepatosplenomegaly, which enhances the danger of regurgitation and aspiration.

Intravenous access is frequently difficult because of the child's thick skin and abnormal anatomy secondary to joint contractures. However, an IV tube should be placed prior to induction of anesthesia. Intravenous induction agents should be administered very slowly. Inhalation induction may be difficult because of the tendency for airway obstruction.[26] Muscle relaxants should not be administered prior to intubation unless the patient can be ventilated easily by mask.

Laryngoscopy may be complicated by the large tongue and small mouth. The tongue can be held forward with forceps or a tongue suture during laryngoscopy. Nasotracheal intubation should not be attempted unless mandated by the nature of the surgery because of the danger of bleeding and the potential for hyperplastic adenoid tissue being impacted in the endotracheal tube. Since the size tube that can be passed is often smaller than would be predicted on the basis of the child's age, various sizes of endotracheal tubes must be readily available. Extubation should be performed with the patient fully awake.

The most common operative procedures performed in these children are myringotomy and placement of PE tubes and umbilical and inguinal hernia repairs. Implantation of fresh human amnion has been attempted in an effort to supply the missing enzymes.[27] It is usually placed extraperitoneally in a pocket deep to the external oblique muscles. If it can be placed superficially, local anesthesia may be adequate. Otherwise, the children will require multiple general anesthetics for repeated amnion transplants.

Type II (Hunter Syndrome)

The Hunter syndrome occurs in severe and mild forms and is the only one of the mucopolysaccharidoses that is inherited as an X-linked recessive trait. The facies are coarse, and mild to moderate dwarfism occurs. Corneal clouding does not occur but retinitis pigmentosa may. Vision and hearing progressively deteriorate. Virtually all patients become deaf. Nodular, ivory-colored skin lesions are characteristic of this disease. Mental retardation and joint disease are less severe than in patients with the Hurler syndrome. Hydrocephalus may be severe and, in some, central nervous system dysfunction leads to early death. Patients with mild forms of the disease survive into adulthood. Valvular and ischemic heart disease are frequent. Although usually less severe, the same airway difficulties may occur as with Hurler syndrome and tracheotomy may be required.[28] In children with hydrocephalus, anesthetic techniques and agents known to increase intracranial pressure must be avoided.

Type III (Sanfilippo Syndrome)

The four biochemically distinct forms of the Sanfilippo syndrome are not clinically distinguishable. Severe, progressive mental retardation is the primary feature of the disorder; the somatic manifestations are relatively mild. Facial features are less coarse than in type I and II mucopolysaccharidoses and joint stiffness is not as severe. Clouding of the cornea does not occur. Patients rarely survive into the second decade. The primary anesthetic consideration is management of a severely retarded, often combative child. In the absence of anticipated airway difficulty, adequate sedation should be administered preoperatively.

Type IV (Morquio Syndrome)

In the Morquio syndrome degradation of keratan sulfate, which is found only in the cornea, cartilage, and nucleus pulposus of the intervertebral discs, is defective. Patients are usually of normal intelligence. Partial deafness is common. The degree of facial coarseness is mild to moderate: the maxilla is usually prominent, the nose short, and the teeth widely spaced. Skeletal abnormalities are severe. The neck and trunk are short and progressive pectus carinatum develops. Genu varum, joint laxity, and severe dwarfism occur. Absence or marked hypoplasia of the odontoid process of the second vertebra and the resulting atlantoaxial instability lead to spinal cord compression.[29] Progressive neurological degeneration, acute quadriparesis,[30] and death due to respiratory arrest occur.

Upper airway obstruction due to collapse of the trachea during head flexion has been reported.[31] Chronic pulmonary disease secondary to the thoracic deformity and repeated pulmonary infection are common.[32] Aortic regurgitation may also accompany the disorder.

Most patients live to adulthood. Prophylactic posterior cervical fusion has been performed in some and may lead to longer survival. The primary anesthetic considerations in patients with this syndrome relate to their cervical spine and chronic pulmonary disease. Preoperative cervical spine x-rays are required. Depending upon the age of the patient and the condition of the cervical spine, awake endotracheal intubation or fiberoptic intubation may be indicated. The absence of symptoms of cervical myelopathy does not mean absence of disease. Patients undergoing major procedures, such as spinal fusions, usually require postoperative observation in an intensive care unit. Postoperative mechanical ventilation is required in those with severe pulmonary disease.

Type VI (Maroteaux-Lamy Syndrome)

The Maroteaux-Lamy syndrome is characterized by short stature, joint stiffness, coarse facial features, and corneal clouding. There is a spectrum of disease severity. Hydrocephalus, cardiac valvular involvement, hypoplasia of the odontoid, lumbar kyphosis, and genu valgum are less consistent features of the disorder. Patients usually die by the second decade. The anesthetic considerations detailed above apply to management of these patients.

Type VII (Sly Syndrome)

Type VII mucopolysaccharidosis is extremely rare and of variable severity. Coarse facies, corneal clouding, hepatosplenomegaly, umbilical and inguinal hernias, pectus carinatum, joint deformities, and aortic disease have been reported. Alterations in anesthetic technique are dictated by the organ systems involved.

Mucolipidoses

Mucolipidosis I (ML I), mucolipidosis II (I-cell disease, ML II), and mucolipidosis III (pseudo-Hurler polydystrophy, ML III) are rare, biochemically related disorders of lysosomal function that primarily affect connective tissue. Most children with ML I have a Hurler-like phenotype, often evident at birth. In addition, cherry-red coloration of the macula and progressive neurodegeneration occur. The clinical manifestations of ML II are similar to those of the Hurler syndrome, but the children are more severely affected and the diagnosis is usually made earlier. Patients with ML III resemble those with Maroteaux-Lamy syndrome. Anesthetic implications have already been discussed.

Glycoprotein Storage Diseases

The clinical phenotypes of the glycoprotein storage diseases generally resemble those of mild mucopolysaccharidoses. The disorders include mannosidosis, fucosidosis, sialidosis, and aspartylglycosaminuria. There is no specific treatment, and anesthetic management depends upon the clinical manifestations.

Acid Lipase Deficiency

A deficiency of lysosomal acid lipase results in massive accumulation of cholesteryl esters and triglycerides in most tissues of the body. Wolman disease is nearly always fatal in the first year. Severe hepatosplenomegaly, steatorrhea, anemia, and failure to thrive are observed within the first few weeks. Adrenal calcification is evident on x-ray. Cholesteryl ester storage disease is more benign and may not be detected in childhood. Hepatomegaly and premature atherosclerosis occur, but adrenal calcification is rare. The diagnosis of both disorders is confirmed by demonstration of acid lipase deficiency in cultured skin fibroblasts or lymphocytes. There is no treatment.

Ceramidase Deficiency

Farber disease is a rare disorder due to acid ceramidase deficiency that results in tissue accumulation of ceramide. The classical clinical triad is subcutaneous nodules, arthritis, and hoarseness. Symptoms are evident between 2 weeks and 4 months of age. The nodules are most prominent around involved joints, which are swollen and painful. Hoarseness usually progresses to aphonia. Dysphagia and respiratory difficulty are due to granuloma formation in the epiglottis and larynx. Macroglossia may compromise the airway. Hepatomegaly, cardiomyopathy, and mental deterioration are less common. The diagnosis can usually be made clinically, but is confirmed by histological examination of a biopsied nodule, assay of enzyme activity in cultured skin fibroblasts or leukocytes, or chromatographic analysis of ceramide in tissue or body fluid. There is no treatment, and affected children usually die by 2 years of age.

Anesthetic experience with children who have Farber disease is extremely limited. It would seem prudent to avoid endotracheal intubation if the operative procedure can safely be performed with general anesthesia administered by mask. When endotracheal intubation is indicated, the tube should be smaller than usually used for a child of the same age to minimize trauma to the vocal cords. The laryngeal inlet may also be markedly decreased in diameter and tracheostomy required.

Sphingomyelin Lipidoses

Niemann-Pick disease is characterized by tissue accumulation of sphingomyelin due to a deficiency of the enzyme sphingomyelinase. There are at least three, and perhaps five, variants of the disorder. Hepatosplenomegaly is a constant feature, and foam cells are found in the bone marrow of all affected children. Involvement of the nervous system and lung is also common. Often a cherry-red spot is evident in the retina. Malnutrition from feeding problems is often seen. Type A disease develops in infancy and is associated with severe nervous system disease. Death occurs by age 3 or 4. Visceral involvement is extensive in type B disease, but nervous system function is normal. Some patients with type B disease have lived into adulthood. Patients with type C disease have both visceral and nervous system involvement and usually die before age 20. Definitive diagnosis of Niemann-Pick disease is made by measuring sphingomyelinase activity in tissue specimens, homogenates of cultured skin fibroblasts, or leukocyte extracts. The disorder affects all ethnic groups, but the majority of children with the classic infantile form of the disease are of Ashkenazi Jewish ancestry. Types B and C do not have the same predilection. Although the spleen is extensively involved, hematological disease is not a prominent feature of the disorder. However, thrombocytopenia and anemia may occur in the terminal stages of the disease. The liver may be massively enlarged, but results of liver function tests are not significantly abnormal.

Children who require anesthesia should be managed with a rapid-sequence induction, because the enlarged spleen and liver render the patient vulnerable to regurgitation and aspiration. Administration of an antacid and cimetidine preoperatively will decrease the potential for aspiration pneumonitis. No anesthetic agents or muscle relaxants are specifically contraindicated.

Glucosylceramide Lipidoses

Gaucher disease is the most common metabolic disorder of glycolipid metabolism. Accumulation of glucocerebroside leads to organ enlargement and dysfunction. The highest incidence (1 in 2500) is found in the Ashkenazi Jewish population. Symptoms of type I disease, also referred to as the adult form, may become manifest at any time from birth to late adulthood. Splenomegaly is the most consistent early finding. Hypersplenism may lead to thrombocytopenia, anemia, and leukopenia, occasionally requiring splenectomy. Hepatomegaly is less pronounced and hepatic function usually remains normal. Bone disease is also a frequent manifestation. Scans reveal decreased bone density in the proximal and distal long bones, hip joints, and vertebrae. Aseptic necrosis of the femoral head and vertebral fractures are common. Severe episodes of bone pain, often accompanied by fever, may be mistaken for osteomyelitis. Pulmonary involvement is common and can lead to pulmonary hypertension and cor pulmonale. The disease usually progresses slowly.

Severe deficiency of enzymatic activity causes accumulation of large amounts of glucocerebroside in patients with type II disease. Neurological signs are usually evident within 6 months, and most patients die within the year from pulmonary infection. Progressive spasticity, hyperreflexia, and pathological reflexes develop. The triad of trismus, strabismus, and retroflexion of the head is classic. Hepatosplenomegaly also occurs.

Hepatosplenomegaly and skeletal and neurological involvement usually begin in adolescence in patients with type III disease. Diagnosis of Gaucher disease is made on the basis of hepatosplenomegaly and demonstration of large lipid-laden histiocytes (Gaucher cells) in bone marrow aspirates. Glucocerebrosidase activity can also be measured in leukocytes or cultured skin fibroblasts.

A full hematological profile should be performed on any child with Gaucher disease who is scheduled for surgery, with special reference to the platelet count and hemoglobin. Platelet counts are often low without clinical manifestations. A mild, compensated anemia is common. Neither platelet concentrates nor packed cells should be administered to treat abnormal numbers found on the blood count unless bleeding is evident or anemia severe. Consultation with a hematologist is recommended. Endotracheal intubation may be difficult in children with type II disease due to trismus and the abnormal head position. This problem is resolved following administration of a muscle relaxant. However, these agents are contraindicated if the child cannot be adequately ventilated by mask.

Galactosylceramide Lipidosis

Krabbe globoid cell leukodystrophy is a rapidly progressive disease usually manifested within 3 to 6 months of age by irritability, hypersensitivity to external stimuli, hypertonicity, vomiting, and failure to thrive. Deficiency of galactosylcerebrosidase results in inability to degrade the glycosphingolipid galactosylceramide in the central nervous system. Progressive mental and motor deterioration and spastic quadriparesis occur, and most children with this disorder die by age 2. Use of succinylcholine is best avoided in children with significant peripheral neuropathy, but no other anesthetic agents are contraindicated.

Sulfatide Lipidoses

There are two disorders involving sulfatase enzymes: metachromatic leukodystrophy and multiple sulfatase deficiency. They are characterized by severe psychomotor retardation and early death. The latter disorder shares several features of the mucopolysaccharidoses, and the same anesthetic considerations apply.

Alpha-Galactosidase A Deficiency

Fabry disease is an X-linked disease in which the neutral glycosphingolipids triglycosylceramide and galactosylceramide accumulate in non-neuronal tissue. The disease is usually manifest in children, but the onset may be delayed until adulthood. The most common presenting symptom is severe, intermittent pain in the extremities that is triggered by exercise, stress, climatic changes, or hyperpyrexia. The typical dermatological lesion is the angiokeratoma, and the disease has been called angiokeratoma corporis diffusum. Hypohidrosis, diarrhea, nausea and vomiting, cardiac conduction defects, cerebrovascular occlusion, and renal disease also occur. Many patients live to adulthood, with death resulting from vascular or renal complications. Definitive treatment is not available; however, painful neuropathy often responds to diphenylhydantoin. Avoidance of exercise in hot weather is important in preventing acute episodes.[33]

The disease should not be confused with malignant hyperthermia. An adequate history should clearly differentiate Fabry disease from malignant hyperpyrexia. Accordingly, administration of the halogenated anesthetic agents is not contraindicated and succinylcholine can be used in the absence of muscle wasting. Patients on chronic diphenylhydantoin therapy should continue to receive the drug in the perioperative period.

Gangliosidoses

The several variants of G_{M1} gangliosidoses differ in severity and onset. The most severe form is evident in the neonate and is characterized by profound motor and mental retardation. The facial features may resemble those of children with the Hurler syndrome.

Tay-Sachs disease is the most common ganglioside storage disease. Testing for the carrier state is recommended in Ashkenazi Jewish populations since the gene incidence is approximately 1 in 27 in this population. An exaggerated startle response is usually noted early. Motor weakness is evident by 6 months and psychomotor deterioration progresses rapidly. Deafness, blindness, and convulsions usually occur. Almost all have cherry-red spots in the macula. There is no treatment, and most children die by 3 to 4 years of age. Feeding gastrostomy may be performed because swallowing becomes progressively ineffective. Such children should be considered at risk for aspiration; either they can be intubated awake or a rapid-sequence induction can be performed. Preoperative antacid therapy and administration of cimetidine may be helpful. Most children already have severe pulmonary disease, and aspiration pneumonitis may be the terminal event.

DISORDERS OF PURINE AND PYRIMIDINE METABOLISM

Lesch-Nyhan Syndrome

This devastating disease is due to virtual absence of hypoxanthine-guanine phosphoribosyl transferase, which is essential for purine metabolism. As a result uric acid accumulates, producing the severe neurological disorders characteristic of the disease. Enzyme activity is assayed using erythrocytes, leukocytes, or cultured skin fibroblasts.

The disorder is inherited in an X-linked recessive manner. The syndrome occurs in approximately 1 in 10,000 males. Partial deficiency of the enzyme occurs in 1 in 100,000 males. Heterozygous females are usually asymptomatic.

Most children with the syndrome are normal at birth, but delayed motor development is evident by 3 to 4 months. Hyperreflexia, extensor plantar reflexes, sustained ankle clonus, and scissoring of the legs are characteristic. Extrapyramidal signs develop between 8 and 12 months and include dystonia, chorea, and athetoid movements of the head and feet. Approximately half of the patients have seizures.

The most severe neurological defect is compulsive self-mutilation. Biting of the lips, buccal mucosa, and fingers is common. The children may also be aggressive toward others. Elevation of uric acid leads to development of subcutaneous tophi and renal calculi. Death usually occurs by the second decade. Allopurinol is administered to decrease serum uric acid levels, but nothing alters the neurological manifestations.

These children may require anesthesia for a variety of operative procedures. Complete dental extractions are often performed to decrease the child's ability to injure himself. Removal of renal calculi may be indicated. If nephrolithiasis is suspected, intravenous pyelography is necessary for diagnosis since the stones are radiolucent.

The anesthesiologist must explain to the operating room personnel what to expect of a child with Lesch-Nyhan syndrome. It may be necessary to administer an induction agent such as intramuscular ketamine or a rectal barbiturate before attempting to transport the child to the operating room. When this technique is employed, suction apparatus and equipment essential for airway management must be available in the room. Once the child is asleep he can be transferred to the operating room and anesthesia can be continued in the conventional manner. Restraints should be replaced before the child emerges from anesthesia.

Xanthinuria

Xanthinuria results from a deficiency of the enzyme xanthine oxidase, which catalzyes the oxidation of hypoxanthine to xanthine and xanthine to uric acid. Diagnosis is made through analysis of enzyme activity in jejunal or liver tissue. At least half of the patients are asymptomatic. Urinary tract calculi develop in a significant percentage. Muscle cramping following exercise and recurring polyarthritis are less common symptoms.

The anesthesiologist must think of malignant hyperthermia in any patient with a history of abnormal muscle cramping. However, there is no reported case of malignant hyperthermia in a patient with this disorder. In the absence of other evidence of susceptibility to malignant hyperthermia, no modification of anesthetic technique is indicated.

Xeroderma Pigmentosum

A disorder of pyrimidine metabolism, xeroderma pigmentosum has an incidence of 1 in 250,000. The disease is usually manifested within the first few years by excessive erythema and blistering following even minimal exposure to sunlight. Keratoses and skin cancers develop at an early age.

Approximately 15 percent of patients have a variant, the De Sanctis-Cacchione syndrome, characterized by microcephaly, mental retardation, ataxia, choreoathetosis, and eventual quadriparesis. Sensorineural deafness and dwarfism also occur.

Avoidance of sunlight is the primary therapy. Despite excision of the lesions and chemotherapy, most patients die before age 20.

Emotional support of these patients is extremely important since they are disfigured by the lesions and as a result of surgery. If extensive head and neck procedures are performed, airway management may be difficult. The chemotherapeutic agents usually employed are not associated with pulmonary toxicity or cardiotoxicity.

SUMMARY

Genetic metabolic diseases continue to be recognized. Some appear to be benign metabolic entities;[34] others have specific anesthetic implications.[35] The anesthesiologist, therefore, must keep abreast of the literature and consult appropriate clinical experts when confronted with anesthetizing a patient with a congenital metabolic disease.

The invaluable editorial and secretarial assistance of Mrs. Diane Coe is gratefully acknowledged.

REFERENCES

1. Stanbury JB, Wyngaarden JB, Fredrickson DS, et al.: The Metabolic Basis of Inherited Disease. 5th ed. New York, McGraw-Hill, 1983.
2. Diseases of the genome — an interview with Victor A. McKusick, MD. JAMA 252:1041, 1984.

3. Ampola MG: Metabolic Diseases in Pediatric Practice. Boston, Little, Brown, 1982.
4. Jackson SH: Inborn errors of metabolism. *In* Katz J, Benumof J, Kadis LB (Eds.): Anesthesia and Uncommon Diseases. 2nd ed. Philadelphia, W. B. Saunders Co., 1981.
5. Brown BB, Watson PD, Taussig LM: Congenital metabolic diseases of pediatric patients: anesthetic implications. Anesthesiology *43:*197, 1975.
6. McKusick VA: Mendelian Inheritance in Man. 6th ed. Baltimore, Johns Hopkins University Press, 1983.
7. Jones AEP, Pelton DA: An index of syndromes and their anaesthetic implications. Can Anaesth Soc J *23:*206, 1976.
8. Steward DJ: Manual of Pediatric Anesthesia. 2nd ed. New York, Churchill Livingstone, 1985. Appendix 1: Anesthetic implications of syndromes and unusual disorders, pp 289–343.
9. Smith DW: Recognizable Patterns of Human Malformation. 3rd ed. Philadelphia, W. B. Saunders Co., 1982.
10. Magalini SI, Scrascia E: Dictionary of Medical Syndromes. 2nd ed. Philadelphia, J. B. Lippincott Co., 1981.
11. Levy HL: Newborn Screening. *In* Avery ME, Taeusch HW (Eds.): Schaffer's Diseases of the Newborn. 5th ed. Philadelphia, W. B. Saunders Co., 1984.
12. Committee on Genetics: New issues in newborn screening for phenylketonuria and congenital hypothyroidism. Pediatrics *69:*104, 1982.
13. Cox JM: Anesthesia and glycogen-storage disease. Anesthesiology *29:*1221, 1968.
14. Grunfeld JP, Ganeval D, Chanard J, et al.: Acute renal failure in McArdle's disease. N Engl J Med *286:*1237, 1972.
15. Coleman P: McArdle's disease. Problems of anaesthetic management for caesarean section. Anaesthesia *39:*784, 1984.
16. Ellis FR: Inherited muscular disease. Br J Anaesth *52:*153, 1980.
17. Edelstein G, Hirschman CA: Hyperthermia and ketoacidosis during anesthesia in a child with glycogen-storage disease. Anesthesiology *32:*90, 1980.
18. Hashimoto Y, Watanabe H, Satou M: Anesthetic management of a patient with hereditary fructose-1,6-diphosphatase deficiency. Anesth Analg *47:*503, 1978.
19. Delaney A, Gal TJ: Hazards of anesthesia and operation in maple-syrup urine disease. Anesthesiology *44:*83, 1976.
20. Crooke JW, Towers JF, Taylor WH: Management of patients with homocystinuria requiring surgery under general anaesthesia. A case report. Br J Anaesth *43:*96, 1971.
21. Baines D, Keneally J: Anaesthetic implications of the mucopolysaccharidoses: a fifteen-year experience in a children's hospital. Anaesth Intens Care *11:*198, 1983.
22. Brosius FC, Roberts WC: Coronary artery disease in the Hurler syndrome. Am J Cardiol *47:*649, 1981.
23. Renteria VG, Ferrans VJ, Roberts WC: The heart in the Hurler syndrome. Am J Cardiol *38:*487, 1976.
24. Perks WH, Cooper RA, Bradbury S, et al.: Sleep apnoea in Scheie's syndrome. Thorax *35:*85, 1980.
25. Brill CB, Rose JS, Godmilow L, et al.: Spastic quadriparesis due to C_1-C_2 subluxation in Hurler syndrome. J Pediatr *92:*441, 1978.
26. Kempthorne PM, Brown TCK: Anaesthesia and the mucopolysaccaridoses: a survey of techniques and problems. Anaesth Intens Care *11:*203, 1983.
27. King DH, Jones RM, Barnett MB: Anaesthetic considerations and the mucopolysaccharidoses. Anaesthesia *39:*126, 1984.
28. Hopkins R, Watson JA, Jones JH, et al.: Two cases of Hunter's syndrome — the anaesthetic and operative difficulties in oral surgery. Br J Oral Surg *10:*286, 1973.
29. Kirkinshaw KJ: Anaesthesia in a patient with an unstable neck — Morquio's syndrome. Anaesthesia *30:*46, 1975.
30. Lipson SJ: Dysplasia of the ondontoid process in Morquio's syndrome causing quadriparesis. J Bone Joint Surg *59A:*340, 1977.
31. Pritzker MR, King RA, Kronenberg RS: Upper airway obstruction during head flexion in Morquio's disease. Am J Med *69:*467, 1980.
32. Jones AEP, Croley TF: Morquio syndrome and anesthesia. Anesthesiology *51:*261, 1979.
33. Scully RE, Mark EJ, McNeely BU: Case records of the Massachusetts General Hospital. N Engl J Med *310:*106, 1984.
34. Levy HL, Coulombe JT, Benjamin R: Massachusetts metabolic disorders screening program: III. Sarcosinemia. Pediatrics *74:*509, 1984.
35. Johnston K, Newth CJL, Shev KR, et al.: Central hypoventilation syndrome in pyruvate dehydrogenase complex deficiency. Pediatrics *74:*1034, 1984.

ORTHOPEDIC DISEASES

14

HELEN M. HOLTBY, M.B. ● *JOHN E. S. RELTON, M.B.*

Uncommon orthopedic problems in patients undergoing surgery include the congenital generalized diseases of bone and a variety of syndromes in which the bony manifestations are secondary to other major disorders. For example, radial aplasia may be associated with thrombocytopenia, facial anomalies, pulmonary and cardiac abnormalities, and Fanconi syndrome.

There are also many acquired bone diseases of significance to anesthetists, such as juvenile rheumatoid arthritis, systemic lupus erythematosus, and the rarer forms of collagen vascular disease.

The purpose of this chapter is to outline some of these rarer problems in orthopedic disease, to simplify the classification and make recommendations regarding management. There are few references in the literature concerning anesthetic management of specific syndromes, but those that are available are listed together with the surgical reports of management.

It must also be remembered that many children with orthopedic disease, particularly those with congenital disease, have had repeated hospitalization with its attendant psychological problems. They usually undergo repeated surgical procedures and have to cope with significant disability in their daily lives.

GENERALIZED CONSTITUTIONAL DISEASES OF BONE AND CARTILAGE

The classification of generalized diseases of bone and cartilage is undergoing constant review and the nomenclature is confusing. It includes a heterogeneous group of disorders whose pathogenesis in many cases remains unknown.

Table 14–1 shows an abbreviated form of the International Nomenclature for Constitutional Diseases of Bone first proposed in 1970[3, 6] and revised in 1977.[7] The classification is based as far as possible on the pathophysiology of the various disorders as demonstrated radiologically; however, there remain many synonyms and eponyms, which add to the difficulties in reviewing the literature. Even within the classification there is great heterogeneity of the various syndromes, especially among the osteochondrodysplasias.

This section will review some of the more common syndromes and outline the problems that may face the pediatric anesthetist in dealing with children with orthopedic disease. General guidelines in dealing with the rarer forms will also be discussed.

Osteochondrodysplasias

The osteochondrodysplasias constitute three major groups (Table 14–1) and include the numerous forms of dwarfism, of which over 70 have thus far been described. Many of these are exceptionally rare, with only one or two cases described; even the most common form, achondroplasia, has an incidence of only 15 per million live births.[8]

The first group, the chondrodystrophies, have been further divided into forms identifiable at birth and those identified in later life. The syndromes identifiable at birth are further subdivided into lethal and nonlethal forms. This is a somewhat artificial distinction, since there are occasional survivors into infancy of the so-called lethal forms. For example, camptomelic dwarfism is classified as a lethal form of dwarfism consisting of skeletal abnormalities, bowing of the femora and tibial micromelia, craniofacial abnormalities, and tracheobronchomalacia. One report describes a case in which the patient survived to the age of 6 years.[9] Frequently, death may occur in patients with a so-called nonlethal disease such as Jeune thoracic dystrophy.

The lethal forms of dwarfism include achondrogenesis, thanatophoric dwarfism, short-rib–polydactyly syndrome (types I and II), type I osteogenesis imperfecta, cerebrocostomandibular syndrome, hypophosphatasia, and usually the camptomelic syndrome. A majority are either stillborn or die within hours of birth and thus are of major interest only to geneticists. The most common cause of death is respiratory insufficiency due to malformation of either the chest wall or the tracheobronchial tree.

The nonlethal forms include achondroplasia and asphyxiating thoracic dystrophy.

Table 14–1. INTERNATIONAL NOMENCLATURE FOR CONSTITUTIONAL DISEASES OF BONE

I. Osteochondrodysplasias
   a. Defects of growth of tubular bones and/or spine
      i. Identifiable at birth, e.g., achondroplasia, asphyxiating thoracic dystrophy, chondrodysplasia punctata
      ii. Identifiable in later life, e.g., spondylometaphyseal dysplasia (McKusick)
   b. Disorganized development of cartilage and fibrous components, e.g., cherubism, neurofibromatosis
   c. Abnormalities of density of cortical diaphyseal structure and/or metaphyseal modeling; e.g., osteogenesis imperfecta, osteopetrosis
II. Dysostoses: malformation of individual bones singly or in combination
   a. Dysostoses with cranial and facial involvement
   b. Dysostoses with predominantly axial involvement
   c. Dysostoses with predominant involvement of extremities
III. Idiopathic osteolyses
IV. Chromosomal aberrations
V. Primary metabolic abnormalities
   a. Calcium and/or phosphorus
   b. Complex carbohydrates
   c. Lipids
   d. Nucleic acids
   e. Amino acids
   f. Metals

Achondroplasia

This is the most common chondrodystrophy, with an incidence of 15 per million live births.[8, 10, 11] It is readily recognizable at birth by the classical clinical features of rhizomelic (proximal) shortening of the limbs, a relatively long trunk, a large head with frontal bossing, depression of the nasal bridge, and a relatively prominent mandible. Characteristically the hands are tridentate, short, and broad.

Achondroplasia is inherited as an autosomal dominant with little clinical variability. Over 80 percent of achondroplastics have no family history of the deformity and are considered new mutations.[11] The disorder may be associated with increased paternal age.

The clinical course of achondroplasia is characterized by neurological, back, and lower limb problems. It is these difficulties that may bring the patient to surgery.

Megalencephaly is a usual finding; mildly dilated ventricles are very common and may be universal.[12] However, only a small proportion of patients develop hydrocephalus.[13] True hydrocephalus must be suspected if the head growth ceases to parallel the normal growth curve, albeit at above the 97th percentile. Hydrocephalus may be due to a small foramen magnum and present with signs of spinal cord compression. Odontoid abnormalities have also been reported and further encroach upon the small foramen magnum.

The signs of cord compression may be subtle or overt. They consist of respiratory difficulties, cyanosis after crying, poor head control, and quadriparesis. The deep tendon reflexes may remain normal.[14] Decompression by means of a suboccipital craniectomy is the treatment of choice. Failure to recognize spinal cord

compression may be the cause of the high mortality in infant achondroplastics.[15–17]

The spine is also affected with bony variations in the vertebrae and an abnormal configuration of the spinal canal, which tapers from top to bottom (in contrast to the normal taper from bottom to top). Thus, the lumbar spinal cord occupies the entire canal in the lumbar spine. The characteristic lumbar lordosis, which may be accompanied by compensatory kyphoscoliosis,[18] does not usually require surgical correction.

The combination of a narrow spinal canal and bony abnormality may result in a neurological deficit in the lower limbs,[19] but this is extremely rare in the pediatric population.[20]

Anesthetic Implications. Reports of the anesthetic management of achondroplastic patients in the literature[21-24] describe a number of actual and potential problems. The first consideration is of airway management. The facial abnormalities do not pose a significant problem, but the cervical spine abnormalities may limit neck extension and make intubation with direct laryngoscopy impossible.[24] Hyperextension or hyperflexion during intubation should be avoided owing to the risk of cervical cord compression. No guidelines are available regarding endotracheal tube size or length. Since the trunk is relatively normal, it is likely that achondroplastic patients will require a tube close to the usual size for age. If there is significant thoracic abnormality or muscular hypotonicity, ventilation should be controlled.

Another consideration is the use of conduction anesthesia. Opinion is divided in case reports regarding the advisability of performing major regional blocks.[21, 22] Although there are no reports of any serious complications, the possibility of neurological impairment following regional techniques must be borne in mind. Technical difficulties with lumbar puncture or epidural techniques are common.

Asphyxiating Thoracic Dystrophy (Jeune Syndrome)

This disease was first described by Jeune in 1954 and is classified as a nonlethal form of dwarfism, although it has a 50 percent mortality in early life. The genetic pattern of this disorder is unclear, but it is likely autosomal recessive.[6, 10] A link may exist between it and the Ellis–van Creveld syndrome (chondroectodermal dysplasia),[25, 26] but there are many differences and it seems likely that they are separate entities.

The clinical manifestations are variable, but the more severely affected infants have a stiff thorax that is small in all dimensions, with very short ribs and a prominent rib rosary in the midaxillary line. The hands and feet are short and broad and there may be postaxial polydactyly. Limb shortening is variable.

This disease is of interest because it has been noted that respiratory function tends to improve with age,[27] and so attempts have been made to support these infants until the child grows sufficiently.[28, 29] Enlargement of the thorax by surgical intervention may increase lung compliance, which, in combination with long-term ventilatory support, may provide substantial improvement. In reported cases it was observed that the underlying lung appeared normal. However, pulmonary hypoplasia, cysts, and other abnormalities have been reported.[30]

Associated problems include pulmonary hypertension and occasional cardiac defects. Renal disease with proteinuria, hypertension, and uremia[31] is a significant cause of death in children surviving infancy.

Anesthetic Implications. Serious difficulty may be encountered in ventilating these infants preoperatively. There is a significant incidence of barotrauma.

Hypoxia and hypercarbia occur frequently. Pulmonary hypertension may contribute to an early demise. The larynx has been noted to be small in both children with the syndrome and their mothers.[29] One case is reported of management by long-term nasotracheal intubation (3½ years!) with surprisingly few complications.[28] In this case, no mention was made of endotracheal tube size.

If surgery to enlarge the thorax is contemplated, major blood loss should be anticipated along with a large flail segment in the postoperative period necessitating, at the very least, short-term ventilatory support.

In older children, regardless of the surgery contemplated, it should be borne in mind that there is limited respiratory reserve. Renal function should be checked preoperatively.

Chondro-Ectodermal Dysplasia (Ellis–van Creveld Syndrome)

This disorder has features in common with asphyxiating thoracic dystrophy but is felt to be a separate entity. It was first described in 1940[32] and is inherited as an autosomal recessive. The largest incidence of the syndrome occurs in the Amish people of Lancaster County, Pennsylvania,[33] although over 40 other cases have been reported worldwide.

Clinical Course. The skeletal abnormalities consist of polydactyly, mesomelic dwarfism, and a long narrow thorax; there are also abnormalities of the nails and teeth.

Respiratory distress is common in the newborn period and is related to absence of cartilage in the tracheobronchial tree, which tends therefore to collapse and cause tension lobar emphysema.[34] Cardiac anomalies have been reported to affect as many as 60 percent of patients, but this may represent an overestimate[33] inasmuch as individuals with cardiac symptoms are more likely to seek medical attention. The most common abnormalities are atrial and ventricular septal defects, often with complete absence of the septum. Cleft mitral valve may also occur.

Dental anomalies are common, and erupted teeth may be present at birth.

Anesthetic Implications. There are no reports of anesthetic experience with these children, and indeed the Amish people treated polydactyly by amputation using string binding without benefit of surgeon or anesthetist!

A major consideration is the cardiorespiratory status. Physical examination may reveal significant heart disease preoperatively, so that antibiotic prophylaxis can be given and management plans formulated. There is a continual problem of airway collapse and emphysema in neonates and infants, particularly if they are allowed to breathe spontaneously. Conversely, high airway pressures during positive-pressure ventilation should be avoided because of barotrauma and gas trapping. Nitrous oxide should be avoided if emphysema is present.

Chondrodysplasia Punctata

Chondrodysplasia punctata describes a heterogeneous group of disorders associated with radiographic stippling of the epiphyses and extraepiphyseal cartilage. There are several synonyms and eponyms (chondrodystrophia calcificans congenita, Conradi disease, stippled epiphyses), and there are probably at least two distinct genetic entities.[10]

Over 100 cases have been described in the literature, revealing a variety of manifestations of multisystem involvement. The most constant characteristics include short stature, typical facies with hypertelorism, saddle nose, frontal bossing, high arched palate, short neck, and tracheal stenosis.[35] Additional findings which are less constant include renal anomalies, congenital heart disease,[36] and neurological abnormalities; in one study all patients examined had major abnormalities of the central nervous system, which included Dandy-Walker malformation of the fourth ventricle.[37] Atlantoaxial instability may also occur.[38]

Anesthetic Implications. The facial abnormalities and tracheal stenosis make difficulty with the airway a distinct possibility. The lower jaw is normal. The presence of atlantoaxial instability demands extreme care at intubation.

Renal function should be checked preoperatively and any evidence of renal impairment noted and investigated. Examination may reveal significant cardiac anomalies, and antibiotic prophylaxis must be used. Hydrocephalus may be present with the concomitant danger of coning of the medulla during anesthesia.

Osteogenesis Imperfecta

This is a connective tissue disorder primarily affecting bone. The earliest known case was probably that of Ivar the Boneless in the 9th century, and there are descriptions dating from the 16th century.[2, 41]

The etiology of the disorder is complex. There is considerable evidence supporting an autosomal dominant inheritance with full penetrance but variable expressivity, but cases occur that would suggest an autosomal recessive inheritance.

There is no consensus regarding its precise pathophysiology.[36] The basic defect appears to involve the synthesis of collagen. There is also evidence that there is some disturbance of high-energy phosphate metabolism[39] because there are abnormalities in platelet aggregation, increased oxygen consumption, evidence of generally elevated metabolic rates,[40] and raised serum thyroxine levels.

Clinical Course. Three clinical forms are recognized, although these may be different manifestations of the same entity. Type I, osteogenesis imperfecta congenita, is usually the most severe form; type II, osteogenesis imperfecta tarda gravis, presents from birth up to 1 year; and type III, osteogenesis imperfecta tarda levis, presents from 1 year onward. The classic triad of blue sclera, multiple fractures, and deafness is not constant,[41] with deafness being present in only about 10 percent of each type.

Osteogenesis imperfecta congenita has an incidence of 1 in 20,000 to 1 in 60,000 live births. It may be recognized prenatally through ultrasound diagnosis. At birth it may present as a stillbirth either from fractures in utero or from intracerebral hemorrhage due to the trauma of delivery on an unossified and fragile skull. If the infant survives, respiratory failure from marked thoracic involvement is a common cause of death in the neonatal period.

Trivial trauma such as changing a diaper or the application of a blood pressure cuff may result in transverse subperiosteal fractures. Over time gross deformity occurs, particularly in the long bones, due to repeated fractures, which are painful and debilitating.

Other clinical findings are dentinogenesis imperfecta (discolored and brittle teeth), ligamentous laxity, scoliosis, cardiovascular anomalies, and an ill-defined bleeding diathesis that is probably secondary to platelet dysfunction.

Scoliosis is a very common finding and is particularly difficult to treat.[42] However, there are case reports of successful surgical management.[41, 42]

The cardiovascular abnormalities include aortic and mitral regurgitation as a result of dilatation of the valvular annulus, abnormalities of the chordae tendineae, and cystic medial necrosis of the aorta.[43]

Management. The medical management of osteogenesis imperfecta has been disappointing. Calcitonin, anabolic steroids, and sodium fluoride do not provide any real benefit.

The surgical management has usually been directed toward correcting any deformity whenever possible, particularly in the lower limbs, which tend to bear the brunt of the disorder. Ambulation is the key aim. The most commonly performed procedures are intramedullary nailing of the femur and Sofield osteotomies with pin fixation[44] to correct tibial deformity. Harrington instrumentations[41] and modified Dwyer procedures[42] have been performed to correct scoliosis.

Anesthetic Implications. These children constitute a major problem if their disease is severe since monitoring, positioning, establishment of IV access, and control of the airway all place them at risk of further fractures. It is important to document old and new fractures preoperatively and check for fractures postoperatively.

The use of a sphygmomanometer cuff to establish IV access may be contraindicated. Control of bleeding in the operative field by tourniquet may also be contraindicated, and this, together with a tendency to bleed, may make surgery technically difficult. Bleeding is a particular problem during correction of scoliosis.

Scrupulous care of the fragile teeth must be exercised when applying the mask and during laryngoscopy. Succinylcholine is relatively contraindicated owing to the danger of fasciculation-induced fractures.

Significant scoliosis causes ventilation-perfusion abnormalities and the potential for hypoxemia, particularly in patients breathing spontaneously. Cardiovascular anomalies, if present, will need appropriate management including antibiotic prophylaxis. Deafness makes communication difficult, and repeated hospitalizations and chronic pain add psychological problems to the considerable practical difficulties.

Prepubertal children with osteogenesis imperfecta tend to show a rise in temperature under anesthesia,[45] but this is not felt to be due to malignant hyperthermia[46] and is easily controlled with surface cooling and cold IV solutions.

One report of anesthetic experience exists[47] in which the satisfactory use of intramuscular ketamine for repeated procedures on a 4-year-old child with severe osteogenesis imperfecta is described. Other reports of open heart surgery on patients with osteogenesis imperfecta make no comment on the anesthesia but do describe problems with bleeding following cardiopulmonary bypass.[48, 49]

Osteopetrosis (Albers-Schönberg Disease)

Albers-Schönberg disease may present either in an autosomal recessive form, which usually results in death in infancy, or in an autosomal dominant form, which does not present until early adulthood.

The usual presentation of the infantile type is a failure to thrive in the first few months of life. Frequently, petechiae or ecchymoses are seen and the infant is pale and unwell. Megalocephaly or true hydrocephalus may be present. Abnormal eye movements are often seen, and examination may reveal optic atrophy. Variable degrees of hepatosplenomegaly may occur.[3, 10, 36]

Radiological examination reveals a generalized skeletal density with disturbed mineralization at the growth plates similar to rickets. There is profound anemia, thrombocytopenia, and neutropenia. Serum calcium is frequently low despite an increase in calcium uptake from the gut. The anesthetic implications are (1) fractures (despite the density, the bones are brittle); (2) pancytopenia, with the implications of anemia, risk of infection, and bleeding disorders; and (3) hypocalcemia, which renders the patient susceptible to arrhythmias, seizures, and possible difficulty in reversing nondepolarizing neuromuscular blockade.

General Guidelines for the Management of Osteochondrodysplasias

Since there are so many different syndromes classified under the general title of osteochondrodystophies, and many of them are rare, it would seem useful to have a general plan for the preoperative assessment and intraoperative management of these patients. This will embrace the significant problems.

There are a number of problems that are common to many of the dwarfing syndromes:

1. Odontoid Hypoplasia and/or Atlantoaxial Instability.[20, 50] Preoperatively patients with these problems should wherever possible have clinical and radiological examination of the cervical spine, and great care should be taken when intubating them.

It should be remembered that the classic pyramidal tract signs and symptoms of cord compression are often not seen in infants and children. Suspicions should be raised by a history of cyanosis after crying or feeding, respiratory difficulties, poor head control, fatigue, and decreased exercise tolerance, all of which may appear before any pyramidal tract signs are detected.[13, 14, 50] Surgical fusion of the cervical vertebrae is recommended for these patients.

The syndromes (or groups of syndromes) in which this is most commonly seen are (1) achondroplasia (these patients may also have stenosis of foramen magnum), (2) mucopolysaccharidoses, (3) spondyloepiphyseal dysplasia (all forms including pseudoachondroplasia), (4) chondrodysplasia punctata, (5) metatropic dwarfism, (6) Kniest syndrome, (7) cartilage-hair hypoplasia (McKusick) (metaphyseal chondrodysplasia) and (8) Dyggve-Melchior-Clausen dysplasia. It should be noted that a majority of patients with abnormalities of the atlantoaxial joint are stable, though they may have limited neck mobility. Patients presenting with quadriparesis may have overt or occult autonomic instability, rendering them susceptible to cardiac arrhythmias and acute changes in blood pressure. It may be difficult to wean such a patient from artificial ventilation.

2. Airway Problems. Many airway problems will be evident on examination of the child; the syndromes mentioned in the preceding paragraph are all complicated by potential airway problems, which may be compounded by micrognathia, cleft palate, and tracheal stenosis. The craniofacial abnormalities are dealt with separately (see Chapter 9), so the following list is far from exhaustive: (1) mesomelic dysplasia, (2) diastrophic dwarfism, (3) Kniest syndrome, and (4) spondyloepiphyseal dysplasia.

3. Thoracic Dystrophy. The asphyxiating thoracic dystrophy of Jeune is an obvious example of thoracic abnormality with short stature, but there are also a number of other syndromes in which the chest cavity is small and may also be noncompliant. Such patients may have problems with repeated chest infections, hypoxemia, increased work of breathing, and ultimately pulmonary vascular changes. Many die in the neonatal period. Conditions involving thoracic dystrophy include: (1) asphyxiating thoracic dystrophy (Jeune), (2) metaphyseal chondrodysplasia (Jansen), (3) metaphyseal dwarfism, (4) achondroplasia, (5) Ellis–van Creveld syndrome, (6) lymphopenic agammaglobulinemia, (7) camptomelic dwarfism, and (8) osteogenesis imperfecta congenita.

4. Kyphoscoliosis. Kyphoscoliosis occurs in a majority of dwarfing syndromes. In some cases, such as in achondroplasia, marked kyphosis and lordosis compound the structural problems of a small spinal canal, leading to neurological impairment. However, this is not common in the pediatric age group.

5. Cardiac Disease. Septal defects, patent ductus arteriosus, and other cardiac anomalies are associated with a number of dwarfing conditions: (1) Ellis–van Creveld syndrome, (2) Holt-Oram (described below), (3) metaphyseal chondrodysplasia, and (4) osteogenesis imperfecta. In addition, many patients with dwarfing syndromes have mental retardation, central nervous system abnormalities with or without hydrocephalus, and seizure disorders.

A careful preoperative assessment should reveal most of the significant problems and enable a plan of management to be formulated. One further consideration is that neither age nor weight[22] gives a reliable prediction of endotracheal tube size or length. No anesthetic drugs are contraindicated because of short stature per se, although airway problems or other complications may dictate a particular technique of management. Doubts have been expressed concerning the use of regional techniques in adult achondroplastics,[12, 22] although such techniques have been used. In view of the rarity of neurological problems in achondroplastic children, caudal block, though possibly technically difficult, is probably not contraindicated.

Dysostoses

The dysostoses are malformations of individual bones arising singly or in combination. The craniofacial dysostoses constitute a single group and are reviewed elsewhere (see Chapter 9). Several of these patients also exhibit axial involvement (for example, in Goldenhar syndrome). Of the dysostoses with predominantly axial involvement the Klippel-Feil syndrome is probably the most common. These disorders may present local problems (for example, intubation difficulties due to severely limited neck mobility) and systemic manifestations such as congenital heart disease and urinary tract abnormalities. These patients frequently require surgery for scoliosis arising from their structural vertebral abnormalities, particularly isolated hemivertebrae.

The dysostoses often present with predominant involvement of the extremities. The most commonly seen examples are syndactyly and polydactyly, which may be seen in combination with craniofacial or other abnormalities, as in Apert syndrome or Carpenter syndrome. Laryngeal abnormalities, particularly atresia, stenosis, or web, may occur.

The syndromes described below illustrate some of the potential general problems that should be kept in mind in treating the child with a peripheral abnormality.

Radial Dysgenesis[51]

There are two types of radial dysgenesis. Either total absence or partial absence (usually of the distal portion) of the radius may occur, and the incidence of each type is about equal. Unilateral cases occur most frequently on the right side and account for about 50 percent of cases. The male:female ratio is about 3:2. This deformity is frequently associated with other defects, such as vascular and musculoskeletal abnormalities of the limb. It is rarely seen as an isolated defect (1 in 55,000 live births).

Radial and thumb aplasia may be associated with several chromosomal aberrations, notably trisomy 18 (1 in 6600 live births), chromosome 13q−, and trisomy 13. The combination of chromosomal abnormalities and radial dysgenesis usually implies multiple other abnormalities, including congenital heart disease[52] and severe mental retardation. The life expectancy is usually less than 3 years. Two other syndromes with mental retardation and radial aplasia that may cause problems for the anesthetist, because of potential airway and intubation difficulties, are bird-headed dwarfism and Cornelia de Lange syndrome. Varying degrees of mental retardation, microcephaly, and a characteristic facies occur in both these rare syndromes.

The association between craniofacial abnormalities and radial dysplasia is quite frequent. Some 7 percent of patients with radial aplasia have a cleft lip and palate. It is also seen in association with Treacher Collins syndrome, Goldenhar syndrome, craniosynostosis, and abnormalities of the tracheobronchial tree, notably laryngeal atresia and laryngeal web.

Cardiac anomalies may also occur in two forms of heart-hand syndrome[53] (Holt-Oram and Lewis upper limb cardiovascular syndrome). Holt-Oram syndrome is an autosomal dominant disorder with variable expressivity (usually worse in females) and consists of mild congenital heart disease (atrial septal defect in 70 percent of patients) combined with radial aplasia and abnormalities of the hand. Cardiac rhythm disturbances, both atrial and ventricular, are occasionally present together with conduction defects. In Lewis syndrome, which is also autosomal dominant, the cardiovascular anomalies are more variable but are usually nonfatal. There are multiple skeletal abnormalities of the upper limb.

Radial aplasia is seen with Fanconi syndrome, which consists of pancytopenia with bone marrow hypoplasia, multiple congenital defects, and renal tubular acidosis usually secondary to cystinosis (see Chapter 7). Seventy percent of patients show abnormalities of the radius, 20 percent are mentally retarded, and a variable number have congenital heart disease and congenital hip dislocation. The pancytopenia does not usually become pronounced with childhood, although this is variable. Preoperative assessment of renal function, avoidance of renally excreted drugs, and correction of metabolic disturbances may be required. The pancytopenia may be severe enough to require reverse isolation and transfusion of blood components either preor intraoperatively.

A second hematological disorder associated with bilateral radial aplasia is the TAR syndrome (thrombocytopenia, absent radius), in which profound thrombocytopenia is seen in infancy. If at all possible, surgery should be avoided in patients with the TAR syndrome until age 1 year, by which time platelet counts have usually risen significantly. Episodic thrombocytopenia may be precipitated by minor illness or stress, and counts as low as 15,000 per μl are not unusual. This syndrome is autosomal recessive and has a high mortality (30 to 40 percent) in the first year of life owing to intracranial hemorrhage.

Finally, radial aplasia is seen as part of the VATER association,[54] which is an unexplained grouping of abnormalities including vertebral segmentation, congenital scoliosis, imperforate anus, tracheoesophageal fistula, renal abnormalities, absent radius, and congenital heart disease. As the radial agenesis is the most obvious defect seen at birth, it should trigger a search for other anomalies. It has been noted that as the number of defects increases, so does the mortality.[55]

METABOLIC DISEASES OF BONE

There are a large number of metabolic disturbances, including the mucopolysaccharidoses, mucolipidoses, and disorders of glycogen synthesis and storage, that show bony abnormalities as part of the disease process.[36] However, the orthopedic problems are rarely if ever of prime importance. Renal and endocrine disorders are also associated with derangements of calcium metabolism and abnormalities in bone growth, but again, these rarely require the attention of the orthopedic surgeon and in any case are secondary to the ongoing primary disease process.

Metabolism and Control of Calcium[36, 56]

Bone is formed from calcium phosphate impregnated onto an organic matrix of collagen fibers and ground substance of glycosaminoglycans and glycoproteins. Calcium is the most prevalent electrolyte in the body, forming about 1.6 percent of the body weight in the adult.

The absolute and relative calcium content of the body increases rapidly from the seventh month in utero to adulthood. At 7 months the calcium content of the fetus is 8 g, and this rises fourfold to some 30 g at term. It reaches 1100 g in the adult. About 99 percent of this calcium is fixed in the skeleton; the remaining 1 percent occurs free as ionized calcium (0.4 percent) or bound to plasma proteins and chelating agents such as citrate (0.6 percent).

Calcium has many important functions; its primary importance (in bulk at least) is in the formation of ossified bone, providing a rigid framework for the body. However, it is also a critical factor in cellular membrane permeability and enzyme function throughout the body.

Calcium levels in the body are governed by intake, excretion, and mobilization of body stores, which can be modified by the hormonal influences of PTH (parathormone), calcitonin, and the active form of vitamin D. Calcium absorption is entirely from the gut and is modified by the activity of a transport protein whose synthesis is inhibited by renal insufficiency and decreased levels of vitamin D. Calcium is eliminated via the kidneys and the gut and to a limited extent through the skin.

Vitamin D is absorbed in the gut and transformed in the body to a number of active metabolites, of which the most significant is 1,25-dihydroxycholecalciferol, which is synthesized by the kidney from 25-hydroxycholecalciferol in response to decreased serum calcium levels. The effects of 1,25-dihydroxycholecalciferol are to increase calcium absorption from the gut, increase phosphate reabsorption in the kidney, and liberate calcium from bone. In turn, the conversion of vitamin D to its active form is regulated by PTH. The normal infant needs about 400 to 800 international units/day of vitamin D to prevent dietary rickets. Hypervitaminosis D (greater than 5000 units daily for several years) results in hypercalcemia with ectopic calcification and hypercalciuria with stone formation and renal damage. In children the hypercalcemia may result in arrested growth with a permanent defect. Hypervitaminosis D during pregnancy may result in supravalvular aortic stenosis in the infant.[57]

Parathormone (PTH) is secreted by the parathyroid gland in response to a decrease in serum calcium. Its exact mechanism of action is unknown, but it increases the cell membrane permeability to calcium, increases levels of cyclic AMP, liberates calcium from bone by stimulation of the formation of osteoclasts, and increases tubular reabsorption of calcium while decreasing phosphate reabsorption. The net effect therefore is to increase serum calcium levels.

The third hormone involved in calcium homeostasis is calcitonin, discovered by Copp in 1962, which is secreted from the parafollicular cells of the thyroid gland. Hypercalcemia stimulates the secretion of calcitonin, which in turn effects direct inhibition of bone resorption. This occurs by a mechanism separate from the action of PTH that affects osteoclast and osteoblast activity.

Thus, there are many factors that influence the maintenance of serum calcium levels within the normal range of 2.2 to 2.7 mmol/L. Derangements in this process lead to abnormalities of bone growth, disturbances of membrane and enzyme function, and renal impairment.

Hypocalcemia

Hypocalcemia is very common in the newborn period, especially if the infant suffers fetal distress during delivery. The stores of calcium in the newborn are very small. A combination of respiratory alkalosis and elevated serum bicarbonate from overzealous resuscitation will tend to decrease further the serum ionized calcium level. Hypocalcemia also occurs with vitamin D deficiency states (whether absolute or relative) and in the various forms of hypoparathyroidism. The DiGeorge syndrome (thymic hypoplasia and hypoparathyroidism) is a rare cause of hypocalcemia.

Acute hypocalcemia decreases the threshold for neuronal excitability, leading to tetany and seizures. Prolongation of atrioventricular conduction in the heart gives rise to heart block. Delayed repolarization leads to a prolonged Q-T interval and ventricular dysrhythmias. Cardiac contractility and vasomotor tone are decreased, resulting in hypotension.

Chronic hypocalcemia may be asymptomatic.

Anesthetic Implications. The use of potent inhalational anesthetics will increase the degree of hypotension and myocardial depression. Halothane may worsen the atrioventricular block and increase the risk of arrhythmia. The tendency for tetanic contracture affects muscle of the vocal cords, so laryngospasm is a likely occurrence. This may be exacerbated by exogenous or endogenous catecholamines. Muscular weakness and difficulty in reversing neuromuscular blockade should be anticipated.

Acute hypocalcemia is treated by the administration of intravenous calcium chloride or calcium gluconate. A continuous infusion may be needed, especially in neonates. The maintenance dose is 2 mmol/kg/24 hours. Hypokalemia and hypomagnesemia both exacerbate the effects of hypocalcemia and hinder efforts to restore normal calcium levels.

Hypercalcemia

Hypercalcemia may arise as a result of hypervitaminosis D or hyperparathyroidism. Occasionally, patients (especially those with sarcoidosis) show hypersensitivity to vitamin D. Hypercalcemia may also be seen with lymphoproliferative disorders such as myeloma. Hyperparathyroidism commonly presents with a vague clinical picture and a history of renal calculi (see Chapter 7). Serum calcium levels of 3.5 mmol/L or higher are associated with abdominal pains, anorexia, nausea and vomiting, polyuria, dehydration, tachycardia, and hypertension (stones, bones, and abdominal groans!).

Treatment should be commenced immediately. It should begin with rehydration of the patient with a sodium containing solution and administration of furosemide 0.5 to 1 mg/kg q 4 to 6 hours to encourage the saline-induced calciuria. Potassium supplements will be required to avoid furosemide-induced hypokalemia. Steroids have been found to be useful in lymphoproliferative disorders and in the management of vitamin D intoxication. The cytotoxic antibiotic mithramycin has also been used and is extremely effective in the longer term, but requires 48 to 72 hours to take effect. Calcium disodium edetate (EDTA) may also be used but it is not recommended owing to the danger of an acute excessive fall in serum calcium.

Anesthetic Implications. Circulating volume must be restored, and an assessment of the degree of dehydration may be difficult owing to hypertension. Care must be taken with drug doses in the child with volume concentration. Potent inhalational agents may unmask a low circulating volume by causing vasodilatation.

Paralytic ileus may cause regurgitation and the possibility of aspiration at induction. A rapid-sequence induction is therefore recommended.

Metabolism and Control of Phosphate

Phosphate is an important constituent of high-energy bonds and modifies calcium concentrations in tissues. It is also a significant buffer of intracellular fluid and plays a primary role in renal excretion of hydrogen ions.

Phosphate is absorbed by an active process from the gut. This is modified by high concentrations of calcium or aluminum, which form insoluble salts and decrease absorption, and by vitamin D, which increases phosphate absorption. It is excreted via the kidneys. In children there is a net positive balance of phosphate and the serum phosphate level is higher than in adults. This relative increase in phosphate increases the affinity of hemoglobin for oxygen, and a hypothesis has been proposed that this explains the physiological anemia of childhood.[58]

Calcium and phosphate levels in blood are inversely related; a reduction in plasma phosphate levels permits increases in calcium levels and inhibits deposition of more bone salt. Conversely, elevated plasma phosphate levels facilitate the effects of calcitonin.

Rickets

Rickets is a disorder of growing bone characterized by a decrease in bone anabolism and minimal mineralization of the new bone. The four principal causes of rickets are vitamin D deficiency, renal tubular insufficiency, chronic renal failure, and hypophosphatasia.

Simple deficiency of vitamin D is well recognized but still remains relatively frequent (compared, for example, with scurvy). Premature infants are particularly at risk because of diminished stores. The major concerns in anesthetizing such infants relate to their poor dentition and their general debility. They may present with muscular hypotonia, a hypochromic anemia, and other deficiency states. If vitamin D deficiency remains untreated, kyphoscoliosis may eventually develop. The serum calcium level is usually normal, but the phosphate level is low because of a compensatory elevation of parathormone levels. There is a high incidence of hyperchloremic acidosis secondary to renal phosphate loss. Supplementation with vitamin D, calcium, and phosphate is required for treatment. It is important not to supplement phosphate alone (despite the often normal serum calcium), since total body calcium is depleted and life-threatening hypocalcemia may occur with acute elevation of the serum phosphate level.

Rickets due to renal tubular insufficiency occurs in a number of disorders that result in either excess phosphate loss (most commonly) or excess calcium loss from the renal tubule. Simple hypophosphatemic vitamin D refractory rickets, hypophosphatemic vitamin D refractory rickets with aminoaciduria, and hypophosphatemic vitamin D refractory rickets with aminoaciduria and acidosis are all treated with large doses of vitamin D and phosphates.[59, 60] The last two syndromes have been referred to as the Fanconi syndrome and are included together in some texts. Close supervision of children with this disorder is necessary to prevent vitamin D toxicity with its attendant risk of renal damage and hypercalcemia (see Chapter 7).

The surgical treatment of these patients includes correction of lower limb and pelvic deformities and treatment of kyphoscoliosis. It is important that vitamin D supplementation be discontinued 4 to 6 weeks preoperatively, since immobilization results in increased demineralization of bone, which may lead to dangerous levels of hypercalcemia and hypercalciuria. Obviously if children with this disorder present for emergency surgery, urinary and serum calcium levels must be followed in the postoperative period and treatment instigated.

DISORDERS OF THE SPINE

Spinal disorders in children may be congenital or acquired. With the widespread use of vaccination against poliomyelitis and the increasing rarity of disseminated tuberculosis in the western world the acquired forms are becoming relatively rare.

Congenital spinal disorders may be classified in several ways: by the resultant deformity (for example, kyphosis, scoliosis), by the location of the apex of the curve produced, or by the anatomical defect causing the deformity.

Associated anomalies are common in congenital disorders of the spine; the VATER association has already been described (see page 366). In a series of 170 patients with congenital spinal deformities 110 anomalies outside the verteberal column were seen.[61] There is an association between congenital cyanotic heart disease and scoliosis.[62, 63]

Some 20 to 30 percent of children with congenital spinal abnormalities have urogenital anomalies. Careful evaluation of the urogenital tract is essential to detect occult renal disease secondary to chronic obstruction.

Other problems that occur include facial anomalies (notably Goldenhar syndrome), lung abnormalities, and gastrointestinal malformations (commonly tracheoesophageal fistula and imperforate anus).

Scoliosis is the most frequent feature of spinal disease and often requires surgical treatment.

Scoliosis

Scoliosis is derived from the Greek word meaning "crooked."[1] It can be defined as lateral deviation and rotation of a series of vertebrae from the midline anatomical position of the normal spinal axis. There are two fundamental types of scoliosis: functional (or postural) scoliosis, in which the curve is flexible and can be corrected by changes in posture, and structural scoliosis, in which the curvature is fixed. The classification of scoliosis on an etiological basis as outlined by Cobb is seen in Table 14–2. This may be further

Table 14–2. CLASSIFICATION OF SCOLIOSIS

Functional (Postural)
Structural
  Congenital
  Acquired
    Idiopathic
      Infantile
      Juvenile
      Adolescent
    Neuromuscular
      Poliomyelitis
      Von Recklinghausen disease
      Friedreich ataxia
      Cerebral palsy
      Syringomyelia
      Myelodysplasias
      Intraspinal tumor
      Muscular dystrophies
      Arthrogryposis multiplex congenita
    Osteogenic
      Postempyema, post-thoracoplasty,
        postirradiation, inflammatory conditions,
        rheumatoid, tuberculotic
      Tumors, e.g., osteoid osteoma
      Osteochondrodystrophies
      Osteogenesis imperfecta
      Scoliosis in congenital heart disease
    Traumatic
    Riley-Day syndrome (familial dysautonomia)
    Congenital indifference to pain

expanded by adding, for example, the different anatomical subsets of congenital vertebral anomalies leading to congenital scoliosis. The basic pathophysiology remains unknown with the exception of those types of scoliosis secondary to neuromuscular disease in which the pathophysiological process may be due to muscular imbalance pulling the spinal column into abnormal configuration.

Congenital scoliosis is a lateral curve of the spine arising as a result of vertebral anomalies. Some anomalies cause so little deformity that they remain undetected, so the true incidence is unknown. Multiple anomalies are usually hereditary, whereas single ones are often sporadic. The scoliosis is often rigid and may be very difficult to treat. It is more common in girls than in boys. The prognosis is variable depending on the nature of the abnormality. The most severe form of scoliosis occurs when there is an unsegmented bar with an isolated contralateral hemivertebra. In such a case the spine deteriorates rapidly and may attain a curvature before 3 years of age.[64]

Some 80 percent of cases requiring surgical correction are idiopathic in etiology, and 80 to 85 percent of these cases are in females. The incidence in North America is 4 per 1000 live births.[65] There is a striking geographical difference between England and North America in the incidence of infantile scoliosis, which is infrequent in North America but almost as common as adolescent scoliosis in England.[66, 67] The infant is usually male (90 percent of cases) with a left-sided curve that often disappears spontaneously,[68] although in some cases there is rapid progression with severe deformity.[69] The adolescent, on the other hand, is usually female (85 percent) with a right-sided curve, but again only about 10 percent require active treatment. However, with an overall incidence of 4 per 1000, this constitutes a significant number of patients.

The neuromuscular forms of scoliosis can demonstrate rapid deterioration and often require both anterior and posterior fixation.[1] Poliomyelitis is now a rare cause of scoliosis, although before the introduction of vaccination the incidence of paralytic scoliosis approached that of the idiopathic type. The curvature usually presents some 2 years after the acute illness and can increase rapidly if this period coincides with a growth spurt.[70]

In 10 percent of children with neurofibromatosis (von Recklinghausen disease) a spinal curvature develops. This bears no relation anatomically to the location of neurofibromas and is most commonly a sharply angled thoracic kyphoscoliosis. These children require careful preoperative assessment to rule out pheochromocytoma, which although still rare is more common in patients with this disease than in the general population. (Pheochromocytoma has an incidence of 1:1000 hypertensive patients. Probably less than 5 percent of pheochromocytomas are associated with neurofibromatosis.) In children sustained hypertension is the rule,[71] rather than the episodic hypertension that is the classic presenting feature of pheochromocytoma.

Death from scoliosis has been recognized since the time of Hippocrates,[4] and is due to cardiorespiratory failure. Associated neuromuscular weakness or congenital cardiac disease may add to this mortality.

Cardiorespiratory Pathophysiology

The most common finding associated with scoliosis is an abnormality in pulmonary function (Fig. 14–1). This is a restrictive pattern of disease, with the most striking reduction occurring in vital capacity and smaller reductions in total lung capacity and functional residual capacity.[72] In children with idiopathic and congenital scoliosis, in contrast to adult patients, thoracic elastance remains normal.[73]

The major abnormalities in gas exchange are alveolar hypoventilation[74] with increased ventilation-perfusion abnormality,[75] leading to an increased alveolar to arterial oxygen gradient and reduced PaO_2.[76] Although V_D/V_T ratios are elevated, the $PaCO_2$ remains normal until late in the disease. Thus elevation of $PaCO_2$ is an ominous sign. However, the response to carbon dioxide is impaired relatively early in the disease.[77] Severe infantile scoliosis results in decreased alveolar development.[78]

Cardiovascular compromise is a later development arising from the sequelae of pulmonary hypertension triggered by low lung volumes and chronic hypoxia. Pulmonary hypertension ultimately progresses to cor pulmonale and death. The signs of pulmonary hypertension (right ventricular enlargement, loud pulmonic second sound, and murmur of pulmonary insufficiency) should be sought in any patient with more than a 65-degree curvature and a long history of scoliosis.

The ECG changes of right ventricular hypertrophy and right atrial enlargement are late developments. Phonocardiography is a more sensitive investigation[79] and demonstrates a prolonged interval between pulmonary valve closure and tricuspid opening before clinical or electrocardiographic changes.

These cardiorespiratory changes may be complicated by neuromuscular disease, resulting in inadequate cough and inability to clear secretions despite a relatively normal vital capacity. Cyanotic congenital heart disease accentuates the arterial hypoxemia and may hasten the onset of pulmonary hypertension. Cardiac failure per se will also complicate management.

Surgical correction of the deformity ideally should be performed before cardiorespiratory compromise has occurred. However, operation is often well tolerated despite striking reductions in vital capacity (below 35 percent of predicted values), particularly in the absence of neuromuscular disease. Patients with a vital capacity less than 30 percent of predicted values usually require postoperative mechanical ventilation.[80, 81]

Surgical treatment of scoliosis generally does not result in any significant change in pulmonary function as determined by lung volume studies,[82] although some improvement may occur in younger patients.[83] Improvement in gas exchange has been demonstrated.[84] Surgery does, however, make a significant contribution to maintaining mobility in these children[1] and arrests the deterioration in pulmonary function.

Anesthetic Considerations

Preoperative Assessment. Preoperatively the etiology of the scoliosis should be assessed and a search made for associated abnormalities. A majority of patients presenting for corrective surgery do not suffer pulmonary impairment. If the spinal curvature is less than 65 degrees (Cobb), lung function can be regarded as "normal" in most cases. Increasing pulmonary dysfunction is found in cases with a greater curvature, particularly if the deformity is compounded by the presence of neuromuscular disease or excessive lordosis. Formal testing of pulmonary function must be performed in all such cases. Patients who demonstrate significant respiratory compromise should be warned about the possibility of postoperative mechanical ven-

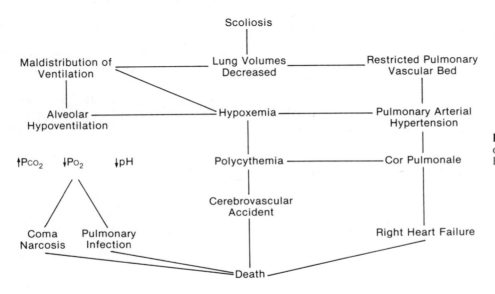

Figure 14–1. Pathophysiology of scoliosis. (Courtesy of Dr. Henry Levison.)

tilation. Narcotic premedication should be avoided in cases of severe respiratory impairment.

Difficulty may be encountered in those patients who have undergone preoperative correction of a curvature by exoskeletal apparatus such as skull halo–pelvic hoop traction or a body cast. In this group of patients muscle relaxants should not be used until control of the airway by intubation is accomplished by one of several alternative techniques.[88] In severe cases of scoliosis tracheal shortening or distortion may occur, and kinking of the pulmonary artery has been reported.[86]

Corrective Surgery by the Posterior Approach

Operative procedures to reduce the deformity by the posterior approach involve spinal fusion following corrective stabilization. This is usually achieved by Harrington or Luque instrumentation. The patient must be in the prone position in order to accomplish the extensive dissection. Severe blood loss may occur. The causes of this blood loss may be summarized as follows:[87]

1. Vertebral venous engorgement. Pressure applied to the anterior abdominal wall may cause partial or complete obstruction of the inferior vena cava, thereby diverting the venous return through Batson's plexus into the vertebral venous plexuses.

2. Surgical factors. These include the nature and extent of the procedure; the ease or difficulty of the dissection; and the time involved in applying the instruments, especially after the vertebrae have been decorticated. In one series of cases[89] operative blood loss varied from 8 to 67 percent of the estimated blood volume depending on the etiology of the disease and the complexity of the surgical procedure. Particularly severe hemorrhage often accompanies surgical correction of scoliosis in patients with Duchenne muscular dystrophy.

Blood loss may be minimized by several methods that do not contribute significantly to the operative risk. Meticulous attention to the positioning of the patient helps to counteract the adverse effects of the prone posture. A suitable scoliosis operating frame may be used that gives satisfactory support without allowing external pressure to be exerted on the anterior abdominal wall.[89] Maintenance of the correct prone-suspended position during surgery is of paramount importance in achieving acceptable operating conditions. In addition to encouraging venous drainage it has been shown to increase the functional residual capacity of the lungs and thereby discourage the development of perioperative atelectasis and hypoxia.

Infiltration of the operative site in depth with a large volume of dilute (1:500,000) epinephrine solution minimizes blood loss from the skin and subcutaneous tissues and eases the dissection by separating tissue planes.

The peripheral vasoconstriction caused by controlled hyperventilation is an aid in achieving hemostasis. A

meticulous surgical technique involving subperiosteal plane dissection, firm packing, and expeditious application of the instruments is most important.

Alternative methods of blood conservation have been advocated such as the staging of complex procedures, autotransfusion,[90] or induced arterial hypotension.[91, 93] All add to the operative risk and increase complexity. In particular, the use of drug-induced arterial hypotension may achieve excellent operating conditions at a potentially high price.[94] Ganglionic blocking agents and other vasodilating drugs cause pooling of the blood in dependent parts and a fall in venous return. If inadvertent obstruction of the inferior vena cava occurs despite careful positioning, circulatory failure may ensue in the absence of compensatory reflexes. In addition, these drugs encourage spinal cord ischemia[94] in circumstances in which, during spinal cord manipulation, a normal arterial blood supply is desirable.

Acute intraoperative hemodilution using crystalloid or colloid solutions has been recommended as a method of blood conservation that does not add substantially to the operative risk.[90] It provides fresh autologous blood with a high hemoglobin content and unimpaired clotting capacity.

Corrective Surgery by the Anterior Approach

In cases requiring an anterior approach, a thoracotomy is performed and the diaphragm is divided near its peripheral attachments to provide access to the vertebral column on the convex side of its curvature. An instrumentation system of the type described by Dwyer[85] or Zielke[92] is used to stabilize the spinal fusion. Severe blood loss does not usually occur during these procedures. However, spinal osteotomy with wedge excision of abnormal vertebrae may cause excessive blood loss because of the proximity of the vertebral and epidural plexuses. Bleeding in these circumstances may be difficult to control.

Postoperative hypoventilation, secretion retention, atelectasis, and pain are more severe following anterior fusion via a thoracotomy than after procedures involving a posterior approach.

Monitoring of Spinal Cord Function

These are two methods of monitoring spinal cord function intraoperatively. The intra-operative "wake-up" procedure is a one-time test of motor tract function. The use of somatosensory cortical evoked potentials provides a continuous record of sensory tract integrity.

Waking patients during the surgery and asking them to move their feet after the distracting rods are in place is a simple method of monitoring spinal cord function.[95] It has an advantage in that it is a definitive test (although it does not rule out paraparesis). Disadvantages include the fact that it is not continuous and that the patient may move excessively, possibly causing extubation, or take a deep breath and entrain air through exposed epidural veins. There is also the vexing problem of an "awake" patient who does not move the lower limbs on request owing to the residual effects of anesthetic drugs.

Somatosensory cortical evoked potentials (SCEP) are recorded from scalp electrodes following stimulation of peripheral nerves of the lower limb. This provides continuous monitoring of spinal cord function.[96] Good correlation has been demonstrated between SCEP and cord injury.[97] However, there are disadvantages, including a longer set-up time, false positives and negatives, technical problems of interference from electrocautery, and cost, inasmuch as a technician and sophisticated equipment are required.

The incidence of neurological problems is low (0.56 percent),[98] but spinal cord damage is so devastating that any incidence is of concern. It must be recognized that the wake-up test involves a certain risk, and it should probably be reserved for patients in whom correction of a severe curve is performed or those who show persistent abnormality in the SCEP.[99]

CONNECTIVE TISSUE DISORDERS

The connective tissue disorders are a diverse group of diseases that include juvenile rheumatoid arthritis (JRA), systemic lupus erythematosus, dermatomyositis, and scleroderma. All show a degree of joint involvement.

Juvenile rheumatoid arthritis (or Still disease in its classic form) is the most common pediatric connective tissue disorder, comprising 75 to 80 percent of rheumatic disorders in two established pediatric rheumatology clinics.[100] Systemic lupus erythematosus accounts for a further 10 percent of cases.

The surgical management of rheumatoid arthritis has become more aggressive in the past 15 years and includes such procedures as osteotomies, joint replacement, and soft tissue releases. Surgery is occasionally required for extra-articular problems such as pericarditis.

Juvenile Rheumatoid Arthritis

The classic modern description of juvenile rheumatoid arthritis was made in 1897 by Still, and the acute systemic form of the disease bears his name. The true incidence is unknown, but it is estimated to be approximately 2 per 100,000 per year. It is seen in all races and all geographic areas. Its etiology is unknown but may be multifactorial. It is rare below 6 months of age, but the frequency then rises rapidly to peak between the ages of 1 and 3 years. The criteria of the American Rheumatism Association for the classification of JRA are listed in Table 14–3, and three distinct types of onset are recognized as listed in Table 14–4.

The disease is a chronic one, with quiescent periods interspaced with acute exacerbations. Both the articular

Table 14–3. CRITERIA FOR CLASSIFICATION OF JUVENILE RHEUMATOID ARTHRITIS

1. Age of onset less than 16 years
2. Arthritis in one or more joints defined as swelling or effusion, or by the presence of at least two of the following:
     Limitation of range of motion
     Tenderness or pain on motion
     Increased heat
3. Duration of disease of 6 weeks
4. Type of onset of disease during the first 6 months identified as:
     Polyarthritis
     Oligoarthritis
     Systemic disease
5. Exclusion of other rheumatic diseases

and extra-articular manifestations and the effects of medical management have significance for the anesthetist.[101, 102]

Airway Problems

Airway problems are caused by at least four mechanisms:

1. Involvement of the temporomandibular joint is common in JRA and limits mouth opening.

2. Mandibular hypoplasia may be extreme. It is related to temporomandibular joint involvement and to growth impairment on the basis of chronic disease, which may be exacerbated by steroid therapy.

3. Active involvement of the synovial joints of the larynx, particularly the cricothyroid articulation or disease of the laryngeal tissues, results in narrowing of the glottis.

4. Cervical spine involvement occurs in as many as 50 percent of cases. It may severely limit neck mobility as a result of apophyseal joint fusion, which is rare in adults. Subluxation of the atlantoaxial joint may also occur with the risk of cord compression, quadriplegia,

Table 14–4. TYPES OF ONSET OF JUVENILE RHEUMATOID ARTHRITIS

	Polyarthritis	Oligoarthritis	Systemic Disease
% cases	50%	40%	10%
Sex (F:M)	2:1	2:1	1:1
Age of onset	Peak 2 years	Early childhood Peak 2 years	Through childhood
Joints	5+	4 or less	Variable
Systemic involvement	Variable	None	Systemic illness
Chronic uveitis	5%	20%	0%
Rheumatoid nodules	10%	Rare	Rare
ANA*	40%	70% (with uveitis)	15%
HLA B27	8%	12%	8%
Prognosis	Good	Excellent	Moderate

*ANA, antinuclear antibodies.
From Cassidy J: Textbook of Pediatric Rheumatology. Copyright © 1982, John Wiley & Sons, Inc., New York. Reprinted by permission of John Wiley & Sons, Inc.

and death. The degree of cervical involvement is related to the duration of the disease and unrelated to age, being much more common after 5 years of disease.[103]

Respiratory Problems

In comparison to adult rheumatoid disease, lung involvement is relatively uncommon and usually consists of pleuritis, pleural effusion, and occasionally pneumonitis. Atypical pneumonia may develop in the immunosuppressed child, and tuberculosis may also occur. Since fever and leukocytosis are frequent manifestations of the disease, diagnosis of superimposed infection can be difficult.

Cardiovascular Problems

Cardiac involvement in the form of pericarditis is relatively common in JRA[104, 105] but usually responds to medical management (in the form of steroids) and only rarely causes significant hemodynamic sequelae. Myocarditis and rheumatoid involvement of either the conducting system of the heart or the valves may occur. In children with systemic involvement, vasculitis may develop into a disseminated necrotizing disease resulting in polyneuropathy and enteropathy with bloody diarrhea.

Renal and Hematological Problems

Renal impairment is common and is related to the duration of the disease. It may arise as a result of amyloid deposit or be secondary to vasculitis. It rarely progresses to overt renal failure, although some impairment of creatinine clearance is common.

Hematological abnormalities include a microcytic hypochromic anemia, which is chronic and refractory to iron therapy (the "anemia of chronic disease"). Occult or overt bleeding as a result of anti-inflammatory agents may be superimposed on this. Children with systemic involvement often have a significant neutrophilia with white cell counts as high as 50,000 μl and may have high fevers. Splenomegaly is also common, especially in the acute phase of the disease. It may be associated with thrombocytopenia (Felty syndrome).

Problems Related to Drug Therapy

The agents most frequently used in the medical management of JRA are salicylates, nonsteroidal anti-inflammatory agents, steroids, gold, and penicillamine. Cytotoxic agents such as cyclophosphamide are used rarely.

The salicylates and nonsteroidal anti-inflammatory agents are associated with gastrointestinal bleeding related to acute gastritis and peptic ulceration and to impairment of platelet function. They are rarely associated with hepatotoxicity. Steroids are a particular problem in JRA, because they cause growth impairment as well as the other well-known side effects of long-term treatment. Gold salts are toxic and may cause renal damage leading to the nephrotic syndrome,

bone marrow depression, and exfoliative dermatitis. A similar picture is seen with penicillamine.

Anesthetic Management

Preoperative assessment of the child with JRA should include physical examination with special emphasis on the airway. Indirect laryngoscopy, flow volume loops, soft tissue views of the neck, and flexion-extension views of the cervical spine may be required. A useful clinical test for atlantoaxial instability is the Sharp and Purser test.[106] The patient is seated with the neck flexed and pressure is applied to the forehead. A finger is placed on the spinous process of C2, and in normal subjects no movement can be felt. In 50 percent of patients with atlantoaxial instability a gliding movement is felt as the subluxation is reduced.

Thorough evaluation of the cardiovascular system should be performed and should include careful auscultation for murmurs, a chest x-ray, and an ECG. Echocardiography may also be indicated to delineate pericardial effusion or valvular involvement.

Laboratory investigation should include a complete blood count with differential and platelet count; measurements of bleeding time, electrolytes, blood urea nitrogen, and creatinine; and urinalysis.

Preoperative steroid supplementation is necessary for those patients on long-term steroid therapy or those with a recent history of steroid therapy within the past 3 months. Preoperative transfusion may be required for symptomatic patients with anemia but not for the compensated chronically anemic child. Children with atlantoaxial instability should come to the operating room in a cervical collar.

Intravenous induction of anesthesia and the use of muscle relaxants are not recommended unless there is certainty about securing the airway. Strategies for intubation may include a blind nasal technique, careful direct laryngoscopy, or use of a fiberoptic laryngoscope (either with the patient awake or following inhalation induction).

The younger child should be intubated while awake only in circumstances of dire necessity, since this approach is fraught with distress and difficulty for all involved. Fiberoptic techniques are also beset with difficulties in the smaller patient because of the poorer resolution and absence of suction with small-diameter bronchoscopes.

Other problems encountered preoperatively include difficulties with vascular access, fragile veins, and an increased bleeding tendency. The skin should be carefully padded and meticulous care taken with positioning because of flexures, thin skin, and osteoporosis associated with steroid therapy. Cardiac and renal reserve may be limited. Agents that depress myocardial function should be used cautiously, and renally excreted agents should be carefully titrated. Anemic patients need a high inspired oxygen concentration and controlled ventilation. Transfusions are started early. Any patient with a difficult airway should be left intubated until full consciousness has returned and he or she is able to maintain adequate ventilation.

In the postoperative period steroid coverage must be tapered to maintenance levels. Nutritional support should be commenced early, because these patients are often malnourished. Intravenous alimentation may be required if there is any delay in reestablishing oral intake. Postoperative analgesics must be carefully titrated to avoid respiratory depression.

Regional techniques have been used successfully in the management of patients with rheumatoid arthritis,[107] although technical difficulties are common because of anatomical deformity. Peripheral neuropathy is a contraindication to regional block.

Ketamine has been advocated for patients with significant airway problems.[108] However, the technique as described relies on spontaneous ventilation and therefore is not suitable for many procedures.

Systemic Lupus Erythematosus[109]

Systemic lupus erythematosus (SLE) is an autoimmune disorder that is frequently a severe or even life-threatening multisystem disease in children.

Twenty percent of cases arise in childhood, usually after the age of 8 years. In younger children it occurs with such predisposing factors as familial lupus or complement defects. The infants of mothers with SLE have a high incidence of congenital complete heart block, and endocardial fibroelastosis has been reported.[109]

Children with SLE may be encountered in the intensive care unit with pulmonary lupus or acute pulmonary hemorrhage. Pleural effusion is common together with cardiac involvement consisting of pericarditis, myocarditis, and Libman-Sacks endocarditis. Coronary vasculitis may also occur.

The neurological sequelae include seizures, strokes, psychoses, and peripheral neuropathies. Renal involvement is common and may progress to the nephrotic syndrome or chronic renal failure. Hepatic failure is rare.

Hematological abnormalities occur in 90 percent of children, some 50 percent having leukopenia and 30 percent a positive Coombs test. Severe hemolysis is unusual. Thrombocytopenia and clotting abnormalities may also occur.

FAT EMBOLISM

Fat embolism is a recognized complication of trauma whether operative or accidental. It was first described in humans by Zenker in 1862, but despite over 100 years of experience with the entity a precise definition is not possible. This is due to controversy regarding both the origin of the fat and the precise pathophysiology of its effects. The presence of fat globules in the lungs and other tissues in patients dying of trauma varies from 46 to 100 percent in different series. However, the clinical incidence of the fat embolism syndrome is very much lower than this, varying from 1 to 6 percent in two reviews quoted by Wilkins.[110]

The fat embolism syndrome follows an initial episode of trauma, most commonly long bone fractures, and progresses within 48 hours to signs of cerebral impairment, fever, tachypnea, hypotension, and tachycardia. The onset of these symptoms in the early postoperative period (especially if a high fever is present) mimics the malignant hyperthermia syndrome. The pulmonary pathophysiological changes result in progressive hypoxia due to shunting and hemorrhagic edema. The clinical picture becomes indistinguishable from adult respiratory distress syndrome. Fat globules can usually be demonstrated in either urine or sputum. At autopsy fat can be seen in the pulmonary capillaries and in the systemic circulation involving the brain, liver, and kidneys. Coagulation abnormalities are common as a secondary event and petechiae may be seen, typically on the upper part of the body.

Treatment of the syndrome includes supportive measures, such as intermittent positive-pressure ventilation with positive end-expiratory pressure. Hypoxic respiratory failure is the usual cause of death. Ethanol, either intravenously or by inhalation, has been advocated in the treatment of this syndrome[111] but its use remains controversial. Heparin has also been administered,[112] although there are no clinical trials supporting its use and the side effects are particularly hazardous in the patient with multiple trauma. Steroids have also been recommended, based on reports of their use in three patients[113] and a prospective study in high-risk patients.[114]

The incidence of fat embolism in the pediatric population is unknown. A report from The Hospital for Sick Children in Toronto suggested an incidence of less than 0.5 percent.[115] The authors regarded as significant the presence of connective tissue disease in three of the nine cases.

Two cases of fat embolism following spinal fusion have been reported,[116, 117] as has another case in an achondroplastic patient.[118]

Pediatric patients at risk for fat embolism include those with major long bone fractures, extensive crush injury, children with collagen vascular disease, or rickets and any child undergoing procedures that involve compression of the intramedullary canal or extensive bony dissection. A high index of suspicion is necessary to make the diagnosis.

REFERENCES

General References
1. Tachdjian MO: Pediatric Orthopedics. 2nd ed. Philadelphia, W.B. Saunders Co., 1976.
2. Behrman RE, Vaughan VC III (Eds.): Nelson Textbook of Pediatrics. 12th ed. Philadelphia, W.B. Saunders Co., 1983.

3. McKusick VA: Heritable Disorders of Connective Tissue. St. Louis, C.V. Mosby Co., 1972.
4. Zauder HL (Ed.): Anaesthesia for Orthopaedic Surgery. Philadelphia, F.A. Davis Co., 1980.
5. Stehling L, Zauder HL: Anesthetic Implications of Congenital Anomalies in Children. New York, Appleton-Century-Crofts, 1980.
6. Bailey JA: Disproportionate Short Stature. Philadelphia, W.B. Saunders Co., 1973.

Generalized Constitutional Diseases of Bone and Cartilage

7. Second International Nomenclature of Constitutional Diseases of Bone. J Pediatr 93:614, 1978.
8. Murdoch JA, Walker BA, Hull JG, et al.: Achondroplasia: a genetic and statistical survey. Ann Hum Genet 33:227, 1970.
9. Spranger J, Langer LO, Maroteaux P: Increasing frequency of a syndrome of multiple osseous defects. Lancet 2:716, 1970.
10. Rimoin DL: The chondrodystrophies. Adv Hum Genet 5:1, 1975.
11. Zellweger H, Taylor B: Genetic aspects of achondroplasia. J Lancet 85:8, 1965.
12. Dennis JP, Rosenberg HS, Alvord EC: Megalencephaly, internal hydrocephalus and other neurological aspects of achondroplasia. Brain 84:427, 1961.
13. Cohen ME, Rosenthal AD, Matson D: Neurological abnormalities in achondroplastic children. J Pediatr 71:367, 1967.
14. Yamada H, Nakamura S, Masutaka T, et al.: Neurological manifestations of paediatric achondroplasia. J Neurosurg 54:49, 1981.
15. Warkany J: Congenital Malformations. Chicago, Year Book Medical, 1971.
16. Potter EL, Coverstone LA: Chondrodystrophy fetalis. Am J Obstet Gynecol 56:790, 1948.
17. Bergstrom K, Laurent U, Lindberg PO: Neurological symptoms in achondroplasia. Acta Neurol Scand 47:59, 1971.
18. Lutter LD, Lonstein GE, Winter RB, et al.: Anatomy of the achondroplastic lumbar canal. Clin Orthop Rel Res 126:139, 1977.
19. Vogl H, Osbourne RL: Lesions of the spinal cord in achondroplasia. Arch Neurol Psychol 61:644, 1949.
20. Bethem D, Winter RB, Lutter L, et al.: Spinal disorders of dwarfism. J Bone Joint Surg 63A:1412, 1981.
21. Cohen SE: Anesthesia for cesarean section in an achondroplastic dwarf. Anesthesiology 52:264, 1980.
22. Watts LF, Finerman G, Wyatt GM: Anesthesia for dwarfs and other patients of pathological small stature. Can Anaesth Soc J 22:703, 1975.
23. Bancroft GH, Lauria JI: Ketamine induction for cesarean section in a patient with acute intermittent porphyria and achondroplastic dwarfism. Anesthesiology 59:143, 1983.
24. Mather JS: Impossible direct laryngoscopy in achondroplasia. Anaesthesia 21:244, 1966.
25. Hanissian AS, Riggs WW Jr, Thomas DA: Infantile thoracic dystrophy—a variant of Ellis–van Creveld syndrome. J Pediatr 71:855, 1967.
26. Kozlowski K, Szmigiel C, Baylak A, et al.: Difficulties in differentiation between chondroectodermal dysplasia and asphyxiating thoracic dystrophy. Aust Radiol 16:401, 1972.
27. Langer LO Jr: Thoracic-pelvic-phalangeal dystrophy. Radiology 91:447, 1968.
28. Zelt BA, LoSasso AM: Prolonged nasotracheal intubation and mechanical ventilation in the management of asphyxiating thoracic dystrophy: a case report. Anesth Analg 51:342, 1972.
29. Barnes ND, Hull D, Miller AD, et al.: Chest reconstruction in thoracic dystrophy. Arch Dis Child 46:833, 1971.
30. Finegold MJ, Katzew H, Genieser NB, et al.: Lung structure in thoracic dystrophy. Am J Dis Child 22:153, 1971.
31. Herdman RC, Langer LO Jr: The thoracic asphyxiant dystrophy and renal disease. Am J Dis Child 116:192, 1968.
32. Ellis RW, van Creveld S: A syndrome characterized by ectodermal dysplasia, polydactyly, chondrodysplasia and congenital morbus cordis. Arch Dis Child 15:65, 1940.
33. McKusick VA, Egeland JA, Eldridge R, et al.: Dwarfism in the Amish. 1. The Ellis–van Creveld syndrome. Bull Johns Hopkins Hosp 115:306, 1964.
34. Moore TC: Chondroectodermal dysplasia (Ellis–van Creveld syndrome) with bronchial malformation and neonatal tension lobar emphysema. J Thorac Cardiovasc Surg 46:1, 1963.
35. Tasker WY, Martin AR, Gold AP: Chondrodysplasia calcificans congenita. Am J Dis Child 119:122, 1970.
36. Maroteaux P: Bone Diseases of Children. Philadelphia, J.B. Lippincott Co., 1979.
37. Nyham WC, Sakati NO: Genetic and Malformation Syndromes in Clinical Medicine. Chicago, Year Book Medical, 1976.
38. Afshani E, Girdany BR: Atlanto-axial dislocation in chondrodysplasia punctata. Report of the findings in two brothers. Radiology 102:399, 1972.
39. Hathaway WE, Johnson CC, Oh JE: Abnormalities of platelet function in osteogenesis imperfecta. Clin Res 18:209, 1970.
40. Cropp GV, Myers DN: Physiological evidence of hypermetabolism in osteogenesis imperfecta. Pediatrics 49:375, 1972.
41. King JD, Bobechko WP: Osteogenesis imperfecta. An orthopaedic description and surgical review. J Bone Joint Surg 53B:72, 1971.
42. Gitelis S, Whiffen J, DeWald RL: The treatment of severe scoliosis in osteogenesis imperfecta. Clin Orthop Rel Res 175:56, 1983.
43. Heppner RL, Babitt HI, Bianchine JW, et al.: Aortic regurgitation and aneurysm of the sinus of Valsalva associated with osteogenesis imperfecta. Am J Cardiol 31:654, 1973.
44. Sofield HA, Millar EA: Fragmentation realignment and intramedullary rod fixation of deformities of long bones in children. J Bone Joint Surg 34A:500, 1952.
45. Jones E, Burnap TK: International symposium on malignant hyperthermia. Anaesthesiology 36:192, 1972.
46. Solomons CC, Yers DN: Hyperthermia of osteogenesis imperfecta and its relationship to malignant hyperthermia. In Gordon RA, Britt BA, Kalow W (Eds.): International Symposium on Malignant Hyperthermia. Springfield, IL, Charles C Thomas, 1973.
47. Oliverio RM: Anaesthetic management of intramedullary nailing in osteogenesis imperfecta. Report of a case. Anesth Analg 52:232, 1973.
48. Wood SJ, Thomas J, Braimbridge MV: Mitral valve disease and open heart surgery in osteogenesis imperfecta tarda. Br Heart J 35:103, 1973.
49. Weisinger B, Glassman E, Spencer FC, et al.: Successful aortic valve replacement for aortic regurgitation associated with osteogenesis imperfecta. Br Heart J 37:475, 1975.
50. Perovic MN, Kopits SE, Thompson RC: Radiological evaluation of the spinal cord in congenital atlanto-axial dislocation. Radiology 109:713, 1973.
51. Goldberg MJ, Meyer M: The radial clubhand. Orthop Clin North Am 7:341, 1970.
52. Goldberg MJ, Ampola MG: Birth defect syndromes in which orthopedic problems may be overlooked. Orthop Clin North Am 7:285, 1976.
53. Noonan JA: Association of congenital heart disease with syndromes or other defects. Pediatr Clin North Am 25:797, 1976.
54. Quan L, Smith DW: The VATER association. Vertebral defects, anal atresia, T-E fistula with esophageal atresia, radial and renal dysplasia. A spectrum of associated defects. J Pediatr 82:104, 1973.
55. Bany JE, Auldist AW: The Vater association: one end of a spectrum of anomalies. Am J Dis Child 128:769, 1974.

Metabolic Diseases of Bone

56. Goodman AG, Gilman LS, Gilman A (Eds.): The Pharmacological Basis of Therapeutics. 6th ed. New York, MacMillan, 1980.

57. Freidman WR, Roberts WC: Vitamin D and the supravalvular aortic stenosis syndrome. Circulation 34:77, 1966.

58. Card RT, Brain MC: The "anemia" of childhood: evidence for a physiological response to hyperphosphatemia. N Engl J Med 288:388, 1972.

59. Parfitt AM: Hypophosphatemic vitamin D refractory rickets and osteomalacia. Orthop Clin North Am 3:653, 1972.

60. Rathburn JC: Hypophosphatasia, a new developmental anomaly. Am J Dis Child 75:822, 1948.

Disorders of the Spine

61. Kulns J, Homel R: Management of congenital scoliosis. Review of 170 cases. Arch Surg 65:250, 1952.

62. Jordan GE, White RJ, Fischer KC, et al.: The scoliosis of congenital heart disease. Am Heart J 84:463, 1974.

63. Roth A, Rosenthal R, Hall JE, et al.: Scoliosis and congenital heart disease. Clin Orthop 93:95, 1973.

64. McMaster MJ, Ohtsuka K: The natural history of congenital scoliosis. A study of 251 patients. J Bone Joint Surg 64A:1128, 1982.

65. Shands AR, Eisberg HB: The incidence of scoliosis in the state of Delaware. J Bone Joint Surg 37A:1249, 1955.

66. James JIP: The etiology of scoliosis. J Bone Joint Surg 52:410, 1970.

67. Wynne Davies R: Familial (idiopathic) scoliosis. J Bone Joint Surg 50B:24, 1968.

68. Lloyd Roberts GC, Pitcher MF: Structural idiopathic scoliosis of infancy. J Bone Joint Surg 7B:520, 1965.

69. Scott JC, Morgan TH: The natural history and prognosis for infantile idiopathic scoliosis. J Bone Joint Surg 37B:400, 1955.

70. Keim HA: Scoliosis. CIBA Foundation Symposium, 1978.

71. Isselbacher KJ, Adams RD, Braunwald E, et al. (Eds.): Harrison's Principles of Internal Medicine. 10th ed. New York, McGraw-Hill, 1983.

72. Kafer ER: Respiratory and cardiovascular functions in scoliosis and the principles of anesthetic management. Anesthesiology 52:339, 1980.

73. Nisbet HIA, Lamarre A, Levison H, et al.: Thoracic elastance and its components in anaesthetized scoliotic children. J Bone Joint Surg 55A:1721, 1973.

74. Bergofsky EH, Turino GM, Fishman AP: Cardiorespiratory failure in kyphoscoliosis. Medicine 38:263, 1959.

75. Bradford DS, Moe JH, Winter RB: Scoliosis and kyphosis. In Rothman RH, Simeone FH (Eds.): The Spine. Philadelphia, W.B. Saunders Co., 1982.

76. Kafer ER: Idiopathic scoliosis. Gas exchange and the age dependence of arterial blood gases. J Clin Invest 58:825, 1976.

77. Kafer ER: Idiopathic scoliosis. Mechanical properties of the respiratory system and ventilatory response to carbon dioxide. J Clin Invest 55:1153, 1975.

78. Davies G, Reid L: Effect of scoliosis on growth of alveoli and pulmonary arteries and on the right ventricle. Arch Dis Child 46:623, 1971.

79. Schmerson JM, Verno A, Prime FJ: A study of pulmonary artery preessure, electrocardiography and mechanocardiography in thoracic scoliosis. Thorax 32:700, 1977.

80. Caro CG, Dubois AB: Pulmonary function in kyphoscoliosis. Thorax 16:282, 1961.

81. Jenkins JG, Bohn DJ, Edmonds JF, et al.: Evaluation of pulmonary function in muscular dystrophy patients requiring spinal surgery. Crit Care Med 10:645, 1982.

82. Westgate DH, Moe JH: Pulmonary function in kyphoscoliosis before and after correction by the Harrington instrumentation method. J Bone Joint Surg 51A:935, 1969.

83. Bjune J, Nachemson A: Non-treated scoliosis. Clin Orthop Rel Res 93:44, 1973.

84. Shannon DC, Riseborough EJ, Kazemi H: Ventilation perfusion relationships following correction of kyphoscoliosis. JAMA 217:579, 1971.

85. Dwyer AF, Schafer MF: Anterior approach to scoliosis. Results of treatment in fifty one cases. J Bone Joint Surg 56B:218, 1974.

86. Abrahamson ML: Pulmocardiac failure associated with deformity of the chest. Lancet 1:449, 1959.

87. Relton JES, Conn AW: Anaesthesia for the surgical correction of scoliosis by the Harrington method in children. Can Anaesth Soc J 10:603, 1963.

88. Relton JES: Anaesthesia in the original correction of scoliosis. In Riseborough EJ, Hendon JH (Eds.): Scoliosis and Other Deformities of the Axial Skeleton. Boston, Little, Brown, 1975.

89. Relton JES, Hall JE: An operation frame for spinal fusion. A new apparatus designed to reduce haemorrhage during operation. J Bone Joint Surg 49B:327, 1967.

90. du Toit G, Relton JES, Gillespie R: Acute haemodilutional autotransfusion in the surgical management of scoliosis. J Bone Joint Surg 60B:178, 1978.

91. McNeill TN, DeWald RL, Kino KN, et al.: Controlled hypotensive anaesthesia in scoliosis surgery. J Bone Joint Surg 56A:1167, 1974.

92. Zielke B: Ventral derotation spondylodesis. Preliminary report of fifty-eight cases. Beitr Orthop Traumatol 85:103, 1978.

93. Jacobs HK, Lieponais VV, Bunch WH, et al.: The influence of halothane and nitroprusside on canine spinal cord haemodynamics. Spine 7:35, 1982.

94. Grundy BL, Nash CL Jr, Brown RH: Arterial pressure manipulation alters spinal cord function during correction of scoliosis. Anesthesiology 54:249, 1981.

95. Hall JE, Levine CR, Sudhir KG: Intraoperative awakening to monitor spinal cord function during Harrington instrumentation and spinal fusion. J Bone Joint Surg 60A:533, 1978.

96. Grundy BL, Nash CL Jr, Brown RH: Deliberate hypotension for spinal fusion. Prospective randomized study with evoked potential monitoring. Can Anaesth Soc J 29:452, 1982.

97. Rowed DW, McLean JAG, Tator CH: Somatosensory evoked potentials in acute spinal cord injury. Prognostic value. Surg Neurol 9:203, 1978.

98. MacEwan GD, Bunnell WP, Krishnaswani S: Acute neurological complications in the treatment of scoliosis. J Bone Joint Surg 57A:404, 1975.

99. Pathak KS, Brown RH, Nash CL, et al.: Continuous opioid infusions for scoliosis fusion surgery. Anesth Analg 62:841, 1983.

Connective Tissue Disorders

100. Cassidy J: Textbook of Pediatric Rheumatology. New York, John Wiley & Sons, 1982.

101. Edelist G: Principles of anesthetic management in rheumatoid arthritis patients. Anesth Analg 43:227, 1964.

102. Jenkins LC, McGraw RW: Anaesthetic management of patients with rheumatoid arthritis. Can Anaesth Soc J 16:407, 1969.

103. Ornilla E, Ansell BM, Swamell AJ: Cervical spine involvement in patients with chronic arthritis undergoing orthopaedic surgery. Ann Rheum Dis 31:364, 1972.

104. Brewer E Jr: Juvenile rheumatoid arthritis—cardiac involvement. Arthritis Rheum 20:217, 1977.

105. Bernstein B: Pericarditis in juvenile rheumatoid arthritis. Arthritis Rheum 20:241, 1977.

106. Sharp J, Purser DW: Spontaneous atlanto-axial dislocation in ankylosing spondylitis and rheumatoid arthritis. Ann Rheum Dis 20:47, 1961.

107. Hodgkinson R: Anesthetic management of a parturient with

severe juvenile rheumatoid arthritis. Anesth Analg 60:611, 1981.

108. D'Arcy EJ, Fell RH, Ansell BM, et al.: Ketamine and juvenile chronic polyarthritis. Anaesthesia 31:624, 1976.

109. Schaller J: Lupus in childhood. Clin Rheum Dis 8:219, 1982.

Fat Embolism

110. Wilkins KE: Fat embolism. In Zauder HL (Ed.): Anaesthesia for Orthopaedic Surgery. Philadelphia, F.A. Davis Co., 1980.

111. Nice GW: Alcohol in fat embolism. J Kans Med Soc 75:306, 1974.

112. Guenter CA, Braun TE: Fat embolism syndrome: changing prognosis. Chest 79:143, 1981.

113. Ashbaugh DG, Petty TL: Use of corticosteroids in treatment of respiratory failure. Surg Gynecol Obstet 123:493, 1966.

114. Schonfeld S, Ploysonyang G, Dilisio R, et al.: Fat embolism prophylaxis with corticosteroids. A prospective study in high risk patients. Ann Intern Med 99:438, 1983.

115. Drummond DS, Salter RB, Boone J: Fat embolism in children. Can Med Assoc J 101:200, 1969.

116. Gittman JE, Buchanan TA, Fisher BJ, et al.: Fatal fat embolism after spinal fusion for scoliosis. JAMA 249:779, 1983.

117. Brown LP, Stehling LH: Fat embolism as a complication of scoliosis fusion. J Bone Joint Surg 56A:1764, 1974.

118. Ganel A, Israeli A, Horozowski H: Fatal complication of femoral elongation in an achondroplastic dwarf. Clin Orthop Rel Res 185:69, 1984.

15 | SKIN AND CONNECTIVE TISSUE DISEASES

MICHAEL F. SMITH, M.D.

This chapter considers diseases of the skin and connective tissue in children. The more severe of these disorders are chronic, multisystemic in nature, and often debilitating. Treatment may involve prolonged medical support and repeated surgical interventions. Successful anesthetic management requires recognition of the relevant pathophysiological implications of each disorder and consideration of the psychological needs of anxious and often intolerant young patients enduring chronic illness.

It is appropriate that skin and connective tissue diseases be discussed in the same chapter. Connective tissue elements appear in the skin and in the stroma of most organ systems of the body and are vulnerable to similar underlying pathological mechanisms; thus, many of these diseases are closely related. The skin is an important diagnostic aid for the internist in recognizing systemic disease, just as observation of the skin is a valuable monitor for the anesthetist in assessing a patient's response during anesthesia and surgery.

For purposes of organization, skin diseases and connective tissue disorders are considered in separate sections within the chapter.

SKIN DISEASES

Structure and Functions of Normal Skin

The outer layer of the skin, the epidermis, is an organized stratified epithelium with appendages, notably hair follicles, sweat glands, and sebaceous glands, that project into the dermis. The squamous cells, or keratinocytes, are continuously renewed in an orderly fashion from basal cell layers, in a transit time of about 28 days.[6] Other cells within the basal epidermis include melanocytes, which synthesize the pigment melanin, and Langerhans cells, which are dendritic

mesenchymal cells, functioning as the initial receptor for the cutaneous immune response to external antigens.

The dermis, interposed between the epidermis and subcutaneous fat, forms a tough viscoelastic supporting structure composed of collagen, elastin, and reticular fibers and an amorphous ground substance. It contains the epidermal appendages, blood vessels, lymphocytes, nerves, arrector pili muscles, and considerable amounts of bound water.[1] The predominant cell is a spindle-shaped fibroblast that synthesizes the fibrillar protein collagen and the mucopolysaccharides of the ground substance. Other cells include phagocytic histiocytes or macrophages, mast cells, and motile leukocytes.

The subcutaneous tissue or panniculus is composed of lobules of fat cells divided by fibrous septa. These help anchor the dermis to the underlying fascia.

Intact, the skin provides an airtight, waterproof, elastic surface cover for the body. It offers protection from physical trauma and ultraviolet light. Sensory organs aid in protection against injury. The surface film of lipid secretions from sebaceous glands creates an antiseptic layer, retarding the growth of microorganisms and reducing moisture loss from the epidermis.

The skin plays a major role in the regulation of body temperature, particularly in infants, who have a large surface area relative to their body mass. The gradient for heat loss by radiation is determined by skin blood flow, which may increase from basal levels of 50 ml/100 g/min to 200 ml/100 g/min under the sympathetic control of arteriovenous shunts in the dermis.[18] Further heat loss results from the evaporation of insensible water loss and of the hypotonic secretion of eccrine sweat glands.

Anesthesia interferes with the functions of the skin in several ways. The protective role of sensation is eliminated, and this may lead to injury such as diathermy burns or nerve damage. Most anesthetic techniques and agents increase skin blood flow and significantly reduce the ability of children to maintain a normal body temperature. The use of anticholinergic drugs may reduce sweating sufficiently to cause hyperthermia.[18]

Neonatal Skin Disorders

Compared with that of the older child or adult, the skin of the neonate is thinner and less hairy, has weaker intercellular attachments, and is more sensitive to external irritants. It produces less sweat and sebaceous gland secretions.[3] Sweating on the face and trunk in a term infant is usually noted on the third to fifth day of life, but in premature infants may be delayed until the 24th day.[2] The increased susceptibility to micrococcal infections may be related to decreased neutrophil and monocyte mobility and to impaired bactericidal activity.[3] Depressed contact allergen reactivity may be explained by low levels of complement C_3 and C_4 in the neonate. The percutaneous adsorption of toxic substances is increased in premature infants and in damaged areas of skin.[3] This combination of deficiencies helps to explain the vulnerability of newborns to skin disease.

Toxic Erythema Neonatorum

Despite its dramatic descriptive name, toxic erythema neonatorum is a benign, asymptomatic, and self-limited cutaneous eruption of erythematous macules, papules, and pustules. It occurs in 50 to 70 percent of term infants.[3] Preterm infants are less affected. The skin lesions usually appear during the first 3 to 4 days of life. They may occur in numbers of a few to several hundred, anywhere on the body except the palms and soles. In more severe cases, urticarial wheals may develop. Smears of the pustular fluid show a predominance of eosinophils. Spontaneous recovery occurs within 2 days, and recurrences are rare. No treatment is required.

Apart from careful aseptic technique, there are no specific anesthetic considerations.

Herpes Simplex Neonatorum

A fetus may acquire herpes simplex virus infection on passage through the birth canal if the mother has an active herpetic cervicitis or vulvitis at the time of delivery. The previously healthy child becomes ill on day 4 to 8 of life and may develop erythematous or vesiculobullous lesions, which may recur, on the face, scalp, or upper trunk.[3] The disseminated infection may initiate devastating hepatitis and encephalitis and may be fatal.[4]

Treatment must be aggressive and may include exchange transfusion from a donor with a history of a herpetic infection of the appropriate type, transfusion of type-specific immune globulin, and donor herpes-virus-sensitive lymphocytes and monocytes. Adenosine arabinoside intravenously, 10 to 20 mg/kg/day, may be helpful.[19]

Anesthetic considerations include a careful assessment of hepatic function and neurological status, especially with respect to intracranial pressure control and anticonvulsant therapy.

Erythema Desquamativum (Leiner Disease)

Leiner disease is a rare, possibly hereditary disorder thought to be a severe form of seborrheic dermatitis. It may occur in the first week of life, but is usually seen in infants age 2 to 4 months who are breast fed; girls are affected more often than boys. It is characterized by the sudden onset of a generalized exfoliative erythemic dermatitis associated with intractable diarrhea, anemia, wasting, and recurrent local and systemic gram negative infections (Fig. 15–1). The etiology is unknown, but in the familial form a defect in the opsonic activity of complement, leading to a functional deficiency of C_5, has been recognized.[4]

Children with Leiner disease require intensive care, with correction of associated hypovolemia, anemia, sepsis, and secondary infections, usually pneumonia and meningitis. Temperature control is impaired. Intravenous access is difficult in infants who have generalized dermatitis and who may have severe cushingoid features. Adhesive tape should be used with caution. Despite aggressive supportive care with parenteral nutrition and fresh frozen plasma, corticosteroids, and antibiotics, the mortality of this disease remains high.[20]

Neonatal Ichthyoses

The ichthyoses represent a heterogeneous group of inherited keratinizing disorders in which there is increased epidermal germinal cell activity and a failure of separation of stratum corneum cells. The hyperkeratosis produces large amounts of scale of varying thickness on the skin surface. Except for ichthyosis vulgaris, which presents in early childhood and is less severe, all forms are usually obvious at birth. The most common neonatal presentation of ichthyosis (1 in 300,000 births),[1] occurs in the collodion baby, often as a manifestation of lamellar ichthyosis. The child is encased in a dry, taut membrane resembling oiled parchment that fissures and then desquamates over the next several weeks.[6] Constriction of the chest and distortion of the face may compromise spontaneous respiration and the ability to feed.

Maintaining a warm, humidified environment is the most efficient means of hydrating the membrane and keeping it pliable.[1, 21] Respiratory function must be monitored and adequate hydration and nutrition must be provided. Intravenous access is difficult. Skin infections at fissure sites and pneumonias must be aggressively treated with antibiotics. Temperature control is impaired.

Figure 15–1. Erythema desquamativum (Leiner disease) in an 8-month-old female infant. Note generalized scaling, weeping lesions, and pronounced cushingoid features.

The most severe presentation of this disorder is the rare harlequin fetus, in which the child is covered by thick plates of stratum corneum separated by fissures. Few survive beyond 1 week.[4, 6]

In the variants such as mild lamellar ichthyosis, ichthyosis vulgaris, or epidermolytic hyperkeratosis, the disorder is limited to the skin and is manifested as a build-up of considerable epidermal scale from massive hyperkeratosis (Fig. 15–2). These variants are seen in older children. Treatment is directed at reducing or softening the scale by the application of lubricants or keratinolytic agents such as retinoic acid or salicylic acid. The oily base in some of these agents prevents adhesives from sticking to the skin. Intravenous cannulas, ECG electrodes, and endotracheal tubes must be tied or sutured in place.

Sclerema Neonatorum

This uncommon disorder occurs in the first few weeks of life in premature, cold-stressed, or debilitated infants who have serious underlying sepsis, respiratory distress, gastroenteritis and dehydration, or congenital heart disease.[3] It is a grave prognostic sign and is characterized by an abrupt onset of diffuse, generalized hardening of the skin, which becomes waxy and stony in consistency, non-pitting, and cold.[6] Joint mobility and respiration are compromised. The child becomes sluggish and feeds poorly. The mortality of affected infants is 50 to 75 percent; death usually results from respiratory failure or secondary infections. In those who survive, the skin findings resolve without sequelae.[3, 22] The etiology is unknown.

Figure 15–2. Epidermolytic hyperkeratosis in a 4-year-old boy. The accumulation of thickened epidermal scale has been softened by keratolytic and lubricant agents.

Management includes treatment of the underlying condition, supportive care in a warm environment with oxygen as required, and aggressive antibiotic control of infections. Systemic corticosteroids have been advocated.[3]

No specific anesthetic experience has been reported.

Subcutaneous Fat Necrosis

This uncommon disorder is accepted as a variant of sclerema neonatorum, but is a benign and self-limited disease affecting healthy full-term infants. Often cases are attributed to birth trauma, asphyxia, overexposure to cold, and maternal diabetes.[6] Subcutaneous fat necrosis is characterized by the early development of sharply circumscribed, firm, irregular, subcutaneous nodules that may be tender, but are infrequently associated with constitutional symptoms. Most lesions resolve spontaneously without scarring, but occasionally, fluctuant lesions require aspiration to prevent rupture.[2]

Fat necrosis can be a complication of hypothermia induced by surface cooling. In such cases the hypothermia may aggravate depression of circulatory and respiratory function in anesthesia. No other direct implications of subcutaneous fat necrosis for anesthesia are recognized.

Figure 15–3. Aplasia cutis congenita in its extreme form in a prone newborn male infant. Note the total absence of cranial vault and dura and the partial infarction of left cerebral cortex.

Developmental Abnormalities of the Skin

Cutaneous Defects

Congenital Localized Absence of the Skin (Aplasia Cutis Congenita). Congenital localized absence of the skin is an uncommon inherited defect in skin development manifested at birth by single or multiple 1- to 2-cm ulcers, usually on the scalp. The depth of the ulcers is variable, but they may infrequently involve tissue deep to the dermis and even extend to the periosteum, skull, and dura. In its extreme, the defect may be staggering (Fig. 15–3). Associated defects are rare, but include cleft lip and palate, vascular malformations, congenital heart disease, defects of the central nervous system, and trisomy 13 syndrome.[6] Bart has described the association of this disorder with epidermolysis bullosa.[23] Congenital localized absence of the skin away from the scalp may in fact be a clinical expression of epidermolysis bullosa.

Small defects reepithelialize spontaneously. Large or multiple lesions may be complicated by secondary infection, massive hemorrhage, and meningitis. The repair may require excision, dural grafting, and rotation flaps to cover the defect.

The anesthetist must be aware of the possible association of this condition with epidermolysis bullosa and with the other congenital anomalies described. Adequate blood products must be available for use during the closure of large defects.

Focal Dermal Hypoplasia (Goltz Syndrome).[1, 6,][17] Focal dermal hypoplasia is a rare, possibly familial disorder occurring principally in girls and characterized by the herniation of fat through thinned, partly deficient dermis, producing multiple papillomas. The papillomas usually involve the periorificial skin and the oral mucous membranes, but lesions in the oropharynx and peritonsillar regions have been described.[17, 24] The skin may also show atrophy and linear hyperpigmentation. Associated anomalies include syndactyly, scoliosis, ocular abnormalities, dental defects, small stature, and mental deficiency.

The airway must be evaluated preoperatively, but no difficulty in laryngoscopy has been reported. Apart from recognizing the associated abnormalities, no specific anesthetic recommendations are made.

Congenital Anhidrotic Ectodermal Dysplasia (Christ-Siemens-Touraine Syndrome). Congenital anhidrotic ectodermal dysplasia is a rare sex-linked recessive disorder seen with full expression only in males, although carrier females may be mildly affected. The ectodermal defect is manifested by the triad of absent sebaceous and sweat glands, partial or complete absence of teeth, and hypotrichosis (absent hair).[1, 6] The skin is dry and heat loss by evaporation is impaired.[18, 26] There may be virtual absence of mucous glands from the respiratory tract and esophagus.[24] Respiratory infections are frequent. Body odor may be lacking.[18, 25] Affected children may demonstrate the characteristic facies, which features a depressed bridge and root of the nose, prominent supraorbital ridges, large deformed ears, thick lips, and an underdeveloped maxilla and mandible.[18, 26, 27]

Affected infants may appear normal early in life and the diagnosis may not be suspected until age 6 to 12 months, when the defective hair and teeth are recognized. The disorder ought to be suspected in a child presenting with pyrexia of unknown origin.[25] The prognosis is good, provided the child can be protected from the risks of hyperpyrexia secondary to infection, hot weather, or vigorous exercise. Survival to adulthood is common.

Several anesthetic considerations are important in the management of affected children. The usual facies and mandibular underdevelopment may make airway management by mask awkward and laryngoscopy and intubation difficult. In some cases, regional anesthesia may be a reasonable alternative. Where general anesthesia is required, fresh gases should be warmed and humidified. Lacrimation may be reduced and the eyes should be protected by an ophthalmic ointment and taped closed. Careful monitoring of body temperature is necessary because of impaired thermoregulation.[27] Measures for cooling the patient such as padded ice bags, cool intravenous solutions, or fans should be available. Anticholinergic medication, although important in children, will reduce any available sweat production further and may contribute to hyperthermia.

In anticipation of postoperative chest infections, preoperative teaching and vigorous postoperative chest physiotherapy should be planned.[28]

Vascular Malformations

Hemangiomas.[1, 5] Hemangiomas are quite common and occur in 10 percent of children under 1 year.[5] They usually appear shortly after birth and may vary considerably in number and size. Despite the marked overlap in their histology, they are usually classified as capillary, those composed of superficial, dilated capillaries with or without endothelial proliferation; as cavernous, consisting of large blood-filled cavities that have compressed single-layered endothelium and involve deeper tissues; or as mixed. They are characterized by an initial proliferative stage, in which there is rapid growth over the first 5 to 7 months of age, and then by an involuting phase, in which there is variable regression of the lesion size with fibrosis and fat deposition. Cavernous hemangiomas are often composed of more mature vascular elements that are less likely to involute.[5]

The *strawberry nevus* is a capillary hemangioma that usually appears at 1 to 2 months of age on the face, scalp, or trunk and is more frequent in girls. These nevi are raised, bright red lesions rarely exceeding 5 cm in size. Spontaneous involution occurs in 95 percent by age 9 years, and fewer than 10 percent of patients have cosmetic defects that require plastic surgery.

Giant hemangiomas are often mixed capillary and cavernous lesions and are usually seen on the face and scalp. They may become very large, ulcerate, become secondarily infected, or bleed, or by compression they may interfere with vital functions. When such complications become severe, systemic corticosteroid therapy with prednisone 2 to 4 mg/kg/24 hours may produce significant regression in 2 to 3 weeks.[6, 29] For more benign lesions, compressive bandaging will often reduce the hemangioma size satisfactorily. Surgery may be advised when involution has not begun by age 4 years and when arteriovenous fistulas have been demonstrated.[1, 29]

There may be significant problems in maintaining an airway by mask in children with distorting facial hemangiomas (Fig. 15–4). Laryngoscopy and intubation may be difficult and may traumatize upper airway components of the lesion. Even minor surgery may precipitate considerable hemorrhage, and a reliable large-bore intravenous cannula is essential. For major procedures, the child must be in optimal hemodynamic and hemostatic condition prior to induction and adequate blood products must be available.

Patients on systemic corticosteroids require additional coverage during the perioperative period.

Kasabach-Merritt Syndrome. In this syndrome infants with giant hemangiomas, usually of the cavernous type, develop thrombocytopenia, hypofibrinogenemia, and a chronic consumption coagulopathy, which can precipitate acute hemorrhage and a sudden increase in the size of the lesion.[1, 5] Platelets entrapped within the cavities are thought to continuously stimulate activation of the clotting mechanism.[30, 31]

Volume resuscitation with blood products may be

Figure 15–4. Mixed cavernous and capillary hemangioma of the face in a 14-month-old child. Remarkably, airway management by mask and laryngoscopy were not difficult.

required, and repeated platelet administrations may be necessary to correct ongoing thrombocytopenia.

Systemic corticosteroid therapy is recommended as the treatment of choice, but radiotherapy has been reported to be successful.[1, 5] Conservative management is preferred to surgical excision, which could precipitate disseminated intravascular coagulation.[10]

Diffuse Neonatal Hemangiomatosis. In this severe multisystemic disorder, multiple hemangiomas develop in the skin and most viscera, producing arteriovenous shunts and high-output congestive cardiac failure, complicated by thrombocytopenia and hemorrhage. The organ systems usually involved are the gastrointestinal tract and liver, central nervous system, and lungs. Few infants survive past 2 to 3 months of age, usually dying of cardiac failure, sepsis, respiratory obstruction, or central nervous system catastrophes.[32] Some response has been reported with systemic corticosteroids and radiotherapy. If cardiac failure cannot otherwise be controlled, some benefit from hepatic artery ligation is reported.[5]

These children are critically ill and deserve aggressive attempts to optimize their circulating blood volume, cardiac and respiratory status, and hemostatic mechanisms preoperatively. Central venous and arterial lines may be necessary for the evaluation of volume resuscitation and cardiovascular function. A reliable intravenous cannula is essential for perioperative blood product and fluid administration, and for postoperative intravenous alimentation when required.

Klippel-Trenaunay-Weber Syndrome. This noninherited condition is characterized by a variety of vascular malformations, including port-wine nevus, venous varicosities, and arteriovenous aneurysms that develop in one or more extremities, usually the legs. Hypertrophy of regional soft tissues and bones occurs secondary to the increased limb blood flow (Fig. 15–5). There may be associated polydactyly and syndactyly. If the functional arteriovenous shunt is significant, high-output cardiac failure may develop.[5] The treatment for this otherwise benign disorder is usually conservative, but occasionally plastic reconstructive surgery and varicectomy are recommended.[33]

It is important to recognize that children with Klippel-Trenaunay-Weber syndrome may have an increased cardiac output and will not tolerate anesthetic agents that decrease myocardial contractility.

Sturge-Weber Syndrome (Encephalotrigeminal Angiomatosis). The diagnostic features of this syndrome are the presence of a port-wine stain on the face in the distribution of the ophthalmic division of the trigeminal nerve and ipsilateral intracranial linear calcifications. Focal seizures and hemiparesis occur contralateral to the facial lesion. The vascular nevus is present at birth, but the neurological signs may not develop until later in childhood.[1, 6] Congenital glaucoma on the affected side is seen in 40 to 50 percent of patients.[5] Mental retardation is occasionally seen. In some cases, excision of the leptomeningeal angiomatosis is practical and of help in the treatment of seizures.[5] Hemispherectomy may be required.

Telangiectasias[1, 4, 6]

Ataxia Telangiectasia (Louis-Bar Syndrome). This autosomal recessive disorder presents as progressive cerebellar ataxia in children 12 to 18 months old. Oculocutaneous telangiectasia appears at about age 3 to 5 years on the conjunctiva and on the skin of the eyelids, face, ears, upper chest, and popliteal and antecubital fossae. Occasionally, café-au-lait spots are seen.[1] Deficiencies in the immune response are manifested by recurrent pulmonary infections and bronchiectasis, which may be fatal. Many children who survive to adolescence develop malignant lymphomas.[4, 6] No specific treatment can be offered.

The principles of anesthetic management are directed at the complications of the disease, namely, the chronic pulmonary infections, bronchiectasis, and the development of lymphoreticular malignant tumors.

Figure 15–5. Klippel-Trenaunay-Weber syndrome in a 7-year-old boy demonstrating cutaneous phlebectasias and regional soft tissue and bone hypertrophy of the lower extremity.

Hereditary Hemorrhagic Telangiectasia (Osler-Weber-Rendu Syndrome). Hereditary hemorrhagic telangiectasia is an autosomal dominant condition manifested by delicate ectatic vascular lesions in the skin, mucous membranes, and viscera. The telangiectasias are found most commonly in the nasal mucosa, lips, tongue, and gastrointestinal tract and less commonly in the bladder, bronchi, liver, and brain. Pulmonary lesions tend to resemble arteriovenous fistulas. The syndrome may present in childhood as repeat episodes of epistaxis. The diagnosis may be missed, in the absence of a positive family history, because only at puberty do the skin lesions develop and subsequently increase in number. Infrequently the disease may present with gastrointestinal hemorrhage in infancy.[34]

Although clotting factors are normal, bleeding may be difficult to control. Hemorrhage is the most serious complication and may result in severe anemia.[1] In an attempt to control mucosal bleeding, skin grafting to the nasal mucosa has been helpful although the telangiectasias continue to develop around the graft site.[35] Estrogen therapy to induce squamous metaplasia has had limited success.

Prior to the induction of anesthesia, significant anemia or hypovolemia must be corrected. Care must be taken not to traumatize oral mucosal lesions during laryngoscopy. Nasal intubation is relatively contraindicated.

Lymphangiomas

Lymphangiomas are hamartomatous malformations composed of dilated lymph channels lined by normal lymph endothelium. The four clinical types—simple lymphangiomas, lymphangioma circumscriptum, cavernous lymphangiomas, and cystic hygromas—may vary greatly in size. The lesions are present at birth or develop in early infancy. They are usually slow-growing, do not spontaneously involute, and are not radiosensitive. Lymphangiomas occur most commonly on the proximal limbs, shoulders, neck, tongue, and buccal mucosa. Symptoms are caused by compression of local structures. Surgical excision is often unsatisfactory, as recurrence of these lesions is frequent.

Cystic hygromas are uncommon, large, cystic lymphangiomas usually occurring on the neck, although the axilla, groin, and popliteal fossa are other reported sites (Fig. 15–6). They are frequently present at birth and grow slowly, infiltrating adjacent vessels, muscles, and nerves.[5] When cystic hygromas occur on the neck intubation may be difficult, and tracheostomy is often required to protect the child from subsequent airway obstruction.[36, 37]

Vesiculobullous Disorders

Common to all the vesiculobullous disorders is a disturbance of intraepidermal or dermoepidermal ad-

Figure 15–6. Recurrent cystic hygroma in the left axilla of a 10-month-old girl positioned for surgical excision.

herence with the subsequent accumulation of serous fluid within the cavities formed by tissue separation. Many pathological mechanisms lead to blister formation. Immunological techniques for diagnosis and for treatment evaluation have suggested that the immune system may feature in the pathogenesis of these disorders and explain their not infrequent association with connective tissue disorders such as systemic lupus erythematosus.[4]

Epidermolysis Bullosa[1, 4, 5, 6]

Epidermolysis bullosa is a rare subgroup of the mechanobullous diseases characterized by blister formation initiated by minor trauma to the skin. A clinical sign common to many of these diseases is Nikolsky sign: the separation of epidermis by lateral finger pressure. The several forms of epidermolysis bullosa are divided into scarring or nonscarring categories. The severity of the disease, however, is determined more by the extent of the bullous lesions and subsequent complications than by the presence of scarring alone, which merely reflects the depth of the cleavage plane.[4]

The nonscarring category includes epidermolysis bullosa simplex, junctional epidermolysis bullosa (letalis), and Bart syndrome.

Epidermolysis bullosa simplex is inherited as an autosomal dominant trait. The generalized form (Koebner) presents in the neonate as intraepidermal blisters on the hands, feet, elbows, knees, legs, and scalp, but any skin surface may be involved. Intraoral lesions are minimal. Affected infants are usually vigorous; the lesions heal quickly without scarring, and exacerbations tend to decrease with age. Life span is normal. In the localized form (Weber-Cockayne), which presents in early childhood to adulthood, the bullae are limited to the hands and feet. There are no oral lesions. The incidence of both forms increases in warmer climates and in summer.[1, 38]

Junctional epidermolysis bullosa (letalis), an autosomal recessive disorder, presents at birth as severe subepidermal blisters on the scalp and extremities, which may eventually involve the entire cutaneous surface, sparing only the palms and soles[1, 6] (Fig. 15–7). Oral lesions are severe and may extend to the esophagus.[4] The lesions heal slowly, often becoming secondarily infected and forming chronic granulomas, which may lead to scarring. A refractory anemia is common. The disease is progressive, and death from septicemia usually occurs in the early months or before age 2 years.

Bart described a syndrome of congenital localized absence of the skin and blistering, usually on the legs, with dystrophic nail changes. This variant may be a form of epidermolysis bullosa and has a good prognosis.[23]

The scarring category includes dystrophic epidermolysis bullosa, which has dominant and recessive forms.

Dystrophic epidermolysis bullosa, autosomal dominant form (Cockayne-Touraine), presents in early infancy as subepidermal bullae, usually limited to the hands, feet, and sacral area, which heal rapidly to leave soft, superficial wrinkled scars. Deformities are uncommon and oral lesions are minor. The general health of children with this form and their prognosis are often good.

Dystrophic epidermolysis bullosa, autosomal recessive form (polydysplastic, mutilans), although rare (1 in 300,000),[1, 39] is the most incapacitating variant of the disorder. It presents at birth or in early infancy as severe, erosive, subepidermal bullae that heal slowly with atrophic scarring. All areas of the skin are vulnerable. Continuous mucous membrane involvement may be unrelenting, involving the mouth, pharynx, esophagus, and anus, and may cause severe feeding problems and nutritional deprivation, even in older children. Anemia and growth retardation are common. Repeat cycles of bullae formation and healing by scarring lead to strictures of the mouth, tongue, larynx, and esophagus and produces the mitten-hand deformity from digital fusion[38, 44] (Fig. 15–8). Joint contractures also occur. The overall prognosis is poor and death usually occurs in the first three decades.

The underlying etiology of this disease is unknown. No specific effective treatment is available. Therapy is supportive and directed at skin care and at the management of complications such as anemia, malnutrition, and infections as they arise. Systemic corticosteroids are used in critical periods and may be palliative for such complications as esophageal strictures.[43] Surgical intervention in these children is usually indicated for dental restorations, reconstructive procedures on the extremities, and the excision and grafting of corneal ulcers. Anesthesia may also be required for diagnostic esophagoscopy or cystoscopy.

Anesthetic Management. Children with epidermolysis bullosa demand careful preanesthetic assessment. They are often debilitated and in poor nutritional states. They may have chronic anemias, respiratory infections, sepsis, or fluid and electrolyte

Figure 15–7. Junctional epidermolysis bullosa in a 3-month-old infant.

Figure 15—8. Dystrophic epidermolysis bullosa (recessive) in a 12-year-old boy demonstrating the classical mitten-hand deformity.

disturbances. Renal disease from secondary amyloidosis has been reported.[45] Hypercoagulable states have been described.[46] The extent of active disease, vulnerable skin areas, and contractures must be carefully identified.

Good rapport with a young patient will encourage cooperation at induction and may avoid a traumatizing struggle. Premedication may be necessary and should be given orally. However, awake patients able to transfer themselves will avoid the potential trauma of even gentle handling.[47] Perioperative steroid supplementation may be necessary.

All personnel caring for these children must recognize the vulnerability of their skin to trauma. Friction is more harmful than perpendicular pressure. The bedding beneath the patient must be smooth and adequate padding must be provided for pressure points when the patient is positioned. The removal of adhesive materials will cause skin loss, and where possible these materials should be avoided.

Monitoring is a considerable challenge and should be adequate but kept to a reasonable minimum. The skin on the arm can be protected from a blood pressure cuff by soft cotton padding. Nonadhesive ECG contacts or plates, axillary temperature probes, and weighted precordial stethoscopes should be used. The use of indwelling temperature probes and esophageal stethoscopes should be avoided. An atraumatic spray antiseptic should be used for invasive procedures; intravenous and arterial lines should be secured in place by sutures and gauze bandaging. The eyes must be protected by an ophthalmic ointment and not taped shut. The operating room must be warm for small children, in whom thermoregulation may be significantly impaired.

Most procedures in children will be done using general anesthesia. Infiltration with local anesthetics is contraindicated because of bulla formation and potential skin slough.[10, 41, 48, 49] Regional blocks are best avoided in view of skin involvement and complications at access points.

Intravenous and intramuscular ketamine has been used with good results for induction or as the sole agent.[47, 49, 50] Induction is smooth and the airway and ventilation are usually maintained adequately.[211] The original reports of close association between epidermolysis bullosa and porphyria[51, 52] have been overemphasized,[45] and more recently the association has been narrowed down to dystrophic epidermolysis bullosa involving skin only and porphyria cutanea tarda.[18, 53] Although barbiturates have been used often and without incident for induction,[37, 54–57] they should be avoided in the latter group of patients.[18] Despite the theoretical risk of hyperkalemia in patients with extensive tissue injury, no complications have been reported using succinylcholine.[37–42, 54–58] There may be increased sensitivity to the nondepolarizing neuromuscular blocking agents.[49] Halothane probably remains the inhalational agent of choice.

When general inhalational anesthesia is required, airway management presents major difficulties. Perioral scarring may restrict the opening of the mouth, the tongue may be distorted by adhesions,[57] and the larynx may be stenosed.[40, 44] The application of a face mask and finger support of the mandible may induce blister formation (Fig. 15–9). Following airway instrumentation, airway obstruction from oropharyngeal bullae and hemorrhage have been reported.[10, 56, 58] However, there are no reports of laryngeal or tracheal bullae during or after anesthesia.[38] James and Wark, in a retrospective study of 113 oral and 18 nasal intubations, reported only three cases of intraoral bulla formation directly attributable to intubation, and none caused postoperative problems.[55]

Figure 15–9. Dystrophic epidermolysis bullosa (recessive) in a 12-year-old boy. Note the ulceration of tongue and lips discovered after the removal of the dental dam following a 90-minute anesthesia for dental restorations.

Inhalational induction may be achieved by delivering warmed and humidified anesthetic agents at high flows from a mask held just above the face. Several noncontact induction hoods or boxes have been proposed.[59, 60] Prior to mask or finger contact, the skin of the face and chin should be protected by 0.5 percent hydrocortisone cream[51, 58] or by cotton sponges soaked in saline, petroleum jelly (Vaseline), or another lubricant.[51, 58] The use of oropharyngeal airways is discouraged by most authors.[10]

When required, intubation should be performed very gently and with the patient sufficiently deeply anesthetized or paralyzed to facilitate the procedure. The MacIntosh blade is preferred, to minimize contact with the epiglottis.[61] The blade and endotracheal tube must be generously lubricated to reduce friction and a smaller tube than usual selected. The tube should be secured by soft flannel ties or by an external fixation device to avoid skin contact.[51] To avoid coughing, the patient may be extubated deep (unless contraindicated) or following intravenous lidocaine, 1 to 1.5 mg/kg.

The patient must be carefully observed for airway problems throughout the postanesthetic recovery period.

Erythema Multiforme[1, 4, 6]

The term erythema multiforme represents a spectrum of acute inflammatory diseases involving the skin and mucous membranes ranging from a mild illness, erythema multiforme minor, to a severe, life-threatening condition, erythema multiforme major or the Stevens-Johnson syndrome.[63] The disorder is relatively common, accounting for up to 1 percent of dermatology outpatient visits. Although the disorder is rare in children under age 3 years, more than 50 percent of patients are under age 20 years; 60 percent are males. Young adults and children, especially boys, present with the more severe forms.

Many etiological factors have been implicated in the precipitation of erythema multiforme. Infections are the best documented and include viral infections with herpes simplex and adenovirus and *Mycoplasma* infections, particularly with *M. pneumoniae*. Drugs are associated with 60 percent of cases, but are often falsely implicated because many are administered for the prodromal symptoms of the infections or of the disease itself.[1] These include the sulfonamides, penicillin, the hydantoin anticonvulsants, barbiturates, salicylates, hydralazine, and many others.[64] Erythema multiforme is seen in association with malignancies, usually lymphomas and some connective tissue diseases, notably systemic lupus erythematosus.[65] The discovery of deposits of IgM, complement, and fibrin in dermal vessels suggests a hypersensitivity or immune complex etiology.[66]

Erythema multiforme minor presents with a nonspecific prodrome of malaise, low-grade fever, arthralgias, and symptoms of an upper respiratory tract infection, often in the spring and fall. The rash is usually symmetrical and distributed over the extensor surfaces of the extremities, including the palms and soles, the conjunctiva, and rarely the oral mucosa. The patient is usually asymptomatic, although the oral lesions may burn. The exanthem begins as dull, red macules that expand and then clear centrally, to form characteristic target or iris lesions (Fig. 15–10). Urticarial plaques may be seen.[1] Occasionally, the macules progress to vesicle formation in more severe cases. Successive crops of lesions may appear, but the rash rarely persists for more than 2 weeks. Apart from symptomatic measures, no specific treatment is required. Short-term corticosteroid therapy may be helpful in the more severe cases.

Erythema multiforme major (Stevens-Johnson Syndrome)[67] is an uncommon but severe disease with a mortality rate, if untreated, of 5 to 15 percent.[1] Prodromal symptoms of malaise, fever, headache, sore throat, cough, chest pain, vomiting and diarrhea, myalgia, and arthralgia occur 1 to 14 days prior to the sudden onset of erosive bullous lesions on the skin and mucous membranes. The oral mucosa, lips, and bulbar conjunctiva are the most frequently and severely involved areas (Fig. 15–11). The painful, erosive bullae may extend from the mouth and lips to the external nares, pharynx, esophagus, larynx, and tracheobronchial tree and involve the genital areas. Eating and breathing are uncomfortable and difficult. The ocular lesions include purulent conjunctivitis, corneal ulcerations, anterior uveitis, and staphylococcal panophthalmitis.[69] Blindness may ensue. Bullae in the visceral pleura may lead to pneumothorax[70] and large pleural effusions may

Figure 15–10. Erythema multiforme minor demonstrating typical iris lesions in the hands.

develop.[71] Gastrointestinal tract ulceration and hemorrhage have occurred.[71] Poor nutrition, anemia, and fluid and electrolyte disturbances are frequent. Acute tubular necrosis, nephritis, and renal failure have been described. Cardiac involvement may be manifested by atrial fibrillation, pericarditis, and myocarditis.[72] Fatal complications usually arise from widespread epidermal necrolysis, respiratory obstruction, pulmonary infection, and septicemia.

The treatment of Stevens-Johnson syndrome is essentially supportive but requires hospital supervision. Precipitating infections and associated diseases should be treated, and implicated medications should be discontinued. Skin lesions are best managed with wet dressings and baths. Fluid and electrolyte disturbances must be corrected quickly. Intravenous alimentation may be required in younger children.[71] Secondary infections must be promptly treated with antibiotics. Systemic corticosteroids are usually administered in high doses during the stage of mucocutaneous extension and slowly tapered during the 1- to 3-week healing phase.[5, 73] Resolution of the disease may take 2 to 7 weeks. Recurrences are seen in all forms of erythema multiforme in 25 percent of cases.

Anesthetic Management. Children with erythema multiforme present a major challenge to the anesthetist. They are usually febrile and toxic and distressed by the painful lesions as described. Hypovolemia, anemia, and electrolyte disturbances must be corrected preoperatively. Percutaneous intravenous cannulation is preferred because cutdown incisions heal poorly and are vulnerable to infection. In very ill patients, no premedication is recommended.

Monitoring is important, but extreme care is required to avoid skin trauma. The arm may be protected from the blood pressure cuff by a soft roll, and a weighted precordial stethoscope may be used. ECG monitoring to identify dysrhythmias is necessary, but the removal of electrodes must be gentle. Temperature should be monitored by an axillary probe; esophageal stethoscopes and nasal temperature probes should not be used. The presence of urethritis should discourage

Figure 15–11. A mild example of Stevens-Johnson syndrome demonstrating the oral lesions and conjunctivitis.

the use of urinary catheters. Appropriate physical means to control pyrexia (for example, cooling blankets) should be available.

If general anesthesia is required, airway maintenance poses many potential problems. If obstructing bullae or edema compromise the upper airway, a tracheostomy (not without its own risks) may be required preoperatively.[10] The application of a face mask may denude affected skin, and the face must be protected by lubricated cotton or gauze sponges. The insertion of oral airways and laryngoscopy and intubation, however gentle, may traumatize existing bullae or laryngeal and tracheal mucosa sufficiently to initiate bleeding or bulla formation.

Induction techniques depend on the surgery planned. Ketamine has been used as the sole agent.[71] Barbiturates should be avoided. Otherwise, a cautious inhalational induction is preferred. There are no reports of adverse reactions to neuromuscular blocking agents. Pancuronium is probably the nondepolarizing agent of choice. Because chest x-rays may not identify pleural bullae, positive-pressure ventilation should be avoided or used with the lowest possible peak airway pressure. Corticosteroid coverage for the operative period will likely be required.

Regional anesthesia may be a useful alternative if the overlying skin is clear and the child is cooperative.

The potential for postextubation airway obstruction is high in these patients, and close postoperative airway monitoring and supervision must be provided.

Toxic Epidermal Necrolysis (Lyell Disease)[1, 4]

Toxic epidermal necrolysis is a rare but extremely severe acute bullous eruption of the skin and mucous membranes that is seen in all age groups. The highest mortality rates (20 to 40 percent) are in young children and the elderly.[4, 10]

A short prodrome of fever, malaise, and conjunctivitis usually precedes the acute development of mildly tender, diffuse erythema, which may be widespread. Nikolsky sign (separation of the epidermis with lateral finger pressure) is present early. Confluent, flaccid bullae develop quickly and rupture, shedding large sheets of epidermis and leaving huge, denuded, erosive areas on the back, shoulders, and face. Severe mucous membrane lesions are common and involve the oropharynx, tongue, larynx, tracheobronchial tree, and esophagus, often resulting in tracheitis, pneumonia, and gastrointestinal hemorrhage.[1] The course may be relentlessly progressive for one or more weeks and may be complicated by high fever, hypovolemia, electrolyte imbalance, secondary infections and septicemia, shock, renal impairment, and disseminated intravascular coagulation.[75, 76] Recovery is slow; healing may lead to scarring contractures of both skin and mucous membranes.

The etiological factors implicated in toxic epidermal necrolysis are similar to those responsible for erythema multiforme: drugs, including barbiturates, analgesics,

and hydantoin anticonvulsants;[64, 77, 78] viral, bacterial, and fungal infections; vaccinations; radiation; and malignancies, notably lymphomas.[1, 6] Some authors believe toxic epidermal necrolysis to represent the most devastating form of erythema multiforme.[79] Histological studies show necrosis of basal epidermal cell layers and subepidermal bulla formation.

The prognosis depends on the adequacy of treatment but is always guarded. High-dose systemic corticosteroid therapy, aggressive antibiotic control of secondary infections, and correction of fluid and electrolyte imbalance are mandatory. Local skin care, particularly of the mouth and eyes, is important.[1, 4]

The principles of anesthetic management in patients with toxic epidermal necrolysis are similar to those for erythema multiforme and epidermolysis bullosa. Careful attention must be paid to thermoregulation in small children.

Staphylococcal Scalded Skin Syndrome (Ritter Disease)

Staphylococcal scalded skin syndrome is an uncommon superficial cutaneous eruption manifested as widespread epidermolysis and intraepidermal desquamation.[1] It occurs in infants and young children either as a localized form, called bullous impetigo, or as a generalized form (Ritter disease).

Following a variable prodrome of malaise, conjunctivitis, or occult upper respiratory tract infection, a periorificial or generalized scarlatiniform rash appears which is exquisitely tender. Nikolsky sign is present early. Within 48 hours large, flaccid intraepidermal bullae develop and sheets of epidermis separate. The moist erythematous base thus exposed usually dries quickly, with superficial desquamation. Mucosal involvement is rare. Healing is usually complete in 5 to 12 days,[1, 81] but a small number of patients may develop cellulitis, pneumonia, and septicemia. The disease still carries a significant mortality rate of 2 to 3 percent.[1]

The syndrome is caused by the exotoxin epidermolysin, which is produced by infections with *Staphylococcus aureus* group II, phage type 71.[1, 4] It is distinct from toxic epidermal necrolysis because basal epidermal cell necrosis does not occur. Treatment requires strict isolation, the administration of penicillinase-resistant antibiotics, attention to hydration and electrolyte balance, and local skin care.[80, 81] The use of corticosteroids is considered only in those patients who become critically ill.[4]

The anesthetic management of children with this disorder requires the preoperative correction of fluid and electrolyte disturbances and the recognition of complicating secondary infections such as pneumonia. Contact with involved skin is painful, and the patient must be handled gently. Anticholinergic agents should be used with caution because thermoregulation may be impaired. Temperature monitoring is mandatory.

No specific anesthetic technique is recommended, but local infiltration should be avoided. When inhalational anesthesia is used, the face must be protected to prevent frictional trauma and bulla formation. Adhesives should be avoided. Instrumentation of the airway must be cautious in the presence of mucosal involvement.

All equipment used should be regarded as septic and cleaned appropriately after use.[10]

Pemphigus, Pemphigoid, Dermatitis Herpetiformis, and Chronic Bullous Dermatosis of Childhood

The term pemphigus refers to a group of bullous diseases involving the skin and mucous membranes, which all demonstrate the presence of serum antibodies directed against squamous epithelial intercellular substance.[82, 83] The subsequent loss of cohesive epidermal cell bridges is called acantholysis and leads to intraepidermal bulla formation at varying depths.[1] Nikolsky sign is frequently seen. Although pemphigus is most common in adults, three forms are recognized as occurring during childhood.

Pemphigus vulgaris most typically presents in the fourth and fifth decades of life and in people of Jewish and Mediterranean origin, but has been reported in all races and in children as young as 3½ years old.[1, 84, 85] A genetic link is suggested, but has not been proved. In children, the disease is first manifested as painful oral ulcers and subsequently as large, flaccid, suprabasal bullae, most commonly on the scalp, face, and trunk. These lesions tend to enlarge and rupture, producing painful denuded areas that heal slowly.[1, 6] Oropharyngeal lesions may compromise adequate nutrition, and laryngeal lesions may cause hoarseness.[10] No other organ systems are primarily affected in children, but progressive disease may produce fluid and electrolyte disturbances or hypoalbuminemia and may be complicated by secondary infection and sepsis. Untreated, the mortality may reach 90 percent.[1] Pemphigus vulgaris has been found in association with thymomas and myasthenia gravis, lymphoid malignancies, and systemic lupus erythematosus.[86, 87] An important differential diagnosis in children is erythema multiforme.

Pemphigus foliaceus is less common and less severe than pemphigus vulgaris. The cleavage plain is higher in the epidermis and the bullae are superficial. They rupture easily to produce shallow erosions with scaling and crusting, which may be intensely pruritic. Common areas of involvement are the scalp, face, and upper chest, although generalized extension of the disease has been seen. Oral lesions are infrequent. A localized variant of this form, pemphigus erythematosus, presents as a lupus-like butterfly rash on the face. The prognosis is generally good.

Familial benign pemphigus (Hailey-Hailey disease) is inherited as an autosomal dominant trait and usually presents in the second decade as small pruritic vesicles on an erythematous base in the axilla, groin, and antecubital fossae. General health is not affected. Remissions occur, but there is little tendency to improvement with age.[1]

The successful treatment of pemphigus vulgaris requires prompt, high-dose systemic corticosteroid therapy, particularly during acute exacerbations. Local skin care with wet compresses is important.[1, 4] During critical periods with patients on steroids, secondary infections and fluid and electrolyte disturbances must be managed aggressively. Supplemental immunosuppressive agents, methotrexate, cyclophosphamide, and azathioprine have reduced maintenance steroid requirements.[1, 4, 89–91] Parenteral gold therapy has been a useful alternative in some patients.[1] Less severe forms of pemphigus respond well to lower doses of steroids; even topical preparations may be adequate.

Bullous pemphigoid is similar to but distinct from pemphigus, from which it is differentiated histologically by the presence of subepidermal bullae. It occurs rarely in children, in whom it presents as large, tense bullae over intertriginous areas, the flexor surfaces of the forearm, the groin, and the lower abdomen.[6, 85, 93] Mucous membrane lesions are reported in 10 to 20 percent of cases and include the mouth, pharynx, esophagus, vagina, and anus.[4] The bullae may rupture, leaving denuded areas, but these tend to heal well. Pruritus is less a feature, and the patient's general condition is good. The disease tends to be chronic, but with remissions and improvement over time.

Treatment includes systemic corticosteroids and immunosuppressive agents, but in lower doses than for pemphigus. Sulfapyridine and dapsone have been helpful.[93]

Dermatitis herpetiformis is a chronic eruptive disease characterized by intensely pruritic, small, tense papules and vesicles grouped symmetrically over the extensor surfaces of the extremities, the buttocks, and the scalp. In the juvenile form, lesions may appear in the axillae and groin.[1] The mucous membranes are usually spared. This disorder occurs in all age groups but most commonly in middle life. The etiology is unknown, but there is a strong association with celiac sprue (gluten-sensitive enteropathy) and an immunodeficiency mechanism is postulated.[4] No cure is available, but effective suppression of the disease is possible by maintenance doses of sulfapyridine or dapsone.[4, 6]

Chronic bullous dermatosis of childhood (linear IgA dermatosis) is a noninherited disorder presenting in preschool children as deep, tense, 1- to 2-cm bullae on the lower trunk, perineum, and thighs and occasionally on the scalp and face. This condition may resemble bullous pemphigoid and dermatitis herpetiformis, but tends to be self-limiting and remits within 1 to 4 years of onset.[5, 6] Treatment includes a combination of corticosteroids, sulfapyridine, and dapsone.

Anesthetic Management. Evidence of the diseases associated with pemphigus must be sought and recognized in the preoperative assessment. These diseases include systemic lupus erythematosus, rheumatoid arthritis, lymphoid malignancies, thymoma, and myasthenia gravis. Each requires additional considerations for anesthetic management.[86, 87] The effects of maintenance medications must be evaluated in relevant systems. Immunosuppressive agents may cause bone marrow suppression, hepatic dysfunction, and infiltrative pneumonitis. Sulfapyridine causes crystalluria and may impair renal function. Dapsone may induce a chronic hemolytic anemia[4] and a peripheral neuropathy.[4, 10] Perioperative corticosteroid coverage will usually be required. In acute exacerbations, children with pemphigus may develop secondary infections, fluid and electrolyte disturbances, and hypovolemia.

No particular anesthetic techniques have been recommended in these patients, but local infiltration is contraindicated because of potential skin slough. In adults, the successful use of regional anesthesia by peridural catheter supplemented by ketamine[95] and of a combination of ketamine and diazepam as sole agents[96] has been reported.

When present, the facial, oropharyngeal, and laryngeal lesions produce difficulties for airway management similar to those in patients with epidermolysis bullosa and the same principles apply. Skin surfaces must be carefully protected, and airway instrumentation, if required, must be cautious and gentle.

Acrodermatitis Enteropathica

Acrodermatitis enteropathica is a rare autosomal recessive disorder of zinc metabolism presenting in the first year of life as an acral and periorificial vesiculobullous eruption followed by alopecia, severe diarrhea, failure to thrive, and progressive cachexia.[4, 97] Associated manifestations include glossitis, stomatitis, and secondary bacterial and candidal infections. Untreated, the course is chronic and relapsing. Acute exacerbations may be fatal.[4]

The metabolic defect appears to be related to the intestinal absorption of zinc, and oral zinc preparations rapidly abolish manifestations of the disease.[98]

Children with acrodermatitis enteropathica may be debilitated, nutritionally deprived, hypovolemic, anemic, and weak from muscle loss. The preoperative correction of treatable parameters should be undertaken. Under anesthesia, these children may show poor tolerance to inhalational agents and sensitivity to narcotics and neuromuscular blocking agents.

Disorders of the Epidermis

Psoriasis

Psoriasis is a chronic papulosquamous dermatosis characterized by epidermal hyperplasia and increased epidermal turnover. The incidence varies from 0.1 to 3 percent with equal frequency in males and females.[1] Presentation before age 16 years is reported in 30 to 45 percent of cases.[99, 100] The onset of psoriasis in childhood (mean age 8.1 years) is associated with a strong family history and is twice as common in girls as in boys.[101] The etiology includes both genetic and environmental factors.

The initial appearance and subsequent outbreaks of the eruption may follow epidermal injury (the Koebner reaction), infections, stress, cold weather, or withdrawal from corticosteroid therapy. The lesions are discrete erythematous papules and plaques covered with silvery scales and occur usually on the scalp, face, elbows, and knees. Pitting of the fingernails is characteristic. Mucosal lesions are rare. The increased blood flow to the subepidermal cutis in the generalized form, psoriatic erythroderma, has caused high-output cardiac failure in adults.[101, 102] Psoriatic lesions are culture positive for *Staphylococcus aureus* in 30 percent of cases.[103] The arthropathy seen in 5 percent of adults with psoriasis is infrequently diagnosed in children and is rarely severe.[104, 105] Temporomandibular joint ankylosis has been reported in a 28-year-old male.[106] Hyperuricemia is seen in more extensive disease, but without gout.[1]

The variant most commonly seen in children is guttate psoriasis, in which the lesions are small, teardrop plaques on the scalp, face, trunk, and proximal limbs (Fig. 15–12). There is frequently a history of prior streptococcal respiratory tract infection. Diaper psoriasis precedes chronic psoriasis in 17 percent of cases.[4] Neonatal psoriasis, although rare, is severe and recalcitrant and may be complicated by early joint involvement.[107] Children rarely develop the unusual manifestations of the disease, such as pustular psoriasis and psoriatic erythroderma.

The management of childhood psoriasis is conservative. Topical therapy with tar preparations, keratolytic agents, and low-dose ultraviolet light precedes the cautious addition of topical corticosteroids. Systemic steroids and methotrexate are avoided in children if possible. Prophylactic penicillin or tonsillectomy may reduce poststreptococcal guttatic flare-ups.[100]

Anesthetic considerations in children with psoriasis include the preoperative evaluation of the activity and extent of the disease, maintenance medications, and the identification of complications such as psoriatic arthropathy or high-output cardiac failure in psoriatic erythroderma.

No specific techniques are recommended, but several points deserve attention. It is important to prevent physical and chemical trauma to the skin, because further lesions may be precipitated. The handling and transfer of patients must be gentle. The use of adhesive tapes and ECG electrodes on areas of involved skin should be avoided if possible. The presence of *Staphylococcus aureus* in psoriatic skin demands careful, aseptic techniques for intravenous cannulation and may contraindicate the use of regional blocks. Anesthetic and operating room equipment should be appropriately cleaned after use.

Disorders of the Dermis

Ehlers-Danlos Syndrome

The Ehlers-Danlos syndrome is a heterogeneous group of inherited disorders of collagen synthesis. The

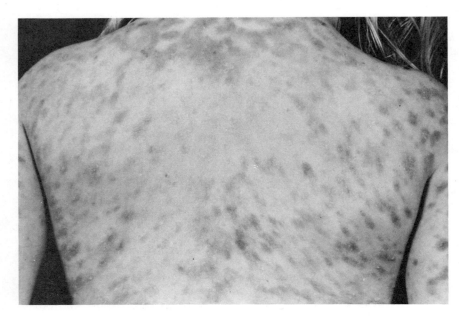

Figure 15–12. Guttate psoriasis in a 6-year-old girl.

clinical manifestations have been classified by Beighton and associates into eight distinct forms.[108] Characteristic clinical signs include hyperextensible skin, hypermobile joints, and excessive bleeding after minor trauma. The usual inheritance is autosomal dominant.

Premature birth is a frequent feature and is secondary to early rupture of the amniotic membranes, which share the connective tissue defect of the child. Transient postnatal hypotonia may predispose to pneumonia.[4] In all types, the skin is thin, hyperextensible, elastic, and very fragile. Minor trauma may result in lacerations that heal poorly, leaving thin atrophic "cigarette paper" scars. Umbilical, femoral, and inguinal hernias are common and develop early. Joint hypermobility is manifested as congenital hip dislocation or later as spontaneous dislocations and kyphoscoliosis. Blood vessel walls are fragile and minor trauma may induce ecchymoses or bleeding. Gastrointestinal hemorrhage and perforation are well-known complications. Varicose veins are common. The excessive bleeding, particularly in the ecchymotic form (type IV), may be explained by decreased collagen-platelet interaction,[109] the failure of vessel constriction, and the absence of effective surrounding tissue tamponade. Coagulation is usually normal, but the bleeding time is prolonged.

Cardiovascular manifestations of the disease may be minor, but are unpredictable and potentially catastrophic in some patients. They include mitral valve prolapse, aortic insufficiency, conduction defects, and sudden death from spontaneous aortic aneurysm rupture.[110] Spontaneous pneumothorax has been reported.[111]

The management of Ehlers-Danlos syndrome is conservative. The potential complications of uncontrolla-

ble hemorrhage and wound dehiscence discourage invasive or surgical procedures unless absolutely necessary. The prognosis of this disorder, in the absence of arterial complications, is good and life span may be normal.[4]

The anesthetist must anticipate complications in managing patients with this disorder.[112] A coagulation screen, including bleeding time, should be obtained to identify the risk of excessive bleeding. Adequate blood products must be available even for minor procedures. Patients with cardiac murmurs should receive prophylactic antibiotics. Intramuscular premedication should be avoided. In the operating room, the patient must be transferred and positioned carefully to prevent skin and skeletal injuries.

Good intravenous access is mandatory, but may be difficult and require surgical cutdown. Severe extravasation of intravenous fluid or hematoma formation may go unnoticed in these patients. Internal jugular or subclavian central venous lines may be complicated by mediastinal or pleural hematomas. Arterial cannulation may lead to aneurysm formation. Such invasive monitoring should be used only when essential.

Regional techniques have been used successfully despite the risk of hematoma, but are best avoided in children.[113] Inhalational anesthesia by mask is the recommended technique for short, minor procedures. When intubation is required, the patient must be adequately relaxed so that airway instrumentation is smoothly accomplished, minimizing the risk of airway hematoma formation and temporomandibular joint dislocation. Peak ventilatory pressures must be kept as low as possible. Hypertension should be avoided or corrected early to reduce hemorrhage and the risk of aneurysm rupture. To minimize coughing at extubation, the endotracheal tube may be removed with the patient under deep anesthesia or after intravenous lidocaine, 1.5 mg/kg, has been administered.

Close postoperative monitoring of the patient's airway, ventilation, and blood pressure is mandatory.

Cutis Laxa

Cutis laxa is a rare congenital disorder of elastin synthesis, affecting the skin and internal organs. Inheritance may be autosomal recessive, X-linked recessive, or dominant. An acquired form, presenting later in life, may follow a febrile illness, a drug eruption, or erythema multiforme.[4, 114] Skin biopsies show deficient and disorganized elastin fibers in the dermis and vascular walls.

In all forms of the disease, the skin hangs on the body in loose pendulous folds like an ill-fitting suit. The child looks prematurely wrinkled and aged. Unlike Ehlers-Danlos syndrome, the skin fails to recoil when released, but it does not bruise easily and heals normally. Hypermobile joints are not a feature. Infants may have a hoarse cry from vocal cord laxity.

Dominant cutis laxa may present only cosmetic problems, but the recessive forms may have multiple system manifestations. These include umbilical, inguinal, and obturator hernias, diaphragmatic atony, gastrointestinal and genitourinary tract diverticula, rectal prolapse, and generalized osteoporosis.[115] Severe cardiorespiratory complications include emphysema, peripheral pulmonary artery stenosis, pulmonary hypertension, cor pulmonale, and aneurysmal aortic dilatation. In the acquired form, severe occlusive coronary artery disease has been described in young children.[114]

No specific treatment is available, although anti-inflammatory agents and steroids may be useful in the acquired form. Complications are treated as they arise.

The chief anesthetic considerations in these children concern the severity of cardiac and pulmonary complications, in particular, cor pulmonale, aortic dilatation with valvular insufficiency, and coronary artery disease.

Pseudoxanthoma Elasticum

Pseudoxanthoma elasticum is a rare degenerative disorder of elastin tissue, involving the skin, eye, cardiovascular system, and gastrointestinal tract. It is inherited by autosomal dominant or recessive patterns and occurs in 1 per 160,000 to 1 per 1,000,000 population.[116] The diagnosis is often made after age 30 years, but many severely affected patients are children, and the disease has been reported in a 6-month-old infant.[117, 118]

The skin lesions usually appear in childhood as small yellow papules in linear or reticular patterns on the neck, axillary and inguinal folds, the umbilical area, and the popliteal and antecubital fossae. The involved skin becomes lax with poor elastic recoil and hangs in folds. Ocular signs present as loss of visual acuity from amyloid streaks and retinal detachment.

The entire cardiovascular system is affected by the degenerative changes and calcification that develop in the arterial media. Peripheral pulses may be absent. Intermittent claudication and ischemic ulcers are frequent findings. Angina pectoris is seen in 8 percent of patients under age 20 years.[116] A triple aortocoronary bypass has been reported in an 18-year-old girl who had angina from age 11 years.[117] Dysrhythmias, renal hypertension, cerebrovascular occlusion, gastrointestinal and uterine hemorrhage, hypothyroidism, and psychotic depression have all been reported.[4, 6, 116]

There is no effective treatment. The prognosis varies considerably; despite reports of sudden death in children,[118] many patients seem to have normal longevity. Vascular surgery has often proved helpful.[119]

The primary anesthetic consideration in patients with pseudoxanthoma elasticum concerns the severity of cardiovascular complications. Even in children, a history of angina must be sought. An oral premedication to tranquilize young patients is desirable. Note that older patients may be taking maintenance tricyclic antidepressants.[116]

Monitoring must include use of an ECG and a precordial stethoscope. Blood pressure is best taken by a cuff and an ultrasonic Doppler probe. Arterial cannulation is difficult and may accelerate distal vascular ischemia, but may be necessary in critically ill patients.[116] Myocardial oxygen supply and demand must be optimized by avoiding tachycardia and hypertension.

No specific anesthetic techniques or drugs are recommended.

Disorders of Subcutaneous Tissue

Lipodystrophy

The rare syndromes of partial and generalized lipodystrophy are characterized by the absence of subcutaneous fat over part of the body surface.

Partial lipodystrophy occurs more commonly in females and presents before the age of 10 years as the progressive loss of subcutaneous fat from the face downward to the arms and upper trunk. The skin is normal, but the facies becomes cadaverous and the muscles and veins of the trunk become prominent. Insulin-resistant diabetes mellitus develops in 20 percent of cases.[1] Many patients develop glomerulonephritis, but the incidence of significant renal disease is unknown.

Congenital generalized lipodystrophy (Seip-Lawrence syndrome) is a progressive multisystemic disorder inherited by an autosomal recessive trait. It may be present at birth as a generalized loss of subcutaneous fat or occur in early infancy. Associated features are prominent veins, hirsutism, and skin pigmentation. Hepatomegaly may be prominent even in infancy, secondary to fatty infiltration and cirrhosis. Skeletal growth is accelerated. With time, insulin-resistant nonketotic diabetes mellitus develops.[1, 6]

There is no treatment for either condition.

Anesthetic management requires attention to the control of associated diabetes mellitus and the recognition of coincident renal and hepatic dysfunction. Infants may become hypothermic easily and are vulnerable to hypoglycemia if glycogen stores are reduced.

Eczema

Eczema (Greek *eczein*, boiling over) is a generic term describing a particular inflammatory reaction pattern in the skin. The important forms of eczema in children are atopic dermatitis, contact dermatitis, and seborrheic dermatitis.

Atopic Dermatitis

Atopic dermatitis is a relatively common skin disorder (affecting 1 to 5 percent of children under age 5 years)[120] characterized by erythema, edema, intense pruritus, exudation, crusting, and scaling. There appears to be a genetic predilection. The onset is usually at age 2 to 3 months, with pruritic erythematous patches on the cheeks and subsequent extension to the face, neck, wrists, hands, and extensor aspects of the extremities. Constant scratching induces weeping and crusting. Secondary infection with staphylococci, beta-hemolytic streptococci, and herpes simplex virus is common and may be severe (Fig. 15–13). There is a tendency to remission at age 3 to 5 years, but the disease may become chronic.[5, 6] With increasing age, the involved areas of skin tend to dry and thicken.

About 80 percent of patients with atopic dermatitis have increased serum IgE levels, but a specific role for allergens, whether foods or inhalants, is disputed.[6] A significant number of children with atopic dermatitis subsequently develop reactive airway disease.[5]

The treatment of atopic dermatitis requires the avoidance of environmental precipitants. During acute flare-ups, therapy includes local care with wet dressings, antihistamines, topical corticosteroid cream, and systemic antibiotics for secondary infections.

Several considerations are important in the anesthetic management of children with atopic dermatitis. A careful history of allergies should be taken. The development of reactive airway disease in older children may favor the use of inhalational agents that reduce bronchomotor tone. Affected skin sites should be avoided for intravenous cannulation, and the face, if actively involved, should be protected from mask pressure by saline-soaked gauze. Supplemental steroid coverage is rarely required.

Contact Dermatitis[5, 6]

Allergic contact dermatitis is a T-cell–mediated hypersensitivity reaction that is provoked by application of an antigen to the skin surface. Sensitization requires several days and becomes manifest as local, erythematous, intensely pruritic, eczematous dermatitis on reexposure to antigen. If the reaction is severe, edema, vesicles, and bullae may develop.

Treatment requires removal of the allergen and the application of cool moist compresses. Antihistamines and topical corticosteroids are usually effective. In the acute massive bullous reactions, such as poison ivy, a short course of systemic corticosteroids is very helpful.

Anesthetic considerations are similar to those for atopic dermatitis.

Seborrheic Dermatitis

Seborrheic dermatitis is a chronic inflammatory disorder that is manifested as dry, scaly, erythematous

Figure 15–13. Atopic dermatitis in a 3-year-old girl complicated by secondary infection with herpes simplex virus.

papular lesions. In children, it is most common in infancy and adolescence. Constitutional symptoms are infrequent and recovery is usual, even without treatment. Its severest clinical manifestation, erythema desquamativa (Leiner disease) was discussed on page 379.

Wiskott-Aldrich syndrome[1, 2, 4] is an X-linked recessive disorder manifested by thrombocytopenia purpura, recurrent infections, and severe seborrheic dermatitis. The thrombocytopenia is present at birth. Bloody diarrhea is common, and a severe anemia develops early. Recurrent infections with pneumococcus, meningococcus, and *Haemophilus influenzae* begin at age 6 months. Recurrent pauciarticular arthritis[7] may be seen. A deficient immune response is postulated as the etiology of this syndrome.

Treatment is mainly supportive. Despite transfer factor therapy and bone marrow transplantations, survival past puberty is rare.[4]

Should these patients require surgery, they present major challenges to the anesthetist, notably chronic debilitation, acute hypovolemia, anemia, coagulopathies, and secondary infections.

Letterer-Siwe disease is an acute, disseminated, and frequently fatal variant of histiocytosis X. It usually presents in infancy with a seborrheic or eczematous eruption on the scalp, postauricular folds, intertriginous areas, and diaper region. Major complications arise from involvement of bone, of the reticuloendothelial system and of the central nervous system.[4, 6] Mandibular hypoplasia may occur and make laryngoscopy and intubation very difficult.

Menkes syndrome is an inherited, neurodegenerative disorder associated with a copper enzyme deficiency state. Seborrheic dermatitis, generalized hypopigmentation, and sparse, kinky hair are frequent cutaneous features. Death from central nervous system complications usually occurs before age 2 years.[1, 4]

Photosensitivity

Photosensitivity denotes a qualitatively or quantitatively abnormal skin reaction to sunlight. Host factors are important, particularly normal melanin pigmentation, which reflects, absorbs, and scatters light. Photosensitivity may be a feature of some diseases, such as the porphyrias, or may be an exacerbating factor in others, such as erythema multiforme and connective tissue disorders, including systemic lupus erythematosus and dermatomyositis.[6]

Xeroderma pigmentosum is a rare autosomal recessive disorder characterized by severe photosensitivity and the subsequent formation of cutaneous malignancies.[1, 4, 6] By age 3 years, exposed skin has become atrophic and scarred and develops telangiectasia and actinic keratoses. Basal and squamous cell carcinomas and malignant melanomas finally appear. Death from metastatic disease usually occurs between ages 7 and 20 years.

The rigorous avoidance of sunlight and the surgical excision of malignancies as they arise is the only treatment available.[121]

Apart from care in handling involved skin and the recognition of metastatic disease, there are no specific anesthetic recommendations.

Disorders with Pigmentary Change

Neurofibromatosis (von Recklinghausen Disease)

Neurofibromatosis is a relatively common (1 per 3200 population)[122] autosomal dominant disorder characterized by café-au-lait spots and the appearance of neurofibromas in the skin, subcutaneous tissue, nervous system, bones, and internal organs. These tumors are overgrowths of the Schwann cells and endoneurium, which cover nervous tissue; their manifestations are greatly varied.

The presence of six or more café-au-lait spots (local areas of cutaneous hyperpigmentation) with a diameter of greater than 1.5 cm is usually diagnostic, but the disease is confirmed by the appearance of cutaneous and subcutaneous neurofibromas later in childhood. These tumors are usually soft, may be pedunculated, and may affect any area of the skin. Plexiform neuromas are less common but may be large and infiltrative and cause considerable disfigurement.[6]

Central nervous system involvement may approach 66 percent of cases and may be associated with an increased incidence of gliomas and meningiomas.[10] Cranial nerves are frequent sites for neurofibromas. Acoustic neuromas cause deafness and vertigo, and optic neuromas may cause visual impairment. Pituitary and hypothalamic dysfunction may be manifested by growth disturbances and by precocious sexual development.[123] Spinal cord neuromas may cause paresis. A thoracic meningocele with vertebral anomalies has been reported.[135] Mild mental impairment is common, and seizure disorders are seen in 5 percent of patients.[6] Pheochromocytoma occurs in 1 percent of adults with neurofibromatosis, a manifestation of autonomic nervous system involvement.[1, 6] Hypertension seen in children with neurofibromatosis is more often secondary to renal artery compression and stenosis.[123, 130]

Skeletal complications occur in 30 to 50 percent of cases. Thoracic scoliosis, being the most common, is seen in 10 to 40 percent of cases.[125] Subperiosteal lesions may lead to pathological long bone fractures.

Neurofibromas arising from the larynx and pharynx are rare, but have been reported in young children.[125, 127, 129] Respiratory distress from airway obstruction, dysphonia, and dysphagia were the usual presentations. Tracheostomy may be required.[127]

Other manifestations of neurofibromatosis include genitourinary tract obstruction with uremia and the development of pulmonary interstitial fibrosis and honeycomb lung cysts. The lung changes usually occur only in adults older than 35 years.[128] Sarcomatous degeneration of neurofibromas occurs in 1 pecent of patients, but is rare in children.[6, 129]

In the absence of malignant change, life span may be normal. Surgical intervention in children with neurofibromatosis is required to correct scoliosis, resect painful subcutaneous nodules, repair renal artery stenosis, correct obstructive uropathy, and reduce pathological fractures.

Several considerations deserve attention in planning anesthetics for these children. The preoperative identification of upper airway lesions is mandatory. If obstructive symptoms have developed, tracheostomy may be required.[127]

Ventilatory function in the presence of scoliosis should be evaluated fully with pulmonary function tests. In patients who are hypertensive, laboratory investigations should include tests of urinary catecholamines, pituitary function, electrolytes, blood urea nitrogen, and creatinine.

The child should be positioned carefully and all pressure points should be adequately protected. All basic monitoring is required. In patients who have pulmonary dysfunction or hypertension, an arterial line may be necessary.

Regional anesthesia has been used in older children, but technical difficulties from occult neurofibroma and back deformities may be encountered.[129]

When general anesthesia is required, no specific drugs are recommended. Of the inhalational agents, halothane may be more likely to cause dysrhythmias in patients with renal hypertension.[143] Patients with neurofibromatosis are reported to have increased sensitivity to both succinylcholine and nondepolarizing agents.[130, 131] High thoracic spinal lesions may predispose some patients to autonomic hyperreflexia.[10] Hypertensive crises should be quickly controlled.

Incontinentia Pigmenti (Bloch-Sulzberger Syndrome)

Incontinentia pigmenti is a rare multisystemic disorder inherited by an X-linked dominant gene, usually lethal in males. Skin lesions may be the only manifestation, but 80 percent of patients have additional neurological, ocular, and skeletal defects.[6, 133]

The skin lesions present in the first 2 weeks of life as erythematous streaks and plaques of vesicles on the trunk and limbs, followed by intermediate verrucous lesions that may persist for 6 months. Subsequently, irregular macules develop that contain patches of brown to slate-gray pigment. The skin lesions usually resolve by adulthood.[133]

The central nervous system manifestations include developmental retardation, cortical atrophy, degrees of spastic paresis, seizures, and hydrocephalus. Ocular complications include strabismus, cataracts, retinal detachment, and optic nerve atrophy. Blindness occurs in over 15 percent of cases.[6] Skeletal anomalies are less

common, but include spina bifida, cleft lip and palate, dwarfism, and chondrodystrophy. Pegged (conical) teeth are characteristic. Despite the partial anodontia, mandibular development is normal.[10]

No anesthetic problems have been reported. Many of the patients are mentally impaired and blind. The operating room must be quiet for induction.

No specific anesthetic drugs or techniques are recommended. Succinylcholine must be used with caution in the presence of spastic paresis. Laryngoscopy and intubation are usually straightforward, but care must be taken because of the anomalous teeth.

Giant Congenital Melanocytic Nevus

These congenital lesions are relatively rare and occur in fewer than 1 in 20,000 newborns. They vary considerably in size, but may cover a major anatomical area of the body, often the back, torso, or "bathing suit" region and occasionally part of an extremity. They contain varying degrees of pigment, are often covered by dark, coarse hair, and have raised, verrucous borders (Fig. 15–14). Distribution on the head and neck is often associated with leptomeningeal melanocytosis, leading to seizure disorders and hydrocephalus.[5]

The major concern in these lesions is their potential for malignant degeneration. Malignant melanomas develop in 6 to 10 percent of these lesions, often in childhood.[4, 134–136] Optimal treatment requires staged, total surgical excision and the application of split-thickness skin grafts.[4]

Urticarial and Hypersensitivity Disorders

Urticarial lesions are well-circumscribed, raised, pruritic, and erythematous areas of edema in the skin, limited to superficial layers of the dermis. When the edematous process is deeper, extending into the lower dermis and subcutaneous tissue, the lesion is referred to as angioedema.

Cold Urticaria

Cold urticaria is an uncommon disorder characterized by abrupt swelling and edema in the skin on exposure to cold stimuli. It may be life-threatening when there is a local reaction to the ingestion of cold foods or when there is associated hypotension and cardiovascular collapse.[1, 137] Cold challenge in these patients induces an IgE-dependent degranulation of mast cells and the release of histamine and other vasoactive mediators.[1] Both acquired and familial forms are described.

A careful history of attack symptoms will identify the usual severity of the patient's reaction. Premedication with H_1 and H_2 histamine antagonists and steroids will not prevent the release of histamine but may attenuate many of its vascular effects.[137, 138] The operating room, as well as the laryngoscope, intrave-

Figure 15–14. Giant congenital melanocytic nevus involving the torso and back of a prone 10-day-old infant.

nous solutions, and anesthetic gases, must be warmed. Warming blankets should be in place.

Inhalational anesthesia is probably the best choice in children. Those drugs known to cause histamine release should be avoided.[139–141, 157] A fentanyl-metocurine combination, with the above premedication, was used in a 47-year-old man with cold urticaria for cardiopulmonary bypass and hypothermia to 31° C.[137]

Hereditary Angioedema

Hereditary angioedema is an uncommon autosomal dominant disorder manifested by attacks of nonpitting edema of the face, upper airway, extremities, and abdominal viscera. These attacks may occur spontaneously or following trauma. The underlying cause is a deficiency of C_1-esterase inhibitor, allowing uncontrolled complement activation and the formation of vasoactive mediators to proceed. Two thirds of patients are symptomatic before age 13 years.[142] The mortality of untreated episodes from laryngeal edema has been reported as high as 30 percent.[142]

Blunt trauma, including tonsillectomy, dental manipulation, and endoscopy, has initiated the syndrome in over half the cases. Emotional upset and anxiety may also provoke attacks.[145] Oropharyngeal and laryngeal edema occur in 64 percent of cases.[142] Abdominal pain is a frequent symptom; accompanying diarrhea may cause hypovolemia. The onset is acute and the edema lasts 24 to 72 hours.

The management of acute attacks requires large doses of epinephrine subcutaneously or by intravenous infusion[146–148] and fresh frozen plasma.[144] Antifibrinolytic agents may also be helpful. Corticosteroids and antihistamines are still used, but are rarely effective alone.[140] Narcotics may be required for abdominal pain. If the airway is compromised, early intubation is advised before emergency tracheostomy becomes necessary.[149]

Long-term prophylactic therapy with an antifibrinolytic agent, epsilon-aminocaproic acid or tranexamic acid, has had modest success.[142] Androgens have also been used.

The major priority in the anesthetic management of these patients is adequate preoperative preparation. For elective surgery, a 2- to 3-day course of an antifibrinolytic agent and an infusion of fresh frozen plasma the day before is recommended. This treatment will restore the levels of C_1-esterase inhibitor to normal for 1 to 4 days.[143, 144] For emergency surgery, an immediately preoperative infusion of fresh frozen plasma may be sufficient.[143, 144] Intraoperative angioedema has been managed with epsilon-aminocaproic acid.[150]

Following preoperative preparation, there are no specific anesthetic recommendations in the literature. Effective premedication to reduce anxiety is important; antihistamines have been used.[146] Local infiltration for dental extractions,[145] a regional spinal block for genitourinary surgery[146] and a hyoscine, thiopentone, succinylcholine induction for cesarean section[144] have been reported without problem.

In children, general anesthesia using a simple technique with inhalational agents may be preferred. Intubation, when required, must be performed gently to avoid upper airway trauma. Throat packs are discouraged.[18] Postoperative observation in an intensive care area is advised for 24 hours.[145]

Mastocytosis

Mastocytosis is a relatively rare disorder characterized by abnormal aggregates of mast cells in the dermis and in various organs of the body. Most cases are sporadic and occur in whites, with equal frequency in both sexes.[1] Local and systemic manifestations are due to the release of vasoactive mediators from the mast cell granules.

Urticaria pigmentosa is the most common form of the disease. It presents in children before the age of 2 years. The lesions are limited to the dermis and appear as yellow to brown macules, papules, or nodules distributed symmetrically over the skin, usually sparing the mucous membranes.[6] Occasionally, recurrent bullae are seen in infants. Pruritus may be intense. Isolated infiltrates (mastocytomas) occur in 10 percent of cases. The prognosis is good; spontaneous involution occurs by puberty in 50 percent of cases.

Systemic mastocytosis occurs in 5 to 10 percent of cases.[1, 6] Bone lesions are painful and may cause pathological fractures. Intestinal malabsorption, peptic ulceration, hepatic dysfunction, hepatosplenomegaly, and infiltrations in the kidneys, lymph nodes, and marrow may occur. Secondary anemia, thrombocytopenia, and coagulopathy are not infrequent. Pulmonary eosinophilic granulomas have been reported.[151] The prognosis of systemic mastocytosis is guarded. Rarely, mast cell leukemia develops; this condition is rapidly fatal.[152]

Episodic systemic symptoms are caused by mast cell degranulation and the release of histamine, prostaglandin D_2[153] and heparin into the circulation. Forty to 50 percent of patients have attacks of flushing, pruritus, headaches, palpitations, abdominal colic, and occasionally vomiting and diarrhea[1, 156] (Figs. 15–15 and 15–16). More severe attacks are accompanied by syncope and profound hypotension, which can progress to refractory shock and death. Bronchospasm is unusual, but has been reported with salicylates.[153] Rarely, grand mal seizures are seen. Heparin release may induce the bleeding diathesis occasionally found in patients without systemic disease. Factors precipitating mediator release include mechanical stimulation of skin lesions, psychological stress, extreme temperature changes, alcohol ingestion, and a variety of histamine-releasing medications such as the opiates, salicylates, atropine, muscle relaxants, and polymycin B, to name a few.

No treatment is available to control the progress of the disease, although single mastocytomas may be excised. Symptomatic therapy provides variable results and includes H_1 and H_2 receptor antagonists, oral disodium cromoglycate, corticosteroids for severe bullous eruptions in infants, and the avoidance of triggering factors. Antimetabolites may have limited use in systemic disease.

Surgical intervention may be required for the excision of isolated skin lesions, the reduction of pathological fractures, intestinal surgery for ulcers, or thoracotomy for pulmonary resection.[10] Even in unrelated and minor procedures, profound cardiovascular collapse has been reported.[154, 156] The primary anesthetic considerations, therefore, are the prevention of vasoactive mediator release and the prompt treatment of hypotension, should it occur.

Anesthetic Management. A preoperative history of vasoactive symptoms and precipitating factors may be very helpful. Investigations must include hemoglobin, platelet count, coagulation screen, and serum electrolytes. Adequate blood products must be available when appropriate. Perioperative steroid coverage may be required. Good rapport with the patient and adequate premedication will reduce anxiety levels in the operating room. Sedation should be given orally, and an antihistamine and cimetidine should be included.[154, 155] Atropine should be avoided; glycopyrrolate may be safe, but no experience is reported.

The operating room must be warm and the temperature not allowed to fluctuate. The patient must be transferred and positioned carefully to avoid stimulation of skin lesions, bone pain, and pathological fractures.

No specific techniques are recommended. Both regional and general anesthesia have been reported.[155–157, 161] Drugs to avoid are atropine, morphine, codeine, D-tubocurarine, metocurine, gallamine, and the salicylates.[155–157] Thiopentone and pancuronium have both been shown to release histamine.[158, 159] Succinylcholine is considered safe,[156] but little experience is published. Rectal methohexital has been used without

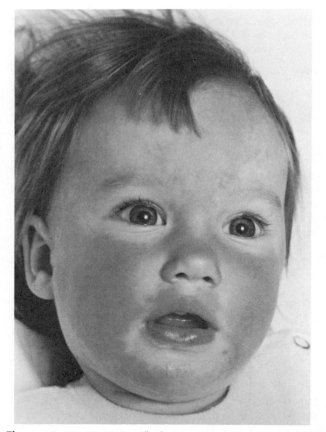

Figure 15–15. Histamine flush in a 14-month-old girl with mastocytosis.

Figure 15–16. Urticarial lesions and flush in a 14-month-old girl with mastocytosis.

incident.[155] Demerol is the recommended analgesic,[155, 156] but fentanyl may also be free of histamine-releasing properties.[157] Inhalational agents do not appear to release histamine.

In elective procedures in children, a cautious inhalational induction with halothane is the best choice. Reliable intravenous access should be obtained early. Intubation, if required, should not be difficult with the patient under halothane anesthesia. Oral lesions, if present, are minor. Muscle relaxants should be avoided, but in an emergency glycopyrrolate and succinylcholine may be required. Monitoring must include use of an ECG, precordial stethoscope, and temperature probe. Blood pressure should be monitored by an arterial line for thoracotomies or major laparotomies.

Should a hypotensive crisis occur, immediate resuscitative treatment with intravenous fluids, antihistamines, and sympathomimetics must be initiated. Epinephrine by infusion is reportedly the most effective vasopressor.[160] Minor hemorrhage has been controlled by protamine.[155] Transfusion reactions may be lethal.[10]

Equally vigilant care must be continued throughout the postoperative period.

Erythema Nodosum

Erythema nodosum is a syndrome characterized by the development of inflammatory cutaneous nodules on the extremities. These nodules represent a hypersensitivity reaction to various antigens and involve the septal vessels of fat lobules. The disease affects females more than males (3:1), usually between the age of 15 and 30 years.[1]

Following a variable prodrome of fever, malaise, and arthralgias, symmetrical crops of painful, indurated, red, hot, raised nodules appear on the extensor surfaces of the limbs, usually over the shins. After 2 to 3 weeks, the induration decreases and the violaceous colors subside, finally leaving a brown residuum. Joint involvement is usually minor, affecting the ankles most frequently with tender swelling and effusions. After 6 to 8 weeks, the disease becomes quiescent and rarely recurs.[1, 6]

Etiological factors include infections with tuberculosis, streptococci, brucellosis, toxoplasmosis, and some viruses. Drugs have also been implicated, in particular the sulfonamides, oral contraceptives, phenytoin anticonvulsants, and salicylates. Erythema nodosum is seen in association with other diseases, notably sarcoidosis (Lofgren syndrome),[162] systemic lupus erythematosus, ulcerative colitis, regional ileitis,[163] and Behçet syndrome.[1]

Treatment is directed at the underlying cause: antibiotics for infections and the discontinuation of precipitating drugs. Bed rest and symptomatic relief with wet dressings and salicylates (if not a cause) are usually adequate. Corticosteroids are relatively contraindicated.[6, 10]

Preoperatively, the underlying cause and associated diseases must be identified. If arthritis is a feature, the temporomandibular joints must be examined to determine whether laryngoscopy will be difficult. Care must be taken in transferring and positioning the patient. No specific anesthetic techniques are recommended. All contaminated anesthetic equipment should be appropriately cleaned.

Miscellaneous Skin Disorders

Behçet Syndrome

Behçet syndrome is traditionally described as a relatively rare mucocutaneous ocular disorder characterized by recurrent uveitis, aphthous stomatitis, and genital ulcerations. It is now well recognized to have serious manifestations in additional organ systems.[1, 164] Males are affected more than females (2.3:1). The average age of onset is 20 to 30 years, but the disease has been described in children.[165, 166] The etiology is uncertain, but an immune mechanism is postulated.[164, 165]

The oral lesions present as recurrent painful ulcers involving the lips, gums, tongue, pharynx, and larynx. Healing by scarring is not a usual complication but has been described.[166] Ocular lesions include recurrent uveitis, conjunctivitis, choroiditis, and optic atrophy; blindness may follow. The skin manifestations include papules, subcutaneous nodules, vesicles, pyoderma, and abscesses.

Central nervous system involvement may relapse and remit, and clinical signs include spastic paresis, ataxia, seizures, coma, and spinal cord lesions.[10] Cardiovascular manifestations include pericarditis, recurrent thrombophlebitis, superior and inferior vena caval obstruction, and arterial aneurysms.[167] A transient inhibition of fibrinolysis is recognized to coincide with the episodes of thrombophlebitis. Hemoptysis and obstructive pulmonary disease have been reported.[168] Arthritic involvement is limited to the large joints and does not cause deformities.[169] Renal dysfunction with anemia may progress to nephrotic syndrome secondary to glomerulonephritis or amyloidosis[165] (see Chapter 7).

The course of the disease is variable but is usually chronic and progressive. Treatment has included corticosteroids, immunosuppressants, and fibrinolytic agents but does not appear to alter the gradual deterioration of the patient's condition.[170]

The anesthetic management of patients with Behçet syndrome requires attention to several points. Multiple systems are involved and each deserves full assessment. Clinical appraisal of the upper airway should include pharyngoscopy with the patient awake to identify oropharyngeal scarring, which may make laryngoscopy and intubation difficult.[166] When this complication is suspected, intubation should be performed with the patient awake, using topical anesthesia and modest sedation, or under deep halothane anesthesia and breathing spontaneously. Once the airway is secured, no specific recommendations are reported. Aseptic techniques must be followed in the presence of active pyoderma.

Malignant Atrophic Papulosis (Köhlmeier-Degos Disease)

Malignant atrophic papulosis is a rare, often fatal, multisystemic disease characterized by multiple infarcts in the skin, gastrointestinal tract, central nervous system, and other organs. It usually occurs in young adults but has been described in children.[171] The underlying pathology is an occlusive vasculitis of unknown etiology.

The skin lesions develop as porcelain white papules, which heal to form atrophic scars. Catastrophic complications arise from gastrointestinal lesions, which may result in bowel perforation and peritonitis, and from central nervous system infarcts, which may cause cerebral edema, increased intracranial pressure, and uncal herniation.[171] Pleural effusions, restrictive pulmonary disease, constrictive pericarditis with effusions, and myocardial infarctions are also reported.[172] No effective treatment is available.[173]

Surgical intervention may be required for acute gastrointestinal perforation and peritonitis and occasionally for pulmonary decortication and pericardiectomy. Patients with this disease are critically ill, and most require aggressive preoperative fluid resuscitation. Invasive cardiovascular monitoring is advised, to provide optimal evaluation of compromised cardiac and pulmonary function. The maintenance of adequate venous return in the presence of constrictive pericarditis and pericardial effusion is mandatory. Those patients with increased intracranial pressure would benefit from a light narcotic with relaxant technique and hyperventilation.[10] Postoperative management should be provided in an intensive care unit.

Fabry Disease (Angiokeratoma Corporis Diffusum Universale)

Fabry disease is a sex-linked recessive inborn error of metabolism (alpha-galactosidase A deficiency), fully penetrant in males and characterized by the deposition of the glycolipid ceramide trihexoside in the blood vessels of skin, mucous membranes, eyes, heart, kidneys, liver, peripheral nerves, and brain (see Chapter 13).[1, 6, 174] The vascular reaction causes ischemia and degenerative change in the affected organs. The skin lesions are angiokeratomas: small ectasias of dermal vessels protruding into the epidermis. They appear at puberty on scrotal, sacral, and umbilical areas, elbows, thighs, fingers, lips, and mucous membranes of the mouth. They may, however, be absent.[175] Hypohidrosis and hypotrichosis may occur.[10] Eye findings occur in late childhood as corneal opacities, conjunctival and retinal vessel tortuosity, and posterior capsular cataracts.

The disease presents in childhood as recurrent febrile episodes associated at first with weakness and then, in adolescence, with agonizing limb pain and paresthesias. The limitation of joint movement, including the temporomandibular joint, is seen but has not been explained. In early adulthood, symptoms of advancing organ system involvement appear. Neurological complications include presenile dementia, seizures, paralyses, and cerebrovascular accidents. Cardiac disease is manifest by angina pectoris, myocardial infarction, hypertension, dysrhythmias, and valvular disease (mitral insufficiency).[10, 176] Progressive renal failure with hypertension is a major cause of death by the fifth decade, but has been reported in a 16-year-old.[177, 178]

There is no specific treatment for this disease. Complications are treated as they arise. The paresthesias and acral pain have been controlled by oral diphenylhydantoin. Renal transplantation has had variable success.[179]

Anesthetic Management. The serious renal and cardiac complications of this disorder may not arise until early adulthood, but these systems must receive thorough evaluation even in children. A history of exercise intolerance or angina may be unlikely, but a chest x-ray and ECG should be obtained and the hemoglobin, electrolytes, blood urea nitrogen, creatinine, and urinalysis should be reviewed. Restriction to mouth opening is uncommon but must be identified preoperatively.

General anesthesia is usually required. Regional techniques in the presence of acral pain, paresthesias, and peripheral neuropathy are discouraged. All routine monitoring, including temperature probes, must be used. Anticholinergic agents may aggravate hypohidrosis and further impair thermoregulation. No specific anesthetic agents are recommended, but tachycardia and large blood pressure changes should be avoided.

Pyoderma Gangrenosum[4]

Pyoderma gangrenosum is an unusual syndrome, affecting any age group, and is characterized by unique skin ulcerations which appear most often on the lower extremities. Oral lesions have been described.[4] The ulcers, which may be large, have purple, raised, tender, undermined borders with purulent granulating bases. There is frequent association with a variety of systemic diseases, notably ulcerative colitis, Crohn disease, rheumatoid arthritis, some hematological malignancies, and Wegener granulomatosis.[10, 299]

Treatment is directed at the control of the underlying disease and local measures. Occasionally systemic corticosteroids and immunosuppressive agents are required.

CONNECTIVE TISSUE DISEASES

The connective tissues of the body arise from the differentiation of embryonic mesoderm and are adapted to a great number of diverse functions. They form the extracellular structures of support and movement—periosteum, bone, cartilage, fascia, and ligaments. They provide body coverings—the dermis, serosa, and internal organ capsules—and are major components in the structures of nourishment—blood vessels, the lymphatics, and the tracheobronchial tree. Connective tissue is composed of the fibrillar proteins collagen, elastin, and reticulin and a ground substance matrix.[1, 4, 7]

Collagen is the most abundant protein in man, constituting one third of total body protein, and is the principal fibrillar component of most connective tissue. The basic peptide is synthesized in fibroblasts and then undergoes postsynthetic, extracellular aggregation and cross-linking to form stable fibers of high tensile strength.[180] Elastin is synthesized in smooth muscle cells.[1] It is a highly branching fiber and lacks the tensile srength of collagen, but displays much greater elasticity. With reticulin, elastin provides the major fibrillar component of connective tissue in blood vessels, muscles, and the parenchyma of internal organs.

The fibrous proteins are set in a ground substance matrix, composed of glycosaminoglycans (mucopolysaccharides), which are long-chain carbohydrate polymers, maintained in stiffly extended configuration from the protein core by highly negatively charged molecular groups. A large amount of water and about half the plasma proteins are held within the spaces created by these molecules.[7]

The constant remodeling of connective tissue by degradation and regeneration is one of the primary reparative functions of the inflammatory process. In connective tissue disease, these tissues become the important focus of destruction or of degenerative change when the directed functions of acute inflammation are disturbed. The etiology and pathogenesis of the connective tissue diseases are not fully understood. They all exhibit a variety of autoimmune phenomena in both the humoral and cellular immune systems, but the causal relationship of these phenomena to the inflammatory process is not always clear.[7, 181] However, in acute fulminant autoimmune disease, the most important therapeutic maneuver remains the use of anti-inflammatory agents.[182]

The connective tissue diseases usually present as clinically distinct entities, but their chronic and multisystemic features may produce considerable overlap in signs and symptoms. Precise diagnostic and laboratory criteria are lacking.

However uncommon these disorders may be, many of the patients require surgical intervention. Pediatric anesthetists must therefore have a good understanding of the several systemic manifestations of each disease and of the secondary effects that medical management might induce (see page 419).

Juvenile Rheumatoid Arthritis (Still Disease)

Juvenile rheumatoid arthritis is a chronic and extremely variable systemic disease characterized by synovitis and associated extra-articular manifestations.[6-8] It is the most common of the pediatric connective tissue disorders. Its annual incidence is 3 to 10 cases per 100,000 population. Childhood onset disease (prior to age 16 years) accounts for 5 percent of all patients with rheumatoid arthritis. Girls are twice as frequently affected as boys. All races and geographical regions are vulnerable. The etiology and pathogenesis are unknown, but infections, autoimmunity, and immunogenetic predisposition are considered possible causes.[7]

The pathology of adult and juvenile rheumatoid arthritis is similar. The synovitis is characterized by chronic, nonsuppurative, proliferative inflammation with hyperemia, edema, and an infiltration with lymphocytes and plasma cells. Joint effusions are common. Continuing synovitis may induce synovial hypertrophy and the progressive erosion and destruction of articular cartilage and contiguous bone. Although joint damage occurs much later and less commonly in juvenile onset disease than in adults, joint subluxation, ankylosis, and deformity still represent end-stage disease in some patients. Rheumatoid nodules are seen less frequently in juvenile disease, and systemic complications over the long term tend to be less severe.

Clinical Manifestations. The presentation of juvenile rheumatoid arthritis rarely occurs before the age of 2 years and usually falls into one of three broad clinical groups defined by the features that develop in the first 6 months of illness, namely polyarticular, pauciarticular, and systemic onset disease.[183, 184]

Polyarticular onset disease accounts for 40 to 50 percent of cases and may present at any time throughout childhood. Rheumatoid factor seronegativity is usual. The initial synovitis affects five or more joints and may be mild or fulminant, in which case the joints are warm, tender, swollen with effusions, painful, and stiff. The large joints are involved first: the knees, ankles, wrists, and elbows, and then the fingers. Hip involvement is frequent and may be severe with destruction of the femoral head.

Cervical spine arthritis occurs in 50 percent of cases and is complicated by early apophyseal ankylosis leading to fusion en bloc, usually of C2 and C3. Flexion deformities, loss of neck extension, and torticollis are common features. Atlantoaxial subluxation is a frequent radiological finding, but the incidence of instability and neurological complications is uncertain in children.[7, 8, 185]

Temporomandibular joint involvement, often manifested as earache, occurs in 65 percent of cases.[186, 187] Grosfeld and associates report that 16 percent of patients develop reduced mouth opening and 5 percent have severe secondary mandibular hypoplasia and retrognathia (Fig. 15–17).[187] Cricoarytenoid arthritis, seen in 26 percent of adults, is uncommon in children,[188, 189] but it may occur with pain, dysphagia, hoarseness, stridor, or dyspnea and has led to airway obstruction.[190]

The systemic manifestations in polyarticular onset disease are variable, but not as acute or persistent as in systemic onset juvenile disease. Irritability, low-grade fever, mild anemia, minor hepatosplenomegaly, and subclinical pericarditis are typical features.

An important subgroup of children, usually girls who are rheumatoid factor seropositive, present with

Figure 15–17. Juvenile rheumatoid arthritis in a 14-year-old boy. Note the fusion of cervical vertebrae from C2 inferiorly and the severe mandibular hypoplasia. Temporomandibular joint involvement was also present.

polyarticular disease in late childhood. Their arthritis is characterized by rheumatoid nodules, erosive synovitis, and a chronic course very similar to that of adult onset disease.

Pauciarticular onset disease accounts for 30 to 40 percent of cases. It usually affects girls and is associated with rheumatoid factor seronegativity. The arthritis usually presents before the age of 4 years in four or fewer joints as a low-grade inflammatory reaction affecting the knees, ankles, and elbows. The hips are spared. Only rarely are the temporomandibular joints, fingers, or neck involved. No systemic features are seen. This type of disease is prone to early remission.

The concern in this group is chronic uveitis, which occurs in 20 to 30 percent of cases and may persist for years. The major ocular sequelae are posterior synechiae, cataracts, glaucoma, visual impairment, and blindness in 10 to 20 percent of children affected.

Systemic onset disease occurs in 10 to 15 percent of cases of juvenile rheumatoid arthritis, with equal frequency among girls and boys. It may present at any time throughout childhood. The systemic manifestations may precede the development of arthritis by months or years. Joint involvement is variable but usually follows the pattern of polyarticular disease. In some cases, the arthritis may become chronic and persist after the remission of systemic symptoms well into adulthood.

The characteristic systemic features are a high daily or twice daily fever associated with the classic rash of juvenile rheumatoid arthritis. It is described as an evanescent, migratory, erythematous macular eruption on the trunk and proximal limbs. Frequently, impressive hepatosplenomegaly and generalized lymphadenopathy develop. Abdominal pain is often a feature. Cardiac involvement occurs in 5 to 10 percent of cases, commonly as pericarditis associated with minor effusions and mild substernal discomfort.[197, 198] It is not usually regarded as a bad prognostic sign in children.[7] Aortic valvular insufficiency has been described but is exceptional. Rarely, severe chest pain, dyspnea, and cardiac failure from pericardial tamponade have been reported.[193, 194]

Pulmonary involvement is usually limited to transient pneumonitis and pleural effusions. Although diffuse interstitial fibrosis is described in children, the classic rheumatoid lung of adult disease is rare.[196, 197] Anemia and transient proteinuria are common during periods of acute disease. Renal impairment is an unusual and late complication of juvenile disease, often occurring in association with amyloidosis. The vasculitis involving small and medium-sized vessels and the central and peripheral nervous system manifestations seen in adults are much less common in children.

The systemic manifestations may be severe in some patients, but usually run a self-limited course of several months. Recurrences are rare once adulthood is reached, although chronic arthritis may persist.

Course and Prognosis. Juvenile rheumatoid arthritis is rarely a life-threatening disease. It follows a course of remissions and exacerbations for several years, often causing little disability. The major morbidity of the polyarticular and systemic onset types is chronic joint disease, which occurs in 10 to 25 percent of patients and may be complicated by severe joint destruction and permanent disability.[6] In pauciarticular onset disease, the major concerns are the complications of chronic uveitis, as described above.

Treatment. There is no cure for juvenile rheumatoid arthritis. The principles of management are to preserve joint function and to control symptoms with as conservative a program as possible.

Aspirin is the single most important drug used in the treatment of this disorder. It reduces the inflammatory arthritis and controls the fever and other systemic manifestations in 70 percent of patients. The chronic administration of salicylates to children is extremely safe.[7] However, the toxic signs of salicylism vary from drowsiness, metabolic acidosis, and ketosis in very young children to hyperventilation and respiratory alkalosis in older children. Salicylates induce irreversible platelet dysfunction, as demonstrated by an increased bleeding time, and may be responsible for unexpected surgical blood loss.[199, 200] Other hemorrhagic and hypersensitivity reactions are rare in children.

Of the nonsteroidal antiflammatory agents, only tolmetin is currently licensed for use in children. It has proved effective in juvenile disease. Acetaminophen is discouraged for long-term use because of possible interstitial nephritis.[7] The antimalarial drug hydroxychloroquine is used less frequently now in view of its retinal toxicity.

Parenteral gold salts provide remissions in some patients unresponsive to other conservative therapy, but the toxic effects of stomatitis, dermatitis, marrow suppression, and renal dysfunction limit its widespread use. Penicillamine is similarly effective but may induce a lupus syndrome, dermatitis, thrombocytopenia, and proteinuria.

Although systemic corticosteroids dramatically suppress symptoms, they do not induce remissions, prevent joint damage, or alter the outcome of the disease in children. They are infrequently used for arthritic manifestations alone; steroids may accelerate avascular necrosis of the femoral head and aggravate growth disturbances. The indications for their use are usually limited to the management of severe, unresponsive systemic complications such as pericarditis and deteriorating chronic uveitis. The lowest effective doses are sought, and gradual withdrawal is begun as soon as possible. The limited use of intra-articular steroid injections may be of help in selected active joints of some patients. Immunosuppressive agents are approved in children only for life-threatening complications.

Chronic uveitis is usually controlled by a mydriatic agent (to prevent posterior synechiae) and dexamethasone eye drops.

Physical and occupational therapy provide essential training and rehabilitation programs to maintain muscle tone and joint function. Orthopedic splints help to reduce joint subluxation and deformity that may complicate chronic, active disease. Surgical intervention is discouraged until the children are older and bone growth has ceased. Prophylactic synovectomies are not beneficial in juvenile rheumatoid arthritis. Once the disease is quiescent, reconstructive procedures such as total joint prosthesis for hips and knees are often very successful.[201, 210]

Anesthetic Management. Juvenile rheumatoid arthritis is a multisystemic disease. Patients with this disease require thorough preoperative assessment.[202–204] The major challenge to the anesthetist in these children is usually airway management. Temporomandibular joint ankylosis, mandibular hypoplasia, and reduced neck extension can make application of a face mask difficult and direct laryngoscopy impossible[205] (Fig. 15–17). Chronic or active cricoarytenoid arthritis can cause glottic narrowing, and if suspected should be confirmed preoperatively by indirect laryngoscopy.[206, 207] Atlantoaxial subluxation is common in children with polyarticular or systemic onset disease, despite the infrequency of symptoms, and must be identified by flexion-extension x-rays of the cervical spine.

Although systemic involvement is not usually as compromising in children as in adults, cardiovascular and respiratory dysfunction can be serious. All patients should have a chest x-ray, ECG, and if indicated, pulmonary function tests. In systemic onset disease, anemia is pronounced and may require correction prior to major surgery. Significant hepatosplenomegaly may compromise ventilation in small children. Hemostasis may be altered in patients on salicylates; a platelet count and bleeding time and coagulation studies will be helpful.[199, 200] Adequate blood products must be available. Renal impairment is seen rarely in children, usually secondary to amyloidosis, but levels of serum electrolytes, blood urea nitrogen, and creatinine should be checked and a urinalysis performed. Perioperative corticosteroid supplementation must be arranged for those children on systemic therapy.

Modest sedative premedication may facilitate the induction of anesthesia in anxious and uncomfortable children. But, in those patients who have potentially difficult airways, conservative doses are advised. Metoclopramide and cimetidine should be included to reduce the acidity and volume of gastric contents.[208, 209]

Patients with active disease may splint their painful joints fearfully. They must be transferred in the operating room gently and supported in a comfortable position with adequate protection for pressure points created by contractures and deformities. The safe position for atlantoaxial instability is extension of this joint. Flexion of the neck must be avoided. All usual noninvasive monitors must be employed for induction. Patients with difficult airways should have an intravenous infusion started prior to induction.

The choice of anesthetic technique in children with difficult airways is determined by the skill and experience of the anesthetist, his assessment of the patient, and the nature of the surgical procedure. It may not be unreasonable for a skilled practitioner to provide inhalational anesthesia by mask for short, minor procedures. This is a judgmental decision, which carries the risk of airway obstruction, regurgitation, and pulmonary aspiration.

Regional blocks have obvious advantages, but are not always suited for young children. These procedures are relatively contraindicated in patients with peripheral neuropathies. D'Arcy and colleagues have reported good success with ketamine, nitrous oxide, and oxygen as the sole anesthetic agents for major joint surgery in patients in whom direct laryngoscopy was not possible.[210] However, ketamine provides no guarantee of reflex laryngeal competence.[211]

In those children who have difficult airways, endotracheal intubation is the best solution to airway management. However, intravenous induction with thiopentone and the use of muscle relaxants prior to intubation is a dangerous practice. The potential for airway obstruction and the loss of spontaneous ventilation in a patient whose larynx cannot be visualized may lead to disaster. Numerous acceptable techniques have been described.[212–226]

The safest approach is blind nasotracheal intubation with the patient awake, relying on cautious sedation or analgesia and the use of topical anesthesia for mucous membranes and glottic structures.[215] Atropine should be given to dry secretions and to protect against vagal reflexes. Small amounts of topical cocaine should be used to shrink the nasal mucosa. A smaller tube than usual must be selected, particularly in patients with cricoarytenoid involvement. To allow passage of the tube, when not tolerated by young patients, inhalational or ketamine anesthesia may be required, maintaining spontaneous ventilation. Hyperventilation, induced by adding 2 to 3 percent inspired carbon dioxide or 1 to 2 mg/kg doxapram intravenously, may facilitate laryngeal intubation in some cases.[216, 217] Cautious manipulation of the head and neck may be required. Fiberoptic laryngoscopy[218–221] and the use of various hooks, introducers, and retrograde catheters have been well described.[222–226] Should all efforts fail, a tracheostomy with use of local anesthesia may be necessary.

Once the airway is secured, several considerations remain. Patients with pulmonary disease or hepatosplenomegaly should have ventilation assisted or controlled.[202, 203] Cardiac reserve is reduced by myocarditis and aortic insufficiency, and agents decreasing myocardial contractility will be tolerated poorly. Patients with secondary muscle atrophy may be sensitive to neuromuscular blocking agents. Gardiner reports low tolerance in adults to narcotics; all central nervous system depressants should be used with care.[204]

Extubation must be delayed until full recovery of neuromuscular function is verified and the child is awake. Postoperatively, close observation of the airway is mandatory and may warrant admission to an intensive care area.

Spondyloarthropathies

Juvenile Ankylosing Spondylitis

Juvenile ankylosing spondylitis is a chronic inflammatory disease characterized by progressive arthritis of the axial and peripheral skeleton with associated extra-articular manifestations. In 8 to 10 percent of adults with ankylosing spondylitis, onset occurred in childhood between the age of 10 and 15 years.[7] The disorder in children may be as common as juvenile rheumatoid arthritis, but in this disease males predominate by a ratio of 6:1. The pathological changes are very similar to those of rheumatoid arthritis. Its strong familial incidence and close association with the antigen HLA B27 suggests a genetically determined immune mechanism as the etiology.

In most children, juvenile ankylosing spondylitis presents in early adolescence, usually with the peripheral arthritis first, affecting the hips, knees, and ankles. Occasionally, the shoulder and temporomandibular joints are involved. Enthesitis (inflammation and pain at the insertion of ligaments and tendons on bone) is a frequent symptom, particularly involving the heel and the tibial tuberosity. Subsequent deformity of the peripheral joints is uncommon, but destructive hip disease may develop and is the most severe peripheral joint complication.[7, 227]

The classic involvement of the sacroiliac joints and lumbodorsal spine produces low back pain and leads to early loss of lumbar spinal mobility. Chest expansion may be reduced by costovertebral and costosternal joint inflammation.[228] The ascending progression of axial skeletal changes to form the "bamboo spine" rigidity does not occur until much later in adulthood. Cervical involvement is rare in children, but atlantoaxial subluxation has been reported.[229]

Systemic symptoms at the disease onset are rare and systemic manifestations develop to significant degrees only in adulthood. However, 20 percent of children develop acute, recurrent uveitis, which fortunately has no ocular sequelae. The cardiac complications seen in 4 to 10 percent of adults, notably pericarditis, conduction defects, and aortitis, are rare in children, but aortic insufficiency has been described.[230, 231] Clinical pulmonary fibrosis is rare in children. Amyloidosis, seen in 8 percent of adults, has not been described in juvenile ankylosing spondylitis.[7, 230]

The course of this disease is usually remitting and is frequently mild. In most cases, the prognosis is favorable if good posture is maintained and treatment begun early. Salicylates are usually effective for relief of pain; tolmetin has proved to be a useful alternative. Systemic corticosteroids are rarely indicated, but local steroid injection of sites of enthesitis may be helpful.

The anesthetic considerations for juvenile ankylosing spondylitis are similar to those for juvenile rheumatoid arthritis. Laryngoscopy is less a problem in children, but particular attention should still be directed to the evaluation of neck mobility and temporomandibular joint function and to the rare complications of atlantoaxial instability and aortic insufficiency.[222, 229, 231]

Acute Rheumatic Fever

Acute rheumatic fever is an inflammatory disease that usually presents with joint and cardiac manifestations but may also affect the central nervous system, skin, and subcutaneous tissue. It occurs as a direct consequence of a prior upper respiratory tract infection with group A beta-hemolytic streptococci. Where antibiotic prophylaxis is available, the disease is now much less common and the annual incidence has dropped to 10 per 100,000 population.[234] The peak incidence of first attacks occur in the 5- to 15-year age group.

The precise pathological mechanism of acute rheumatic fever is not known. Host factors and hypersensitivity reactions may be important. Antistreptococcal antibodies have been shown to cross-react with antigens found in cardiac muscle and valves, suggesting an autoimmune etiology.[235] A subsequent exudative inflammatory reaction involves the connective tissue of each target organ.

Clinical Manifestations. The major clinical manifestations include arthritis, carditis, chorea, subcutaneous nodules, and erythema marginatum.

Joint symptoms are the most frequent presenting complaint and occur in 75 percent of cases as a migratory polyarthritis usually affecting the knees, ankles, elbows, and wrists. Pain may be severe, but no permanent deformities develop and the arthritis resolves in 3 to 4 weeks.

Carditis occurs in 40 to 50 percent of initial attacks, with the highest frequency in young children. Rheumatic valvular disease represents the only long-term morbidity from rheumatic fever. Carditis may be asymptomatic, but may still lead to permanent valvular damage. Less frequently it is severe, and it has been fatal in acute disease. Suggestive findings are tachycardia, cardiomegaly, a gallop rhythm, and the appearance of organic murmurs, usually a pansystolic murmur of mitral valvulitis and less commonly a murmur of aortic insufficiency. Pericarditis may produce chest pain, friction rubs, and effusions. Congestive failure may present as dyspnea, abdominal pain, and hepatomegaly.[6, 7] The manifestations of carditis may persist for 6 weeks to 6 months.

Chorea occurs in 10 to 15 percent of patients and is characterized by involuntary, purposeless movements associated with emotional lability (St. Vitus dance). Treatment with barbiturates may be helpful. It usually subsides in 3 months. Painless, mobile, subcutaneous nodules appear over body prominences in 5 to 10 percent of cases and last 1 to 2 weeks. The classical rash, erythema marginatum, occurs in less than 5 percent of patients.

Minor clinical manifestations include fever, arthralgia, prolongation of the P-R interval, positive antistreptolysin O titer, and a previous history of rheumatic fever or heart disease. The Jones criteria for diagnosis require the presence of two major or one major and two minor clinical manifestations.[236] Skin biopsies may help in the diagnosis.[237]

Treatment. Bed rest is important until the rheumatic process is quiescent, particularly in patients with carditis. Salicylates alone control the fever and arthritis dramatically. But in patients with carditis and cardiomegaly, prednisone 2 mg/kg/24 hours is preferred for 2 weeks and then gradually withdrawn and replaced by salicylates. Congestive failure is usually controlled by fluid restriction, but diuretics and digoxin may be needed. Penicillin is often begun in the acute attack and continued as long-term prophylaxis against streptococcal infections.

Surgical intervention is rarely indicated in first attacks, but may subsequently be required for the correction of rheumatic mitral valvular disease even in children. Both closed mitral valvotomy and mitral valve replacement, the latter usually for valvular insufficiency, have been reported in large series of children.[238]

Anesthetic Management. Of major importance in the anesthetic management of children with acute rheumatic fever is the preoperative evaluation of cardiac function. Although uncommon, severe congestive cardiac failure may be precipitated by pericardial effusions, myocarditis, and valvular dysfunction. Recurrent disease may produce a variety of valvular lesions: mitral stenosis, mitral insufficiency, and aortic insufficiency. Atrial fibrillation may complicate mitral valve disease.[238] A cardiologist's consultation should be obtained and a chest x-ray and ECG should be reviewed. The management of specific cardiac lesions is discussed in Chapter 6.

The presence of active arthritis, chorea, and the medical therapy of each must be noted. Supplemental corticosteroid therapy may be required. Prophylactic antibiotic coverage is mandatory. Laryngoscopy is not a reported problem in acute rheumatic fever. No specific recommendations of anesthetic drugs or technique have been made.

Reiter Syndrome

Reiter syndrome refers to the classical triad of urethritis, arthritis, and conjunctivitis. Other manifestations may include gastroenteritis and a mucocutaneous eruption. It is uncommon in children. Boys are affected more than girls by a 4:1 ratio. The disease often follows an enteritis caused by *Shigella*, *Yersinia*, or *Salmonella* infections in young children or following sexual contact in older children and adults.[239] There is a strong association with HLA B27.[240] Reiter syndrome has been described as a postinfectious or reactive arthritis.[7]

Joint involvement is generally pauciarticular and affects the large joints, usually the knees and ankles. The severity of the arthritis may be remarkable. Enthesitis is common. Occasionally, the temporomandibular, cervical spine, sacroiliac, and cricoarytenoid joints are affected.[241] The arthritis, urethritis, and conjunctivitis usually resolve within a few months. Joint complications are infrequent, but occasionally recurrent chronic arthritis may persist. Uncommonly children may develop painless erythematous patches or ulcerations in the oropharynx. Scarring is not a feature.

The treatment for Reiter syndrome is directed at the relief of symptoms by salicylates and at the preservation of joint function with physiotherapy.

Apart from the evaluation of neck mobility and temporomandibular joint movement, there are no specific anesthetic considerations.

Arthritis of Inflammatory Bowel Disease

Between 10 to 20 percent of children with chronic ulcerative colitis or regional ileitis develop a spondylitis or a peripheral joint arthropathy, often coinciding with periods of active bowel disease.[7, 242] The affected children are usually over the age of 10 years.

The peripheral arthropathy is pauciarticular and involves the knees and ankles most commonly, although the temporomandibular joints and hands may be affected. The arthritis rarely lasts more than 2 months and responds well to salicylates or to prednisone, if required for control of the bowel disease. Functional loss is most unusual. In contrast, the sacroiliac and lumbar spine disease tends to progress, despite good control of the bowel disorder. The spondylitis behaves very much like ankylosing spondylitis and may be accompanied by destructive hip disease.

The anesthetic considerations are similar to those for juvenile rheumatoid arthritis.

Psoriatic Arthropathy

Although psoriasis is relatively common in children, psoriatic arthropathy is rarely seen. The arthritis may precede the skin manifestations by several years and early cases are frequently misdiagnosed. Girls affected outnumber boys by a ratio of 2.5:1. The usual age at onset of the joint symptoms is 9 to 10 years.[7, 105]

The arthritis is often pauciarticular, usually involving the distal interphalangeal joints of the hands, and is associated with flexor tendinitis of the wrists. The knees and small joints of the feet may be affected. Of children with the arthropathy, 25 percent develop sacroiliitis. Cervical spine involvement, when it occurs, is not functionally restricting in children. The prognosis is generally good.

Symptomatic control is usually achieved with salicylates or tolmetin. Parenteral gold salts or systemic corticosteroids may occasionally be required.

The anesthetic considerations are similar to those for juvenile ankylosing spondylitis.

Arthritis of Immune Deficiency

The immunodeficiency diseases, in particular X-linked agammaglobulinemia, selective IgA deficiency, and complement component deficiencies, are associated with various forms of arthritis and connective tissue disorders. The incidence may be as high as 30 percent.[7] The usual pattern of arthropathy is similar to juvenile rheumatoid arthritis, and the most common connective tissue disorder seen is systemic lupus erythematosus. The etiological implications of the close association of immune deficiency with the autoimmune diseases is currently of intense interest.

The treatment of connective tissue disorders in patients with immune deficiency is the same as for uncomplicated disease, but corticosteroids and immunosuppressive agents must be used with extreme caution.

Systemic Lupus Erythematosus

Systemic lupus erythematosus is a multisystemic disease characterized by widespread inflammatory changes in the blood vessels and connective tissues of many organs. The annual incidence of the disease is 0.6 to 1 per 100,000 population. Eighteen to 20 percent of cases present in childhood after the age of 8 years. Females are affected more often than males by an 8:1 ratio. The disease seems to be more prevalent in dark-skinned races. The disease in children is usually more acute and more severe than in adults; although unpredictable, it is usually progressive and often fatal if untreated.

The etiology of the disease is probably multifactorial. Although an altered immune response of genetic predisposition is a central feature,[243] intercurrent viral infections, the hormonal changes of pregnancy, and environmental factors such as sunlight are associated with exacerbations of the disease. A transient, lupuslike syndrome may develop following exposure to some drugs, notably hydralazine, isoniazid, the sulfonamides, procainamide, penicillamine, and the hydantoin anticonvulsants.[251]

The pathological lesions in systemic lupus include an immune complex–initiated necrotizing vasculitis, inflammatory cellular infiltrates of serosal tissues, and degenerative connective tissue changes.

Clinical Manifestations. The onset of the disease in children may be insidious and episodic, or acute and rapidly fatal from cardiac, pulmonary, renal, and neurological complications or from secondary infection.[245, 246] Presenting features vary greatly, depending on which organ systems are involved. The usual constitutional symptoms of acute disease include fever, malaise, weakness, arthralgias, anorexia, and weight loss.

The mucocutaneous manifestations occur in most children at some stage. An erythematous butterfly rash over the nose and cheeks is highly suggestive of the disease. It may extend over the face, neck, shoulders, and trunk and may become bullous and secondarily infected. Erythematous macules, secondary to dermal vasculitis, may appear anywhere on the skin.[6] Oral and nasal ulcerations occur in 50 percent of patients.[7] Raynaud phenomenon, purpura, erythema nodosum, and erythema multiforme are associated skin features.

Arthralgias and migratory arthritis, affecting the small joints of the hands, wrists, elbows, shoulders, knees, and ankles, are common. The arthritis may be severely painful, but is transient and almost never destructive. However, ischemic necrosis of the femoral heads does occur. Cricoarytenoid joint ankylosis is described in an adult.[247]

Cardiac involvement may be severe. Pericarditis with friction rubs is most common. Myocarditis occurs in 25 percent of patients and is manifested as cardiomegaly, congestive failure, and dysrhythmias.[248] Verrucous endocarditis (Libman-Sacks), usually affecting the mitral valve, may develop in acute crises. Myocardial infarction is rare, but has been described in children.[249] Pleuritic chest pain, pleural effusions, pulmonary infiltrates, pneumonitis, and secondary pneumonias may lead to later fibrosis.[197, 250] The necrotizing vasculitis may cause spontaneous pneumothorax or severe pulmonary hemorrhage[6, 7] (Fig. 15–18).

Central nervous system involvement is manifested as personality changes, seizure disorders, cerebrovascular accidents, and peripheral neuropathies.[251] Acute abdominal pain from inflammatory serositis may occur

Figure 15–18. Chest x-ray of an 11-year-old girl with systemic lupus erythematosus in crisis, whose pulmonary vasculitis has produced a deteriorating pneumonitis complicated by spontaneous pneumothorax and pneumomediastinum (*arrows*).

with vomiting and diarrhea. Mesenteric vasculitis, complicated by the infarction of bowel, may require emergency laparotomy.[252] Moderate hepatosplenomegaly and generalized lymphadenopathy occur in active disease. Anemia, with a hematocrit of less than 30, is seen in 50 percent of affected children. Leukopenia, thrombocytopenia, and coagulopathies occur frequently in active disease.[253] Idiopathic thrombocytopenic purpura may be the initial presentation of systemic lupus.

Significant clinical renal involvement occurs in 75 percent of children. It is more severe than that seen in adults and develops within 2 years of the disease onset. The more severe forms of lupus nephritis, identified by renal biopsy, are diffuse proliferative glomerulonephritis and membranous glomerulonephritis. Nephrotic syndrome and hypertension are not uncommon. Renal failure may eventually occur in almost half the affected patients.[7]

Systemic lupus erythematosus may mimic many other rheumatic diseases. The diagnosis is based on clinical findings and confirmed by laboratory tests. Antinuclear antibodies are always present but are not specific. Antibodies to DNA are specific but present only in active disease. Serum hemolytic complement components are decreased in active disease and provide a good guide to the adequacy of treatment and remission.

Neonatal Lupus Erythematosus. Some infants of mothers with active disease will have transient lupus manifestations caused by the transplacental transfer of IgG autoantibodies. The most frequent clinical finding is a malar erythema, similar to adult discoid lupus. Transient thrombocytopenia, hemolytic anemia, and leukopenia have been described.[6, 7] No treatment is required; the abnormalities resolve spontaneously in a few months.

Congenital complete heart block is described in infants born to mothers with systemic lupus and some other rheumatic diseases.[262] Neonatal endocardial fibroelastosis has also been reported.[6]

Sjögren Syndrome. Sjögren syndrome is a multisystemic disorder, characterized by the triad of the sicca syndrome (dry eyes and mouth), a connective tissue disease, usually systemic lupus erythematosus, and high titers of autoantibodies, which are often rheumatoid factors and antinuclear antibodies. Although it is rare in children, it usually presents as recurrent parotid swelling and as complaints of the sicca syndrome.[254] Lymphocytic infiltration is seen in the lacrimal and salivary glands; this may extend to involve the upper respiratory tract, larynx, stomach, and genitourinary tract. Systemic manifestations include achlorhydria, pancreatitis, chronic active hepatitis, nephropathy, lymphoma, and anemia.

The treatment of Sjögren syndrome is symptomatic and includes artificial tears and increased air humidity.

Treatment. No specific treatment for lupus erythematosus is available. Patients should avoid excessive exposure to sunlight and the drugs associated with exacerbations. The objectives of medical treatment are to maintain clinical well-being and to slow the disease progression by suppressing the inflammatory process and the formation of immune complexes.

In mild disease without nephritis, salicylates and occasionally antimalarial drugs may be quite effective. Topical steroids often control the skin rash. In acute lupus crises, systemic corticosteroids are required in high doses (prednisone 1 to 2 mg/kg/24 hours) for the control of carditis, neurological manifestations, and nephritis. Withdrawal to maintenance doses is not attempted for 4 weeks. The immunosuppressive agents azathioprine, cyclophosphamide, and chlorambucil are used with extreme caution when the nephritis is unresponsive to steroids.

Secondary infections during periods of active disease may be lethal and, when identified, must be treated aggressively.

Although remissions may occur in children, the usual course is one of chronic disease, extending over many years. The 5-year survival has now improved to 90 percent.[256] The major causes of death are secondary sepsis, nephritis, gastrointestinal hemorrhage and perforation, pulmonary hemorrhage, malignant hypertension, and carditis.[7]

Anesthetic Management. Systemic lupus erythematosus represents a chronic disease with potentially severe multiple organ dysfunction. Children with this disease may be acutely ill, febrile, weak, and debilitated and have secondary infections. Careful evaluation must be made of renal, cardiac, and pulmonary function and central nervous system manifestations. Joint mobility, particularly of the neck and temporomandibular joints, must be assessed. Erosive lesions of the nasal or oropharyngeal mucosa may make passage of an endotracheal tube difficult or traumatic and may compromise the airway. Patients with active disease are usually anemic and thrombocytopenic and may have a coagulopathy. Cross-matching for blood products may be difficult because of erythrocyte antibodies, but adequate blood products must be available.[6] Perioperative steroid coverage will likely be required. Antibiotic prophylaxis will be necessary in patients with endocarditis.

For general anesthesia, all usual monitors should be used. The anesthetic gases must be warmed and humidified. For patients with Sjögren syndrome the eyes should be protected by an ophthalmic ointment. Airway maintenance and laryngoscopy are not a reported problem in children, but care must be exercised in patients with facial bullae and erosive oropharyngeal mucous membrane lesions.

No specific anesthetic agents or techniques are recommended, but those drugs excreted via the kidney should be used with caution in the presence of renal impairment. Agents that depress myocardial contractility will be poorly tolerated in patients with carditis. Ventilation should be controlled in children with pulmonary involvement. The use of anticholinergic (drying) agents is discouraged in Sjögren syndrome. Regional blocks are relatively contraindicated in patients with peripheral neuropathies.

Dermatomyositis

In dermatomyositis, the skin and striated muscles are affected by a diffuse, nonsuppurative inflammatory process which may be acute or chronic. The incidence of the disease is 1 per 2,000,000 population. Childhood onset usually occurs between ages 4 to 10 years and accounts for 15 to 20 percent of cases.[7] Girls are affected twice as frequently as boys. Polymyositis, the same disease without cutaneous manifestations, is rare in children.

The etiology is unknown, but a cell-mediated immunological disturbance is responsible for some of the disease features. Photosensitivity, drug hypersensitivity, and infections have also been implicated. A necrotizing vasculitis of vessels in the skin, muscle, and subcutaneous tissue and occasionally in the gastrointestinal tract is the usual pathological finding in childhood dermatomyositis.

Clinical Manifestations. In children, the usual presenting feature is the insidious development of muscle weakness involving the proximal muscles of the hip and shoulder girdle. Muscle pain, tenderness, and stiffness are commonly associated with gait disturbances, fever, malaise, and weight loss.[257, 258] In 10 percent of cases, weakness of the palatal and pharyngeal muscles may cause dysphonia and dysphagia and lead to incompetent swallowing mechanisms and pulmonary aspiration.[259] Intercostal involvement may impair adequate ventilation. The healing of affected muscles by fibrosis may lead to incapacitating contracture deformities.

The hallmark of dermatomyositis is the skin rash, seen in 75 percent of affected children[257] (Fig. 15–19). The violaceous discoloration of the eyelids and occasionally the cheeks associated with periorbital and facial edema is pathognomonic. Generalized erythema may develop. Symmetrical, erythematous, atrophic changes are found over the extensor surfaces of joints of the hands, elbows, and knees. Nonpitting edema of the skin and subcutaneous tissue may be present. Mucosal ulcerations may develop secondary to local vasculitis. With resolution of the rash, varying pigmentation changes are subsequently observed in the skin. Raynaud phenomenon is not seen in children.

Subcutaneous deposition of calcium (calcinosis) in response to tissue injury and fibrosis is a feature in 40 percent of children. The accumulations may be large and may ultimately protrude through the skin, producing sizable ulcerated and denuded areas. A transient, nondeforming arthritis develops occasionally. Modest hepatosplenomegaly and lymphadenopathy may be found. Infrequently, gastrointestinal ulceration and hemorrhage may cause anemia. Apart from aspiration pneumonitis, pulmonary involvement with interstitial fibrosis is rare in children.[260] Myocarditis and pericarditis are described, but are also rare.[7]

The diagnosis is confirmed by the combination of muscle weakness, characteristic skin rash, elevated serum enzymes, notably the transaminases and creatine phosphokinase, and an abnormal electromyogram.

The course may be acute, with a mortality rate of 40 percent in untreated patients from complications of palatorespiratory weakness and gastrointestinal hemorrhage, or may become slowly inactive over several years. Subsequent exacerbations are unusual. The associated malignancies (carcinomas) seen in 20 percent of adults do not occur in children.

Treatment. Functional recovery depends on the preservation of muscle strength and the prevention of deforming contractures. Ongoing physical therapy is important. In the acute phase, close scrutiny of the competence of swallowing and the adequacy of respiratory function is mandatory. Intubation and ventilatory support may be required.

Corticosteroids effectively suppress the inflammatory process and have reversed the earlier grim prognosis. Prednisone, 1 to 2 mg/kg/24 hours, is usually continued for 2 to 4 weeks before reduction to a maintenance dose is attempted. Steroids are often necessary for 1 to 2 years. Salicylates may be helpful in the relief of joint symptoms and myalgias. Rarely, immunosuppressive agents are required.

Anesthetic Management. The preoperative assessment of muscle weakness is mandatory. Palatal and pharyngeal weakness with incompetent swallowing may leave considerable mucus in the upper airway. The loss of respiratory reserve through muscle weakness may be complicated by aspiration pneumonitis. A forced vital capacity should be obtained and the chest x-ray reviewed. The presence of a facial rash, edema, and oral ulcerations must be identified. Patients with dermatomyositis may be anemic and generally debilitated. Perioperative corticosteroid coverage will usually be required.

Because of potential pharyngeal incompetence, gen-

Figure 15–19. Rash of dermatomyositis on the scalp in a 7-year-old girl.

eral anesthesia with intubation is usually recommended.[10] Facial and oropharyngeal contractures do not occur and laryngoscopy should not be difficult. In the presence of active myositis, succinylcholine should probably be avoided, although in a recent case report its use in a child was not associated with problems.[261] There may be heightened sensitivity to nondepolarizing muscle relaxants; these agents should be used only if necessary. Intolerance to narcotics may be pronounced; all sedatives must be used in modest doses. Ventilation should be assisted or controlled throughout the anesthetic.

Prior to extubation, the full return of neuromuscular function must be verified if relaxants were used and the patient should be awake. If preoperative pulmonary function was significantly reduced, short-term postoperative ventilatory support should be planned in an intensive care area following major surgery.

Scleroderma

Scleroderma is a chronic, multisystemic disorder of connective tissue affecting the skin, heart, lungs, kidneys, gastrointestinal tract, and synovium. The disease is very uncommon in children, who account for only 1 to 3 percent of the total cases. The usual age of onset is 3 to 15 years; girls are predominantly affected, by a 5:1 ratio. In childhood, scleroderma usually presents as localized skin involvement alone, either in focal patches, *morphea*, or in linear patterns of distribution, *linear scleroderma*. Uncommonly seen in children is *progressive systemic sclerosis*, manifested by symmetrical skin involvement and severe visceral complications.

The affected tissues show perivascular infiltration with mononuclear cells and edema. Collagen fibers are thickened and have increased density. The disease progresses through stages of inflammation, fibrosis, and atrophy.[262] The etiology is unknown but may include an immune mechanism and an abnormality in collagen tissue.[263]

Clinical Manifestations. The skin and subcutaneous tissue involvement in morphea is patchy and often found on an extremity. The lesions are initially erythematous with nonpitting edema and a shiny atrophic appearance. Subsequent induration and scarring binds the skin to underlying structures. If extensive, this "hide-binding" may limit growth of the extremity or cause crippling contractures.

In systemic disease the cutaneous features are similar, but distribution is symmetrical and involves the fingers, toes, distal extremities, trunk, and face. The indurative phase produces the characteristic masklike facies with the loss of skin folds, a pinched nose, small contracted mouth, and prominent teeth. Mouth opening is significantly reduced in 28 percent of adult patients.[264] Telangiectases of the face, lips, tongue, chest, and hands may develop. Accumulations of subcutaneous calcification may enlarge to ultimately ulcerate through the skin. Raynaud phenomenon is a complaint in most patients.

Diffuse pulmonary fibrosis occurs in 60 percent of adults and children and presents as a dry cough or as exertional dyspnea.[7] Accompanying small airway disease is identified by a decreased maximal mid-expiratory flow rate and increased closing capacities.[265] Twenty-nine percent of patients have restrictive pulmonary disease, which may be complicated by pulmonary hypertension, cor pulmonale, and cardiac failure.[266–269]

Cardiac disease in adults with scleroderma is manifested by myocardial fibrosis with secondary conduction defects, dysrhythmias, right and left ventricular hypertrophy, and congestive failure. Angina pectoris with normal coronary arteries from presumed vasospastic phenomena is described.[270, 271] The above features are not seen in children often, but pericardial effusions and cardiac failure do occur.

Renal dysfunction, presenting as proteinuria, hypertension, and azotemia, develops in 45 percent of patients within 3 years of the onset of disease. The underlying pathology is a microangiopathy.[7] Malignant hypertension develops in 7 percent of patients secondary to increased renin production.[7] The prognosis of renal complications is usually dismal.

Abnormalities in esophageal motility are found in the majority of patients and present as retrosternal dysphagia and pharyngeal reflux. Associated gastroesophageal reflux may be complicated by esophageal strictures in 25 percent of patients. Duodenal and small bowel pathology may cause diarrhea, constipation, and a malabsorption syndrome.

An inflammatory polyarthritis with juxta-articular osteoporosis, fibrosis, and contractures may develop involving the fingers (sclerodactyly), wrists, ankles, knees, and elbows. The mandible may be involved.[272] About 25 percent of children are anemic either from chronic disease or from repeat hemorrhage from telangiectasia. The malabsorption of vitamin K may lead to a coagulopathy.

Two similar disorders should be mentioned at this time:

Scleredema. This rare disorder is characterized by edematous induration of the face, neck, shoulders, thorax and upper arms. In children, the disease is often preceded by a streptococcal infection. Systemic manifestations are uncommon, but minor cardiac abnormalities may occur. These include a diastolic gallop without failure and nonspecific ECG changes.[1, 7] Spontaneous resolution of the disease usually occurs within 6 months to 2 years.

Mixed Connective Tissue Disease. This uncommon overlap syndrome includes features of scleroderma, systemic lupus erythematosus, and dermatomyositis.[4, 7] Common clinical manifestations include the edematous phase of scleroderma skin changes, the rash of dermatomyositis, Raynaud phenomenon, myositis, anemia and thrombocytopenia, myocarditis, pericarditis, pleurisy, and Sjögren syndrome. Severe renal disease is rare.[7, 273] High titers of antibodies to ribonucleoprotein are invariably found. Most manifestations of the disease respond rapidly to corticosteroids, and the prognosis of most patients is good.

Treatment. There is no specific treatment for scleroderma. Patients are advised to avoid cold and trauma. Joint mobility must be maintained by exercise and positions of function maintained by the use of splints. Lubricant creams may improve skin pliability.

Raynaud's phenomenon may be improved by sympathetic blocking agents such as reserpine, phenoxybenzamine, or methyldopa. Gastroesophageal reflux often requires antacids and cimetidine. Esophageal strictures may need surgical intervention. Cardiac failure can usually be controlled by digoxin and pericardial effusions by diuretics, although pericardiocentesis may be necessary. Some encouraging results from early treatment of renal failure with dialysis and transplantation have been reported.[274] Hypertension is usually managed with renin-suppressing agents such as captopril.[275]

Systemic corticosteroids are used for the suppression of the inflammatory contribution to pulmonary fibrosis and for acute myositis when it occurs. Very little response to steroids is seen in other features of the disease.

The prognosis of progressive systemic sclerosis depends on the severity of visceral organ involvement; the long-term outlook in children is guarded. Cardiac, renal, and pulmonary complications may cause death in 6 months to 10 years after the diagnosis is made.[7]

Anesthetic Management. Children with scleroderma may have severe multisystemic disease and require thorough preoperative assessment.

Of particular importance is the evaluation of the upper airway. Contracted perioral skin and a reduced mouth opening will make laryngoscopy difficult. Oropharyngeal telangiectasia should be identified. Pulmonary function tests should be obtained prior to major procedures. The cardiac complications of cor pulmonale, congestive failure, or pericardial effusion may have developed and a history of angina pectoris in older children should be sought. A chest x-ray and ECG should be reviewed and renal and hepatic function assessed. Patients may be anemic and have a vitamin K dependent coagulopathy secondary to malabsorption. Joints affected by active arthritis should be noted.

These patients may be on a variety of medications, notably antihypertensive drugs, sympathetic blocking agents, and systemic corticosteroids. Perioperative steroid supplementation may be required. Hypertensive patients may be volume contracted and will benefit from preoperative hydration. Premedication should include cimetidine and an antacid in the presence of gastroesophageal reflux.

The operating room should be kept warm and the patient transferred carefully. In the presence of esophageal reflux, a relatively head-up position is advised.

Regional blocks have proved very successful in adults.[276–279] The prolonged analgesic effects reported may be useful in children for postoperative pain relief even if general anesthesia was required.[277]

When general anesthesia is required, all usual monitors should be applied. Blood pressure is best taken by cuff and Doppler probe. An arterial line may aggravate vasospastic phenomena and should be used only if necessary. Intravenous access may be difficult, but should be obtained prior to induction. Intravenous injections may be painful and may provoke Raynaud phenomenon.[279]

Patients who have limited mouth opening should be intubated awake with modest sedation as for patients with juvenile rheumatoid arthritis (see page 404). No relaxants should be used prior to successful intubation. In some children, an inhalational induction may be preferred. When laryngoscopy is performed in patients with a small mouth opening, avoid excessive retraction force as the corner of the mouth may tear.[280] Cricoid pressure and a head-up position is recommended even in elective operations.[212] Ketamine may be useful in some patients.[281]

With the airway under control, several recommendations remain. The anesthetic gases should be warmed and humidified. Ventilation should be assisted or controlled where pulmonary reserve is reduced. Hypovolemia and hypotension must be corrected quickly, particularly in hypertensive children, because any fall in renal blood flow may seriously compromise renal function.[7] Patients who were difficult to intubate should not be extubated until they are awake and have fully competent laryngeal reflexes.

Systemic Vasculitis Syndromes

The inflammatory degeneration of vascular tissues produces a great variety of disease patterns that are determined by the location and the size of affected vessels. There may be considerable overlap among these syndromes and with connective tissue diseases in which vasculitis is a feature, notably systemic lupus erythematosus, dermatomyositis, scleroderma, and less commonly rheumatoid arthritis.

The most common vasculitis syndrome in childhood is Henoch-Schönlein purpura, which affects small, nonmuscular blood vessels. The involvement of small and medium muscular vessels, referred to as polyarteritis nodosa, includes the variants infantile polyarteritis nodosa, Kawasaki disease, and probably Wegener granulomatosis; these are rare in children. Takayasu arteritis affects the aorta and great vessels and is extremely rare in children.

Henoch-Schönlein Purpura (Anaphylactoid Purpura)

Henoch-Schönlein purpura is an acute, necrotizing vasculitis of small nonmuscular blood vessels clinically manifested as nonthrombocytopenic purpura, arthritis or arthralgias, abdominal pain, gastrointestinal hemorrhage, and nephritis. This syndrome is not rare and occurs most commonly in previously healthy children between the ages of 2 and 10 years. Boys are affected twice as frequently as girls.[7] The etiology is unknown, but important associations with allergies, drug sensitivities, and prior upper respiratory streptococcal infections are recognized. The vasculitis involves capillaries, small arterioles, and venules, which are surrounded by an acute inflammatory exudate of polymorphonuclear cells. Local edema and hemorrhage may occur at any site affected.

Clinical Manifestations. The onset is usually acute and presents with a purpuric rash over the buttocks and lower legs, which may extend to the arms and less commonly, the face. The lesions appear in crops, and they are seen at different stages of resolution (Fig. 15–20). Nonpitting edema may involve the hands, feet, and upper face. Erythema multiforme and erythema nodosum may be associated conditions.[6]

Most children develop concurrent gastrointestinal symptoms, usually colicky abdominal pain and vomiting. Stools may show evidence of gross bleeding, and hematemesis may occur. Intestinal intussusception,

Figure 15–20. Henoch-Schönlein purpura in a 4-year-old boy. Note the purpuric lesions at different stages of resolution.

infarction, and perforation are complications in less than 5 percent of cases, but develop rapidly.[7] Most patients are anemic, but coagulation is normal.

Renal involvement occurs in about half the patients and is manifested by hematuria and proteinuria. In 5 percent of patients, the nephritis is complicated by progressive renal failure and hypertension. The central nervous system is affected infrequently, but this involvement is serious. Seizure disorders, paresis from intracranial hemorrhage, and coma may occur. Pulmonary involvement is most unusual, but has been described in an adult.[282]

Arthritis or arthralgia occurs in 75 percent of patients, usually affecting knees and ankles, but elbows and hands may be involved. Joint swelling and tenderness is marked, but is transient and nondeforming. Nonspecific constitutional symptoms of fever and malaise are usually present.

Treatment. No specific therapy is available; treatment is supportive and symptomatic. Identified allergens should be removed and streptococcal infections treated with antibiotics. Symptomatic relief of the arthralgias and fever by salicylates is usually adequate. Systemic corticosteroids are indicated only for life-threatening gastrointestinal hemorrhage or obstruction and for severe central nervous system manifestations.

In most children, resolution of the disease occurs within 4 weeks and the prognosis is excellent. Exacerbations may recur within 2 years. A major cause of morbidity is severe nephritis, which may progress to renal failure. In acute disease, death may occur from gastrointestinal hemorrhage or perforation, renal failure, or central nervous system complications.

Anesthetic Management. These children may be acutely ill and require careful preoperative assessment. The gastrointestinal complications of obstruction, intussusception, hemorrhage, perforation, and peritonitis demand aggressive resuscitation to correct anemia and hypovolemia. Adequate blood products must be available. Peripheral intravenous access may be difficult. Renal dysfunction, central nervous system signs, and acute arthropathies must be identified.

No specific anesthetic agents or techniques are recommended. However, when general anesthesia is required for such procedures as laparatomy, a rapid-sequence induction and intubation should be planned. Patients who are hypovolemic will not tolerate potent myocardial depressants, nor peripheral vasodilatation. Intraoperative hypovolemia and hypotension must be corrected quickly; any fall in renal blood flow may seriously jeopardize renal function in children with nephritis. In patients with cerebral vasculitis and increased intracranial pressure, a technique incorporating hyperventilation should be used. Postoperative care in an intensive care area is recommended.

Polyarteritis Nodosa

In polyarteritis nodosa, a necrotizing vasculitis involves the entire vessel wall thickness of medium and small muscular arteries of many organs. This manifests as tissue necrosis, vessel thrombosis, or aneurysm formation.[6, 7, 283] The clinical presentation and course of the disease may be extremely variable and is determined by the sites of the vascular disease. The most severe complications arise from involvement of the gastrointestinal tract, heart, kidneys, and central nervous system. The etiology is unknown, but associations with drug exposures, hepatitis B antigen, and streptococcal infections are described.[6, 7] It is a rare disease in children; boys are affected three times more commonly than girls.

The onset of polyarteritis nodosa in children is often insidious, with vague constitutional symptoms of fever, malaise, weakness, and weight loss, but its ultimate progression is usually severe. Various purpuric or petechial skin lesions and joint symptoms may develop early. Gastrointestinal tract manifestations can result in an acute abdomen with colicky pain, hemorrhage, infarction, and perforation.[252] Anemia is frequent. The nephritis is usually severe and is complicated by hypertension and early renal failure. Coronary vasculitis and myocarditis precipitate myocardial infarctions and congestive failure. Central nervous system involvement and peripheral neuropathies occur in 50 to 70 percent of patients.[7] Organic psychoses, seizures, hemiparesis, and coma are not uncommon. Pulmonary infiltrates from parenchymal vasculitis initiate coughing and occasionally wheezing, and pharyngeal edema has been described in adults.[284]

Corticosteroids may suppress acute manifestations of the disease and prolong survival, but the overall prognosis is poor. Death usually results from renal failure, myocardial infarctions, or complications of hypertension.

Infantile Polyarteritis Nodosa. This variant of polyarteritis is a rare condition, but presents in infants less than 1 year of age with a characteristic clinical pattern. The illness begins similar to a persistent viral upper respiratory tract infection with fever, rhinitis, conjunctivitis, and a macular erythematous skin rash, but subsequent internal organ involvement develops quickly. Cardiac manifestations include aneurysmal coronary artery vasculitis with myocardial infarction, cardiomegaly, congestive failure, and pericarditis. Severe nephritis with hypertension and renal failure, peripheral and central nervous system complications, and gastrointestinal crises reflect the severe widespread vasculitis.[6, 7, 285]

No effective treatment is available. Corticosteroids have not been beneficial; antiplatelet and antithrombotic agents may be more appropriate. Death often occurs within 1 month of the onset of disease from myocardial infarction and renal complications.[7]

Anesthetic Management. These children are usually critically ill with multiple organ system dysfunction and demand careful preoperative assessment. Medical therapy may include corticosteroids, antihypertensive agents, and supportive treatment for myo-

cardial failure with digoxin and diuretics. The correction of anemia and hypovolemia will be necessary.

Basic anesthetic considerations in children with polyarteritis nodosa are similar to those for Henoch-Schönlein purpura. However, several additional points should be stressed. Aggressive, invasive monitoring may be indicated. Small infants with acute abdomens are most safely intubated awake. Pulmonary involvement can be severe and ventilation should be controlled. In view of the risk of coronary artery disease, myocardial oxygenation should be optimized by avoiding tachycardia and large swings in blood pressure. Lead II and/or V_5 should be monitored on the ECG.

Postoperative support in an intensive care area should be considered.

Mucocutaneous Lymph Node Syndrome (Kawasaki Disease)

The mucocutaneous lymph node syndrome is an acute febrile illness characterized by a systemic vasculitis of small and medium muscular arteries affecting primarily infants and children. Although this syndrome is much less severe, many features are similar to those of infantile polyarteritis nodosa. The latter may represent an extreme expression of this disease. Kawasaki disease is uncommon, but is seen most frequently in Japanese children. An increasing incidence is now being recognized in North America.[7] Boys are affected more than girls by a ratio of 1.5:1; the peak age of onset is 1 to 4 years. The etiology is unknown; various viral and bacterial infecions have been associated with the disease, but none are proven to cause it.

Clinical Manifestations. The classical features of its presentation include an acute, high, and remittent fever that may cause febrile convulsions, accompanied by a skin rash that is usually erythematous and macular. Characteristic mucocutaneous changes include dry, red, fissuring lips, erythema of the oropharynx, and a strawberry tongue. Bilateral conjunctivitis is common. Painful, edematous induration of the hands and feet with subsequent desquamation of local skin during recovery is seen in 65 percent of patients.[7] Transient lymphadenopathy, usually involving the anterior cervical nodes, is common.[286–289]

Other clinical features may include a prodromal upper respiratory tract infection and variable pulmonary infiltrates. Abdominal pain from mesenteric vasculitis may be accompanied by watery diarrhea and dehydration. Central nervous system involvement may range from minor personality changes to the severe manifestations of aseptic meningitis. Large joint arthralgias are frequent. Hepatic dysfunction occurs in 10 percent of patients, but renal involvement is mild.

Cardiac complications represent the most serious manifestations of the disease and may be identified to some degree in 70 percent of patients.[287] Overt clinical myocarditis with conduction defects, dysrhythmias, pericarditis, mitral insufficiency, and congestive failure may be seen in 10 percent of patients. During the recovery period, coronary artery aneurysms are diagnosed in 20 percent of patients by two-dimensional echocardiography[288, 289] (Figs. 15–21 and 15–22). Myocardial infarction, coronary thrombosis, or rupture of the coronary aneurysms probably accounts for the early death described in 1.5 to 2.0 percent of affected children. The long-term prognosis of cardiac involvement is unknown.

The acute febrile stage lasts for 7 to 10 days and is followed by a subacute stage over the next 2 to 4 weeks. The subsequent recovery period may continue for months and possibly years.

Treatment. In the acute stage, careful monitoring of cardiac function is required in the hospital. High-dose salicylate therapy is used for its antiplatelet effects and to control the arthritis. In the acute phase, gammaglobulin may decrease aneurysm formation.[288] Dipyridamole, a vasodilator, may be used in combination with salicylates. Corticosteroids may accelerate the development of coronary aneurysms and are generally contraindicated except for cautious use in patients with severe myocarditis. Successful aortocoronary bypass grafting has been performed for severe coronary disease in a 4-year-old boy.[290]

Anesthetic Management. Of critical importance is the preoperative assessment of cardiac function and the identification of congestive failure, dysrhythmias, conduction defects, myocardial ischemia, coronary artery disease, and valvular dysfunction. The other major organ systems involved require careful review as well. Dehydration and electrolyte disturbances secondary to diarrhea must be corrected. The implications of maintenance medications, which may include salicylates, digoxin, diuretics, narcotics for pain, and steroids, must be recognized. Cautious premedication may be required to facilitate a quiet induction.

No specific anesthetic drugs or techniques are recommended, but the approach should be similar to that for patients with coronary artery disease.[291] Induction should be smooth. Myocardial oxygen supply and demand should be optimized by avoiding tachycardia and acute swings in blood pressure. All usual monitors should be used at induction. EEG leads II and V_5 should be monitored to identify ischemic change in the myocardium. In some patients and for major procedures full invasive monitoring may be required. Laryngoscopy must be gentle to avoid trauma to inflamed lips, tongue, and oropharynx. Ventilation should be controlled, and if significant central nervous system manifestations exist, hyperventilation may be indicated.

Postoperative care for these patients may be best provided in an intensive care area.

Takayasu Arteritis (Pulseless Disease)

This uncommon disorder is characterized by a segmental arteritis involving the aorta, its major branches, and the pulmonary arteries. It predominantly affects young women more than men by an 8:1 ratio. Twenty percent of patients are less than 20 years of age, and the disease has been descibed in young children.[292] The etiology is unknown.

The characteristic pathology is a focal or diffuse loss of muscular and elastic tissue in the arterial wall with subsequent, extensive fibrosis of the media. Giant cells are frequently seen in the areas of destruction. Aneurysmal dilatation, rupture, stenosis, and occlusion may occur in affected vessels. Pulses to the upper exremity may be absent and the blood pressure in the legs may exceed that in the arms (hence, the terms pulseless disease and reverse coarctation). Seventy-five percent of patients develop myocardial failure, ventricular strain, or coronary artery involvement.[294] The impair-

Figure 15–21. Kawasaki disease in a 4-year-old boy. Note the aneurysmal dilatation of the right and left coronary arteries (*arrows*).

Figure 15–22. Severe, occlusive aortic and peripheral vascular disease in a 4-year-old boy with Kawasaki disease. Note the femoral artery aneurysms (*arrows*).

ment of renal blood flow leads to secondary hypertension; the interruption of cerebral blood flow may cause neurological disturbances.

Over half of affected children present with an acute onset of fever and hypermetabolic symptoms including night sweats, anorexia, and weight loss. Arthritis and anemia are frequent features. The disease may, however, be asymptomatic; in these cases, disorders of peripheral pulses or hypertension may be the first indications of its presence.[292]

Treatment. Anti-inflammatory agents usually alleviate symptoms of the disease; corticosteroids may have a beneficial effect in acute periods. Hypertension may require aggressive medical management with renin-inhibiting agents and vasodilators. Anticoagulants may be useful in the chronic, occlusive phase. Surgical endarterectomy, bypass grafting, and radiological dilatation angioplasty have had good reported success, but these procedures are not advised in patients with acute disease.[293] The prognosis of the disease is variable, but slow progression is the usual rule.

Anesthetic Management. The cardiovascular system must be evaluated preoperatively to identify the cardiac complications of failure and myocardial ischemia and to assess the extent of reduced peripheral pulses. Secondary renal hypertension and its medical management should be noted. Coincident anemia may require correction prior to surgery.

All usual monitors are required.[294, 295] ECG leads II and V_5 best identify ischemic changes. The true blood pressure may be difficult to measure in extremities with reduced peripheral pulses whether a Doppler flowmeter or indwelling cannula is used. Warner and associates recommend the use of a balloon-tipped flow-directed pulmonary artery catheter for major surgery in patients with absent pulses. Cardiac output, wedge pressures and mixed venous gases can then be measured.[294]

Anesthetic techniques and drugs should be chosen that will preserve the balance of myocardial oxygen supply and demand and are appropriate for patients with hypertension and coronary artery disease. Premedication will be helpful. Diazepam, fentanyl, and pancuronium have been used in adults.[294] A careful inhalation induction may be more suitable for some children. Care should be taken to prevent, or quickly correct, hypovolemia and secondary hypotension, which will jeopardize vital organ perfusion.

Wegener Granulomatosis

Wegener granulomatosis is a rare syndrome in children. Destructive granulomatous lesions in the upper airway and lungs are associated with a necrotizing angiitis most prominent in the lungs and kidneys. In a more widespread form, the skin, heart, central nervous system, gastrointestinal tract, and joints may be involved. When the lesions are limited to the upper respiratory tract and the vasculitis is minimal, the disorder is called *lethal midline granuloma*. The onset usually occurs between ages 25 and 50 years, but it has been described in children 1 year old. It occurs predominantly in males by a ratio of 2:1.[296] The etiology is unknown, but an association with drug sensitivity and allergy is reported.[6]

Clinical Manifestations. The clinical presentation usually begins with nasal congestion and discharge and respiratory symptoms of cough, hemoptysis, and pleuritic chest pain. Fever, malaise, and weight loss are frequent. The progressively destructive lesions may cause obliteration of the nasal sinuses, perforation of the orbit and palate, and ulcerations or narrowing of the pharynx, larynx, and trachea. A complicating tracheoesophageal fistula is described in an adult.[297] Pulmonary infiltrates due to granuloma formation in conjunction with obstructive airway disease and reduced lung volumes are common.[298] Pleural effusions, pneumothorax, and massive pulmonary hemorrhage are described.[7]

In the presence of necrotizing glomerulonephritis, uremia and renal failure may develop rapidly without hypertension. Cardiac involvement with coronary vasculitis, conduction defects, valvular distortion, and congestive failure has been described, but is uncommon. Arthritis involving the larger joints, splenomegaly, anemia, and peripheral neuropathy may be seen.

The prognosis of untreated disease is grim. Death from pulmonary complications or renal failure may occur in months. However, the immunosuppressive agents cyclophosphamide, azathioprine, and chlorambucil may arrest the disease and permit long-term survival. Corticosteroids may also suppress the vasculitis if used in early stages.

Anesthetic Management. The preoperative evaluation of mid-facial anatomy and the upper airway to identify ulcerations and obstructing lesions is imperative. Preoperative tracheostomy may rarely be required. Pulmonary complications must be recognized and pulmonary function tests should be obtained where indicated. Renal impairment and cardiac dysfunction must be noted. The complications of immunosuppressive agents, namely anemia, leukopenia, thrombocytopenia, and hepatic dysfunction with coagulopathy, should be corrected if possible. Perioperative steroid coverage may be required.

In the operating room, intravenous access should be obtained early and all usual monitors should be used. In patients with upper airway lesions, Lake recommends the use of regional techniques where appropriate.[301] When general anesthesia is required in children with lesions obstructing the airway, intubation must be performed gently, avoiding trauma to the lesions. A smaller tube than usual may be required. Laryngoscopy should be done with the patient awake, cautiously sedated, or under inhalational anesthesia with spontaneous ventilation maintained.

An anesthetic technique appropriate for patients with ischemic myocardial disease should be used, avoiding tachycardia and large swings in blood pressure. Intraoperative blood loss and hypovolemia must be corrected quickly. Ventilation should be controlled, but pressures must be kept as low as possible.

Careful postoperative observation for airway obstruction is mandatory.

Goodpasture Syndrome

Patients with Goodpasture syndrome develop episodic intra-alveolar pulmonary hemorrhage in association with glomerulonephritis. The disorder is probably a distinct clinical entity but may have some overlap with polyarteritis nodosa, although generalized vasculitis is not a feature. The pulmonary lesion is thought to be the primary defect; electron microscopy has demonstrated endothelial cell gaps and thickened alveolar septa. The renal disease arises secondary to the development of cross-reactive anti–basement membrane antibodies. The etiology is unknown, but the syndrome has occurred in association with drug sensitivities, hepatitis, rheumatoid arthritis and scleroderma.[7] Young adult men are predominantly affected; 90 percent of cases occur in males. Goodpasture syndrome is unusual in patients less than 16 years of age, but has been described in children.[302, 303]

The early clinical presentation may be insidious, but is eventually characterized by hemoptysis, nephritis and anemia. Dyspnea, wheezing, fever, malaise, and weakness are usual associated symptoms. The chest x-ray demonstrates perihilar flocculent infiltrates, which may extend out to the peripheral lung fields. In time, pulmonary fibrosis may develop.[303] The nephritis is usually complicated by azotemia and renal failure, but hypertension is rare.[7] The recurrent pulmonary hemorrhages lead to a chronic anemia in most patients.

The progression of the disease is variable, but often rapid; death usually occurs from pulmonary hemorrhage, asphyxia, or uremia. Corticosteroids and immunosuppressive agents may prolong survival in some patients; plasmapheresis has been shown to be of some benefit in others.[302]

Anesthetic Management. Particular attention should be directed to the evaluation of pulmonary and renal function. A chest x-ray should be reviewed; arterial blood gases, hemoglobin, electrolytes, blood urea nitrogen, and creatinine should be measured; and a urinalysis should be obtained. Preoperative transfusion may be required if the anemia is severe, and adequate blood products must be available for the operating room. Elective surgery should be postponed during periods of pulmonary hemorrhage. Perioperative corticosteroid supplementation may be necessary.

No specific anesthetic techniques or drugs are recommended. If pulmonary fibrosis has produced significant restrictive disease, ventilation should be controlled with an increased FIO_2, small tidal volumes, and an increased ventilatory rate.

Miscellaneous Connective Tissue Disorders

Marfan Syndrome

The Marfan syndrome is a familial disorder of connective tissue inherited as an autosomal dominant trait with prominent manifestations in the skeletal, ocular, cardiovascular, and pulmonary systems.[4, 7, 304] The prevalence of the syndrome is about 4 to 6 cases per 100,000 population. The underlying defect involves collagen synthesis or maturation and results in connective tissue elements of decreased tensile strength and elasticity. An inborn error of metabolism is presumed, but not yet identified; the etiology remains unknown.

Clinical Manifestations. There is considerable variance in the clinical expression of the Marfan syndrome; the diagnosis may be made in infancy or not recognized until later in life.

Skeletal abnormalities may be pathognomonic. Patients are usually tall and thin from excessive longitudinal bone growth and have long "spidery" fingers (arachnodactyly). Body segments are disproportionate, and arm span usually exceeds body height. The face is long, narrow, and asymmetrical, often with a prognathic jaw; a high-arched palate is common. Atlantoaxial instability, thoracolumbar scoliosis, pectus excavatum and carinatum, slipped epiphysis of the femoral head, and talipes equinovarus may occur with varying degrees of severity.

Joint hypermobility is a relatively consistent feature. Pain, effusions, and even dislocation may occur after minor trauma. Peripheral muscular hypotonia may account in part for the high frequency of inguinal, umbilical, femoral, and even diaphragmatic hernias.

The most important ocular complication (seen in 50 to 80 percent of patients) is dislocation of the lens from weakened suspensory ligaments. This may be complicated by secondary glaucoma. Most patients are myopic and may develop retinal detachments. Visual impairment is frequent.

The cardiovascular manifestations represent the greatest threat to patients with Marfan syndrome. These complications result from the degeneration of elastic fibers in the vascular media, referred to as cystic medial necrosis. Subsequent dilatation of the mitral annulus, aortic root, and aortic arch leads to valvular dysfunction and to aneurysm formation, which may be complicated by dissection and rupture. Aortic root dilatation can be identified early in childhood and variably progresses to aortic regurgitation in later years. Mitral valve prolapse is equally common in children. Mitral regurgitation may be severe and require prosthetic valvular replacement; it is the leading cause of cardiovascular morbidity in these children.[305] Sixty percent of patients have auscultatory evidence of aortic or mitral regurgitation or systolic clicks. Ventricular strain, cardiomegaly, congestive failure, or angina pectoris may develop before the fourth decade.[4]

Restrictive pulmonary disease may result from severe kyphoscoliosis or pectus excavatum. The forced vital capacity is consistently low in these patients.[304] Diffuse and bullous emphysema with a "honeycomb" appearance on the chest x-ray may be complicated by spontaneous pneumothorax.[306] Compression of the left mainstem bronchus by an enlarged left atrium has been described in children.[307]

Skin manifestations (striae) are minor. Wound healing and scar formation are normal.

Treatment. No specific treatment is available. Beta-adrenergic blockade with propranolol has been used to reduce cardiac and great vessel wall tension and thereby to limit dilatation complications, but the results have not been encouraging. The indications for surgical intervention vary greatly, but include hernia repairs, scoliosis correction, retinal detachment procedures, thoracotomy for pneumothorax,[306] aneurysm repairs, and prosthetic valvular replacements.

Anesthetic Management. These children require careful preoperative assessment to identify the cardiac complications of valvular dysfunction, cardiac failure, and aortic aneurysm and the pulmonary complications of emphysema, bronchogenic bullae, and decreased respiratory reserve. Medications for cardiac failure and propranolol therapy should be continued if good control has been established.[10] Prophylactic antibiotic coverage should be arranged for those patients with cardiac lesions.

The patient must be transferred gently in the operating room and positioned carefully to avoid stress on joints and to prevent intraoperative dislocations. All usual monitors are required for induction. Intravenous access should be obtained early. Additional invasive monitors should be reserved for major cases and high-risk patients because of the potential for vascular complications.

No specific anesthetic recommendations are reported, but the induction and maintenance technique used should avoid hypertension and tachycardia to prevent aneurysm rupture and preserve myocardial oxygenation. When intubation is required, laryngoscopy must be gentle to avoid soft tissue trauma and temporomandibular joint damage. Ventilation may have to be assisted or controlled, but peak airway pressures should be kept as low as possible. The appropriate equipment to treat a pneumothorax should be readily available.

Sarcoidosis

Sarcoidosis is a multisystemic disorder of variable clinical severity characterized by the development of noncaseating granulomas in the lungs, liver, spleen, lymph nodes, bones, eyes, and skin. It occurs in all races and regions of the world, but in North America is more common in rural communities and among blacks; women are more frequently affected than men. The diagnosis is usually made between the ages of 20 and 50 years. It does occur in children, but is uncommon under the age of 10 years.

The etiology of sarcoidosis is unknown, but evidence suggests a host reaction pattern determined by an abnormal immune response to some initiating factor. The reactive granulomas do not undergo central necrosis, but heal by fibrosis. The original granuloma contracts and becomes hyalinized to leave a small, dense scar.[309]

Clinical Manifestations. The disease onset is usually insidious; many patients are asymptomatic despite extensive organ involvement. Constitutional symptoms in more acute presentations include fever, malaise, anorexia, weight loss, and abdominal pain.

Pulmonary involvement is most common and eventually develops in 85 to 90 percent of patients.[310, 311] Even in asymptomatic patients, pulmonary function tests show early changes of restrictive disease with decreased vital capacity and functional residual capacity. Ventilation and perfusion abnormalities develop, compliance falls as fibrosis increases, and finally a progressive obstructive component complicates the clinical picture. A dry cough and exertional dyspnea are common complaints in late disease. Typical chest x-ray findings are bilateral hilar and paratracheal lymphadenopathy with scattered parenchymal infiltrates. The pulmonary adenopathy may compress and partially obstruct large bronchi.[310] In severe cases, pulmonary fibrosis may be complicated by cor pulmonale and right ventricular failure.

Upper airway involvement has been reported in 1 to 5 percent of adults as mucosal infiltration of the nose, pharynx, tonsils, and larynx.[309] Laryngeal lesions are usually supraglottic and present with symptoms of obstruction rather than hoarseness.

Disseminated disease may affect almost every organ system. Significant cardiac involvement occurs in 5 percent of cases; conduction defects, paroxysmal tachyarrhythmias, and congestive failure may develop. Hepatic dysfunction, splenomegaly, and generalized lymphadenopathy can occur. Painless parotid gland enlargement is not uncommon. Other manifestations described include skin lesions very similar to erythema nodosum, interstitial nephritis, renovascular hypertension, central nervous system symptoms and peripheral neuropathies, chronic uveitis, and a peripheral arthritis that may be destructive and usually involves the ankles, knees, wrists, and hands.[7]

The characteristic features of rare cases under the age of 1 year include arthritis, skin lesions and uveitis.

Laboratory findings may include anemia and thrombocytopenia, a polyclonal hypergammaglobulinemia, positive rheumatoid factor (which correlates with the degree of pulmonary involvement[10]), hypercalciuria, and hypercalcemia. The diagnosis is confirmed by tissue biopsy and often by a positive Kveim test.

The treatment of sarcoidosis is symptomatic and supportive. Anti-inflammatory agents, particularly corticosteroids, may be required to suppress acute manifestations. The prognosis in children is unpredictable; remissions do occur, but the course is often chronic with slowly progressive obstructive pulmonary disease.[6, 312]

Anesthetic Management. Although some patients are symptom-free, significant systemic disease may be established and careful preoperative assessment is important. The upper airway must be evaluated for obstructing nasal or laryngeal lesions and ankylosis of the temporomandibular joints. A history of exertional dyspnea, auscultation of the chest, and a review of the chest x-ray are important. Pulmonary function tests may be required to quantitate lung volumes and the relative degree of restrictive and obstructive respiratory disease. Preoperative arterial blood gases on room air may be very helpful. Cardiac involvement in children is uncommon, but an ECG should be obtained. Hepatic and renal dysfunction should be identified. Perioperative corticosteroid supplementation may be required.

No specific anesthetic drugs or techniques are recommended. All usual monitors including the ECG must be used for induction. If a difficult laryngoscopy is anticipated, relaxants should be avoided until the airway is secured. If laryngeal or epiglottic lesions are found, a smaller endotracheal tube than predicted may be required. Anesthetic gases must be warmed and humidified.

In the presence of significant pulmonary disease, ventilation should be assisted or controlled and an increased FIO_2 used. Patients with restrictive disease may require small tidal volumes and an increased respiratory rate.

Relapsing Nodular Nonsuppurative Panniculitis (Weber-Christian Disease)

This rare, recurrent, febrile illness is characterized by subcutaneous and visceral fat necrosis. The foci of fatty tissue inflammation and degeneration heal with fibrosis and occasionally with calcification. The etiology is unknown, but infections, drug reactions (bromides and iodides), and hypersensitivity are suggested. The disorder may represent a vasculitis or be the presenting sign of a connective tissue disease. It has been associated with pancreatic disease and with corticosteroid withdrawal. A similar but localized and transient disorder, subcutaneous fat necrosis, is seen in some neonates on exposure to cold (see page 381). Adults are predominantly affected, but Weber-Christian disease has been reported in all age groups, including infants.[313]

Clinical Manifestations. Weber-Christian disease may present with crops of subcutaneous nodules that are tender, erythematous, and warm and appear on the thighs, abdomen, and arms. Fever, associated with arthralgias and myalgias, is a common feature. Individual lesions regress without scarring over days or weeks, leaving brown atrophic areas, but recur. The disorder may continue in this fashion for months.

Systemic features depend on the severity of the visceral sites affected. Pericardial fat involvement with subsequent fibrosis can lead to constrictive pericarditis with a fixed, low cardiac output. Mesenteric disease may cause abdominal pain and tenderness. Hepatosplenomegaly has been reported.[6] An association with coagulopathy and hemolytic anemia has been reported.[314] Central nervous system or meningeal fat necrosis may provoke a seizure disorder. Acute adrenal insufficiency from adrenal infarction has been reported secondary to retroperitoneal panniculitis.[10]

The treatment is symptomatic and supportive. Anti-inflammatory agents and corticosteroids are usually effective for most manifestations of the disease.

Anesthetic Management. The preoperative identification of systemic complications is mandatory. Constrictive pericarditis, seizure disorders, and adrenal insufficiency must be recognized. Perioperative corticosteroid supplementation may be required for some patients.

Care must be taken to protect the patient's subcutaneous tissue and skin from heat, cold, trauma, and pressure, which may precipitate new lesions. The operating room, intravenous solutions, and anesthetic equipment should be warm. Anesthetic gases should be warmed and humidified.

Patients who have constrictive pericarditis require high venous filling pressures. Adequate preoperative hydration and volume resuscitation are critically important. Reliable intravenous access must be available for operative and postoperative fluid administration. Bradycardia and agents that depress myocardial contractility will be tolerated poorly. Invasive cardiovascular monitoring may be required in patients with severe disease.

No specific anesthetic drugs or techniques are recommended. No contraindications to the use of inhalational agents, whose biodegradation releases bromide and fluoride ions, have been reported.[10]

Eosinophilic Fasciitis

This unusual and rare syndrome is characterized by painful inflammation and induration of the skin, subcutaneous tissue, and fascia of the upper or lower extremities. The inflammation may occasionally extend to the trunk and face. The characteristic feature on biopsy is a thickened fascia with perivascular infiltration by eosinophils, histiocytes, and lymphocytes.[7] The disorder has frequently followed heavy physical exertion. It is most often seen in adults, but has been reported in children.[315] Some clinicians feel this syndrome is a variant of scleroderma.[315]

There are no systemic manifestations, although musculoskeletal contractures may develop.[6] Raynaud phenomenon is absent. Small doses of corticosteroids markedly improve symptoms. The disorder is usually self-limited; spontaneous resolution often occurs in less than 3 to 4 years, but the long-term prognosis is unknown.

Children with eosinophilic fasciitis may require perioperative corticosteroid supplementation. Significant facial involvement may reduce the mobility of the temporomandibular joint and create a small mouth opening. As a result, laryngoscopy and intubation may be difficult. In this situation, the recommended approach to airway management is similar to that described for juvenile rheumatoid arthritis (see page 404).

IMPLICATIONS OF CORTICOSTEROID THERAPY

The corticosteroid drugs are the most potent anti-inflammatory agents used in the treatment of skin and connective tissue diseases. The beneficial effects of topical and systemic steroid therapy must be weighed against the potentially serious complications that may arise from their use. The manipulation of perioperative steroid management is a shared responsibility of the pediatrician and the anesthetist and deserves special attention at this time.

The anti-inflammatory and immunosuppressive actions of the corticosteroids are multiple and complex.[14, 316–321] Steroids maintain the integrity of capillary endothelium, reducing edema and cellular infiltration, and stabilize cellular and lysosome membranes. They inhibit the migration of cells to areas of inflammation. Steroids interfere with phagocytosis and antigen processing by lymphocytes and macrophages. The inflammatory response of the antigen-antibody complex is also reduced. Cell-mediated immunity is modified substantially.

Prolonged, suppressive therapy with corticosteroids in the supraphysiological dose range is associated with many complications and side effects that have significant anesthetic implications (Table 15–1). The more important of these in children include growth retardation, osteoporosis, protein wasting, iatrogenic Cushing syndrome, sodium and water retention, hypertension, metabolic alkalosis, gastrointestinal irritation, susceptibility to infections, and carbohydrate intolerance. Accelerated coronary artery disease may be seen after 10 years of therapy.[7] Cataracts, myopathies, and psychoses are not infrequent. Surgical patients on steroids have increased morbidity and prolonged recovery times. Typical problems include poor tissue healing complicated by wound dehiscence, hematomas, and infections. The latter may present as localized abscesses or as septicemia and shock.

One of the most common and potentially hazardous complications of corticosteroid therapy is the suppression of the hypothalamic-pituitary-adrenal (HPA)

Table 15–1. COMPLICATIONS OF CORTICOSTEROID THERAPY

Endocrine
  Suppression of hypothalamic-pituitary-adrenal axis
  Growth disturbances
Metabolic
  Glucose intolerance; diabetes mellitus
  Hyperosmolar nonketotic coma
  Hyperlipidemia
  Centripetal obesity
Gastrointestinal
  Gastric hemorrhage
  Gastric and duodenal ulceration
  Intestinal perforation
  Pancreatitis
Suppression of Immune Response
  Secondary bacterial, viral, and fungal infections
    and parasitic infestation
Renal
  Sodium and water retention and edema
  Hypokalemic alkalosis
Cardiovascular
  Hypertension
  Accelerated coronary artery disease
Musculoskeletal
  Myopathy
  Osteoporosis, vertebral compression fractures
  Aseptic necrosis, especially of femoral head
Ophthalmological
  Posterior subcapsular cataracts
  Glaucoma
Inhibition of Fibroplasia
  Impaired wound healing
  Subcutaneous tissue atrophy
Central Nervous System
  Steroid-induced neuroses, psychoses

axis. Biochemical evidence of HPA axis suppression has been demonstrated within 5 days to 2 weeks of therapy and has been shown to persist for up to 12 months.[316–318]

The degree of HPA axis suppression is determined by duration of treatment, dose of steroid required, potency of the drug used, and schedule of administration. The reduction of the dose and discontinuance of therapy, as permitted by the disease response, is attempted as early as possible. Alternate-day therapy has been shown to allow recovery of the HPA axis and an improvement of some other complications.[316, 317] Suppression of the HPA axis in children has been described following the systemic absorption of topical steroids when the area of application is large and when potent agents are used, especially under occlusive dressings.[322, 323]

An often quoted study by Graber and colleagues (1965) defined the recovery of the HPA axis after withdrawal of therapy in patients who had been on steroids for at least 1 year.[325] For the first month after withdrawal, depressed function of both the pituitary and adrenal glands persists. During the second to fifth months, corticotropin levels rise to above normal, but the adrenal output of cortisol remains low. From the fifth to ninth months cortisol output is normal, but only with continuing high corticotropin levels. After 9 months, full recovery of adrenal function can be demonstrated.

During periods of stress, such as infection, trauma, and major surgery, the endogenous production of cortisol normally rises from two to seven fold above basal levels for at least 72 hours.[326, 339, 347] If this demand is not met, acute adrenal insufficiency may be precipitated. The patient's depressed stress response may progress to cardiovascular collapse and death. Such perioperative catastrophes have been reported.[327, 328]

The role that corticosteroid hormones play in cardiovascular homeostasis is not clearly defined. Steroids appear to be involved in synthesis and release of endogenous catecholamines and in the cardiovascular response to these catecholamines.[329] They also influence the homeostatic fluid shift response to acute hemorrhagic challenge.[330]

However, cortisol is not the prime factor in the maintenance of arterial pressure in the perioperative period in glucocorticoid-treated patients.[331, 332] Postoperative cardiovascular collapse has rarely been associated with low plasma cortisol, and a low plasma cortisol level alone is not a sufficient condition to produce hypotension.[333–335] Provided adequate fluid and electrolyte homeostasis is maintained perioperatively, circulatory collapse is rarely encountered even when steroid coverage is omitted.[336] Meyers has reported depressed neuromuscular transmission in patients with adrenocortical insufficiency.[338]

Despite the controversy described above, supplemental corticosteroids are provided to prevent the risk of unrecognized acute adrenal insufficiency. Most authors recommend steroid coverage for patients who have been treated with supraphysiological steroid doses for more than 5 days in the previous 9 months, or who currently require maintenance therapy. If there is time preoperatively, the functional reserve of the HPA axis should be evaluated by the patient's response to the rapid ACTH stimulation test or metyrapone test. If this reserve is normal, no steroid coverage is necessary. If it is borderline, coverage is preferred. Acute, supplemental steroids, even if unnecessary, can be withdrawn without difficulty as the acute stress resolves.

Many protocols for steroid coverage have been proposed.[339–348] Work with adults by Plumpton and associates (1969) formed the basis of earlier practice and advocated the use of high-dose steroid supplementation in the range of 400 mg per 24 hours.[339]

Current recommendations for adults call for more moderate doses as described by Baxter and Tyrell.[345] For major procedures, hydrocortisone hemisuccinate 100 mg is given intramuscularly on call to the operating room and continued intravenously at 50 mg every 6 hours for 24 hours. The dose is then reduced to 25 mg every 6 hours for 24 hours and finally withdrawn slowly over the following 3 to 5 days. For minor procedures, the same initial protocol is followed, but discontinued after 24 hours. For short diagnostic procedures, a single dose of hydrocortisone hemisuccinate 100 mg preoperatively should be adequate. If at any time postoperatively hypotension, fever, or other complications arise, then the full supplemental coverage of 200 to 400 mg per 24 hours should be reinstituted immediately (Table 15–2).

Two recent studies have recommended a low dose schedule for steroid supplementation of hydrocortisone 125 mg per 24 hours. No problems were encountered and plasma cortisol levels were considered more physiological.[347, 348]

Intramuscular cortisone acetate has been used frequently and without problems to provide steroid coverage. However, the administration of this preparation should be commenced at least 48 hours preoperatively because plasma cortisol levels by the intramuscular route are very slow to rise.[339, 349]

Table 15–2. PERIOPERATIVE STEROID REPLACEMENT FOR MAJOR SURGERY (IN ADULTS)

1. Hydrocortisone hemisuccinate, 100 mg IM, 1 hour preoperatively
2. Hydrocortisone hemisuccinate, 50 mg IV, q6h for 24 hours
3. If postoperative course is satisfactory, reduce dose to 25 mg IV q6h for 24 hours, then taper dose to maintenance level over next 5 days
4. If hypotension, fever, or other complications arise, increase hydrocortisone dosage to 200 to 400 mg per 24 hours
5. Approximate doses for children may be calculated proportionate to body surface area

Kenny has demonstrated that daily cortisol production rates (11.8 ± 2.5 mg/m^2/24 hours) are equivalent in children and adults when corrected for body surface area.[350] An approximate dose for steroid coverage in children can be extrapolated from the adult protocol by comparing body surface areas.[351] The use of body weight to calculate steroid doses may provide inadequate coverage in younger children and infants.

SUMMARY

Children with skin diseases and connective tissue disorders are often suffering from chronic and multisystemic illnesses. They present complex and diverse problems to the anesthesiologist should they require surgical intervention.

In this chapter, attention has been directed to the clinical presentation, pathophysiology, and treatment of these conditions and to the anesthetic management of affected children. With this information, it is hoped that anesthesiologists will be better prepared to provide these patients with safe and effective perioperative care.

The author would like to thank his wife, Connie, for her tolerance and support during the preparation of this chapter and his father, Dr. Foster Smith, for his continuing interest in anesthesia and his example.

He is also indebted to Ms. Pearl Pal for her help in producing the manuscript.

REFERENCES

Skin and Connective Tissue Disorders—General

1. Fitzpatrick TB, Eisen AZ, Wolff K, et al. (Eds.): Dermatology in General Medicine. Textbook and Atlas. 2nd ed., New York, McGraw-Hill, 1979.
2. Rook A, Wilkinson DS, Ebling FJG: Textbook of Dermatology. 3rd ed. Oxford, Blackwell Scientific Publications, 1979.
3. Maibach HI, Boisits EK (Eds.): Neonatal Skin. Vol. 1. Structure and Function. New York, Marcel Dekker, Inc., 1982.
4. Moschella SL (Ed.): Dermatology Update. Reviews for Physicians. New York, Elsevier/North Holland, 1979.
5. Rasmussen JE (Ed.): Symposium on pediatric dermatology. Pediatr Clin North Am 30 (3 and 4), 1983.
6. Behrman RE, Vaughan VC III (Eds.): Textbook of Pediatrics. 12th ed. Philadelphia, W.B. Saunders Co., 1983.
7. Cassidy JT: Textbook of Pediatric Rheumatology, New York, John Wiley and Sons, 1982.
8. Ansell BM: Rheumatic Disorders in Childhood. London, Butterworth and Co. Ltd., 1980.
9. Resnick D, Niwayama G: Diagnosis of Bone and Joint Disorders, Philadelphia, W.B. Saunders Co., 1981.
10. Katz J, Benumof J, Kadis LB (Eds.): Anesthesia and Uncommon Diseases: Pathophysiologic and Clinical Correlations. 2nd ed. Philadelphia, W.B. Saunders Co., 1981.
11. Gregory GA (Ed.): Pediatric Anesthesia. New York, Churchill Livingstone, 1983.
12. Stoelting RK, Dierdorf SF (Eds.): Anesthesia and Co-Existing Disease. New York, Churchill Livingstone, 1983.
13. Smith RM (Ed.): Anesthesia for Infants and Children. 4th ed. St. Louis, C.V. Mosby Co., 1980.
14. Felig P, Baxter JD, Broadus AE, et al. (Eds.): Endocrinology and Metabolism. New York, McGraw-Hill, 1981.
15. Kaplan SA (Ed.): Symposium on pediatric endocrinology. Pediatr Clin North Am 26(1), 1979.
16. Smith CA (Ed.): The Critically Ill Child. Diagnosis and Management. 2nd ed. Philadelphia, W.B. Saunders Co., 1977.
17. Gorlin RJ, Pinborg JJ, Cohen MM (Eds.): Syndromes of the Head and Neck. 2nd ed. New York, McGraw-Hill, 1976.
18. Smith GB, Shribman AJ: Anaesthesia and severe skin disease. Anaesthesia 39:443, 1984.

Neonatal and Developmental Abnormalities

19. Amstey MS, Lewin EB, Meyer MR: Herpesvirus infection in the newborn. Its treatment by exchange transfusion and adenosine arabinoside. Obstet Gynecol 47(Suppl):33, 1976.
20. Weston WL, Humbert JR: Failure of fresh plasma in Leiner disease. Arch Dermatol 113:233, 1977.
21. Rane RE, Baden HP: The ichthyoses—a review. J Am Acad Derm 8:285, 1983.
22. Benedek TG, Rodnan GP: The early history and nomenclature of scleroderma and its differentiation from sclerema neonatorum and scleroedema. Semin Arth Rheum 12:52, 1982.
23. Bart BJ: Epidermolysis bullosa and congenital localized absence of skin. Arch Dermatol 101:78, 1970.
24. Goltz RW, Henderson RR, Hitch JM, et al.: Focal dermal hypoplasia syndrome. A review of the literature and report of two cases. Arch Dermatol 101:1, 1970.
25. Rietschel RL: Anhidrotic ectodermal dysplasia and heat loss: management. Dermatology 18:370, 1979.
26. Capitanio MA, Chen JT, Arey JB, et al.: Congenital anhidrotic ectodermal dysplasia. Am J Roentgenol 103:168, 1968.
27. Ramchander V, Jankey N, Ramkissoon R, et al.: Anhidrotic ectodermal dysplasia in an infant presenting with pyrexia of unknown origin. Clin Pediatr 17:51, 1978.
28. Beahrs JO, Lillington GA, Rosan RC, et al.: Anhidrotic ectodermal dysplasia: predisposition to bronchial disease. Ann Intern Med 74:92, 1971.
29. Edgerton MT: The treatment of hemangiomas: special reference to the role of steroid therapy. Ann Surg 183:517, 1976.
30. Meeks EA, Jay JB, Heaton LD: Thrombocytopenic purpura occurring with large hemangioma. Am J Dis Child 90:349, 1955.
31. Kasabach HH, Merritt KK: Capillary hemangioma with extensive purpura. Am J Dis Child 59:1063, 1940.
32. Keller L, Bluhm JF: Diffuse neonatal hemangiomatosis. Cutis 23:295, 1979.
33. Gloviczki P, Hollier LH, et al.: Surgical implications of Klippel-Trenaunay syndrome. Ann Surg 197:353, 1983.
34. Mestre JR, Andres JM: Hereditary hemorrhagic telangiectasia causing hematemesis in an infant. J Pediatr 101:577, 1982.
35. Ulso C, Vase P, Stoksted P: Long-term results of dermatoplasty in the treatment of hereditary haemorrhagic telangiectasia. J Laryngol Otol 97:223, 1983.
36. Weller RM: Anaesthesia for cystic hygroma in a neonate. Anaesthesia 29:588, 1974.
37. MacDonald DJF: Cystic hygroma. Anaesthesia 21:66, 1966.

Epidermolysis Bullosa

38. Reddy ARR, Wong DHW: Epidermolysis bullosa. A review of anaesthetic problems and case reports. Can Anaesth Soc J 19:536, 1972.

39. Davison BCC: Epidermolysis bullosa. J Med Genet 2:223, 1965.
40. Cohen SR, Landing BH, Isaacs H: Epidermolysis bullosa associated with laryngeal stenosis. Ann Otol Rhinol Laryngol 87:25, 1978.
41. Milne B, Rosales JK: Anaesthesia for correction of esophageal stricture in a patient with recessive epidermolysis bullosa dystrophia: case report. Can Anaesth Soc J 27:169, 1980.
42. Becker MH, Swingard CA: Epidermolysis bullosa dystrophica in children. Radiological manifestations. Radiology 90:124, 1968.
43. Katz J, Gryboski JD, Rosenbaum HM, et al.: Dysphagia in children with epidermolysis bullosa. Gastroenterology 52:259, 1967.
44. Ramadass T, Thangavelu TA: Epidermolysis bullosa and its E.N.T. manifestations. Two case reports. J Laryngol Otol 92:441, 1978.
45. Malaga S, Fernandez Toral J, Santos F, et al.: Renal amyloidosis complicating a recessive epidermolysis bullosa in childhood. Helv Paediatr Acta 38:167, 1983.
46. Tio TH, Waardenburg PJ, Vermeulen HJ: Blood coagulation in epidermolysis bullosa hereditaria. Arch Derm 88:76, 1963.
47. Hamann RA, Cohen PJ: Anesthetic management of a patient with epidermolysis bullosa dystrophica. Anesthesiology 34:389, 1971.
48. Kubota Y, Norton ML, Goldenberg S, et al.: Anesthetic management of patients with epidermolysis bullosa undergoing surgery. Anesth Analg 40:244, 1961.
49. Lee C, Nagel EL: Anesthetic management of a patient with epidermolysis bullosa dystrophica. Anesthesiology 43:122, 1975.
50. LoVerme SR, Oropollo AT: Ketamine anesthesia in dermolytic bullous dermatosis (epidermolysis bullosa). Anesth Analg 56:398, 1977.
51. Marshall BE: A comment on epidermolysis bullosa and its anaesthetic management for dental operations. A case report. Br J Anaesth 35:724, 1963.
52. Dundee JW, Riding JE: Barbiturate narcosis in porphyria. Anaesthesia 10:55, 1955.
53. Price DG, Swart E: Epidermolysis bullosa. Anaesthesia 23:707, 1968.
54. Tomlinson AA: Recessive dystrophic epidermolysis bullosa. The anaesthetic management of a case for major surgery. Anaesthesia 38:485, 1983.
55. James I, Wark H: Airway management during anesthesia in patients with epidermolysis bullosa dystrophica. Anesthesiology 56:323, 1982.
56. Pratilas V, Biezunski A: Epidermolysis bullosa manifested and treated during anesthesia. Anesthesiology 43:581, 1975.
57. Young DA, Hardwick PB: Anaesthesia for epidermolysis bullosa dystrophica. A report of multiple anaesthetics in one patient. Anaesthesia 23:264, 1968.
58. Berryhill RE, Benumof JL, Saidman LJ, et al.: Anesthetic management of emergency cesarean section in a patient with epidermolysis bullosa dystrophica polydysplastica. Anesth Analg 57:281, 1978.
59. Fisk GC, Kern IB: Anaesthesia for oesophagoscopy in a child with epidermolysis bullosa—a case report. Anaesth Intens Care 1:297, 1973.
60. Petty WC, Gunther RC: Anesthesia for nonfacial surgery in polydysplastic epidermolysis bullosa (dystrophic). Anesth Analg 49:246, 1970.
61. Wilson F: Epidermolysis bullosa: a rare disease of anaesthetic interest. Br J Anaesth 31:26, 1959.
62. Haber RM, Ramsay CA, Boxall LBH: Assessment of a treatment for epidermolysis bullosa. Can Med Assoc J 131:10, 1984.

Erythema Multiforme

63. Chandra JJ, Callen JP: Erythema multiforme and the Stevens-Johnson syndrome. South Med J 71:566, 1978.
64. Pollack MA, Burk PG, Nathanson G: Mucocutaneous eruptions due to antiepileptic drug therapy in children. Ann Neurol 5:262, 1979.
65. Rallison ML, Carlisle JW, Lee RE Jr, et al.: Lupus erythematosus and Stevens-Johnson syndrome. Am J Dis Child 101:725, 1961.
66. Kazmierowski JA, Wuepper KD: Erythema multiforme: immune complex vasculitis of superficial cutaneous microvasculature. Clin Res 25:282 (abstract), 1977.
67. Stevens AM, Johnson FC: A new eruptive fever associated with stomatitis and ophthalmia. Am J Dis Child 24:526, 1922.
68. Costello MJ: Erythema multiforme exudativum. J Invest Dermatol 8:127, 1947.
69. Taaffe AG: The Stevens-Johnson syndrome. Br J Clin Pract 29:169, 1975.
70. Broadbent RV: Stevens-Johnson disease presenting with pneumothorax. Rocky Mount Med J 64:69, 1967.
71. Cucchiara RF, Dawson B: Anesthesia in Stevens-Johnson syndrome: report of a case. Anesthesiology 35:537, 1971.
72. Schartum S: Stevens-Johnson syndrome with cardiac involvement: report of two cases. Acta Med Scand 179:729, 1966.
73. Rasmussen JE: Erythema multiforme in children: response to treatment with systemic corticosteroids. Br J Dermatol 95:181, 1976.
74. Alexander MK, Cope S: Erythema multiforme exudativum major (Stevens-Johnson syndrome). J Pathol Bacteriol 68:373, 1954.

Toxic Epidermal Necrolysis

75. Krumlowsky FA, Del Greco F, Herdson PB, et al.: Renal disease associated with toxic epidermal necrolysis. Am J Med 57:817, 1974.
76. Lyell A: Toxic epidermal necrolysis (the scalded skin syndrome): a reappraisal. Br J Dermatol 100:69, 1979.
77. Stuttgen G: Toxic epidermal necrolysis provoked by barbiturates. Br J Dermatol 88:291, 1973.
78. Hunter JAA, Davison AM: Toxic epidermal necrolysis associated with pentazocine therapy and severe reversible renal failure. Br J Dermatol 88:287, 1973.
79. Orfanos CE, Schaumberg-Lever G, Lever WF: Dermal and epidermal types of erythema multiforme. Arch Dermatol 109:682, 1974.
80. Rasmussen JE: Toxic epidermal necrolysis: a review of 75 cases in children. Arch Dermatol 111:1135, 1975.
81. Melish ME, Glasgow LA: Staphylococcal scalded skin syndrome: the expanded clinical syndrome. J Pediatr 78:958, 1971.

Pemphigus

82. Beutner EH, Jordon RE: Demonstration of skin antibodies in sera of pemphigus vulgaris patients. Proc Soc Exp Biol Med 117:505, 1964.
83. Schiltz JR, Michel B, Papay R: Pemphigus antibody interaction with human epidermal cells in culture. J Clin Invest 62:778, 1978.
84. Berger BW, Maier HS, Kantor I, et al.: Pemphigus vulgaris in a 3½ year old boy. Arch Dermatol 107:433, 1973.
85. Bean SF, Jordon RE: Chronic non-hereditary blistering diseases in children. Arch Dermatol 110:941, 1974.
86. Krain LS: The association of pemphigus with thymoma or malignancy: a critical review. Br J Dermatol 90:397, 1974.

87. Chorzelski TP, Jablonska S, Blaszczyk M: Immunopathological investigations in the Senear-Usher syndrome. Br J Dermatol 80:211, 1968.
88. Izumi AK, Shmunes E, Wood MG: Familial benign chronic pemphigus. Arch Dermatol 104:177, 1971.
89. Lever WF: Immunosuppressants and prednisone in pemphigus vulgaris. Arch Dermatol 113:1236, 1977.
90. Lever WF: Methotrexate and prednisone in pemphigus vulgaris. Arch Dermatol 106:491, 1972.
91. Roenigk HH, Deodhar S: Pemphigus treatment with azathioprine. Arch Dermatol 107:353, 1973.
92. Cotterill JA, Barker DJ, Millard LG: Plasma exchange in the treatment of pemphigus vulgaris. Br J Dermatol 98:243, 1978.
93. Piamphongsant T, Chaikittisilpa S, Kullavanijaya P: Bullous pemphigoid in childhood: report of three cases and a review of literature. Int J Dermatol 16:126, 1977.
94. Hamilton DV, McKenzie AW: Bullous pemphigoid and primary biliary cirrhosis. Br J Dermatol 99:447, 1978.
95. Jeyaram C, Torda TA: Anesthetic management of cholecystectomy in a patient with buccal pemphigus. Anesthesiology 40:600, 1974.
96. Vatashsky E, Aronson HB: Pemphigus vulgaris: anaesthesia in the traumatized patient. Anaesthesia 37:1195, 1982.
97. Neldner KH, Hagler L, Wise WL, et al.: Acrodermatitis enteropathica. A clinical and biochemical survey. Arch Dermatol 110:711, 1974.
98. Portnoy B, Molokhia M: Acrodermatitis enteropathica treated by zinc. Br J Dermatol 91:701, 1974.

Epidermal and Dermal Disorders
99. Farber EM, Nall ML: The natural history of psoriasis in 5600 patients. Dermatologica 148:1, 1974.
100. Nyfors A, Lemholt K: Psoriasis in children. A short review and a survey of 245 cases. Br J Dermatol 92:437, 1975.
101. Fox RH, Shuster S, et al.: Cardiovascular, metabolic and thermoregulatory disturbances in patients with erythrodermic skin diseases. Br Med J 1:619, 1965.
102. Shuster S: High-output cardiac failure from skin disease. Lancet 1:1338, 1963.
103. Aly R, Maibach HI, Mandel A: Bacterial flora in psoriasis. Br J Dermatol 95:603, 1976.
104. Bachmann E, Clemmensen OJ, Dyrbye M, et al.: Joint involvement in psoriasis: scintigraphic, radiologic and clinical findings. Dermatologica 166:250, 1983.
105. Lambert JR, et al.: Psoriatic arthritis in children. Clin Rheum Dis 2:339, 1976.
106. Stimson CW, Leban SG: Recurrent ankylosis of the temporomandibular joint in a patient with chronic psoriasis. J Oral Maxillofac Surg 40:678, 1982.
107. Lerner MR, Lerner AB: Congenital psoriasis—report of 3 cases. Arch Dermatol 105:598, 1972.
108. Beighton P, Price A, Lord J, et al.: Variants of the Ehlers-Danlos syndrome. Am Rheum Dis 28:228, 1969.
109. Karaca M, Cronberg L, Nilsson IM: Abnormal platelet-collagen reaction in Ehlers-Danlos syndrome. Scand J Haematol 9:465, 1972.
110. Cabeen WR Jr, Reza MJ, Kovick RB, et al.: Mitral valve prolapse and conduction defects in Ehlers-Danlos syndrome. Arch Intern Med 137:1227, 1977.
111. Smit J, Alberts C, Balk AG: Pneumothorax in Ehlers-Danlos syndrome. Consequence or coincidence? Scand J Resp Dis 59:239, 1978.
112. Dolan P, Sisko F, Riley E: Anesthetic considerations for Ehlers-Danlos syndrome. Anesthesiology 52:266, 1980.
113. Abouleish E: Obstetric anaesthesia and Ehlers-Danlos syndrome. Br J Anaesth 52:1283, 1980.
114. Muster AJ, Bharati S, Herman JJ, et al.: Fatal cardiovascular disease and cutis laxa following acute febrile neutrophilic dermatosis. J Pediatr 102:243, 1983.
115. Sakati NO, Nyhan WL: Congenital cutis laxa and osteoporosis. Am J Dis Child 137:452, 1983.
116. Krechel SL, Ramirez-Inawat RC, Fabian LW: Anesthetic considerations in pseudoxanthoma elasticum. Anesth Analg 60:344, 1981.
117. Bete JM, Banas JS Jr, Moran J, et al.: Coronary artery disease in an 18 year old girl with pseudoxanthoma elasticum: successful surgical therapy. Am J Cardiol 36:515, 1975.
118. Wilhelm K, Pauer K: Sudden death in pseudoxanthoma elasticum. Med J Aust 2:1363, 1972.
119. Carter DJ, Woodward DA, Vince FP: Arterial surgery in pseudoxanthoma elasticum. Postgrad Med J 52:291, 1976.
120. Walker RB, Warin RP: The incidence of eczema in childhood. Br J Dermatol 68:182, 1956.
121. Lynch HT, Frichot BC, Lynch JF: Cancer control in xeroderma pigmentosum. Arch Dermatol 113:193, 1977.

Disorders with Pigmentary Changes
122. Riccardi VM: Pathophysiology of neurofibromatosis. IV. Dermatologic insights into heterogeneity and pathogenesis. J Am Acad Dermatol 3:157, 1980.
123. Wander JV, Das Gupta TK: Neurofibromatosis. Curr Probl Surg 14:11, 1977.
124. Leech RW: Intrathoracic meningocele and vertebral anomalies in a case of neurofibromatosis. Surg Neurol 9:55, 1978.
125. Chaglassian JH, Riseborough EJ, Hall JE: Neurofibromatous scoliosis. Natural history and results of treatment in thirty-seven cases. J Bone Joint Surg 58:695, 1976.
126. Cohen SR, Landing BH, Isaacs H: Neurofibroma of the larynx in a child. Ann Otol Rhinol Laryngol 87:29, 1978.
127. Chang-Lo M: Laryngeal involvement in von Recklinghausen's disease: a case report and review of the literature. Laryngoscope 87:435, 1977.
128. Sagel SS, Forrest JV, Askin FB: Interstitial lung disease in neurofibromatosis. South Med J 68:647, 1975.
129. Fisher MM: Anaesthetic difficulties in neurofibromatosis. Anaesthesia 30:648, 1975.
130. Yamashita M, Matsuki A, Oyama T: Anaesthetic considerations on von Recklinghausen's disease. Abnormal response to muscle relaxants. Anaesthetist 26:317, 1977.
131. Magbagbeola JAO: Abnormal responses to muscle relaxants in a patient with von Recklinghausen's disease. Br J Anaesth 42:710, 1970.
132. Krishma G: Neurofibromatosis, renal hypertension and cardiac dysrhythmias. Anesth Analg 54:542, 1975.
133. Carney RG: Incontinentia pigmenti. A world statistical analysis. Arch Dermatol 112:535, 1976.
134. Hendrickson MR, Ross JC: Neoplasms arising in congenital giant nevi. Am J Surg Pathol 5:109, 1981.
135. Greeley PW, Middleton AG, Curtin JW: Incidence of malignancy in giant pigmented nevi. Plast Reconstr Surg 36:26, 1965.
136. Rhodes AR, Sober AJ, Day CL, et al.: The malignant potential of small congenital nevocellular nevi. J Am Acad Dermatol 6:230, 1982.

Urticarial and Hypersensitivity Disorders
137. Johnston WE, Moss J, Philbin DM, et al.: Management of cold urticaria during hypothermic cardiopulmonary bypass. N Engl J Med 306:219, 1982.
138. Philbin DM, Moss J, Akins CW, et al.: The use of H1 and H2 histamine antagonists with morphine anesthesia: a double-blind study. Anesthesiology 55:292, 1981.
139. Moss J, Rosow CE, Savarese JJ, et al.: Role of histamine in the hypotensive action of d-tubocurarine in humans. Anesthesiology 55:19, 1981.

140. Lorenz, W, Doenicke A, Meyer R, et al.: Histamine release in man by propanidid and thiopentone: pharmacological effects and clinical consequences. Br J Anaesth 44:355, 1972.

141. Gerecke WB, Imasato Y, Keats AS: Histamine release by drugs used in association with anesthesia in man. Abstracts of Scientific Papers. Annual Meeting of the American Society of Anesthesiologists, 1969, p. 127.

142. Frank MM, Gelfand JA, Atkinson JP: Hereditary angioedema: the clinical syndrome and its management. Ann Intern Med 84:580, 1976.

143. Jaffe CJ, Atkinson JP, Gelfand JA, et al.: Hereditary angioedema: the use of fresh frozen plasma for prophylaxis in patients undergoing oral surgery. J Allergy 55:386, 1975.

144. Hopkinson RB, Sutcliffe AJ: Hereditary angioneurotic oedema. Anaesthesia 34:183, 1979.

145. Gibbs PS, LoSasso AM, Moorthy SS, et al.: The anesthetic and perioperative management of a patient with documented hereditary angioneurotic edema. Anesth Analg 56:571, 1977.

146. Abada RP, Owens WD: Hereditary angioneurotic edema, an anesthetic dilemma. Anesthesiology 46:428, 1977.

147. Cohen G, Peterson A: Treatment of hereditary angioedema with fresh frozen plasma. Ann Allergy 30:690, 1972.

148. Roth M, Schreier L, Cutter R: Adrenalin treatment for hereditary angioneurotic edema. Ann Allergy 35:175, 1975.

149. Hamilton AG, Bosley ARJ, Bowen DJ: Laryngeal oedema due to hereditary angioedema. Anaesthesia 32:265, 1977.

150. Johns ME, Vanselow MA, Boles R: Hereditary angioneurotic edema. Treatment with epsilon-aminocaproic acid during surgery. Arch Otolaryngol 99:388, 1974.

151. Wyre HW, Henrichs WD: Systemic mastocytosis and pulmonary eosinophilic granuloma. J Am Med Assoc 239:856, 1978.

152. Cooper AJ, Winkelmann RK, Wiltsie JC: Hematologic malignancies occurring in patients with urticaria pigmentosa. J Am Acad Dermatol 7:215, 1982.

153. Roberts LJ, Sweetman BJ, Lewis RA, et al.: Increased production of prostaglandin D_2 in patients with systemic mastocytosis. N Engl J Med 303:1400, 1980.

154. Scott HW, Parris WCV, Sandidge PC, et al.: Hazards in operative management of patients with systemic mastocytosis. Ann Surg 197:507, 1983.

155. Coleman MA, Liberthson RR, Crone RK, et al.: General anesthesia in a child with urticaria pigmentosa. Anesth Analg 59:704, 1980.

156. Rosenbaum KJ, Strobel GE: Anesthetic considerations in mastocytosis. Anesthesiology 38:398, 1973.

157. Rosow CE, Moss J, Philbin DJ, et al.: Histamine release during morphine and fentanyl anesthesia. Anesthesiology 56:93, 1982.

158. Brown TP: Thiopentone anaphylaxis—case report. Anaesth Intens Care 3:257, 1975.

159. Buckland RW, Avery RF: Histamine release following pancuronium. A case report. Br J Anaesth 45:518, 1973.

160. Roberts LJ, Turk JW, Oates JA: Shock syndrome associated with mastocytosis: pharmacological reversal of the acute episode and therapeutic prevention of recurrent attacks. Adv Shock Res 8:145, 1982.

161. Parris WCV, Sandidge PC, Petrinely G: Anaesthetic management of mastocytosis. Anesthesiol Rev 8:32, 1981.

162. Hannuksela M: Erythema nodosum with special reference to sarcoidosis. Ann Clin Res 3(Suppl 7):1, 1971.

163. Jacobs WH: Erythema nodosum in inflammatory disease of the bowel. Gastroenterology 37:286, 1959.

Miscellaneous Disorders

164. Lehner T: Progress report: oral ulcerations and Behçet's syndrome. Gut 18:491, 1977.

165. Penza R, Brunetti L, Franciosa G, et al.: Renal amyloidosis in a child with Behçet's syndrome. Int J Pediatr Nephrol 4:35, 1983.

166. Turner ME: Anaesthetic difficulties associated with Behçet's syndrome. Br J Anaesth 44:100, 1972.

167. Roguin N, Haim S, Reshef R, et al.: Cardiac involvement and superior vena caval obstruction in Behçet's disease. Thorax 33:375, 1978.

168. Ahonen AV, Stenius-Aarniala BSM: Obstructive lung disease in Behçet's syndrome. Scand J Respir Dis 59:44, 1978.

169. Mason RM, Barnes CG: Behçet's syndrome with arthritis. Ann Rheum Dis 28:95, 1969.

170. Chajeh T, Fainarn M: Behçet's disease: report of 41 cases and review of literature. Medicine 54:179, 1975.

171. Horner FA, Myers GJ, Stumpf DA, et al.: Malignant atrophic papulosis (Kohlmeier-Degos disease) in childhood. Neurology 26:317, 1976.

172. Pierce RN, Smith GJW: Intrathoracic manifestations of Degos' disease. Chest 73:79, 1978.

173. Black MM: Malignant atrophic papulosis (Degos' disease). Int J Dermatol 15:405, 1976.

174. Taaffe A: Angiokeratoma corporis diffusum. The evolution of a disease entity. Postgrad Med J 53:78, 1977.

175. Flynn DM, Lake BD, Boothby CB, et al.: Gut lesions in Fabry's disease without a rash. Arch Dis Child 447:26, 1972.

176. Rowe JW, Caralis DG: Accelerated atrioventricular conduction in Fabry's disease. Angiology 29:562, 1978.

177. Sheth KJ, Roth DA, Adams MB: Early renal failure in Fabry's disease. Am J Kidney Dis 2:651, 1983.

178. Gubler MC, Lenoir G, Grünfeld JP, et al.: Early renal changes in hemizygous and heterozygous patients with Fabry's disease. Kidney Int 13:223, 1978.

179. Bühler FR, Theil G, Dubach UC, et al.: Kidney transplantation in Fabry's disease. Br Med J 3:28, 1973.

Connective Tissue Disease

180. Prockop J, Kiviriko KI, Tuderman L, et al.: The biosynthesis of collagen and its disorders. N Engl J Med 301:13,77, 1979.

181. MacKay IR, Burnet FM: Autoimmune Diseases: Pathogenesis, Chemistry and Therapy. Springfield, IL, Charles C Thomas, 1964, p 16.

182. Rees AJ: Autoimmunity and autoimmune disease. Br J Anaesth 51:13, 1979.

Juvenile Rheumatoid Arthritis

183. Schaller JG: The diversity of juvenile rheumatoid arthritis: A 1976 look at the subgroup of chronic arthritis. Arth Rheum 20(Suppl):52, 1977.

184. Calabro JJ, Katz RM, Malty BA: A critical appraisal of juvenile rheumatoid arthritis. Clin Orthop 74:101, 1971.

185. Smith PH, Sharp J, Kellgren JH: Natural history of rheumatoid cervical subluxations. Ann Rheum Dis 31:222, 1972.

186. Martis CS, Kara Kasis DT: Ankylosis of the temporomandibular joint caused by Still's disease. Oral Surg 35:462, 1973.

187. Grosfeld O, Czarnecka B, Drecka-Kuzan K, et al.: Clinical investigations of the temporomandibular joint in children and adolescents with rheumatoid arthritis. Scand J Rheum 2:145, 1973.

188. Lofgren RH, Montgomery WW: Incidence of laryngeal involvement in rheumatoid arthritis. N Engl J Med 267:193, 1962.

189. Montgomery WW: Cricoartenoid arthritis. Laryngoscope 73:801, 1963.

190. Jacobs JC, Hui RM: Cricothyroid arthritis and airway obstruction in juvenile rheumatoid arthritis. Pediatrics 59:292, 1977.
191. Svantesson H, Bjorkhem G, Elborgh R: Cardiac involvement in juvenile rheumatoid arthritis. A follow-up study. Acta Paediatr Scand 72:345, 1983.
192. Brewer E: Juvenile rheumatoid arthritis—cardiac involvement. Arth Rheum 20(Suppl):231, 1977.
193. Majeed HA, Kvasnicka J: Juvenile rheumatoid arthritis with cardiac tamponade. Ann Rheum Dis 37:273, 1978.
194. Scharf J, Levy J, Benderly A, et al.: Pericardial tamponade in juvenile rheumatoid arthritis. Arth Rheum 19:760, 1976.
195. Zvaifler NJ, Weintraub AM: Aortitis and aortic insufficiency in the chronic rheumatic disorders—a reappraisal. Arth Rheum 6:241, 1963.
196. Walker WC, Wright V: Rheumatoid pleuritis. Ann Rheum Dis 26:467, 1967.
197. Divertie MB: Lung involvement in the connective-tissue disorders. Med Clin North Am 48:1015, 1964.
198. Conn DL, McDuffie FC, Dyck PJ: Immunopathologic study of sural nerves in rheumatoid arthritis. Arth Rheum 15:135, 1972.
199. Davies DW, Steward DJ: Unexpected excessive bleeding during operation: role of acetyl salicylic acid. Can Anaesth Soc J 24:452, 1977.
200. Amrein PC, Ellman L, Harris WH: Aspirin-induced prolongation of bleeding time and perioperative blood loss. JAMA 245:1825, 1981.
201. Ansell BM, Arden GP, McLennan I: Valgus knee deformities in children with juvenile polyarthritis treated by epiphyseal stapling. Arch Dis Child 45:388, 1970.
202. Jenkins LC, McGraw RW: Anaesthetic management of the patient with rheumatoid arthritis. Can Anaesth Soc J 16:407, 1969.
203. Edelist G: Principles of anesthetic management in rheumatoid arthritic patients. Anesth Analg 43:227, 1964.
204. Gardiner DL, Holmes F: Anaesthetic and postoperative hazards in rheumatic arthritis. Br J Anaesth 33:258, 1961.
205. Taylor RC, Way WL, Hendrixson R: Temporomandibular joint problems in relation to the administration of general anesthesia. J Oral Surg 26:327, 1968.
206. Funk D, Raymon F: Rheumatoid arthritis of the cricoarytenoid joints: an airway hazard. Anesth Analg 54:742, 1975.
207. Phelps JA: Laryngeal obstruction due to cricoarytenoid arthritis. Anesthesiology 27:518, 1966.
208. Goudsouzian N, Cote CJ, Liu LM, et al.: The dose-response effects of oral cimetidine on gastric pH and volume in children. Anesthesiology 55:533, 1981.
209. Salem MR, Wong AY, Mani M, et al.: Premedicant drugs and gastric juice pH and volume in pediatric patients. Anesthesiology 44:216, 1976.
210. D'Arcy EJ, Fell RH, Ansell BM, et al.: Ketamine and juvenile chronic polyarthritis (Still's disease). Anaesthesia 31:624, 1976.
211. Carson IW, Moore J, Balmer JP, et al.: Laryngeal competence with ketamine and other drugs. Anesthesiology 38:128, 1973.
212. Salem MR, Wong AY, Fizzotti GF: Efficacy of cricoid pressure in preventing aspiration of gastric contents in paediatric patients. Br J Anaesth 44:401, 1972.
213. Salem MR, Mathrubhutham M, Bennett EJ: Difficult intubation. N Engl J Med 295:879, 1976.
214. France NK: Management of the difficult intubation. In Gregory GA (Ed.): Pediatric Anesthesia. New York, Churchill Livingstone, 1983, p 825.
215. Pelton DA, Daly M, Cooper PD, et al.: Plasma lidocaine concentrations following topical aerosol application to the trachea and bronchi. Can Anaesth Soc J 17:250, 1970.
216. Davies JAH: Blind nasal intubation using doxapram hydrochloride. Br J Anaesth 40:361, 1968.
217. Salem MR, Wong AY, Kiam D, et al.: Difficult intubation in children: evaluation of two techniques. Abstracts of scientific papers. American Society of Anesthesiologists Meeting, 1977.
218. Rucker RW, Silva WJ, Worcester CC: Fiberoptic bronchoscopic nasotracheal intubation in children. Chest 76:56, 1979.
219. Stiles CM: A flexible fiberoptic bronchoscope for endotracheal intubation of infants. Anesth Analg 53:1017, 1974.
220. Alfery DD, Ward CF, Harwood IR, et al.: Airway management for a neonate with congenital fusion of the jaws. Anesthesiology 51:340, 1979.
221. Fan LL: Transnasal fiberoptic endoscopy in children with obstructive apnea. Crit Care Med 12:590, 1984.
222. Munson ES, Cullen SC: Endotracheal intubation in a patient with ankylosing spondylitis of the cervical spine. Anesthesiology 26:365, 1965.
223. Rosenberg MB, Levesque PR, Bourke DL: Use of the LTA kit as a guide for endotracheal intubation. Anesth Analg 56:287, 1977.
224. Waters DJ: Guided blind endotracheal intubation. Anaesthesia 38:128, 1963.
225. Berry FA: The use of a stylet in blind nasotracheal intubation. Anesthesiology 61:469, 1984.
226. Stone DJ, Stirt JA, Kaplan MJ, et al.: A complication of lightwand-guided nasotracheal intubation. Anesthesiology 61:780, 1984.

Spondyloarthropathies

227. Ladd JR, Cassidy JT, Martel W: Juvenile ankylosing spondylitis. Arch Rheum 14:579, 1971.
228. Schaller J, Bitnum S, Wedgwood RJ: Ankylosing spondylitis with childhood onset. J Pediatr 74:505, 1969.
229. Reid GD, Hill RH: Atlantoaxial subluxation in juvenile ankylosing spondylitis. J Pediatr 93:531, 1978.
230. Applerouth D, Gottlieb NL: Pulmonary manifestations of ankylosing spondylitis. J Rheumatol 2:446, 1975.
231. Reid GD, Patterson MWH, Patterson AC, et al.: Aortic insufficiency in association with juvenile ankylosing spondylitis. J. Pediatr 95:78, 1979.
232. Calin A, Porta J, Fries JF, et al.: Clinical history as a screening test for ankylosing spondylitis. JAMA 237:2613, 1977.
233. Brewerton DA, Hart FD, Nicholls A, et al.: Ankylosing spondylitis and HL-A27. Lancet 1:904, 1973.
234. DiSciascio G, Taranta A: Rheumatic fever in children: A review. Am Heart J 99:635, 1980.
235. Van de Rijn I, Zabriskie JB, McCarty M: Group A streptococcal antigens cross-reactive with myocardium. J Exp Med 146:579, 1977.
236. Stollerman GH, Markowitz M, et al.: Jones criteria (revised) for guidelines in the diagnosis of rheumatic fever (Committee report). Circulation 32:664, 1965.
237. Troyer C, Grossman ME, Silvers DN: Erythema marginatum in rheumatic fever: early diagnosis by skin biopsy. J Am Acad Dermatol 8:724, 1983.
238. John S, Bashi VV, Jairaj PS, et al.: Mitral valve replacement in the young patient with rheumatic heart disease. J Thorac Cardiovasc Surg 86:209, 1983.
239. Felman YM, Nikitas JA: Reiter's syndrome. Cutis 31:152, 1983.
240. Brewerton DA, Caffrey M, Nicholls A, et al.: Reiter's syndrome and HL-A27. Lancet 2:996, 1973.
241. Singsen BH, Bernstein BH, et al.: Reiter's syndrome in childhood. Arth Rheum 20(Suppl):402, 1977.
242. Lindsley CB, Schaller JB: Arthritis associated with inflammatory bowel disease in children. J. Pediatr 84:16, 1974.

Systemic Lupus Erythematosus

243. Brunner CM, Davis JS: Immune mechanisms in the pathogenesis of systemic lupus erythematosus. Bull Rheum Dis 26:854, 1976.
244. Lee SL, Chase PH: Drug-induced systemic lupus erythematosus: a critical review. Semin Arth Rheum 5:83, 1975.
245. Fish AJ, Blau EB, Westberg NG, et al.: Systemic lupus erythematosus within the first two decades of life. Am J Med 62:99, 1977.
246. Koster-King K, Kornreich HK, et al.: The clinical spectrum of systemic lupus erythematosus in childhood. Arth Rheum 20(Suppl):287, 1977.
247. Sourander LB, Pulkinen K: Simultaneous occurrence of ankylosis of cricoarytenoid joints with dyspnea and lupus erythematosus syndrome in rheumatoid arthritis. Acta Rheum Scand 8:255, 1962.
248. del Rio A, Vazquez JJ, Sobrino JA, et al.: Myocardial involvement in systemic lupus erythematosus. Chest 74:414, 1978.
249. Ishikawa S, Segar WE, Gilbert EF, et al.: Myocardial infarct in a child with systemic lupus erythematosus. Am J Dis Child 132:696, 1978.
250. Matthay RA, Schwarz MI, Petty TL, et al.: Pulmonary manifestations of systemic lupus erythematosus: review of twelve cases of acute lupus pneumonitis. Medicine 54:397, 1975.
251. Bennahum DA, Messner RP: Recent observations on central nervous system lupus erythematosus. Semin Arth Rheum 4:253, 1975.
252. Zizic TM, Classen JN, Stevens MB: Acute abdominal complications of systemic lupus erythematosus and polyarteritis nodosa. Am J Med 73:525, 1982.
253. Davis S, Furie BC, Griffin JH, et al.: Circulating inhibitors of blood coagulation associated with procainamide-induced lupus erythematosus. Am J Hematol 4:401, 1978.
254. Bernstein B, Koster-King K, et al.: Sjögren's syndrome in childhood. Arth Rheum 20:361, 1977.
255. Esscher E, Scott JS: Congenital heart block and maternal systemic lupus erythematosus. Br Med J 1:1235, 1979.
256. Walravens PA, Chase HP: The prognosis of childhood systemic lupus erythematosus. Am J Dis Child 130:929, 1976.

Dermatomyositis

257. Winkelmann RK: Dermatomyositis in childhood. Clin Rheum Dis 8:353, 1982.
258. Rose AL: Childhood polymyositis. A follow up study with special reference to treatment with corticosteroids. Am J Dis Child 127:518, 1974.
259. Metheny JA: Dermatomyositis. A vocal and swallowing disease entity. Laryngoscope 88:147, 1978.
260. Olsen GN, Swenson EW: Polymyositis and interstitial lung disease. Am Rev Respir Dis 105:611, 1972.
261. Johns RA, Finholt DA, Stirt JA: Anesthetic management of a child with dermatomyositis. Can Anaesth Soc J 33:71, 1986.

Scleroderma

262. Siegel RC: Scleroderma. Med Clin North Am 61:283, 1977.
263. Fleischmajer R: The pathophysiology of scleroderma. Int J Dermatol 16:310, 1977.
264. Weisman RA, Calcaterra TC: Head and neck manifestations of scleroderma. Ann Otol 87:332, 1978.
265. Guttadauria M, Ellman H, Emmanuel G, et al.: Pulmonary function in scleroderma. Arth Rheum 20:1071, 1977.
266. Ritchie B: Pulmonary function in scleroderma. Thorax 19:28, 1964.
267. Iliffe GD, Pettigrew NM: Hypoventilatory respiratory failure in generalized scleroderma. Br Med J 286:337, 1983.

268. Russell DC, Maloney A, Muir AL: Progressive generalized scleroderma: respiratory failure from primary chest wall involvement. Thorax 36:219, 1981.
269. Young RH, Mark GJ: Pulmonary vascular changes in scleroderma. Am J Med 64:998, 1978.
270. Bulkley BH, Ridolfi RL, Salyer WR, et al.: Myocardial lesions of progressive systemic sclerosis. Circulation 53:483, 1976.
271. Clements PJ, Furst DE, Cabeen W, et al.: The relationship of arrhythmias and conduction disturbances to other manifestations of cardiopulmonary disease in progressive systemic sclerosis. Am J Med 71:38, 1981.
272. Caplan HI, Benny RA: Total osteolysis of the mandibular condyle in progressive systemic sclerosis. Oral Surg 46:362, 1978.
273. Singsen BH, Bernstein BH, Kornreich HK, et al.: Mixed connective tissue disease in childhood. J Pediatr 90:893, 1977.
274. LeRoy EC, Fleischmann RM: The management of renal scleroderma—experience with dialysis, nephrectomy, transplantation. Am J Med 64:974, 1978.
275. Lopez-Ovejero JA, Saal SD, D'Angelo WA, et al.: Reversal of vascular and renal crises of scleroderma by oral angiotensin-converting-enzyme blockade. N Engl J Med 300:1417, 1979.
276. Thompson J, Conklin KA: Anesthetic management of a pregnant patient with scleroderma. Anesthesiology 59:69, 1983.
277. Neill RS: Progressive systemic sclerosis. Prolonged sensory blockade following regional anaesthesia in association with reduced response to systemic analgesics. Br J Anaesth 52:623, 1980.
278. Lewis GBH: Prolonged regional analgesia in scleroderma. Can Anaesth Soc J 21:495, 1974.
279. Eisele JH, Reitan JA: Scleroderma, Raynaud's phenomenon and local anesthetics. Anesthesiology 34:386, 1971.
280. Davidson-Lamb RW, Finlayson MCK: Scleroderma. Complications encountered during dental anaesthesia. Anaesthesia 32:893, 1977.
281. Birkhan J, Heifetz M, Haim S: Diffuse cutaneous scleroderma: an anaesthetic problem. Anaesthesia 27:89, 1972.

Systemic Vasculitis Syndromes

282. Kathuria S, Chejfec G: Fatal pulmonary Henoch-Schönlein syndrome. Chest 82:654, 1982.
283. Reimold EW, Weinberg AG, Fink CW, et al.: Polyarteritis in children. Am J Dis Child 130:534, 1976.
284. Martin TH: Pharyngeal edema associated with arteritis. Can Med Assoc J 101:229, 1969.
285. Roberts FB, Fetterman GH: Polyarteritis nodosa in infancy. J Pediatr 63:519, 1963.
286. Kawasaki T, Kosaki F, Okawa S, et al.: A new infantile acute febrile mucocutaneous lymph node syndrome (MLNS) prevailing in Japan. Pediatrics 54:271, 1974.
287. Melishe ME: Kawasaki syndrome (the mucocutaneous lymph node syndrome). Ann Rev Med 33:569, 1982.
288. Rowe RD, Rose V: Kawasaki disease: Canadian update. Can Med Assoc J 132:25, 1985.
289. Bell DM, Brink EW, Nitzin JL, et al.: Kawasaki syndrome: description of two outbreaks in the United States. N Engl J Med 304:1568, 1981.
290. Wada J, Endo M, Takao M, et al.: Mucocutaneous lymph node syndrome. Successful aortocoronary bypass homograft in a 4 year old boy. Chest 77:443, 1980.
291. McNiece WL, Krishna G: Kawasaki disease—a disease with anesthetic implications. Anesthesiology 58:269, 1983.
292. Feld LG, Weiss RA, Weiner S, et al.: Takayasu's arteritis. Asymptomatic presentation in a two-year-old boy. NY State J Med 83:229, 1983.

293. Pokrovsky AV, Sultanaliev TA, Spiridonov AA: Surgical treatment of vasorenal hypertension in nonspecific aortoarteritis (Takayasu's disease). J Cardiovasc Surg 24:111, 1983.

294. Warner MA, Hughes DR, Messick JM: Anesthetic management of a patient with pulseless disease. Anesth Analg 62:532, 1983.

295. Ramanthan S, Gupta V, Chalon J, et al.: Anesthetic considerations in Takayasu arteritis. Anesth Analg 58:247, 1979.

296. Beckman A, Grahne B, Holopainen B, et al.: Wegener's granulomatosis in childhood. A clinical report based on 3 cases. Int J Pediatr Otorhinolaryngol 1:145, 1979.

297. Kulis JC, Nequin ND: Tracheo-esophageal fistula due to Wegener's granulomatosis. JAMA 191:148, 1965.

298. Fauci AS, Haynes BF, Katz P, et al.: Wegener's granulomatosis: prospective clinical and therapeutic experience with 85 patients for 21 years. Ann Intern Med 98:76, 1983.

299. Thomas RHM, Payne CMER, Black MM: Wegener's granulomatosis presenting as pyoderma gangrenosum. Clin Exp Dermatol 7:523, 1982.

300. Landman S, Burgener F: Pulmonary manifestations in Wegener's granulomatosis. Am J Roentgenol Radium Ther Nucl Med 122:750, 1974.

301. Lake CL: Anesthesia and Wegener's granulomatosis: case report and review of the literature. Anesth Analg 57:353, 1978.

302. Simonsen H, Brun C, Thomsen OF, et al.: Goodpasture's syndrome in twins. Acta Med Scand 212:425, 1982.

303. Proskey AJ, Weatherbee L, Easterling RE, et al.: Goodpasture's syndrome. A report of five cases and review of the literature. Am J Med 48:162, 1970.

Miscellaneous Connective Tissue Disorders

304. Pyeritz RE, McKusick VA: The Marfan syndrome: diagnosis and management. N Engl J Med 300:772, 1979.

305. Sisk HE, Zahka KG, Pyeritz RE: The Marfan syndrome in early childhood: analysis of 15 patients diagnosed at less than 4 years of age. Am J Cardiol 52:355, 1983.

306. Hall JR, Pyeritz RE, Dudgeon DL, et al.: Pneumothorax in the Marfan syndrome: prevalence and therapy. Ann Thorac Surg 37:500, 1984.

307. Bolande RP, Tucker AS: Pulmonary emphysema and other cardiorespiratory lesions as part of the Marfan syndrome. Pediatrics 33:356, 1964.

308. Newbold SG, Shafer AD, Goodwin CD, et al.: Stage III Wilm's tumour of a solitary kidney in a patient with Marfan's syndrome: a 5-year survival. J Pediatr Surg 17:841, 1982.

309. Miglets AW, Viall JH, Kataria YP: Sarcoidosis of the head and neck. Laryngoscope 87:2038, 1977.

310. Snider GL, Doctor LR: The mechanics of ventilation in sarcoidosis. Am Rev Respir Dis 89:897, 1964.

311. Johnson RL, Lawson WH, Wilcox WCN: Alveolar capillary block in sarcoidosis. Clin Res 9:196, 1961.

312. Kendig EL, Brummer DL: The prognosis of sarcoidosis in children. Chest 70:351, 1976.

313. Hendricks WM, Ahmad M, Gratz E: Weber-Christian syndrome in infancy. Br J Dermatol 98:175, 1978.

314. Spivak JL, Lindo S, Coleman M: Weber-Christian disease complicated by consumption coagulopathy and microangiopathic hemolytic anemia. Johns Hopkins Med J 126:344, 1970.

315. Britt WJ, Duray PH, Dahl MV, et al.: Diffuse fasciitis with eosinophilia: a steroid responsive variant of scleroderma. J Pediatr 97:432, 1980.

Corticosteroid Therapy

316. Axelrod L: Glucocorticoid therapy. Medicine 55:39, 1976.

317. Melby JC: Systemic corticosteroid therapy: pharmacology and endocrinologic considerations. Ann Intern Med 81:505, 1974.

318. Thorn GW: Clinical considerations in the use of corticosteroids. N Engl J Med 274:775, 1966.

319. Kaplan SR, Calabresi P: Immunosuppressive agents. N Engl J Med 289:952, 1973.

320. Chabner BA, Myers CE, Coleman CN, et al.: The clinical pharmacology of antineoplastic agents. N Engl J Med 292:1107 and 1159, 1975.

321. Schein PS, Winokur SH: Immunosuppressive and cytotoxic chemotherapy: longterm implications. Ann Intern Med 82:84, 1975.

322. Munro DD: The effect of percutaneously absorbed steroids on hypothalamic-pituitary-adrenal function after intensive use in in-patients. Br J Dermatol 94(Suppl 12):67, 1976.

323. Wilson L, Williams DI, Marsh SD: Plasma corticosteroid levels in out-patients treated with topical steroids. Br J Dermatol 88:373, 1973.

324. Laaksonen AL, Sunell JE, Westeren H, et al.: Adrenocortical function in children with juvenile rheumatoid arthritis and other connective tissue disorders. Scand J Rheumatol 3:137, 1974.

325. Graber AL, Ney RL, Nicholson WE, et al.: Natural history of pituitary-adrenal recovery following long-term suppression with corticosteroids. J Clin Endocrinol Metab 25:11, 1965.

326. Cope CL: The adrenal cortex in internal medicine (I). Br Med J 2:47, 1966.

327. Fraser CG, Preuss FS, Bigford WD: Adrenal atrophy and irreversible shock associated with cortisone therapy. JAMA 149:1542, 1952.

328. Roberts JC: Operative collapse after corticosteroid therapy—a survey. Surg Clin North Am 50:363, 1970.

329. Kehlet H, Nikki P, et al.: Plasma catecholamines during surgery in unsupplemented glucocorticoid treated patients. Br J Anaesth 46:73, 1974.

330. Barton RN, Passinghem BJ: Early responses to hemorrhage in the conscious rat: effects of corticosterone. Am J Physiol 243:R416, 1982.

331. Weatherill D, Spence AA: Anaesthesia and disorders of the adrenal cortex. Br J Anaesth 56:741, 1984.

332. Kehlet H, Binder C: Adrenocortical function and clinical course during and after surgery in unsupplemented glucocorticoid-treated patients. Br J Anaesth 45:1043, 1973.

333. Oyama T: Hazards of steroids in association with anaesthesia. Can Anaesth Soc J 16:361, 1969.

334. Gordon NH, Scott DB, Percy Robb IW: Modification of plasma corticosteroid concentrations during and after surgery by epidural blockade. Br Med J 1:581, 1973.

335. Bovill JG, Sebel PS, Fiolet JW, et al.: The influence of sufentanil on endocrine and metabolic response to cardiac surgery. Anesth Analg 62:391, 1983.

336. Ishihara H, Ishida K, Matsuki A, et al.: Adrenocorticol response to general anaesthesia and surgery. Can Anaesth Soc J 26:186, 1979.

337. Traynor C, Hall GM: Endocrine and metabolic changes during surgery: Anaesthetic implications. Br J Anaesth 53:153, 1981.

338. Meyers EF: Partial recovery from pancuronium neuro-muscular blockade following hydrocortisone administration. Anesthesiology 46:148, 1977.

339. Plumpton FS, Besser GM, Cole PV: Corticosteroid treatment and surgery. Anaesthesia 24:3, 1969.

340. Black GW, Montgomery DAD: Adrenal disease. In Vickers MD (Ed.): Medicine for Anaesthetists. Oxford, Blackwell Scientific Publications, 1982, p 451.

341. Fass B: Glucocorticoid therapy for non-endocrine disorders: withdrawal and "coverage." Pediatr Clin North Am 26:251, 1979.

342. Olin R: When should you consider a cortisone prep? Medical Times 100:64, 1972.

343. Morse WI: Carrying the patient on steroids through surgery. NS Med Bull 45:185, 1966.
344. Solem JH, Lund I: Surgery in patients treated with cortisone or cortisone-like steroids. Oslo City Hosp J 19:3, 1969.
345. Baxter JD, Tyrell JB: The adrenal cortex. In Felig P, Baxter JD, Broadus AE, et al. (Eds.): Endocrinology and Metabolism. New York, McGraw-Hill, 1981, p 462.
346. Gran L, Pahle JA: Rational substitution therapy for steroid-treated patients. Anaesthesia 33:59, 1978.
347. Kehlet H: A rational approach to dosage and preparation of parenteral glucocorticoid substitution therapy during surgical procedures. Acta Anaesth Scand 19:260, 1975.
348. Symreng T, Karlberg BE, Kågedal B, et al.: Physiological cortisol substitution of long-term steroid-treated patients undergoing major surgery. Br J Anaesth 53:949, 1981.
349. Fariss BL, Hane S, Shinsako J, et al.: Comparison of absorption of cortisone acetate and hydrocortisone hemisuccinate. J Clin Endocrinol Metab 47:1137, 1978.
350. Kenny FM, Preeyasombat C, Midgeon CJ: Cortisol production rate. II. Normal infants, children and adults. Pediatrics 37:34, 1966.
351. Cassidy JT: Basic concepts of drug therapy. In Cassidy JT (Ed.): Textbook of Pediatric Rheumatology. New York, John Wiley and Sons, 1982, p 118.

IMMUNE AND ALLERGIC DISORDERS | 16

FREDERICK A. BURROWS, M.D. ● *JERROLD LERMAN, M.D.*

INTRODUCTION

T Cells
B Cells
Immunoglobulins

Normal Antibody Function
General Anesthetic Considerations in
Immunodeficiency Syndromes

The host defense mechanism is a multicomponent system consisting of physical components (such as integument and motile cilia) serving as the initial defense against foreign substances, and the immune response. The immune response is mediated by cellular elements (macrophages, leukocytes, lymphocytes) and the complement system of soluble proteins. As a consequence of the immunological system allergic response, autoimmune phenomenon, and transplant rejection occur.

Dysfunction of immune response has several consequences for the patient and implications for the anesthetist. Understanding of these anesthetic implications requires some understanding of normal development and function of the immune system.

In the immune system are organs and two principal cell types, T and B cells. Products of these cells include lymphokines and antibodies, which recruit macrophages, neutrophils, eosinophils, basophils, mast cells, and natural killer cells to participate in the immune response.

T CELLS

T cells arise from pluripotent stem cells of mesenchymal origin (Fig. 16–1). Precursor cells differentiate and mature after entering the thymus. On leaving the thymus, T cells travel throughout the body in the bloodstream and seed the spleen, lymph nodes, intestinal Peyer's patches, and appendix. T cells remain only transiently in these locations and then leave through the efferent lymphatic vessels, reentering the circulation. Mature T cells express surface antigens acquired in the thymus; this permits the identification of subpopulations of T cells. T4 and T8 antigens are important as these enable the distinction of T cells with so-called helper or inducer functions (T4) from those with suppressor or cytotoxic functions (T8).

Helper T cells undergo blast transformation and cell division when they interact with complementary antigens presented on the surface of macrophages, dendritic cells, and Langerhans' cells in the skin. The activated T helper cells produce soluble factors (inter-

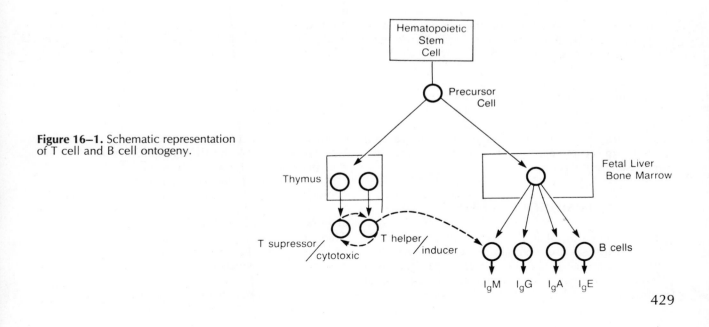

Figure 16–1. Schematic representation of T cell and B cell ontogeny.

429

leukins and lymphokines) that are responsible for macrophage chemotaxis and activation, B cell growth and differentiation, and interferon production. T suppressor cells can be activated by contact with the appropriate antigen or by interaction with T helper cells. In either case, an interleukin produced by the T helper cell is required to convert the T suppressor cells into cytotoxic cells. The activated T suppressor cells release soluble factors that in turn suppress the T helper cells, thus modulating the immune response.

In this manner then, T cells produce soluble factors that engage other T and B cells in the immune response. This response, established by the T helper cell, is countered by activation of the T suppressor cell, which dampens the immune response. T cells alone can control viral and fungal infections, reject grafts of foreign tissues, and cause delayed hypersensitivity reactions. These immune responses are referred to as "cellular immunity."

B CELLS

The multipotent stem cells that give rise to the T cells also give rise to the B cell lineage (Fig. 16–1). Development begins in the fetal liver and continues in the bone marrow after the shift of hematopoiesis to that site with later development. During this development immunoglobulin gene rearrangement occurs, determining the specific immunoglobulin the cell will produce.

After formation, B cells enter the circulation and migrate to form lymphoid follicles in the spleen, lymph nodes, Peyer's patches, and other lymphoid tissues. Like T cells, they recirculate through the lymphatic and circulatory system, but unlike the T cells, they are short-lived. This is compensated for by a high B cell production.

The B cell has surface antigens that enable recognition of and thereby interaction with T cells. Such interaction is a requirement for antigen activation of the resting B cell. Activation of a B cell occurs both after antigen interaction with B cell surface antibody molecules and on interaction with a T helper cell. The B cell then enlarges and undergoes differentiation to the plasma cell capable of secreting thousands of identical antibodies per second. These plasma cells rarely divide and are short-lived. This "humoral immunity" includes elimination of bacteria, prevention of viral reinfection, neutralization of toxins, and immediate allergic reactions.

IMMUNOGLOBULINS

Immunoglobulin M is the first immunoglobulin to be formed in response to an antigenic challenge and is distributed primarily in the vascular space. It is a polymer, a pentamer consisting of five individual immunoglobulins linked by disulfide bonds and a J,

or joining, chain. IgM does not cross the placenta. It is extremely efficient in activating complement in agglutination, and in opsonic activity.

Immunoglobulin G (IgG) is the major immunoglobulin in blood. It has a long life and is the only immunoglobulin that can cross the placenta and thus is suited for passive immunization. There are four subgroups of IgG (IgG$_1$, IgG$_2$, IgG$_3$, IgG$_4$), each of which has a unique biological behavior. IgG$_1$ and IgG$_3$ respond to Rh antigens, and IgG$_2$ responds to polysaccharide antigens. IgG$_4$, unlike the other subgroups, does not fix complement.

Immunoglobulin A (IgA) exists in two forms. In blood it exists as a monomer (IgA$_1$). IgA, however, serves its primary function in secretions (IgA$_2$), where it exists as a dimer joined by a J chain and protected by proteolysis by a secretory component, a peptide acquired from the epithelial cells through which it must pass to reach the duct or lumen into which it is secreted. IgA protects mainly the secretory surfaces of the gastrointestinal tract and eyes. IgA functions by immobilizing microorganisms or by preventing their attachment to mucosal surfaces, or both. It can also activate C3 of the complement system directly by the alternative pathway, producing cellular destruction.

Immunoglobulin E (IgE) is bound to surface receptors on mast cells and basophils such that its antigen binding sites are exposed. Interaction of antigen with these receptors results in the release of pharmacologically active mediators from the cell. This release can cause asthma, hay fever, and anaphylaxis.

Immunoglobulin D (IgD) functions as a receptor on B cell surfaces. It is felt to be important in directing antigen to the B cell surfaces facilitating initial immunization.

With the administration of antigen to an individual, IgM is seen to appear first. This is followed in a few days by IgG. If the individual is reexposed to the same antigen, an amnestic response is obtained: the IgM response is similar to that of the initial response, but the IgG antibody appears sooner and rises to a higher level. The speed of the secondary response explains why infections often are minimal or do not occur at all.

NORMAL ANTIBODY FUNCTION

Antibodies function to bind antigen. This binding has several different possible results, depending upon the particular antibody and/or antigen.

Antibodies can produce a precipitative reaction or agglutination. This occurs because antibodies have at least two binding sites while antigens have many. This enables complexes of antigen and antibody to form. These complexes exclude water and will eventually precipitate. Agglutination is an identical process except that the antigen is a larger structure, such as a cell.

Antibodies function in neutralization of toxic substances. For example, tetanus toxin is neutralized by antibodies as it happens to be an antigenic determinant. Antibodies that facilitate phagocytosis of particulate antigens are important in opsonization. In opsonization antibodies combine with the foreign antigenic determinant. The free portion of the antibody then combines with receptors on the surface of phagocytes, thus greatly enhancing the ability to ingest the antigen. Antibodies can also facilitate complement activation by either the classical or the alternative pathway (see page 454). Such complement activation can result in release of factors that facilitate chemotaxis, function as anaphylatoxins, or assist in cell lysis.

GENERAL ANESTHETIC CONSIDERATIONS IN IMMUNODEFICIENCY SYNDROMES

Current understanding of the mechanisms by which the human body resists microbial agents has been accrued over the last 25 years. The effects of anesthetic agents and surgery on the immune system of the normal patient have been described in the literature, but very little investigation has been done into the effects of anesthesia and surgery on the immune system with an underlying defect. Because of this, it is largely impossible to recommend specific anesthetic techniques by virtue of their less depressant effect on an already compromised immune system. Many of the immunological syndromes do have associated abnormalities that may have anesthetic implications. These will be discussed in relation to the particular syndrome in question. There are, however, essentials of anesthetic management of immunosuppressed patients that can be discussed together. These relate to the increased susceptibility of these patients to infection. The particular risk of infection involved varies considerably among syndromes and within a given syndrome (Table 16–1).

Patients with immunodeficiency disorders have an increased susceptibility to infection and, even prior to anesthesia and surgery, may harbor microbial agents resistant to antibiotic therapy. Recently acquired acute infections are common. Such infective processes may dictate the surgical procedure, such as a diagnostic lung biopsy or drainage of an abscess.

If surgery is required, the preoperative preparation is aimed at optimizing the patient's condition. This should be handled in consultation with the physician managing the immunodeficient state.

The respiratory system is frequently involved in the infectious process occurring in these patients (Table 16–1). The diseases can range from mild recurrent upper respiratory infections to recurrent pneumonias and bronchiectasis. Assessment of the status of the respiratory system is therefore very important. Acute infections should be aggressively treated and eradicated if time and antibiotic sensitivities permit. Preoperative teaching regarding physiotherapy, incentive spirometry, coughing, deep breathing, and bronchodilator

therapy should be instituted to familiarize the child with the techniques that will be necessary postoperatively. Pulmonary function tests should be used to establish baseline values and assess the adequacy of therapy.

Viral infections may increase airway resistance, and these changes may persist for up to 5 weeks after infection. Thus, if possible, surgery should be delayed for such a period of time, especially in view of the adverse effect of the viral infection on the respiratory defense mechanisms against bacteria.

Chronic respiratory disease may produce right-sided heart failure. Therefore, cardiac status needs assessment prior to anesthesia and surgery, and appropriate drug therapy should be instituted if necessary.

Treatment with antibiotics can result in renal insufficiency, and the possibility of impaired renal function must be assessed.

The involvement of other organ systems, such as in liver or cerebral abscesses, must be evaluated in regard to possible effects on anesthetic management. It should be emphasized that involvement of one organ can produce effects in other organs, especially when cardiac disease is present.

The preanesthetic use of prophylactic antibiotics has been advocated, particularly when bacteremia is possible (such as in airway manipulation or abscess drainage). Because of the increased susceptibility of patients with immune disorders to infections and the difficulty

Table 16–1. SYNDROMES PREDISPOSING TO INCREASED SUSCEPTIBILITY TO INFECTION

Host Deficiency	Predominant Infections
X-linked agammaglobulinemia	Pyogenic bacterial
Immunodeficiency with increased IgM (and IgD)	Pyogenic bacterial
Selective IgA deficiency	Respiratory or none
Selective IgM deficiency	Pneumococcal and meningococcal
Severe combined immunodeficiency	All*
Ataxia-telangiectasia syndrome	Sinopulmonary
Thymic hypoplasia (DiGeorge syndrome)	Viral, fungal, mycobacterial
Chronic granulomatous disease	Catalase-producing bacterial, fungal
Myeloperoxidase deficiency	Candidal, bacterial, or none
Hyperimmunoglobulin E syndrome	*Staphylococcus aureus*
Lazy leukocyte syndrome	Upper respiratory, stomatitis
Chédiak-Higashi syndrome	Gram positive coccal
Primary deficiency of complement C3	Pyogenic bacterial
Primary deficiency of complement C5	*Staphylococcus aureus*, *Saccharomyces* (yeast), and gram negative bacillary

*All: includes viral, bacterial, fungal, and protozoan infections.

in treating them, such preanesthetic treatment is mandatory.

Meticulous antiseptic technique is required for all techniques requiring skin puncture, such as intravenous access, invasive monitors, and bladder catheterization. Such monitors and lines should be discontinued as soon as possible to minimize the risk of infection at these sites. Anesthetic equipment coming in direct contact with the patient should be sterile. The anesthetist should use full aseptic technique in handling these patients.

The use of regional anesthetic techniques in immunosuppressed patients is controversial. Guidelines have been established regarding the use of such techniques in the presence of infection, but no recommendations concerning their use in an immunosuppressed patient have been made.

I do not recommend against the use of regional anesthetic techniques in immunosuppressed patients where indicated. Meticulous antiseptic technique will minimize the risk of inducing infection. However, an indwelling catheter may increase this risk and should be removed as soon as possible.

Postoperatively, immunodeficient patients require protective or reverse isolation. This does not protect the patient against infection by endogenous organisms but decreases the patient's risk of acquiring infections from others in the postanesthetic recovery room or the ward.

Many immunodeficient patients presenting for anesthesia and surgery harbor organisms that are resistant to antibiotic therapy. These patients may pose a hazard to operating room personnel and patients to be operated on later in the same operating room. The use of disposable circuits and bacterial filters will aid in prevention of contamination of the anesthetic equipment. Postoperatively, these patients will require isolation.

REFERENCES

Cantor H, Gershon RK: Immunological circuits, cellular composition. Fed Proc 38:2058, 1979.

deFreitas AA, Coutinho A: A very rapid decay of mature B lymphocytes in the spleen. J Exp Med 154:994, 1981.

Engleman EG, Benike CJ, Grumet FC, et al.: Activation of human T lymphocyte subsets: helper and suppressor/cytotoxic T cells recognize and respond to distinct histocompatibility antigens. J Immunol 127:2124, 1981.

Gathings WE, Lawton AR, Cooper MD: Immunofluorescent studies of the development of pre-B cells, B lymphocytes and immunoglobulin isotype diversity in humans. Eur J Immunol 7:804, 1977.

Gillis S: Interleukin 2: biology and chemistry. J Clin Immunol 3:1, 1983.

Howard JC, Hunt SV, Gowans JL: Identification of marrow-derived and thymus-derived small lymphocytes in the lymphoid tissue and thoracic duct lymph of normal rats. J Exp Med 130:200, 1972.

Julius MH: Cellular interactions involved in T-dependent B-cell activation. Immunol Today 3:295, 1982.

Krensky AM, Burakoff SJ: Cytotoxic T-lymphocyte response to HLA antigens. J Pediatr 102:814, 1983.

Lachman LB: Human interleukin 1: purification and properties. Fed Proc 42:2639, 1983.

Reinherz EL, Kung PC, Goldstein G, et al.: Discrete stages of human intrathymic differentiation: analysis of normal thymocytes and leukemic lymphoblasts of T-cell lineage. Proc Natl Acad Sci 77:1588, 1980.

Rosen FS, Cooper MD, Wedgwood RJ: The primary immunodeficiencies I. N Engl J Med 311:235, 1984.

Rosen FS, Wedgwood RJ, Aiuti F, et al.: The primary immunodeficiency diseases: report prepared for the WHO by a Scientific Group on Immunodeficiency. Clin Immunol Immunopathol 28:450, 1983.

Thomas Y, Rogozinski L, Irigoyen OH, et al.: Functional analysis of human T cell subsets defined by monoclonal antibodies. IV. Induction of suppressor cells within the OKT4+ population. J Exp Med 154:459, 1981.

Tonegawa S: Somatic generation of antibody diversity. Nature 302:575, 1983.

Weissman IL: Thymus cell migration: studies on the origin of cortisone-resistant thymic lymphocytes. J Exp Med 137:504, 1973.

General Anesthetic Consideration in Immunodeficiency Syndromes

Altemeier WA (Ed.): Committee on Control of Surgical Infections: Manual of Control of Infection in Surgical Patients. Philadelphia, J. B. Lippincott Co., 1976.

Appel GB, Neu HC: The nephrotoxicity of antimicrobial agents. N Engl J Med 296:663, 722, 784, 1977.

Committee on Infections within Hospitals, American Hospital Association: Infection control in the hospital. Chicago, American Hospital Association, 1979.

Green GM, Jakob GJ, Low RB, et al.: Defense mechanisms of the respiratory membrane. Am Rev Respir Dis 115:479, 1977.

Hall WJ, Douglas RG, Hyde RW, et al.: Pulmonary mechanics after uncomplicated influenza A infection. Am Rev Respir Dis 113:141, 1976.

Levine AS, Seigel SE, Schreiber AD, et al.: Protected environments and prophylactic antibiotics: a prospective controlled study of their utility in the therapy of acute leukemia. N Engl J Med 288:477, 1973.

Schimpff SC, Greene WH, Young VM, et al.: Infection prevention in acute nonlymphocytic leukemia. Ann Intern Med 82:351, 1975.

PRIMARY IMMUNODEFICIENCY DISEASES

Predominant Antibody Defects (Antibody Deficiency Syndromes)
X-Linked Agammaglobulinemia
X-Linked Hypogammaglobulinemia with Growth Hormone Deficiency
Autosomal Recessive Agammaglobulinemia
Immunoglobulin Deficiency with Increased IgM (and IgD)
Selective Immunoglobulin A Deficiency
Selective Deficiency of Secretory Component
Selective Immunoglobulin M Deficiency
Immunoglobulin G Deficiencies
Transient Hypogammaglobulinemia of Infancy
Medical Management of Antibody Deficiency Syndromes

Predominant Defects of Cell-Mediated Immunity
Severe Combined Immunodeficiency
Severe Combined Immunodeficiency with Adenosine Deaminase Deficiency
Purine Nucleoside Phosphorylase Deficiency
Combined Immunodeficiency with Predominant T Cell Defect
Immunodeficiency Associated with Other Defects
Wiskott-Aldrich Syndrome
Ataxia-Telangiectasia Syndrome
Thymic Hypoplasia (DiGeorge Syndrome)
Chronic Mucocutaneous Candidiasis
Acquired Immunodeficiency Syndrome
Graft-versus-Host Disease

Syndromes of immunological dysfunction may involve solely B or solely T cells or both cell types. Generally T cell disorders present a more unfavorable prognosis than B cell disorders, and the prognosis of combined disorders is even worse.

In this section primary and secondary disorders of immunological function will be considered and anesthetic experience will be presented when possible. The classification and nomenclature of diseases used in this discussion conforms to that accepted by the World Health Organization.

PREDOMINANT ANTIBODY DEFECTS (ANTIBODY DEFICIENCY SYNDROMES)

X-Linked Agammaglobulinemia

Panhypogammaglobulinemia is a term that describes a deficiency of the three major classes of immunoglobulins, IgG, IgM, and IgA. Several forms of the disease present: autosomal recessive, sporadic, and late onset. Congenital X-linked agammaglobulinemia (Bruton disease) is the best defined of these syndromes and is discussed here in more detail.

Affected males demonstrate a lack of IgA and IgM in their serum and IgA in their secretions. IgG levels are normal at birth due to placental transfer, but these levels decrease as maternal IgG is diluted and catabolized. Levels of IgG are low thereafter.

These patients have been demonstrated to lack B cells in their blood and plasma cells in their blood and tissues. Investigation of their bone marrow demonstrates the presence of B lymphocyte precursors, implying the defect is one involving failure of differentiation to mature B cells. T cell function as assessed

by in vitro techniques and by delayed hypersensitivity skin responses is normal.

Patients appear normal until 4 months of age, during which time their underlying immune deficiency has been hidden by placentally transferred maternal IgG. After this period, recurrent infections are common. The respiratory tract is most often affected. Recurrent otitis media and sinusitis occur in the upper airway, which is also characterized by a decreased amount of pharyngeal lymphoid tissue with small or absent tonsils and adenoids. Lower airway diseases include bouts of pneumonia and bronchitis producing a chronic pulmonary disease with bronchiectasis, pulmonary fibrosis, and eventual cor pulmonale. Common infecting organisms include *Streptococcus pneumoniae, Haemophilus influenzae,* and staphylococci. With normal T cell system function most patients recover promptly from viral infections. There are exceptions to this, however; of note is the ECHO virus, which affects 10 percent of patients. It can produce an acute fatal encephalitis or a prolonged deterioration with chronic viremia.

Other systems may be involved less commonly. *Giardia lamblia* infection of the gastrointestinal tract may occur and produce severe diarrhea with lack of weight gain. Treatment with metronidazole is usually effective, but about 10 percent of all patients develop an enteropathy that resembles Crohn disease. Significant amounts of protein may be lost into the gut from this enteropathy, the etiology of which is uncertain. It has been suggested that it may occur as the result of a bacterial overgrowth, as antibiotic therapy seems helpful in some cases.

A dermatomyositis-like syndrome is also described in these patients. This is thought to be of viral etiology and is characterized by transient rashes that lack the normal distribution of dermatomyositis, and by a firm peripheral edema.

Elevation of serum IgE occurs frequently in this condition and is associated with eczema, recurrent skin infections, and an increased incidence of allergic phenomena.

An autoimmune disease resembling rheumatoid arthritis is present in about 10 percent of patients. This is distinguishable from true rheumatoid arthritis by a lack of rheumatoid factor. The presence of *Ureaplasma* species in effusions suggests an infectious etiology. Knees and ankles are most commonly affected. In some patients with gastrointestinal manifestations the spine may be involved as well. The symptoms usually respond to IgG replacement.

Anesthetic Considerations. Patients with panhypogammaglobulinemia are at increased risk of bacterial infection, and require reverse isolation and strict sterile technique in their anesthetic management. Chronic pulmonary disease is common and may result in severe debilitation with cor pulmonale. The cardiopulmonary system requires careful evaluation and optimization of pulmonary and cardiac status prior to surgery. The presence of otitis media and sinusitis may contraindicate use of nitrous oxide. Preoperative prophylactic antibiotic therapy is advised.

Autoimmune features of the disease may result in difficulty in positioning. Although temporomandibular joints and the cervical spine are rarely involved, their function should be assessed. Patients with spinal dysfunction require assessment of serum protein and electrolyte levels, as enteropathy frequently accompanies spinal involvement. This results in significant loss of serum into the gut, and hypoproteinemia can affect drug disposition. Bowel infections should be treated appropriately.

Musculoskeletal and skin involvement may occur with a resultant dermatomyositis-type lesion. The use of succinylcholine might then produce acute rises in serum potassium.

Viral CNS infections are not uncommon, and any change in level of consciousness should alert the physician to possible CNS infection and elevation of intracranial pressure. Anesthetics in this instance should be chosen to avoid further increases in ICP.

As these patients suffer from chronic infections including *Staphylococcus, Streptococcus pneumoniae,* and *Haemophilus influenzae,* anesthetic equipment requires appropriate cleaning or disposal.

X-Linked Hypogammaglobulinemia with Growth Hormone Deficiency

A defect with B cell dysfunction is currently described in only one family: Panhypogammaglobulinemia is present in three members, while the fourth demonstrates some B cell function with normal IgM and IgA. Cellular immunity and T cell function are normal. The growth hormone defect is manifested by short stature, retarded bone age, small phallus, and delayed onset of puberty. The basic defect is unknown but may be a block in B cell differentiation. The reason for the association of growth hormone defect is unclear.

Autosomal Recessive Agammaglobulinemia

This name has been applied to a form of agammaglobulinemia presenting in female patients that is indistinguishable from X-linked agammaglobulinemia. The disorder is believed to be the same as X-linked agammaglobulinemia, a defect of precursor to B cell differentiation.

Immunoglobulin Deficiency with Increased IgM (and IgD)

The occurrence of this disease suggests an X-linked inheritance, but the etiology of this disorder is unclear. Affected boys have decreased levels of IgG but elevated levels of IgM and in some instances elevated levels of IgD. The syndrome is characterized by severe pyogenic infections, autoimmune disorders, and lymphoproliferative disorders. T cell function is normal. Acquired forms of the disease and its occurrence in females have been demonstrated. Treatment is with IgG replacement.

Selective Immunoglobulin A Deficiency

IgA is the major immunoglobulin protecting the respiratory system, gastrointestinal tract, and other secreting areas. Deficiency of IgA is the most common primary defect of specific immunity. The incidence is reported as 1 in 400 to 1 in 3000 depending upon the ethnic group. Its inheritance has been variously reported as autosomal dominant and autosomal recessive and it has also been reported as a rare complication of the congenital rubella syndrome. Its occurrence is primarily sporadic, however.

IgA-deficient patients possess normal serum levels of IgG and IgM, and have been demonstrated to possess IgA-bearing B cells in their blood. In vitro lymphocyte testing reveals that these cells are able to differentiate into plasma cells but fail to synthesize and release normal amounts of IgA. The etiology is not entirely clear, but some patients have been demonstrated to have T cells suppressing the production of IgA but not IgG or IgM.

Most patients with IgA deficiency are healthy. Others usually have symptoms that relate to infections, autoimmunity, allergy, or malignancy.

Recurrent respiratory infections may occur in the form of sinusitis, bronchitis, or pneumonia. Diarrhea due to *Giardia* or other infection may occur, and some patients become chronic salmonella carriers. Suscepti-

Table 16–2. AUTOIMMUNE SYNDROMES ASSOCIATED WITH SELECTIVE IgA DEFICIENCY

Autoimmune Syndromes	Percent Affected
Rheumatoid arthritis	30
Systemic lupus erythematosus	15
Thyroiditis	10
Pernicious anemia	10
Dermatomyositis	<1
Sjögren syndrome	<1
Addison disease	<1
Pulmonary hemosiderosis	<1
Hemolytic anemia	<1
Thrombocytopenia	<1

bility to viral infections is less well documented. Many patients have no excess infections, and this is most likely related to the potential of IgG and IgM antibodies to protect mucosal surfaces. Another possibility is associated changes in other immunoglobulins. Patients with associated low IgG$_2$ levels and normal total serum IgG tend to have an increased susceptibility to infections as compared with those patients with IgA deficiency but normal IgG$_2$ levels.

There is a high incidence of autoimmune syndromes in patients with IgA deficiency (Table 16–2). This apparently is due to the absorption of dietary proteins through IgA-unprotected intestinal mucosae. This results in a stimulus to antibody production against normally nonabsorbed antigen. Some of the antibodies can be of importance in the etiology of major transfusion reactions.

There is a positive correlation of low IgA levels with atopic disorders. This correlation is possibly due to decreased presence of IgA, which normally would incorporate foreign antigens into antigen-antibody complexes. Failure of this to occur enables their incorporation into IgE and IgG complexes.

There is also an increased risk of malignancy in these patients. Primarily of gastrointestinal and lymphoreticular origin, malignancies occur at a rate of two to four times normal.

Anesthetic Considerations. As with panhypogammaglobulinemia, patients with selective IgA deficiency exhibit increased susceptibility to infections. The respiratory system and gastrointestinal tract are commonly involved, and management is as described previously. Similarly, there is a high incidence of autoimmune syndromes (Table 16–2) and all patients should be carefully assessed. The presence of Addison disease requires steroid supplementation. Dermatomyositis is more common in children than in adults and is a contraindication to use of succinylcholine. Hemolytic anemia and thrombocytopenia occur and require assessment.

Patients demonstrate a higher incidence of atopic disorders than the normal population. A complete history must be obtained and appropriate management undertaken (see page 431). In many cases, owing to the underlying nature of the disease, the agents producing allergic reactions will be unknown to the patient or parents, and careful vigilance is thus necessary.

Antibodies to IgG and IgM as well as IgA may be present in as many as 40 percent of patients. This is of particular importance as their presence, especially that of IgA antibodies, can induce severe transfusion reactions. Matching of blood can be extremely difficult and may require a longer period than usual for a safe cross match to be established. The emergency administration of type O, Rh negative blood is dangerous for this reason.

Selective Deficiency of Secretory Component

As described previously, secretory component is a protein produced by epithelial cells in secretory surfaces. Its function is believed to be one of assisting transport of IgA from its site of synthesis in plasma cells at the lamina propria and possibly in preventing it from proteolysis during its transport to the secretory surface. There are at least two clinical situations in which deficiency of secretory component may be important (as distinct from IgA deficiency states due to lack of IgA on secretory surfaces). The first of these is a state of chronic diarrhea, which may produce dehydration and electrolyte imbalance in poorly managed patients. The second situation is suggested by a study that demonstrated a deficiency of component in 62.5 percent of children with sudden infant death syndrome (SIDS).

Patients with a selective deficiency of secretory component lack IgA in their secretions but serum IgA levels are normal. Because of this lack on secretory surfaces, these patients also exhibit signs and symptoms of infection and atopic disorders similar to those seen in patients with selective IgA deficiency.

Anesthetic Considerations. The presence of chronic diarrhea necessitates evaluation of the state of hydration and serum electrolyte balance. Intravenous hydration is advisable during any period of fasting prior to surgery. The occurrence of SIDS in patients with this disorder requires careful postoperative monitoring for apnea in an intensive care unit or other area with personnel trained in the field of apnea management.

These patients are subject to infections and atopic disorders and must be managed as discussed in IgA deficiency.

Selective Immunoglobulin M Deficiency

Deficiency of IgM is defined to be present in any individual with serum IgM levels lower than two standard deviations below the normal for age. It does not require a complete absence of IgM. This deficiency is called selective when it is associated with otherwise normal serum immunoglobulin levels and with normal cell-mediated immunity. It occurs with a frequency of 1 in 1000, usually in males. Although in adults it is most commonly secondary to lymphoma, primary cases are well described. Present evidence suggests a genetic etiology, as relatives, especially fathers, have been demonstrated to have decreased levels of serum IgM. There are several hypotheses for the decreased serum IgM. It may represent T cell suppression of differentiation of B cells to mature plasma cells: B cells bearing IgM have been demonstrated in the blood of some patients. It may represent selective failure of IgM monomers to polymerize or a premature switch of IgM to IgG and IgA production.

Affected infants are extremely prone to septicemia, particularly with encapsulated organisms, such as pneumococci and meningococci. Each patient differs in susceptibility, and this difference is due to varying ability to produce IgM. These patients must receive aggressive antibiotic therapy at the first sign of infection and possibly should have continuous prophylactic antibiotics. Associated with this disorder is an increased frequency of Whipple disease, regional enteritis, and lymphoid nodular hyperplasia.

Anesthetic Considerations. Patients with this disorder are extremely susceptible to infection, and septicemia is not uncommon. This requires very careful sterile technique and reverse isolation. Prophylactic antibiotic therapy is advisable and should be commenced preoperatively. Associated regional enteritis may result in hemoglobin and protein loss and serum electrolyte imbalance. These need to be assessed and managed.

Immunoglobulin G Deficiencies

As discussed previously there are at least four subgroups of IgG—IgG_1, IgG_2, IgG_3, and IgG_4. A complete lack of all IgG components is not seen, but selective subgroup deficiencies do occur.

In normal individuals, IgG_1 predominates and IgG_4 levels may normally be low enough to be undetected. In IgG subgroup deficiency total serum IgG is normal but subgroup deficiencies can be detected as abnormalities of electrophoretic mobility.

Although selective deficiencies of a particular subclass are not associated with particular clinical syndromes, some antibodies are preferentially made in a particular subclass, and clinically these patients manifest an increased susceptibility to infections as is characteristic of that seen in panhypogammaglobulinemia.

Anesthetic Considerations. Sterile techniques and reverse isolation are advised during perioperative management with the administration of prophylactic antibiotics.

Transient Hypogammaglobulinemia of Infancy

By definition, this is a transient condition that resolves by the first to second year of life. Although common, occurring in 18 percent of patients with a primary immunodeficiency, it is rare as a clinical problem and is found in less than 0.01 percent of patients studied for immune disorders.

The disorder is characterized by a lower than normal serum immunoglobulin G level. IgM and IgA levels are frequently normal. On antigenic stimulation good antibody responses are usually demonstrated but T cell function is depressed, as shown by a deficient response of B cells to T cell–dependent stimulation. It is believed that the syndrome may represent delayed maturation of the normal humoral response. Clinically the patients suffer recurrent infections, which will vary in frequency or severity with the individual patient.

There are two groups of patients with transient hypogammaglobulinemia, those with and those without immunodeficient relatives.

As stated, all patients recover by the first to second year of life. Since patients recover spontaneously, treatment with immunoglobulins is usually reserved for those demonstrating severe recurrent infections.

MEDICAL MANAGEMENT OF ANTIBODY DEFICIENCY SYNDROMES

Acute bacterial infections require antibiotic therapy; this treatment must be aggressive in IgM-deficient patients because of their tendency to develop septicemia.

Prophylaxis may consist of continuous treatment with an antibiotic such as cotrimoxazole, and this has been advocated in the IgM deficiency states. Prophylaxis, however, depends primarily upon IgG replacement by intramuscular injection of immune serum globulin (ISG), which contains 150 mg IgG per ml. This is administered with an initial loading dose of 1.4 ml/kg followed every 4 weeks by 0.7 ml/kg. In big patients, the administered volume becomes very large and it may be necessary to increase the frequency of injections so as to decrease the volume of the injectate. The aim of this treatment is to achieve a serum level of 300 mg/100 ml.

ISG can be administered intravenously but it then requires additional processing so as to be aggregate-free. The presence of such aggregates may activate complement, causing anaphylaxis by the production of vasoactive kinins. Processing of ISG by physical and chemical means is available, and a variety of products are now available. These permit the administration of large amounts of immunoglobulin to achieve nearly normal blood levels which are not obtainable with intramuscular injections. The recommended dose is 100 mg/kg per month, which provides an increase of about 200 mg/100 ml in serum IgG level after equilibration. The IgG level decreases progressively until the time of the next injection, but it is possible by increasing the dose to maintain a normal level even at the nadir.

An alternative to the use of ISG is the use of plasma. Plasma contains 10 mg/ml of IgG and provides protection at a dose of 1.5 ml/kg every 21 days. In addition, plasma provides IgA and IgM, which are not provided by ISG, and for patients with associated malabsorption syndromes plasma has the advantage of providing a range of proteins. The main disadvantage to plasma is the risk of serum hepatitis. This risk can be minimized by restricting the number of donors and by careful screening of plasma.

Approximately 20 percent of patients receiving intramuscular ISG develop reactions at some stage. Complement activation from aggregates in the injectate, which produce vasoactive kinins, is considered the most likely etiology. These reactions vary in severity from mild limb and back pain to anaphylaxis. They usually occur within 30 minutes of administration. Mild reactions resolve spontaneously within 3 to 4 hours and require no treatment.

It is important to realize that the optimal dose and optimal serum levels of ISG have yet to be determined. Likewise, there is no information available on the efficacy of ISG in prevention of long-term complications of immunoglobulin deficiency, such as chronic sinopulmonary disease.

PREDOMINANT DEFECTS OF CELL-MEDIATED IMMUNITY

There are few diseases of deficiency of cell-mediated immunity in which antibody production by B cells is normal. This is due to the requirement of interaction of T helper cells and B cells for most antibody responses in man. Because of this association, T cell compromise produces deficient antibody production by B cells and, as such, clinical features of combined T and B cell disease.

Severe Combined Immunodeficiency

The disorder is inherited as an autosomal recessive or X-linked recessive trait, and consequently most of the patients (75 percent) are male. The etiology appears to be a primary T cell abnormality that secondarily produces a failure of normal embryogenesis of the thymic epithelium. Infants become ill during the first few months of life, with marked failure to thrive. Moniliasis of the oropharynx, larynx, and skin can be extensive, but systemic candidiasis is rare. Pneumonitis is frequent, usually interstitial and due to *Pneumocystis carinii*. These two features plus intractable diarrhea form the characteristic triad of findings in this disease.

Patients are extremely vulnerable to overwhelming viral infections such as varicella, herpes, and cytomegalovirus, which are fatal if contracted by an untreated patient. Smallpox vaccination is contraindicated. Many infants in the first few days of life have a morbilliform rash due to an abortive graft-versus-host reaction (see page 443) from maternally transferred lymphocytes. A profound lymphopenia is common (less than 1000 lymphocytes per cubic millimeter). Other hematological abnormalities include thrombocytosis and anemia. Monocytosis and eosinophilia may occur in response to overwhelming infection, such as occurs with *Pneumocystis* pneumonia. The disorder is usually fatal in the first few years of life.

Current treatment consists of transplants of fetal liver cells, or of implants of fetal thymus or thymic epithelium. Most successful has been bone marrow transplantation with HLA-identical donors. This originally required HLA-identical siblings as donors, but it is now possible to use parental haploidentical marrow. This depends upon removal of the T cells from donated marrow to prevent the recipient from developing graft-versus-host disease caused by T cells. Thus the therapeutic possibilities for bone marrow transplantation have been extended.

Anesthetic Considerations. Patients are extremely vulnerable to infection and are frequently chronically infected. The pulmonary and nutritional status must be assessed. Strict aseptic technique must be applied to these patients, and sterile anesthetic equipment should be used. Sites for intravenous access and access sites for other invasive monitors should be very carefully prepared with antiseptic solutions. Postoperatively monitoring lines and intravenous lines should be discontinued as early as possible to decrease the risk of infection.

The use of blood products adds the risk of graft-versus-host disease. Since lymphocytes in blood from blood banks are viable for 3 weeks, blood being transfused into such patients should be irradiated prior to transfusions in order to kill the lymphocytes. If anemia is present irradiated blood may be required preoperatively.

Serum proteins and electrolytes must be checked if the patient has diarrhea. Intravenous therapy may be necessary to prevent dehydration during fasting prior to surgery.

The presence of certain pathogens will necessitate the disinfection of the room and anesthetic equipment postoperatively. Disposable equipment should be used whenever possible.

Severe Combined Immunodeficiency with Adenosine Deaminase Deficiency

This is a variant of severe combined immunodeficiency and results from a deficiency of the enzyme adenosine deaminase. The disorder is inherited in an autosomal recessive pattern.

Adenosine deaminase converts adenosine and deoxyadenosine to inosine and deoxyinosine, thus functioning as a purine salvage pathway enzyme. It is present in most cells, including erythrocytes and lymphocytes. In its absence, ATP, cyclic AMP, and their deoxy analogues increase to toxic levels. This results in inhibition of ribonucleotide reductase, which impairs reduction of other nucleoside diphosphates and causes inhibition of DNA synthesis. No other organ system is affected by this deficiency, and the reason for this specificity is unclear.

Features of the disorder are similar to that of severe combined immunodeficiency, except that at birth lymphocyte function is usually normal. After birth, a gradual deterioration of lymphocyte function occurs. Definitive diagnosis is by means of enzyme level determination in erythrocytes. Without treatment most patients die by 2 years of age.

The disease is most satisfactorily treated by bone marrow transplantation. In the absence of a suitable bone marrow donor, transfusions of frozen irradiated red blood cells have been used as a source of adenosine deaminase. This is believed to be effective by supplying sufficient enzyme to protect the lymphocytes from the accumulation of products to toxic levels.

Purine Nucleoside Phosphorylase Deficiency

Purine nucleoside phosphorylase (PNP) deficiency is a rare enzyme defect. Deficiency results in the intracellular accumulation of deoxyguanosine triphosphate, which inhibits ribonucleotide reductase, in turn limiting cell division. The urine and blood of these patients contain increased amounts of inosine, guanosine, deoxyguanosine, and guanosine triphosphate.

PNP deficiency causes a much more severe defect in T cell function (because T cells divide more rapidly) than in B cell function. Immunoglobulins and the percentage of B cells are usually normal. As disease increases in severity B cells become affected, owing to a decrease of normal B cell–T cell interactions, and immunoglobulin function may become impaired.

This immunodeficiency may not be demonstrated at birth. Neonates and infants may demonstrate normal lymphocyte counts and in vitro function and yet become symptomatic with decreasing T cell function before 18 months of age.

Symptoms occur between 7 months and 7 years of age. Early problems include recurrent upper respiratory infections and a Coombs positive hemolytic anemia, suggesting beginning of impaired regulation of antibody responses. Later, if vaccinia or varicella infections occur they may be fatal. Graft-versus-host disease may occur if nonirradiated blood is administered.

Laboratory confirmatory findings demonstrate a deficiency of PNP in red cell lysates. Mutant forms of the enzyme may be present. Spot or 24-hour urine studies to demonstrate purine excretion also help to confirm the diagnosis.

The response to therapy is uncertain. Irradiated red cell infusions, injections of thymus extracts, and uridine or deoxycytidine treatments have been tried.

Anesthetic Considerations. The problems of immunodeficiency have been discussed previously. Hemoglobin levels may be low because of an autoimmune hemolytic process. If transfusions are required the blood should be irradiated to kill donor lymphocytes; otherwise graft-versus-host disease may result. Death due to transfusion with nonirradiated blood has been reported in a patient with PNP deficiency.

Combined Immunodeficiency with Predominant T Cell Defect

First described in 1964, this disorder is also known as Nezelof syndrome. It consists of a predominant T cell defect with essentially normal B cell function and normal serum immunoglobulins. It has been observed in children with congenital viral infections (for example, cytomegalovirus). It is not as rapidly fatal as severe combined immunodeficiency, but affected persons have a poor long-term prognosis. This disease may represent a prodromal stage to acquired immunodeficiency syndrome (see page 441).

IMMUNODEFICIENCY ASSOCIATED WITH OTHER DEFECTS
Wiskott-Aldrich Syndrome

The Wiskott-Aldrich syndrome is an X-linked recessive disorder with an incidence of 4 per 1 million live births. It is characterized by thrombocytopenia, eczema, and recurrent infections.

The immunodeficiency is progressive, so that abnormal immunological findings become increasingly common with increasing age. Serum IgG is usually normal, IgM reduced, and IgA and IgE elevated. Normal antibody responses with IgG and IgA are usually present, while IgM demonstrates impaired ability to form antibody active against bacterial polysaccharides. With time, increases in IgA and decreases in IgM occur and abnormalities of the lymphoid tissues develop.

Deficiencies of cell-mediated immunity are variable, depending upon the age of the patient. A mild T cell dysfunction is apparent, but this is less than that ascribed to other T cell deficient states. With increasing age patients become anergic and are slow to reject foreign skin grafts.

Thrombocytopenia is present (less than $50,000/\mu l$); the platelets are small in size and are deficient in ADP, so they fail to aggregate normally. The abnormalities of platelet size are secondary features as they disappear after splenectomy.

Clinically, patients with Wiskott-Aldrich syndrome demonstrate early onset eczema with an unusual atopic distribution. Thrombocytopenia may lead to bloody diarrhea and intracranial hemorrhage. These patients are susceptible to a wide range of infections, including otitis media and externa, pneumonitis, and septicemia. They are particularly susceptible to infections by herpes simplex as well as other opportunistic organisms. Twenty percent experience renal problems including hematuria, proteinuria, increased blood urea nitrogen, and decreased creatinine clearance.

Few patients survive into their teens. Infection is responsible for 60 percent of deaths, bleeding for 27 percent, and malignancy for 5 percent.

Medical Management. Bone marrow transplantation has been successful but, unlike in combined immunodeficiency diseases, it is necessary to destroy the recipient's own stem cell population. This requires the use of large doses of cyclophosphamide or high-level irradiation prior to transplantation. This increases the mortality and morbidity of the procedures.

Those patients without tissue type—matched siblings have undergone therapy with intravenous transfer factor or thymosin. Although increased anergic response, increased platelet counts, and decreased bleeding tendencies have provided symptomatic improvement, survival does not appear to be prolonged.

Splenectomy is successful in decreasing the risk of bleeding, particularly that due to intracranial hemorrhage. This improvement is due in part to an increase in platelet number and in part to improved function. However, splenectomy also increases susceptibility to infection (particularly pneumoccocal), and this increased susceptibility in patients with an underlying immunodeficiency is an indication for long-term prophylactic antibiotic therapy.

Anesthetic Considerations. Patients present with a combined immunodeficiency picture. Antibiotic prophylaxis is necessary preoperatively, and the use of sterile technique is necessary to minimize the risk of infection.

Thrombocytopenia with platelet counts less than $50,000/\mu l$ is frequently present, and this level is insufficient for even minor surgical procedures, particularly when combined with failure of proper platelet aggregation. The patients may be anemic as well as thrombocytopenic and require transfusions of red blood cells and platelets prior to surgery. Since these patients demonstrate dysfunction of cell-mediated immunity, blood products should be irradiated prior to transfusion to prevent graft-versus-host disease.

The presence of bloody diarrhea, as well as serving as a focus for blood loss, may produce electrolyte imbalance, which should be assessed and corrected prior to surgery. Twenty percent of patients demonstrate decreased renal function with an elevated blood urea nitrogen and decreased creatinine clearance. Renal function should be adequately evaluated preoperatively.

Patients suffer from chronic and recurrent pulmonary infections because of their immunodeficient status. Pulmonary status should be optimized, and the presence of chest infections may be an indication to delay surgery should the infection be expected to improve with therapy and the surgery not be urgent.

Ataxia-Telangiectasia Syndrome

The ataxia-telangiectasia syndrome is an autosomal recessive disorder with an incidence of 2 to 3 per 100,000 live births. The disorder is characterized by a progressive ataxia, chronic sinopulmonary disease, ocular and cutaneous telangiectasia, endocrine abnormalities, and a variable B and T cell deficiency. An embryological fault producing abnormalities in mesodermal-entodermal interactions causing telangiectasia, lymphoid abnormalities, and neurological disease underlies the disorder.

The ataxia is a result of progressive neuronal degeneration in the cerebellar cortex. Purkinje cells, granular cells, and the neurones of the dentate and olivary nuclei are particularly affected. Anterior horn cell degeneration and posterior column demyelination characterize spinal cord involvement. The Schwann cells of the peripheral nerves degenerate and this, in conjunction with spinal cord involvement, produces a progressive muscle weakness.

The telangiectases are venous rather than arterial, and bleeding is rarely a significant problem. The bulbar conjunctivae, the bridge of the nose, the ears, and the shoulders are the areas primarily affected by telangiectatic involvement. Other dermatological changes include progeric changes with premature graying of hair, skin atrophy, pigmentary changes with vitiligo or café au lait spots, multiple senile keratoses, and basal cell carcinoma.

Endocrine abnormalities, such as ovarian hypoplasia, elevated gonadotropins, and cytoplasmic vacuoles in the anterior pituitary, also occur.

Biochemically, ataxia-telangiectasia cells have increased susceptibility to breakage upon exposure to X-radiation or ultraviolet light. There appears to be a defect of DNA excision repair as well, but the etiology of this failure of repair is not yet established.

The immunological defect is a variable and progressive B and T cell defect. The B cell defect consists of low or absent serum IgE and IgA. IgG is usually normal, and IgM levels are elevated. T cell defects result in lymphopenia. Cell-mediated immunity is often normal in younger children, but by 12 years of age there is a decrease in delayed hypersensitivity, which continues to worsen with time.

Clinical Features. Cerebellar ataxia is usually the presenting symptom, becoming apparent as the child begins to walk. Later there is progressive muscle weakness, dysarthria, nystagmus, intention tremor, increased drooling, and choreoathetosis. Intellectual development is normal until the age of 9, after which development ceases. Patients with this syndrome generally have placid and agreeable temperaments.

Recurrent infections are common, affecting particularly the respiratory tract. Bronchiectasis and pneumonia are the most common cause of death.

Malignancies are the second leading cause of death in these patients, and most commonly affect the lymphoreticular system.

Treatment. Treatment of this disorder is at present unsatisfactory. Some improvement in lymphoctye function has been demonstrated following thymus grafting or thymosin treatment, but the neurological course of the disease has remained unaffected.

Anesthetic Considerations. Patients present a variable B and T cell defect. As they are immunodepressed, preoperative prophylactic antibiotic therapy and sterile technique to prevent infection are suggested. Chronic and recurrent pulmonary infections are common, and the pulmonary status should be optimized prior to surgery. Similarly, hemoglobin and hematocrit should be assessed.

Excessive drooling is a problem in these patients, and an anticholinergic premedicant may be of benefit.

Emotionally, the patients are usually agreeable and cooperative although their mental age tends to plateau at 9 years of age and they will show an apprehension to needles in spite of an older chronological age.

These patients suffer from progressive muscle weakness due to peripheral nerve and anterior horn cell degeneration, and are subject to marked elevations in serum potassium with the administration of depolarizing muscle relaxants; succinylcholine should be avoided.

Thymic Hypoplasia (DiGeorge Syndrome)

Embryologically, the thymus and the parathyroids are derived from the third and fourth pharyngeal pouches. The DiGeorge syndrome is characterized by failure of normal development of the third and fourth pouches and subsequent failure of development of the thymus and parathyroids. To confirm the diagnosis T cell dysfunction and parathyroid hormone deficiency must be demonstrated. Other features that are variably present include abnormalities of the heart and great vessels, micrognathia, low-set ears, and short philtrum.

The hypoplastic parathyroid glands result in low parathormone levels and hypocalcemia. There is a spectrum of clinical expressions of the immunological problem ranging from minimal thymic involvement to B cell deficiency. The patients are at increased risk for infections by *Candida, Pneumocystis* and numerous other organisms that may produce chronic diarrhea.

Diagnosis may be made as early as the first week of life, when tetany or evidence of cardiac failure may become apparent. If the symptoms are mild, diagnosis may not be made until cardiac evaluation is carried out or until surgery, when the absence of a thymus is apparent.

Treatment of the disorder depends upon the severity. In those with minimal thymic hypoplasia, spontaneous acquisition of normal T cell function is possible. Thymic transplantation and transplantation of thymus cells in a millipore chamber have also been effective and suggest the involvement of soluble factors in normal T cell function. Hypocalcemia may respond to enteral calcium supplementation with vitamin D.

Anesthetic Considerations. Patients with thymic hypoplasia present anesthetic challenges. The presence of decreased serum ionized calcium has several implications. Management of such patients requires ready access to serum calcium and arterial blood gas determinations. The low initial serum ionized calcium and reduced ability of the patient to respond to further decreases in serum ionized calcium (due to parathyroid deficiency) make these patients susceptible to develop symptomatic hypocalcemia. This may be secondary to citrate in blood transfusions or alkalosis induced by hyperventilation. Hypocalcemia can produce tetanic seizures, cardiac depression, and prolonged nondepolarizing neuromuscular block. Treatment of low calcium levels requires the administration of intravenous calcium. Flashburg and colleagues reported low normal serum ionized calcium levels throughout the anesthetic course of management of such a patient, but were able to manage the problem with appropriate monitoring of acid-base balance and serum ionized calcium.

Cardiovascular anomalies may involve both the heart and the great vessels, and cardiac status needs to be assessed carefully. Common abnormalities include transposition of the great vessels, interrupted aortic arch, truncus arteriosus, tetralogy of Fallot, and anomalous pulmonary venous drainage. Cardiac anomalies may be manifested as cardiac failure, which may be accentuated in the presence of low serum ionized calcium.

Upper airway problems may occur because of the small jaw and, in the presence of a vascular ring anomaly, which is not uncommon in this syndrome, tacheomalacia may be present and become apparent following repair of the vascular ring.

Although infections in these patients with intact immunoglobulins are usually viral or fungal, severe forms of the syndrome may present with associated B cell dysfunction. In this case susceptibility to bacterial infections may be a problem. Such patients are subject to chronic interstitial pneumonitis, and the pulmonary status requires careful assessment. It may not be possible to eradicate pulmonary infections fully prior to surgery.

Prevention of infection requires the use of sterile technique (reverse isolation) to minimize the risk of introducing a source of infection. The need for invasive monitoring should be carefully considered, and all lines should be removed as soon as they are no longer necessary. Perioperative prophylactic antibiotic therapy is advised. Blood for transfusion should be irradiated to prevent graft-versus-host disease.

Chronic Mucocutaneous Candidiasis

Chronic mucocutaneous candidiasis comprises a group of diseases all of which demonstrate chronic infection of the skin and mucosa with *Candida albicans.*

There are various subdivisions of this group of diseases based upon the presence or absence of endocrinopathy and laboratory abnormalities.

Endocrine abnormalities, which may manifest themselves at any time, include hypothyroidism, hypoadrenalism, hypoparathyroidism, hypopituitarism, and pernicious anemia. The presence of autoantibodies in some patients implies a possible autoimmune mechanism to the endocrine disorders.

Patients may demonstrate normal serum immunoglobulins or selective IgA deficiency. Anti-candidal antibodies are usually high. T cell numbers and function are usually normal except for a decreased reactivity to *Candida*.

Clinical Features. Onset occurs in infancy with either endocrine abnormalities or the appearance of candidal lesions as the first symptom. The mouth, lips, scalp, eyelashes, vagina, and nails are the most common sites of involvement; systemic spread of *Candida* is very rare.

Treatment. Patients demonstrate an abnormality of iron metabolism, and the resultant anemia shows improvement after treatment with oral or intravenous iron. Most patients require intravenous antifungal agents. Amphotericin and ketoconazole are extremely effective; ketoconazole is less toxic than amphotericin and is currently replacing it as the most commonly used therapeutic agent. Recurrences are frequent with discontinuation of treatment. Such relapses can frequently be treated with topical ketoconazole or clotrimazole. Transfer factor, leukocyte infusions, and thymosin have all been used in treatment with variable success.

All patients must be investigated for endocrinopathies, and appropriate therapy must be initiated. Cases of sudden death during minor infections have been reported and these are likely to be due to an adrenal crisis.

Anesthetic Considerations. Patients suffer from a very mild immunodeficiency affecting B cells and T cells. Infections with organisms other than *Candida* are rare. However, the utilization of sterile technique is recommended in handling these patients. As a selective IgA deficiency may be present, these patients are at risk for transfusion reactions if blood products containing IgA are given. Because of this, full crossmatching of blood is required and may be difficult.

Patients must be carefully assessed for the presence of endocrinopathies and treated appropriately. Endocrinopathies can become manifest at any time, so previously normal assessments must be discounted and further studies performed.

Many of these patients will be on or will have received amphotericin for treatment of the candidiasis. There are several effects of this drug that may complicate perioperative management. Acute administration may produce anaphylaxis. Long-term treatment can produce thrombocytopenia and leukopenia, which are not usually present in chronic mucocutaneous candidiasis. A normochromic normocytic anemia may be present owing to a decrease in erythropoietin activity. Amphotericin may produce hepatic toxicity; however, more recent work has raised questions about whether this is directly related to therapy with this drug. Amphotericin produces a decrease in renal function in 80 percent of patients. Function usually returns to normal upon completion of therapy, but some individuals who have received a complete course have residual glomerular dysfunction. In those currently undergoing treatment, mild renal tubular acidosis and hypokalemia are frequently present and supplemental potassium may be required to correct serum potassium levels prior to anesthesia. Hypomagnesemia is also observed and may require supplementation.

ACQUIRED IMMUNODEFICIENCY SYNDROME

Acquired immunodeficiency syndrome (AIDS) was first recognized in 1981. Since that time many cases have been identified worldwide and the incidence is increasing.

The immunodeficiency in AIDS is an acquired alteration in cell-mediated function; immunoglobulin function and complement activity remain normal. T cell function is abnormal, patients exhibit anergy to skin test antigens, and a decreased lymphocyte response to various mitogens and antigens is demonstrated. Natural killer T cell activity is present and there is an absolute increase in T-suppression lymphocytes. Patients are capable of producing immunoglobulins, as stated above, but with time and progression of disease some patients lose this ability.

The syndrome was first recognized in homosexual men and intravenous drug abusers. Other groups at risk include Haitians, persons with hemophilia receiving factor VIII concentrates, transfusion recipients, prison inmates, female sexual partners of men with AIDS, and infants in high-risk households. This list is constantly expanding.

AIDS is uncommon in pediatric patients. The syndrome has been identified in children with hemophilia and in infants delivered to at-risk mothers. Transfusion-associated AIDS has also been reported in children having received blood products from patients who subsequently developed AIDS. Pediatric patients with AIDS present with recurrent or chronic opportunistic infection (Table 16–3). The malignant neoplasms associated with AIDS (Kaposi sarcoma, diffuse undifferentiated non-Hodgkin lymphoma, Burkitt lymphoma) generally occur late, but have been reported in infants. Other features include failure to thrive, hepatosplenomegaly, generalized lymphadenopathy, pneumonia, and encephalitis. Laboratory evidence of T cell dysfunction is present.

This immune deficiency in this disease is due to infection by a retrovirus known as lymphadenopathy-associated virus (LAV) or human T-lymphotropic virus III (HTLV-III).

Table 16–3. OPPORTUNISTIC INFECTIONS OF ACQUIRED IMMUNODEFICIENCY SYNDROME

Viral Agents	Fungal Agents
Herpes simplex	*Candida*
Herpes zoster	*Cryptococcus*
Cytomegalovirus	*Histoplasma*
Polyomavirus (JC virus)	*Aspergillus*
Progressive multifocal	*Zygomycetes*
leukoencephalopathy	*Petriellidium*
Protozoal Agents	**Bacterial Agents**
Pneumocystis	*Nocardia*
Toxoplasma	*Mycobacterium*
Cryptosporidium	*M. tuberculosis* Non-
Isospora	*tuberculosis* mycobacteria

If such an agent is involved, transmission would appear to require direct intimate contact involving mucosal surfaces (such as sexual contact) or parenteral spread (such as occurs among intravenous drug abusers and during blood transfusions). Airborne spread and interpersonal spread through casual contact seem unlikely. (These resemble the pattern of spread and the modes of spread of the hepatitis B virus.) Additionally in infants, it has been suggested that transplacental, perinatal, and postnatal transmissions of the infectious agent may occur.

The prognosis of pediatric AIDS is not known currently but at best appears to be poor. Some pediatric patients, after contracting the disease in infancy, have lived to 4 years of age, whereas others have died early of overwhelming infection.

There is no specific treatment for AIDS at present. Opportunistic infections should be treated with appropriate agents when available. These patients have T-cell dysfunction, and prophylactic trimethroprim and sulfamethoxazole should be given. Patients who do not make antibodies should receive gamma-globulin. Experimental treatment with interferon, thymic factors, and transplantation of immunologically competent cells has not been extensively evaluated.

More recently, concern has been raised that cases of prolonged unexplained lymphadenopathy may be a prodrome to AIDS. Immunological changes have been demonstrated in children with hemophilia A, especially those who have received factor VIII replacement from commercial concentrates as compared with those who received cryoprecipitate. The commercial concentrates are prepared from pooled plasma from up to 20,000 donors. Thus the average patient with severe hemophilia using commercial concentrate is exposed to many thousands of blood donors, whereas patients receiving cryoprecipitate are exposed to products of the plasma of individual donors. The possibility that cumulative doses of cryoprecipitate are less likely to predispose to lymphocyte abnormalities or that the changes seen with commercial factor VIII concentrate portend the development of AIDS cannot be excluded. However, various investigators have proposed that until these suggestions are confirmed there be no change in the current management of hemophilia.

The anesthetic and operative management of AIDS patients requires care to prevent infection of the patients as well as protection of the staff involved. It is recommended that strict sterile technique be followed when establishing intravenous access and inserting invasive monitors and that these invasive techniques be discontinued as soon as possible. Sterile endotracheal tubes and disposable sterile circuits should be used. These should be of the nonrebreathing type to facilitate cleaning of the anesthetic machine.

Blood products require irradiation to kill donor lymphocytes and prevent graft-versus-host disease. Because of potential for decreased B cell production of immunoglobins, prophylactic antibiotic therapy is advised in the perioperative period.

Although no cases of the acquired immunodeficiency syndrome have as yet been reported in clinical or laboratory health care workers, this will likely occur in the future. Guidelines for protection have been suggested by the Centers for Disease Control and are presented here.

1. Extraordinary care must be taken to avoid accidental wounds from sharp instruments contaminated with potentially infectious material and to avoid contact of open skin lesions with material from AIDS patients.

2. Gloves should be worn when handling blood specimens, blood-soiled items, fluids, excretions, and secretions, as well as surfaces, materials, and objects exposed to them.

3. Gowns should be worn when clothing may be soiled with body fluids, blood, secretions, or excretions.

4. Hands should be washed after removing gowns and gloves and before leaving the rooms of known or suspected AIDS patients. Hands should also be washed thoroughly and immediately if they become contaminated with blood.

5. Blood and other specimens should be labeled prominently with a special warning, such as "Blood Precautions" or "AIDS Precautions." If the outside of the specimen container is visibly contaminated with blood, it should be cleaned with a disinfectant (such as 1:10 dilution of 5.25 percent sodium hypochlorite [household bleach] with water). All blood specimens should be placed in a second container, such as an impervious bag, for transport. The container or bag should be examined carefully for leaks or cracks.

6. Blood spills should be cleaned up promptly with a disinfectant solution, such as sodium hypochlorite (see above).

7. Articles soiled with blood should be placed in an impervious bag prominently labeled "AIDS Precautions" or "Blood Precautions" before being sent for reprocessing or disposal. Alternatively, such contaminated items may be placed in plastic bags of a particular color designated solely for disposal of infectious wastes

by the hospital. Disposable items should be incinerated or disposed of in accord with the hospital's policies for disposal of infectious wastes. Reusable items should be reprocessed in accord with hospital policies for hepatitis B virus–contaminated items. Lensed instruments should be sterilized after use on AIDS patients.

8. Needles should not be bent after use, but should be promptly placed in a puncture-resistant container used solely for such disposal. Needles should not be reinserted into their original sheaths before being discarded into the container, since this is a common cause of needle injury.

9. Disposable syringes and needles are preferred. Only needle-locking syringes or one-piece needle-syringe units should be used to aspirate fluids from patients, so that collected fluid can be safely discharged through the needle, if desired. If reusable syringes are employed, they should be decontaminated before reprocessing.

10. A private room is indicated for patients who are too ill to use good hygiene, such as those with profuse diarrhea, fecal incontinence, or altered behavior secondary to central nervous system infections. Precautions appropriate for particular infections that concurrently occur in AIDS patients should be added to the above, if needed.

GRAFT-VERSUS-HOST DISEASE

Graft-versus-host disease (GVHD) occurs in patients with severely impaired cell-mediated immunity who have received allogenic immunocompetent lymphocytes. In the recipient the donor lymphocytes attack the recipient's major histocompatibility antigens. GVHD can be subdivided into acute and chronic forms, the features of which are similar.

Symptoms generally begin within 5 to 30 days after administration of immunocompetent lymphocytes to an immunodeficient patient. Initially there is skin involvement with lymphocytes infiltrating the dermis and epidermis, resembling the "scalded skin syndrome." Later there is liver involvement with periportal necrosis of hepatocytes, fever, gastrointestinal mucosal degeneration with diarrhea, hemolytic anemia, granulocytopenia with aplastic anemia, cough, and pulmonary infiltrates as a result of lymphocyte infiltration and necrosis of the bronchial mucosa. The outcome depends on the degree of incompatibility, the patient's age, the number of cells received, and the primary pathology. In infants the administration of 50 ml of blood containing completely mismatched lymphocytes may be fatal. Those receiving incompletely but partially matched lymphocytes do better.

Chronic GVHD is characterized by scaling erythroderma, alopecia, and failure to thrive.

In both forms of disease there is increased susceptibility to both bacterial and viral infections. Latent infections such as cytomegalovirus may become active and fulminant. *Pneumocystis carinii* pneumonia also is common.

Treatment of established GVHD has consisted of use of antithymocyte or antilymphocyte globulin, but success with this approach has been limited. Lymphocytes in blood from blood banks are viable for 3 weeks. Blood being transfused into patients with T cell dysfunction should be irradiated prior to transfusion to kill the lymphocytes.

REFERENCES

X-Linked Agammaglobulinemia

Fu SM, Hurley JN, McCune JM, et al.: Pre-B cells and other possible precursor lymphoid cell lines derived from patients with X-linked agammaglobulinemia. J Exp Med *152*:1519, 1980.

Hoffman T, Winchester R, Schulkind M, et al.: Hypogammaglobulinemia with normal T cell function in female siblings. Clin Immunol Immunopathol 7:364, 1977.

Mease PJ, Ochs HD, Wedgwood RJ: Successful treatment of echovirus meningoencephalitis and myositis-fasciitis with intravenous immune globulin therapy in a patient with X-linked agammaglobulinemia. N Engl J Med *304*:1278, 1981.

Ochs HD, Ament ME, Davis SD: Giardiasis with malabsorption in X-linked agammaglobulinemia. N Engl J Med 287:341, 1972.

Ochs HD, Davis SD, Wedgwood RJ: Immunologic responses to bacteriophage φX 174 in immunodeficiency diseases. J Clin Invest 50:2559, 1971.

Pearl ER, Vogler LB, Okos AJ, et al.: B lymphocyte precursors in human bone marrow: an analysis of normal individuals and patients with antibody deficient states. J Immunol *120*:1169, 1978.

Saulsbury FT, Bernstein MT, Winkelstein JA: *Pneumocystis carinii* pneumonia as the presenting infection in congenital hypogammaglobulinemia. J Pediatr 95:559, 1979.

Saulsbury FT, Winkelstein JA, Yolken RH: Chronic rotavirus infection in immunodeficiency. J Pediatr 97:61, 1977.

Schwaber J, Lazarus H, Rosen FS: Bone marrow–derived lymphoid cell lines from patients with agammaglobulinemia. J Clin Invest 62:302, 1978.

Stuckey M, Quinin PA, Gelfand EW: Identification of *Ureaplasma urealyticum* (T-strain *Mycoplasma*) in a patient with polyarthritis. Lancet 2:917, 1978.

Wedgwood RJ: X-linked agammaglobulinemia. *In* Seligson D (Ed.): CRC Handbook Series in Clinical Laboratory Science. Section F, Vol. 1, Part 1. West Palm Beach, Fla., CRC Press, 1978, p 41.

Wright PF, Hatch MH, Kasselberg AG, et al.: Vaccine-associated poliomyelitis in a child with sex-linked agammaglobulinemia. J Pediatr 91:408, 1977.

X-Linked Agammaglobulinemia with Growth Hormone Defect

Fleisher TA, White RM, Broder S, et al.: X-linked agammaglobulinemia with isolated growth human defect. N Engl J Med *302*:1429, 1980.

Autosomal Recessive Agammaglobulinemia

Hoffman T, Winchester R, Schulkind M, et al.: Hypogammaglobulinemia with normal T-cell function in female siblings. Clin Immunol Immunopathol 7:364, 1977.

Rosen FS, Cooper MD, Wedgwood RJ: The primary immunodeficiencies I. N Engl J Med *311*:235, 1984.

Immunoglobulin Deficiency with Increased IgM (and IgD)

Schwaber JF, Lazarus H, Rosen FS: IgM-restricted production of immunoglobulin by lymphoid cell lines from patients with immunodeficiency with hyper IgM (dysgammaglobulinemia). Clin Immunol Immunopathol 19:91, 1981.

Selective Immunoglobulin A Deficiency

Atwater JS, Tomasi TB: Suppressor cells and IgA deficiency. Clin Immunol Immunopathol 9:379, 1978.

Cunningham-Rundles C, Brandeis WE, Good RA, et al.: Milk precipitins, circulating immune complexes and IgA deficiency. Proc Natl Acad Sci USA 75:3387, 1978.

Cunningham-Rundles C, Pudefin DJ, Armstrong D, et al.: Selective IgA deficiency and neoplasia. Vox Sang 38:61, 1980.

Frommel D, Moullec J, Lambin P, et al.: Selective IgA deficiency. 25:513, 1973.

Koistinen J: Selective IgA deficiency in blood donors. Vox Sang 29:192, 1975.

Lawton AR, Royal SA, Self K, et al.: IgA determinants on B lymphocytes in patients with deficiency of circulating IgA. J Lab Clin Med 80:26, 1972.

Ogra PA, Coppola PR, MacGillivray MH, et al.: Mechanisms of mucosal immunity to viral infections in A immunoglobulin deficiency syndromes. Proc Soc Exp Biol Med 145:811, 1974.

Oxelius VA, Laurell AB, Lindquist B, et al.: IgG subclasses in selective IgA deficiency. N Engl J Med 304:1476, 1981.

Paganelli R, Levinsky RS, Atherton DJ: Detection of specific antigen within immune complexes. Validation of the assay and its application to food antigen antibody complexes in healthy and food allergic complexes. Clin Exp Immunol 36:44, 1981.

Soothill JF, Hayes K, Dudgeon JA: The immunoglobulins in congenital rubella. Lancet 1:1385, 1966.

Taylor B, Norman AP, Orgel HA, et al.: Transient IgA deficiency and pathogenesis of infantile atopy. Lancet 2:111, 1973.

vanLoghem E: Familial occurrence of isolated IgA deficiency associated with antibodies to IgA. Evidence against a structural gene defect. Eur J Immunol 4:57, 1974.

Vyas GN, Fudenberg HH: Immunobiology of human anti-IgA: a serologic and immunogenetic study of immunization to IgA in transfusion and pregnancy. Clin Genet 1:45, 1970.

Waldman TA, Broder S, Krakauer R, et al.: Defect in IgA secretion and in IgA specific suppressor cells in patients with selective IgA deficiency. Trans Assoc Am Phys 89:215, 1976.

Selective Deficiency of Secretory Component

Strober W, Krakauer R, Klaeveman HL, et al.: Secretory component deficiency. N Engl J Med 294:351, 1976.

Selective Immunoglobulin M Deficiency

Faulk WP, Kiuasu WS, Cooper MD, et al.: Deficiency of IgM. Pediatrics 47:399, 1971.

Hobbs JR: IgM deficiency. In Bergsma D, et al. (Eds.): Immunodeficiency in Man and Animals. Sunderland, MA, Sinauer Press, 1975.

Hobbs JR, Melner RDG, Watt PJ: Gamma-M deficiency predisposing to meningococcal septicaemia. Br Med J 4:583, 1967.

Immunoglobulin G Deficiencies

Spiegelberg HL: Biological activities of immunoglobulins of different classes and subclasses. Adv Immunol 19:259, 1974.

Transient Hypogammaglobulinemia of Infancy

Hayakawa H, Iwata T, Yata J, et al.: Primary immunodeficiency syndrome in Japan. I. Overview of a nationwide survey on primary immunodeficiency syndrome. J Clin Immunol 1:31, 1981.

Rieger CHL, Nelson LA, Peri BA, et al.: Transient hypogammaglobulinemia of infancy. J Pediatr 91:601, 1977.

Tiller, TL Jr, Buckley RH: Transient hypogammaglobulinemia of infancy: review of the literature, clinical and immunologic features of 11 new cases, and long-term follow-up. J Pediatr 92:347, 1978.

Medical Management of Antibody Deficiency Syndromes

Ammann AJ, Ashman RF, Buckley RH, et al.: Use of intravenous γ-globulin in antibody immunodeficiency: results of a multicenter controlled trial. Clin Immunol Immunopathol 22:60, 1982.

Buckley RH: Replacement therapy in immunodeficiency. In Thompson R (Ed.): Recent Advances in Clinical Immunology I. Edinburgh, Churchill Livingston, 1977.

Norman ME, Hansell JR, Holtzapple PG, et al.: Malabsorption and protein losing enteropathy in a child with X-linked agammaglobulinaemia. Clin Immunol Immunopathol 4:157, 1975.

Nydegger UE (Ed.): Immunotherapy: A Guide to Immunoglobulin Prophylaxis and Therapy. New York, Academic Press, 1981.

Soothill, JF: Reactions to immunoglobulin. In Hypogammaglobulinaemia in the United Kingdom. MRC Special Report Series 310. London, Her Majesty's Stationery Office, 1975.

Severe Combined Immunodeficiency

Gatti RA, Meuwissen HJ, Allen HD, et al.: Immunological reconstruction of sex-linked lymphopenic immunological deficiency. Lancet 2:1366, 1968.

Githens JH, Fulginiti VA, Suvatte V, et al.: Grafting of fetal thymus and hematopoietic tissue in infants with immune deficiency syndromes. Transplantation 15:427, 1973.

Haynes BF, Warren RW, Buckley RH, et al.: Demonstration of abnormalities in expression of thymic epithelial surface antigens in severe cellular immunodeficiency diseases. J Immunol 130:1182, 1983.

Hong R, Santosham M, Schulte-Wisserman H, et al.: Reconstruction of B and T lymphocyte function in severe combined immunodeficiency disease after transplantation with thymic epithelium. Lancet 2:1270, 1976.

Keightley RG, Lawton AR, Cooper MD, et al.: Successful fetal liver transplantation in a child with severe combined immunodeficiency. Lancet 2:850, 1975.

Levey RH, Klemperer MR, Gelfand EW, et al.: Bone-marrow transplantation in severe combined immunodeficiency syndrome. Lancet 2:571, 1971.

O'Reilly RJ, Dupont B, Pahwa S, et al.: Reconstruction in severe combined immunodeficiency by transplantation of marrow from an unrelated donor. N Engl J Med 297:1311, 1971.

Rádl J, Dooren LJ, Eijsvoogel VP, et al.: An immunological study during post-transplantation follow-up of a case of severe combined immunodeficiency. Clin Exp Immunol 10:367, 1972.

Reinherz EL, Geha R, Rappaport JM, et al.: Reconstitution after transplantation with T-lymphocyte-depleted HLA haplotype-mismatched bone marrow for severe combined immunodeficiency. Proc Natl Acad Sci USA 79:6047, 1982.

Reisner Y, Kapoor N, Kirkpatrick D, et al.: Transplantation for severe combined immunodeficiency with HLA-A, B, D, Dr incompatible parenteral marrow cells fractionated by soybean agglutinin and sheep red blood cells. Blood 61:341, 1983.

Severe Combined Immunodeficiency with Adenosine Deaminase Deficiency

Carson DA, Kaye J, Seegmiller JE: Lymphospecific toxicity in adenosine deaminase deficiency and purine nucleoside phosphorylase deficiency: possible role for nucleoside kinases. Proc Natl Acad Sci USA 74:5677, 1977.

Chen SH, Ochs SD, Scott CR, et al.: Adenosine deaminase deficiency. J Clin Invest 62:1386, 1978.

Hirschorn R: Clinical delineation of adenosine deaminase deficiency. In Enzyme Defects and Immune Dysfunction. Ciba Foundation Symposium 68. Amsterdam, Excerpta Medica, 1979.

Hirschorn R, Beratis N, Rosen FS, et al.: Adenosine deaminase deficiency in a child diagnosed prenatally. Lancet 1:73, 1978.

Hirschorn R, Roegner-Maniscalco V, Kuritsky L, et al.: Bone marrow transplantation only partially restores purine metabolites to normal in adenosine deaminase–deficiency patients. J Clin Invest 68:1387, 1981.

Ito K, Sakura N, Usui T, et al.: Screening for primary immuno-deficiencies associated with purine nucleoside phosphorylase or adenosine deaminase deficiency. J Lab Clin Med 90:844, 1977.

Parkman R, Gelfand EW, Rosen FS, et al.: Severe combined immunodeficiency and adenosine deaminase deficiency. N Engl J Med 292:714, 1975.

Polmer SH: Enzyme replacement and other biochemical approaches to the therapy of adenosine deaminase deficiency. In Enzyme Defects and Immune Dysfunction. Ciba Foundation Symposium 68. Amsterdam, Excerpta Medica, 1979.

Polmar SH, Wetzler EM, Stern RC, et al.: Restoration of in vitro lymphocyte responses with exogenous adenosine deaminase in a patient with severe combined immunodeficiency. Lancet 2:743, 1975.

Purine Nucleoside Phosphorylase Deficiency

Cohen A, Coyle D, Martin DW Jr, et al.: Abnormal purine metabolism and purine overproduction in a patient deficient in purine nucleoside phosphorylase. N Engl J Med 295:1449, 1976.

Cohen A, Guidas LJ, Ammann AJ, et al.: Deoxyguanosine triphosphate as a possible toxic metabolite in the immunodeficiency associated with purine nucleoside phosphorylase deficiency. J Clin Invest 61:1405, 1978.

Gelfand EW, Dosch HM, Biggar WD, et al.: Partial purine nucleoside phosphorylase deficiency: studies on lymphocyte function. J Clin Invest 61:1071, 1978.

Gelfand EW, Lee JJ, Dosch HM: Selective toxicity of purine deoxynucleosides from human lymphocyte growth and function. Proc Natl Acad Sci USA 76:1998, 1979.

Giblett ER, Ammann AJ, Sandman R, et al.: Nucleoside phosphorylase deficiency in a child with severely defective T cell immunity and normal B cell immunity. Lancet 1:1010, 1975.

Rich KC, Arnold WJ, Palella T, et al.: Cellular immune deficiency with autoimmune hemolytic anaemia in purine nucleoside phosphorylase deficiency. Am J Med 67:172, 1979.

Sandman R, Ammann AJ, Grose C, et al.: Cellular immunodeficiency associated with nucleoside phosphorylase deficiency: immunologic and biochemical studies. Clin Immunol Immunopathol 8:247, 1977.

Staal GEJ, Stoop JW, Zegers BJM, et al.: Erythrocyte metabolism in purine nucleoside phosphorylase deficiency after enzyme replacement by infusion of erythrocytes. J Clin Invest 65:103, 1980.

Stoop JW, Zegers BJM, Hendricks GFM: Purine nucleoside phosphorylase deficiency associated with selective cellular immunodeficiency. N Engl J Med 296:651, 1977.

Combined Immunodeficiency with Predominant T Cell Defect

Ammann AJ: Is there an acquired immune deficiency syndrome in infants and children? Pediatrics 72:430, 1983.

Lawlor GJ Jr, Ammann AJ, Wright WC Jr, et al.: The syndrome of cellular immunodeficiency with immunoglobulins. J Pediatr 84:183, 1974.

Nezelof C, Jammet ML, Lortholary P, et al.: L'Hypoplasie hereditaire du thymus: sa place et sa responsibilité. Arch Fr Pediatr 21:897, 1964.

Schimke RN, Bolano C, Kirkpatrick CH: Immunologic deficiency in the congenital rubella syndrome. Am J Dis Child 118:626, 1969.

Wiskott-Aldrich Syndrome

Cooper MD, Chase HP, Lowman JT, et al.: Immunologic defects in patients with Wiskott-Aldrich syndrome. In Bergsma D (Ed.): Immunologic Deficiency in Man. New York, National Foundation, March of Dimes, 1968.

Kuramoto, A, Steiner M, Baldine MG: Lack of platelet response to stimulation in the Wiskott-Aldrich syndrome. N Engl J Med 282:475, 1970.

Lum, LG, Tubergan DG, Blaese RM: Splenectomy and prophylactic antibiotics in the management of Wiskott-Aldrich syndrome. N Engl J Med 302:892, 1980.

Parkman R, Rappaport J, Geha R, et al.: Complete correction of the Wiskott-Aldrich syndrome by allogenic bone marrow transplantation. N Engl J Med 298:921, 1978.

Perry GS, Spector BD, Schuman LM, et al.: The Wiskott-Aldrich syndrome in the United States and Canada. J Pediatr 97:72, 1980.

Spitler LE: Transfer factor therapy in the Wiskott-Aldrich syndrome. Results of long term follow-up in 32 patients. Am J Med 67:59, 1979.

Ataxia-Telangiectasia Syndrome

Biggar WD, Good RA: Immunodeficiency in ataxia telangiectasia. In Bergsma D, et al. (Eds.): Immunodeficiency in Man and Animals. Sunderland, MA, Sinauer Press, 1975.

Boder E: Ataxia-telangiectasia: some historic, clinical and pathologic observations. In Bergsma D, et al. (Eds.): Immunodeficiency in Man and Animals. Sunderland, MA, Sinauer Press, 1975.

McFarlen DE, Strober W, Waldmann TA: Ataxia telangiectasia. Medicine 51:281, 1972.

Paterson MC, Smith PJ: Ataxia telangiectasia: an inherited human disorder involving hypersensitivity to ionizing radiation and related DNA-damaging chemicals. Ann Rev Genet 13:291, 1979.

Trompeter RS, Layward L, Hayward AR: Primary and secondary abnormalities of T cell subpopulations. Clin Exp Immunol 34:388, 1978.

Thymic Hypoplasia

Cleveland WW: Immunological reconstitution in the DiGeorge syndrome by fetal thymic transplant. In Bergsma D, et al. (Eds.): Immunodeficiency in Man and Animals. Sunderland, MA, Sinauer Press, 1975.

Conley ME, Beckwith, JB, Maneer JFK, et al.: The spectrum of DiGeorge syndrome. J Pediatr 94:883, 1979.

Delinger JK, Nahrwold ML, Gibbs PS, et al.: Hypocalcemia during rapid blood transfusion in anaesthetized man. Br J Anaesth 48:995, 1976.

DiGeorge AM: Congenital absence of the thymus and its immunological consequences. Concurrence with congenital hypoparathyroidism. Birth Defects Original Article Series 4:116, 1968.

Flashburg MH, Dunbar BS, August G, et al.: Anesthesia for surgery in an infant with DiGeorge syndrome. Anesthesiology 58:479, 1983.

Freedom RM, Rosen FS, Nadas AS: Congenital cardiovascular disease and abnormalities of the third and fourth pharyngeal pouch. Circulation 46:165, 1972.

Hong R, Ammann AJ, Huang SW, et al.: Cartilage-hair hypoplasia: effect of thymus transplants. Clin Immunol Immunopathol 7:15, 1972.

Kahn RC, Jascott D, Carlon GC, et al.: Massive blood replacement: correlation of ionized calcium, citrate, and hydrogen ion concentration. Anesth Analg 58:274, 1979.

Kelley RI, Zakai EH, Emanuel BS, et al.: The association of DiGeorge anomalad with partial monosomy of chromosome 22. J Pediatr 101:197, 1982.

Lobdell DH: Congenital absence of the parathyroid glands. Arch Pathol 67:412, 1959.

Lux SE, Johnston RB, August CS, et al.: Chronic neutropenia and abnormal cell mediated immunity in cartilage-hair hypoplasia. N Engl J Med 282:231, 1970.

McKusick VC, Cross HE: Ataxia telangiectasia and Swiss type agammaglobulinemia. JAMA 195:119, 1966.

Steele RW, Limas C, Thurman GB, et al.: Familial thymic

hypoplasia. (Attempted reconstruction with fetal thymus in a millipore diffusion chamber.) N Engl J Med 287:787, 1972.

Waud BE, Waud DR: Interaction of calcium and potassium with neuromuscular blocking agents. Br J Anaesth 52:863, 1980.

Chronic Mucocutaneous Candidiasis

Arulanantham K, Dwyer JM, Genel M: Evidence for defective immunoregulation in the syndrome of familial candidiasis endocrinopathy. N Engl J Med 300:164, 1979.

Fischer A, Ballet JJ, Griscelli C: Specific inhibition of in vitro candida-induced lymphocyte proliferation by polysaccharide antigens present in the serum of patients with chronic mucocutaneous candidiasis. J Clin Invest 62:1005, 1978.

Higgs JM, Wells RS: Chronic mucocutaneous candidiasis, associated abnormalities in iron metabolism. Br J Dermatol 86(S8):88, 1972.

Kirkpatrick CH: Transfer factor and defense against infectious disease. In Amos DB, Schwartz RS, Janicki BW (Eds.): Immune Mechanisms and Diseases. New York, Academic Press, 1979.

Sande MA, Mandell GA: Antimicrobial agents: miscellaneous antibacterial agents; antifungal and antiviral agents. In Gilman AG, Goodman LS, Gilman A (Eds.): The Pharmacological Basis of Therapeutics. 6th ed. New York, MacMillan, 1980.

Valdimarsson H, Higgs JM, Wells RS, et al.: Immune abnormalities associated with chronic microcutaneous candidiasis. Cell Immunol 6:348, 1973.

Acquired Immunodeficiency Syndrome

Acquired immune deficiency syndrome (AIDS): precautions for clinical and laboratory staffs. Morbid Mortal Wkly Rep 31:577, 1982.

Acquired immunodeficiency syndrome (AIDS): precautions for health care workers and allied professionals. Morbid Mortal Wkly Rep 32:450, 1983.

Ammann AJ: Is there an acquired immune deficiency syndrome in infants and children? Pediatrics 72:430, 1983.

An evaluation of the acquired immunodeficiency syndrome (AIDS) reported in health-care personnel—United States. Morbid Mortal Wkly Rep 32:358, 1983.

Bove JR: Transfusion-associated AIDS—a cause for concern. N Engl J Med 310:115, 1984.

Curran JW, Lawrence DN, Jaffe H, et al.: Acquired immunodeficiency syndrome (AIDS) associated with transfusions. N Engl J Med 310:69, 1984.

Gill JC, Minitove JE, Wheeler D, et al.: Generalized lymphadenopathy and T cell abnormalities in hemophilia A. J Pediatr 103:18, 1983.

Gordon EM, Berkowitz RJ, Strandjord SE, et al.: Burkitt lymphoma in a patient with classic hemophilia receiving factor VIII concentrates. J Pediatr 103:75, 1983.

Gottlieb MS, Groopman JE, Weenstein WM, et al.: The acquired immunodeficiency syndrome. Ann Intern Med 99:208, 1983.

Landay A, Poon MC, Abo T, et al.: Immunologic studies in asymptomatic hemophilia patients. J Clin Invest 71:1500, 1983.

Oleske JM, Minnefor AB: Acquired immune deficiency syndrome in children. Pediatr Infect Dis 2:85, 1983.

Rubinstein A: Acquired immunodeficiency syndrome in infants. Am J Dis Child 137:825, 1983.

Scott GB, Buck BE, Leterman JG, et al.: Acquired immunodeficiency syndrome in infants. N Engl J Med 310:76, 1984.

Speck WT: Acquired immune deficiency syndrome. J Pediatr 103:161, 1983.

Update on acquired immune deficiency syndrome (AIDS)—United States. Morbid Mortal Wkly Rep 31:509, 1983.

Graft-versus-host Disease

Beschomer WE, Saral R, Hutchins GM, et al.: Lymphocytic bronchitis associated with graft versus host disease in recipients of bone marrow transplants. N Engl J Med 299:1030, 1978.

Grebe SC, Streilein SW: Graft versus host reaction. A review. Adv Immunol 22:119, 1974.

Lerner KG, Kao GF, Storb R, et al.: Histopathology of graft versus host reaction in human recipients of marrow from HL-A matched siblings donors. Transplant Proc 6:367, 1974.

Tsoi MS, Storb R, Jones E, et al.: Deposition of IgM and complement at the dermatoepidermal junction in acute and chronic graft versus host disease in man. J Immunol 120:1485, 1978.

THE PHAGOCYTIC SYSTEM AND ASSOCIATED DISEASES

Disorders of Polymorphonuclear Leukocytes
Disorders of Bactericidal Function

Disorders of Chemotaxis
Mixed Functional Defects
Disorders of Mononuclear Leukocytes

Phagocytes are either mononuclear or polymorphonuclear. They arise from a pluripotent stem cell in the bone marrow and other hemopoietic tissue (Fig. 16–2). Phagocytes are produced in numbers equal to those of erythrocytes, but they have a much shorter half-life, accounting for their lower absolute numbers.

Mononuclear phagocytes (monocytes) have a circulating half-life of 70 hours. There exists a large reserve of monocytes in the bone marrow and marginated in the circulation. Monocytes are released immature and after a period in the circulation they leave the blood compartment to become the fixed macrophages of the spleen, liver, lungs, lymph nodes, intestine, and central nervous system. With maturation their phagocytic activity increases. Fixed macrophages demonstrate morphological and metabolic characteristics that are unique and dependent upon the resident organ system. Circulating mononuclear cells migrate into areas of inflammation and are responsible for "walling off" an infectious process and for granuloma formation.

Polymorphonuclear leukocytes (PMNs) (neutrophils, basophils, eosinophils) have a circulating half-life of 6 to 10 hours. As with monocytes, there is a large reservoir of PMNs stored in the bone marrow and marginated in the circulation. PMNs are released into the circulation as highly differentiated mature cells,

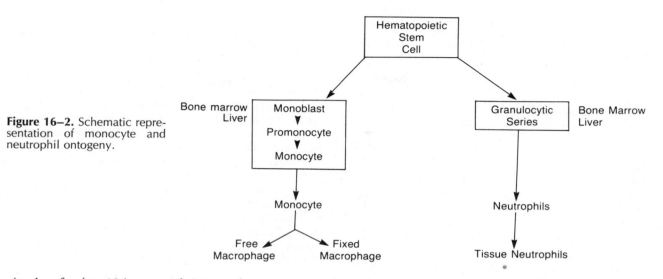

Figure 16–2. Schematic representation of monocyte and neutrophil ontogeny.

circulate for 4 to 10 hours, and then, as do monocytes, migrate into tissues.

Inflammation results in mobilization of the store of phagocytes and their absolute numbers can increase rapidly. Inflammation also stimulates rapid multiplication of precursor cells and rapid differentiation.

The functions of phagocytes are complex. They enter the circulation from the bone marrow or marginated pool in response to inflammatory stimuli, producing a sharp increase in absolute numbers. In the area of inflammation phagocytes adhere to the vascular endothelium and enter the tissues by diapedesis. Once in the tissues, they migrate toward the affected area by moving up a concentration gradient of chemotactic substances (chemotaxis).

Once the phagocytes reach the affected area and contact with the infecting organism occurs, adherence, endocytosis, and killing occur. Properties of the foreign particles may contribute to the activity of phagocytes, including spontaneous activation of complement by the alternate pathway as occurs with some yeasts, a hydrophobic surface, a surface charge, and surface sugars. Opsonins are specific antibacterial antibodies and components of complement that neutralize antiphagocytic factors on bacterial surfaces and serve as ligands binding bacteria to phagocytes. Interaction of

bacteria with such opsonins enhances phagocytosis. Phagocytic cells have membrane receptors for portions of the antibodies and for the activated fragments of complement.

Once such recognition and adherence occurs, endocytosis follows by the activation of certain contractile proteins, which results in pseudopod formation surrounding the organism. With complete surrounding of the particle by the cell membrane, a phagocytic vacuole is formed. Cytoplasmic granules contribute their contents into this phagosome, resulting in the stimulation of oxidative metabolism.

Phagocytosis is associated with a burst of oxygen consumption. This is associated with a tenfold increase in glucose utilization by the hexose monophosphate pathway. Oxygen is univalently reduced to form superoxide radical, then to produce hydrogen peroxide and hydroxyl radicals, and finally to water (Fig. 16–3). Halides are oxidized. Interaction of reactive oxygen molecules, myeloperoxidase (which originates from the cytoplasmic granules), and halides produces the rapid killing of most bacterial and fungal organisms. Oxygen-reduced pyridine nucleotides and oxidases are essential for this response.

Defects in phagocytic function, either singly or in combination, may occur at one or more of the above

Figure 16–3. Oxidative response of the hexose monophosphate pathway with phagocytosis demonstrating the production of hydrogen peroxide (H_2O_2) and superoxide radical (O_2^-), which are responsible for the bactericidal activity of the cells. ADP = adenosine diphosphate; GSH = reduced glutathione; ATP = adenosine triphosphate; GSSG = oxidized glutathione; NAD^+ = oxidized nicotinamide adenine dinucleotide; NADH = reduced nicotinamide adenine dinucleotide; $NADP^+$ = oxidized nicotinamide adenine dinucleotide phosphate; NADPH = reduced nicotinamide adenine dinucleotide phosphate.

Table 16–4. INCREASED SUSCEPTIBILITY WITH
SPECIFIC DEFECTS

Bactericidal Defects	
Chronic granulomatous disease	Catalase-producing bacterial and fungal infections
Myeloperoxidase deficiency	Candidiasis, bacterial infections, or none
Defects of Chemotaxis	
Hyperimmunoglobulin E (Job syndrome)	*Staphylococcus aureus* infection of skin and nodes
Lazy leukocyte syndrome	Upper respiratory tract infections and stomatitis
Mixed Disorders	
Chédiak-Higashi syndrome	Gram positive coccal infections
Other	
Neutropenia, congenital or acquired	Bacterial infections

steps. Table 16–4 describes the susceptibilities to infection with different defects.

DISORDERS OF POLYMORPHONUCLEAR LEUKOCYTES

Disorders of Bactericidal Function (Table 16–5)

Chronic Granulomatous Disease of Childhood

Chronic granulomatous disease (CGD) is a genetic disorder characterized by recurrent and chronic bacterial or fungal infections. It is a disorder of phagocytic cells in which bactericidal capacity is defective owing to an abnormal oxidative metabolic response during phagocytosis. Humoral and cell-mediated responses are unaffected and the cells are morphologically normal.

The inheritance pattern of CGD appears to be X-linked. In males, patients are either normal or affected. In females, heterozygous and homozygous states occur. As a group, female heterozygotes have low levels of bactericidal activity, but there is considerable variability and normal levels of bactericidal activity do not exclude heterozygosity.

The onset of CGD may occur at any age from infancy to adulthood, and diagnosis can now be made in utero from fetal cells obtained at amniocentesis. The presentation of the syndrome is variable, and Table 16–6 lists some of the clinical manifestations that may occur.

Patients demonstrate increased susceptibility to both

Table 16–5. DISORDERS OF BACTERICIDAL
FUNCTION

Chronic granulomatous disease
Myeloperoxidase deficiency
Glucose-6-phosphatase deficiency
Glutathione peroxidase deficiency
Down syndrome
Bilobed PMN nucleus
Chédiak-Higashi syndrome

bacterial and fungal infections. *Staphylococcus aureus*, *Serratia marcescens*, and *Klebsiella* are common infecting organisms. The syndrome is characterized by recurrent and chronic microabscesses of lymph nodes and liver, osteomyelitis, and chronic pneumonitis.

Pneumonitis is frequent, with *Staphylococcus aureus*, gram negative bacilli, and *Aspergillus fumigatus* as causative agents. In spite of appropriate therapy, chronic infiltrates and residual pulmonary changes are frequent. The presence of circulating immune complexes is common and can produce arthralgias, urticaria, and costochondritis. Female heterozygotes demonstrate an increased incidence of systemic lupus erythematosus.

Pathogenesis. As previously described, neutrophils normally metabolize oxygen to produce superoxide anion and hydrogen peroxide. After ingestion of a foreign organism production of oxygen metabolites by

Table 16–6. CLINICAL MANIFESTATIONS OF
CHRONIC GRANULOMATOUS DISEASE

System	Disease
Skin	Eczematous dermatitis Granulomas Pyoderma
Ear-nose-throat	Otitis Rhinitis Sinusitis
Cardiopulmonary	Pericarditis Mediastinitis Pneumonia Focal lung abscess Diffuse persistent pulmonary infiltrates
Gastrointestinal	Ulcerative stomatitis Esophagitis Antral granuloma or thickening with obstruction Subphrenic abscess Focal liver abscess Miliary liver abscesses Granulomatous ileitis/colitis Vitamin B_{12} malabsorption Steatorrhea Perianal fistulas
Genitourinary	Renal abscess Pyelonephritis Cystitis Dysuria of unknown cause
Endocrine	Septic thyroiditis with thyrotoxicosis
Neurological	Meningitis Epidural abscess
Hematological	Granulocytosis Hypochromic/microcytic anemia
Immunological	Diffuse hypergammaglobulinemia Lymphadenopathy Suppurative lymphadenitis Splenomegaly Urticaria, arthralgias, costochondritis
Musculoskeletal	Osteomyelitis Septic arthritis Pyomyositis

the hexose monophosphate pathway and their accumulation occurs in the phagosome. Myeloperoxidase, delivered into the phagosome by degranulation, and hydrogen peroxide kill the phagocytized microbe. Many microorganisms produce catalase, which is capable of catabolizing hydrogen peroxide, but neutrophils normally produce hydrogen peroxide in amounts sufficient to overwhelm this catalase and enable normal bactericidal capacity. In patients with chronic granulomatous disease the oxygen metabolites including hydrogen peroxide are not produced by the neutrophils. Although some microorganisms produce hydrogen peroxide themselves, those that produce catalase (catalase positive) are able to catabolize the produced hydrogen peroxide and therefore are not killed. Catalase-negative cells such as *Streptococcus* are unable to break down hydrogen peroxide produced by the microbe itself, which, in association with the myeloperoxidase delivered, is sufficient to enable its own destruction.

The disorder is termed "granulomatous" because the phagocytosed bacteria elicit a granulomatous response, common to intracellular pathogens, in tissues such as lymph nodes, liver, bone marrow, and lung that contain many macrophages. Histologically the lesions consist of polymorphonuclear, lymphocytic, macrophage, and plasma cell infiltration.

Medical Management. Currently there is no satisfactory treatment available to correct the defect in bactericidal activity, and management is aimed at the prophylaxis of infections. Many infections, if detected and treated early, respond to conservative therapy such as oral antibiotics. More severe infections require hospitalization and intravenous antibiotics; frequently broad-spectrum antibiotic coverage is used when the offending organism cannot be identified. Once phagocytosed into neutrophils, the bacteria are segregated from most antibiotics. Agents such as chloramphenicol and rifampin have been advocated in many of these cases because of their ability to diffuse into neutrophils and kill phagocytosed bacteria.

Granulocyte transfusion therapy has been used with success in these patients, but such therapy is difficult. This is due to a lack of the normally present Kell antigens on the erythrocytes and leukocytes of these patients, increasing their susceptibility to develop transfusion reactions.

Glucocorticoid therapy has been tried but appears to offer no advantages.

Medical and surgical management have considerably improved the course and prognosis of this disorder over the past few years.

Anesthetic Considerations. Careful attention must be paid to aseptic techniques. Patients with CGD frequently harbor chronic infections or abscesses and may have draining sinuses from previous surgery. The high incidence of resistant organisms in these individuals who have been treated with numerous antibiotics makes isolation necessary.

The cardiopulmonary status needs assessment. Pericarditis has been reported, and pneumonitis and chronic pulmonary changes are common. Pulmonary function tests, arterial blood gases, and a current chest radiograph must be obtained preoperatively.

Obstruction of the gastric antrum by granuloma formation is frequent. Such obstruction may produce nausea and vomiting and may delay gastric emptying; thus, patients with CGD must be managed to avoid potential aspiration during induction of anesthesia.

The lack of the normally present Kell antigens on the erythrocytes and leukocytes complicates blood transfusion. There is a high risk for transfusion reactions, and the use of blood products containing red blood cells and/or leukocytes requires careful crossmatching. Such matching may require a longer than normal period. Similarly, emergency blood (type O, Rh negative) should be used only when absolutely necessary and then with extreme caution. Concurrent drug therapy must be assessed for potential interactions with anesthetic agents. Many antibiotics are known to interact with muscle relaxants.

The considerations mentioned above are some of the more common problems associated with chronic granulomatous disease. Table 16–6 delineates some of the other clinical manifestations of chronic granulomatous disease that have been reported.

Myeloperoxidase Deficiency

Myeloperoxidase deficiency is an autosomal recessive disorder characterized by the absence of myeloperoxidase from the granules of neutrophils and monocytes. This enzyme potentiates the bactericidal effectiveness of hydrogen peroxide, and its absence produces a bactericidal defect in neutrophils. The impairment is less severe than occurs in chronic granulomatous disease. This syndrome may be relatively common in the population, but because patients may not appear as unusually susceptible to infections it may not be as readily recognized as is chronic granulomatous disease.

Glucose-6-Phosphate Dehydrogenase Deficiency

Glucose-6-phosphate dehydrogenase (G6PD) deficiency is a relatively common inborn error of metabolism primarily affecting erythrocytes. Profound deficiencies of the enzyme (values less than 5 percent of normal) are rare, however, and it is only these profound deficiencies that affect neutrophil function. Such a deficiency produces a defect similar to chronic granulomatous disease with recurrent infections and granulomatous lesions. G6PD generates reduced pyridine nucleotide NADPH by the hexose monophosphate pathway, which is necessary for conversion of oxygen to superoxide and for maintaining intracellular levels of reduced glutathione.

Glutathione Peroxidase Deficiency

This enzyme is involved in the glutathione-dependent reduction of H_2O_2 to H_2O. Its deficiency results

Table 16–7. CELLULAR DEFECTS OF CHEMOTAXIS

Chédiak-Higashi syndrome
Shwachman syndrome
Panhypogammaglobulinemia
Lazy leukocyte syndrome
Hyperimmunoglobulin E and A
Down syndrome
Wiskott-Aldrich syndrome
Chronic renal failure
Acrodermatitis enteropathica
Mannosidosis
Leukemia
Kartagener syndrome
Anchor disease
Ichthyosis

in intracellular accumulation of H_2O_2 after the initial increase in hexose monophosphate pathway activity following phagocytosis. This accumulation results in injury or death of cells, producing neutropenia.

Disorders of Chemotaxis

Movement of PMNs to the site of infection within the first few hours is critical for the elimination of invading bacteria. Abnormal locomotion has been identified in many patients with recurrent serious infections. Such abnormal movement may result from cellular abnormalities or conditions with abnormal PMN chemotaxis, which are listed in Table 16–7.

Hyperimmunoglobulin E Syndrome (Job Syndrome)

Abnormal PMN chemotaxis has been identified in patients with extremely elevated levels of IgE. These patients present with recurrent severe staphylococcal infection, cellulitis, or subcutaneous or deep muscle abscesses. Eczema and atopic dermatitis is common. The association of staphylococal infections, defective phagocytic cell chemotaxis, eczema, and hyperimmunoglobulin E is common in this disease, although the degree of each individual abnormality is variable. Patients with Job syndrome frequently, but not always, have red hair. They generally develop severe bacterial infections within the first months of life. Pulmonary involvement is common, and pneumatoceles may develop and require surgical removal.

Although *Staphylococcus aureus* is the most commonly seen organism, others such as *Cryptococcus* and *Pneumocystis carinii* may be present and produce serious infection, suggesting an associated dysfunction of cell-mediated immunity.

Immotile Cilia Syndrome (Kartagener Syndrome)

Patients with this disorder demonstrate abnormal ciliary function and abnormal polymorphonuclear leukocyte motility. It is an autosomal recessive trait with an incidence of 1 in 4000. There are several consequences of this disorder, most of which are related to the abnormal ciliary function. Chronic otitis media and sinusitis are common in children due to impaired clearance from the sinuses, middle ear, and eustachian tubes. Males are sterile due to inadequate spermatozoal movement. Chronic bronchitis due to abnormal mucociliary clearance is common in children. Bronchiectasis is usually a late complication. Wheezing is common and is due to inadequate clearance of antigens from the lungs. Situs inversus is a usual finding in these patients and may be due to failure of ciliary-like activity during embryonal development. The presence of abnormal neutrophil chemotaxis further increases the susceptibility to infection. Associated abnormal ciliary function and neutrophil locomotion suggests a common physiological basis for these cellular activities.

Medical Management. Currently treatment is symptomatic and includes aggressive treatment of otitis media, sinusitis, and pulmonary infections with antibiotics, physiotherapy, and bronchodilators. *Haemophilus* and *Pneumococcus* are common infecting organisms. Prognosis is unknown, but morbidity due to bronchiectasis is considerable.

Anesthetic Considerations. Patients with Kartagener syndrome are at an increased risk of infection and are likely to be harboring pathogens. Their pulmonary status is of primary concern and must be optimized prior to surgery. Physiotherapy, bronchodilator therapy, and antibiotic coverage must be provided.

The presence of chronic otitis media and sinusitis may represent a contraindication to the use of nitrous oxide.

The presence of chronic infective processes demands that these patients be isolated to prevent cross contamination. Careful cleaning of the room and equipment after the procedure and utilization of disposable equipment when possible are indicated.

The neutrophil dysfunction increases susceptibility to infection even at sites that are not influenced by the ciliary dysfunction. Strict aseptic techniques are therefore necessary.

Shwachman Syndrome

Patients with Schwachman syndrome suffer pancreatic insufficiency and metaphyseal dyschondroplasia and are susceptible to recurrent infections, having depressed neutrophil chemotaxis. It is rare and is inherited in an autosomal recessive pattern. It is, however, the second most common cause of pancreatic insufficiency in children, after cystic fibrosis. Unlike in cystic fibrosis, the secretions are normal in Shwachman syndrome. In addition to impaired chemotaxis, neutropenia, thrombocytopenia, and hypoplastic anemia are present. The latter two are rarely a problem. The decreased number of cells seems to represent an arrest of maturation in the bone marrow.

Musculoskeletal abnormalities are common with metaphyseal dyschondroplasia producing short stature. Ribs may also be affected, and in some patients the thoracic cage may be sufficiently narrow to impair respiration.

Medical Management. There is no specific treatment available. Early in life patients require pancreatic supplements, but this may not be necessary for life as the malabsorption syndrome may improve. Most patients survive infancy, and their subsequent prognosis is usually good.

Infants suffer from malabsorption, and serum proteins may be depressed; these factors may affect drug distribution. Thrombocytopenia and anemia may be present and require correction prior to surgery. The musculoskeletal abnormalities may produce problems with positioning and the involvement of the rib cage may decrease chest wall compliance and compromise ventilatory parameters intraoperatively. The presence of neutrophil dysfunction requires consideration.

Lazy Leukocyte Syndrome

Patients with this syndrome have normal neutrophils in the bone marrow, but these cells display defective locomotion. This affects migration from the bone marrow to the circulation, producing neutropenia, and from the circulation to sites of inflammation. These patients are susceptible to upper respiratory infections and stomatitis.

Inhibitors of Chemotaxis

Patients with circulating inhibitors of chemotaxis present a similar clinical picture as those with cellular defects of chemotaxis. Table 16–8 lists conditions in which circulatory inhibitors have been demonstrated. Circulating inhibitors include a lymphocyte-derived chemotactic factor that is found in the serum of patients with Wiskott-Aldrich syndrome. Inhibitors of chemotaxis are present in normal plasma, but their levels are elevated in certain conditions such as Hodgkin disease. Polymeric IgA may inhibit normal chemotaxis in individuals with elevated levels of this immunoglobulin.

Deficiency of Chemotactic Factors

The absence of normal chemotactic factors can affect the efficiency of chemotaxis. The majority of these factors are derivatives of the complement system of proteins and have been discussed previously. Other causes are presented in Table 16–9; all are rare.

Mixed Functional Defects

Chédiak-Higashi Syndrome

The Chédiak-Higashi syndrome (CHS) is an autosomal recessive immunological disorder of neutrophil

Table 16–8. CIRCULATING INHIBITORS OF CHEMOTAXIS

Wiskott-Aldrich syndrome
Chronic mucocutaneous candidiasis
Rheumatoid arthritis
IgA myeloma
Hodgkin disease

Table 16–9. DEFICIENT PRODUCTION OF CHEMOTACTIC FACTOR

Absent C5
Hageman factor abnormality
Abnormal activation of C3
Systemic lupus erythematosus
Immunoglobulin deficiency

function. The immunological disorder consists of defects in chemotaxis, lysosomal degranulation, and intracellular killing. Giant cytoplasmic lysosomes are identified in leukocytes, lymphocytes, erythrocytes, and fibroblasts as well as in neurons and renal tubular epithelium. In neutrophils these granules appear to contain normal lysosomal enzymes, peroxidase, and acid phosphatase. Phagocytosis is normal, but degranulation of the lysosomes into the phagosome is inhibited. It has been suggested that microtubular function, necessary for normal chemotaxis and degranulation, may be altered in these patients, producing the abnormalities seen.

Patients with CHS are characterized by abnormal pigment of skin, hair, and eyes (partial oculocutaneous albinism), photophobia, and nystagumus. Neurological abnormalities may be present and include long tract signs, cerebellar involvement, peripheral neuropathies, and mental retardation.

The defect in neutrophil function results in frequent bacterial or fungal infections of the upper and lower respiratory tract and skin. Viral infections are handled normally.

Initially in infancy infections are minor and respond to appropriate antibiotic therapy. Later an accelerated phase occurs associated with lymphoid infiltration of all tissues, anemia, neutropenia, refractory infections, and hemorrhage associated with thrombocytopenia and defective platelet function, all of which require supportive therapy. Infections require aggressive antibiotic management, and many become refractory to therapy. Steroids, cytotoxic drugs, and splenectomy are utilized to attempt to induce remission but are rarely successful. The disease is commonly fatal in early childhood and death is most often secondary to infection.

Recently it has been demonstrated that normal microtubular function is regulated by 3′,5′ guanosine monophosphate (cyclic GMP). Agents that increase neutrophil cyclic AMP have been demonstrated to improve neutrophil function and have been used successfully in patients with CHS, but the long-term implications are unclear.

Anesthetic Considerations. Patients with CHS present several potential problems. Their susceptibility to recurrent respiratory infections may have left them with compromised pulmonary status. Chronic respiratory infections may be present and may be resistant to therapy. Vigorous therapy is required postoperatively to prevent serious complications. During progression of the disease and particularly during the accelerated phase, anemia and thrombocytopenia with defective platelet function may be present and require therapy. This may contraindicate certain techniques (for example, epidural anesthesia, intramuscular injections). The presence of peripheral neuropathies due to the disease or its treatment (see below) is a contraindication to the use of depolarizing muscle relaxants. Renal function may be impaired due to the involvement of the renal tubular epithelium. Concurrent antibiotic medication must be assessed, optimized, and evaluated for possible interaction with anesthetic agents. Supplemental steroid therapy may be required. The implications of cytotoxic agents if in use should be considered. Vincristine is commonly used and may produce a peripheral neuropathy, different in etiology from that described above, and may produce an autonomic dysfunction. Because of the susceptibility to infections, aseptic techniques are mandatory, and it is best to avoid techniques (such as epidural anesthesia) in which any complicating infection is likely to be devastating. The presence of chronic infections, many of which are resistant to antibiotic therapy, requires that anesthetic equipment be carefully cleaned prior to use with other patients and that, when possible, disposable equipment be utilized.

Postoperatively these patients require reverse isolation and isolation to prevent the spread of their chronic infections.

Actin Dysfunction

A defect in the actin filaments has been associated with recurrent bacterial infections with the formation of pus. The PMNs exhibited profoundly depressed chemotactic and phagocytic abilities. Bactericidal abilities are normal.

Bilobed PMN Nucleus

A bilobed PMN nucleus, intermittent neutropenia, deficient specific granules, defective bactericidal activity against *Staphylococcus aureus*, and impaired chemotaxis form the constellation of features of this rare disorder. Phagocytosis and other bactericidal activity are normal.

DISORDERS OF MONONUCLEAR LEUKOCYTES

Few functional defects of mononuclear leukocyte cells have been identified or well characterized. Those that have been described are similar to those seen in PMNs. Mononuclear leukocytes demonstrate depressed chemotaxis in conditions in which PMN chemotaxis is depressed. This includes allergic conditions with elevated immunoglobulin E, and the Wiskott-Aldrich syndrome (see Table 16–7). The anesthetic considerations are the same as described for defects of PMNs.

REFERENCES

Introduction

Babior BM: Oxygen-dependent microbial killing by phagocytes. N Engl J Med 298:659, 1978.

Fleidner TM, Cronkite EP, Killmann SA, et al.: Granulopoiesis. II. Emergence and pattern of labelling of neutrophilic granulocytes in human beings. Blood 24:683, 1964.

Mauer AM, Athens JW, Ashenbrucker H, et al.: Leukokinetic studies. II. A method for labelling granulocytes in vitro with radioactive de-isopropyl-fluorophosphate (DFP$_{32}$). J Clin Invest 39:1482, 1960.

Metcalfe D: Transformation of granulocytes into macrophages in bone marrow colonies in vitro. J Cell Physiol 77:277, 1971.

Nathan CF, Murray HW, Cohn ZA: The macrophage as an effector cell. N Engl J Med 303:622, 1980.

Quesenberry P, Levitt L: Hematopoietic stem cells. N Engl J Med 301:755, 1979.

Stossel TP: Phagocytosis. N Engl J Med 290:774, 1974.

Chronic Granulomatous Disease of Childhood

Ament ME, Ochs HD: Gastrointestinal manifestations of chronic granulomatous disease. N Engl J Med 288:382, 1973.

Boxer LA, Baehner RL: Defects in neutrophil leukocyte function. In Franklin EC (Ed.): Clinical Immunology Update. New York, Elsevier/North-Holland, 1981, p 357.

Clark RA, Klebanoff SJ: Chronic granulomatous disease. Studies of a family with impaired neutrophil chemotactic, metabolic and bactericidal function. Am J Med 65:941, 1978.

Curnette JT, Whitten DM, Babior BM: Defective superoxide production by granulocytes from patients with chronic granulomatous disease. N Engl J Med 290:1527, 1973.

Dupree E, Smith CW, MacDougall NLT, et al.: Undetected carrier state in chronic granulomatous disease. J Pediatr 81:770, 1972.

Gold SB, Hanes DM, Stites DP, et al.: Abnormal kinetics of degranulation in chronic granulomatous disease. N Engl J Med 291:332, 1974.

Griscom NT, Kirkpatrick JA Jr, Girdany BR, et al.: Gastric antral narrowing in chronic granulomatous disease of childhood. Pediatrics 54:456, 1974.

Johnston RB Jr, Baehner RL: Chronic granulomatous disease: correlation between pathogenesis and clinical findings. Pediatrics 48:730, 1971.

Lazarus GM, Neu HC: Agents responsible for infection in chronic granulomatous disease of childhood. Pediatrics 86:415, 1975.

Lobo, MC, Mandell GL: Treatment of experimental staphylococcal infection with rifampicin. Antimicrob Agents Chemother 2:195, 1972.

March WL, Oyen R, Nichols ME, et al.: Chronic granulomatous disease and the Kell blood group. Br J Haematol 29:247, 1975.

Melts, EL, Rholl KS, Quie PG: X-linked inheritance in females with chronic granulomatous disease. J Clin Invest 66:332, 1980.

Newberger PE, Cohen HJ, Rothchild SB, et al.: Prenatal diagnosis of chronic granulomatous disease. N Engl J Med 300:178, 1979.

Philippart AI, Colodny AH, Baehner RL: Continuous antibiotic therapy in chronic granulomatous disease: preliminary communication. Pediatrics 50:923, 1972.

Quie PG, White JG, Holmes B, et al.: In vitro bactericidal capacity of human polymorphonuclear leukocytes: diminished activity in chronic granulomatous disease of childhood. J Clin Invest 46:668, 1967.

Raubitschek AA, Levin AS, Stites DP, et al.: Normal granulocyte infusion therapy for aspergillosis in chronic granulomatous disease. Pediatrics 51:230, 1973.

Windhorst DB, Page AR, Holmes B, et al.: The pattern of genetic transmission of the leukocyte defect in fatal granulomatous disease of childhood. J Clin Invest 47:1026, 1968.

Myeloperoxidase Deficiency

Lehrer RI, Cline MJ: Leukocyte myeloperoxidase deficiency and disseminated *Candida*: the role of myeloperoxidase in resistance to *Candida* infection. J Lab Clin Med 93:232, 1979.

Salmon SE, Cline MJ, Schultz J, et al.: Myeloperoxidase deficiency: immunologic study of a genetic leukocyte defect. N Engl J Med 282:250, 1970.

Glucose-6-Phosphatase Deficiency

Cooper MR, DeChatelet LR, McCall CE, et al.: Complete deficiency of leukocyte glucose-6-phosphate dehydrogenase with defective bactericidal activity. J Clin Invest 51:768, 1972.

Glutathione Peroxidase Deficiency

Boxer LA, Oliver JM, Spielberg SP, et al.: Protection of granulocytes by vitamin E in glutathione synthetase deficiency. N Engl J Med 301:901, 1979.

Oliver JM, Spielberg SP, Pearson CB, et al.: Microtubule assembly and function in normal and glutathione synthetase-deficient polymorphonuclear leukocytes. J Immunol 120:1181, 1978.

Spielberg SP, Boxer LA, Oliver JM, et al.: Oxidative damage to neutrophils in glutathione synthetase deficiency. Br J Haematol 42:215, 1979.

Hyperimmunoglobulin E Syndrome

Gallin JI: Abnormal chemotaxis: Cellular and humoral components. *In* Bellanti JA, Dayton DH (Eds.): Phagocytic Cell in Host Resistance. New York; Raven Press, 1975, pp 227–248.

Gallin JI, Wright DG, Malech HL, et al.: Disorders of chemotaxis. Ann Intern Med 92:520, 1980.

Hill HR, Quie PG: Raised serum IgE levels and defective neutrophil chemotaxis in three children with eczema and recurrent bacterial infections. Lancet 1:183, 1974.

Miles AA, Miles EM, Burke J: The value and duration of defence reactions of the skin to the primary lodgement of bacteria. Br J Exp Pathol 38:79, 1957.

Schopfer K, Boerlocher K, Price P, et al.: Staphylococcal IgE antibodies, hyperimmunoglobulin E and staphylococcal infection. N Engl J Med 300:835, 1979.

Snyderman R, Pike MC: Disorders of leukocyte chemotaxis. Pediatr Clin North Am 24:377, 1977.

Steerman RL, Snyderman R, Leiken SL, et al.: Intrinsic defect of the polymorphonuclear leukocyte resulting in impaired chemotaxis and phagocytosis. Clin Exp Immunol 9:939, 1971.

Immotile Cilia Syndrome

Afzellius B: A human syndrome caused by immotile cilia. Science 193:317, 1976.

Eliasson R, Mossberg B, Camner P, et al.: The immotile cilia syndrome. N Engl J Med 297:1, 1977.

Fischer TJ, McAdams JA, Entis GN, et al.: Middle ear ciliary defect in Kartagener's syndrome. Pediatrics 62:443, 1978.

Pedersen H, Mygend N: Absence of axonemal arms in nasal mucosa cilia in Kartagener's syndrome. Nature 262:494, 1976.

Rooklin AR, McGeady SJ, Mikaelian DO, et al.: The immotile cilia syndrome: a cause of recurrent pulmonary disease in children. Pediatrics 66:526, 1980.

Sturgess JM, Chao J, Wong J, et al.: Cilia with defective radial spokes: a cause of human respiratory disease. N Engl J Med 300:53, 1979.

Shwachman Syndrome

Aggett PJ, Cavanagh NPC, Matthew DJ, et al.: Shwachman's syndrome. Arch Dis Child 55:331, 1980.

Burke V, Colebatch JH, Anderson CM, et al.: Association of pancreatic insufficiency and chronic neutropenia in childhood. Arch Dis Child 42:147, 1967.

Schussheim A, Choi SJ: Exocrine pancreatic insufficiency with congenital anomalies. J Pediatr 89:782, 1976.

Shmerling DH, Prader A, Hitwig WH, et al.: The syndrome of exocrine pancreatic insufficiency, neutropenia, metaphyseal dysostosis and dwarfism. Helv Pediatr Acta 24:547, 1969.

Lazy Leukocyte Syndrome

Miller ME, Oski FA, Harris MB: Lazy-leukocyte syndrome: a new disorder of neutrophil function. Lancet 1:665, 1971.

Deficiency of Chemotactic Factors

Gallin JI, Quie PG (Eds.): Leukocyte Chemotaxis: Methods, Physiology and Clinical Implications. New York, Raven Press, 1978.

Gallin JI, Wright DG, Malech HL, et al.: Disorders of chemotaxis. Ann Intern Med 92:520, 1980.

Hill HR, Quie PG: Raised serum IgE levels and defective neutrophil chemotaxis in three children with eczema and recurrent bacterial infections. Lancet 1:183, 1974.

Schopfer K, Baerlocher K, Price P, et al.: Staphylococcal IgE antibodies, hyperimmunoglobulinemia E and *Staphylococcus aureus* infections. N Engl J Med 300:835, 1979.

Synderman R, Pike MC: Disorders of leukocyte chemotaxis. Pediatr Clin North Am 24:377, 1977.

Chédiak-Higashi Syndrome

Blume RS, Wolff SM: The Chédiak-Higashi syndrome. Studies in four patients and a review of the literature. Medicine 51:247, 1972.

Boxer LA, Watanabe AM, Rister M, et al.: Correction of leukocyte function in Chédiak-Higashi syndrome by ascorbate. N Engl J Med 295:1041, 1976.

Clark RA, Kimball HR: Defective granulocyte chemotaxis in the Chédiak-Higashi syndrome. J Clin Invest 50:2645, 1971.

Dent PB, Fish LA, White JG, et al.: Chédiak-Higashi syndrome. Observations on the nature of the associated malignancy. Lab Invest 15:1634, 1966.

Gallin JI, Elin RJ, Hubert RT, et al.: Efficacy of ascorbic acid in Chédiak-Higashi syndrome (CHS): studies in humans and mice. Blood 53:226, 1979.

Leader RW: The Chédiak-Higashi anomaly—an evolutionary concept of disease. Nat Cancer Inst Monogr 32:337, 1969.

Malawista SE: Microtubules and the mobilization of lysosomes in phagocytizing human leukocytes. Ann NY Acad Sci 253:738, 1975.

Oliver JM: Impaired microtubule function correctable by cyclic GMP and cholinergic agonists in the Chédiak-Higashi syndrome. Am J Pathol 85:395, 1976.

Rausch PG, Pryzwansky KB, Spitznagel JK: Immunocytochemical identification of azurophilic and specific granule markers in the giant granules of the Chédiak-Higashi syndrome. N Engl J Med 286:120, 1972.

Root RK, Rosenthal AS, Balestra DJ: Abnormal bactericidal metabolic and lysosomal functions of Chédiak-Higashi syndrome leukocytes. J Clin Invest 51:649, 1972.

Stossel TP, Root RK, Vaughan M: Phagocytosis in chronic granulomatous disease and the Chédiak-Higashi syndrome. N Engl J Med 286:120, 1972.

Actin Dysfunction

Boxer LA, Hedley-Whyte ET, Stossel TP: Neutrophil actin dysfunction and abnormal neutrophil behavior. N Engl J Med 291:1093, 1974.

Bilobed PMN Nucleus

Komyama A, Morosawa H, Nakahata T, et al.: Abnormal neutrophil maturation in a neutrophil defect with morphologic abnormality and impaired function. J Pediatr 94:19, 1979.

Strauss RG, Boue KE, Jones JF, et al.: An anomaly of neutrophil morphology with impaired function. N Engl J Med 290:478, 1974.

Disorders of Mononuclear Leukocytes

Altman LC, Synderman R, Blaese RM: Abnormalities of chemotactic lymphokine synthesis and mononuclear leukocyte che-motaxis in Wiskott-Aldrich syndrome. J Clin Invest 54:486, 1974.

Rogge JL, Hanifin JM: Immunodeficiencies in severe atopic dermatitis: depressed chemotaxis and lymphocyte transformation. Arch Dermatol 112:1391, 1977.

Synderman R, Buckley RH: Defects of monocyte chemotaxis in patients with hyperimmunoglobulinemia E and undue susceptibility to infection. J Allergy Clin Immunol 55:102, 1975.

THE COMPLEMENT SYSTEM AND ASSOCIATED DISEASES

The Complement System
  Classical Pathway Activation
  Alternate Pathway Activation
  Regulatory Mechanisms

Inherited Disorders of the Complement System
  Autoimmune Phenomenon
  Bacterial Infections
  Hereditary Angioneurotic Edema
Secondary Disorders of the Complement System

THE COMPLEMENT SYSTEM

The complement system is a system of soluble proteins that interact with each other in a sequential fashion. It serves as the primary humoral effector system of inflammation against infection (Table 16–10). The complement system works via either the classical or the alternate pathway (Fig. 16–4). There are 20 components and regulators composing the complement system, all are proteins, and together they make up 10 percent of the globulin fraction of serum.

The components of the classical pathway are assigned numbers corresponding to the order of their discovery, not necessarily the same as their order of activation. Fragments of the component proteins resulting from their cleavage are assigned small letters (a, b, c, d, or e). With the exception of C2, released fragments are designated by "a" and the part of the component retained in the protein complex is assigned "b." An activated component is designated by a bar, for example, $\overline{C1}$. Components of the alternate pathway have been assigned letters B, D, and P (properdin). Factor 8 has an active form $\overline{Bb}$. The common feature of these pathways is that they both serve to activate C3.

Complement in association with antibody is necessary for the bactericidal capacity of serum. This is demonstrated by the fact that when complement is destroyed by heating serum, bactericidal capacity is lost even when antibody remains active.

Classical Pathway Activation (Fig. 16–4)

The combination of antigen with antibody produces a conformational change in the antibody exposing a binding site for the C1 component of the cascade. C1 is a trimolecular complex. It is bound by the C1q subunit to the Fc portion of the antibody. This produces a conformational change in the C1 component that results in the activation of the C1s component, an esterase. The third subunit (C1r) acts to bind the two reactive subunits. A second substance, C-reactive protein, can also initiate the binding of C1. Elevated in certain inflammatory states, C-reactive protein is not an antibody but a protein that can react with C-carbohydrates on microorganisms. It can combine with only a few organisms, but it does have the potential of initiating inflammation in the absence of antibody.

C4 and C2 are next bound, producing $\overline{C14b2a}$. C4a is released. This is an anaphylatoxin that induces mast cells to release mediators of immediate hypersensitivity. With the binding of C2, a kinin-like peptide is

Table 16–10. ACTIVITIES OF COMPLEMENT IN HOST DEFENSE AGAINST INFECTION

Components or Fragments	Functional Activity
C14, C1423	Neutralization of viruses
C4a, C3a, C5a	"Anaphylatoxin" (capillary dilation)
C5a	Chemotaxis of neutrophils, monocytes, eosinophils
C3b	Opsonization
C3b	Enhancement of cell-mediated cytotoxicity
C3b	Stimulation of production of B cell lymphokines
C3b, C3d	Enhanced induction of antibody formation
C3e	Induction of granulocytosis
Bb	Macrophage adherence and spreading
C5	Opsonization of fungi
C1–6 (? additional components)	Inactivation of endotoxin
C1–9	Lysis of viruses, virus-infected cells, tumor cells, mycoplasma, protozoa, spirochetes, and bacteria

From Johnston RB Jr: Complement and associated diseases. *In* Behrman RE, Vaughan VC III (Eds.): Nelson Textbook of Pediatrics. 12th ed. Philadelphia, W.B. Saunders Co., 1983.

Figure 16–4. Sequence of activation of the components of the classical pathway of complement and interaction with the alternate pathway. Regulator proteins are each enclosed in a box. Ag = antigen (bacterium, virus, tumor cell, or erythrocyte); Ab = antibody (IgG or IgM classes only); C-CRP = C carbohydrate–C-reactive protein; C1 INH = C1 inhibitor; C3b INA = C3b inactivator; C4-bp = C4-binding protein. (*From* Johnston RB Jr: Complement and associated diseases. *In* Behrman RE, Vaughan VC III (Eds.): Nelson Textbook of Pediatrics. 12th ed. Philadelphia, W. B. Saunders Co., 1983.)

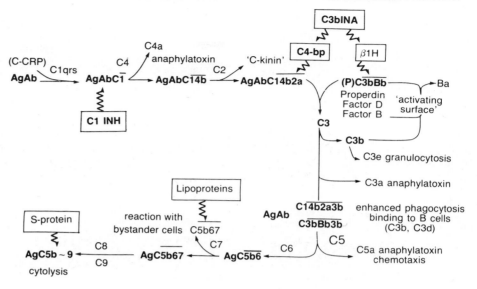

released that can increase vascular permeability and edema via action on postcapillary venules. C4b enables immune adherence of the complex to neutrophils, monocytes, and erythrocytes (known as immune adherence). C3 is activated next. The fixation of C3b enables adherence of the antibody-antigens to cells with C3b receptors, including neutrophils, monocytes, macrophages, B lymphocytes, and erythrocytes. This fixation is extremely important in phagocytosis by the phagocytic cells. The released C3a fragment has anaphylatoxin activity. C3b is broken down by C3b inactivator to produce C3d, which remains bound, and C3c, which is released. C3c is cleaved to C3e, which induces the release of granulocytes from the bone marrow.

C3 may also be activated by C3bBb of the alternate pathway (see below). The action of C14b2a3b or C3bBb3b on C5 releases C5a, an anaphylatoxin and chemoattractant for neutrophils, monocytes, and macrophages. C6 is bound to C5b but serves to stabilize the complex, not undergoing cleavage. The C5b6 complex next dissociates from the parent complex (C5 convertase) and combines with C7. The C5b67 complex attaches to the cell membrane and binds C8 and C9. The complex breaks the integrity of the cell membrane by forming a hole, producing cell lysis.

Alternate Pathway Activation (Fig. 16–4)

There are several mechanisms by which the alternate pathway can be activated. C3b can bind to B to form C3bB, which is then cleaved by D to form C3bBb. This becomes an efficient C3 convertase producing more C3b. C3 alone may bind to B to be cleaved to C3Bb, which is analogous to but less active than

C3bBb. Cleavage of B releases Ba, which has chemotactic activity. P (properdin) can bind to C3bBb, preventing decay-disassociation of B.

Other mechanisms for alternate pathway activation include activation of thrombin, plasmin, trypsin, or leukocyte proteases.

Regulatory Mechanisms (Fig. 16–4)

Regulatory mechanisms exist to protect the host. C1 inhibitor (C1 INH) inhibits C1s activity and therefore the cleavage of C2 and C4. The short half-life of C2 effectively limits the activity of the complexes in which it takes a part. The C3bBb of the alternate pathway has a short half-life, but this is increased by binding to properdin. C3a and C5a activity is controlled by a deactivating enzyme. C3b inactivator (C3b INA) is important in that it serves as a means of controlling both pathways. $\beta 1H$ increases the inactivation of C3b by C3b INA, and C4 binding protein accelerates cleavage of C4b by C3b INA.

INHERITED DISORDERS OF THE COMPLEMENT SYSTEM

Deficiencies or dysfunction of all components of the complement system have been described (Table 16–11). Not all of the deficiencies are associated with increased susceptibility to infection. Depending upon the particular component, patients may present with histories of (1) autoimmune disease, (2) recurrent bacterial infection, or (3) angioedema. Overlap of symptoms does occur.

Table 16–11. CONGENITAL DEFICIENCIES OF THE COMPLEMENT SYSTEM

Deficient Component*	Probable Inheritance†	Associated Clinical Findings‡
C1q	Not known	Recurrent infections, dermatitis, CGN
C1q dysfunction	AR (CD)	SLE syndrome
C1r	AR (CD)	CGN, SLE syndrome
C1s	Not known	SLE
C4	AR (CD)	SLE or SLE syndrome, discoid lupus erythematosus
C2	AR (CD)	SLE or SLE syndrome; MPGN; H-S purpura; dermatomyositis; septicemia, especially pneumococcal
C3	AR (CD)	Pyogenic infections, absence of expected neutrophilia; CGN
C5	AR (CD)	SLE; pyogenic infections; gonococcal, meningococcal infections
C5 dysfunction	AD	Pyoderma, septicemia, Leiner disease
C6	AR (CD)	Gonococcal, meningococcal infections, SLE syndrome
C7	AR (CD)	Sclerodactyly; chronic nephritis; gonococcal, meningococcal infections
C8	AR (CD)	Gonococcal, meningococcal infections; SLE syndrome
C8 dysfunction	Not known	Meningococcal infections
C9	AR (CD)	Meningococcal infections
C1 INH×	AD	Angioedema, SLE
C3b INA×	AR (CD)	Pyogenic infections

Abbreviations:

*INA = inactivator; INH = inhibitor.

†AD = autosomal dominant; AR = autosomal recessive; AR (CD) = autosomal recessive, co-dominant (heterozygotes have approximately half-normal serum levels).

‡CGN = chronic glomerulonephritis; H-S = Henoch-Schönlein; MPGN = membranoproliferative glomerulonephritis; SLE = systemic lupus erythematosus.

From Johnston RB Jr: Complement and associated diseases. *In* Behrman RE, Vaughan VC III (Eds.): Nelson Textbook of Pediatrics. 12th ed. Philadelphia, W. B. Saunders Co., 1983.

Autoimmune Phenomenon

Deficiencies of certain components of the classical activities pathway are associated with an increased incidence of rheumatic diseases. Patients with C1q, C1r, C1s, C2, C4, and C1 INH deficiencies present with rheumatic diseases but with less increased susceptibility to bacterial infection as occurs in other component deficiencies. This implies that alternate pathway activation may be sufficient for host protection. This results in C3 activation, which is required for opsonization of foreign organisms, which in turn promotes phagocytosis by neutrophils and macrophages. Deficiencies of C5, C6, C7, and C8 cause an increased susceptibility to bacterial infection as well as an increased incidence of rheumatic diseases. This susceptibility to infection is likely to be due to impairment of complement mediated cytolysis by the C5–C9 complex, decreasing resistance to infections (especially with *Neisseria*).

The etiology of the increased incidence of rheumatic diseases is unclear. It has been postulated that the classical activating pathway is in some way responsible for the clearance of immune complexes and that impairment of this function may predispose to rheumatic disease. A genetic basis linking complement genes with histocompatibility genes has also been suggested as a possible mechanism for the association.

Bacterial Infections

Complement factor 3 can be activated by either the classical or alternative pathways and, because of this, a defect in either pathway can be compensated for to some extent. Defects or deficiencies in C3 or beyond, however, result in a significant increase in the susceptibility to bacterial infection. Congenital absence of C3 is associated with recurrent pyogenic infections such as pneumococcal pneumonia and meningococcal meningitis. C3 is required for the opsonization of foreign organisms through production of C3b. Likewise, production of C3e causes an increase in neutrophil count, and C3 activation of C5 produces C5a, which is a chemotactic factor. Therefore, the lack of C3 reduces the efficiency of phagocytosis. Patients with deficiencies of C5, C6, C7, or C8 appear to be unusually susceptible to systemic *Neisseria* infections. This implies that complement-mediated serum bacteriolysis is an important factor in resistance to these organisms. Patients with a deficiency of C3b inactivator have a congenital deficiency of the regulatory protein of the C3 convertase of the alternate pathway. Such a deficiency allows continuous activation of C3 convertase, causing a decrease of C3 owing to its high rate of catabolism. These patients suffer the same symptoms as those that occur in C3 deficiency.

Medical Management. Certain complement defects

may be treated by plasma infusions to replace components. C5 abnormalities are due to a dysfunction rather than a deficiency, and repeated plasma infusions may be used to deter infections. In those with deficiencies rather than dysfunction of components, infusions of foreign complement components introduces a risk of antibody formation to these complement factors if long-term replacement therapy is attempted. Although replacement therapy may be used for a short period, most of the primary diseases of the complement system can receive only supportive management. The exact diagnosis of the defect is important. Patients with some defects (Table 16–11) are extremely susceptible to infections and require earlier and more aggressive intervention than others. Such patients should be immunized against bacterial antigens when possible.

Anesthetic Considerations. Because most of the disorders of complement result in some increase in susceptibility to infection, these patients should be treated with careful aseptic technique as previously described. Although many of the disorders can be treated only in supportive fashion, it is important to determine the specific defect. Associated disorders (Table 16–11) may have significant anesthetic implications that may demand varying techniques.

Hereditary Angioneurotic Edema

Hereditary angioneurotic edema (HAE) is a rare genetically determined (autosomal dominant) disorder of complement regulation. This disorder involves deficiency of the alpha globulin (C1 inhibitor) that inhibits the activated first component of complement (Fig. 16–4). Consequently, there is excessive consumption of C4 with low levels of this component during and between attacks. Clinical presentations are episodic and are characterized by swelling of the extremities, face, and bowel wall, leading to severe morbidity in many patients. Involvement of the upper airway with resultant asphyxia is a major cause of mortality.

Onset of the disorder is usually in the second or third decade, although symptoms may present at an advanced age. Diagnosis is established by demonstrating low levels of C1 inhibitor (5 to 30 percent of normal) and of C4. During attacks levels of C2 are also depressed. In about 15 percent of cases C1 inhibitor levels are reported to be normal by immunological measurements but low by functional assays. Inhibitor is present but functionally inactive.

Attacks can occur spontaneously (without an apparent cause) but more commonly can be attributed to physical or emotional trauma. During an attack, levels of C1 inhibitor and C4 and C2, the substrates of C1s, are depressed. The levels of other complement components are normal. A vasoactive peptide that increases local vascular permeability is generated during the attack and accounts for the development of the subepithelial edema. The nature of the peptide produced is not clear. It may be derived by the breakdown of C2, which produces the "C-kinin." It has also been postulated that trauma may activate the Hageman factor, which interacts with other cofactors initiating fibrinolysis, converting plasminogen to plasmin (Fig. 16–5). Plasmin activates C1 with subsequent breakdown of C2 and release of "C-kinin." Recently, however, it has been suggested that activation of the plasma kallikrein system may induce attacks of HAE. C1 inhibitor also normally inhibits activated Hageman factor and kallikrein, enzymes that participate in the generation of bradykinins. Minor damage to the vas-

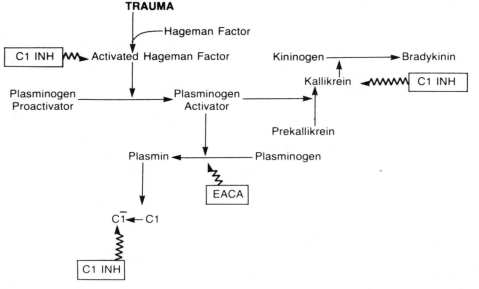

Figure 16–5. Schematic representation of the pathogenesis of hereditary angioneurotic edema by the production of bradykinin and activated complement factor 1. The sites of action of C1 INH and EACA are demonstrated. C1 INH = complement factor 1 inhibitor; EACA = epsilon aminocaproic acid; C1 = complement factor 1; C̄1 = activated complement factor 1.

cular interna may first facilitate the formation of activated Hageman factor locally and promote the activation of plasma kallikrein and the release of kinins, such as bradykinin, which can enhance vascular permeability and produce edema.

The cutaneous edema is not painful or itchy, nor is it accompanied by redness of the skin. Edema of the small bowel causes severe abdominal cramps and bilious vomiting. Colonic involvement produces a profuse watery diarrhea. Laryngeal edema is the most severe manifestation, and in the past up to 25 percent of patients with laryngeal involvement have suffered death from respiratory obstruction.

Medical Management. For patients who suffer infrequent and mild attacks, no ongoing therapy may be indicated. In more severe cases prophylaxis was, for many years, carried out by utilization of plasmin inhibitors such as epsilon-aminocaproic acid (EACA) or the use of anabolic steroids such as methyltestosterone. However, side effects made therapy with these agents unsatisfactory. EACA therapy is associated with muscle discomfort associated with a reversible elevation of serum enzymes, creatinine phosphokinase, and aldolase. The drug is also an antifibrinolytic agent, and as such may cause thrombotic episodes that may lead to serious consequences. Side effects of methyltestosterone include cholestatic jaundice, suppression of endogenous androgen production, and masculinization in women.

Danazol and stanozolol have been found to be extremely effective in preventing attacks of HAE. They suppress the pituitary ovarian axis by inhibiting the output of gonadotropins from the pituitary gland and interfere with hormonal target tissue interactions. The only hormonal activity other than pituitary inhibition is mild androgenic activity, which is dose-related. It is the androgenic activity that stimulates the synthesis of normal C1 inhibitor in patients with C1 inhibitor deficiency, without the side effects of methyltestosterone.

By raising levels of C1 inhibitor, these agents provide more effective regulation of C1 activation, Hageman factor, and kallikrein. Adverse effects of treatment with such attenuated steroids include impairment of growth rate in children (this has resulted in the preferential use of EACA in children in some centers), masculinization in women, and a reversible disturbance of liver function.

Management of ongoing episodes can be difficult. Often patients with involvement of the head and neck do not require hospitalization. Many episodes will resolve without treatment, and most others will respond to measures such as antihistamines and/or adrenergic agents. Failure of response or progression of symptoms will require hospitalization. Suggestion of airway involvement necessitates close observation, as these patients are in a high-risk category for mortality, and airway support by tracheostomy or intubation may be necessary.

The use of fresh frozen plasma (FFP) to supply active C1 inhibitor has for many years been debated as a treatment for ongoing episodes of HAE. The use of FFP has reportedly been sufficient to arrest an attack of HAE in progress, but well controlled studies have not been performed. The controversy arises in the treatment of ongoing attacks, because, in addition to C1 inhibitor, C2 and C4 are also supplied, and these may serve as additional substrates during an attack. The use of FFP also carries the risks associated with transfusion, such as hepatitis.

Recently, trials evaluating the replacement of C1 inhibitor protein partly purified from pooled plasma were carried out. In asymptomatic patients the administration of C1 inhibitor protein produced increases in C4 activity, indicating biological activity of the infused C1 inhibitor. Of greatest interest is that the administration of the C1 inhibitor during acute abdominal or laryngeal attack of HAE resulted in abatement of symptoms in addition to increased C4 activity. The initial treatment of the pooled plasma in preparing the concentrate is with 20 percent polyethylene glycol, which serves to precipitate C1 esterase, C2 and C4, and hepatitis B virus if present. Therefore the risk of transfusion-associated hepatitis B is minimized. This preparation, then, may offer safe effective replacement therapy and may provide a means of controlling an attack of HAE that is in progress.

Anesthetic Considerations. The problem faced in the management of patients is that attacks of HAE may be induced by physical or emotional trauma, both of which are present in the perioperative period.

Preoperatively, several aspects of these patients require special attention. The upper respiratory tract requires careful evaluation so that any evidence of edema in the early postoperative period may be quickly identified. Many patients require intubation that can produce local trauma, which, even if minimal, may be sufficient to induce an attack of HAE. The importance of this is demonstrated by the mortality rate of 25 to 30 percent with upper airway involvement. Attacks involving the gastrointestinal tract may produce a watery diarrhea, which necessitates careful evaluation of fluid and electrolyte status. Concurrent medications may involve drugs with attenuated androgen function. These drugs may affect hepatic function, and liver function tests should therefore be included preoperatively.

Levels of C1 inhibitor and C4 should be assessed preoperatively. Fifteen percent of patients have normal C1 inhibitor levels, but this C1 inhibitor is nonfunctional, and this can be demonstrated by depressed C4 levels in the presence of normal C1 inhibitor levels. In long-term management, because many of the side effects of androgen therapy can be annoying to patients, such as virilization in females, doses are generally reduced to the lowest level required to prevent attacks regardless of the measured C1 inhibitor.

For surgery, the ideal is to have the C1 inhibitor

and C4 as near as possible to normal levels. For elective surgery, the full therapeutic dose of androgen (danazol 200 mg orally t.i.d.) should be resumed for 7 to 10 days preoperatively with monitoring of C1 inhibitor and C4 levels. Such androgen treatment also results in the formation of a functional C1 inhibitor in patients with the variant form of the disease with an antigenically intact but functionally inactive C1 inhibitor. Plasmin inhibitors such as epsilon-aminocaproic acid and tranexamic acid also provide effective prophylactic treatment but due to their significant toxicities are rarely used today.

If an untreated patient requires emergency surgery, the administration of 5 to 10 ml/kg of FFP is recommended to supply C1 inhibitor. As discussed, if an attack of HAE has already started, FFP administration is controversial because it provides not only C1 inhibitor but also complement compounds that could worsen the attack. Partly purified C1 inhibitor is effective in acutely elevating C1 inhibitor levels without the addition of further complement compounds. It is also very effective in terminating ongoing episodes of HAE. Various doses have been suggested; interruption of attacks of HAE has been successful with infusions of 1000 plasma equivalents of C1 inhibitor, although up to 3000 plasma equivalents have been used.

The ability to elevate C1 inhibitor and C4 to normal levels has greatly assisted our management of the airway of these patients. Danazol pretreatment and FFP have been demonstrated to prevent attacks of HAE in patients undergoing oral surgery. Thus general anesthesia with an endotracheal tube may be safe when C1 inhibitor and C4 levels have been demonstrated to be normal. If concern exists the avoidance of oropharyngeal airways and endotracheal tubes is suggested. Conduction anesthesia has been successfully carried out in these patients.

Postoperatively, patients require monitoring in the intensive care unit for a period of time depending upon the type and extent of surgery. C1 inhibitor levels and C4 levels drop toward pretreatment levels by 36 hours and patients require early recommencement of androgen therapy or intravenous supplementation. Vital signs need to be closely monitored. With acute attacks use of the partly purified C1 inhibitor may be successful in their treatment. The development of eminent pharyngeal edema requires endotracheal intubation or tracheotomy.

Associated Conditions. Systemic lupus erythematosus and lymphoid cancers have been described in association with HAE.

SECONDARY DISORDERS OF THE COMPLEMENT SYSTEM

Defects in complement are seen in other conditions in which they occur secondary to or in association with the primary disorder.

The association of rheumatic disorders with certain complement deficiencies has been discussed. The presence of primary systemic rheumatic disorders is frequently associated with depressed concentrations of serum C1q, C4, and C3. In those conditions response to therapy may be demonstrated by return of complement levels to normal. In more localized rheumatic disorders, the serum levels of complement are frequently normal but synovial fluid will demonstrate decreased complement levels.

Certain renal diseases demonstrate alterations of serum complement levels. Poststreptococcal glomerulonephritis demonstrates depression of C3. An immunoglobulin G autoantibody termed nephritic factor is present in these cases. It serves to stabilize the $\overline{C14b2a}$ complex (the classical pathway C3 convertase) resulting in C3 deficiency due to catabolism. A similar situation is demonstrated in patients with chronic membranoproliferative glomerulonephritis and partial lipodystrophy. In these cases, the nephritic factor is once again an IgG autoantibody but is directed against $\overline{C3bBb}$ (the alternate pathway 3 convertase), again producing a C3 deficiency. Increased susceptibility to infection occurs when C3 levels decrease to below 10 percent of normal.

The frequency of pneumococcal infections in association with sickle cell disease and in patients who have undergone splenectomy can be explained in part by an as yet not fully defined defect of the alternate pathway.

Anesthetic Considerations. The anesthetic considerations in these patients are related to their primary disease, but additionally they demonstrate increased susceptibility to infection.

REFERENCES

Hereditary Angioneurotic Edema

Abada RP, Owens WD: Hereditary angioneurotic edema, an anesthetic dilemma. Anesthesiology 46:428, 1977.

Donaldson VH, Rosen FS, Bing DH: Role of the second component (C2) and plasmin in kinin release in hereditary angioneurotic edema (H.A.N.E.) plasma. Trans Assoc Am Phys 90:174, 1977.

Frank MM, Gelfand JA, Atkinson JP: Hereditary angioedema: the clinical syndrome and its management. Ann Intern Med 84:580, 1976.

Gadek JE, Hosea SW, Gelfand JA, et al.: Replacement therapy in hereditary angioedema: successful treatment of acute episodes of angioedema with partly purified C₁ inhibitor. N Engl J Med 302:542, 1980.

Gelfand JA, Sherins RJ, Alling DW, et al.: Treatment of hereditary angioedema with danazol: reversal of clinical and biochemical abnormalities. N Engl J Med 295:1444, 1976.

Gibbs PS, LoSasso AM, Moorthy SS, et al.: The anesthetic and perioperative management of a patient with documented hereditary angioneurotic edema. Anesth Analg 56:571, 1977.

Hosea SW, Santaella KL, Brown EJ, et al.: Long-term therapy of hereditary angioedema with danazol. Ann Intern Med 93:809, 1980.

Jaffe CJ, Atkinson JP, Gelfand JA, et al.: Hereditary angioedema: the use of fresh frozen plasma for prophylaxis in patients undergoing oral surgery. J Allergy Clin Immunol 55:386, 1975.

Landerman NS: Hereditary angioneurotic edema. I. Case report and review of the literature. J Allergy 33:316, 1962.

Michel RG, Hudson WR, Pope TH: Angioneurotic edema: a review of modern concepts. Arch Otolaryngol 101:544, 1975.

Ohela K, Rasanen JA, Wager O: Hereditary angioneurotic edema. Genealogical and immunological studies. Ann Clin Res 5:174, 1973.

Pence HL, Evans R, Gurnsey LH, et al.: Prophylactic use of epsilon aminocaproic acid for oral surgery in a patient with hereditary angioneurotic edema. J Allergy Clin Immunol 53:298, 1974.

Rothbach C, Green RL, Levine MI, et al.: Prophylaxis of attacks of hereditary angioedema. Am J Med 66:681, 1979.

Schapira M, Silver LD, Scott CF, et al.: Prekallikrein activation and high-molecular-weight kininogen consumption in hereditary angioedema. N Engl J Med 308:1050, 1983.

Secondary Disorders of the Complement System

Berkel AI, Loos M, Sanal O, et al.: Clinical and immunologic studies in a case of selective complete C1q deficiency. Clin Exp Immunol 38:52, 1979.

Colten HR: Biosynthesis of complement. Adv Immunol 22:67, 1976.

Corry JM, Polhill RB Jr, Edmonds SR, et al.: Activity of the alternate complement pathway after splenectomy: comparison to activity in sickle cell disease and hypogammaglobulinemia. J Pediatr 95:964, 1979.

Fearon DT: Complement. J Allergy Clin Immunol 71:520, 1983.

Fearon DT, Austin KF: The alternate pathway of complement: a system for host defense to microbial infection. N Engl J Med 303:259, 1980.

Halbwachs L, Leveillé M, Lesavre PH, et al.: Nephritic factor of the classical pathway of complement: immunoglobulin G autoantibody directed against the classical pathway C3 convertase enzyme. J Clin Invest 65:1249, 1980.

Hyatt AC, Altenburger KM, Johnston RB Jr, et al.: Increased susceptibility to severe pyogenic infections in patients with an inherited deficiency of the second component of complement. J Pediatr 98:412, 1981.

Johnston RB Jr: Complement and associated diseases. In Behrman RE, Vaughan VC III (Eds.): Nelson Textbook of Pediatrics. 12th ed. Philadelphia, W. B. Saunders Co., 1983, pp 516–518.

Johnston RB Jr, Stroud RM: Complement and host defense against disease. J Pediatr 90:169, 1977.

Lachman PJ, Rosen FS: Genetic defects of complement in man. Semin Immunopathol 1:339, 1978.

Sissons JGP, West PJ, Fallows J, et al.: The complement abnormalities of lypodystrophy. N Engl J Med 294:461, 1976.

URTICARIA AND ANGIOEDEMA

Pathophysiology
Etiology
Management

Urticaria and angioedema are cutaneous disorders that may result in fulminant cardiorespiratory collapse during anesthesia. In addition, the anesthesiologist may be called on to assist in the management of acute medical emergencies in these patients.

Urticaria is a cutaneous eruption characterized by diffusely distributed, raised wheals of varying size, shape, and number, which are red or pale and blanch under pressure. Urticarial lesions (commonly known as hives) are intensely pruritic and appear within minutes after a trigger stimulus. They usually resolve in 24 hours or less.

Angioedema is a generalized cutaneous eruption characterized by a single giant wheal that is neither erythematous nor pruritic. This lesion may cause a stinging, burning, or tingling sensation. In angioedema, the lesion appears slowly, evolving over a few hours, and resolves slowly over hours or days. Angioedema may occur on any part of the body, but is most common on the face, extremities, and genitalia. It may affect the mucous membranes of the upper airway, larynx, bronchi, gastrointestinal tract, and genitourinary tract. If laryngeal edema develops, the presenting signs may include hoarseness, stridor, dyspnea, and respiratory failure. Laryngeal edema, however, is a rare complication of urticaria and angioedema. Angioedema rarely affects the brain and meninges, conjunctiva, cornea, or uveal tract. Systemic angioedema may cause vomiting, diarrhea, and fluid sequestration. Severe fluid and electrolyte imbalance may result in cardiovascular instability and seizures.

The incidence of urticaria and angioedema in infants and children is about 3.4 percent. Up to 20 percent of young adults experience at least one episode of urticaria or angioedema by college age. Urticaria occurs more frequently in patients with a history of eczema and hay fever, and 2.5 times more frequently in patients with a history of asthma.

Urticaria and angioedema may occur either individually or together. When they appear together, urticaria is the predominant skin disorder. The "acute" form of these disorders is defined arbitrarily as an isolated episode lasting less than 6 weeks. The "chronic" form is defined as involving lesions that last 6 weeks or longer. The acute form is commonly a single, nonrecurrent episode that occurs more frequently in atopic children. The chronic form occurs as infrequently as once or twice per year or as often as many times per day. Eighty percent of all cases of urticaria and angioedema are idiopathic, without any known etiology, and 70 percent resolve completely within 1 year (90 percent within 5 years).

The lesions of urticaria and angioedema result from the triple response described by Lewis: first, a red reaction results from precapillary sphincter dilatation; second, an axon reflex results in an erythematous flare from arteriolar dilatation; and third, a wheal is formed by a serum transudate. The triple response is a result of the release of histamine and other mediators from the mast cells and basophils. Many mediators are capable of producing a triple response, including histamine liberators such as anaphylatoxin, trypsin, and acetylcholine and direct effectors such as serotonin, bradykinin, and kallikrein. Histamine is the most important mediator for the formation of urticarial lesions, although acetylcholine is predominant in cholinergic urticaria. In urticaria the lesions occur principally in the dermis, whereas in angioedema the lesions occur in the deep dermal and subcutaneous layers. In urticaria, irritation of the superficial cutaneous nerve endings results in pruritus, whereas in angioedema this does not occur.

PATHOPHYSIOLOGY

The wheals of urticaria and angioedema are transient evanescent lesions mediated by substances that produce edema, erythema, and pruritus. The most common mediators include histamine, serotonin, bradykinin, eosinophil chemotactic factor of anaphylaxis (ECF-A), arachidonic acid metabolites, and C3 and C5 fragments.

Histamine is released from preformed granules within mast cells and basophils, and causes erythema (vasodilation), edema (increased vascular permeability), and pruritus (irritation of the nerve endings). Histamine is also chemotactic for eosinophils. Other factors, such as the metabolites of arachidonic acid, are synthesized and released after the mast cells are stimulated. SRS-A (slow reacting substance of anaphylaxis), causes bronchial smooth muscle constriction and increases vascular permeability. PGE_1 or PGE_2 may cause both pain and the triple response.

Platelet activating factor (PAF) is also released from mast cells. PAF increases vascular permeability and, more importantly, stimulates the release of serotonin from platelets present at the site of action.

Serotonin is present in platelets in high concentrations. It is released after activation of PAF, which itself is derived from mast cells. Serotonin probably amplifies the principal mast cell degranulation and directly causes erythema.

The importance of SRS-A and PAF in these reactions in humans is not completely understood.

Acetylcholine causes vasodilatation and erythema when injected into the dermis. It may modulate mediator release from mast cells, although its role in humans has not been fully elucidated.

The activation of complement is responsible in part for the genesis of the lesions in urticaria and angioedema. Both C3a and C5a are products of complement

activation and are potent anaphylatoxins. They adhere to the surface of mast cells (even in the absence of antibodies) and cause the mast cells to degranulate and release histamine. C5a is a more potent anaphylatoxin than C3a. C5a also increases vascular permeability and is a chemotactic factor for neutrophils, eosinophils, and mononuclear cells.

Bradykinin is another important mediator that is released during urticaria and angioedema. Bradykinin is the end product of a chain of converting enzymes and their products. When a small quantity of Hageman factor is activated, it in turn activates kallikrein. Kallikrein converts kininogen to the vasoactive peptide, bradykinin. Bradykinin is a potent vasodilator and increases vascular permeability to the same extent as histamine. At high serum concentrations, bradykinin may cause profound hypotension. It also irritates nerve endings, causing a burning pain in the area of the lesions.

The vasoactive mediators may be released by one of two mechanisms: immunological or nonimmunological. The immunological mechanism includes the classic type I, II, or III allergic reactions. Type I reactions, the immediate hypersensitivity reactions, are those in which an inhaled, ingested, or parenterally administered trigger binds to IgE on the surface and results in the release of histamine and other mediators.

Type II reactions, the cytotoxic mechanism, occur when IgG or IgM binds to an antigen on a cell surface and activates complement. ABO blood type incompatibility is an example of such a reaction. Type III reactions are those in which antigen-antibody complexes (IgG, IgM, or IgA) deposit in target tissues, activate complement, and release mast cell mediators through the action of C3a and C5a. Serum sickness is mediated by such a mechanism.

Nonimmunological stimuli are very important in the pathogenesis of urticaria and angioedema. Table 16–12 lists those important factors considered responsible for this mechanism of action.

Table 16–12. NON-IMMUNOLOGICAL CAUSES OF URTICARIA

Drugs
Food
Physical urticarias
  Cold
  Cholinergic
  Pressure
  Dermographia
  Solar
  Vibratory
Mastocytosis
Hereditary diseases
  Hereditary angioedema
  C3b inactivator deficiency
  Familial cold urticaria
  Urticaria, deafness, amyloidosis syndrome
Malignancy
Idiopathic

The final common pathway for mediator release is degranulation of the mast cells. The message from cell surface to degranulation follows a series of steps which likely involve changes in membrane potential, cyclic nucleotide concentrations, and sodium and calcium transmembrane fluxes. This is important in the drug management of this disorder.

ETIOLOGY

The etiology of urticaria and angioedema is diverse. The following is a brief description of some of the more relevant causes:

Drugs. The most common cause of urticaria and angioedema is the administration of drugs: oral, rectal, or parenteral. Drugs cause urticaria and angioedema by one of five possible mechanisms: (1) type I IgE hypersensitivity reaction, (2) type III antigen-antibody reaction, (3) direct histamine release from mast cells, (4) complement activation, and (5) alteration in arachidonic acid metabolism.

Those drugs commonly responsible for urticaria and angioedema include codeine, morphine, demerol, penicillin, aspirin and nonsteroidal anti-inflammatory drugs, diuretics, and hormones.

The drug responsible for the urticaria or angioedema is identified by a careful history. Because more than one drug may be taken concurrently, this may be difficult. All drugs must be stopped if possible and then reintroduced one at a time to determine which is responsible. Skin testing is useful only for IgE-mediated urticaria and angioedema and has many false positive reactions. The radioallergosorbent test (RAST) measures IgE concentration following administration of a drug. However, this test is available only on a limited basis and has many false negative results.

Blood. Urticaria and angioedema may occur in response to a blood transfusion, because of (1) ABO incompatibility, (2) type II complement-mediated cytotoxic reaction, (3) type I and III reactions, particularly following administration of fresh frozen plasma, factor VIII, and cryoprecipitate, and (4) trace concentrations of haptens in the blood.

Food. Food may cause urticaria and angioedema by type I (IgE-mediated) hypersensitivity reaction or through a direct effect on histamine release. Food dyes (tartrazine) and additives such as sodium benzoate are responsible for urticaria in up to 15 percent of patients.

Infections and Infestations. Urticaria and angioedema have been reported after most bronchial, viral, fungal, and parasitic diseases. Viral respiratory infections are a major cause of urticaria in children. Approximately 25 percent of patients with hepatitis and 6 percent with infectious mononucleosis have urticaria during their illnesses. Most infections cause acute urticaria and angioedema; only rarely do infections cause chronic manifestations. Infections may induce urticaria through type III and, less commonly, type I allergic reactions.

Physical Urticarias. Physical stimuli may cause urticaria by releasing histamine, and this effect is reproducible. Other mediators that may be responsible for this type of urticaria include serotonin and ECF-A.

Cold Urticaria and Angioedema. Cold-induced urticaria and angioedema are precipitated by changes in temperature, either warm or cold. The mediators responsible for the reaction include histamine and ECF-A. Cold-induced urticaria and angioedema may occur as isolated lesions or in association with other diseases such as cold agglutination, cryoglobulinemia, cryofibrinogenemia, and paroxysmal hemoglobinemia of the Donath-Landsteiner type. The lesions in cold-induced urticaria may be either focal or diffuse and can be associated with systemic symptoms such as nausea, vomiting, headache, tachycardia, and syncope. To test for cold urticaria, an ice cube is placed on the volar aspect of the forearm for 4 minutes, and the site is observed for 10 minutes. The therapy for cold-induced urticaria is the use of cryoprecipitate (periactin), an antihistamine, in a dose of 0.2 mg/kg/day.

Cholinergic Urticaria. In this type of urticaria, stimuli such as exercise, sweating, heat, and anxiety cause acetylcholine release from parasympathetic (and sympathetic) nerve fibers. Acetylcholine causes the release of vasoactive mediators such as histamine and ECF-A. Intradermal injection of 100 μl of methacholine will produce a wheal and flare response in patients with cholinergic urticaria. Effective therapy includes hydroxyzine (Atarax), 1 to 3 mg/kg/day in divided doses.

Pressure Urticaria and Angioedema. Pressure-induced urticaria and angioedema occur under the pressure points of the body. Lesions may begin within minutes or up to 24 hours after stimulation. Fever, chills, and nausea may occur in the delayed form. The diagnosis is verified by the appearance of lesions at the sites of pressure. The therapy is to avoid pressure on bony points by such techniques as the use of padding. Antihistamines are relatively ineffective, although theophylline and corticosteroids do work in some patients.

Dermographia. This variety of urticaria results from stroking the skin. The wheal and flare response occurs immediately after stroking and resolves within 30 minutes. In approximately 50 percent of patients dermographia is IgE-mediated. It is seen in 5 percent of normal patients, in some patients with chronic idiopathic urticaria, and in mastocytosis. Therapy for dermographia includes antihistamines.

Melkersson Syndrome. This rare syndrome is associated with angioedema of the face, peripheral facial nerve palsy, and lingua plicata.

Urticaria-Deafness-Amyloidosis Syndrome. This very rare inherited syndrome begins in adolescence with frequent but brief attacks of an urticaria-like rash. This syndrome is associated with progressive nerve deafness, hyperglobulinemia, nephropathy, and amyloidosis.

Systemic Diseases. There are a small number of systemic diseases that may be associated with urticaria and angioedema.

Urticaria and angioedema are often associated with serum sickness, a type III allergic reaction. Among the many causes of serum sickness are drugs, including penicillin, cephalosporins, and sulfonamides. Serum sickness is usually self-limiting and resolves once the drugs are discontinued.

The connective tissue disorders, juvenile rheumatoid arthritis, acute rheumatic fever, and lupus erythematosus may be associated with the skin lesions of urticaria and angioedema. The patients have multisystemic signs and symptoms associated with the connective tissue disorder, which simplifies the diagnosis of the urticarial lesions.

Urticaria and angioedema may be associated with lymphomas and carcinomas, but there are relatively few cases in the pediatric literature. Urticaria is rarely associated with thyrotoxicosis. Urticaria pigmentosa and systemic mastocytosis are discussed on page 476.

Idiopathic Urticaria and Angioedema. Thorough investigation will result in a diagnosis in only 5 to 20 percent of patients. The remainder have chronic urticaria or angioedema of unknown etiology. This disease occurs most frequently in women in their third or fourth decade, and is benign without associated systemic manifestations or complications. It is rare in childhood.

MANAGEMENT

Acute self-limited urticaria in patients under anesthesia does not usually require therapy. However, if the urticaria is generalized, immediate management may be required to prevent circulatory and respiratory collapse. This most commonly occurs in hereditary angioneurotic edema. Therapeutic management includes epinephrine, H_1 and H_2 antihistamines, theophylline, and other sympathomimetics. For the drug doses required, refer to the sections on Anaphylaxis and Asthma later in this chapter. H_1 and H_2 blockers may act synergistically to reduce the size of the wheal and flare response to intradermal histamine. However, up to 50 percent of patients do not respond completely to combined H_1 and H_2 antihistamine therapy. Antihistamines bind to the histamine receptors or the effector cells. They reduce the severity of pruritus and the evolving lesions. However, antihistamines do not speed the resolution of lesions that are already present. Steroids have been used with varying success.

Urticaria may occur at the site of intravenous blood transfusion. This reaction may be treated with parenteral H_1 antihistamines. The blood transfusion may be continued. If signs of the systemic manifestations of a transfusion reaction develop, such as fever, cyanosis, hypotension, and oliguria, then the blood transfusion should be stopped and returned to blood bank for further cross-matching. Resuscitation should include oxygen, H_1 and (if necessary) H_2 antihistamines, sympathomimetics, and fluids.

Preoperative Assessment. The diagnosis of urticaria and angioedema is often made before the anesthetist contacts the patient. The precipitating causes and the local and systemic manifestations of the lesions must be carefully enumerated and recorded. Most of the nonsystemic forms manifest local reactions only and do not present life-threatening problems during anesthesia. However, if any of the systemic disorders are responsible for the skin lesions, then a careful history and physical examination for the stigmata of rheumatoid arthritis, lupus erythematosus, lymphoma, carcinoma, and systemic mastocytosis must be performed. In all cases, previous medical records must be obtained to examine the course of the previous anesthetics. Careful questioning to elicit a history of recent steroid administration must be documented on the preoperative record.

Intraoperative Course. The principal goal of the management of patients with urticaria and angioedema under anesthesia is to avoid all trigger stimuli. Those drugs that are known to trigger urticaria should be avoided. Furthermore, it is advisable to avoid those drugs that may release histamine (see the section on Anaphylaxis later in this chapter). If temperature is the trigger of urticaria, then the operating room should be warmed before the patient arrives, and all facilities for maintaining temperature control should be made available. All pressure points should be padded. Specific considerations for patients with systemic illness associated with urticaria depend on the individual disease.

REFERENCES

Beall GN: Urticaria: a review of laboratory and clinical observations. Medicine *43*:131, 1964.

Benveniste J, Kamoun P, Polonsky J: Aggregation of human platelet activating factor from human and rabbit basophils (abstract). Fed Proc *34*:985, 1975.

Champion RH, Roberts SOB, Carpenter RG, et al.: Urticaria and angio-oedema. Br J Derm *81*:588, 1969.

Clark RAF, Gallin JI, Kaplan AP: The selective eosinophilic chemotactic activity of histamine. J Exp Med *172*:1462, 1975.

Collins-Williams C. Urticaria and angioedema. *In* Kelley VC (Ed.): Practice of Pediatrics. Vol. 2. Philadelphia, Harper & Row, 1984.

Harvey RP, Schocket AL: The effect of H_1 and H_2 blockade on cutaneous histamine release in man. J Allergy Clin Immunol *65*:136, 1980.

Kaplan AP. Urticaria and angioedema. *In* Middleton E, Reed CE, Ellis EF (Eds.): Allergy: Principles and Practice. Vol 2. St. Louis, C. V. Mosby Co., 1983.

Kettel K: Melkersson's syndrome: report of 5 cases, with special reference to pathologic observations. Arch Otolaryngol *46*:341, 1947.

Plant M: Histamine, H_1 and H_2 antihistamines, and immediate hypersensitivity reactions. J Allergy Clin Immunol *63*:371, 1975.

Schneider SB, Atkinson JP: Urticaria and angioedema. *In* Fitzpatrick TB, Eisen AZ, Wolff K, et al. (Eds.): Update: Dermatology in General Medicine. New York, McGraw-Hill, 1983, p 61.

Sheffer AL: Urticaria and angioedema. Pediatr Clin North Am 22:193, 1975.

Sly RM: Urticaria and angioedema. *In* Berman, BA, MacDonnell KF (Eds.): Differential Diagnosis and Treatment of Pediatric Allergy. Boston, Little, Brown, 1981.

Smith GB, Shribman AJ. Anaesthesia and severe skin disease. Anaesthesia 39:443, 1984.

Twarog FJ: Urticaria in childhood: pathogenesis and management. Pediatr Clin North Am 30:887, 1983.

Voss MJ, O'Connell EJ, Hick JF, et al.: Association of acute urticaria in children with respiratory tract infections. J Allergy Clin Immunol 69:134, 1982.

Warin RP, Champion RH. Urticaria. London, W. B. Saunders Co., 1974, p 10.

ASTHMA

Etiology
Pathogenesis
Pathophysiology
Preoperative Management
    History

Physical Examination
Laboratory Tests
Drug Therapy
Anesthetic Management

Asthma is a chronic disorder of the tracheobronchial tree characterized by paroxysmal increases in airway resistance of varying degree and duration that are partially or totally reversible either spontaneously or pharmacologically. The defect in asthma is a hyper-responsiveness of the airways to both endogenous and exogenous stimuli. The clinical spectrum of asthma ranges from occasional wheezing to chronic debilitating episodes of airway obstruction and shortness of breath, which may progress in some cases to respiratory failure (status asthmaticus).

Asthma is one of the most common chronic diseases afflicting children. The prevalence varies with age: it is most common in young children, less common in adolescents, and again more common in adults. Asthma affects 0.06 to 12 percent of children in different populations, with a predominance in males. This large variation may be attributable to differences in geographic location (0.06 percent in Sweden) and in the criteria for diagnosis (12 percent includes those children who wheeze only during respiratory infections). Asthma accounts for 11 percent of all chronic diseases in children under 17 years of age and for approximately 23 percent of all school days missed because of chronic diseases in the United States. About 70 percent of asthmatic children experience wheezing by 3 years of age. Of those children with mild asthma beginning before 10 years of age, most will be symptom-free by adulthood. In contrast, of those children with moderate to severe asthma beginning between 3 and 10 years of age, approximately one third will continue to wheeze during adulthood. Some of this latter group may then become incapacitated. The number of hospital admissions for asthma is greatest in infants and children and decreases with increasing age. Mortality is approximately 1.1 per 100,000 children, and is 1 to 2 percent in children with chronic severe asthma. Mortality is more frequent in those under 5 years or between 10 and 14 years of age. In these older children death is often attributable to relative drug overdoses.

ETIOLOGY

Asthma may be classified into the following groups based on its causes: (1) extrinsic (allergic), (2) intrinsic (nonallergic, infectious, idiopathic), (3) exercise-induced, (4) aspirin-induced, (5) occupational, and (6) mixed.

Extrinsic Asthma. Extrinsic asthma is caused by either IgE or cytotoxic IgG activated mast cell and basophil mediator release (type I allergic reaction). In infants and children, extrinsic asthma may be heralded by atopic dermatitis (eczema), allergic rhinitis, and food intolerance. It is reported to occur in up to 50 percent of infants and children with a history of eczema. Furthermore, of those children with two mildly atopic parents, 50 percent will have mild atopy, 25 percent will have severe atopy, and 25 percent will be spared. This suggests an autosomal codominant pattern of inheritance. Although skin testing is used to detect allergic tendencies it may be unreliable, particularly in children under 4 years of age.

Intrinsic Asthma. Intrinsic asthma is a diagnosis of exclusion, in which no allergic etiology is detectable. Intrinsic asthma occurs more commonly in adolescents and adults than in children, and is often associated with respiratory tract infections. Asthmatic bronchitis refers to wheezing associated with viral infections, usually in children under 3 years of age. The viruses responsible for these infections in younger children are the respiratory syncytial virus and the parainfluenza B virus; in older children and adults the most common causative viruses are the rhinovirus and influenza A virus.

The mechanism of wheezing during a viral respiratory infection is unclear. Asthmatic bronchitis presents with signs of an upper respiratory infection (rhinorrhea and nasal congestion) that progresses to coughing and wheezing. The characteristic upper respiratory infection usually lasts longer than expected, and is more debilitating than expected. Bacterial infections have never been demonstrated as the cause of asthmatic bronchitis in children. Inflammation of the nasal passages and systemic signs such as fever may be present. A significant percentage of children with asthmatic bronchitis progress to asthma.

Intrinsic asthma causes reflex bronchoconstriction, which may be attenuated by inhaled atropine. This suggests that intrinsic asthma may be mediated by a reflex cholinergic pathway. Airways are hyperresponsive to inhalational challenges with methacholine and histamine.

Exercise-Induced Asthma. Exercise-induced asthma (EIA) occurs in 90 percent of children with asthma and 40 percent of children with allergic rhinitis. EIA can occur after as little as 5 minutes of exercise and lasts between 20 minutes and several hours. The mechanism postulated for EIA is a decrease in the temperature of the airways and possibly hyperventilation. This results in the release of mediators and reflex bronchospasm. Patients respond well to cromolyn sodium, beta-adrenergic inhalers, and theophylline.

Aspirin-Induced Asthma. This syndrome is a triad of aspirin sensitivity, hyperplastic rhinitis (associated with polyps and sinus infections), and asthma. It is more frequent in adults than in children. Some patients manifest only part of the triad of symptoms. Aspirin tolerance extends to all nonsteroidal anti-inflammatory agents, including tartrazine. Tartrazine (yellow dye No. 5) is present in many foods (ice cream, gelatins, beverages) and drugs. It is prudent to check the contents of all drugs prior to administration in any patient with a known sensitivity to aspirin. The mechanism of aspirin-induced wheezing is unclear, but may be mediated through increased synthesis of prostaglandins (PGF_{2a}, PGD_2) and leukotrienes (including slow-reacting substance of anaphylaxis, SRS-A).

Occupational Asthma. This rare form of asthma is seen infrequently in pediatric practice. Once the patient is removed from the stimulus, the asthma resolves.

Mixed Asthma. Any combination of the preceding forms of asthma may be found in any one individual. Treatment follows the general therapeutic guidelines.

PATHOGENESIS

Airway hyperresponsiveness is the hallmark of asthma. It causes bronchoconstriction in response to a challenge of inhaled, physical, or pharmacological stimuli. There is evidence to suggest that airway hyperreactivity may originate from either an imbalance of the autonomic neural control or mast cell dysfunction. Neural control of the tracheobronchial tree influences the bronchomotor tone through four possible pathways: (1) beta$_2$-adrenergic hyperreactivity or (2) nonadrenergic inhibitory pathways decreasing bronchomotor tone, or (3) alpha-adrenergic hyperreactivity or (4) cholinergic hyperreactivity increasing bronchomotor tone.

Although the sympathetic innervation of the tracheobronchial tree is scant, the sympathetic nervous system has a strong influence on bronchomotor tone through the first messenger pathway, hormones. Epinephrine is the most important circulating hormone in asthma. The beta$_2$-adrenergic receptor activates membrane-bound adenyl cyclase to produce $3'5'$ cyclic AMP (cAMP) (second messenger). An increase in cAMP exerts two effects on bronchomotor tone: (1) it diminishes the release of mediators from the mast cells and basophils, and (2) it decreases the tone of the smooth muscle of the airways. cAMP is metabolized by phosphodiesterase, a pathway that may be pharmacologically important in the mechanism of action of theophylline. It has been suggested that beta$_2$-hyporeactivity may be responsible for bronchial hyperreactivity in asthmatics. Although the cAMP response to beta$_2$-agonist stimulation in some atopic and asthmatic models is blunted, there is no evidence in humans that beta$_2$-hyporesponsiveness is the mechanism responsible for bronchial hyperreactivity.

The nonadrenergic nervous system is an incompletely defined alternate nervous pathway that was recognized first for its ability to relax the gastrointestinal smooth muscle. Activation of this nervous pathway relaxes the smooth muscle of the airway. Although inhibition of this pathway may cause an increase in bronchomotor tone, there is no experimental evidence linking the nonadrenergic pathway to the pathogenesis of asthma in humans.

Alpha-adrenergic stimulation causes a small increase in bronchomotor tone. Airway hyperreactivity in asthma may be in part dependent on an alpha-adrenergic hyperresponsiveness.

The cholinergic pathway, carried by vagal fibers in the lung, primarily controls the tone of the central airways (larynx and bronchi). Stimulation of the cholinergic receptors increases cytoplasmic cGMP (a second messenger). The effects of cGMP are opposite to those of cAMP: cGMP increases the release of mediators from mast cells and basophils, and it increases bronchomotor tone. Inhalation of methacholine (a cholinergic agonist) has been shown to increase bronchomotor tone in the asthmatic.

The afferent and efferent pathways for the cholinergic fibers have been well defined. The vagal afferent pathway begins at the irritant receptors in the lung, synapses in the central nervous system, and returns through vagal efferent pathways. This afferent irritant pathway may be important in understanding the mechanism by which drugs and foreign bodies (for example, endotracheal tubes) precipitate rapid reflex increases in bronchomotor tone.

Mast cell dysfunction may result in hyperresponsive airways in allergic patients or in patients with intrinsic asthma. When the membrane surface is activated, a number of intermediary events begin that culminate in the release of the mediators of anaphylaxis: histamine, eosinophil chemotactic factor (ECF-A), neutrophil chemotactic factor (NCF-A), kallikrein, and in the synthesis and release of the leukotrienes (including slow-reacting substance of anaphylaxis, SRS-A). Platelet activating factor (PAF) is released not only from the mast cell but also from polymorphonuclear leukocytes.

In the asthmatic, arachidonic acid is liberated by either phospholipase A_2 or by the resultant action of phospholipase C from membrane phospholipids. Adrenal corticosteroids may reduce bronchospasm by preventing the activation of phospholipase A_2 and thus the release of arachidonic acid. Prostaglandins may be synthesized after activating cyclo-oxygenase, lipoxygenase, H_1 receptors, bradykinin, leukotrienes, prostaglandin generating factor, and smooth muscle bronchoconstriction. Cyclo-oxygenase metabolizes arachidonic acid into a number of prostaglandins. PGD_2 is the major prostaglandin synthesized in mast cells, and PGE_2 is the major prostaglandin from polymorphonuclear white cells. PGI_2 (prostacyclin) is synthesized in vascular endothelium, and thromboxane A_2 originates in platelets. PGD_2, PGF_2, and thromboxane A_2 cause bronchoconstriction, whereas PGE_2 causes bronchodilatation. PGD_2 causes vasodilatation. In a parallel pathway, lipoxygenase metabolizes arachidonic acid into leukotrienes C, D, and E. These three combine to form SRS-A, an important mediator of bronchoconstriction. In addition, leukotriene D increases vascular permeability and is a vasodilator, and leukotriene B has chemotactic activity for granulocytes.

Increased cytoplasmic calcium may in part cause bronchial hyperreactivity, although supportive evidence is weak. Verapamil or nifedipine may prove to be of value in the treatment of pediatric asthma.

Mediator Action. Histamine (via H_1 receptors), bradykinin, leukotrienes C, D, and E, PGD_2, PGF_2 and thromboxane A_2 all produce bronchoconstriction. Histamine, bradykinin, leukotrienes C, D, and E, and PGE increase capillary permeability, which reduces intravascular volume and may produce edema, syncope, and, if severe, cardiac arrest. Histamine can stimulate the submucosal glands (via cholinergic receptors). In decreasing order of potency, leukotriene D, leukotriene C, PGF_2, PGD_2, PGI_2, and PGE_1 stimulate secretions of the mucous glands. With prolonged mucus production and bronchoconstriction, desquamated cells of the tracheobronchial tree and secretions may become inspissated (forming Charcot-Leyden crystals) and plug the airways. This may worsen ventilation/perfusion mismatch. Inspissated secretions in the mold of bronchioles (Curschmann spirals) may be seen if the sputum is examined.

PATHOPHYSIOLOGY

The clinical signs and symptoms of asthma result from a triad of pathophysiologic changes in the tracheobronchial tree: (1) a reduction in the diameter of the airways, (2) inflammatory thickening of the bronchial mucosa, and (3) the accumulation of tenacious secretions. Bronchospasm results from smooth muscle constriction and causes narrowing of the central airways; it is responsible for most acute episodes of asthma. Chronic inflammation and the accumulation of tenacious secretions also narrow the diameter of the peripheral airways and are responsible for the chronic changes seen in asthma. Because both the pathophysiological changes in the tracheobronchial tree and the primary site of airway involvement vary from child to child, the therapeutic management must be carefully individualized.

The pathophysiological changes in asthma affect all indices of pulmonary function. Because of physiological differences in the respiratory system, children are more susceptible than adults to the effects of asthma on respiratory function. Bronchospasm and the inflammatory airway changes of asthma increase the resistance to airflow. This, together with a faster respiratory rate, causes air trapping and an increase in static lung volumes (residual volume, functional residual capacity, and total lung capacity).

Approximately 50 percent of the total airway resistance in infants resides in the peripheral airways, in contrast to only 20 percent in adults. Thus, small changes in the caliber of the peripheral airways will significantly affect the airway resistance in infants; furthermore, the smooth muscle present in the terminal bronchioles of infants may not be responsive to therapeutic drugs or other interventions. Air trapping transiently compensates for the constricted airways by keeping airways open (that is, increasing functional residual capacity above closing volume). Closing volume, however, is proportionally greater in infants than in adults because of the increased chest wall compliance (noncalcified horizontal ribs) and the decreased lung compliance (reduced elastin, a reduced number of alveoli, and compression of the lung by a protuberant abdomen). Because the functional residual capacity is similar in infants and adults, infants are at a disadvantage compared with adults because they are prone to early airway closure, V/Q mismatch, and intrapulmonary shunting.

Air trapping results in a reduced chest compliance and an increased physiological dead space. It increases the lung volumes and shifts ventilation up the compliance curve where compliance is reduced. This increases the work of breathing, which is compensated to some extent by activation of the accessory muscles of respiration and augmented diaphragmatic activity. The accessory muscles of respiration, however, are poorly developed in the infant and may not respond adequately. In infants, the diaphragm works at a mechanical disadvantage because it is flat and has few fatigue-resistant fibers. As a consequence, the diaphragm of the infant may fatigue much more rapidly than that of the adult. These factors all reduce the pulmonary reserve for gas exchange, predisposing infants and children to pulmonary insufficiency during asthma. The increased work of breathing also increases oxygen consumption and carbon dioxide production. All of these problems tend to increase the arterial carbon dioxide tension, worsen ventilation/perfusion mismatch, and decrease arterial oxygenation.

Ventilation/perfusion mismatch results from an altered distribution of ventilation (because of bronchospasm), air trapping, atelectasis from retained secretions, and an increased pulmonary artery pressure. Atelectasis may be prominent in children with asthma because children have smaller airways and a greater concentration of mucous glands than adults. Furthermore, interalveolar and interlobar gas exchange may be impaired because the pores of Kohn and canals of Lambert are poorly developed. The proportionately greater metabolic rate and decreased surface area for gas exchange in infants and children reduce their capacity to tolerate significant increases in ventilation/perfusion mismatch.

Pulmonary artery pressure becomes elevated secondary to the increased pulmonary arteriolar resistance (alveolar vessels) that results from marked air trapping. The increased pulmonary artery pressure may reverse hypoxic pulmonary vasoconstriction and worsen the ventilation/perfusion mismatch. Furthermore, pulmonary hypertension may cause right ventricular strain and cor pulmonale. The reduced cardiac output during hypoxemia and hypercarbia may prove fatal.

PREOPERATIVE MANAGEMENT

History

The purposes of the preoperative assessment are to develop a clear understanding of the severity of the asthma, to determine whether the child is currently experiencing bronchospasm, and to ascertain whether further therapeutic intervention is warranted before proceeding with anesthesia. All this information is necessary for planning an optimal anesthetic regimen. As in most pediatric cases, it is imperative that a full history of the child's illness be obtained from the parents.

The anesthesiologist should determine the age of onset of wheezing, the periodicity of the wheezing, and factors associated with the wheezing (such as viral respiratory infections, exercise, cold weather, and eczema). A history of eczema, allergies to food, and allergies to drugs (particularly aspirin) should be obtained; this history should extend back to infancy. If respiratory infections are a recurrent problem, a history of these infections should be taken indicating their periodicity, the date and duration of the last infection, whether hospital admission was required, and whether continued cough and sputum were present. If cough or sputum is persistent, it is important to know whether either of these symptoms has changed or worsened recently. The association of drug administration with the onset of wheezing should be clarified.

It is important to document the severity of bronchospasm during each attack and the therapy required to relieve the bronchospasm. This should include information on whether the child visited or was admitted to the hospital, was placed in intensive care, received drug treatment (with or without parenteral drugs), or required artificial ventilation or intubation.

It is important to review previous anesthetic records, to determine the severity of the asthma prior to and the reactivity of the airways during anesthesia. It is also important to determine whether there were any intraoperative or postoperative anesthetic complications attributable to the asthma.

A detailed history of all recent drug therapy should be obtained. One should determine time course, dose, side effects, and efficacy of all drug therapy. For those children taking aminophylline, monitoring of the blood concentration of theophylline (normal range is 10 to 20 μg/ml) is preferred for judging the adequacy of the therapy. The use of steroids by inhalation or orally must be included in the drug history.

Physical Examination

The physical examination should focus on the respiratory and cardiovascular systems. The child with acute asthma may breathe with nasal flaring, be tachypneic, and be sitting upright, unable to lie down because of shortness of breath. Respiratory effort may be labored and requiring the use of the sternomastoid accessory muscles. Lower rib flaring may be present. The chest appears hyperinflated with an increased anteroposterior diameter, and is hyperresonant to percussion. On auscultation, breath sounds are diminished. High-pitched expiratory wheezing is heard throughout the chest. Occasionally, compression of the chest between the stethoscope and a hand placed on the back produces wheezing in the patient with latent asthma. As the severity of the bronchospasm increases, inspiratory breath sounds disappear, and expiratory wheezing decreases until no air movement is audible. Bronchial breathing may indicate a pneumonic process. The complete absence of air entry on one side of the chest with hyperresonance suggests a pneumothorax. The signs of severe acute asthma with impending respiratory failure (hypoxia and hypercapneic narcosis) include central nervous system depression (manifest by glassy-eyed staring, a slow response to auditory or visual stimuli, and confusion) and shallow respirations without audible air entry. Peripheral cyanosis may be present.

The cardiovascular responses to asthma include tachycardia and a weak, thready pulse. Dehydration is not uncommon during an acute asthmatic attack. Pulsus paradoxus (greater than 10 mmHg decrease in systolic blood pressure during inspiration) is present with the more severe cases. Occasionally bradycardia occurs.

Chronic hypoxemia and pulmonary hypertension may result in right ventricular strain, cor pulmonale, and cardiovascular collapse. These are rare in children. The signs of right heart failure include an elevated jugular venous pressure, hepatomegaly, hepatojugular reflux, peripheral edema, and pleural effusion. Dehydration, manifested by depressed fontanelles, sunken eyes, dry mouth, loss of skin turgor, and oliguria, may complicate a protracted episode of asthma or chronic respiratory infection.

Laboratory Tests

Hemoglobin and hematocrit are increased in proportion to the degree of chronic hypoxemia and the extent of dehydration. An eosinophil concentration between 5 and 40 percent may be present. A sample for urinalysis may be difficult to obtain because of oliguria. However, if one can be obtained it usually has a high specific gravity and often contains protein as a result of infections and fever.

Chest x-rays will indicate hyperinflation (flat diaphragm) and increased lung markings (peribronchial cuffing) and may demonstrate prominent pulmonary arteries, which are indicative of pulmonary hypertension. X-rays are not usually helpful in the diagnosis of acute exacerbations of asthma. They may, however, be useful in the diagnosis of complications of asthma—atelectasis, pneumonia, pneumothorax, pneumomediastinum, or pleural effusions.

In mild asthma the arterial blood gas levels may indicate mild hypocapnia and hypoxemia at rest. In severe cases hypercapnia, respiratory acidosis, and occasionally metabolic acidosis may occur.

The electrocardiogram may indicate right bundle branch block, atrial or ventricular premature beats, right ventricular hypertrophy pattern, or cor pulmonale.

Pulmonary function testing (PFT) is usually restricted to children over 6 years of age, and often involves only spirometry. Such testing in asthma will indicate an obstructive pattern during episodes of acute asthma with increases in lung volumes (RV, FRC, TLC) and decreases in flow rates (FEV_1, FVC) and lung compliance. A minimum increase of 10 to 15 percent in flow rates after bronchodilator therapy indicates reversibility of the disease. Flow volume loops may be used to indicate reductions in both static lung volumes and flow rates and to differentiate wheezing of other causes.

Drug Therapy

Bronchodilators may be administered by four routes: orally, rectally, parenterally, or by inhalation. Oral administration is restricted to therapy for chronic asthma. This route of drug administration suffers from the problems of incomplete gastrointestinal absorption and the first pass effect of the liver. Parenteral administration is useful during anesthesia. Aminophylline, isoproterenol, and steroids are the only bronchodilators currently administered by this route. Bronchodilators may also be delivered to their site of action by inhalation. This path is direct, maximizes the concentration of drug at the site of action, and minimizes systemic side effects. Inhalants are available in either a prepared aerosol delivered via a fluorocarbon propellant generator or a liquid form delivered by jet nebulizer. The prepared aerosol is more difficult to administer to smaller children, but both preparations may be used during anesthesia.

Methylxanthines, sympathomimetics, and steroids are the major drugs in the treatment of asthma. Recently, cromolyn and ketotifen have been added for the management of chronic asthma. Anticholinergics may be used to treat some cases of asthma.

Theophylline

Theophylline, a dimethylated xanthine, is a principal drug in the treatment of asthma. It has been suggested that theophylline may relieve bronchospasm by relaxing bronchial smooth muscle. Four possible mechanisms of action have been proposed: (1) inhibition of phosphodiesterase (increasing cAMP), (2) translocation of intracellular calcium, (3) inhibition of adenosine bronchoconstriction, and (4) antagonism of prostaglandin synthesis. However, theophylline does not act by the first two pathways at serum levels less than 50 μg/ml. Adenosine inhibition is currently believed to be the primary mechanism in bronchodilation. Theophylline affects many organ systems. It increases diaphragmatic contractility and sensitizes the brain stem to carbon dioxide. This latter effect is used to prevent apnea in premature infants. Theophylline increases cerebrovascular resistance, decreases cerebral blood flow, and stimulates the central nervous system, causing irritability, tremors, and seizures. At serum concentrations greater than 15 μg/ml, theophylline triggers the vomiting center.

Theophylline affects the cardiovascular system by increasing chronotropy, and at high serum concentrations by inducing arrhythmias. It dilates both the coronary vessels and peripheral arteriolar and venous vessels, and also increases both right and left ventricular contractility. It dilates the renal arteries and causes a transient diuresis. At the neuromuscular junction, theophylline antagonizes the nondepolarizing blockade by pancuronium.

Serum concentrations above 20 μg/ml are toxic. The toxic side effects increase in proportion to the serum concentration. At concentrations below 20 μg/ml, theophylline induces minor gastrointestinal upset and central nervous system irritation. These minor disturbances usually subside within 7 to 10 days of therapy. At concentrations between 20 and 35 μg/ml, toxic side effects including headache, nausea, irritability, insomnia, vomiting, gastric bleeding, and diarrhea are seen. Above 35 µg/ml, seizures, cardiac arrhythmias, and death are not uncommon.

Severe toxicity and death may occur in the pediatric age group in sick children receiving excess intravenous or rectal theophylline. The symptoms of irritability may suddenly progress to seizures and brain damage. However, seizures may occur without prior signs of impending toxicity. The mechanism of brain damage may be severe cerebral vasoconstriction and the associated neuronal hypoxia. These toxic effects are enhanced in the presence of ephedrine.

Mild seizures may respond to diazepam, dilantin, phenobarbital, or thiopentone. However, at higher serum concentrations, theophylline-induced seizures may be resistant to all forms of therapy. The definitive preventive management is to maintain serum levels below 20 µg/ml.

Markedly increased serum concentrations should be treated first by stopping the aminophylline. Whether the aminophylline was administered orally or intravenously, the stomach may be lavaged with charcoal every 4 hours to remove the theophylline. A persistently increased serum concentration may be reduced by charcoal hemoperfusion or, less efficiently, by peritoneal dialysis. Protracted vomiting from toxic concentrations of theophylline may result in dehydration in children. Vomiting, dehydration, and a renal diuresis together suggest toxicity.

Cardiac arrhythmias occur less commonly in children than in adults. Tachycardia, ventricular ectopic beats, and severe hypotension (especially following infusion through a central venous line) may occur. Ventricular ectopic beats respond to cessation of the theophylline and intravenous lidocaine.

The pharmacokinetics of theophylline are well known. The optimal bronchodilator effect of theophylline occurs between serum concentrations of 10 and 20 µg/ml, although some patients have full therapeutic benefit from serum concentrations as low as 5 µg/ml, particularly following acute loading doses. The volume of distribution is fairly constant: 0.6 L/kg in neonates and premature infants, and 0.45 L/kg in children and adults. Theophylline freely crosses the placenta, and reaches 90 percent of the serum concentration in the cerebrospinal fluid of premature infants. Approximately 40 percent is albumin-bound in neonates as compared with 60 percent in the older age groups. Ninety percent is eliminated by the microsomal mixed function oxidase enzyme system in the liver. Metabolism is reduced in prematures and neonates to approximately 50 percent and is greatest in older children and adolescents. There is no first pass effect by the liver. The remaining 10 to 15 percent is excreted unchanged by the kidney.

Theophylline clearance is reduced in neonates, in patients with heart and liver failure or severe pneumonia, and in association with the administration of cimetidine, propranolol, erythromycin, and macrolide antibiotics. In animals, hypercapnia or hypoxia reduces metabolism. In patients in whom clearance is decreased, the dose should be reduced. In contrast, in patients receiving phenobarbital or intravenous infusions of isoproterenol, the clearance of theophylline may be increased. However, this latter effect may not be of major clinical importance.

Theophylline is available in a wide variety of preparations for oral, rectal, and intravenous administration. Slow-release oral preparations (elixirs, uncoated tablets, and bead-filled capsules [50 or 60 mg each]) and rectal solutions may be administered every 6 to 8 hours to infants or every 4 to 6 hours to children and adults with high metabolic rates. Children may use the elixirs or the bead-filled capsules sprinkled over their food. Uncoated tablets should only be given to older children. If the tablets are crushed, the absorption of theophylline may be increased. Rectal solutions are useful because they are packaged with a calibrated syringe for accurate dosing. They may be used preoperatively in patients who are fasting or vomiting and can be repeated, but should be stopped after 36 hours of continuous therapy because of the mucosal irritation that may occur from the alkaline pH of the solutions. Suppositories of theophylline are erratically and incompletely absorbed and are not recommended.

If theophylline is required during anesthesia to relieve bronchospasm in a patient who had not received the drug recently, then 7.5 mg/kg should be given intravenously over 15 to 30 minutes. This will provide a serum concentration of approximately 15µg/ml. If the loading dose is administered too rapidly, transient toxic serum concentrations may result. If the patient had received theophylline recently and still develops bronchospasm, then a blood sample should be taken for serum concentration, and 2.5 mg/kg should be administered over 30 minutes. After an appropriate loading dose is administered, therapeutic serum concentrations should be maintained by infusion at the rates listed in Table 16–13.

Serum theophylline concentrations should be monitored serially after 4 to 6 hours of therapy, and every 12 hours until stable serum concentrations are achieved.

Sympathomimetic Drugs

The beta agonist sympathomimetics are among the most commonly used bronchodilators. Beta agonist drugs combine with the membrane-bound receptors to activate magnesium-dependent cAMP and convert ATP to cAMP. This prevents the release of the stored mediators of bronchoconstriction. Beta receptors are divided into two types: $beta_1$, responsible for chronotropy, inotropy, and lipolysis; and $beta_2$, responsible for smooth muscle relaxation (bronchodilatation, vasodilatation), attenuating histamine release, increasing mucociliary clearance, and skeletal muscle tremor.

The preferred bronchodilators should activate $beta_2$ receptors and exert minimal effects on the $beta_1$ recep-

Table 16–13. INFUSION RATES TO MAINTAIN THERAPEUTIC SERUM THEOPHYLLINE LEVELS

Age	Theophylline (mg/kg/hr)
Neonates	0.13
Infants (2–6 mos)	0.4
Infants (6–11 mos)	0.7
Children (1–9 yrs)	0.8
Children (9–16 yrs) to adults (smokers)	0.6
Adults (nonsmoking, healthy)	0.4
Elderly and adults with cor pulmonale	0.25
Cardiac failure, liver dysfunction	0.1

tors. Sympathomimetic bronchodilators are divided into several categories: catecholamines, noncatecholamines, resorcinols, saligenins, and others.

Catechols. Epinephrine, isoproterenol, and isoetharine are 3,4-dihydroxybenzene rings with substituted amine side chains. Bulky substitutions on the N-terminus of the side chain increases their beta activity and decreases their alpha activity. Bulky substitutions on the carbons on the side chains decrease $beta_1$ activity more than $beta_2$ activity. The catechols are inactivated by reuptake into the presynaptic membrane and metabolized to a lesser extent by the monoamine oxidase (MAO) enzymes and catechol-O-methyl transferase (COMT). Because of the presence of MAO in the gastrointestinal tract, catechols are inactivated by metabolic pathways when the drugs are ingested.

Epinephrine has alpha, $beta_1$, and $beta_2$ activity, although $beta_2$ activity is the primary beta effect in vivo. In addition to the beta activity, the alpha activity shrinks mucosal congestion. The *l*-isomer is considered to be the active form. The dose of epinephrine for adults is 0.1 to 0.3 ml of 1:1000 solution and for children, 0.02 to 0.10 ml/kg of 1:10,000 solution administered subcutaneously. This dose can be repeated every 30 minutes. The onset of bronchodilatation occurs with 5 to 10 minutes and lasts up to 60 minutes. Subcutaneous epinephrine is reserved for acute severe asthmatic episodes and allergic reactions. Epinephrine should not be administered intravenously for the treatment of acute bronchospasm because of the high risk of ventricular fibrillation and cardiac arrest.

Isoproterenol is a catechol devoid of alpha activity because of the bulky N-terminus substitutions. It has both $beta_1$ and $beta_2$ properties, but is dose-limited because of its $beta_1$ chronotropic stimulation. Its short duration of action is caused by reuptake and metabolism by COMT. Isoproterenol may be administered by inhalation (0.5 ml of 0.5 to 1 percent solution); in this form it has an onset of action within 1 to 2 minutes, peaks within 5 minutes, and lasts for 10 to 30 minutes. When it is administered by the intravenous route to children, an initial infusion dose of 0.1 μg/kg/min is recommended (see Table 16–18). The dose is increased until either the bronchospasm is

relieved or the heart rate reaches 200 beats per minute. The intravenous regimen for isoproterenol has been found to be very effective in children with severe asthmatic episodes and borderline respiratory failure within the intensive care setting. Caution must be exercised when using isoproterenol by inhalation since rebound bronchospasm, ventricular fibrillation, and death have been reported.

Isoetharine, which contains a substituted side chain, has one tenth of the $beta_2$ activity and one three-hundredth of the $beta_1$ activity of isoproterenol. It is metabolized primarily by COMT and is resistant to MAO. It is available by aerosol only (340 μg/puff). One to four puffs every 4 hours should provide a therapeutic response. Peak activity is at 15 minutes and duration is less than 2 hours.

Noncatecholamines. Ephedrine is a noncatecholamine sympathomimetic with alpha, $beta_1$, and $beta_2$ activity. Because its mechanism of action is predominantly indirect (through the release of norepinephrine), the effects of ephedrine decrease with frequently repeated doses. It is associated with a significant incidence of side effects, including central nervous system irritability (headaches, tremors, restlessness, and weakness), palpitations, tachycardia, and hypertension. Although ephedrine is currently used, newer $beta_2$ selective bronchodilators are slowly replacing it. The dosage of oral ephedrine ranges from 15 to 45 mg, depending on the age of the patient. The time of action is from 30 minutes to 3 hours. Seventy percent of ephedrine is excreted in the urine unchanged.

Resorcinols. The resorcinols are metaproterenol, terbutaline, and fenoterol. Metaproterenol (Alupent or orciprenalin) is a 3,5-dihydroxyphenyl group with a bulky amine substituted side chain. This combination confers $beta_2$ receptor selectivity, although the overall beta activity is 10 to 40 times less than that of isoproterenol. Metaproterenol may be taken orally (10 to 20 mg for an adult) with a duration of action of 2 to 5 hours, or by inhalation from a pressurized cannister (640 μg/puff) and up to 8 puffs per day to an adult. The puff delivery has a very rapid onset of action. This drug, like all resorcinols, is resistant to metabolism by COMT and MAO. Metaproterenol has equivalent bronchodilating activity as isoproterenol but produces more cardioacceleration than other $beta_2$ selective agents.

Terbutaline is a synthetic resorcinol that is similar in structure to metaproterenol. The tertiary butyl substitution on the N-terminal side chain further reduces the $beta_1$ activity. Compared with metaproterenol, terbutaline is twice as potent a bronchodilator with double the duration of action and fewer side effects. Terbutaline has been effective in combination with theophylline, although seizures have been reported. Terbutaline causes skeletal muscle tremor and sinus tachycardia, and if given parenterally myocardial ischemia, ventricular tachycardia, and pulmonary edema. Terbutaline is available for oral use (2.5 to 5 mg per day for children over 12 years of age) or for subcutaneous use (0.25 mg every 30 minutes to a maximum of 0.5 mg within 4 hours).

Fenoterol hydrobromide (Berotec) is a synthetic sympathomimetic similar to metaproterenol with a 4-hydroxyphenyl substitution on the N-terminal side chain. Compared with ephedrine, fenoterol has a faster onset of action and a longer duration of activity, and is a more potent bronchodilator. It acts primarily in the smaller airways of children, with optimal bronchodilation after 5 mg is given by mouth. Oral fenoterol has a peak action of 2 hours and a duration of 6 hours. Side effects include tachycardia and tremor.

Saligenins. Salbutamol (Ventolin, albuterol) has a molecular structure similar to isoproterenol with a $CH_2(OH)$ substitution at position 3 of the benzene ring. This has the effect of reducing the beta activity, $beta_1$ more than $beta_2$. Salbutamol is devoid of alpha activity. It is almost as potent a bronchodilator as isoproterenol and has only 10 to 20 percent of the chronotropic effect. Salbutamol may be administered by inhalation 100 μg per puff, 1 to 2 puffs every 4 hours (maximum 8 puffs per day) with a maximum effect within 15 minutes and a duration up to 5 hours, or orally (1 to 4 mg every 6 to 8 hours in adults) with a maximum effect after 2 to 4 hours. Nebulized salbutamol appears to be effective in children over 20 months of age.

Salbutamol has minimal chronotropic side effects. However, when it is administered orally, it may cause tremor, loss of appetite, headache, and nausea. Excessive use or overdose may cause electroencephalographic abnormalities and convulsions.

In studies comparing salbutamol, terbutaline, and metaproterenol, all three were found to be effective when taken orally, although metaproterenol exhibited less $beta_2$ selectivity than the other two. Skeletal muscle tremors were reported after all three drugs when they were given orally but not after they were given by the inhalational route; this direct $beta_2$ effect varies among patients and the three drugs.

Steroids

Corticosteroids are second line drug therapy for the treatment of asthma and are indicated for failure of conventional therapy (optimal aminophylline and inhaled aerosols), acute exacerbations of asthma (including status asthmaticus), or chronic asthma (1 to 10 percent of children with asthma) or to reduce the dose of the first line bronchodilators. They modify bronchospasm by four possible mechanisms: (1) potentiating the beta-adrenergic system, (2) inhibiting the release of the mediators of bronchoconstriction and inflammation, (3) changing leukocyte kinetics and function, and (4) thinning mucus and reducing mucosal edema. The importance of steroids in asthma and anesthesia relates to (1) the treatment of severe asthma in the perioperative period and (2) protection against relative hypoadrenalism during anesthesia.

Corticosteroids may be administered to children by three routes: oral, inhalation, and parenteral. Oral administration of steroids may be indicated for one of two reasons: daily steroids for a brief period after an acute exacerbation and alternate-day oral therapy for continued use. The oral steroid preparation is usually prednisone, which is available in a syrup (1 mg/ml) for children. It is administered in the morning as a single daily dose to minimize adrenal suppression. The usual dose for acute exacerbations is about 30 mg (1 to 2 mg/kg) for a 10-year-old for 1 week and then gradually tapered over a 10-day period. Although prednisone, 7.5 mg/m^2/day, usually causes minimal side effects, doses as small as 4 to 6 mg/m^2/day have been reported to cause growth suppression.* Alternate-day prednisone in a single morning daily dose is less likely to suppress adrenal function or cause growth retardation, osteoporosis, or cushingoid symptoms.

Beclomethasone dipropionate (BD) (Beclovent) is the most commonly used steroid aerosol. BD is administered by inhalation to the tracheobronchial tree and is rapidly absorbed. Approximately 59 μg of BD is available per puff, and of this 50 percent reaches the airways. The other 50 percent is swallowed, and may be absorbed through the gastrointestinal tract. There is a significant first-pass metabolism in the liver. It has been suggested that less than 1000 μg daily is required for the maximum steroid effect. Systemic absorption is reported to be minimal with BD, with few systemic effects when the dose is restricted to less than 1000 μg. However, adrenal-hypothalamic axis suppression has been reported with doses between 400 and 800 μg daily in children. A similar degree of adrenal suppression is seen with 20 to 40 mg of prednisone every other day. It has been suggested that doses less than 13 μg/kg/day of BD do not suppress the adrenal-hypothalamic axis. Local side effects commonly reported include oral and esophageal moniliasis and hoarseness. It is the author's opinion that additional preoperative steroids should be used in children receiving steroids by inhalation.

Parenteral steroids may be useful in the treatment of acute asthma and status asthmaticus. However, the effect of steroids may take at least 3 to 4 hours for the onset of action, and up to 24 hours to improve pulmonary function (FEV_1). The delayed onset of action is consistent with the time that may be required for protein synthesis. Steroid therapy for an acute attack should begin with a short-acting form such as hydrocortisone 1 to 2 mg/kg bolus, and be followed by 0.5 mg/kg/hr, or methylprednisolone 2 to 3 mg/kg/day in four divided doses. Therapy should be continued for 24 hours, at which time an oral preparation should be introduced (1 to 2 mg/kg prednisone) as one daily dose in the morning. This should be continued for 5 to 7 days and then tapered over 7 to 10 days.

---

*A 10-year-old child has a surface area of about 1 m^2.

Prophylactic steroids should be administered in the perioperative period if the child: (1) is currently receiving steroids, or (2) has taken steroids for at least 1 week in the previous 6 months. During the stress of surgery, adrenal steroid production may increase two- to sevenfold. Patients who are receiving steroids or recently (less than 1 year ago) received steroids may be unable to mount an adrenal response to surgery, and develop relative adrenal insufficiency. To prevent hypotension and shock, parenteral steroids should be administered. One successful regimen is 1.5 mg/kg hydrocortisone as a slow intravenous infusion in the perioperative period, followed by the same dose q8h. Recently, this dose of steroids has been reduced to hydrocortisone 0.4 mg/kg in the preoperative period followed by an intravenous infusion of 1.5 mg/kg over 24 hours. This infusion is then tapered over the subsequent 72 hours.

Steroids are required because the adrenergic receptors of vascular smooth muscle are hyporesponsive to catecholamines. Consequently, if the blood pressure falls, the vascular smooth muscle is unable to compensate by constricting. Parenteral steroids enhance the vascular smooth muscle response to catecholamines, and prevent or reverse the hypotension.

Cromolyn

The mechanism of action of cromolyn is not well understood. Cromolyn sodium, a sodium salt of the bis-cromones, prevents bronchospasm by inhibiting mediator release from mast cells. It has no direct bronchodilating properties nor direct sympatho-mimetic activity, and is effective only when given prophylactically prior to mediator release. Because cromolyn is not lipid-soluble, it is poorly absorbed (approximately 1 percent) by the gastrointestinal tract. It is administered by inhalation only in asthma. Two vehicles are available: the turbo-inhaler and the pressurized cannister. The turbo-inhaler delivery system is difficult for young children with asthma to use; therefore it had limited application until a nebulized form of cromolyn solution (20 mg in a 1 percent solution) became available.

Approximately 10 percent of cromolyn is absorbed from the distal airways in the lung. It has an onset of action of 10 to 20 minutes, and a duration of action of approximately 6 hours. Its action is terminated by excretion of the unchanged drug in the urine (50 percent) and in the liver (50 percent). Cromolyn is optimally effective when administered 10 minutes prior to the stimulus.

Cromolyn is a very safe drug with a very low incidence of side effects, which include hyperventilation, hoarseness, dry mouth, nasal congestion, and rarely bronchospasm. Other rare side effects include nausea, vomiting, facial dermatitis, and joint swelling. Hypersensitivity to cromolyn powder may present as laryngeal edema, urticaria, angioedema, or anaphylaxis. There have been no reports of hematological, renal, or hepatic dysfunction from its use in children.

Cromolyn is indicated for prophylaxis against exercised-induced, IgE-mediated, and intrinsic asthmas as well as type III delayed reactions. Although cromolyn reduces the theophylline requirement in children with asthma, it is not indicated for the treatment of acute asthma or status asthmaticus already in evolution.

Contraindications to cromolyn sodium include known hypersensitivity to the drug and eosinophilic pneumonitis.

Ketotifen

Ketotifen is an antiasthmatic and antianaphylactic drug that is effective as a prophylactic agent only. Ketotifen may act by antagonizing histamine, inhibiting phosphodiesterase, blockade of calcium channels, inhibiting mediator release, or antagonizing slow reacting substance of anaphylaxis (SRS-A). It is effective in reducing bronchoconstriction in patients with allergic and aspirin-induced asthma. In children, 1 mg/kg of ketotifen may be effective when administered orally twice daily. In one study, there were no side effects or complications from this drug. Ketotifen appears to be effective in preventing asthma in children.

Anticholinergics

The use of anticholinergic agents in pediatric asthma is limited. They may reduce bronchomotor tone in the central airways (as described earlier), mucous gland secretions, and the size of the bronchial vascular bed. To effect these changes, anticholinergic drugs are administered by intravenous or intramuscular injection or by inhalation. Intravenous or intramuscular atropine (0.01 to 0.02 mg/kg) is commonly used by pediatric anesthetists for preventing bradycardia and drying secretions in the airways. However, the parenteral use of atropine in the treatment of chronic asthma is both impractical because of its short half-life and complicated with extensive side effects. Anticholinergic agents for bronchospasm are available by inhalation (Sch 1000 or ipratropium bromide) and these have fewer side effects than parenteral atropine. Ipratropium bromide has been shown to be effective for asthma triggered by irritant inhalation and in 50 percent of patients with exercise-induced asthma. Glycopyrrolate has also been used by inhalation in asthma with similar success.

Atropine causes a dose-related toxicity leading to tachycardia, restlessness, headache, constipation, urine retention, dry hot skin, delirium, coma and arrhythmias, which may culminate in death. Ingestion of 10 mg of atropine has been fatal in children. The author believes an absolute maximum dose of oral or parenteral atropine in children is approximately 50 μg/kg in divided doses.

The dose of nebulized ipratropium bromide is about 50 μg/kg in children. Ipratropium bromide produces comparable bronchodilatation when compared to isoproterenol and metaproterenol by inhalation. The side effects of ipratropium are fewer compared to parenteral atropine. Xerostomia is a common complaint. Ipratropium bromide, in contrast to the beta blockers, does not cause tremor or restlessness in recommended doses.

ANESTHETIC MANAGEMENT

During the preoperative visit, a decision about whether or not to proceed with surgery is made. If the surgery is elective and the child has not been optimally treated for asthma, then surgery must be delayed and therapy optimized. If the surgery is a life-saving emergency procedure, the relative risks of surgery and anesthesia must be discussed with both the parents and the surgeon, with therapy for control of the asthma instituted immediately. If surgery can be delayed a short while, immediate therapy for cases of severe asthma may be effective. If surgery cannot be delayed, as safe an anesthetic as possible must be administered.

Premedication may be administered for bronchodilatation and/or sedation. Children should receive their routine oral bronchodilators on the morning of surgery with a sip of water. Inhaled bronchodilators should also be given on the morning of surgery and if necessary, repeated just prior to transfer to the operating room. If the child is either currently receiving steroids, or has received steroids for at least 1 week in the past 6 months, an intravenous infusion of hydrocortisone hemisuccinate (1.5 mg/kg) should be commenced about 1 hour before surgery. Atropine (0.02 mg/kg) or glycopyrrolate (0.01 mg/kg) may be administered intramuscularly 45 minutes before surgery for antisialorrhea, bronchodilatation, and suppression of the afferent irritant vagal pathways in the lung.

Sedation may be indicated for those children in whom asthma is precipitated by anxiety. Diazepam (0.15 to 0.2 mg/kg) syrup or pentobarbital (2 mg/kg) may be given orally 1 to 2 hours before surgery. Alternatively, pentobarbital may be given per rectum at the same dose. If the child is extremely anxious, methohexital (15 mg/kg of a 1 percent solution with 0.02 mg/kg atropine) may be given per rectum 10 minutes before surgery. In adolescents and adults, the major tranquilizer promethazine (Phenergan) has been suggested as a premedication (25 mg/70 kg intramuscularly) for both its sedating and antisialogogue effects. Although controversial, the combination of a narcotic such as meperidine and promethazine has been recommended for premedication of the older patients with lung disease. The preoperative use of H_2 antagonists such as cimetidine or ranitidine may be theoretically contraindicated in asthma, because H_2 receptors are thought to inhibit the feedback control of mediator release and may result in increased bronchoconstriction.

The choice of anesthetic technique includes local, regional, and general. In pediatrics, local infiltration for surgery is often extremely difficult. Regional anesthesia is becoming increasingly popular: caudal, spinal, and axillary blocks may be used. A spinal block may be effective for lower abdominal or lower extremity surgery. If, however, preservation of an adequate vital capacity for an effective cough is important, then there is evidence to suggest that regional techniques may not have advantages over general anesthesia.

If general anesthesia is undertaken, intubation of the trachea should be avoided if possible, since a foreign body in the airway is one of the most potent triggers for bronchospasm. Therefore, anesthesia should be given by mask whenever possible.

Anesthesia may be induced by either an intravenous or inhalational route. Thiopentone theoretically releases more histamine than methohexitone or ketamine, although there are no controlled clinical studies in asthmatics to support this theory. In clinical doses, thiopentone does not block against irritant-induced reflex bronchoconstriction, although there is evidence that thiopentone is relatively safe in asthmatics. Methohexitone does not release histamine in vitro, and may be useful as an induction agent in asthmatics, although one anaphylactoid reaction to rectal methohexital has been reported. Ketamine relaxes the airways through activation of the sympathetic system (beta-adrenergic agonist action), blockade of endogenous catecholamine reuptake, and depression of afferent irritant vagal pathways. In the dog model, ketamine protects against antigen-induced bronchospasm better than thiopentone.

The inhalational agents halothane, enflurane, and isoflurane all prevent and reverse bronchospasm. The mechanism is thought to involve blockade of the irritant vagal pathways within the central nervous system. It is therefore important that a deep level of anesthesia is established before the trachea is intubated. Although it has been suggested that halothane produces bronchoconstriction by its $beta_2$ agonist action, there is no evidence to support this theory. Halothane is, however, associated with an increased incidence of arrhythmias in dogs pretreated with aminophylline, compared with enflurane or isoflurane in the same model. Despite this caution, halothane remains the most commonly used inhalational agent in pediatric asthma. Isoflurane is associated with an increased incidence of breath-holding, coughing, and laryngospasm as compared with halothane and enflurane in children, and may be less desirable for use in asthmatics for these reasons. Ventricular arrhythmias may occur in children with high therapeutic blood levels of theophylline during halothane anesthesia, and in this situation isoflurane may be the preferred agent.

Narcotics release histamine, which may be responsible for narcotic-induced bronchospasm, and should be avoided. Although H_1 antihistamines block the hypotensive effects of narcotics, they are ineffective in preventing narcotic-induced bronchospasm. For a complete discussion of narcotic and histamine release, see the following section on Mastocytosis.

Neuromuscular blocking drugs may release histamine and some cause bronchoconstriction. Pancuronium is probably the best relaxant for asthmatics. A detailed discussion is found in the section on Masto-cytosis.

If possible, endotracheal intubation should be performed while the patient is at a deep level of general anesthesia. This blocks the irritant reflex afferent vagal pathways from the lung. Deep anesthesia may be accomplished with high concentrations of an inhalational agent or during a lighter level of anesthesia supplemented with intravenous lidocaine. Lidocaine blocks the irritant reflex vagal pathways from the lungs and, as suggested by studies in animals, may directly relax bronchial smooth muscle. Intravenous lidocaine is preferred to aerosol lidocaine because it removes the need for prior laryngoscopy and avoids use of a high-pressure gas propellant.

During anesthesia ventilation may become difficult, and then the asthmatic may quite quickly become dusky and cyanotic. This may necessitate differentiating a tight chest as a result of light anesthesia from that due to bronchospasm. The former is relieved after administration of muscle relaxants or deep anesthesia, whereas the latter is unaffected by muscle relaxants but is relieved by a deeper level of anesthesia.

Anesthetic gases should be humidified, particularly in smaller children, in whom inspissated secretions may plug the small diameter endotracheal tube. Humidification is also recommended for prolonged anesthesia, and in those children with chest infections in whom suctioning and chest physiotherapy are required to remove secretions.

At the end of anesthesia, neuromuscular blockade must be completely reversed. Although neostigmine may increase bronchomotor tone, the addition of an anticholinergic agent such as atropine or glycopyrrolate will minimize this effect. The trachea should be extubated while the child is deeply anesthetized and breathing spontaneously or when the child is wide awake. There have been controlled clinical studies comparing these two extubation techniques. The decision to extubate the child under deep anesthesia or awake depends on the expertise of the anesthetist, the severity of the asthma, and preexisting problems that may predispose the child to regurgitation.

In the postanesthetic room, children should receive humidified oxygen. Careful attention should be paid to auscultating the chest for evidence of bronchospasm. If bronchospasm develops, then ventolin should be administered by inhalation. If this treatment is insufficient, consideration should be given to parenteral theophylline. Postoperative sedation should be used with caution, particularly if ventilation or oxygenation is impaired. Regional anesthesia may be used to prevent postoperative pain.

If bronchospasm occurs during anesthesia, the differential diagnosis outlined in Table 16–14 should be considered.

If the child is not intubated, management includes assisted ventilation with 100 percent oxygen and increasing concentrations of halothane. If the diagnosis

Table 16–14. DIFFERENTIAL DIAGNOSIS OF WHEEZING

	Intraoperative	Nonoperative
Upper airway obstruction	Endobronchial intubation	Foreign body in the airway
	Obstructed endotracheal tube	Croup
		Epiglottitis
	Carinal irritation	Tracheal stenosis or malacia
	Secretions in the airway	
	Foreign body in the airway	Extrinsic compression of trachea (tumor, cyst, nodes, vascular)
	Aspiration	
Lower airway disease	Pneumothorax	Bronchiolitis
	Aspiration	Bronchiectasis
		Cystic fibrosis
		Pneumonia
Cardiac	Pulmonary edema	Pulmonary edema

is most certainly asthmatic bronchospasm and the bronchospasm is severe, the child should be ventilated with 100 percent oxygen. In cases of severe asthmatic bronchospasm, inhalational therapy is often ineffective, and parenteral therapy is then required. Severe bronchospasm requires endotracheal intubation in order to ensure adequate alveolar ventilation, and supplementation with parenteral bronchodilators such as theophylline or isoproterenol.

If the child is intubated and the diagnosis is asthmatic bronchospasm, the child should be hyperventilated with 100 percent oxygen and increasing concentrations of halothane. If the bronchospasm is not relieved, aerosol ventolin should then be administered through the inspiratory limb of the anesthetic circuit as close to the endotracheal tube as possible. Further therapy with intravenous theophylline or isoproterenol may be required. Isoproterenol in doses beginning with 0.1 μg/kg/min may be administered intravenously (see Table 16–18). Subcutaneous, slow intravenous, or endotracheal epinephrine must be administered cautiously in the presence of halothane.

REFERENCES

Andersson KE, Persson CG: Extrapulmonary effects of theophylline. Eur J Respir Dis *61*(Suppl 109):17, 1980.

Aranda JV, Turmen T: Methylxanthines in apnea of prematurity. Clin Perinatol 6:87, 1979.

Aublier M, DeTroyer A, Sampson M, et al.: Aminophylline improves diaphragmatic contractility. N Engl J Med *305*:249, 1981.

Avner SE: Beta-adrenergic bronchodilators. Pediatr Clin North Am *22*:121, 1975.

Bernstein IL, Johnson CL, Tse CST: Therapy with cromolyn sodium. Ann Intern Med *89*:228, 1978.

Berstrand H: Phosphodiesterase inhibition and theophylline. Eur J Respir Dis *61*(Suppl 109):37, 1980.

Bierman CW, Pearlman DS: Asthma. *In* Kendig EL Jr, Chernick V, (Eds.): Disorders of the Respiratory Tract in Children. 4th ed. Philadelphia, W.B. Saunders Co., 1983.

Bory C, Baltassat P, Rorthault M, et al.: Metabolism of theophylline to caffeine in premature newborn infants. J Pediatr *94*:988, 1981.

Boutros AR, Weisel M: Comparison of effects of three anaesthetic techniques on patients with severe pulmonary obstructive disease. Can Anaesth Soc J 18:296, 1971.

Bukowskyj M, Nakatsu K, Munt PW: Theophylline reassessed. Ann Intern Med 101:63, 1984.

Bundgaard A, Bach-Mortensen N, Schmidt A: The effect of sodium cromoglycate delivered by Spinhaler and by pressurized aerosol on exercise-induced asthma in children. Clin Allergy 12:601, 1982.

Chang TMS, Espinosa-Melendez E, Francoeur TE, et al.: Albumin-collodion activated charcoal hemoperfusion in the treatment of severe theophylline intoxication in a 3-year-old patient. Pediatrics 65:811, 1980.

Church MK: The role of basophils in asthma. 1. Sodium cromoglycate on histamine release and content. Clin Allergy 12:223, 1982.

Crago RR, Bryan AC, Laws AK, et al.: Respiratory flow resistance after curare and pancuronium measured by force oscillation. Can Anaesth Soc J 19:607, 1972.

Dawson A, Simon RA: Bronchospastic disorders: an overview. In Dawson A, Simon RA (Eds.): The Practical Management of Asthma. Orlando, Grune and Stratton, 1984.

Dees SC: Asthma. In Kendig EL Jr, Chernick V, (Eds.): Disorders of the Respiratory Tract in Children. 3rd ed. Philadelphia, W.B. Saunders Co., 1977.

Delaney JC: The effect of ketotifen on aspirin-induced asthmatic reactions. Clin Allergy 13:247, 1983.

Dorow P, Schiess W: Influence of ketotifen on the airway responsiveness in asthmatics. J Asthma 21:81, 1984.

Downes H, Gerber N, Hirshman CA: I.V. lignocaine in reflex and allergic bronchoconstriction. Br J Anaesth 52:873, 1980.

Downes H, Hirshman CA: Lidocaine aerosols do not prevent allergic bronchoconstriction. Anesth Analg 60:28, 1981.

Downes JJ, Wood DW, Harwood I, et al.: Intravenous isoproterenol infusion in children with severe hypercapnia due to status asthmaticus: effects on ventilation, circulation and clinical. Crit Care Med 1:65, 1973.

Ellis EF: Asthma. In Scarpelli EM, Auld PAM, Goldman HS (Eds.): Pulmonary Disease of the Fetus, Newborn and Child. Philadelphia, Lea and Febiger, 1978, pp 286.

Ellis EF: Theophylline and derivatives. In Middleton E, Reed CE, Ellis EF (Eds.): Allergy: Principles and Practice. St. Louis, C.V. Mosby Co., 1978.

Ellis EF, Koysooko R, Levy G: Pharmacokinetics of theophylline in children with asthma. Pediatrics 58:542, 1976.

Ellul-Micallef R, Fenech FF: Effect of intravenous prednisolone in asthmatics with diminished adrenergic responsiveness. Lancet 2:1269, 1975.

Falliers CJ: Cromolyn sodium (disodium cromoglycate) prophylaxis. Pediatr Clin North Am 22:141, 1975.

Falliers CJ: Corticosteroids for childhood asthma: systemic and topical treatment. J Asthma 20:475, 1983.

Fanta CH, Rossing TH, McFadden ER: Glucocorticoids in acute asthma—a critical controlled trial. Am J Med 74:845, 1983.

Feldman CH, Sher TN, Hutchinson VE, et al.: Fenoterol dose-response study in children with asthma. J Allergy Clin Immunol 73:356, 1984.

Friedman MS: Psychological factors associated with pediatric asthma death: a review. J Asthma 21:97, 1984.

Gal P, Roop C, Robinson H, et al.: Theophylline-induced seizures in accidentally overdosed neonates. Pediatrics 65:547, 1980.

Gal TJ, Suratt PM, Lu J: Glycopyrrolate and atropine inhalation: comparative effects on normal airway function. Am Rev Respir Dis 129:871, 1984.

Geller-Bernstein C, Sneh N: The management of bronchial asthma in children under the age of 3½ years using Intal (sodium cromoglycate) administered by Spinhaler. Clin Allergy 10:503, 1980.

Giacoia G, Jusko WJ, Menke J, et al.: Theophylline pharmacokinetics in premature infants with apnea. J Pediatr 89:829, 1976.

Godfrey S: The place of a new aerosol steroid, beclomethasone dipropionate, in the management of childhood asthma. Pediatr Clin North Am 22:147, 1975.

Gran L, Pahle JA: Rational substitution therapy for steroid-treated patients. Anaesthesia 33:59, 1978.

Greenwood C: The pharmacology of ketotifen. Chest 82:45S, 1982.

Gross NJ, Skomedin MS: Anticholinergic, antimuscarinic bronchodilators. Am Rev Respir Dis 129:856, 1984.

Hardy CC, Robinson C, Tattersfield AE, et al.: The bronchoconstrictor effect of inhaled prostaglandin D₂ in normal and asthmatic men. N Engl J Med 311:209, 1984.

Hendles L, Weinberger M: Theophylline. In Middleton E, Reed CE, Ellis EF (Eds.): Allergy: Principles and Practice. Vol I. St. Louis, C. V. Mosby Co., 1983, p 535.

Henderson WR, Shelhamer JH, Reingold DB, et al.: Alpha-adrenergic hyper-responsiveness in asthma: analysis of vascular and pupillary responses. N Engl J Med 300:642, 1979.

Hirshman CA: Airway reactivity in humans. Anesthesiology 58:170, 1983.

Horrobin DF, Manku MS, Franks DJ, et al.: Methylxanthine phosphodiesterase inhibitors behave as prostaglandin antagonists in a perfused rat mesentery artery preparation. Prostaglandins 13:33, 1977.

Jacobs MH, Senior RM, Kessler G: Clinical experience with theophylline: relationship between dosage, serum concentration and toxicity. JAMA 235:1983, 1976.

Katz RM, Rachelefsky GS, Siegel SC, et al.: Theophylline administration in children with asthma: optimal pulmonary function and possible tolerance to chronic administration. Ann Allergy 50:23, 1983.

Kemp JP: Adrenergic bronchodilators, old and new. J Asthma 20:45, 1983.

Kingston HGG, Hirshman CA: Perioperative management of the patient with asthma. Anesth Analg 63:844, 1984.

Kline LE: Sympathomimetic agents. In Dawson A, Simon RA (Eds.): The Practical Management of Asthma. Orlando, Grune and Stratton, 1984.

Konig P: The use of cromolyn in the management of hyperreactive airways and exercise. J Allergy Clin Immunol 73:686, 1984.

Landay RA, Gonzalez MA, Taylor JC: Effect of phenobarbital on theophylline disposition. J Allergy Clin Immunol 62:27, 1978.

Letarte L, duSouich P: Influence of hypercapnia and/or hypoxemia and metabolic acidosis on theophylline kinetics in the conscious rabbit. Am Rev Respir Dis 129:762, 1984.

Levy G, Koysooko R: Pharmacokinetic analysis of the effect of theophylline on pulmonary function in asthmatic children. J Pediatr 86:789, 1975.

Lichtenstein LM, Gillespie E: Inhibition of histamine release controlled by the receptor. Nature 244:287, 1973.

Lonnerholm G, Foucard T, Lindstrom B: Dose, plasma concentration, and effect of oral terbutaline in long-term treatment of childhood asthma. J Allergy Clin Immunol 73:508, 1984.

McFadden ER Jr.: Pathogenesis of asthma. J Allergy Clin Immunol 73:413, 1984.

McLaughlin ET, Bethea LN, Wittig HJ: Comparison of the bronchodilator effect of oral fenoterol and ephedrine in asthmatic children. Ann Allergy 49:191, 1982.

Menendez R, Kelly HW: Theophylline therapy. J Asthma 20:455, 1983.

Middleton E Jr: The biochemical basis for the modulation of allergic reactions by drugs. Pediatr Clin North Am 22:111, 1975.

Mislap RL, Krauss AN, Auld PAM: Oxygen consumption in apneic premature infants after low-dose theophylline. Clin Pharmacol Ther 28:536, 1980.

Mitenko PA, Ogilvie RI: Rational intravenous doses of theophylline. N Engl J Med 289:600, 1973.

Mueller RA: Recent developments in the physiology of bronchomotor tone and the pharmacology of bronchodilators. Int Anesthesiol Clin 15:137, 1977.

Nathan RA, Segall N, Glover GC, et al.: The effects of H_1 and H_2 antihistamines on histamine inhalation challenges in asthmatic patients. Am Rev Respir Dis 120:1251, 1979.

Oyama T: Hazards of steroids in association with anaesthesia. Can Anaesth Soc J 16:361, 1969.

Patel KR: Sodium cromoglycate in histamine and methacholine reactivity in asthma. Clin Allergy 14:143, 1984.

Pollock J, Kiechel F, Cooper D, et al.: Relationship of serum theophylline concentration to inhibition of exercise-induced bronchospasm and comparison with cromolyn. Pediatrics 60:840, 1977.

Popa VT: Clinical pharmacology of adrenergic drugs. J Asthma 21:183, 1984.

Prenner BM: Safety, efficacy and bronchodilator sparing effects of nebulized cromolyn sodium solution in the treatment of asthma in children. Ann Allergy 49:186, 1982.

Ravin MB: Comparison of spinal and general anesthesia for lower abdominal surgery in patients with chronic obstructive pulmonary disease. Anesthesiology 35:319, 1971.

Schuhl JF, De Cuesta DH: A double-blind trial comparing disodium cromoglycate (DSCG), and ketotifen in extrinsic children. Clin Allergy 11:401, 1981.

Selcow JE: Cromolyn therapy in children. J Allergy 20:361, 1983.

Shapiro GG: Corticosteroids in the treatment of allergic disease: principles and practice. Pediatr Clin North Am 30:955, 1983.

Sherman B, Weinberger M, Chen-Walden H, et al.: Further studies of the effects of inhaled glucocorticoids on pituitary-adrenal function in healthy adults. J Allergy Clin Immunol 69:208, 1982.

Shnider SM, Paper EM: Anesthesia for the asthmatic patient. Anesthesiology 22:886, 1961.

Siegel SC: Bronchial asthma. In Kelley VC (Ed.): Practice of Pediatrics. Philadelphia, Harper and Row, 1984.

Simons FER, Friesen FR, Simons KJ: Theophylline toxicity in term infants. Am J Dis Child 134:39, 1980.

Sly RM: Current theories of the pathophysiology of asthma. J Asthma 20:419, 1983.

Somani SM, Khanna NN, Bada HS: Caffeine and theophylline serum/CSF correlation in premature infants. J Pediatr 96:1091, 1980.

Stevenson DD: Anticholinergic agents. In Dawson A, Simon RA (Eds.): The Practical Management of Asthma. Orlando, Grune and Stratton, 1984.

Symreng T, Karlberg BE, Kagedal B, et al.: Physiological cortisol substitution of long-term steroid-treated patients undergoing major surgery. Br J Anaesth 53:949, 1981.

Szefler SJ: Practical considerations in the safe and effective use of theophylline. Pediatr Clin North Am 30:943, 1983.

Tinkelman DG: The scope and state of pediatric asthma. J Asthma 20:331, 1983.

Tserng K, King KC, Takieddine FN: Theophylline metabolism in premature infants. Clin Pharmacol Ther 29:594, 1981.

Urthaler F, James TN: Both direct and neurally mediated components of the chronotropic actions of aminophylline. Chest 70:24, 1976.

Webb-Johnson DC, Andrews JL: Bronchodilator therapy. (Part I). N Engl J Med 297:476, 1977.

White VA, Kumagai LF: Preoperative endocrine and metabolic considerations. Med Clin North Am 63:1321, 1979.

Weinberger M, Hendles L, Ahrens R: Clinical pharmacology of drugs used for asthma. Pediatr Clin North Am 28:61, 1981.

Weinberger MM: Use of ephedrine in bronchodilator therapy. Pediatr Clin North Am 22:121, 1975.

Weinberger MM, Bronsky EA: Evaluation of oral bronchodilator therapy in asthmatic children. J Pediatr 84:421, 1974.

Weinberger MM, Bronsky EA: Interaction of ephedrine and theophylline. Clin Pharmacol Ther 17:585, 1975.

Wyatt R, Waschek J, Weinberger M, et al.: Effects of inhaled beclomethasone dipropionate and alternate-day prednisone on pituitary-adrenal function in children with chronic asthma. N Engl J Med 299:1387, 1978.

Zeiger RS: Special considerations in the approach to asthma in infancy and early childhood. J Asthma 20:353, 1983.

Zwillich CW, Sutton FD, Neff TA, et al.: Theophylline-induced seizures in adults: correlation with serum concentrations. Ann Intern Med 82:784, 1975.

MASTOCYTOSIS

Diagnosis
Pathophysiology
Treatment
    Symptomatic Therapy

Curative Therapy
Therapy of Malignant Complications
Anesthetic Management

Mastocytosis, a disorder of unknown etiology, is defined histologically as an abnormal proliferation of mast cells in the skin (urticaria pigmentosa) or less frequently, in both the skin and systemic tissues (systemic mastocytosis). This rare disorder (0.01 to 0.1 percent of new dermatology clinic patients) presents with cutaneous signs at birth in 11 percent of cases, and by 2 years of age in 50 to 80 percent of the cases. The inheritance pattern for mastocytosis is thought to be multifactorial, although autosomal dominant patterns with variable penetrance have been suggested. The prognosis of the disease in the pediatric age group is excellent, with resolution of the disease in 50 percent of the children by puberty. Mast cell leukemia is a rare complication of systemic mastocytosis, usually of the adult-onset type.

Urticaria pigmentosa is the most common form of mastocytosis in the pediatric age group. This disorder is characterized by a single or multifocal eruption of reddish-brown macules, papules, or nodules 1 to 3 cm in diameter on the trunk or, less commonly, on the extremities. These lesions appear and disappear over a period of time. They can coalesce and give the appearance of "leopard skin." In infancy, vesicular or bullous lesions are characteristic. Mastocytomas may also appear in early infancy in as many as 10 percent of all patients with urticaria pigmentosa as solitary reddish-brown or yellow nodules on the trunk or extremities. Rarely, yellow papules (xanthelasmoidea) resembling xanthomas are also present in infants with urticaria pigmentosa. The erythrodermic and diffuse cutaneous forms of mastocytosis are rare and suggest the possibility of systemic involvement, particularly in the adult age group.

Systemic mastocytosis, which occurs in approximately 10 percent of all cases, complicates urticaria pigmentosa infrequently in infants and children. However, when present it can involve bone (15 percent of pediatric cases), the gastrointestinal tract, the liver (48 percent of cases), the spleen, and to a lesser extent lymph nodes, thymus, and pancreas. Systemic mastocytosis rarely involves cardiac, renal, pulmonary, and meningeal tissues. Systemic complications of mastocytosis result from the dense proliferation of large numbers of mast cells, which engorge the organ and compromise function. When bone is involved, local bone pain and tenderness is common. Invasion of the bone marrow (myelolisthesis) may replace bone marrow precursors and result in pancytopenia. Direct infiltration of the gastric, small bowel, and rectal mucosae may cause anorexia, nausea, vomiting, diarrhea, and hematemesis. A resultant malabsorption syndrome can cause vitamin B_{12} deficiency and hypocalcemia. Peptic ulcers are present in 5 percent of patients with systemic mastocytosis. Extensive infiltration of the liver can produce hepatic dysfunction, resulting in a decrease in the serum concentrations of the liver-dependent coagulation factors, albumin, and cholesterol. If portal hypertension develops, splenomegaly, anemia, and bleeding may ensue. The hematological manifestations include anemia and decreased eosinophil chemotaxis. Bleeding may occur because of a reduced concentration of the liver-dependent coagulation factors, thrombocytopenia, or from systemic heparin released from mast cells during degranulation. Infrequently, polycythemia rubra vera is associated with urticaria pigmentosa.

DIAGNOSIS

Urticaria pigmentosa is usually diagnosed by the characteristic skin lesions, the presence of circumferential erythema when the lesions are firmly stroked (Darier sign is positive in 92 percent of cases), dermographism (wheals in 50 percent of cases), or the presence of vesicles and bullae in infants and children when uninvolved skin is firmly stroked. The diagnosis is confirmed by a skin biopsy, which reveals densely packed mast cells (in addition to eosinophils, plasma cells, and lymphocytes) in the perivascular regions of the dermis. The peripheral blood smear usually shows a leukocytosis; mast cells are rarely present.

The local and systemic manifestations of mastocytosis result from the clinical effects of the products of degranulation: histamine, heparin, and possibly prostaglandin D_2 (Table 16–15). Two thirds of those patients with isolated urticaria pigmentosa are asymptomatic. However, approximately one third of these patients experience pruritus and intermittent episodes of flushing of the face and upper torso. Less commonly bruising, blistering, and bleeding occur. These symp-

Table 16–15. MAST CELL MEDIATORS

Mediator	Pharmacological Effect
Preformed mediators	
Histamine (H_1)	Bronchoconstriction, increased capillary permeability
Eosinophil chemotactic factor (ECFA)	Eosinophil chemotaxis
Neutrophil chemotactic factor (NCFA)	Neutrophil chemotaxis
Heparin	Anticoagulation, inhibition of complement activation
Immediately synthesized mediators	
Leukotrienes C, D, E (slow reacting substance)	Bronchoconstriction, increased capillary permeability
PGD_2, PGF_2	Bronchoconstriction
Thromboxane A_2, PGE_1, PGE_2	Bronchodilation, increased capillary permeability
Platelet activating factor (PAF)	Platelet aggregation and degranulation

toms may be precipitated by exercise, stress, wide swings in temperature, or drugs such as aspirin and codeine.

Systemic mastocytosis should be thought of when the symptoms described above complicate either isolated mastocytosis or extensive cutaneous infiltrations (with bullous, erythrodermic, or diffuse cutaneous forms). Furthermore, systemic mastocytosis should be suspected when the mastocytosis syndrome of headache, fever, flushing, dyspnea, palpitations, syncope, nausea, vomiting, diarrhea, hepatosplenomegaly, or bone pain occurs alone or in combination with cutaneous lesions such as isolated mastocytoma, extensive bullae, erythroderma, or diffuse cutaneous eruptions.

Histamine concentrations have been measured in both the urine and serum of patients with mastocytosis. Urine concentrations of histamine and 1-methyl-4-imidazolacetic acid (the major metabolite of histamine) may be significantly increased in these patients. However, urine concentrations may fluctuate and do not remain consistently increased. The severity of mastocytosis does not correlate with the urine concentration of histamine. The serum concentration of histamine is not usually increased in patients with mastocytosis except during sudden degranulation of mast cells. During this period, the serum concentration does not reliably correlate with the severity of the disease nor does it reflect the tissue concentration of histamine.

Carcinoid syndrome is the major differential diagnosis from systemic mastocytosis. Patients with carcinoid syndrome present with symptoms similar to those of systemic mastocytosis—palpitations, diarrhea, syncope, and flushing. However, carcinoid syndrome differs from systemic mastocytosis in that the major urinary metabolite in carcinoid syndrome, 5-hydroxyindoleacetic acid, is rarely present in urticaria pigmentosa, and a skin biopsy in carcinoid syndrome reveals extensive argentaffin cell (rather than mast cell) infiltration in the dermis. Additionally, antiserotonin drugs are therapeutic in carcinoid syndrome and not mastocytosis. Right-sided heart disease may be present in carcinoid syndrome but not in mastocytosis.

PATHOPHYSIOLOGY

The local and systemic manifestations of mastocytosis result from the extensive degranulation of mast cells producing histamine, heparin, and prostaglandin D. In mastocytosis, the concentrations of mediators in mast cells and the extent of degranulation of the mast cells are similar to those of mast cells from unaffected individuals. The local and systemic effects of mastocytosis result from the degranulation of a large number of mast cells. The mediators released (Table 16–15) cause both local (cutaneous) and systemic effects. The local effects are described on page 477. Systemic effects include respiratory (bronchoconstriction and increased mucous secretions), cardiovascular (hypotension, arrhythmias, increased capillary permeability, and shock) and gastrointestinal (vomiting, diarrhea, and bleeding).

Mast cells release mediators in response to either immunological or nonimmunological triggers. The immunological triggers may be either a type I (IgE) hypersensitivity reaction or a complement-mediated reaction. Although immunological triggers may be present, there is no evidence that allergy, atopy, or asthma is associated with either urticaria pigmentosa or mastocytosis. Nonimmunological triggers of mast cell degranulation (Table 16–16) are probably responsible for the release of mast cell mediators in mastocytosis. The mechanism responsible for the release during a nonimmunological trigger is unclear, but drugs, wide fluctuations in temperature, vomiting, psychogenic stimulation, and skin irritation have been implicated. Drugs remain the most common nonimmunological trigger of mast cell degranulation in mastocytosis.

Anesthetic drugs must be carefully selected to minimize the risk of mast cell degranulation. In the experimental model, the extent of mast cell degranu-

Table 16–16. NONIMMUNOLOGICAL TRIGGERS OF MAST CELL DEGRANULATION

Physical stimuli
    Temperature fluctuations
    Cutaneous stimulation
    Trauma
Psychogenic stimulus
Calcium ionophor A23187
Drugs
    Codeine, morphine
    D-Tubocurarine, gallamine, dexamethonium
    Polymyxin B, dextran
    Adenosine phosphate
    Alcohol
    Radiographic dyes

lation by drugs is proportional to the peak serum concentration of histamine. Incremental doses of drugs release histamine in a graded response. The release of histamine has been shown to be proportional to the logarithmic concentration of a number of drugs, including morphine and D-tubocurarine. This graded response suggests that all drugs should be administered in small incremental doses to minimize the release of histamine. Although this model may not accurately reflect the response to these drugs "in vivo," the serum concentration of histamine remains the only method currently available for comparing the effects of drugs on mast cell degranulation.

The release of histamine in response to intravenous drugs varies with age. Three groups of children, ages 1 to 4, 5 to 9, and 10 to 15 years, were challenged with D-tubocurarine. There was a highly significant increase in local histamine release with increasing age. This suggests that older children (10 to 15 years) are more likely to release histamine in response to a trigger than are younger children.

General anesthetic drugs have a varied effect of histamine release. The inhalational agents halothane, enflurane, and isoflurane do not release histamine and actively relax the airways in a dose-dependent manner. Rare episodes of bronchospasm have been reported following exposure to enflurane. Of the intravenous drugs currently available for induction of anesthesia, both thiopentone and methohexitone are reported to release histamine in at least 75 percent of responders within 10 minutes of administration, although recent data suggest that methohexital releases significantly less histamine from mast cells in vitro. Ketamine and etomidate are the only intravenous agents that do not release histamine.

Anticholinergic drugs theoretically attenuate mast cell degranulation by decreasing cytoplasmic cGMP concentration. Atropine and glycopyrrolate do not increase the serum concentration of histamine. In contrast, scopolamine is reported to induce mast cell degranulation.

Muscle relaxants have a variable effect on histamine release. D-Tubocurarine causes a moderate release of histamine in a dose-dependent manner. Succinylcholine, metocurine, and atracurium mildly stimulate release of histamine, whereas gallamine, pancuronium, and vecuronium do not to any extent.

Neostigmine in doses up to 0.4 mg/kg does not release histamine from mast cells.

The effect of narcotics is unclear. Demerol has been the narcotic of choice for many years in allergic and asthmatic patients because it does not release clinically significant quantities of histamine. Morphine, however, is avoided in allergic patients because it does release histamine and thus may precipitate bronchospasm. In contrast, fentanyl and sufentanil do not release significant quantities of histamine in doses of 100 μg/kg and 15μg/kg, respectively, and recent research suggests that butorphanol also does not. There are no studies on alfentanil and histamine. Demerol, fentanyl, and sufentanil are probably safe to use in these patients.

TREATMENT

There is no known cure for urticaria pigmentosa or mastocytosis. Therapy is often unnecessary in children with asymptomatic skin lesions. If, however, the lesions cause persistent pruritus or wheals or are bothersome in some other way, or if systemic manifestations of mastocytosis occur, then therapy is indicated. This may be divided into three categories: (1) symptomatic, (2) curative, and (3) therapy for malignancies.

Symptomatic Therapy

The systemic manifestations of mastocytosis result from the release of large quantities of mediators, most commonly histamine. Histamine exerts its physiological effects through two functional receptors, H_1 and H_2. Stimulation of H_1 receptors results in contraction of smooth muscle (as in bronchoconstriction), an increased spacing between the tightly packed endothelial cells (as in increased vascular permeability and edema), and stimulation of nerve end organs (as in pruritus). Stimulation of H_2 receptors results in changes in the cellular cyclic nucleotides, increased gastric acid secretion, and reduced leukocyte function. The overall effect of histamine on a particular organ depends on which histamine receptor is more dominant in that organ.

Antihistamines block the systemic manifestations of histamine by blocking its tissue uptake. They are most effective when given prophylactically. There is recent evidence that antihistamines may stabilize the mast cell membrane and thereby attenuate the release of histamine.

H_1 and H_2 antihistamines may be used in combination to attenuate the systemic manifestations of mastocytosis. H_1 antihistamines alone are unsatisfactory. The H_2 antihistamines, cimetidine (4 mg/kg) and ranitidine (not currently available for pediatrics) have each been successful in controlling the gastrointestinal problems. The combination of H_1 and H_2 antihistamines appears more effective than either drug used singularly to control the systemic manifestations. Anecdotal reports vary concerning this combination therapy for symptomatic control. There have been no controlled studies comparing combination antihistamine therapy to the individual therapies.

Both H_1 and H_2 antihistamines may cause side effects and toxicity even within the dose range recommended for children. H_1 antihistamines produce drowsiness, incoordination, dizziness, tinnitus, blurred vision, and tremor. Some children become hyperactive, irritable, and excitable and rarely progress to convulsions. Toxic doses of antihistamines may disturb the autonomic nervous system, resulting in cardiorespiratory arrest. The treatment of an overdose of an H_1 antihistamine includes supportive therapy, gastric emptying and lavage, anticonvulsants, and, if necessary, hemodialysis.

Although H_2 antihistamines have not been used for an extended period of time in pediatrics, there are data available from studies in adults. H_2 antihistamines cause gastrointestinal disturbances, headache, and rash in less than 2 percent of adults. Cimetidine may lower the threshold for histamine-induced bronchospasm. Hepatic and renal complications have been reported in addition to leukopenia and altered moods. The latter complications appear to be reversible upon cessation of the drug.

Disodium cromoglycate is a membrane-stabilizing drug that has been used with moderate success in patients with urticaria pigmentosa and systemic mastocytosis. The dose of oral disodium cromoglycate is in the range of 300 mg/day to 100 mg/kg/day. Large doses of cromoglycate are required since only 1 percent of the oral preparation reaches the systemic circulation. The oral preparation of cromoglycate appears most effective for the gastrointestinal symptoms of mastocytosis, but is also reported to relieve both the cutaneous and central nervous system manifestations.

Ketotifen is a new antihistamine and antianaphylactic drug currently under investigation for use in patients with urticaria pigmentosa and mastocytosis. Preliminary data suggest that ketotifen acts by inhibiting mediator release, blocking calcium channels, and indirectly by activating beta-agonist receptors. Studies suggest that ketotifen may be as effective as disodium cromoglycate in preventing histamine release in mastocytosis.

The indications for aspirin and other nonsteroidal anti-inflammatory drugs in the treatment of mastocytosis are unclear. Both drugs inhibit prostaglandin synthesis and may attenuate systemic manifestations but have been contraindicated because of reports of severe hypotension following their use. The current recommendations are that aspirin and other noninflammatory drugs may be used with mastocytosis provided they are administered only after the patients are adequately blocked with H_1 and H_2 antihistamines, and only in small incremental doses.

Curative Therapy

Isolated skin lesions in infancy and children usually resolve spontaneously but may require surgical excision. PUVA (a combination of oral 8-methoxypsoralen and long-wave ultraviolet radiation) has been used with moderate success.

Therapy of Malignant Complications

Malignancy is extremely rare in mastocytosis, particularly in pediatric patients. If a malignancy occurs, it may be either leukemia or a benign neoplasm that became malignant. Because these lesions are rare and quite variable, no specific chemotherapeutic regimen has been recommended.

ANESTHETIC MANAGEMENT

Preoperative

A careful history of the signs and symptoms of the systemic manifestations of mastocytosis is important. Because massive amounts of histamine may be released in any patient with urticaria pigmentosa or urticaria, specific triggers such as drugs, anxiety, and others listed in Table 16–16 must be identified and carefully avoided.

Physical examination should begin with the dermatological system, noting the areas of skin involvement and in particular the presence of vesicular or bullous lesions on the face. The respiratory, cardiovascular, hepatic, and neurological systems should be examined for the systemic manifestations of mastocytosis. Laboratory investigations should include a routine hemoglobin assay, urinalysis, platelet count, and a coagulation screen (prothrombin time and partial thromboplastin time).

Premedication should include an H_1 and an H_2 antihistamine (Table 16–17). H_1 and H_2 antihistamines have been effective in attenuating the clinical manifestations of mastocytosis in chronically treated children. These drugs should be administered orally about 1½ hours prior to surgery. There is evidence that disodium cromoglycate (100 mg/kg/day) or ketotifen (0.05 mg/kg) may also be effective in preventing mast cell degranulation when administered orally 1½ hours prior to surgery. For children who are anxious about the surgery, diazepam, 0.2 mg/kg, should be administered orally 2 hours before surgery.

Intraoperative

The anesthetic technique must be tailored to the patient, the surgery, and the anesthetist. The three anesthetic techniques are local, regional, and general anesthesia. There are reports of mast cell degranulation with local and regional techniques. General anesthesia is the technique most commonly used.

To manage these patients successfully during surgery, regardless of anesthetic technique, it is imperative to avoid all the triggers of mast cell degranulation. Because large changes in temperature may precipitate mast cell degranulation, the operating room should be warmed to a comfortable temperature before the patient arrives. Ancillary warming equipment, including a blood warmer, heater humidifier, and warming blanket, should be available. The routine anesthetic monitors, including an electrocardiogram, blood pressure cuff, core temperature probe, and precordial stethoscope, must be present. Nonallergenic tape should be used where possible in these children to avoid dermographism, wheals, and bullae.

Resuscitation equipment and drugs must be available in the operating room before induction of anesthesia. The life-threatening complications of mastocytosis are profound hypotension (shock) and intense bronchospasm. Profound hypotension must be treated immediately with a balanced salt solution (Ringer lactate or normal saline, 10 to 20 ml/kg initially), epinephrine infusion, and diphenhydramine (Table 16–18). If the response to this is poor, then repeated boluses of balanced salt solution or colloid may be infused, as well as further doses of epinephrine. Isolated mild bronchospasm may respond to halothane or a beta$_2$ agonist by inhalation. Intense bronchospasm may require further beta$_2$ agonist by inhalation in 100 percent oxygen, intravenous aminophylline, and isoproterenol (see Table 16–18 and the section on Asthma earlier in this chapter).

The drugs used during general anesthesia in these patients should have either no effect or only a minimal effect on histamine release. Nevertheless, we recommend that general anesthesia be induced with either an inhalational induction (halothane, nitrous oxide, and oxygen) or an intravenous induction (methohexital or ketamine). If an intravenous cannula is not in place before induction of anesthesia, then an intravenous should be started immediately after induction of anesthesia and intravenous atropine, 0.02 mg/kg, should be administered. Pancuronium, vecuronium, or succinylcholine may be used to provide muscle relaxation. If there are no lesions on the face, anesthesia may be maintained with an inhalational agent administered by a soft mask. However, if there are bullous or vesicular lesions on the face, endotracheal intubation can be used to avoid exacerbations of these lesions caused by physical irritation by the mask. The endotracheal tube should be secured with a 2-inch wide flannel tie around the endotracheal tube and the patient's neck. For premature infants, neonates, and older infants, the caliber of the endotracheal tubes is too small to secure with a flannel tie. In these cases, we recommend that nonallergenic tape be used and the tube supported with a bite block. Supplemental narcotics, including meperidine, fentanyl, or sufentanil, may be used safely during surgery. All neuromuscular blockade should be reversed at the completion of anesthesia, with extubation when the patient is completely awake.

Table 16–17. ANTIHISTAMINES IN PEDIATRICS

Drug	Dose*	$t_{1/2}$ (Hours)	t_{max} (Hours)
Diphenhydramine (Benadryl)	5 mg/kg/day in divided doses	3.4†	2.5†
Chlorpheniramine (Chlor-Trimeton)	0.35 mg/kg/day in divided doses	9.6–13	2.5
Promethazine (Phenergan)	0.3 mg/kg/day in divided doses		
Hydroxyzine (Atarax)	2–4 mg/kg/day in 4 divided doses	7	2

*Oral drug dose
†Adult data.

Table 16–18. RESUSCITATION REGIMEN

Drug	Dilution	Dose	Maximum Dose	Frequency
Epinephrine (Adrenalin)	1:10,000	0.02–0.1 ml/kg Sc or IV or in ETT (2–10 μg/kg)	0.5 mg	q 5–10 min
Diphenhydramine (Benadryl)	50 mg/ml	1–2 mg/kg IV	50 mg	Bolus
		5 mg/kg/day IV or PO		q 6 h
Isoproterenol (Isuprel)	1 mg in 250 ml Ringer lactate	3 μg/kg IV	100 μg	Bolus
		0.05–0.5 μg/kg/min IV	2 μg/kg/min	Continuous
Aminophylline	500 mg in 500 ml of D5W/0.2%	5–7 mg/kg	Serum levels <20 μg/ml	Infusion over 20 minutes
		1 mg/kg/hour		Infusion
Atropine		20 μg/kg IV, IM, or SL*	1.0 mg	q 20 min

*SL = sublingual
Adapted from Edmonds, J, Surh, L, Banks J: Resuscitation Card. Resuscitation Committee 1984, The Hospital for Sick Children, Toronto.

Postoperative

In the postoperative period, analgesia must be restricted to small doses of those drugs that do not release histamine: meperidine, acetaminophen, and fentanyl. Codeine, which is commonly used in the postoperative period for analgesia in children, should not be given. If fentanyl is used, it should be given as an infusion only in the postanesthetic recovery room or intensive care unit where continuous monitoring of respiratory rate is possible.

Postoperative fever may be treated with either oral or rectal acetaminophen (10 mg/kg for infants and young children). Although aspirin had been considered contraindicated in these patients, its use has been recommended recently. However, aspirin should be used cautiously in the immediate postoperative period since it may cause postoperative bleeding.

REFERENCES

Ammann RW, Vetter P, Deyhle P, et al.: Gastro-intestinal involvement in systemic mastocytosis. Gut 17:107, 1976.

Basta SJ, Savarese JJ, Ali HH, et al.: Histamine-releasing potencies of atracurium besylate (BW 33A), metocurine, and d-tubocurarine. Anesthesiology 57:A261, 1982.

Bristow MR, Ginsburg R, Harrison DC: Histamine and the human heart: the other receptor system. Am J Cardiol 49:249, 1982.

Broitman SA: Mastocytosis and intestinal malabsorption. Am J Med 48:382, 1970.

Businco L, Cantani A, Businco E, et al.: Systemic mastocytosis in a 5-year-old child: successful treatment with disodium cromoglycate. Clin Allergy 14:147, 1984.

Campbell EW, Hector D, Gossain V: Heparin activity in systemic mastocytosis. Ann Intern Med 90:940, 1979.

Caplan RM: The natural course of urticaria pigmentosa. Analysis and follow-up of 112 cases. Arch Dermatol 87:146, 1963.

Christophers E, Honigsmann H, Wolff K, et al.: PUVA—treatment of urticaria pigmentosa. Br J Dermatol 98:701, 1978.

Coleman MA, Liberthson RR, Crone RK, et al.: General anaesthesia in a child with urticaria pigmentosa. Anesth Analg 59:704, 1980.

Colten HR: Mediators of allergic response. In Kelley VC (Ed.): Practice of Pediatrics. Vol 2. Philadelphia, Harper and Row, 1984.

Czarnetzki BM, Behrendt H: Urticaria pigmentosa: clinical picture and response to oral disodium cromoglycate. Br J Derm 105:563, 1981.

Demis DJ: The mastocytosis syndrome: clinical and biological studies. Ann Intern Med 59:194, 1963.

Demis DJ: Walton MD, Higdon RS: Histaminuria in urticaria pigmentosa: a clinical study and review of the literature with definition of mastocytosis syndrome. Arch Derm 83:127, 1961.

DiBacco RS, De Leo VA: Mastocytosis and the mast cell. J Am Acad Dermatol 7:709, 1982.

Ellis JM: Urticaria pigmentosa: report of a case with autopsy. Arch Pathol 48:426, 1949.

Fine J: Mastocytosis. Int J Dermatol 19:117, 1980.

Flacke JW, Van Etten A, Flacke WE: Greatest histamine release from meperidine among four narcotics: double-blind study in man. Anesthesiology 59:A51, 1983.

Galletly DC, Treuren BC: Anaphylactoid reactions during anaesthesia: seven years' experience of intradermal testing. Anaesthesia 40:329, 1985.

Gay MW, Noojin RO, Finley WH: Urticaria pigmentosa discordant in identical twins. Arch Dermatol 102:29, 1970.

Gerrard DM, Ko C: Urticaria pigmentosa: treatment with cimetidine and chlorpheniramine. J Pediatr 94:843, 1979.

Greenwood C: The pharmacology of ketotifen. Chest 82:45S, 1982.

Hermens JM, Ebertz JM, Hanifin JM, et al.: Comparison of histamine release in human skin mast cells induced by morphine, fentanyl, and oxymorphone. Anesthesiology 62:124, 1985.

Hirschowitz BI, Groarke MB: Effect of cimetidine on gastric hypersecretion and diarrhea in systemic mastocytosis. Ann Intern Med 90:769, 1979.

Hirshman CA, Edelstein RA, Eastman CL, et al.: Histamine release by barbiturates in human mast cells. Anesthesiology 61:A352, 1984.

Karlin JM: The use of antihistamines in allergic disease. Pediatr Clin North Am 22:157, 1975.

Klaus SN, Winkelman RK: Course of urticaria pigmentosa in children. Arch Dermatol 86:86, 1962.

Lewis RA, Austen KF: Mastocytosis—clinical mediators and therapeutic intervention. In Fitzpatrick TB, Eisen AZ, Wolff K, et al. (Eds.): Update: Dermatology in General Medicine. New York, McGraw-Hill, 1983, p 197.

Lorenz W, Doeniche A: Anaphylactoid reactions and histamine release by IV drugs used in surgery and anesthesia. In Watkins J, Ward AM, (Eds.): Adverse Response to IV Drugs. New York, Grune and Stratton, 1978, p 83.

Lucaya J, Perez-Candela V, Aso C, et al.: Mastocytosis with skeletal and gastrointestinal involvement in infancy. Radiology 131:363, 1979.

Manchikanti L, Kraus JW, Edds SP: Cimetidine and related drugs in anesthesia. Anesth Analg 61:595, 1982.

Miller RD, Rupp SM, Fisher DM, et al.: Clinical pharmacology of vecuronium and atracurium. Anesthesiology 61:444, 1984.

Mishima S, Yamamura T: Anaphylactoid reaction to pancuronium. Anesth Analg 63:865, 1984.

Moss J, Rosow CE: Histamine release by narcotics and muscle relaxants in humans. Anesthesiology 59:330, 1983.

Moss J, Rosow CE, Savarese JJ, et al.: Role of histamine in the hypotensive action of d-tubocurarine in humans. Anesthesiology 55:19, 1981.

Nightingale DA, Bush GH: A clinical comparison between d-tubocurarine and pancuronium in children. Br J Anaesth 45:63, 1973.

Orkin M, Good RA, Clawson CC, et al.: Bullous mastocytosis. Arch Dermatol 101:547, 1970.

Parker F, Odland GF: The mastocytosis syndrome. In Fitzpatrick TB, Eisen AZ, Wolff K, et al. (Eds.): Dermatology in General Medicine. New York, McGraw-Hill, 1979, p 772.

Philbin DM, Moss J, Akins CW, et al.: The use of H₁ and H₂ histamine antagonists with morphine anesthesia: a double-blind study. Anesthesiology 55:292, 1981.

Roberts LJ II, Sweetman BJ, Lewis RA, et al.: Increased production of prostaglandin D₂ in patients with systemic mastocytosis. N Engl J Med 303:1400, 1980.

Rockoff AS: Urticaria pigmentosa in identical twins. Arch Dermatol 114:1227, 1978.

Rosenbaum KJ, Strobel GE: Anesthetic considerations in mastocytosis. Anesthesiology 38:398, 1973.

Rosow CE, Moss J, Philbin DM, et al.: Histamine release during morphine and fentanyl anesthesia. Anesthesiology 56:93, 1982.

Rosow CE, Philbin DM, Keegan CR, et al.: Hemodynamics and histamine release during induction with sufentanil or fentanyl. Anesthesiology 60:489, 1984.

Sagher F, Even-Paz Z: Mastocytosis and the Mast Cell. Chicago, Year Book Medical, 1967, pp 14–120, 148–338.

Schachner L, Press S: Vesicular bullous and pustular disorders in infancy and childhood. Pediatr Clin of N Am 30:609, 1983.

Scott RPF, Savarese JJ, Basta SJ, et al.: Atracurium: clinical strategies for preventing histamine release and attenuating the hemodynamic response. Br J Anaesth 57:550, 1985.

Siler JN, Mager JG, Wyche MQ: Atracurium: hypotension, tachycardia and bronchospasm. Anesthesiology 62:645, 1985.

Simone JV, Hayes WT: Bullous urticaria pigmentosa with bleeding. J Pediatr 78:160, 1971.

Soter NA, Austin KF, Wasserman SI: Oral disodium cromoglycate in the management of systemic mastocytosis. N Engl J Med 30:465, 1979.

Sutter MC, Beaulieu G, Birt AR: Histamine liberation by codeine and polymyxin B in urticaria pigmentosa. Arch Dermatol 86:217, 1962.

Watkins J: Adverse anaesthetic reactions. Anaesthesia 40:797, 1985.

Williams JG: H₂ receptor antagonists and anesthesia. Can Anesth Soc J 30:264, 1983.

Wyre HW, Hendrichs WD: Systemic mastocytosis and pulmonary eosinophilic granuloma. JAMA 239:856, 1978.

ERYTHEMA MULTIFORME

Erythema Multiforme Minor
Erythema Multiforme Major (Stevens-Johnson Syndrome)

Treatment
Anesthetic Management

Erythema multiforme is an inflammatory cutaneous syndrome that occurs in all age groups. This syndrome is usually benign, although in the more severe form of the disease (Stevens-Johnson syndrome) death has been reported in as many as 18 percent of cases. Death results from extensive respiratory, skin, and infectious complications.

Erythema multiforme is classified into two types: (1) erythema multiforme minor, which is a self-limiting mild cutaneous syndrome, and (2) erythema multiforme major (or Stevens-Johnson syndrome). The latter may present with the same cutaneous findings as the minor type, but is distinguished by the sudden onset of a febrile illness associated with severe lesions of the mucocutaneous membranes (stomatitis and conjunctivitis) and possibly toxic epidermal necrolysis. Toxic epidermal necrolysis is associated with approximately 50 percent mortality.

ERYTHEMA MULTIFORME MINOR

In one third of patients the onset of the minor form of erythema multiforme is heralded by an upper respiratory tract infection. The characteristic skin lesion is a target lesion, which begins as a round erythematous macule and evolves into a papule with circumferential pallor within a few days. The center of the papule undergoes epidermal necrosis leaving a pale center and an erythematous ring. The papules may coalesce into plaques with a central vesicle, bulla, or dry skin. The skin lesions are symmetrically distributed over the dorsal surfaces of the hands, nailfolds, and extensor surfaces (elbows and knees), and are particularly prominent in areas of sun exposure and physical trauma (Koebner phenomenon). These lesions may cause pruritus and burning and usually resolve within 2 to 4 weeks, leaving areas of hyperpigmentation.

ERYTHEMA MULTIFORME MAJOR (STEVENS-JOHNSON SYNDROME)

The major form is a much more severe disease having systemic manifestations including fever, malaise, headache, sore throat, cough, chest pain, vomiting, and diarrhea, which occur up to 2 weeks before the onset of mucocutaneous lesions. The characteristic lesion is a bullous one that appears quite suddenly on the oral mucosa, lips, and conjunctiva. Other ocular problems include bilateral purulent conjunctivitis, corneal ulcers, and panophthalmitis. Atrial fibrillation and myocarditis may also be present.

The skin lesions may evolve into large bullae or extensive areas of toxic epidermal necrolysis, which have a tendency to become infected and slough. They develop slowly and may take up to 6 weeks to heal completely.

Mucosal involvement may include the oropharynx, nasopharynx, tracheobronchial tree, esophagus, and genitourinary tract. Extensive ulceration of the respiratory tree has been reported. This has been complicated by pneumonia, pleural effusions, and bronchopleural fistulas.

Histological examination reveals an accumulation of mononuclear cells in the upper dermis. In the major form, there may be severe epidermal skin damage with necrosis and exfoliation of large areas of full-thickness epidermis.

Erythema multiforme is associated with four underlying causes: (1) drugs, (2) *Mycoplasma pneumoniae* infections, (3) recurrent herpes simplex viral infections, and (4) neoplasms.

The major form is one of the most severe cutaneous reactions associated with drugs. Sulfa drugs (such as thiazides), barbiturates, penicillins, and diphenylhydantoin have been implicated. The eruption may occur from hours to weeks after exposure.

Antecedent infections are the second most common cause of erythema multiforme major. *Mycoplasma pneumoniae* or recurrent herpes simplex may herald an eruption.

Two mechanisms have been proposed to explain the pathogenesis of this disorder: (1) an immune complex response or (2) a generalized hypersensitivity reaction.

TREATMENT

Treatment of the minor form of erythema multiforme includes topical soaks with hydrogen peroxide and antihistamines for pruritus, although antihistamines may trigger the major form. There is no indication for topical or systemic steroids in the treatment of the minor form of erythema multiforme.

The major form must be managed more aggressively with special consideration given in the presence of toxic epidermal necrosis, bullous lesions, and ocular complications. This includes control of fluids, temperature, and infections (avoiding penicillin). High-dose steroids have been used in cases of Stevens-Johnson syndrome with extensive exfoliative epidermal necrosis, although the indications for this therapy remain controversial. Prednisone, 1 to 2 mg/kg, may be administered orally (or a comparable dose parenterally) and then tapered quickly over a short period of time.

ANESTHETIC MANAGEMENT

Preoperative assessment should include a careful inquiry for a recent chest infection and for drug reactions or allergies. Reduced exercise tolerance, shortness of breath, or chest pain suggests respiratory or cardiovascular involvement. Recent administration of systemic steroids will require parenteral steroids preoperatively.

The physical examination should assess the severity of the cutaneous and mucosal lesions. If extensive epidermal necrolysis is present, intravenous access may be difficult to establish, the fluid balance and electrolyte concentrations may be abnormal, and the patient's temperature may be difficult to control. If the epidermis is diffusely necrotic, sterile precautions must be used. When extensive oral mucosal lesions are present, care must be exercised in manipulating the airway. In this case, intubation should be avoided if possible. Specific findings in the respiratory system include evidence of lower airway infection, bullous lung disease, or bronchopleural fistulas. Chest tubes may be present in patients with the latter two findings. The cardiac system should be examined for evidence of arrhythmias or cardiac decompensation (myocarditis or pericarditis). Evidence of systemic illness, including fever, dehydration, and electrolyte imbalance, may predispose to renal insufficiency.

Laboratory investigations should include hematocrit, urinalysis, and electrolytes. Depending on the severity of systemic involvement a chest x-ray, blood gas measurement, and an electrocardiogram may be indicated.

Premedication, if required, should be administered orally, rectally, or intravenously. Intramuscular or subcutaneous injections should be avoided because of the risk of bullous epidermal reactions. Preoperative steroids are indicated if the patient is currently receiving them or has received them in the previous 6 months.

All patients with Stevens-Johnson syndrome are susceptible to exfoliative skin reactions from minimal trauma. As a result, all monitors must be adapted to minimize this. The blood pressure cuff should be well padded and the electrocardiogram fitted with needles rather than sticky pads. A precordial stethoscope should be gently placed on the chest without strong adhesives during the induction period. An esophageal stethoscope may be used to monitor the heart sounds and air entry if the trachea is intubated. All pressure points (for example, elbows, heels) should be well padded after the patient is positioned.

The airway should be maintained with minimal intervention. Consideration should be given to local or regional anesthetic techniques, although direct infiltration of drugs may result in bullous formation. Anesthesia may be maintained with a neurolept or inhalational technique. If an inhalational technique is used, gentle application of a padded mask is suggested.

Padding for the mask in such cases may include soft cotton or muslin soaked with hydrocortisone cream.

Endotracheal intubation is sometimes necessary. In these cases care should be taken to avoid trauma to pharyngeal and glottic structures. An uncuffed endotracheal tube, a half size smaller than required, will help minimize the laryngeal trauma. The tube may be secured with a flannel strip around the neck. In those cases in which the larynx cannot be visualized and airway obstruction develops, a tracheotomy may be required.

Anesthesia may be induced with an inhalational induction or ketamine. All barbiturates must be avoided. If the oral lesions are extensive, visualization of the laryngeal inlet may be difficult. In this case, an inhalational induction with halothane and oxygen would be indicated. Anesthesia may be maintained with any combination of inhalational agents (halothane, isoflurane, enflurane, or nitrous oxide), intravenous agents (excluding barbiturates), and neuromuscular blocking drugs. The administration of penicillin, sulfonamides, streptomycin, and chloramphenicol must be carefully avoided at all times.

Mild postoperative pain may be controlled with rectal acetaminophen. If the pain is severe, an intravenous bolus or infusion of narcotics may be required. Salicylates should not be used because they may trigger reactions and cause platelet dysfunction and postoperative bleeding.

REFERENCES

Bean SF, Quezada RK: Recurrent oral erythema multiforme: clinical experience with 11 patients. JAMA 249:2810, 1983.

Bedi TR, Pinkus H: Histopathologic spectrum of erythema multiforme. Br J Dermatol 95:243, 1976.

Collins-Williams C: Urticaria and angioedema. In Kelley VC (Ed.): Practice of Pediatrics. Vol. 2. Philadelphia, Harper and Row, 1984.

Cucchiara RF, Dawson B: Anesthetic in Stevens-Johnson syndrome: report of a case. Anesthesiology 35:537, 1971.

Edmond BJ, Huff JL, Weston WL: Erythema multiforme. Pediatr Clin North Am, 30:631, 1983.

Ginsburg CM: Stevens-Johnson syndrome in children. Pediatr Infect Dis 1:155, 1982.

Lever WF, Schaumburg-Lever G: Histopathology of the skin. 6th ed. Philadelphia, J. B. Lippincott Co., 1983, p 122.

Lyell A: A review of toxic epidermal necrolysis in Britain. Br J Dermatol 79:662, 1967.

Smith GB, Shribman AJ: Anaesthesia and severe skin disease. Anesthesia 39:443, 1984.

Szefler SJ, Ellis EF: Adverse reactions to drugs. In Kelley VC (Ed.): Practice of Pediatrics. Vol. 2. Philadelphia, Harper and Row, 1984.

ANAPHYLAXIS

Etiology
Clinical Manifestations
Pathological Findings

Differential Diagnosis
Pathogenesis
Management during Anesthesia

Anaphylaxis is a clinical syndrome resulting from the sudden release of cytoplasmic mediators from mast cells and basophils. It may be immune-mediated or nonimmunologically mediated. Immune-mediated anaphylaxis is either IgE-mediated or complement-mediated (by C3 and C4 or the alternate pathway). Nonimmunological anaphylaxis (often referred to as anaphylactoid) depends on either arachidonic acid metabolites or direct release of cytoplasmic mediators. Regardless of etiology, anaphylaxis commonly involves four organ systems: skin, cardiovascular, respiratory, and gastrointestinal. The spectrum ranges from a minor reaction involving only the skin to fatal anaphylaxis with cardiovascular and/or respiratory collapse.

The reported incidence of anaphylaxis varies. The incidence of anaphylaxis to drugs at induction of anesthesia ranges from 1 in 1000 to as low as 1 in 30,000. Reactions to penicillin, one of the most common triggers, may occur as frequently as 7 per 1000 patients with a fatality rate of approximately 0.1 per million cases. Anaphylaxis causing death occurs in approximately 0.4 per million patients. The risk of anaphylaxis increases with the duration and frequency of exposures to the triggering agent. Parenteral administration is more likely to induce problems than oral or rectal administration. Recent data suggest that a history of atopy does not predispose patients to anaphylaxis.

ETIOLOGY

IgE-Mediated Anaphylaxis. The immunoglobulin IgE is synthesized in B lymphocytes and comprises less than 0.001 percent of the circulating immunoglobulins in healthy individuals. Between 1000 and 5000 IgE molecules are fixed to the surfaces of mast cells and basophils. When an antigen bridges two IgE molecules, cell membrane receptors are approximated. This activates a membrane-bound methyltransferase enzyme that, with the aid of cAMP, facilitates the transmembrane influx of calcium ions. An increased cytoplasmic concentration of calcium induces degranulation of the mast cells and basophils, with the release of cytoplasmic mediators.

The serum concentration of IgE depends on age. IgE is present in only trace concentrations in the fetus. After birth, the serum concentration of IgE increases very slowly for the first 2 or 3 years of life (to 10 percent of the serum concentration in adults), and then increases to a maximum between 10 and 15 years of age. It then decreases gradually between 20 and 80 years of age.

IgE-mediated anaphylaxis is responsible for most reactions to antibiotics (for example, penicillin, cephalosporin, and vancomycin), some anesthetic drugs (for example, thiopentone, local anesthetics, muscle relaxants, steroids), foreign proteins (for example, insulin, chymopapain, protamine, vasopressin, ACTH), and foods. This type of anaphylaxis occurs in both atopic and nonatopic individuals with similar frequencies.

Immune Complex–Mediated Anaphylaxis. This type of anaphylaxis occurs after the administration of blood or plasma or their byproducts, or other volume expanders such as dextran and other collodion substitutes. Protein complexes in blood may activate complement, which degranulates mast cells and basophils.

Arachidonic Acid Metabolism. Aspirin and the nonsteroidal anti-inflammatory drugs (NSAIDs) may trigger anaphylaxis. Although the mechanism of this is unclear, it has been suggested that these drugs act either by inhibiting cyclo-oxygenase and therefore prostaglandin synthesis, or by disruption of the enzymes in the lipoxygenase pathway involved in arachidonic acid metabolism. The serum concentration of histamine is normal, and complement is usually decreased. Anaphylaxis, urticaria, and angioedema following ingestion of aspirin or NSAIDs may occur in up to 1 percent of the general population, with a possible familial predisposition. The incidence of these reactions in asthmatics is between 1 and 20 percent, also with a possible familial predisposition. Such patients are also cross-sensitive to NSAIDs, tartrazine, and benzoate-containing compounds. An anaphylactic reaction in the asthmatic begins slowly with rhinorrhea and flushing of the upper torso, and progresses to the development of bronchospasm, hypotension, and rarely cyanosis. Symptoms may continue for several hours before abating.

Direct Mast Cell Degranulating Drugs. Anaphylaxis following administration of some drugs results in direct degranulation of mast cells and basophils, causing a massive release of histamine and activation of complement in otherwise normal patients. Drugs reported to cause anaphylaxis in this manner include muscle relaxants (D-tubocurarine, gallamine, succinylcholine, and pancuronium), narcotics (morphine, codeine, and meperidine), thiopentone, methohexitone, alfaxalone (Althesin), local anesthetics (para-aminobenzoic acid esters), steroids (hydrocortisone and methylprednisolone), and radiocontrast media.

Miscellaneous Causes. Idiopathic anaphylaxis is defined as recurrent anaphylaxis of unknown etiology. Exercise-induced anaphylaxis is a recently defined syndrome in which anaphylaxis occurs after exercise if affected patients ingest trigger foods before exercising. Neither of these two syndromes is well defined.

CLINICAL MANIFESTATIONS

The clinical signs and symptoms of anaphylaxis vary from individual to individual, and from attack to attack. Symptoms may occur almost immediately or up to 1 hour after exposure to the trigger. The more acute the onset, the more severe is the reaction. The signs and symptoms may begin with erythema, pruritus, cramps, and presyncope. Urticaria and angioedema may also occur and last up to 24 hours. Early upper respiratory symptoms, which include hoarseness, dyspnea, and in the older child and adult, the sensation of a lump in the throat, may herald laryngeal edema and impending upper airway obstruction. Laryngeal edema is a major cause of fatal anaphylaxis, and respiratory complications are responsible for up to 70 percent of cases of fatalities. Early lower respiratory tract symptoms include dyspnea, wheezing, and bronchospasm.

In some cases, severe and intractable bronchospasm leads to hypoxia and cardiac arrest, which are frequently fatal. Death may occur within minutes of the attack or as long as days or weeks later. Cardiovascular complications alone are responsible for 24 percent of fatal anaphylaxis. Gastrointestinal symptoms include nausea, vomiting, acute cramps, and severe diarrhea. Minor associated problems include nasal, ocular, and palatal pruritus, fecal or urinary incontinence, sneezing, diaphoresis, and disorientation.

PATHOLOGICAL FINDINGS

The triad of pathological findings in severe anaphylaxis include angioedema of the upper airway, bronchospasm of the lower airway, and vasodilatation and circulatory collapse. Approximately 66 percent of cases of fatal anaphylaxis develop angioneurotic or laryngeal edema and upper airway obstruction. Laryngeal edema results from interstitial swelling in the lamina propria of the hypopharynx, larynx, and epiglottis. In cases of delayed death pathological findings in the lower airway are common, with 25 to 50 percent of patients showing changes of pulmonary hyperinflation. Less commonly, atelectasis, pulmonary hemorrhage, and edema are found.

Circulatory collapse is attributed to marked peripheral vasodilatation, which leads to reduced venous return and hypotension. Occasionally, cardiac arrhythmias and myocardial ischemia may occur.

Anaphylaxis may also affect other organs. Congestion of the liver, spleen, and stomach has been reported.

Laboratory and radiological tests for anaphylaxis are

nonspecific. The serum concentration of histamine is increased, clotting times may be prolonged, and the serum concentration of complement is abnormal in some patients. However, none of these tests is diagnostic.

Investigations may be performed to detect allergy to drugs. Intradermal skin testing is commonly used. Pediatric patients will not accept repeated skin punctures. Furthermore, the results of intradermal testing are quite variable in children. During an anaphylactic reaction, blood may be taken for measurement of the serum concentration of histamine, IgE antibody, and the C_3 and C_4 complement fractions.

The passive transfer test provided a very accurate means to detect allergies by transferring serum from an allergic patient to a second individual and then testing that individual for the Prausnitz-Küstner reaction. However, the risk of transferring hepatitis has made this test obsolete.

An assay for detecting antibodies to the trigger may be used. The coprecipitation test and the radioallergosorbent test (RAST) are two such tests. Other studies that may be done are the leukocyte histamine release and IgE inhibition tests.

DIFFERENTIAL DIAGNOSIS

The syndrome of a precipitous eruption of urticaria or angioedema and paroxysmal airway obstruction and circulatory collapse is virtually diagnostic of anaphylaxis. A vasovagal episode, as may occur after injection of a drug in an awake patient, may mimic anaphylaxis without the signs of urticaria or angioedema. In such a case, the patient often feels faint, perspires, and becomes pale. Laryngeal edema is rare and the blood pressure does not change. Patients with hereditary angioedema (HAE) (see page 457) do not commonly exhibit urticaria or hypotension, and there is usually a family history of the disease. The definitive diagnosis of HAE is based on the isolation of C1a inhibitor, the slow response to androgens, and resistance to treatment with epinephrine. Less common syndromes that must be differentiated from anaphylaxis include serum sickness, cold urticaria, insulin anaphylaxis, adrenal insufficiency, and massive hemorrhage. Serum sickness usually has a slow onset—1 to 3 weeks after antigenic exposure—and is associated with fever, edema, lymphadenopathy, nephritis, arthritis, and neuritis. Cold urticaria is associated with a history of cold exposure and the development of urticaria. Insulin anaphylaxis must be differentiated from hypoglycemic shock; during anesthesia, this can be done only on the basis of the serum glucose concentration or the presence of urticaria and angioedema. Occasionally an occult massive hemorrhage may be difficult to distinguish from anaphylaxis; urticaria and angioedema, if present, suggest anaphylaxis.

PATHOGENESIS

Histamine is the principal endogenous mediator responsible for the signs and symptoms of anaphylaxis in humans. It causes bronchoconstriction, vasodilatation, and increased leak of serum from venules (see page 478).

Other mediators may be involved in the pathogenesis of anaphylaxis. SRS-A, slow reacting substance of anaphylaxis, is important in animal models of anaphylaxis but as yet has an indefinite role in humans. SRS-A is composed of leukotrienes C, D, and E and potentiates histamine action, constricting the bronchial airways. Leukotriene C is a vasoconstrictor, and leukotriene D is a potent vasodilator.

Platelet activating factor (PAF, acetyl glyceryl ether phosphorylcholine) is also important in animal models of anaphylaxis. Platelet factor 4 is released after antigen-induced bronchospasm in humans. Other mediators that may be involved include eosinophil and neutrophil chemotactic factors, heparin, and digestive lysozymal enzymes.

Non–IgE-mediated anaphylaxis depends upon complement activation and the release of C3a and C5a, but the precise mechanism remains to be elucidated. C3a and C5a cause bronchospasm, hypotension, and vasogenic edema.

MANAGEMENT DURING ANESTHESIA

When anaphylaxis occurs during anesthesia, it is usually unexpected. Severe reactions culminate in cardiorespiratory collapse and may rapidly prove fatal. Every effort must be made to preclude such an attack. If anaphylaxis develops, the diagnosis should be made quickly so that treatment may begin since the longer the delay, the more likely it is that the outcome will be fatal.

Preoperative evaluation of every patient must include a careful history of allergies to either prescribed or over-the-counter drugs. A review of the previous anesthetic record and medical chart may reveal information about previous anaphylactic reactions. A Medic-Alert bracelet may be the only information available in the unconscious patient.

For those patients at high risk for anaphylaxis because of previous reactions to the same drug or trigger, prophylactic preoperative treatment is indicated. H_1 antihistamines (0.5 to 1.0 mg/kg diphenhydramine orally or subcutaneously) together with H_2 antihistamines (4 to 6 mg/kg cimetidine orally) have been effectively used to attenuate allergic reactions. These antihistamines block the peripheral manifestations of systemic histamine release, as may be demonstrated in the case of histamine release following morphine administration. Cromolyn may also be effective by limiting histamine release. High-dose steroids

(30 mg/kg methylprednisolone sodium succinate) will prevent histamine release from mast cells and mediators. Steroids have been used in combination with antihistamines for prophylaxis against anaphylactic reactions. Steroids may also act by reducing the arachidonic acid metabolites that are responsible for non-immunological anaphylaxis. There is also evidence that the administration of NSAIDs (such as ibuprofen) together with steroids further prevents the release of histamine from mast cells.

If a drug known to cause anaphylaxis must be administered, it should be administered slowly. This will minimize peak serum levels and thus minimize the release of histamine from mast cells and basophils and attenuate an anaphylactic response. Whenever possible another drug should be substituted for one known to cause anaphylaxis.

Life-threatening anaphylaxis presenting as paroxysmal angioneurotic edema (laryngeal edema), bronchospasm, or cardiorespiratory collapse following administration of a trigger must be immediately recognized. The dose of the trigger must be minimized. If the trigger has been administered via an extremity, placement of a tourniquet may help to prevent further absorption until the reaction is under control. If the reaction is life-threatening, the anesthetic and the surgery should be stopped. The goals of initial therapy include maintenance of adequate alveolar ventilation and oxygenation, attenuation of mediator release, and restoration of cardiac output. Angioneurotic edema and laryngeal edema are immediate life-threatening risks since patency of the airway may be lost. The trachea should be intubated, and the lungs should be ventilated with 100 percent oxygen.

Epinephrine is the principal drug for the treatment of anaphylaxis, and should be administered intramuscularly or by slow intravenous infusion in a dose of 0.02 to 0.1 ml/kg, up to a maximum volume of 0.5 to 1.0 ml of a 1:10,000 solution. Epinephrine attenuates the release of mediators and restores the cardiac output and blood pressure. It probably acts by increasing cAMP and thereby decreasing the release of mediators. H_1 antihistamines such as diphenhydramine (0.5 to 1.0 mg/kg) may be effective for persistent or slowly developing angioneurotic edema. H_2 antihistamines may also work. Antihistamines appear to act by blocking the binding of histamine to histamine receptors. The role of steroids in the treatment of laryngeal edema and anaphylaxis remains controversial.

If bronchospasm develops, immediate therapy is required. One hundred percent oxygen should be administered with assisted positive-pressure ventilation. Epinephrine is the drug of choice in the dose indicated above. In those cases in which bronchospasm is not immediately reversed, 5 to 6 mg/kg of aminophylline should be infused over 15 to 30 minutes and followed by a continuous infusion of 0.9 mg/kg/hour or less (see Table 16–13). The use of aminophylline in these cases must be carefully monitored by measurement of the serum concentration of theophylline, particularly in the presence of cimetidine, which blocks hepatic metabolism of the drug. Ranitidine does not appear to inhibit the metabolism of theophylline to the same extent as does cimetidine. To attenuate persistent bronchospasm, hydrocortisone, 3 to 4 mg/kg intravenously, should be given.

Circulatory collapse may result in cardiac arrest from severe hypotension, myocardial ischemia, or arrhythmias. Anaphylaxis causes extreme vasodilatation and peripheral edema with an acute decrease in blood volume. Therapy includes the administration of 100 percent oxygen, placing the patient in the Trendelenburg position, and administration of large volumes of crystalloid or colloid solutions to restore the blood volume. The immediate therapy for hypotension includes parenteral epinephrine, as discussed above. If bradycardia occurs atropine, 0.02 mg/kg intravenously, should be administered. The same dose should be given intramuscularly if venous access is not available. A vasopressor such as metaraminol (0.5 mg intravenously for children less than 10 kg, and 1.0 mg of those over 10 kg) may be required to support the blood pressure, particularly if there is concern over administering repeated doses of epinephrine in the presence of halothane. Although alpha agonists may theoretically cause mediator release by increasing intracellular cGMP, the need for these agents to maintain the circulation overrides this theoretical disadvantage. Secondary therapy includes steroids and H_1 antihistamines for persistent anaphylaxis, although their contribution to a successful outcome remains to be established.

Occasionally, drugs that are known allergens must be administered to very allergic patients. This may precipitate an acute anaphylactic reaction. The severity of allergic and anaphylactic reactions may be attenuated if the trigger agent is administered orally rather than parenterally. However, anaphylactic reactions to oral drugs have been reported. If the patient is very allergic, a small "test" dose may be administered and the patient observed before administering the full drug dose. Both H_1 antihistamines and prednisone may prevent anaphylactic reactions to radiocontrast dyes, protamine, and chymopapain.

REFERENCES

Anderson JR, Poblis A, Slavin R: Fatal case of aminophylline intoxication. Arch Intern Med 143:559, 1983.

Barnard JH: Studies of 400 Hymenoptera sting deaths in the United States. J Allergy Clin Immunol 52:259, 1973.

Beaupre PN, Roizen MF, Cahalan MK, et al.: Hemodynamic and two-dimensional transesophageal echocardiographic analysis of an anaphylactic reaction in a human. Anesthesiology 60:482, 1984.

Beavan MA: Anaphylactoid reactions to anesthetic drugs. Anesthesiology 55:3, 1981.

Bleecker ER, Smith PL, Kagey-Sobotka A: Physiologic manifestations of human anaphylaxis. J Clin Invest 66:1072, 1980.

Burman D, Hodson AK, Wood CBS, et al.: Acute anaphylaxis, pulmonary edema, and intravenous hemolysis due to cryoprecipitate. Arch Dis Child 48:483, 1973.

Chafee FH, Sertipane GA: Aspirin intolerance. I. Frequency in allergic population. J Allergy Clin Immunol 53:193, 1974.

Clarke RSJ, Dundee JW, Garrett RT, et al.: Adverse reactions to intravenous anaesthetics. Br J Anaesth 47:575, 1975.

Criep LH, Wochler TR: The heart in human anaphylaxis. Ann Allergy 29:399, 1971.

Delage C, Irey NS: Anaphylactic deaths: a clinicopathologic study of 43 cases. J Forensic Sci 17:525, 1972.

Driggs RL, O'Day RA: Acute allergic reaction associated with methohexital anaesthesia: report of six cases. J Oral Surg 30:906, 1972.

Edde RR, Burtis BB: Lung injury in anaphylactoid shock. Chest 63:639, 1973.

Evans JM, Keogh JAM: Adverse reactions to intravenous anesthetic induction agents. Br Med J 2:735, 1977.

Fisher MM: Severe histamine mediated reaction to intravenous drugs used in anaesthesia. Anaesth Intens Care 3:180, 1975.

Fisher MM: Intradermal testing after severe histamine reactions to intravenous drugs used in anaesthesia. Anaesth Intens Care 4:97, 1976.

Fisher MM: The management of acute anaphylaxis. In Watkins J, Ward AM (Eds.): Adverse Response to Intravenous Drugs. New York, Grune and Stratton, 1978, p 145.

Fisher MM, Munro I: Life-threatening anaphylactoid reactions to muscle relaxants. Anesth Analg 62:559, 1983.

Frank MM, Gelfand JA, Atkinson JP: Hereditary angioedema: the clinical syndrome and its management. Ann Intern Med 84:580, 1976.

Goldberg M: Systemic reactions to intravascular contrast media. Anesthesiology 60:46, 1984.

Greenberger PA, Patterson R, Simon R, et al.: Pre-treatment studies of high-risk patients requiring radiographic contrast media studies. J Allergy Clin Immunol 67:185, 1981.

Hammerschmidt DE, Harris PD, Wayland H, et al.: Complement-induced granulocyte aggregation in vivo. Am J Pathol 102:146, 1981.

Hammerschmidt DE, White JG, Cradoch PR, et al.: Corticosteroids inhibit complement-mediated granulocyte aggregation: a possible mechanism for their efficacy in shock states. Clin Invest 63:798, 1979.

Haneshiro PK, Weil MH: Anaphylactic shock in man: report of two cases with detailed hemodynamics and metabolic studies. Arch Intern Med 119:129, 1967.

Heimlich EM, Siegel SC: Anaphylaxis. In Kelley VC (Ed.): Practice of Pediatrics. Philadelphia, Harper and Row, 1984.

Henry DA, MacDonald IA, Kitchingham G, et al.: Cimetidine and ranitidine: comparison of effects on hepatic drug metabolism. Br Med J 281:775, 1980.

Horowitz L: Atopy as a factor in penicillin reactions. N Engl J Med 292:1243, 1975.

James LP, Austen KF: Fatal systemic anaphylaxis in man. N Engl J Med 270:597, 1964.

Kelly JF, Patterson R: Anaphylaxis—course, mechanisms and treatment. JAMA 227:1431, 1974.

Kelly JF, Patterson R, Lieberman, P, et al.: Radiographic contrast media studies in high-risk patients. J Allergy Clin Immunol 62:181, 1978.

Knauer KA, Adkinson NF Jr: Clinical significance of IgE. In Middleton E, Reed CE, Ellis EF (Eds.): Allergy: Principles and Practice. St. Louis, C. V. Mosby Co., 1983, p 673.

Knauer KA, Lichtenstein LM, Adkinson NF Jr, et al.: Platelet activation during antigen-induced airway reactions in asthmatic subjects. N Engl J Med 304:1404, 1981.

Larsen EC, Walters AJ, Lang JH: An experimental basis for histamine release in contrast material reactions. Radiology 110:49, 1974.

Levy JH, Rockoff MA: Anaphylaxis to meperidine. Anesth Analg 61:301, 1982.

Lorenz W, Doenicke A: Anaphylactoid reactions and histamine release by intravenous drugs used in surgery and anaesthesia. In Watkins J, Ward AM (Eds.): Adverse Response to Intravenous Drugs. New York, Grune and Stratton, 1978, p 83.

McManus LM, Hannahan DJ, Demopoules CA, et al: Pathobiology of the intravenous infusion of acetyl glyceryl ether phosphorylcholine (AGEPC), a synthetic platelet activating factor (PAF), in the rabbit. J Immunol 124:2919, 1980.

Miller WL, Doppman JL, Kaplan AP: Renal arteriography following systemic reaction to contrast material. J Allergy Clin Immunol 56:291, 1975.

Moss J, McDermott DJ, Thisted RA, et al.: Anaphylactic/anaphylactoid reactions in response to Chymodiactin (chymopapain). Anesth Analg 63:253, 1984.

Orange RP, Donsky GJ: Anaphylaxis. In Middleton E, Reed CE, Ellis EF (Eds.): Allergy: Principles and Practice. St. Louis, C. V. Mosby Co., 1978.

Philbin DM, Moss J, Atkins CW, et al.: The use of H_1 and H_2 histamine antagonists with morphine anesthesia: a double-blind study. Anesthesiology 55:292, 1981.

Ring J, Messmer K: Incidence and severity of anaphylactoid reactions to colloid volume substitutes. Lancet 1:466, 1977.

Settipane GA, Klein DE, Boyd GK: Relationship of atopy and anaphylactic sensitization: a bee sting allergy model. Clin Allergy 8:259, 1978.

Sheffer AL, Austen KF: Exercise-induced anaphylaxis. J Allergy Clin Immunol 66:106, 1980.

Small P, Satin R, Palayew MJ, et al.: Prophylactic antihistamines in the management of radiographic contrast reactions. Clin Allergy 12:289, 1982.

Stechschulte DJ, Orange RP, Austen KF: Detection of slow reacting substance of anaphylaxis (SRS-A) in plasma in guinea pigs during anaphylaxis. J Immunol 111:1585, 1973.

Stoelting RK: Allergic reactions during anesthesia. Anesth Analg 62:341, 1983.

Szefler SJ, Ellis EF: Adverse reactions to drugs: In Kelly VC (Ed.): Practice of Pediatrics. Philadelphia, Harper and Row, 1984.

Tannenbaum H, Ruddy S, Schur PH: Acute anaphylaxis associated with serum complement depletion. J Allergy Clin Immunol 56:226, 1974.

Wasserman SI: Anaphylaxis. In Middleton E Jr, Reed CE, Ellis EF (Eds.): Allergy—Principles and Practice. Vol. 2. p 689, St. Louis, C. V. Mosby Co., 1983.

Watkins J, Udnoon S, Taussig PE: Mechanisms of adverse response to intravenous agents in man. In Watkins J, Ward AM (Eds.): Adverse Response to Intravenous Drugs. New York, Grune and Stratton, 1978, p 71.

Westacott P, Ramachandran PR, Jancelewicz Z: Anaphylactic reaction to thiopentone. Can Anaesth Soc J 31:434, 1984.

DISEASES OF BLOOD 17

WILLIAM R. HAIN, M.D.

Aplastic Anemias
Chronic Renal Failure
Iron Deficiency Anemia
Megaloblastic Anemias
    Vitamin B$_{12}$ Deficiency
    Folic Acid Deficiency
    Megaloblastic Anemia and Nitrous
        Oxide

Marrow Infiltrations: The Leukemias
Hemolytic Anemias
    Hemoglobinopathies
    Spherocytosis
    Glucose-6-Phosphate Dehydrogenase
        Deficiency
Coagulopathies
    Hemophilia
    Thrombocytopenia
Polycythemia

Diseases of the blood are so diverse in etiology, pathophysiology, treatment, and prognosis that a text devoted to them must range widely in approach.

Four aspects of diseases of the blood have special implications for the anesthetist: reduced oxygen carriage, hemolysis of red cells, bleeding diathesis, and susceptibility to thrombosis.[1]

In any particular disorder one or more of these features may require attention in preoperative planning, in choice of agents and techniques for anesthesia, and in postoperative care. The anesthetic management appropriate to each is in some cases well documented (as in sickle cell disease). In others (for example, aplastic anemia), recommendations given below are based upon the known features of the disease, considered in conjunction with accepted anesthetic practice and known drug activity.

The normal range of hemoglobin concentrations for a particular subject differs according to sex, age, race, and the laboratory concerned. A patient with a hemoglobin concentration below the range accepted as normal is suffering from anemia.

Classification of anemias may be based upon etiology,[2, 3] as summarized in Table 17–1.

APLASTIC ANEMIAS

Aplastic anemias are rare and may be congenital or, more frequently, acquired. The incidence of fatal

Table 17–1. CLASSIFICATION OF ANEMIAS

1. Impaired production of red cells
   a. Stem-cell, e.g., aplastic anemias, chronic renal failure
   b. Disturbance of proliferation and maturation of differential erythroblasts, e.g., iron deficiency anemia, vitamin B$_{12}$/folic acid deficiency, marrow infiltrations
2. Shortened red cell survival
   a. Red cell abnormalities, e.g., sickle cell disease, spherocytosis
   b. Extrinsic factors: splenomegaly, toxic agents, bacterial agents
3. Anemia of blood loss
   a. Acute
   b. Chronic

aplastic anemia has been estimated as 1.1 per million up to the age of 9.[4]

The low hemoglobin concentration is due to the absence or reduction in number of erythroblasts. Most often other formed elements of blood are also deficient, so that neutropenia and thrombocytopenia are usually present. Pure red cell aplasia occurs but is exceedingly rare.

Aplastic anemia is associated with other congenital defects of the Fanconi variety,* which is believed due to a recessive autosomal character with a variable degree of expression. Aplastic anemia without associated congenital abnormalities is rare.

Acquired forms of aplastic anemia may result from drugs, toxic agents, or infections. Antimetabolites and cytotoxic agents cause marrow depression in all individuals, but other drugs will only do so in some patients. Among acquired aplastic anemias, that due to chloramphenicol is the most common, accounting for half the cases in one survey.[4] Indeed, patients receiving chloramphenicol are at a risk 13 times greater than the population at large of developing aplastic anemia. The inhalation of aromatic hydrocarbons, such as "glue sniffing," can also be causative.[2] Frank aplastic anemia may occur during viral hepatitis.

Clinical Manifestations. The pancytopenia of constitutional aplastic anemia does not usually appear until 4 to 7 years of age in boys and 6 to 10 years in girls. Exceptions have, rarely, been recorded. A relatively low birth weight is usual, but anemia is not present at birth or in the neonatal period.

Activity is usually normal during the insidious onset of the disease, and bruising, purpura, and hemorrhage are often the presenting symptoms.[4] There is no associated splenomegaly, hepatomegaly, or lymphade-

---

*Hyperpigmentation of genitalia, nipples, and upper trunk; short stature; microcephaly; strabismus, ptosis, and nystagmus; increased tendon reflexes; mental retardation; abnormalities of ears, often causing deafness; skeletal abnormalities, including anomalies of thumbs, radii, and long bones, congenital dysplasia of the hip, and syndactyly; renal defects, including aplasia or reduplication and occasionally hydronephrosis; and cardiac defects, commonly causing murmurs and sometimes frank congenital heart disease. Siblings may show some of these abnormalities even if anemia is not inherited. Leukemia is relatively frequent among relatives.[5]

nopathy.[6] There is often liability to infection. Radiological investigation may show retarded bone age.

Treatment. Blood transfusions, if the hemoglobin level is very low (less than 9 g/100 ml) may be required at intervals of 2 to 3 weeks until improvement occurs. Conservation of veins is important; capillary samples are used whenever possible for blood tests.

Specific therapy consists of corticosteroids and androgens. Androgens are required permanently in constitutional aplastic anemia, and temporarily in acquired forms. Forty to 50 percent of patients survive 10 years on treatment for the constitutional aplastic anemia,[7] but far fewer (approximately 10 percent) survive with acquired varieties. Septicemia and hemorrhage are the principal causes of death.[5]

Anesthetic Management. Bone marrow puncture will be required to establish the diagnosis, and general anesthesia of brief duration is often needed. Affected patients receiving therapy may require incidental surgery.

Preoperative assessment should establish the presence or absence of any other congenital defects and their nature and severity. Any intercurrent infections should be defined, and appropriate therapy instituted. The duration and dosage of steroid hormones must be noted. The degree of cardiovascular compensation for a low hemoglobin level requires assessment. Cardiac murmurs require elucidation, and possible congenital heart disease should be investigated. Consultation with a hematologist, a full blood picture, and a coagulogram should all be obtained before any but the most urgent operation is undertaken. Severe neutropenia alone may warrant prophylactic antimicrobial therapy.

Preoperative blood transfusion should be undertaken only if absolutely required, because sudden rises in blood oxygen content may further depress the marrow and discourage erythropoiesis.[8, 9] Nevertheless, generous allowance should be made when ordering crossmatched blood to replace perioperative blood losses. When repeated transfusions of blood or platelets have previously been given, the patient should be screened for antibodies. Should an adverse reaction (for example, urticaria or angioneurotic edema) appear, intravenous doses of antihistamines and corticosteroids may be beneficial.

Thrombocytopenia (see page 505) usually coexists, and platelet concentrates should be readily available.

Whenever coagulation defects are present, intramuscular injections should be avoided and premedication by alternative routes should be chosen. It is also important to avoid the risk of respiratory depression. Although there are isolated reports of blood dyscrasia related to diazepam[10] and falls in the white cell counts of patients on regular phenothiazine therapy are common,[11] such drugs are probably not contraindicated if given for oral premedication. A distressed struggling child utilizes oxygen rapidly, and hence suitable premedication is often indicated.

Steroid therapy may require supplementation perioperatively. Patients with congenital heart disease will require prophylactic antibiotic therapy.

A smooth induction of anesthesia is desirable. Instrumentation of the airway, with the attendant risk of trauma and hemorrhage, should be avoided whenever possible. However, a reliable airway is essential, and endotracheal intubation should be gently performed whenever it is advantageous. Many local analgesic techniques, especially spinal and epidural analgesia, are contraindicated if a bleeding diathesis is present. For bone marrow puncture and for other short procedures patients may be allowed to breathe spontaneously, but high concentrations of inspired oxygen should be assured.

Nitrous oxide depresses the bone marrow even after relatively short exposures,[12] and it might be desirable to avoid this agent in patients with known or suspected aplastic anemia (see page 493). An oxygen-air mixture is probably the ideal vehicle for inhalation agents, and monitoring transcutaneous oxygen saturation may be helpful, particularly in smaller infants, in ensuring appropriate arterial oxygenation while avoiding any potential bone marrow depressant effects of hyperoxia.

For more major surgery in which intermittent positive-pressure ventilation is required, careful endotracheal intubation is essential. Modest positive end-expiratory pressure should secure optimal hemoglobin saturation at minimum FIO_2. Normocarbia is desirable.

Optimal cardiovascular performance should be maintained, such that oxygen transport is maintained despite a low hemoglobin level. In general, fluid replacement therapy should be adequate to maintain blood volume and cardiac output. Circulatory overload must be avoided, however, especially in patients with coexisting cardiac defects.

Induced hypotension cannot be recommended in anemic patients, despite any potential for reduction in operative blood loss.[13]

Postoperative analgesia should be achieved by intravenous drugs initially, and orally thereafter. Postoperative blood investigations must include hemoglobin estimation. Special care must be taken to promote postoperative cardiovascular stability and to avoid impaired pulmonary function. Postoperative hypoxemia should be anticipated and oxygen therapy administered using a mask, nasal prongs, or head box (Fig. 17–1) as appropriate and tolerated.

CHRONIC RENAL FAILURE

Chronic renal failure affects two to three children per million of total population per year in Britain.[14] This condition involves a normochromic, normocytic anemia that is due to a decreased rate of production and a shortened lifespan of red cells. Iron deficiency, megaloblastic, and hemolytic anemias may also be

Figure 17–1. Infant headbox. Ports allow ingress of air/oxygen mixture and of leads for oxygen partial pressure monitoring. Transparent material is used to maintain visibility. The lid is readily removed if urgent access is required.

present. Folic acid and iron may be prescribed. Androgens may also be indicated.[4]

Blood transfusions are avoided whenever possible. Besides the risk of antibody production, there are possible hazards from hepatitis B and cytomegalovirus. The use of red cells stored in liquid nitrogen and washed prior to transfusion reduces this risk. However, it is often possible to manage patients with chronic renal insufficiency despite hemoglobin levels as low as 4 g/100 ml. Compensatory increases in 2,3-diphosphoglycerate levels and cardiac output permit adequate tissue oxygenation.[3, 15]

Thus, in planning anesthetic management of patients with chronic renal failure the anemia must be considered. However, management will be principally dictated by other aspects of the patient's disorder (see Chapter 7).

IRON DEFICIENCY ANEMIA

The most common anemia of childhood is that due to iron deficiency. Thirty-two percent of British children aged 3 years or younger may show mild anemia, and this incidence increases to 59 percent in lower socioeconomic groups.[5] Significant anemia was noted in 6 percent of a general population of preschool children in the United States, but in 28 percent of impoverished blacks and 44 percent of hospitalized infants.[4] Children from developing countries are frequently anemic, and any nutritional deficiency in these children may be compounded by hookworm infestation.[16]

Iron deficiency anemia may be due to deficient intake of iron (nutritional), deficient absorption (secondary), and excessive blood losses (from infestation or associated with a bleeding tendency).

Children over 3 years of age in Western countries usually have adequate iron intake; if an iron deficiency anemia is diagnosed beyond this age, gastrointestinal investigation is warranted once overt blood loss (such as in hemophilia, epistaxis, or hemoglobinuria) is excluded.[5]

Clinical Manifestations. Anemia may be discovered incidentally by the anesthetist in reviewing the results of preoperative screening tests. Direct questioning of parents may reveal that the patient dislikes iron-rich foods or is anorexic. Other symptoms may include irritability, listlessness, gastrointestinal upsets, pica, or susceptibility to infections. The nails, palms, conjunctivae, and mucous membranes may reveal extreme pallor, and slight splenomegaly may be found. Cardiac enlargement or a "hemic" murmur may be present.

Atrophic glossitis, angular cheilitis, and postcricoid dysphagia may be present early in iron deficiency, even without overt anemia.[17]

Treatment. Simple nutritional iron deficiency anemia is treated by attention to diet and by oral iron therapy. Other nutritional deficiencies (such as vitamin B_{12} and folate deficiencies) may coexist and require supplementary therapy. Noncompliance or gastrointestinal problems from oral therapy may be indications for parenteral iron (iron dextran or iron sorbitol). These may be given intramuscularly or intravenously, but complications have been reported with these techniques.

Response to treatment depends upon the capacity of the marrow to produce hemoglobin, not upon the dosage of any iron medication. A reticulocytosis occurring within 1 week and becoming maximal at about 2 weeks indicates a satisfactory response to therapy. Hemoglobin levels may rise 1 to 1.5 g/100 ml per week.[18] Where iron deficiency is secondary to another disease, treatment must be directed also at the primary cause; this may include diet therapy for celiac disease or chemotherapy for hookworm. In later childhood a peptic ulcer, polyp, or hemangioma may be responsible for the anemia and require anesthesia for surgical treatment.

The child whose anemia is severe, producing fatigue, dyspnea on exertion, palpitations, sustained tachycardia, or frank heart failure requires urgent but cautious infusion of packed red cells. Furosemide may be required concurrently to minimize the risk of cardiovascular overload.

Anesthetic Management. Elective surgery should be postponed until the anemia has been satisfactorily investigated and treated.

Management of the urgent or emergency case may include preoperative infusion of plasma-reduced blood to begin correction of the anemia.

No precise hemoglobin level has been established below which it is unsafe to anesthetize the anemic patient.[3] An oxygen-carrying capacity of 50 percent of normal may be satisfactory, providing other factors affecting tissue oxygenation are optimal.[19]

Cyanosis is usually discernible when more than 5 g/100 ml circulating hemoglobin is in the reduced form. It follows that in patients with very low hemoglobin levels absence of cyanosis cannot be regarded as a sign of adequate oxygenation of the blood. Furthermore, serious iron deficiency anemia is found more frequently among populations with heavy skin pigmentation in whom the recognition of cyanosis is often difficult. Blood gas analysis intraoperatively and postoperatively may be needed to monitor adequacy of oxygenation, particularly in major surgery.

Premedication should not cause respiratory depression. Induction of anesthesia may be by any appropriate means, providing hypoxia is avoided; preoxygenation is desirable. A head box may be the vehicle of choice for preoxygenation in infants (Fig. 17–1). The hyperkinetic circulation, which compensates for serious anemia, is associated with delay in reaching required alveolar concentrations of inhalation agents.[9] Halothane and some narcotics (for example, fentanyl) have a slowing effect on the heart and may depress this hyperkinetic circulation.

During maintenance inspired oxygen concentrations of 50 percent are recommended; higher concentrations of oxygen will not increase the blood oxygen content significantly.

Cardiovascular performance should be closely monitored and preserved at optimal levels. Operative blood losses may be replaced by whole blood transfusion, though plasma-reduced blood may be more desirable because it allows a more rapid restoration of oxygen carrying capacity with less risk of circulatory overload.

The patient with simple iron deficiency anemia presents no particular contraindication to the use of local analgesic techniques, since no bleeding tendency or neurological sequelae need be anticipated. Hence the risk of respiratory depression following narcotic analgesic drugs can be avoided by the substitution, when practicable, of local analgesic techniques both to supplement light general anesthesia and to prevent postoperative pain.

Severe anemia can delay wound healing and increase susceptibility to infection. Serial hemoglobin investigations in the few days postoperatively may indicate any need to give further blood transfusions.

MEGALOBLASTIC ANEMIAS

Vitamin B$_{12}$ Deficiency

Juvenile pernicious anemia is very rare. It may result from (1) genetic inability to secrete intrinsic factor (which may be present from 7 months of age onward; (2) the formation of antibodies to intrinsic factor, with gastric atrophy and possibly other exocrine gland abnormality; (3) a specific defect of vitamin B$_{12}$ absorption associated with proteinuria; (4) extensive surgical resection of the terminal ileum; or (5) infestation by *Diphyllobothrium latum* (fish tape worm).[20]

Clinical Manifestations. Pallor, fatigue, and glossitis may be present, though their occurrence and severity will depend upon the age of the patient and the duration of the anemia. The splenomegaly and slight jaundice seen in adult pernicious anemia is usually absent in childhood. Subacute combined degeneration of the cord may supervene.[21] Treatment consists of parenteral hydroxycobalamin. The dose depends on the etiology.

Folic Acid Deficiency

Infants who are premature or fed only on goat's milk or other folate-poor diet (such as the diet for patients with phenylketonuria) may develop megaloblastic anemia. Malabsorption syndromes and leukemic and hemolytic anemias may also be associated with folic acid deficiency. However, iron deficiency is the usual cause of the anemia of celiac disease.[4]

Folate deficiency can accompany the dialysis of patients with chronic renal disease, severe infection and diarrhea, and co-trimoxazole therapy.[22]

Drugs associated with folic acid deficiency also include the anticonvulsants sodium phenytoin and primidone, barbiturates, methotrexate, and pyrimethamine.

Clinical Manifestations. Symptoms of folic acid deficiency include anorexia, failure to thrive, weakness, liability to infection, and gastrointestinal disturbances. The sore tongue and mouth of tropical sprue are seldom seen in temperate climates. Hemorrhagic manifestations can occur secondary to thrombocytopenia, and infection can occur from neutropenia.

Treatment with folic acid is usually given by mouth but can be given parenterally. No improvement in hemoglobin concentration is expected in the first week of therapy. Blood transfusion may be needed, and in severe cases exchange transfusion may be undertaken.[23] Any other accompanying deficiencies require diagnosis and treatment.

Anesthetic Management. Patients known to be receiving a folate-poor diet, suffering from malabsorption, or receiving therapy with the drugs mentioned above should be particularly carefully assessed for their hematological status. Pallor and gingival hypertrophy may alert the anesthetist to megaloblastic anemia.

Diagnosis and successful treatment should precede nonurgent surgery.

For urgent surgery a small blood transfusion may be needed to initiate treatment. Severely affected patients may have heart failure and pulmonary edema; particular care in transfusion is necessary.

Close attention should be paid to plasma potassium levels pre-, peri-, and postoperatively in the child who is in the early days for treatment of megaloblastic anemia. Falls of nearly 1.0 mEq/L on average have been noted in patients during vitamin B_{12} or folate treatment, with levels as low as 2.5 mEq/L in some cases.[24] The hypokalemia is not universally believed to be of clinical significance.[25] However, based on comparison of patients with megaloblastic anemia with a group of patients with iron deficiency anemia, it has been concluded that megaloblastic anemia is a much more dangerous condition, possibly since purine synthesis is deranged throughout the body.[24, 25]

The management of anesthesia for the child with megaloblastic anemia will be governed by the foregoing and by the general considerations that apply also to patients with anemia. In particular, any bleeding tendency contraindicates intramuscular injections and many local analgesic techniques.

Megaloblastic Anemia and Nitrous Oxide

The administration of nitrous oxide is associated with inhibition of methionine synthetase activity. There is consequent impairment of DNA synthesis with inactivation of vitamin B_{12} and a risk of megaloblastic anemia. Chemical changes indicative of this tendency have been demonstrated after as little as 1 to 2 hours of nitrous oxide administration.[12] The changes are related to the duration of exposure to nitrous oxide and were more common in sick patients than in others who had had uncomplicated surgery,[26] but were not seen at all in patients who had not been given anesthesia.

Folinic acid is effective in preventing the development of bone marrow toxicity when given repeatedly in large amounts. The dose suggested for adults is 60 mg in divided doses, at the beginning and 12 hours after the start of anesthesia.[27]

Such protection notwithstanding, it might be prudent to avoid nitrous oxide in patients whose bone marrow function is depressed, providing alternative agents are available to produce anesthesia that is at least equally safe and effective.

MARROW INFILTRATIONS: THE LEUKEMIAS

Although many different types of marrow infiltration are described,[2] the vast majority presenting in childhood appear as acute leukemia. Acute lymphoblastic leukemia (ALL) is more common in childhood than the acute myeloblastic variety (AML) in an approximate ratio of 14 to 3.[5] Other, rare, varieties occur, including a "leukemic transformation" seen in 30 percent of children with lymphomas.

Leukemias are second only to accidents as a cause of death in the first 4 years of life[28] and make up approximately one third of all childhood malignancies.[29] The risk of developing acute leukemia before the age of 14 is 65 in 100,000 boys and 46 in 100,000 girls. White children are twice as frequently affected as black children.[30] There is a peak incidence at about 2 to 4 years of age, with little variation from country to country.

The etiology of human leukemia is probably multifactorial and remains uncertain despite animal work implicating infection, radiation, and hereditary causes in some species.[5] There is malignant proliferation of hemic precursor cells, primarily affecting the bone marrow but also involving the peripheral blood and other tissues, especially the reticuloendothelial system.

Clinical Manifestations. Although marked differences in specific clinical features in response to therapy and in prognosis distinguish the different leukemias, the general features are similar, as all involve profound disruption of bone marrow function.

The presentation is nonspecific, usually within 6 weeks of onset of signs and symptoms. Failure to "throw off" a mild respiratory infection, pallor, irritability, lassitude, anorexia, fever, and a bleeding tendency with bruising or bone pain are common features. There may be generalized lymphadenopathy, hepatomegaly, or splenomegaly (unlike a typical aplastic anemia). Sepsis, even septicemia, may be the presenting feature.

Pallor and lack of activity reflect the anemia that develops from the disturbed erythropoiesis. Occult or overt hemorrhage due to thrombocytopenia may contribute significantly to the anemia. Mucous membranes and the skin are particularly affected. Characteristic retinal changes that accompany the thrombocytopenia of leukemia are not seen with other forms of thrombocytopenia.

Diagnosis and Treatment. Bone marrow aspiration essentially supplements the blood picture in confirming the diagnosis. The cornerstones of treatment are steroids in combination with intravenous and intrathecal cytotoxic agents initially given at weekly intervals to secure remission. Radiotherapy may additionally be required to reduce the likelihood of meningeal metastases. Response to therapy is gauged by repeated blood and bone marrow examinations.

The treatment pattern is initially intensive but can usually be offered on an outpatient, ambulatory basis after relatively few days of hospitalization. Treatment may extend over a number of years.

Severe anemia may be present at diagnosis or during treatment and is treated with blood transfusions. Severe thrombocytopenia may necessitate temporary cessation of therapy.

Infection may be present at diagnosis. It may also seriously complicate the management of the leukemia. Prophylactic antibiotics and immunoglobulins are often warranted. Fungal infections must receive vigorous treatment.

The basic pattern of leukemia treatment is shown in Table 17–2. The uncertain prognosis, the nauseat-

Table 17–2. A TYPICAL PLAN OF THERAPY IN ACUTE LYMPHOCYTIC LEUKEMIA

Remission	CNS Prophylaxis	Intensification	Reinduction
Induction 3–4 weeks	3–4 weeks or weeks 9–11	5th–6th weeks (Patients unwell for days following)	2–4 years
Steroids	Steroids	Steroids	Steroids
Cytotoxics	Intrathecal cytotoxics	Cytotoxics	Cytotoxics
Vincristine		Etoposide	(As at induction)
Daunorubicin		6-Mercaptopurine	
L-Asparaginase	Radiation	Methotrexate	
		Cytosine arabinoside + reinduction agents	
Treat any intercurrent illness		Co-trimoxazole (Given indefinitely as prophylaxis against *Pneumocystis*)	Co-trimoxazole

ing, debilitating, and disfiguring effects of therapy, and the frequency of follow-up hospital attendances for medical interventions combine to produce stresses in affected families, with marital strain and anxieties compounding those of the patient. Experienced personnel within a dedicated team of physicians, nurses, and social workers are important factors in securing compliance with therapy and ensuring appropriate psychological adjustments.

Testicular metastases sometimes occur despite therapy. Biopsies and sometimes prophylactic orchiectomy may be necessary.

Anesthetic Management. The anesthesiologist may become involved with leukemia patients at diagnosis, during therapy, or for related or unrelated surgery. In British pediatric practice bone marrow aspirations and some other painful medical procedures are often performed with patients under general anesthesia. Thus, the first contact of anesthetist and leukemic child may be at presentation, before confirmation of the diagnosis. Should the diagnosis be confirmed, repeated anesthetics may be requested frequently over the next few weeks and intermittently for a period of perhaps several years. It is therefore advantageous that an anesthetist be part of an identified team of clinicians involved in pediatric hematological and oncological practice and that every effort be made by him or her to secure for the child not only the safest but the most agreeable experience of anesthesia possible. The anesthetic management of the child with leukemia, even when minor intervention only is envisaged, can be critical to the child's acceptance of treatment.

Anesthesia for Investigative and Treatment Procedures. The preoperative visit assesses both the status of the child and the personality of the parents. Explanations of the role of the anesthetist "to stop it hurting" are given. The treatment area of the relevant children's ward can be equipped with facilities for anesthesia and resuscitation. The older child is given explanations and is invited, with parents, to view the apparatus and to try on a face mask. Assessment of the child's willingness to cooperate either on a parent's knee or on the treatment table is assessed, but on this

occasion as a rule no anesthetic is administered. Premedication is prescribed if deemed essential but is rarely required.

Later, when the pediatrician and hematologist are in attendance and the child is adequately fasted, an inhalation induction is performed. (For children with an intravenous infusion already in progress, or those experienced children expressing a preference for "a needle," induction is performed by the intravenous route). Halothane and oxygen are given together with nitrous oxide if the hemoglobin level seems appropriate (more than 9 g/100 ml). When light surgical anesthesia is achieved children aged 2 years or older are turned onto the left side and positioned to facilitate bone marrow puncture from a posterior iliac crest. Tibial specimens suffice in the very young. If required and not already undertaken, an intravenous infusion is set up and blood samples are taken. Sometimes lumbar puncture is also performed on this occasion. The period of anesthesia required rarely exceeds 15 to 20 minutes, and work in progress suggests that no impairment of respiratory exchange due to the extreme posture need be anticipated (unpublished observations). The patient's condition, anesthetic, and mood at induction of anesthesia are recorded together with the relevant anesthetic history both in the case records and on file in the treatment area. Mood is assessed on a five-point scale (A, cheerful and cooperative; B, apprehensive but cooperative; C, tearful, cooperates with difficulty; D, uncooperative; E, terrified and virtually unmanageable).

Once the diagnosis of leukemia is confirmed treatment begins, usually within 24 hours. A request for general anesthesia may be made for this and subsequent occasions. An anesthetic routine is established by the anesthetist in accord with the child's reactions and expressed views. Where inhalation induction proves stormy, C or worse on the mood scale, an intravenous approach is essayed on a subsequent occasion. Any apparent or expressed preference for route of induction is adhered to. Older children are invited to compare the scent of enflurane 1 percent with halothane 0.5 percent, both in oxygen, and this preference is recorded and granted for later anesthetics. Fears of hepatitis from repeat halothane anesthesia in children are almost certainly groundless.[31]

Radiotherapy and cytotoxic therapy both promote nausea and vomiting. Antiemetics, such as prochlorperazine, may be administered prophylactically while the anesthetic is still in progress. Thrombocytopenia is common in leukemic children, and intramuscular drug administration should be avoided.

Using this informal ward-based interactive approach it is found among older children particularly that cooperation without premedication can be achieved, maintained, and even improved, as can be seen from Figures 17–2 and 17–3.

The Hickman Catheter. The hematological, antibiotic, and nutritional support essential to the leukemic child under therapy may necessitate direct access to the central circulation on a long-term basis. The insertion of a Hickman right atrial catheter can be used to secure such access, and general anesthesia may be required.[32] In older children the cephalic vein may be used and a simple inhalation anesthetic with appropriate F_IO_2 may be given as for other minor procedures as described above. In children under 5 the diameter of the cephalic vein is insufficient, however, and the internal jugular vein is used. Endotracheal intubation is then advisable and particular care should be taken, including transfusion of platelets, if there is thrombocytopenia. There is a possibility of lowered plasma cholinesterase prolonging suxamethonium apnea. Infection is an important hazard of indwelling catheters and cannulas, particularly in immunosuppressed patients. Rigorous precautions should be taken by the anesthetist to avoid contamination of the operative site.

Anesthesia and Leukemia Therapy. There are a large number of cytotoxic drugs used in various combinations to treat leukemia and other malignancies in both adults and children. All cause bone marrow suppression, and anemia, thrombocytopenia, and neutropenia are regular complications of therapy. These agents can adversely affect virtually all systems of the body, with different classes of agent acting adversely on particular organs.[33]

Patients receiving therapy currently or in the past should be minutely screened for adverse effects. Selvin has identified seven classes of agents.[34] Some examples of each class—by no means an exhaustive list—are given in Table 17–3.

Armed with a knowledge of what class(es) of agent the patient has received, the anesthetist must proceed to consider each body system in turn, directing particular attention to any problems known to accompany such therapy.

Table 17–4 shows some of the known system lesions complicating therapy with particular classes of agents. Of critical concern to the anesthetist will be the

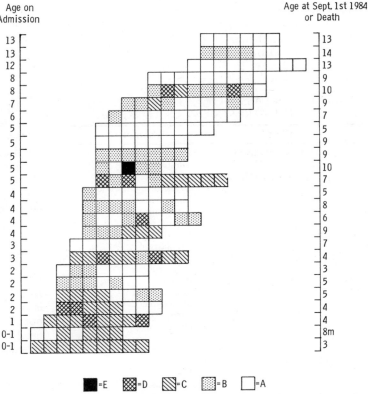

Figure 17–2. Mood at induction of anesthesia in 25 patients receiving 6 to 10 anesthetics, May 1980 to August 1984, at Nottingham Pediatric Oncology/Anesthesia Clinic. Serial anesthetics for each patient are represented by blocks adjacent horizontally. Patients are ranked vertically according to date of birth, with the most recently born at the lowest level. The greatest density of print, indicating the least cooperative behavior (see text), is seen in the youngest patients at the start of treatment. Maintenance or improvement of cooperation is seen most readily in older patients. (From Hain WR, Tomlinson JH, Barbor PRH: Anaesthesia for minor procedures in children with malignant disease. J Roy Soc Med 78:715–720, 1985. Reproduced by permission of the Editor.)

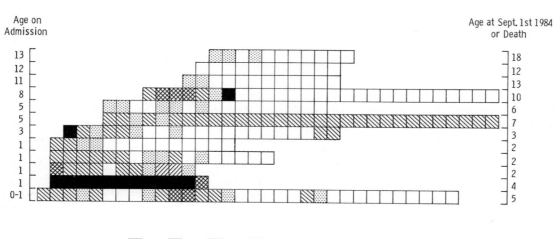

Figure 17–3. Mood at induction of anesthesia in 12 patients receiving more than 10 anesthetics, May 1980 to August 1984, at Nottingham Pediatric Oncology/Anesthesia Clinic. See legend of Figure 17–2 for discussion. (From Hain WR, Tomlinson JH, Barbor PRH: Anaesthesia for minor procedures in children with malignant disease. J Roy Soc Med 78:715–720, 1985. Reproduced by permission of the Editor.)

association of bleomycin therapy with pulmonary toxicity, cardiopathy, and ECG abnormalities. Muscle relaxants may prove unpredictable, especially since electrolyte abnormalities are common, often in combination with dehydration. The central nervous system may be depressed in some patients, and there may be seizures complicating, for example, cisplatin therapy. Liver function and renal function will require specific investigation and attention. It is essential to consider blood transfusion, platelet concentrates, and measures to combat infection for all patients with antecedent or current cytotoxic therapy.

Anesthetic Considerations in Bone Marrow Transplantation. Patients in first remission with AML and

Table 17–3. CLASSES OF CYTOTOXIC AGENTS USED IN TREATMENT OF LEUKEMIA

Class	Examples
Alkylating agents (AA)	Cyclophosphamide
	Thiotepa
Antimetabolites (AM)	Methotrexate
	Cytosine arabinoside
	Thioguanine
	6-Mercaptopurine
	Fluorouracil
Plant alkaloids (PA)	Vincristine
	Vinblastine
Antibiotics (AB)	Adriamycin
	Daunorubicin
	Bleomycin
	Mithramycin
	Mitomycin C
Nitrosoureas (NU)	Carmustine
	Lomustine
	Streptozocin
Enzyme (EZ)	L-Asparaginase
Random synthetics (RS)	Cisplatin
	Dacarbazine
	Procarbazine

second or later remission with ALL may be considered for bone marrow transplantation (BMT), a form of therapy also given preferentially to children with severe combined immunodeficiency disease and aplastic anemia.[35]

Ideally, syngeneic grafting from an identical twin would be performed, but this is rarely possible. Allogeneic grafting, however, is commonly feasible, usually between the patient and a nonidentical sibling or another near relative, but sometimes using a nonrelated donor with compatible human lymphocytic antigens.

Filshie and colleagues[36] have described their anesthetic management for harvest for BMT. Securing consent from a suitable donor for anesthesia is not usually a problem; parental consent is obtained only after full discussion if the prospective donor is a minor, and older children may also be asked to sign the form of consent.

ANESTHESIA FOR DONORS. Anesthesia is indicated for the donor, since multiple bone marrow punctures are performed anteriorly and posteriorly. The program of management commences with a physical examination by a specialist physician. Problems are discussed with the anesthetist. Full blood count, chest x-ray, and electrocardiogram are performed. Adult patients may have 1 unit of blood removed and stored for reinfusion during harvest.

Donors are admitted to the hospital the day before BMT. Further physical examinations are undertaken and, if autologous blood is not already in store, blood is cross-matched. Intercurrent disease in the donor may not contraindicate the procedure. Donors may be needed for more than one attempted graft. Particular attention must therefore be paid to ensure the least disagreeable experience possible, particularly as the patient derives no direct benefit from the procedure.

Premedication may follow the anesthetist's prefer-

Table 17–4. ADVERSE EFFECTS OF CYTOTOXIC THERAPY

Organ/System and Effect	Class of Drug*	Specific Example (Where Appropriate)	Comment/Anesthetic Implications
Bone Marrow Suppression	All		Anemia, leukopenia, and thrombocytopenia occur to variable degree with all classes of agent
	AA		Hemolytic component to anemia
Nonthrombocytopenic bleeding tendency	AB	Mithramycin	
	EZ		Hemorrhagic pancreatitis may occur
Lungs			
Fibrosis and/or pneumonitis	AA		
	AB	Bleomycin	Particularly associated. O₂ toxicity enhanced
			Postoperative ARDS reported
			? Synergistic with radiotherapy
		Mitomycin C	
	NU		
	RS	Procarbazine	
Heart			
Cardiopathy, ECG abnormalities	AA	Cyclophosphamide	
	AB	Adriamycin	Cardiopathy months after therapy
		Daunorubicin	ECG changes may accompany therapy
	RS	Cisplatin	Rarely
Nervous System			
Central	AM	Fluorouracil	Cerebellar ataxia
	PA		Encephalopathy
	EZ		Impaired sensorium, lethargy
	RS	Cisplatin	
		Procarbazine	
Peripheral neuropathy	PA		
	RS	Cisplatin	
		Procarbazine	
Autonomic	PA		Can lead to surgical abdominal emergency
Liver			
Dysfunction	AM	6-Mercaptopurine especially	
	AB	Mithramycin	
	NU	Streptozocin especially	
	EZ		
	RS	Decarbazine	Rarely
Kidneys			
Dysfunction	AA		Uric acid nephropathy at start of treatment if prophylactic allopurinol and fluid therapy omitted
	AM		Tubular necrosis
	PA		Inappropriate antidiuretic hormone secretion
	AB	Mithramycin	
	NU		
	RS	Cisplatin	
Gastrointestinal Epithelium	AM	Methotrexate	Stomatitis, diarrhea, cachexia, mucous membrane ulceration
		Fluorouracil	
	AB	Bleomycin	
Skin	AA		
	AB	Bleomycin	Severity of eruption may parallel pulmonary toxicity
Immune Status			
Suppression	AM		Possible increased requirement for nondepolarizing relaxant
Endocrine System	AA		Inhibition of plasma cholinesterase, increased apnea from suxamethonium
	AB	Mithramycin	Electrolyte disturbances
	NU	Streptozocin	Hypoinsulinism
	RS	Cisplatin	Hypercalcemia
General	RS	Procarbazine	MAO inhibitor status: care with vasopressors, avoid sedatives, narcotics
	RS	Procarbazine	"Influenzal" symptoms can present

*See Table 17–3 for abbreviations.
Data from Selvin BL: Cancer chemotherapy: implications for the anesthesiologist. Anesth Analg 60:425, 1981.

ence. Filshie notes a trend to benzodiazepines. In adults anesthesia may be induced intravenously, fentanyl 200 μg and droperidol 5 mg being given intravenously immediately before a "sleep" dose of thiopental. Lidocaine 4 percent (up to 4 ml) sprayed to the vocal cords allows easy insertion of a cuffed endotracheal tube using alcuronium to secure muscular relaxation. (Other nondepolarizing relaxants can be used.)

Children may have anesthesia induced with nitrous oxide–oxygen–enflurane (or halothane) by inhalation followed by suxamethonium (1.5mg/kg) for intubation. Fentanyl (3 μg/kg) may be given to supplement the anesthetic.

Maintenance of anesthesia includes the provision of intravenous access and standard monitoring facilities. The length of the procedure is extremely variable (15 minutes to 2 hours and 15 minutes). Further increments of fentanyl and relaxants may be required. Care should be taken to avoid heat loss, and transfused fluid should be warmed. Adult patients may be managed with spinal anesthesia using 1.2 to 1.6 ml heavy dibucaine (Cinchocaine, Nupercaine) or similar agents (for example, tetracaine), without general anesthesia.[36]

Once anesthetized, the patient is carefully turned prone and immediately preharvest heparin 1500 IU/m² is injected intravenously. After harvest from the posterior iliac crest the patient is returned to the supine position and further harvest is made from anterior iliac crests and the sternum. Further increments of heparin are given if clotting starts to occur at the site of bone marrow puncture during the harvest. Mixed blood and marrow are aspirated, 750 to 1,000 ml or up to a third of the circulating volume in children. Sequential cell counts determine the volume aspirated. Fluids should be given to cover losses and maintenance. Donors bled 1 week prior to harvest have their stored blood reinfused during the procedure. Cross-matched, irradiated blood is alternatively given, but only after the harvest is complete to avoid harvest of the transfused graft. The irradiation avoids infusion of viable lymphocytes, which could complicate further donations.

Reversal of neuromuscular blockade is undertaken with atropine and neostigmine. Oxygen and fluid therapy are continued into the postoperative period. Analgesia is seldom required.

Nausea, vomiting, and mild pyrexia are reported as minor complications. Patients should be warned in advance and treated appropriately. Iron supplements are given to donors for up to 2 months.

Fat embolism of variable degree is a possible complication of the aspiration of large volumes of bone marrow from multiple sites, though heparin may be protective against this. Filshie[36] reports greater cardiovascular instability in a group of patients who did not receive heparin prior to harvest. He also reports reductions in diffusing capacity of the lungs 24 hours postoperatively; these reductions are similar whether a general or spinal anesthetic is given. The possibility that nitrous oxide may be a hazard to the function of the harvested bone marrow is discounted on present evidence.

HEMOLYTIC ANEMIAS

Hemoglobinopathies

Hemoglobinopathies are inherited as autosomal codominant traits. Over 100 such disorders have been detected and described. Disordered function usually follows from the abnormal structure of the hemoglobin. A familiar example is sickle cell hemoglobin (Hb S), which is less soluble than normal hemoglobin (Hb A) when deoxygenation occurs. Crystals then form, leading to deformation and increased rigidity of the cells; this process is known as "sickling."

Sickle Cell Disease

Hb S is produced under the influence of a single gene that, when present, affects the constitution of the beta chain of hemoglobin, substituting valine for glutamic acid at position 6. The gene is allelomorphic with that for Hb A, and those for many other hemoglobin variants. The proportion of Hb S within a red cell is greater in the Hb S homozygote than in the heterozygote.

The severity of the disease is directly related to the proportion of Hb S within the cell but is also influenced by other factors, notably the proportions of Hb A and fetal hemoglobin (Hb F) and interaction with beta thalassemia.[37]

Other alleles may complicate the picture. The genes for Hb C, Hb D, Hb Punjab, and Hb E may be inherited. Allelomorphic pairs may thus include:

Hb A/Hb A—normal
Hb A/Hb S—sickle cell trait (SCT)
Hb S/Hb S —sickle cell anemia (SCA) (SCD)*
Hb C/Hb S—sickle cell Hb C disease
Hb C/Hb C—Hb C disease

Many other combinations occur; some, such as Hb E/Hb E, also have clinical manifestations.[39]

The Hb S gene is present in about 10 percent of the black population of Britain and North America (Table 17–5) and in 20 to 40 percent of the black African populations. It is also found in the Middle East, the Mediterranean basin, the hill tribes of the Indian subcontinent and in South America.[37, 39] Infants with Hb S appear to have relative immunity from falciparum malaria, probably accounting for the prevalence of SCD within Africa.

In West Africa 1 to 2 percent of the population is

---

*In this text SCD denotes conditions in which sickling may arise.[37, 38] SCA denotes the clinical expression of the homozygous state for Hb S and SCT that of the heterozygous, Hb S/Hb A, genotype. Some other authors[3, 5] restrict SCD to the homozygous state for Hb S.

Table 17–5. INCIDENCE OF COMMON HEMOGLOBINOPATHIES IN THE UNITED KINGDOM, UNITED STATES, AND JAMAICA

Location	Total Births	% Black Births	% of All Infants with Genotype: AS	AC	SS	SC	CC
UK: London	3,165	22.0	2.8	0.9	0.15	0.09	0.090
Birmingham	43,500	10.0	1.19	0.46	0.06	0.06	—
Manchester	7,691	3.8	0.38	—	—	—	—
USA: New York	106,223	35.0	3.26	0.83	0.18	0.12	0.002
Jamaica	8,000	95.0	8.60	2.89	0.30	0.20	0.003

From Henthorn J, Anionwu E, Brozovic M: Screening cord blood for sickle haemoglobinopathies in Brent. Br Med J 289:479, 1984.

homozygous for Hb S, and of those 80 percent die before the age of 2 years.[3] Improved health care is presumed to account for a better prognosis in the United States.

Low cost programs for cord blood electrophoretic screening for families at risk have been established in many centers.[40] Anesthesiologists should have an interest in encouraging the growth of such programs.

Sickle Cell Anemia (SCA). In the homozygous genotype the high proportion of Hb S within the red cells leads to sickling. This process, which occurs when the hemoglobin is deoxygenated, is initially reversible with restoration of oxygenation but becomes irreversible as membrane changes occur.

Sickling has two important clinical effects: an abnormally high rate of hemolysis and the formation of sickle cell aggregates, with microembolic vaso-occlusion leading to organ infarctions.

A severe hemolytic anemia (Hb 5 to 7 g/100 ml) is the consequence of the rapid clearance of sickled cells from the circulation by the reticuloendothelial system. Splenic enlargement, jaundice, bone marrow cavity enlargement, and reticulosis are common sequelae. Pigment gallstones can also occur.

The manifestations of vaso-occlusion are widely varied. The kidneys and spleen are especially liable to repeated infarction with transient pain and fever but permanent loss of function. Lungs, bone, brain, and liver are also prone to this complication.

Clinical Manifestations. While hemolysis and infarctions represent the basic features of SCA at any age, there are differences in presentation characteristic of different age groups.[37] True hemolytic crises are rare and occur predominantly in those patients who also have glucose-6-phosphate dehydrogenase deficiency[5] (see page 503).

INFANCY. Seventy percent of the hemoglobin in a neonate is Hb F, and although this proportion falls in the first few months of life, it exerts a protective effect on the patient with SCA, so that clinical problems are rare in small babies.

Dactylitis from vaso-occlusion is a common presentation, and the "hand-foot syndrome," which involves the dorsum of hands and/or feet, may develop. Growth of the metacarpals and metatarsals may be impaired.

Splenomegaly occurs in most babies with SCD. In SCA episodic infarction of the spleen, accompanied by pain and audible "splenic rubs" on auscultation, can lead eventually to autosplenectomy by 4 to 5 years of age.[37] Prior to autosplenectomy, death from peripheral circulatory failure may ensue from acute splenic sequestration. This condition has a peak incidence between 6 and 18 months of age and is heralded by such nonspecific symptoms as cough, fever, diarrhea, vomiting, pallor, and drowsiness. There is acute splenic enlargement and a fall in hemoglobin concentration exceeding 2 g/100 ml from erythrocyte trapping within the spleen.

CHILDHOOD. Acute episodes of vaso-occlusion (sickling crises) develop and pain, usually of the limbs, may demand hospitalization. Anorexia and constitutional upset with pyrexia and tachycardia compound mild dehydration, which aggravates vascular sludging.

Episodes of bone marrow hypoplasia (aplastic crises) can also occur, with falls in hemoglobin level of 2 g/100 ml without reticulocyte response. Various infections and folic acid deficiency have been incriminated. Indeed, infections, particularly osteomyelitis and meningitis, are recurring problems usually involving *Streptococcus pneumoniae.*

Progressive loss of concentrating power of the kidney develops rapidly in the early years. Polyuria with enuresis occurs. Transfusion may restore kidney function temporarily in the young, but by age 15 the condition is irreversible. Mild hematuria is seen and commonly is due to bleeding from one kidney, occurring four times more frequently on the left than on the right. Renal blood flow, glomerular filtration rate, and the ability to produce dilute urine are all unaffected. Progress to serious renal disease is rare during childhood.[41]

CNS disturbances can arise with seizures and temporary or permanent intellectual impairment.

ADOLESCENCE. Sickling crises and susceptibility to infection continue into adolescence and beyond. Growth problems are seen, with reduced height and weight due to delayed puberty. A characteristic "sickle habitus" includes overgrowth of the maxillae from depression of the bridge of the nose. Chest pain and cough may indicate "sickle chest syndrome" in which signs and x-ray changes of lung consolidation, unilateral or bilateral, may be found to develop over 10 days. Spreading leg ulcers and also priapism, often leading to impotence, may develop in this age group.

Treatment. Repeated blood transfusions, especially in aplastic crises, form the mainstay of medical management of patients with SCA. The benefit is twofold. Anemia is corrected with cells containing a high proportion of Hb A and, since erythropoietin drive is consequently lowered, there is suppression of formation of Hb S–laden cells. Urea and cyanate therapy, once believed useful in the prevention of sickling, are no longer recommended.[42, 43]

Prophylactic penicillin therapy in patients with SCA up to the age of 3 years has been shown to decrease the incidence of *Streptococcus pneumoniae* infections in this age group, and such therapy beyond this age is recommended.[44]

In infancy, despite the subsequent increased risk from infection, splenectomy may be indicated. After even only one episode of splenic sequestration, one third of survivors develop hypersplenism.[45] Patients with painful sickling crises may require bed rest in the hospital, analgesics, intravenous hydration, and, in the presence of infection, antibiotics. Folic acid therapy and prompt treatment of infections may prevent or reduce the occurrence of aplastic crises.

Any infections developing in SCA patients, especially "sickle chest syndrome," demand vigorous antibiotic therapy and consideration of exchange transfusion.

Anesthetic Management. Patients with SCA present relatively frequently for surgery. Operation may be required to remove pigment gallstones. While priapism may respond to hospitalization, analgesics, and exchange transfusion, some sufferers require surgical drainage or shunt procedures. Other surgical procedures directly related to SCA include grafting for leg ulcers and cautery procedures for epistaxis. Orthodontic treatment may be required for excessive growth of maxillary teeth in adolescents.

Patients with SCA may additionally be considered for surgery, however, when vaso-occlusive incidents give pain mimicking, particularly frequently, osteomyelitis and acute abdominal emergencies. Increasing surgical awareness of these presentations in SCA can reduce the incidence of unnecessary surgery.[46] However, many unrelated surgical conditions can also arise in patients with SCA. Umbilical hernia is particularly prevalent in black populations.

GENERAL CONSIDERATIONS. The hazards of general anesthesia for patients with SCD appears to have diminished as awareness of the disease has led to increased preoperative recognition and to assessments of the factors that precipitate sickling crises.

Hypoxia and vascular stasis are the principal dangers. It is relatively easy to avoid hypoxia from respiratory causes in patients intraoperatively while an anesthetist is present. However, general anesthesia predisposes to hypoxia, and local techniques can seldom be used alone in children. Complications arise more frequently in the postoperative period than intraoperatively.[47]

Vascular stasis is favored by the increased viscosity of blood carrying sickle cells, particularly if that blood cools, and by other factors reducing tissue blood flow—dehydration, reduced cardiac output, and hypovolemia.

Over the years several regimens have been recommended to reduce the likelihood of sickling during anesthesia, but some have now been abandoned. Urea and cyanate therapy are no longer advised (see above) and alkalinization of the urine, once recommended,[48–50] is now believed unnecessary and of doubtful efficacy.[46, 51, 52] Alkalosis from oral alkalis over days before surgery will lead to changes in 2,3-DPG and counter any expected benefit from pH change.[36]

Magnesium sulfate prevents the formation of a permanent thrombus and may mobilize sludged erythrocytes, but has dangers and is no longer used prophylactically.[36, 46]

The use of dextrans in sickle cell crises is controversial.[3, 38, 46] The author of this chapter uses dextran 70 to produce a well-filled circulation at the start of anesthesia, providing tissue hydration is assured beforehand. Preoperative blood transfusions were once discouraged unless anemia was very severe. The dangers of reduced oxygen carriage were believed outweighed by potential dangers of blood transfusion.[39] However, the potential value of reducing the proportion of Hb S–laden cells has led many centers to advise routine preoperative blood transfusion. For elective surgery circulating Hb S levels of below 30 percent and hemoglobin levels of at least 10 g/100 ml are recommended.[46, 53] If the last transfusion is given 3 days before surgery the red cell 2,3-DPG levels should be normal.[3]

For emergency cases exchange transfusion may be indicated. When an unlimited supply of cross-matched blood is present, this approach has obvious attraction. Nevertheless, both in Jamaica and in Ghana, where SCA is very prevalent, only a few patients (some 20 percent) are given blood preoperatively, and there appears to be no discernible added risk to the others.[47, 52] If preoperative blood transfusion is indicated for more major surgery, alternative schemes have been suggested.[38] These include a two-volume exchange transfusion, repeated transfusions in the 2 weeks prior to surgery,[46] or a single transfusion of 15 to 20 ml/kg type-specific, sickle-negative packed erythrocytes to any child with a major hemoglobinopathy.[54]

Spinal anesthesia has been discouraged by some workers[39, 46] because of the danger of hypotension and consequent decreased tissue perfusion. However, local infiltration techniques and regional blocks can be considered.

Vascular stasis increases arteriovenous oxygen tension differences and therefore favors sickling, leading to a vicious cycle of sickling–stasis–tissue hypoxia–sickling. Some authors recommend avoidance of tourniquets,[46, 55] whereas others believe that proper application and careful exsanguination can permit safe use of tourniquets.[39, 56] Danger from the use of tourniquets in SCA has not been proven.

SPECIFIC RECOMMENDATIONS. All black children should be screened for SCD. Antenatal diagnosis is possible at certain centers in Europe, America, Israel, and Australia, but is rarely requested.[57] More usually, the presence of Hb S is identified in a small sample of blood. Under a microscope such a sample may be seen to demonstrate sickling when a reducing agent is added. The "Sickledex" test is a very reliable method, but is qualitative only and does not distinguish SCA from SCT. If the test is positive, genotyping by hemoglobin electrophoresis should be undertaken. In an emergency SCA should be assumed when anemia, a positive sickle cell test, the history, and clinical findings are all compatible with that diagnosis.

An immediate preoperative hemoglobin estimation is advisable whether or not transfusion has been used in the preparation for surgery. Changes in hemoglobin levels can occur rapidly, particularly when sequestration occurs.[46] Surgical procedures undertaken during a sickling crisis are nearly always fatal.[58]

All patients should have a thorough physical examination before operation. Any infection should be rigorously treated and prophylactic antibiotic therapy instituted.[46]

Premedication regimens have varied widely or been omitted without observed problems.[47, 52] However, promethazine appears to offer specific advantages for these patients: it does not depress respiration, it produces some drying of the mouth, it is soporific and antiemetic, it can be given by mouth, and it has a fairly prolonged length of action in children. Moreover, promethazine has an antihistamine effect, which may help prevent a transfusion reaction, and it may inhibit the reduction of Hb S.[3] A suitable dose is 1 mg/kg 1 to 2 hours preoperatively by mouth.

Operative management is summarized in Table 17–6.

The choice of agents seems not to be critical. A supposition that suxamethonium fasciculations may be associated with local hypoxia and hence precipitate a sickling crisis appears to be theoretical, and this effect is evidently not seen in practice.[47]

Postoperative Management. Treatment in an intensive care unit is highly desirable. Hypoxia must be avoided. In the immediate recovery phase oxygen should be given by face mask. In later stages of recovery few children tolerate this without excessive sedation, and nasal prongs or catheter or a head box (see Fig. 17–1) may prove more acceptable. FIO$_2$ should be measured and adjusted to 30 to 50 percent. Oxygen tents (Isolettes, Croupettes) are very useful in postoperative care in SCA. Condensation must not be allowed to hide the patient. Postoperative care should be explained to patients and demonstrated preoperatively to elective cases, to ease anxiety. Oxygen therapy should be continued for at least 24 hours in all cases. Thereafter, early mobilization decreases risks from

Table 17–6. OPERATIVE MANAGEMENT IN SICKLE CELL ANEMIA

Problem	Management
Hypothermia	Warm OR, blankets, humidification
Dehydration	Perioperative intravenous infusions
Blood loss	
Minor	Dextrans and/or crystalloid solutions IV
Major	Prompt replacement, fresh blood
Hypoxia	
Induction	Preoxygenate—difficult in small children, but 2 minutes will suffice if mask fit is airtight[60] Hyperventilate with oxygen/halothane prior to intubation, smooth induction, minimum doses/concentrations
Intraoperative	F_IO_2 30–50% $F_IO_2 \propto \dfrac{1}{F_IN_2O}$; hence more supplements needed with high F_IO_2
At extubation	Ventilate with 100% oxygen
Acidosis	Mild hyperventilation, counter hypocapnis vasoconstriction with judicious volatile agent administration
Vascular stasis	Maintain or increase circulating blood volume, maintain cardiac output, avoid peripheral vasodilatation

Modified from Howells TA, et al: Anaesthesia and sickle cell haemoglobin. Br J Anaesth 44:975, 1972.

vascular stasis. Prolonged oxygen therapy may depress erythropoiesis.[3]

After hypoxia, infection is the major hazard. Careful aseptic techniques must be practiced for intravenous cannulation.[46] Attention to hydration is required since oral intake may be restricted, while reduced renal function may impose an obligatory urine volume of as much as 2000 ml/24 hours.[41]

Sickle Cell Trait (SCT). Patients heterozygous for Hb A and Hb S rarely present serious clinical problems. Hb S levels within the red cells are less than 50 percent. Although sickling is very rare, extreme conditions such as flying at altitude in unpressurized aircraft have been reported to induce sickling crises in some individuals.

Recognition of SCT patients will usually depend upon routine testing. If SCT patients are seriously anemic, the cause is unlikely to be related, and an additional cause should be sought and treated appropriately. There is, however, an age-dependent, progressive fall in the concentrating power of the kidney,[41] although during childhood the clinical significance of this must be slight.

Increased risk from anesthesia for SCT patients has not been demonstrated except in extreme situations and in major interventions such as thoracotomy.[3, 39, 52, 55, 60, 61] In such cases, and where such doubts exist concerning the heterozygous status of the patient, or if thalassemia coexists (see below), the recommendations for SCA patients should be followed. Otherwise, no specific plan for anesthesia need be envisaged. The patient's general condition should be optimal before elective surgery, and if anemia is present it should be corrected by transfusion. Appropriate premedication, smooth induction, eucapnic and nonhypoxic maintenance, with special attention to maintenance of cardiovascular performance and adequate hydration, and a well supervised recovery form the basis of safe management.

Oxygen therapy in the postoperative period after major surgery should follow the recommendations given earlier for SCA. After minor surgery the child who resists the imposition of oxygen therapy is probably in no further need of it and will rest better without it. SCT patients would not normally be considered for anesthesia and surgery on an outpatient basis.

A distinguished expert in this field has stated "The same conditions which would cause crisis in patients with SCA could, if pushed to a further unphysiological degree, cause in vivo sickling in patients with SCT."[62]

It would thus be a foolhardy anesthetist who, either during or after surgery, ignored the possibility of catastrophe affecting the patient with SCT. Close attention will always be required. If indicated, intervention as for SCA must be prompt.

Thalassemia

Unlike SCD and many other hemoglobinopathies, thalassemia does not result from amino acid substitution but from a retarded synthesis of either the alpha chain or the beta chain, leading to imbalance (alpha and beta thalassemia, respectively). The synthesis is governed by a pair of allelomorphic autosomal codominant genes, so that both homozygous (major) and heterozygous (minor) forms occur, presenting clinical features of differing severity. The disease has spread well beyond the geographical confines of countries bordering the Mediterranean Sea.

Alpha thalassemia occurring in heterozygotes is relatively common and presents as a mild anemia in American and African blacks. Jaundice and slight splenomegaly may be present, and occasionally episodes of severe anemia may require blood transfusion. Severe homozygous disorders of the alpha chain cause intrauterine death, since they affect Hb F production.

Therefore, the major thalassemias that present clinical problems in childhood are disorders of the beta chain.[57]

Clinical Manifestations of Beta Thalassemia. The homozygous form of beta thalassemia (Cooley or Mediterranean anemia) presents with very severe anemia (hemoglobin less than 7 g/100 ml) in children over 6 months old. Chronic hemolysis and defective erythropoiesis lead to gross marrow hyperplasia. Extramedullary erythropoiesis can lead to characteristic deformities, especially of the skull and face. Growth is impaired and, in survivors, puberty is delayed.

Untreated children die after 1 to 6 years of chronic illness. While transfusion therapy maintains good health in the short term, the consequent iron overload can lead to death from intractable heart failure in early childhood. Nightly subcutaneous infusions of desferrioxamine can control the overload, but there is difficulty in securing compliance with this treatment. Hemosiderosis, with brown pigmentation of the skin and cirrhosis of the liver, may develop in patients receiving frequent transfusions. Anemic crises from aplasia or folic acid deficiency can occur.

Hypersplenism (the combination of gross splenomegaly, excessive erythrocyte destruction, and thrombocytopenia) may require splenectomy to reduce transfusion requirements. The subsequent increased risk of infection necessitates prolonged prophylactic antibiotic therapy.

The heterozygous form, thalassemia minor, presents little clinical problem, and Hb C thalassemia is relatively mild. However, association with a sickling genotype may result in severe problems. Hb E thalassemia is associated with very severe anemia.

Anesthetic Management. Particular attention must be paid to the severity of the anemia in patients with thalassemia major. Iron therapy is absolutely contraindicated. Preoperative transfusion to adequate levels should be performed. Liver function and cardiac status must be carefully assessed preoperatively, and any deficiency must be borne in mind in designing the anesthetic technique. If present, cardiac failure must be treated. Hypoxia, cardiovascular depression, and hemoglobinuria should be avoided.

Preoperative blood transfusions may be augmented intraoperatively during splenectomy by autotransfusion of some of the blood sequestrated within the spleen. The splenic artery is clamped first, and epinephrine is injected provided halothane has not been used.[15]

Uncomplicated thalassemia minor may require no specific precautions from the anesthetist beyond the general duty to assess thoroughly, to take care, to monitor, and to treat incidents meticulously and promptly. Any association of Hb S with thalassemia indicates the full precautionary approach detailed for SCA in the preceding section.

Spherocytosis (Acholuric Jaundice)

This hemolytic anemia is believed to be due to an abnormality of the red cell membrane affecting sodium ion entry into the cell. Energy- and glucose-consuming processes may fail during splenic stagnation, and the cell loses viability.

Clinical Features.[5] Many cases are manifested in the neonatal period, mimicking hemolytic disease of the newborn, but most commonly spherocytosis is first diagnosed in school children. Jaundice (1 to 4 ml/100 ml unconjugated bilirubin) is often slight and intermittent in older children. Kernicterus is reported in the newborn.

Anemia is also moderate and episodic. There may be aplastic or hemolytic "crises" with marked anemia, dyspnea, vomiting, abdominal pain, extreme lassitude, and fever. Such crises may be precipitated by infection or folic acid deficiency. Chronic anemia may be accompanied by impaired growth and mental retardation.

Splenomegaly is usual. After infarction or hemolytic crises, the spleen may be tender.

Treatment. Most frequently this consists of splenectomy, usually deferred until the child is 3 to 4 years old. Folic acid and blood transfusions may be needed to treat crises. Steroids have no place in treatment.

Anesthetic Management. Preoperative transfusion should seldom be required, since anemia is usually moderate and accompanied by increases in 2,3-DPG, facilitating oxygen delivery to the tissues. Careful conduct using standard modern anesthetic techniques is recommended.

Glucose-6-Phosphate Dehydrogenase (G-6-PD) Deficiency

Black, Mediterranean, and North European races demonstrate different clinical pictures in response to glucose-6-phosphate dehydrogenase (G-6-PD) deficiency, which is a congenital defect of the pentose shunt pathway. All forms are inherited as sex-linked characteristics with intermediate dominance.

Racial incidence varies greatly from 10 percent in American blacks to 1 to 35 percent in the different Mediterranean races. It is believed that at least 100 million persons in the world are G-6-PD deficient.[63]

Clinical Features. Hemolytic anemia may follow ingestion of drugs and chemicals, including antimalarials, sulfonamides, nitrofurans, analgesics (notably aspirin), and para-aminosalicylic acid (PAS) (Table 17–7). There is a variable mild chronic hemolytic anemia in affected patients.

Anesthetic Management. Great care must be taken to avoid administration of any of the drugs that have been implicated as causing hemolysis in G-6-PD deficient patients[4, 63–66] (Table 17–7). Prilocaine is contraindicated,[19] but with careful conduct of anesthesia, on present evidence, no specific problem need be anticipated. Folic acid supplementation may be desirable perioperatively.

COAGULOPATHIES

Hemophilia

Hemophilia exists throughout the world, with an estimated incidence in developed countries approximating 1 in 10,000.[57] Hemophilia A (factor VIII deficiency), is clinically indistinguishable from the much rarer hemophilia B (factor IX deficiency). Both disorders occur as X-linked recessive traits. The disease thus affects only males but is carried by heterozygous females.

Table 17–7. AGENTS THAT MAY CAUSE HEMOLYSIS IN G-6-PD DEFICIENT SUBJECTS

Aminoquilones	Sulfones
Primaquine	Dapsone
Pamaquine	Sulfoxone
Chloroquine	Thiazosulfone
Pentraquine	Diaminodiphenylsulfone
Quinocide	
Quinacrine	**Miscellaneous**
Plasmoquine	Vitamin K (water-soluble analogues)
	Naphthalene
Analgesics and Antipyretics	Probenecid
Acetylsalicylic acid	Nalidixic acid
Acetanilid	Dimercaprol
Aminopyrine*	Methylene blue
Phenacetin	Trinitrotoluene*
	Acetylphenylhydrazine
Nitrofurans	Phenylhydrazine
Nitrofurantoin	Isoniazid
Furazolidone	Para-aminosalicylic acid
Nitrofurazone*	Tolbutamide
Furaltadone	Neoarsphenamine
	Diabetic acidosis
Sulfonamides	Fava beans*
Sulfanilamide	Infections (Respiratory
Sulfacetamide	viruses, infectious
Sulfasoxazole	hepatitis, infectious
Sulfamethoxypyridazine	mononucleosis, bacterial
N^2-Acetylsulfanilamide	pneumonias)
Sulfisoxazole	Quinine*
Sulfapyridine	Quinidine*
Sulfasalazine	Chloramphenicol*

*Not believed hemolytic in blacks.

A level of factor VIII activity below 3 percent of normal is associated with severe hemophilia, but in 5 to 10 percent of cases the deficiency is less marked, to 5 percent or more, and a milder form is seen.

Factor VIII deficiency also occurs in von Willebrand disease, together with abnormal capillary fragility. The rare homozygous form is manifested as a grave bleeding disorder.

Clinical Manifestations.[5] Patients with severe forms of hemophilia usually manifest a bleeding tendency within the first year of life, sometimes at circumcision. Hemarthroses may develop in the first 3 years. Spontaneous hemorrhages characterize childhood and, in contrast to those developing in platelet and capillary disorders, the deeper tissues are more usually involved: intramuscular hematomas in the psoas, retroperitoneal bleeding, hemarthroses, and hematuria.

Early manifestations and joint involvement may not be seen in the milder form, hematomas developing only after more severe trauma. Excessive bleeding follows dental extraction or other surgery.

Treatment. The diagnosis may be made antenatally, when it may be followed by midterm abortion,[57] or may be presumed at birth from a family history of affected males. However, 30 percent of males show no family history.[54] Screening coagulation tests on capillary samples are used in small children. The clotting time is prolonged with a normal bleeding time. Full hematological investigation and factor VIII assay must follow any positive or borderline result.

Replacement Therapy. Prior to any surgical procedure factor VIII levels should be augmented. This implies the administration as needed of factor VIII. One unit of factor VIII (antihemophilic globulin, AHG) is the activity present in 1 ml of fresh pooled normal plasma. One guide to dosage is that the number of units of factors required equals

$$\frac{\text{Body weight (kg)} \times \text{Desired increase in activity}}{1.5}$$

Therapeutic materials used in hemophilia management[5, 67, 68] are listed in Table 17–8.

Fifty percent of severely affected hemophiliacs in the United Kingdom are now on home therapy.[67] For minor spontaneous hemorrhages nonspecific measures, such as bed rest, immobilization, sedation, and analgesics (but not aspirin) are used, but replacement therapy is given at home or in the hospital if these measures are ineffective.

Even minor cuts will warrant hospital management. Topical thrombin application by light pressure dressings is advised. If sutures are required, if mild hemorrhage is continuing, or if recurrence would endanger structure or function (for example, of the orbit), replacement therapy, 15 units/kg, is given every 12 hours, usually for several days. The aim is to maintain factor VIII activity at greater than 20 percent of normal.

More severe hemorrhages command more generous therapy, comparable with that recommended to cover major surgery (see below).

Anesthetic Management. Patients with hemophilia may present for related surgery (for example, for hemarthrosis), for dental extraction, or for unrelated surgical conditions.

In the following, hemophilia A is considered. The principles apply also to hemophilia B. Full consultation with a hematologist is mandatory in the management of surgery in hemophiliacs. *At no time should intramuscular injections be given.* Care should always be taken to preserve veins for further use when required.

All patients should be tested for the presence of antibody to factor VIII. In patients whose test results are positive, only life-threatening conditions should be treated surgically, although porcine factor VIII can sometimes be used to provide cover. If this is used, full facilities for treating an anaphylactic reaction must be instantly available.[67]

Patients should also be tested for the presence of hepatitis B surface antigen (HBsAg). Fifty percent of hemophiliacs managed at Oxford, England, are carriers of hepatitis, being HBsAg positive. Vaccines exist, and anesthetists having regular contact with patients known to be HBsAg positive are advised to seek protection.[69, 70]

In recent years it has become clear that many who have received multiple blood transfusions, notably hemophiliacs, carry the HTLV III virus, which in some individuals leads to the acquired immunodeficiency syndrome (AIDS).

At the time of writing there is no clear consensus as to whether all hemophiliacs should be tested for HTLV III antibodies. However, despite its relatively low infectivity, it would appear advisable to take all

Table 17–8. THERAPEUTIC MATERIALS FOR HEMOPHILIA MANAGEMENT

Material	Trade Names	Activity (Approximately)	Comments
Fresh-frozen plasma		0.7 μ/ml	Large volumes may lead to circulatory overload
Dried Factor VIII Fraction BP	Hemofil Koate Factorate Kryobulin Profilate Humanate	25 μ/ml (after reconstitution)	Easily soluble, use isotonic saline. Low reaction rate
Cryoprecipitate		75 to 100 μg/bag	For mild cases, infrequently transfused. For hepatitis risk cases (1 bag/10 kg body weight increases factor VIII activity 15%)
Porcine Factor VIII	Hyate C		For cases with antibodies to human factor VIII. Less problems than with earlier animal preparations, but reactions occur, occasionally severe.
Dried factor IX fraction BP	Prothromplex Proplex		For Hemophilia B
Desmopressin (DDAVP)			Increases factor VIII level in blood 3 to 6 fold Tachyphylaxis occurs Useful in mild cases only
Tranexamic acid	Cyklokapron		Inhibits plasminogen activation, interferes with fibrinolysis
Epsilon-aminocaproic acid (EACA)	Epsikapron		Contraindicated in hematuria

From Rizza CR: Haemophilia A & B. Prescribers' Journal 24:71, 1984.

possible precautions, similar to those taken when hepatitis B subjects are to be anesthetized, to avoid self- or cross-inoculation with the blood of a hemophiliac. Advice currently given by the Department of Health and Social Security in the United Kingdom[70a] emphasizes that the anesthetist should cover any open cut or abrasion with a waterproof dressing, wear gown and gloves for all invasive procedures, and wear goggles or glasses if blood or other body fluid could otherwise enter the anesthetist's conjunctiva. All equipment used in anesthetizing a hemophiliac should be disposable or able to be autoclaved prior to reuse. Handling of equipment must be meticulous so that sharp edges do no harm. All current evidence suggests that even accidental self-innoculation is unlikely to transmit the infection.

Preoperative anemia can be corrected by slow infusion of whole blood or packed red cells, but the hemostatic defect should first be corrected by infusion of a factor VIII concentrate. In an emergency, if factor VIII concentrates are not available, recently thawed fresh frozen plasma (20 ml/kg) should be administered preoperatively.

Hemarthrosis. Prompt home or hospital therapy has reduced the incidence of severe arthroses. Occasionally in young children joint aspiration, prior to pressure bandaging, may indicate general anesthesia. Pain and distress require attention. Oral, rectal, or intravenous routes may be used to administer selected analgesics and sedatives, as needed. Replacement therapy is given prior to aspiration. No special technique of anesthesia is required, but particular care in handling the patient and avoidance of any airway trauma are desirable. If their use is essential, artificial airways should be well lubricated and inserted and removed gently.

Dental Surgery. Even single dental extractions may occasionally command prolonged replacement therapy. Fifteen to 20 units/kg have been recommended.[5] Two to 3 days of treatment will usually suffice, but up to 7 days may be needed. Larger initial doses of factor VIII may be associated with a need for less prolonged therapy.[67] Preoperatively tranexamic acid, 10 mg/kg, may be given intravenously, and further doses (15 mg/kg thrice daily orally) continued for 10 days. Epsilon-aminocaproic acid (0.1 g/kg every 6 hours) may alternatively be used. The objective is to maintain factor VIII levels at or above 20 percent of normal activity.

Penicillin V or other antibiotic may be given to reduce any risk of infection leading to secondary hemorrhage.

Single tooth extractions need not necessarily command the full panoply of nasoendotracheal intubation frequently used for more extensive dental surgery. The patient may be placed in a convenient lateral position, head down, following deep inhalation induction with high F_IO_2. One assistant should have as his or her sole task the prompt aspiration of any secretions or shed blood. The extraction should be performed expeditiously at the highest level of competence available.

Patients with mild hemophilia and some with von Willebrand disease may, when undergoing minor surgery, be treated with desmopressin, a vasopressin analogue. This obviates the use of factor VIII concentrates. A three- to sixfold rise in factor VIII activity follows administration of 0.4 to 0.5 μg/kg intravenously. Desmopressin is of no value in the management of severe hemophilia.[67]

Major Surgery. For more extensive dental or other surgery, more intensive and prolonged therapy is required. Anesthesia should not begin until the level of factor VIII activity is 50 percent of normal, and factor VIII activity must be maintained at or above the 30 percent level for several days, by infusions of factor VIII concentrates every 12 hours.

Assays of factor VIII activity as well as the clinical course of the patient will dictate management, since the activity of the therapeutic materials is not wholly dependable. Sequestration and consumption of infused factor VIII are also unpredictable variables. Daily infusions may be needed from the seventh to the twentieth day postoperatively.

Despite the provision of adequate factor VIII levels possible today, the anesthetist will wish to avoid inflicting damage that could later lead to hemorrhage. Instrumentation of the upper airway should be avoided whenever possible. Artificial airways, endotracheal tubes, and monitoring probes should be generously lubricated and extreme care used in their placement and removal. Nasal intubation is usually traumatic and should be avoided whenever possible in patients with a bleeding disorder.

Thrombocytopenia (Platelet Deficiency)

Hemostasis becomes defective when the level of circulating platelets falls below 100,000/μl. Normal levels range between 150,000 and 500,000/μl.[5, 20] Spontaneous widespread purpura seldom occurs at a level of 25,000/μl or more.[5]

In contrast to hemophilia, the ability of plasma to coagulate at sites of vascular damage is unimpaired in thrombocytopenia. Once active bleeding is arrested (for example, by pressure), coagulation can proceed and recurrence of bleeding is unlikely.

Causes. Reduced platelet production occurs in many blood disorders, including aplastic anemia, megaloblastic anemia, and marrow infiltrations. These conditions are discussed earlier in this chapter.

Increased peripheral destruction of platelets is seen in childhood in idiopathic thrombocytopenia, in hypersplenism (see page 502), and in consumption coagulopathies. Dilutional thrombocytopenia can result from massive blood transfusion or cardiopulmonary bypass.

Idiopathic Thrombocytopenic Purpura (ITP)

"In pediatric practice ITP and acute leukemia constitute the two most frequent [medical] causes of significant thrombocytopenia and the incidence of the two diseases is very similar."[5]

ITP appears to have an immunological basis, and a history of recent infection of the upper respiratory tract is obtained in two thirds of patients.

Clinical Features. Patients present with widespread purpura, particularly over the bony prominences. Petechiae are found in the lax skin. There may be bleeding from the nose or mouth. Hematuria and gastrointestinal bleeding may occur.

Diagnosis is made based on the history and clinical signs, a full blood count, and bone marrow puncture.

Treatment. Mild cases without serious bleeding and with a platelet count exceeding $25,000/\mu l$ usually resolve spontaneously within a few weeks. More severe and persistent cases are treated with oral steroid therapy. Prednisolone, 15 mg every 6 hours for 10 days and then reduced at 10-day intervals over the next month, is a typical regimen (smaller amounts are used in patients under 2 years of age). The course is then stopped, although a second course may be given if improvement is not sustained. About 10 percent of patients fail to respond to medical management;[15] splenectomy is then advised.

Anesthetic Management. Until bone marrow aspirates are examined the diagnosis usually remains uncertain and acute leukemia may be suspected. Anesthetic management for such patients requiring diagnostic bone marrow puncture is fully described in the section on Marrow Infiltrations earlier in this chapter.

Patients may also present for splenectomy or for unrelated surgery. Preoperative preparation of the patient must take into account any steroid therapy given. Extra cover may be considered desirable prophylactically, or it may be deferred to any indication arising later in management, according to circumstance.

As in hemophilia, all intramuscular injections are contraindicated. The anesthetic technique chosen and application of monitoring devices should avoid risk from trauma to the upper airway. Endotracheal tubes or other tubes should be well lubricated, and both placement and removal should be secured as atraumatically as possible. Bleeding from attempted venipuncture sites responds to light pressure maintained for 4 minutes.

Platelet concentrates should be available and can be given in a dose of 1 unit/5 kg, when indicated, to correct thrombocytopenia.[69] Cross-matching for ABO compatibility is necessary. Microfilters remove platelets and should therefore not be used for platelet infusions. When splenectomy is to be performed, platelet infusion is reserved until after the splenic pedicle is clamped.

Postoperatively intramuscular injections should probably be avoided if possible. Further platelet infusions are given only if specifically indicated.

Overwhelming infection is a recognized hazard following splenectomy in childhood. Severe meningitis and septicemia may develop insidiously following splenectomy.[71] Prophylactic antibiotic therapy (for example, oral penicillin) should be given. Vaccines exist and are being evaluated.[44] Parent and patient education should seek to promote recognition of and prompt attention to any signs of infection.

Patients who have had splenectomy in the past may present for unrelated surgery. The anesthetist must take particular care not to add to any risk of infection, and perioperative antibiotic therapy should be considered.

POLYCYTHEMIA

The diagnosis of polycythemia implies a hemoglobin concentration persistently greater than 17 g/100 ml in childhood or 22 g/100 ml in the neonate.

Both primary and secondary forms occur, but polycythemia rubra vera, which has surgical implications,[72] is a disease limited to middle age. Polycythemias are indeed extremely rare in childhood, save those secondary to prolonged arterial oxygen desaturation. Cyanotic congenital heart disease (CHD) is the usual cause, but chronic pulmonary disease as well as residence at high altitude can also lead to enhanced erythropoietin production and consequent polycythemia.

Cyanotic Congenital Heart Disease

The anesthetic management of patients with cyanotic CHD is discussed in Chapter 6.

In severe cases the polycythemia is characterized by absence of the usual postnatal fall in hemoglobin concentration. Anemia develops a few months later, but if it is treated with iron therapy, the hematocrit may rise to 75 percent or more, with accentuation of symptoms.

Red cell mass increases disproportionately as the hematocrit rises and an increased blood volume ensues. The increase in oxygen-carrying capacity and cardiac output are potential advantages. However, above a critical hematocrit of 70 percent these are offset by a marked increase in blood viscosity, which hinders blood flow.

Leachman and associates[73] demonstrated that systemic pulmonary anastomosis prior to correction, leading to a reduction of hemoglobin level to below 18 g/100 ml, considerably reduced surgical mortality. Polycythemia in CHD is commonly accompanied by thrombocytopenia.

Pulmonary Disease

In the absence of heart disease, children found to be polycythemic should undergo pulmonary function investigation. The anesthetic management of children with disease of the respiratory system is discussed in Chapter 5.

Neonatal Polycythemia

Polycythemia in neonates may result from twin-to-twin or other intrauterine transfusion, or from fetal hypoxia. Severe cases may present convulsions, heart failure, and respiratory distress. Thrombosis of peripheral blood vessels or of the renal vein, brain damage, and necrotizing enterocolitis are serious complications.

The condition is more commonly seen in babies small for gestational age, in Down syndrome, and in babies with gastroschisis.

Whether symptoms are present or not, if the hematocrit exceeds 60 percent hypovolemia should be corrected by infusions free of red cells,[75] while both normovolemia and the more characteristic hypervolemia should be treated with partial exchange transfusion using fresh frozen plasma or 5 percent albumin solution.[4, 74]

$$\text{Volume of exchange} = \frac{\dfrac{\text{Blood volume}}{(100 \text{ ml/kg})} \times (\text{Observed hematocrit} - \text{Desired hematocrit})}{\text{Observed hematocrit}}$$

REFERENCES

1. Harrison MJ, Healy TEJ, Thornton JA: Aids to Anaesthesia. Vol. 2. Clinical Practice. Edinburgh, Churchill-Livingstone, 1984.
2. Brain MC: The anemias. *In* Beeson JB, McDermott W, Wyngaarden JB (Eds.): Cecil Textbook of Medicine. 15th ed. Philadelphia, W.B. Saunders Co., 1979.
3. Kaufman L, Sumner E: Medical Problems and the Anaesthetist. London, Edward Arnold, 1979, pp 139–151.
4. Willoughby MLN: Paediatric Haematology. Edinburgh, Churchill-Livingstone, 1977.
5. Willoughby MLN: Disorders of the Blood and Reticuloendothelial System. *In* Forfar JO, Arneil GC (Eds.): Textbook of Paediatrics. 2nd ed. Edinburgh, Churchill-Livingstone, 1978, pp 796–841.
6. Shahidi NT, Diamond LK: Testosterone induced remission in aplastic anemia of both acquired and congenital types. N Engl J Med 264:953, 1961.
7. Li FP, Alter BP, Nathan DG: The mortality of acquired aplastic anemia in children. Blood, 40:153, 1972.
8. Birkhill FR, Maloney MA, Levenson SM: Effect of transfusion polycythaemia upon bone marrow activity and erythrocyte survival in man. Blood 6:1021, 1951.
9. Emlinger PJ, Huff RL, Oda JM: Depression of red cell iron turnover by transfusion. Proc Soc Exp Biol Med 79:16, 1952.
10. Roche Products Ltd. *In* Bailey AJM, Taylor W (Compilers): A.B.P.I. Data Sheet Compendium 1984–85. London, Datapharm Publications Ltd.
11. Jarvik EM: Drugs used in the treatment of psychiatric disorders. *In* Goodman LS, Gilman A: The Pharmacological Basis of Therapeutics. 4th ed. New York, Macmillan, 1970.
12. Amos RJ, Amess SAL, Hinds CJ, et al.: Incidence and pathogenesis of acute megaloblastic bone marrow change in patients receiving intensive care. Lancet 2:835, 1982.
13. Donald JR: Induced hypotension and blood loss during surgery. J Roy Soc Med 75:149, 1982.
14. Arneil GC: Disorders of the urogenital system. *In* Forfar JO, Arneil GC (Eds.): Textbook of Paediatrics. 2nd ed. Edinburgh, Churchill-Livingstone, 1978, pp 853–939.
15. Brown TCK, Fisk GC: Anaesthesia for Children. Oxford, Blackwell Scientific, 1979.
16. Wharton B: Nutrition and nutritional disorders. *In* Forfar JO, Arneil GC (Eds.): Textbook of Paediatrics. 2nd ed. Edinburgh, Churchill-Livingstone, 1978.
17. Rennie JS, MacDonald DG, Dagg JH: Iron and the oral epithelium: a review. J Roy Soc Med 77:602, 1984.
18. Howells TH, Pettit JE: Haematological disorders. *In* Vickers MD (Ed.): Medicine for Anaesthetists. 2nd ed. London, Churchill-Livingstone, 1982, pp 335–385.
19. Howells TH: Anaesthesia and blood diseases. *In* Hewer CL, Atkinson RS (Eds.): Recent Advances in Anaesthesia and Analgesia. Vol. 12. London, Churchill-Livingstone, 1975, pp 120–130.
20. Rendle-Short J, Gray OP, Dodge JA: A synopsis of children's diseases. Bristol, John Wright & Sons Ltd., 1978, p 523.
21. Barltrop D: Nutrition and nutritional disorders. *In* Forfar JC, Arneil GC (Eds.): Textbook of Paediatrics. 2nd ed. Edinburgh, Churchill-Livingstone, 1978.
22. Co-trimoxazole and blood (Editorial). Lancet 2:950, 1973.
23. Herbert V: Megaloblastic anaemias. *In* Beeson PB, McDermott W, Wyngaarden JB (Eds.): Cecil Textbook of Medicine. 15th ed. Philadelphia, W.B. Saunders Co., 1979, pp 1719–1729.
24. Lawson DH, Murray RM, Parker JLW: Early mortality in the megaloblastic anaemias. Q J Med 41:1, 1972.
25. Megaloblastic anaemia and sudden death (Editorial). Br Med J 1:525, 1972.
26. Amess JAL, Burman JF, Rees JM, et al.: Megaloblastic haemopoiesis in patients receiving nitrous oxide. Lancet 2:339, 1978.
27. Amos RJ, Amess JAL, Nancekievill DG, et al.: Prevention of nitrous oxide–induced megaloblastic changes in bone marrow using folic acid. Br J Anaesth, 56:103, 1984.
28. Lascari AD: Leukemia in Childhood. Springfield, IL, Charles C Thomas, 1973.
29. Malpas JS: Childhood cancer. Hosp Update 9:401, 1983.
30. Mauer AM, Simone JV: The current status of the treatment of childhood acute lymphoblastic leukemia. Cancer Treat Rev 3:17, 1976.
31. Wark HJ: Postoperative jaundice in children: the influence of halothane. Anaesthesia 38:237, 1983.
32. Thomas M: The use of the Hickman catheter in the management of patients with leukaemia and other malignancies. Br J Surg 66:673, 1979.
33. Chung F: Cancer chemotherapy and anaesthesia. Can Anaesth Soc J 29:364, 1982.
34. Selvin BL: Cancer chemotherapy: implications for the anesthesiologist. Anesth Analg 60:425, 1981.
35. Serota FT, August CS, Koch PA, et al.: Pulmonary function in patients undergoing bone marrow transplantation. Med Pediatr Oncol 12:137, 1984.
36. Filshie J, Pollock AN, Hughes RG, et al.: The anaesthetic management of bone marrow harvest for transplantation. Anaesthesia 39:480, 1984.
37. Davies SC, Hewitt PE: Sickle cell disease. Br J Hosp Med 31:440, 1984.
38. Salem MR: Anesthesia for orthopedic surgery. *In* Gregory GA (Ed.): Pediatric Anesthesia. Vol. 2. New York, Churchill-Livingstone, 1983, pp 851–898.
39. Howells TA, Huntsman RG, Boys JE, et al.: Anaesthesia and sickle cell haemoglobin. Br J Anaesth 44:975, 1972.
40. Henthorne J, Anionwu E, Brozovic M: Screening cord blood for sickle haemoglobinopathies in Brent. Br Med J 289:479, 1984.
41. Berry FA: Anesthesia for Genitourinary Surgery. *In* Gregory GA (Ed.): Pediatric Anesthesia. Vol. 2. New York, Churchill-Livingstone, 1983, pp 727–771.
42. Treatment of sickle-cell crises (Editorial). Lancet 2:762, 1974.
43. Huntsman RG, Lehman H: Annotation: treatment of sickle cell disease. Br J Haematol 28:437, 1974.

44. John AB, Ramlal A, Jackson H, et al.: Prevention of pneumococcal infection in children with homozygous sickle cell disease. Br Med J 288:1567, 1984.

45. Topley JM, Rogers DW, Stevens MCG et al.: Acute splenic sequestration and hypersplenism in the first five years in homozygous sickle cell disease. Arch Dis Child 56:765, 1981.

46. Bentley PC, Howard ER: Surgery in children with homozygous sickle cell anaemia. Ann Roy Coll Surg Engl, 61:55, 1979.

47. Homi J, Reynolds J, Skinner A, et al.: General anaesthesia in sickle cell disease. Br Med J 1:1599, 1979.

48. Greenberg MS, Kass EH: Studies on the destruction of red blood cells. Arch Intern Med 101:355, 1958.

49. Hugh-Jones K, Lehman H, McAlister JM: Some experiences in managing sickle-cell anaemia in children and young adults, using alkalis and magnesium. Br Med J 2:226, 1964.

50. Gilbertson AA: The management of anaesthesia in sickle-cell states. Proc Roy Soc Med 60:631, 1967.

51. Ho PK, Alleyne GA: Acid base status of adults with sickle-cell anaemia. Br Med J 3:271, 1969.

52. Oduro KA, Searle JF: Anaesthesia in sickle cell states—a plea for simplicity. Br Med J 4:596, 1972.

53. Furman EB: Blood and fluid replacement for paediatric patients. In Steward DJ (Ed.): Some Aspects of Paediatric Anaesthesia. Amsterdam, Excerpta Medica, 1982.

54. Atkinson RS, Rushman GB, Lee JA: A Synopsis of Anaesthesia. 8th ed. Bristol, John Wright, 1977.

55. Janik J, Seeler RA: Perioperative management of children with sickle hemoglobinopathy. J Pediatr Surg 15:117, 1980.

56. Browne RA: Anaesthesia in patients with sickle cell anaemia. Br J Anaesth 37:181, 1965.

57. Modell B, Mibashan RS: Antenatal diagnosis of haemoglobinopathies. In Willoughby M, Siegel SE (Eds.): Hematology and Oncology. London, Butterworth, 1982, pp 162–195.

58. Letsky EA: Inherited red cell defects which may complicate surgical treatment. In Wilkinson AW (Ed.): Recent Advances in Paediatric Surgery. Vol. 3. London, Churchill-Livingstone, 1975, pp 11–20.

59. Berthoud M, Read DH, Norman J: Preoxygenation—how long? Anaesthesia 38:96, 1983.

60. Huehns ER: Diseases of haemoglobin synthesis. In Baron DN, Compston N, Dawson AM (Eds.): Recent Advances in Medicine. London, Churchill-Livingstone, 1972.

61. Searle JF: Anaesthesia in sickle cell states. Anaesthesia 28:48, 1973.

62. Konotey-Ahulu FI: Anaesthetic deaths and the sickle cell trait. Lancet 1:267, 1969.

63. Jacob HS: Hemolysis due to intracorpuscular abnormalities. In Beeson PB, McDermott W, Wyngaarden JS (Eds.): Cecil Textbook of Medcine. 15th ed. Philadelphia, W.B. Saunders Co., 1979, pp 865–869.

64. Keller DF: G-6-PD Deficiency. London, Butterworth, 1971.

65. Wintrobe MM (Ed.): Clinical Hematology. 7th ed. Philadelphia, Lea & Febiger, 1974, p 785.

66. Weatherall DJ: Haemolytic anaemias. In Weatherall DJ, Ledingham JG, Warrell DA (Eds.): Oxford Textbook of Medicine. Oxford, Oxford University Press, 1983.

67. Rizza CR: Haemophilia A & B. Prescribers' Journal 24:71, 1984.

68. Chessells JM: Management of haemophilia and allied disorders. In Wilkinson AW (Ed.): Recent Advances in Paediatric Surgery. Vol. 3. London, Churchill-Livingstone, 1975, pp 22–30.

69. Horsey PJ: Blood transfusion. In Atkinson RS, Langton Hewer C: Recent Advances in Anaesthesia. Vol. 14. London, Churchill-Livingstone, 1982.

70. Trimmer EJ: Hepatitis B immunisation. Br J Parenteral Therapy 5:135, 1984.

70a. Department of Health and Social Security (U.K.) 1986: Guidance for surgeons, anaesthetists, dentists and their teams dealing with patients infected with HTLV III. CMO (86) 7.

71. Eraklis AJ: Spleen and portal circulation. In Welch B (Ed.): Complications of Pediatric Surgery. Philadelphia, W.B. Saunders Co., 1982, pp 264–273.

72. Fitts WTJ, Erde A, Peskin GW, et al.: Surgical implications of polycythemia vera. Ann Surg 152:548, 1960.

73. Leachman RD, Hallman GL, Cooley DA: Relationship between polycythemia and surgical mortality in patients undergoing total correction for tetralogy of Fallot. Circulation 32:65, 1965.

74. Rowe MI: Shock and resuscitation. In Welch B (Ed.): Complications of Pediatric Surgery. Philadelphia, W.B. Saunders Co., 1982, p 20.

NEUROMUSCULAR DISEASES   18

PETER G. DUNCAN, M.D.

Neuromuscular diseases in infants and children are relatively rare, yet their presentation to the pediatric anesthesiologist is not that unusual, since the need for diagnostic procedures or palliative orthopedic surgery occurs with many of these entities. While some of the diseases have profound and well-described anesthetic implications, others, because of their rarity, do not. Consequently, discussion of anesthetic management must be based on the medical description of the pathogenesis and extrapolation of anesthetic implications of related diseases.

Numerous classifications of neuromuscular diseases exist depending on the interest of the writer.[1,2] From the anesthesiologist's viewpoint, diseases are best classified according to the site of the anatomical lesion and hence the likely nature of any adverse occurrence during an operative procedure.[3]

DISEASES OF THE SPINAL CORD AND ANTERIOR HORN CELLS

Primary diseases of the anterior horn cells or the motor nuclei of the cranial nerves present a uniform clinical syndrome of profound weakness, neurogenic muscle atrophy, absent deep tendon reflexes, and fasciculations in the region of the denervated muscle groups. They are differentiated from peripheral nerve damage by the normality of sensation. In infants, the fasciculations and muscle atrophy may be difficult to recognize because of generous subcutaneous fat, and marked hypotonia may be the predominant sign. Segmental involvement of the spinal cord with disease may present with regional signs of the lower motor neuron disease at the level of involvement combined with upper motor signs below the level of the lesion. In the latter situation, the clinical implications to the anesthetist will depend upon the extent of cord involvement.

In any lesion involving the motor nuclei of the spinal cord, the anesthesiologist must be concerned about compromised respiratory reserve secondary to muscle weakness, positioning difficulty due to muscle atrophy and contractures, aspiration due to pharyngeal muscle involvement, and altered effects of neuromuscular blocking drugs. While experience has not been reported with relaxants in all clinical entities,[4] there have been numerous case reports of life-threatening hyperkalemia following succinylcholine administration to paraplegics[5] or patients with lower motor neuron disease.[6] Experimentally the susceptibility begins 14 days after cord or peripheral nerve transection and is present up to 1 year after injury.[7] Beyond a year in patients with stable neurological lesions the induced hyperkalemia is less marked, probably owing to reduction of the muscle bulk.[8] Prior administration of nondepolarizing relaxants does not consistently protect against the phenomenon.[9]

Primary anterior horn cell disease of long-standing duration may also be associated with a potentiation of nondepolarizing muscle relaxants.[10] It has been suggested that there is collateral branching or sprouting by residual nerve fibers to muscles denervated by disease. The new axonal branches produce additional junctions with the muscle membrane and extend the area that responds to acetylcholine beyond the neuromuscular junction until it involves the entire muscle fiber. This phenomenon, called extrajunctional chemosensitivity, is common to all denervated muscle.[4] These newly formed branches and their motor contacts have less reserve for neuromuscular transmission.[10] A normal dose of relaxant may represent a gross overdose in lower motor neuron disease. While nondepolarizing relaxants are preferable to the depolarizing drugs (with their attendant hyperkalemia), judicious tempering of the dose and appropriate monitoring are essential for safety.

Syringomyelia

This is a slowly progressive, degenerative disease involving the spinal cord, the medulla (syringobulbia), or both. A progressive cavitation occurs, usually in the cervical and lumbar segments of the cord, and primarily in the anterior white commissure. Initially there is loss of pain and temperature sensations as the crossed fibers of the lateral spinothalamic tract are disrupted. As the cavitation extends it may involve the long motor tracts, including the corticospinal tract. The lower motor neurons of the medulla and cord are similarly secondarily affected. Progressive dilatation in the cervical region may lead to impaired CSF drainage, elevation of intracranial pressure, and hydrocephalus.

The pathophysiology of the lesion is unknown. It could be due to incomplete closing of the neural tube in the fourth week of gestation. Alternatively, fluid accumulation in the fourth ventricle may result from failure of the foramen of Magendie to open in prenatal life. Most likely, there is a defect in the intermedullary vascular supply, leading to infarction or hemorrhage. The inadequate circulation results in cavitation. Occasionally the syndrome occurs secondary to trauma or infection, but such a relationship is rare in children.

The onset seldom occurs before 15 years of age. Most commonly there is pain and temperature alteration in the fingers, with secondary trophic ulcers. Muscle wasting initially occurs in the small muscles of the hands, and fasciculations are common. Papilledema may accompany the elevated intracranial pressure. Associated physical findings include cervical ribs, kyphoscoliosis, and the Klippel-Feil syndrome (see Table 9–4).

The primary management has been surgical, either laminectomy or suboccipital craniotomy, but the results have been variable and have included mortality of up to 15 percent. Orthopedic surgery may also be used to control the scoliosis. Anesthetic concerns in such procedures include a possibility of raised intracranial pressure, inadequacy of bulbar reflexes protecting the airway, the degree of impairment of ventilatory function due to the kyphoscoliosis, and the extent of preexisting debility of a chronically ill patient. Defective sweating mechanisms may result from autonomic nervous system compromise, and thermal regulation perioperatively may be difficult.

Diastematomyelia

In this entity a mesodermal septum divides the cord laterally into equal portions. The septum, composed of cartilage, fibrous tissue, and bone, is attached to the posterior aspect of the vertebral bodies and passes through the neural canal to the posterior arch. The lesion may occur in the thoracic or lumbar area and may be associated with skeletal changes such as spinal bifida or kyphoscoliosis. Skin lesions, including lipomas, sacrococcygeal sinus, meningomyelocele, nevi, and hemangiomas may occur over the spine.

Clinically the patient presents with signs and symptoms in the lower legs and feet, together with bladder atony. Disruption of the anterior horn cells results in weakness and atrophy, while interference with crossing fibers may impair pain and temperature sensations.

The treatment of the lesion is surgical to prevent or retard progression of symptoms. Specific anesthetic implications have not been reported.

Spinal Cord Lesions

Spinal cord injury in children can result from several causes. It can occur from birth injury or at any age from falls, car accidents, or direct blows to the spine. Vascular injury may result in decreased flow in the anterior spinal artery, as occasionally happens during repair of coarctation of the aorta. Inflammatory lesions may result in transverse myelitis secondary to viral infections or hyperimmune response to immunization. Whatever the etiology, the patient is left in the initial phase of spinal shock with distal flaccidity and loss of bladder and bowel function, followed in a later phase by spasticity and secondary contracture. Sensation is impaired below the lesion, and autonomic regulation of temperature and circulatory dynamics is compromised.

The anesthesiological implications depend on the duration of the lesion.[11] During the acute phase (less than 3 weeks) there may be considerable cardiovascular instability due to impaired sympathetic reflexes and fluctuating vascular volumes. In the intermediate phase (3 days to 3 months) excessively high serum potassium levels occur with the use of depolarizing muscle relaxants (denervation hypersensitivity).[5,12] In the chronic state the patients are prone to secondary musculoskeletal abnormalities, which may compromise positioning for surgery, restrict pulmonary function, and contribute to the development of decubitus ulcers through impairment of sensation over bony prominences. Renal complications, including infection and calculi, are common in patients with long-standing cord lesions.

The level of the lesion is the critical factor determining anesthetic problems. Patients with lesions affecting sympathetic outflow may have significant cardiovascular, thermal, and respiratory difficulties.

Autonomic hyperreflexia may occur in response to stimulation such as pain or a distended bladder. Control of this potentially fatal complication can be attempted by ensuring adequate depths of anesthesia and the use of vasodilating drugs such as sodium nitroprusside to treat hypertension.[13, 14] Hypotensive responses can be controlled by correcting hypovolemia and by the use of vagal blocking drugs to abolish unopposed vagal tone causing bradycardia or heart block. Lack of sympathetic control of sweating and cutaneous blood flow compromises body temperature control, demanding prudent monitoring and maintenance of temperature perioperatively. Finally, lesions in the thoracic cord or above may decrease the function of accessory respiratory muscles, lowering vital capacity and expiratory reserve volumes and predisposing to postoperative pulmonary complications.

Progressive Infantile Spinal Muscle Atrophy

This disease, also known as *Werdnig-Hoffman disease,* is an autosomal recessive degenerative disease of the anterior horn cells and cranial nerve motor nuclei. Clinically the course of the illness varies according to the age of onset. Patients presenting as neonates or in the first 6 months of life experience a rapidly progressive course, with death from respiratory complications by the age of 2 years. Those who become symptomatic after 1 year experience a less fulminating course and may survive into the second decade. No medical treatment is available, although orthopedic surgery may be attempted to stabilize the unsupported spine and thus slow the progression to respiratory failure.

The clinical picture is uniform in these patients. They demonstrate generalized muscle weakness and hypotonia, although sparing of the facial and extraocular muscles allows an alert facial expression to be maintained. Secondary skeletal changes of pectus excavatum and kyphoscoliosis invariably occur. Sensation remains intact despite a marked atrophy of the skeletal muscles. Later bulbar involvement develops and leads to problems with secretion control and recurrent aspiration pneumonia.

Numerous syndomes have been described with similar hereditary degeneration of anterior horn cells. Juvenile proximal hereditary muscular atrophy *(Kugelberg-Welander disease)* has its onset in the first or second decade and progresses slowly over the next 20 to 40 years to total debility. Cardiac arrhythmias and congestive heart failure may occur.[15] *Facioscapulohumeral neurogenic atrophy, scapuloperoneal atrophy,* and *chronic spinal muscular atrophy* are inherited syndromes with predominantly regional involvement beginning in the first decade of life. Progressive bulbar paralysis of childhood *(Fazio-Londe disease)* is a progressive degeneration of the anterior horn cells in the bulbar nuclei and cervical and upper thoracic cord. *Möbius syndrome,* on the other

hand, is a nonprogressive deterioration of the motor nuclei of cranial nerves VI and VII.

Amyotrophic lateral sclerosis is a progressive degenerative disease affecting the cortical spinal tracts, motor nuclei of the lower medulla, and anterior horn cells of the spinal cord. While mainly a disease of adults, it may begin in the first two decades of life and then rapidly progresses. Death usually occurs within several years after diagnosis as a result of bulbar involvement.

The anesthesia literature relative to these degenerative entities is sparse. There are numerous documented reports of succinylcholine-induced hyperkalemia[6, 9] with subsequent cardiovascular collapses, and this drug is therefore contraindicated. Motor nerve degeneration and subsequent recruitment by neighboring fibers may cause a change in the neuromuscular junction, resulting in increased sensitivity to all nondepolarizing relaxants.[4] Hence all relaxants of this type should be used in reduced doses with appropriate monitoring. While there is no evidence that respiratory drive is impaired in these diseases, respiratory reserve is definitely reduced from muscle weakness and skeletal changes. Aspiration is a clear danger in the presence of pharyngeal involvement, particularly in the anesthetic and postoperative periods when muscular deficits may be exaggerated.[16] If there is any doubt as to the ability of the patient to protect his airway or sustain an adequate minute ventilation, mechanical support should be continued well into the postoperative period. Whenever possible, relaxants are best avoided, and any muscle relaxation that is needed should be achieved by use of volatile anesthetics that have significant relaxant properties.

Arthrogryposis Multiplex Congenita

Arthrogryposis is a syndrome present from birth that is characterized by multiple contractures of the arms and legs. The mechanism of inheritance is unknown. In some cases the contractures may be secondary to degeneration of nerve roots or myopathies, but the most common form stems from profound reductions in the number of anterior horn cells in the cervical and lumbar enlargements of the cord.[1] The weak, hypotonic musculature results in multiple deformities of the limbs and permanent contractures. Associated abnormalities include cardiac malformations, inguinal hernias, cleft palate, scoliosis, and rigidity of the temporomandibular joints.

Patients with this rare syndrome present frequently for anesthesia because of the need for release of contractures or correction of associated defects. Preoperatively the ability to open the mouth and control the airway must be assured. Clinical and radiographic examination of the mandible and upper airway may be indicated, and ancillary devices for intubation may be needed. Slow induction by mask with oxygen and volatile agents rather than precipitous intravenous induction is preferred. While adverse reaction to relaxants has not been reported, apprehension exists as to the safety of depolarizing drugs with all anterior horn cell diseases.

Positioning for surgery may pose a considerable problem because of the extensive flexion contractures. Care must be taken to protect skin over bony points and to prevent pathological fractures.

Poliomyelitis

Fortunately less common since the introduction of immunization, the infective destruction of anterior horn cells by the polio virus leaves a clinical picture similar to that of the degenerative diseases of the anterior horn cells. Anesthetic concerns are similar, with sensitivity to depolarizing drugs to be expected. If nondepolarizing relaxants are used, one must be careful to monitor respiratory musculature carefully and avoid erroneous conclusions drawn from assessment of noninvolved muscle groups.[4]

DISORDERS OF PERIPHERAL NERVES AND SPINAL NERVE ROOTS

Guillain-Barré Syndrome

Usually following a nonspecific illness or infection, this syndrome consists of a gradual onset of symmetrical paralysis ascending from the feet. In half the cases the disease involves the cranial nerves, with resultant compromise of respiratory and bulbar function. Patchy sensory loss occurs as well, although it is less prominent than the motor deficit. Autonomic dysfunction is common, with variable heart rates, labile blood pressures, and ECG changes.[17] Pathologically there is demyelination of the axons with lymphocyte infiltration. IgM antibodies in the myelin sheaths suggest an immunological mechanism.

The clinical course is variable, with slow progression over days or weeks or rapid progression to flaccid quadriplegia. Recovery occurs in 2 to 8 weeks, being complete in 65 percent of those afflicted and leaving residual weakness in the remainder. Mortality is quoted at 3 to 4 percent of cases, mainly from complications of respiratory muscle paralysis. Treatment is supportive only; steroid therapy is of equivocal value.

Anesthetic considerations in Guillain-Barré syndrome revolve around the instability of the cardiovascular system and impaired respiratory reserve. Techniques should be employed that cause minimal disruption of compensatory cardiovascular reflexes, intravascular volumes must be carefully maintained, and drugs potentiating catecholamine-induced arrhythmias must be avoided.[18] During positive-pressure ventilation

the cardiovascular system must be carefully monitored to detect alterations in cardiac output.

Traumatic Polyneuropathies

While any nerve or plexus of the body can be damaged by trauma, the brachial plexus is anatomically the most vulnerable. The plexus may be completely avulsed at any age, or individual nerve roots damaged. Birth injury can result in *Erb palsy* (upper trunk injury, C5–6 deficit) or *Klumpke palsy* (lower trunk injury, C8–T1 deficit). The *Parsonage-Turner syndrome* is a paralytic brachial neuritis that can occur at any age. The etiology is unknown.

No specific implications of traumatic polyneuropathy for anesthetic practice have been described, save that improper positioning during operation may be causative. Damage to the sciatic nerve during intramuscular injection represents another iatrogenic neuropathy.

Toxic Polyneuropathies

Postimmunization neuropathies have been reported after use of virtually all preparations, and can affect any of the peripheral nerves. Following rubella immunization the syndrome develops after a latency of 7 to 99 days, usually as a painful sensation in the arm or leg. Recovery is usually complete.

Heavy metal intoxication can similarly result in peripheral neuropathies. Lead intoxication usually produces an encephalopathy, but may be associated with a motor neuropathy with minimal sensory changes. Arsenic, as found in insecticides, produces acute gastrointestinal distress but chronic paresthesias, weakness, and tropic skin changes. Treatment is with chelating drugs.

The bacterial infections of *diphtheria* and *botulism* may each be responsible for a neuropathy in susceptible children. In unimmunized subjects *Corynebacterium diphtheriae* produces weakness classically beginning with swallowing difficulty (paralysis of palate), blurred vision (paralysis of ciliary muscles), and diplopia (paralysis of the extraocular muscles). Subsequently weakness and paresthesias develop in the trunk and extremities. Diphtheritic myocarditis will cause ECG changes varying from slow conduction to AV block. Therapy includes use of antibiotics and antitoxin and supportive management. Botulism is caused by acute food poisoning with the toxin of *Clostridium botulinum;* in infants this classically results from ingestion of home-preserved honey. Progressive weakness beginning in the cranial nerves results in swallowing and respiratory problems requiring medical support. Autonomic nervous system involvement results in ileus and delayed gastric emptying. Recovery is usually complete but may take months.

Metabolic Neuropathies

Diabetes is associated with several peripheral neuropathic syndromes, ranging from a slowly progressive symmetrical distal sensory neuropathy to single or multiple polyneuropathies. Autonomic neuropathy may lead to impaired compensatory cardiovascular reflexes. Such syndromes usually occur in adults but have been noted in up to 10 percent of diabetic children, particularly when disease control is poor.

Acute intermittent porphyria is an autosomal dominant inherited disorder of porphyrin metabolism.[19] Increased levels of delta-aminolevulinic acid synthetase results in increased delta-aminolevulinic acid and porphobilinogen excretion. The former causes patchy demyelination of peripheral nerves, and axonal degeneration results in flaccid paralysis or weakness of skeletal muscle. The disease usually has its onset about the time of puberty, and may present either as a "surgical emergency" with severe, colicky abdominal pain or with psychiatric disturbances. Many drugs, including barbiturates, have been associated with enzyme induction that worsens the syndrome; these drugs must be avoided. While some authors have noted that thiopental has been used inadvertently without problems in the latent periods,[20] others have noted a deterioration in symptoms if it is used during an acute episode. In a review of anesthetic exposures to patients with inducible porphyrias, Mustajoki and Heinonen[21] report that it is rare indeed for any anesthetic drug, including thiopental, to induce symptoms in latent porphyria. During acute attacks it is probable that drugs may be harmful only in association with other factors precipitating the development of symptoms—surgery may worsen an acute attack even without the administration of precipitating drugs. In experimental animals, numerous anesthetics have been shown to induce porphyria synthesis, including barbiturates (thiopental and methohexital), steroids, alfaxalone (Althesin), etomidate, chlordiazepoxide, pentazocine, enflurane, and methoxyflurane. Ketamine is without effect in the rat, but induces delta-aminolevulinic acid synthetase in the chick embryo liver. It has been used without adverse sequelae in humans. It is probably advisable on a theoretical basis to avoid these drugs if alternative agents are available. No harmful effect is expected with opiates, local anesthetics, or inhalational anesthetics (nitrous oxide, halothane, isoflurane). Regional anesthetic techniques may be appropriate during an acute attack, although the etiology of residual neurological deficits may be obscured by major conduction techniques.

Disorders of fat metabolism are associated with various syndromes of peripheral nerve impairment. Abetalipoproteinemia, or *Bassen-Kornsweig syndrome,* is a deficiency of low-density lipoprotein and chylomicrons. Peripheral sensory neuropathy is associated with cardiac failure, arrhythmia, or diarrhea. Familial alphalipoprotein deficiency, or *Tangier disease,* is a deficiency of high density lipoproteins with excessive accumulation of cholesterol ester and triglycerides. The syndrome of *metachromatic leukodystrophy* is characterized by demyelination and intracellular storage of sulfatide in the brain, nerves, liver, and kidney. *Refsum disease* represents a disorder of fatty acid metabolism resulting in excessive storage of phyantic acid in brain, nerves, liver, kidney, and heart. Globoid cell leukodystrophy, or *Krabbe disease,* is a primary deficiency of the enzyme galactocerebrosidase resulting in demyelination and the presence of inclusion bodies in Schwann cells. This disease results in a progressive development of spasticity from infancy, then ultimately a flaccid paralysis and death.

There is no information regarding the effect of anesthesia on these metabolic conditions or on the safety of anesthetic drugs in their presence. Speculatively, positioning and protection of the patient's skin may be difficult during prolonged procedures. Cardiovascular tolerance may be reduced owing to infiltrative involvement of the myocardium and abolition of compensatory sympathetic reflexes. Potent cardiac depressants are best avoided, and hydration must be watched carefully. Respiratory muscle innervation may be affected, and compensation for respiratory embarrassment reduced; if doubt exists, ventilation should be controlled until adequate. Involvement of liver or kidney by fat accumulation may predispose to fasting hypoglycemia, as well as altered fixed drug metabolism and excretion. Careful monitoring for the residual effects of narcotics and relaxants is essential. Although the neuromuscular junction is not primarily affected, denervation hypersensitivity will exist to depolarizing drugs, while reduced reserves exist for nondepolarizing substances.[4]

Hereditary Neuropathies

Hereditary neuropathies are often found associated with other degenerative disorders. The lesions are primarily in the peripheral nerves, resulting in a mixed picture of lower motor neuron disease and sensory deprivation. Secondary neurogenic muscle atrophy occurs, while denervation hypersensitivity can be expected to cause a hyperkalemic response to succinylcholine.

Charcot-Marie-Tooth disease (peroneal muscle atrophy) is an autosomal dominant disorder with its onset in the secondary decade. Weakness is confined to the limbs, particularly the legs and feet. Involvement of the sympathetic postganglionic fibers impairs autonomic function, particularly the control of temperature by sweating. While the primary lesion is demyelination of the peripheral axon, secondary loss of anterior horn cells and degeneration of the posterior columns occur. Life expectancy is not affected, although the degree of debility may be severe.

Hypertrophic interstitial neuritis (*Déjérine-Sottas disease*) has its onset in infancy with delayed motor development and an undulating but progressive course. Weakness and atrophy involve the entire motor system, including bulbar muscles, while sensory changes are more profound. Autonomic changes with thermal lability and mottled cyanosis of the extremities are common. A similar entity, but associated with more severe demyelination, is congenital hypomyelination neuropathy.

Friedreich ataxia is an autosomal recessive disease often with onset in childhood, resulting in progressive degeneration throughout the central nervous system. Clinically there is mental deterioration, ataxia from degeneration of the spinocerebellar tract, and loss of the large myelinated fibers and cells from the dorsal root ganglia. Skeletal abnormalities such as scoliosis and hammer toe are common. The myocardium is involved in 30 percent of cases, with necrosis and degeneration of muscle causing arrhythmias and murmurs.[22]

Numerous syndromes, the hereditary sensory neuropathies, have been described in which the sensory modality is affected without significant muscle weakness. Patients with these disorders are prone to skeletal and cutaneous injury, and also to thermal lability. The lesion usually lies in the dorsal root ganglion or in the myelination of sensory nerves.

One clinical entity with a significant sensory neuropathy is familial dysautonomia (*Riley-Day syndrome*). Occurring predominantly in Ashkenazi Jews, it presents a clinical complex of deficient tear production, absent corneal and deep tendon reflexes, hypotonia, lability of the cardiovascular system, insensitivity to pain, and emotional lability. Absence of fungiform papillae on the tongue may suggest the diagnosis. Pathologically there is focal demyelination of the posterior columns of the spinal cord and degeneration of dorsal root ganglion. The defect in the autonomic nervous system is unknown, although it may represent an imbalance between sympathetic and parasympathetic tone or insufficiency of acetylcholine and catecholamine release. A defect in the formation of norepinephrine from levodopa has also been postulated.

The anesthetic management of Riley-Day syndrome has been described by several authors.[23-27] The fundamental difficulty is the lack of compensatory cardiovascular reflexes, especially in the presence of potent cardiovascular depressant anesthetic drugs. Hypovolemia is also not compensated, and blood volumes must be carefully monitored. Insensitivity to pain may reduce the anesthetic requirement, although lack of cardiovascular signs of blood pressure and pulse rate changes make assessment of anesthetic depth difficult. Careful monitoring and control of body temperature are imperative.

Emotional lability with severe perioperative anxiety is common, and appropriate sedation preoperatively is recommended. Phenothiazines have been recommended because of their alpha-adrenergic blocking effect, which makes it possible to avoid the denervation receptor hypersensitivity to the episodic release of catecholamines that may result in hypertension. Preoperative use of propranolol has been similarly advocated. Difficulty assessing anesthetic depth, in addition to possible disturbed control of ventilation,[28] leads one to advocate controlled ventilation during general anesthetics. No abnormality has been reported with the use of muscle relaxants. Vomiting and aspiration is a significant hazard postoperatively.

One disease of significance to anesthetic practice is neurofibromatosis (*von Recklinghausen disease*).[29,30] Its incidence is 1 in 3000 live births, although the mode of inheritance is uncertain. The syndrome consists of café au lait spots, moles, and benign neurocutaneous tumors. Such neurofibromas can achieve considerable size, causing secondary compromise of nerve or organ function. Lesions in the larynx have been associated with anesthetic disasters. Lesions impinging on bones cause erosion. Fifty percent of patients have kyphoscoliosis. Associated findings may include honeycomb cystic lung changes[31] and renal artery dysplasia with hypertension.[32] Because of common embryonic origins there is an association of this disease with medullary thyroid tumors and pheochromocytoma; such tumors occur in up to 25 percent of cases and may be undetected preoperatively. Anesthetic management of patients with von Recklinghausen disease must include preoperative calcium and blood pressure determinations, as well as a chest x-ray to rule out related abnormalities. The conduct of the anesthetic should be similar to that for a patient with a pheochromocytoma, avoiding physiological trespass and monitoring closely for unexpected blood pressure changes. Prolonged paralysis with depolarizing relaxants has been reported, although the reasons have not been investigated.[33, 34]

Neuropathies Associated with Other Conditions

Connective tissue or collagen vascular diseases have frequently been associated with central nervous system findings, probably owing to interference with nervous blood supply. In *polyarteritis nodosa* there are signs of peripheral neuropathy in up to 50 percent of patients. *Systemic lupus erythematosus* is commonly associated with central nervous system signs in adults, although such are rare in children.

Tumors and neoplasms may cause neuropathies in any age group. *Leukemia*, the most common malignant disease in children, may infiltrate the cranial and peripheral nerves. *Neuroblastoma*, the most common solid tumor, may be associated with a diffuse nervous syndrome consisting of bewildering, athetoid movements. Any other tumor may locally infiltrate peripheral nerves or nerve roots, leading to sensory or motor neuropathies.

DISORDERS OF THE NEUROMUSCULAR JUNCTION

Myasthenia Gravis

Myasthenia gravis is a neuromuscular disorder manifested by weakness and fatigability of voluntary muscles. The ocular muscles are most commonly involved, causing ptosis and diplopia. Cranial nerve problems are usual, resulting in dysarthria and dysphagia. Respiratory muscle weakness is less common but may be profound during a crisis. The symptoms fluctuate and are worsened by exercise and improved by rest. Similarly, electrical stimulation of involved musculature shows fatigue of contraction on repeated stimulation and exhaustion after a tetanic burst.[35]

The basic mechanism of the disease appears to be autoimmune, with a reduction in the number of available acetylcholine receptors at the neuromuscular junction. Antibodies to the receptors have been demonstrated.[36] There is an association with other immunological diseases, particularly thyroid disease. However, a poor relationship of the antibody titers to the clinical state has been documented. The muscles are small, probably owing to neurogenic atrophy, but are structurally normal. Aggregations of lymphocytes about the neuromuscular junctions are again perceived as support for the hypothesis of an autoimmune etiology.

The incidence of the disease is 3 per 100,000, and about 10 percent of patients are under 16 years of age. Pediatric cases are described as one of three types:

1. *Neonatal transient myasthenia,* affecting the infant of a mother with the disease. Symptoms persist for 1 to 8 weeks, and consist of weakness and difficulty in feeding. The severity of the disease in the infant does not correlate with the mother's symptoms, and only 10 to 15 percent of newborns of affected mothers will be affected; however, medical therapy with an anticholinesterase drug may be needed.

2. *Congenital myasthenia gravis,* affecting an infant in the first few months of life. The mother does not have the disease, and the child will persist with symptoms, which are usually mild for life.

3. *Juvenile myasthenia gravis,* affecting those over the age of 10 years, usually girls, with a presentation similar to that in adults. Cases in juvenile and adult patients have been classified by involvement as "ocular," affecting the eye only, or "generalized," affecting all voluntary muscles.

The treatment of myasthenia gravis consists of elevating the level of acetylcholine at the neuromuscular junction by the inhibition of cholinesterase.[37] The most commonly used preparations are oral pyridostigmine and neostigmine. These drugs improve the symptoms but also increase airway secretions and potentiate the effects of narcotics.[38] They will also inhibit the degradation of succinylcholine and ester-type local anesthetics. Steroid hormones are used to suppress the immune response, and although the patients may feel subjectively better, the sensitivity to nondepolarizing muscle relaxants may persist.[39]

Much debate has existed in the anesthetic literature concerning the optimal medical regimen in the perioperative period. It is suggested that if the patient does not absolutely require the anticholinesterase medication (ocular disease only) one should omit treatment on the day of surgery to avoid interaction with anesthetic drugs, potentiated vagal tone, and copious bronchial secretions. If patients are dependent on anticholinesterase therapy and have more than just ocular symptoms, it is appropriate to continue their usual therapy preoperatively. In those cases in which the therapeutic requirement is expected to change following thymectomy, it is suggested that withdrawal of anticholinesterase drugs with bed rest for at least 24 hours preoperatively is the preferred regimen.[40] Postoperative anticholinesterase therapy is then based on the results of repeated edrophonium tests (0.2 mg/kg) as the requirements change in the postoperative period.

The best results of thymectomy for myasthenia are seen in young females with a short history of the disease and no evidence of thymoma. Complications of the procedure are diminished if anticholinesterase therapy is discontinued preoperatively.[37] Improvement can be expected in most cases, with up to 25 percent requiring no further drug therapy. Leventhal and associates[41] predicted that the need for postoperative mechanical ventilation after this procedure would depend upon the duration of the disease, the presence of pulmonary complications, pyridostigmine dosage, and vital capacity. However, others[42] have suggested these predictors are valid only after thymectomy and unreliable after other surgery. Given the sensitivity of these patients to postoperative narcotics and their fluctuating postoperative anticholinesterase requirements, it is usually more appropriate to allow the patient to demonstrate adequate neuromuscular strength (head lift), vital capacity (greater than 15 ml/kg) and inspiratory force (greater than 30 cm H_2O) before assuming that ventilation will be sufficient. The need for continued use of an artificial airway postoperatively will be predicted by the patient's ability to handle secretions, especially with the involvement of bulbar muscles.

It is preferable to omit preoperative sedation because of the risk of potentiated effects. Induction can be performed with thiopentone, although preservation of spontaneous respiration during mask induction will avoid the need for relaxants for intubation. Halothane, as opposed to newer drugs with more potent muscle relaxant effects (enflurane, isoflurane) is preferred until the airway is secured. If really necessary, muscle relaxants can be used with recognition of their altered action in these patients: The patient may be "resistant" to succinylcholine to induce muscle paralysis[43] but more susceptible to dual block from anticholinesterase therapy, while nondepolarizing drugs should be given in doses that are one twentieth of normal with careful monitoring.[40] However, it is preferable to avoid their use altogether by using one of the volatile agents to secure any relaxation needed for surgery.[44] Narcotics are to be used with caution owing to the described respiratory sensitivity,[38] and are better titrated to requirement in the postoperative period. While reversal of the anesthetic drugs and relaxants may be attempted postoperatively, it must be remembered that these patients may require ventilation even after peripheral surgery (and even without relaxants) owing to changing anticholinesterase requirements. It must be noted that hypothermia, by increasing ventilatory requirements, and hypokalemia, by affecting resting membrane potentials, will further impair marginal respiratory function.

General anesthesia can be safely used, but regional or local anesthesia should be considered whenever possible, although it may be difficult to secure cooperation in many pediatric patients. Under such circumstances management will depend on the severity of the disease, with postoperative care following the above principles.

Myasthenic Syndrome

Myasthenic syndrome, also called Eaton-Lambert syndrome, is characterized by a reduction of acetylcholine release at the motor nerve end-plate, presumably due to impaired acetylcholine esterase activity. Associated diseases are common, including hyper- or hypothyroidism. In adults there is an association with small cell carcinoma of the lung, while in children it may occur with leukemia, neuroblastoma, systemic lupus erythematosus, or rheumatoid arthritis.

Clinically myasthenic syndrome differs from myasthenia gravis in that in the former, proximal limb muscles and rarely the bulbar or ocular muscles are involved, and the muscles become stronger with activity. These patients are extremely sensitive to both nondepolarizing and depolarizing relaxants, and such are best avoided by the use of volatile anesthetics to produce any relaxation required.

The anesthetic considerations are similar to those for myasthenia gravis.

Organophosphate Poisoning

The insecticides parathion and malathion are potent inhibitors of cholinesterase throughout the body. They can be rapidly absorbed by the skin or respiratory tract and produce essentially a cholinergic crisis throughout the body. Respiratory support may be necessary owing to profound weakness. Treatment consists of large doses of atropine to inhibit muscarinic effects and 2-pyridine aldoxime methylchloride (2-PAM chloride), which reactivates the inhibited cholinesterase and binds and inactivates the poison.

PROGRESSIVE MUSCULAR DYSTROPHIES

Myopathies are primary diseases of striated muscles in which biochemical, morphological, or neurophysiological changes occur singly or in combination. Dystrophies are hereditary myopathies characterized by progressive muscle degeneration and weakness. Little is known of the primary defects in these disorders, and classification is based on historic descriptions or clinical similarities. Many eponyms have been given to the entities, and the most common are listed in Table 18–1.

Duchenne Muscular Dystrophy

The most common form of muscular dystrophy, Duchenne or pseudohypertrophic muscular dystrophy, is inherited as an X-linked recessive characteristic. Incidence is reported as 3 per 10,000 births. While defects can be found as early as the second trimester in the fetus, the usual presentation is at age 3 to 5 years. The child develops a waddling gait, lumbar lordosis, and difficulty climbing stairs. Gower sign, the use of the arm to assist in standing up, reflects the pronounced weakness of the hip girdle. The proximal muscles are affected first, while the distal muscles may appear hypertrophied, particularly the calves. Contractures develop in the limbs, and progressive kyphoscoliosis restricts pulmonary function. The patient is usually wheelchair-bound by the early teens, with death occurring before 20 years of age. Respiratory weakness, often combined with difficulty swallowing secretions from pharyngeal involvement, often leads to pneumonia as a terminal event. Cardiac involvement

Table 18–1. SYNONYMS FOR PROGRESSIVE MUSCULAR DYSTROPHIES

Duchenne muscular dystrophy
   Aran-Duchenne dystrophy
   Progressive muscular dystrophy
   Pseudohypertrophic muscular dystrophy
Late-onset, X-linked dystrophy
   Becker dystrophy
Facioscapulohumeral dystrophy
   Landouzy-Déjérine dystrophy
Limb-girdle muscular dystrophy
   Erb dystrophy
   Erb limb-girdle dystrophy
   Juvenile dystrophy of Erb
   Leyden-Möbius dystrophy
Myotonic dystrophy
   Steinert disease
   Steinert dystrophy
   Hoffman disease
   Batten-Curschmann disease

occurs in up to 70 percent of cases, although it is clinically significant in only 10 percent—usually during the terminal stages. Arrhythmias and impaired contractility due to involvement of the muscle of the left ventricle may lead to heart failure and sudden death.[45]

Pathological findings are similar in the muscular dystrophies. Muscle bulk is reduced, to be replaced by fat and connective tissue. The basic defect is unknown, although altered muscle membrane permeability leads to large elevations of serum enzymes (particularly creatine phosphokinase [CPK]) and myoglobin. The enzyme concentration is highest early in the disease, then falls as muscle atrophy occurs. The cardiac muscle component (MB) is also increased, although the level correlates poorly with cardiac involvement. The female carriers of the condition also show elevated serum enzymes, although they are asymptomatic.

There is no specific treatment for the disease. Physiotherapy and activity as is possible are suggested to prevent contractures; the disease deteriorates with bed rest. Surgical treatment may be recommended for contractures, while stabilization of the spine may slow the compromise of pulmonary function secondary to kyphoscoliosis.[46] It appears that the rate of deterioration of pulmonary function, as assessed by vital capacity measurements, can be reduced from 20 percent to 5 percent per year by spinal fusion. The risk of surgery varies with vital capacity. If vital capacity is greater than 45 percent of predicted, mechanical ventilation is not needed postoperatively; if it is less than 30 percent of predicted, serious postoperative complications ensue even with mechanical support. Similar predictive figures have been produced by others.[47] The presence of obesity or cardiovascular involvement implies greater risk.

Anesthetic experiences have been reported in Duchenne muscular dystrophy with a wide variety of anesthetic agents and techniques.[48, 49] Anesthetic difficulties seem to parallel the severity of illness, particularly the degree of restrictive lung disease. The earlier literature also warned of the appearance of acute gastric dilatation with cardiovascular compromise, suggesting the routine insertion of a nasogastric tube.[50]

More recently numerous reports have questioned the safety of succinylcholine in Duchenne muscular dystrophy; acute rhabdomyolysis, myoglobinuria, hyperkalemia, and cardiac arrest have been reported after its administration.[51, 52] Similar events have occurred even in the absence of a clinical myopathy[53] and in the distant relative of an affected patient.[54] These events were not associated with a temperature elevation. In addition, the presence of malignant hyperthermia has been proved by biopsy in Duchenne-type muscular dystrophy, although early therapy prevented significant temperature elevations in the reported cases.[55, 56] Undoubtedly the muscle membrane in these patients is damaged by depolarizing relaxants, and their use therefore is contraindicated. Whether halothane alone can elicit a similar response is not yet demonstrated, although the similarity to the syndrome of malignant hyperthermia suggests the volatile agents should be used with caution. The occurrence of hyperkalemia with cardiac arrest in the recovery room after uneventful surgery[51] suggests that continued vigilance is necessary for some hours postoperatively. Routine prophylaxis with dantrolene sodium is not indicated for all patients with muscular dystrophy, and indeed might cause serious weakness. The drug in parenteral form should be available to treat malignant hyperpyrexia if it should present. Preoperative sedation, if used, should include only very small doses of opiates or barbiturates. Atropine and scopolamine are to be avoided if possible. Induction and maintenance of anesthesia with barbiturates, opiates, nitrous oxide, and pancuronium (if necessary) is the preferred technique. Postoperative ventilation may be required.

Late-Onset X-Linked Muscular Dystrophy

This syndrome resembles Duchenne muscular dystrophy but has a later onset, usually in the second decade, and a slower progression of debility. While most patients can still walk by the late teens, only 50 percent survive to age 40. Anesthetic experiences have not been outlined but the considerations should resemble those in Duchenne muscular dystrophy.

Limb-Girdle Muscular Dystrophy

This is a group of clinical syndromes inherited as an autosomal recessive trait and affecting primarily the hips and shoulders. The onset is in the second decade, presenting as weakness in the neck, pectoral, and arm muscles with loss of muscle mass. Later the legs are affected, resulting in wheelchair dependence by age 30. Involvement of the myocardium is variable.

Facioscapulohumeral Dystrophy

An autosomal dominant disease, facioscapulohumeral dystrophy has its onset in the second decade with inability to raise the arms, drooping shoulders, winging of the scapulae, and weakness of the facial musculature. Later involvement of the hips and back may cause kyphoscoliosis. The course is long and insidious, with a normal life span in many cases. Cardiac involvement is less common than in Duchenne muscular dystrophy, but atrial paralysis (absent atrial electrical activity that cannot be paced) with severe bradycardia has been reported. Ventricular pacing may be required. Involvement of the accessory muscles of respiration may cause reduced vital capacity and recurrent respiratory infections, predisposing to perioperative complications.

Ocular Muscular Dystrophy

This form of muscular dystrophy presents before the age of 30 with weakness of the extraocular muscles and ptosis but rarely diplopia. The muscle pathology resembles that of other dystrophies, but progression is slow and involvement of other muscles is limited. In addition, patients with ocular muscular dystrophy have a similarity to myasthenics in their exquisite sensitivity to curare—doses of 10 percent of the usual may result in complete paralysis.[57]

Myotonic Dystrophy

Myotonia implies an abnormal persistence of induced or voluntary muscle contractions, and may appear as part of several syndromes such as periodic paralysis, hypothyroidism, or polymyositis. The syndrome of myotonic dystrophy is inherited as an autosomal dominant trait with a frequency of 5 per 100,000 births. The myotonia affects predominantly the limb muscles, but extraocular and facial muscles are also involved. The myotonia is thought to be due to a generalized membrane defect in which biological membranes have normal resting potentials but increased resistance to electrical conduction. The myotonia persists even after denervation or paralysis.

The clinical picture varies with the age of the subject. The neonate may show poor sucking or swallowing, facial weakness, ptosis, and arthrogryposis. The older child may have muscle atrophy, poor gait, and atrophy of the distal limb muscles. In older subjects cataracts, baldness, gonadal atrophy, and mental retardation form the symptom complex. Swallowing difficulties may lead to aspiration; at all stages CPK is elevated in the serum, while the electromyogram shows high-frequency repetitive discharges. The myotonia is made worse by exercise or cold.

Many of these patients have abnormal electrocardiograms, with bradycardias and delayed intraventricular conduction. Death from arrhythmias is common, and the degree of cardiac abnormality does not correlate with the severity of skeletal muscle involvement. Carbon dioxide retention due to a depressed CO_2 response curve, together with pulmonary hypertension, may complicate anesthetic management. Relative resistance to insulin may result in hyperglycemia. Treatment depends upon stabilization of muscle membranes; phenytoin, procainamide, and quinine are the drugs of choice.

A related progressive myotonic dystrophy called *Schwartz-Jampel syndrome* (myotonic chondrodystrophy) is an autosomal recessive trait characterized by dwarfism, skeletal abnormalities, and muscle stiffness. Thermal regulatory dysfunction with a picture resembling malignant hyperpyrexia has been reported following administration of curare.[58] No evidence exists for similar predisposition to malignant hyperthermia in other myotonic diseases.[63]

Two other myotonic syndromes that are not progressive are myotonia congenita (Thomsen disease) and paramyotonia. In *myotonia congenita* there is myotonia and hypertrophy of some voluntary muscles. The myotonia is most severe following rest and decreases with exercise. There is no dystrophic change, and no involvement of cardiac muscle. The disease begins in childhood, with little progression through life. Inheritance is autosomal dominant.

Paramyotonia is the rarest of the myotonic syndromes, with signs similar to myotonia congenita but with myotonia appearing only on exposure to cold. Both forms of nonprogressive myotonia respond to quinidine therapy.

Anesthetic experience with myotonic syndromes has been reported only with myotonic dystrophy.[59–61] The initial hazard is inability to secure the airway due to spasm of the muscles of the jaw, or inability to ventilate due to respiratory muscle myotonic spasm. The patient may be markedly sensitive to the effects of respiratory depressants including narcotics, thiopentone, halothane, and diazepam, with apnea from low doses and delayed recovery common.[59, 61] Succinylcholine should be avoided, as it may induce a myotonic response. While general anesthesia, spinal anesthesia, and depolarizing relaxant drugs cannot break a myotonic contracture, the effect of using a nondepolarizing relaxant for surgery appears to be normal.[61] While theoretically the reversal of relaxation with neostigmine and atropine might cause a myotonic spasm, the response was normal in the only documented instance.[61]

No preoperative sedatives or analgesics should be given to patients with myotonic dystrophy without close, continuous observation. If necessary, the airway should be secured with the patient in the awake state under topical anesthesia. Otherwise, induction can be achieved with thiopental, anesthesia continued with halothane, and the airway secured without relaxants. While halothane can be safely used, apnea will occur at low concentrations and ventilation must be supported. Cardiac monitoring[62] and avoidance of cold stress are essential. Postoperatively the ventilation and airway must be supported until the patient demonstrates adequate recovery. Provision must be made for prolonged recovery from fixed drugs. Myotonia may compromise the ability to cough effectively and thus create a predisposition to pulmonary complications.

CONGENITAL DEFECTS OF MUSCLES

Congenital myopathies are a group of diseases defined by a pathological defect or a clinical picture of profound weakness and hypotonia from birth. In many cases the pathogenesis is incompletely understood. Weakness is usually of the proximal muscle groups, particularly the hips and shoulder girdle. In most cases the disease is not progressive, but muscle wasting and weakness are associated with secondary skeletal changes or dysmorphic features.

Central Core Disease

Central core disease is a nonprogressive congenital myopathy inherited as an autosomal dominant trait. Intellect is normal. Weakness of the proximal muscles leads to difficulty climbing stairs or rising from chairs. Muscles supplied by the cranial nerves are not involved. Secondary skeletal changes include hip dislocation, kyphoscoliosis, funnel chest, mandibular hypoplasia, and a short neck. Serum enzymes are usually normal.

Pathologically there is aberration of type I fibers with a central core of abnormal fibrillary material. Biochemically there is reduced phosphorylase activity, as well as reduced actomyosin and magnesium-activated ATPase activity and calcium-dependent ATPase activity of the sarcoplasmic reticulum. The net effect is a reduction in the rate of calcium uptake by the sarcoplasmic reticulum, leading to an elevated calcium concentration in the muscle fiber.

The importance of recognizing this entity in anesthesia results from its known association with malignant hyperthermia.[63, 64] While the association of many myopathic disorders with the syndrome remains to be established, patients with central core disease are most certainly at risk. The increased calcium level within the muscle fiber probably leads to a plasmalemmal susceptibility to triggering drugs. All precautions to avoid malignant hyperthermia must be taken when anesthetizing individuals with this diagnosis.

Nemaline Myopathy

Named for the unique rodlike or threadlike structures that run in biopsied muscles, this disease is inherited as an autosomal dominant. The infants are born weak and hypotonic at birth, and may develop respiratory difficulty. The weakness persists into adult life, and is associated with dysmorphic skeletal features. Occasionally the weakness is severe enough to cause recurrent pneumonias or seriously limit respiratory reserves. No cardiac or smooth muscle involvement has been described. In the sole reported anesthetic experience there was a slight resistance to succinylcholine with no abnormal hyperkalemia and a normal response to pancuronium.[65]

Numerous other myopathies due to defects in the sarcolemmal structure have been described.[1] However, their occurrence is rare indeed and anesthetic experience is not available.

Lipid Myopathies

Several disease states have been described in which biochemical abnormalities in lipid metabolism result in excessive storage of material in skeletal muscles. *Carnitine* is required as a cofactor in the transport of long-chain fatty acids into mitochondria for oxidation. A deficiency state has been described that results in reduced fatty acid oxidation and excessive formation of triglycerides. Progressive weakness begins in the first or second decade, and may be associated with a cardiomyopathy. A potentially fatal systemic form with hepatomegaly and episodic acidosis has also been described. Treatment is by dietary supplement and steroids.

Episodic muscle cramps and myoglobinemia characterize *carnitine palmityl transferase deficiency*, particularly after exercise. Weakness is not remarkable. The biochemical lesion results in elevated cholesterol, triglyceride, and free fatty acid concentrations in the serum and muscles.

Pyruvate decarboxylase deficiency causes a syndrome of intermittent ataxia associated with choreoathetosis, particularly with stress or febrile illness.

No anesthetic experience has been reported. Avoidance of prolonged fasting (and hence dependence on lipids for metabolism) and excessive muscle activity such as fasciculations and shivering would appear to be prudent.

Mitochondrial Myopathies

Several myopathies have been described that involve abnormalities of the mitochondria. Indeed, 12 percent of all patients with clinical myopathies have mitochondrial abnormalities, but their significance in the pathogenesis is unknown. The syndromes usually present as a long-term myopathy, usually beginning at birth or in childhood.

In *Luft disease* there is an increased number of mitochondria with an increased amount of cristae, resulting in increased muscle enzyme activity. The increased mitochondrial respiration with loosely coupled oxidative phosphorylation results in the clinical signs of hypermetabolism. Excessive sweating, polydipsia, polyphagia, and heat intolerance present a clinical picture resembling that of hyperthyroidism. Treatment is with chloramphenicol, which reduces mitochondrial synthesis. Anesthetic experiences have not been documented, but the high metabolic rate with high oxygen consumption suggest the importance of maintaining maximal oxygenation, preserving cardiac output and minute ventilation, and carefully monitoring temperature to recognize hyperthermia with its metabolic consequences.

Other mitochondrial myopathies have been described with structural mitochondrial abnormalities, but the metabolic consumption of oxygen was normal. Anesthetic experiences have not been documented, but minimal muscular reserve with stress would be expected in view of the muscle fatigue with exercise.

Glycogen Storage Disease

Glycogen storage diseases are a group of diseases characterized by the accumulation of glycogen of normal or abnormal configuration in various tissues. Each type of disease is caused by the inherited deficiency or absence of a specific enzyme in the metabolic pathway of glycogen. The signs and symptoms result from the excessive glycogen storage, plus the secondary free glucose deficiency with ensuing hypoglycemia. Many of the diseases do not primarily involve muscle; nevertheless, they may be associated with an unexplained weakness and hypotonia. Only those types primarily involved with muscle will be considered here.

1. *Acid maltase deficiency (Pompe disease, Cori type II disease)* is characterized by hypotonia and cardiac involvement in the neonate. Difficulty swallowing secretions, respiratory distress from the large tongue and weak muscles, and congestive cardiac failure lead to death by 1 year of age. Late infantile and adult forms have also been described in which the enzyme deficiency is incomplete, the myopathy is slower to develop, and involvement of the heart and tongue is absent. There is no effective treatment.

2. *Amylo-1,6-glucosidase deficiency (Forbes disease, or Cori type III disease)* results in neonatal symptoms of hypotonia, failure to thrive, hepatomegaly, and hypoglycemia. An adult type with chronic progressive myopathy has also been described. Fasting creates severe hypoglycemia due to limitation of glycogen breakdown, and glucose supplies are then dependent on gluconeogenesis. Ketonuria and hyperlipemia are frequently present.

3. *Amylo-1,4−1,6-transglucosidase deficiency, Anderson disease, Cori type IV disease)* results in diffuse glycogenesis with hepatic failure and cirrhosis. Glycogen accumulates in the tongue and diaphragm disproportionately to other muscles, resulting in weakness and atrophy.

4. *Muscle glycogen phosphorylase deficiency (McArdle disease, Cori type V disease)* causes rapid exhaustion with exercise of otherwise normal muscles. Myoglobinuria may follow moderate or strenuous exercise, while lactic acid cannot be produced with exertion. Cardiac muscle may be involved with bradycardia, increased amplitude of QRS complex, and T wave inversion. CPK elevation occurs with exercise.

5. *Muscle phosphofructokinase deficiency (Tauri disease), phosphoglucomutase deficiency (Thomson disease), and phosphohexoisomerase deficiency (Satoyoshi disease)*, all produce exercise intolerance due to pain and fatigue without further abnormalities of muscle. Lactic acid cannot be produced. The clinical significance of these abnormalities is equivocal.

Little is known of the effect of anesthesia on these entities.[66, 67] The major consideration involves the biochemical abnormalities, particularly hypoglycemia with fasting. Reduced tolerance to exercise implies a reduced respiratory reserve, which dictates careful monitoring and support of ventilatory function periop-eratively. There are no data available on the effects of muscle relaxants in these diseases. Cardiac and hepatic involvement, when present, will influence the choice of pharmacological agents for anesthesia. The inability to withstand exercise implies that ischemia is poorly tolerated, and operative tourniquets should not be used. Myoglobinuria must be treated when it occurs, and succinylcholine must be avoided to prevent simulating severe exercise. For similar reasons shivering triggered by inadvertent hypothermia or halothane administration should be prevented if possible.

Familial Periodic Paralysis

Episodic weakness can occur with several clinical diseases. Often it is associated with a reduced plasma potassium concentration, as is seen in thyrotoxicosis, renal disease, diabetic acidosis, or diuretic ingestion. Hyperaldosterone excess, as occurs with primary hyperaldosteronism (*Conn syndrome*), or pseudoaldosteronism from licorice ingestion may also cause episodic weakness. Periodic weakness is also common in McArdle disease, paramyotonia congenita, and certain mitochondrial myopathies, although no potassium deficit is documented.

Familial periodic paralysis is inherited as an autosomal dominant trait. Two forms have been described depending upon serum potassium levels. In the *hypokalemic* form weakness begins in the second decade and tends to be made worse by high-carbohydrate meals or salt loading or after a period of rest following strenuous exercise. The flaccid paralysis may be severe and may last up to 36 hours, but it spares the cranial and respiratory musculature. Hypokalemia is usually present with serum levels of 2 to 3 mEq/L, and ECG manifestations occur including sinus arrhythmia and QRS and T wave changes. The severity of the weakness correlates poorly, however, with the level of potassium in the serum. Acute attacks can be treated by potassium infusions, while prevention depends on avoiding large meals and salt. Drug therapy with spironolactone or acetazolamide is helpful in maintaining serum potassium levels.

Anesthetic management depends upon the recognition that, no matter how minor the operative procedure, anesthesia and surgery do something (as yet undefined) to initiate an episode of weakness. To minimize occurrence of the event, preoperative electrolytes must be carefully checked. The patient must be instructed not to overeat, and infusions of glucose and sodium are kept to a minimum. Hypothermia can precipitate an attack, so temperature monitoring is critical. The relationship between muscle relaxants and this disease is unknown, so they are best avoided if possible. Prolonged postoperative monitoring is essential even in the presence of a benign intraoperative course and normal serum potassium levels.[68–70]

Hyperkalemic periodic paralysis is also an autosomal dominant trait with onset usually below the age of 10 years. Attacks are similar to these in the hypokalemic form but tend to be shorter-lasting (1 to 2 hours) and are often related to exercise and cold. While patients may have difficulty swallowing or coughing, their respiratory muscles are usually spared. Myotonia may be present. Biochemically the elevation of serum potassium may be transient and mild, and probably represents a hypersensitivity of the muscle membrane to acetylcholine or mechanical stimulation. The treatment of the acute attack is infusion of calcium and insulin/glucose therapy, while acetazolamide paradoxically is effective in prophylaxis.

Three anesthetic exposures have been reported in patients with the hyperkalemic form, with two instances of paralysis lasting several hours postoperatively.[71] It is most essential to prevent carbohydrate depletion by starting a dextrose infusion the night before. All intravenous solutions should be dextrose-rich and potassium-free. ECG monitoring is essential. Muscle relaxants should be avoided, since succinylcholine may induce a hyperkalemic response and neostigmine to reverse nondepolarizing drugs may induce myotonia from excessive acetylcholine elevation. Thermal control is essential.

A third, *normokalemic* form of periodic paralysis has been described in early childhood with severe weakness and loss of a cough reflex. The attack may last many days, and is associated with cardiac tachyarrhythmias. The same anesthetic concerns pertain as suggested for the hypokalemic form.

Myositis Ossificans

This familial disease starts in childhood, with cyst-like nodules developing under the skin after minor trauma. Later bone develops in the area, hardening the muscle. The disease becomes widespread, with death occurring in the second to fourth decade. Terminally the patients develop severe limitation in the motion of the chest with secondary respiratory and cardiac failure. Associated skeletal abnormalities are common.

Anesthetic problems relate to the difficulty in opening the mouth or bending the neck, which are fixed by ossification of muscle. Tracheostomy or blind nasotracheal intubation may be necessary. Limitation of thoracic wall compliance can become a problem in later stages of the disease.

INFLAMMATORY MYOPATHIES

Myositis defines a group of conditions characterized by inflammation of muscles. While it may be related to specific diseases such as scleroderma, lupus erythematosus, polyarteritis, or rheumatoid arthritis, myositis may also occur as the primary presentation.

Dermatomyositis is a relatively rare condition affecting the skin and muscles. It occurs in both children and adults; the childhood form is generally more severe. Commonly pain, fever, and weakness begin in the hips, and the weakness may progress to involve the pharyngeal muscles. Swallowing difficulties may prove fatal, and perforation of the gastrointestinal tract is a common cause of death. Myocardial insufficiency with arrhythmias may occur. Recovery may leave residual atrophy with calcification of involved muscles.

Pathologically there is a diffuse angiopathic process involving the skin, muscle, gastrointestinal tract, and small nerves. Obstruction of the intima of arteries leads to cellular necrosis with elevation of muscle enzymes. The disease is probably immunological in etiology, perhaps triggered by a virus of the myxovirus or picornavirus group. Treatment is with steroid hormones and immunosuppression. The association with malignancy seen in adults is uncommon in children.

No information is available as to the implications for anesthesia. However, the inflammatory process of the musculature with leakage of enzymes would suggest caution with all muscle relaxant drugs. Depolarizing relaxants may be expected to increase membrane leakage, leading to hyperkalemia and myoglobinuria.

RHABDOMYOLYSIS AND MUSCLE DISEASE

Rhabdomyolysis with myoglobinuria is a condition of diverse etiology characterized by the sudden onset of muscle pain and weakness followed by passage of dark urine. There is extreme necrosis of muscle cells without an interstitial inflammatory reaction, and alteration of muscle membrane permeability to intracellular enzymes and proteins. The muscles become swollen and tender, and systemic signs of fever, chills, and general malaise ensue. Therapy is based upon prevention of complications such as renal failure, sudden death from arrhythmias secondary to electrolyte disturbances or myocardial involvement, and respiratory failure from respiratory muscle involvement. The clinical entities associated with rhabdomyolysis-myoglobinuria are listed in Table 18–2.[72] It should be noted that while up to 40 percent of normal children will demonstrate myoglobinemia after a single dose of succinylcholine,[73] there is the occasional case of severe rhabdomyolysis induced by such a dose in the absence of temperature change.[74, 75] Whether this situation represents a variant of malignant hyperpyrexia, or the unmasking of an occult myopathy, remains to be determined.

Malignant Hyperthermia

The syndrome of malignant hyperthermia is a rare but lethal complication of anesthetic drug administration. After administration of inciting drugs the patient develops a rapid rise in temperature, a hypermetabolic state outstripping oxygen delivery, and diffuse rhabdomyolysis usually with muscle rigidity. While the

Table 18–2. CLASSIFICATION OF
RHABDOMYOLYSIS

Defined enzymatic defects
    Muscle phosphorylase deficiency
    Phosphofructokinase deficiency
    Carnitine palmityl transferase deficiency
Presumed metabolic defects
    Fasting/exercise precipitant
    Malignant hyperthermia
    Familial periodic paralysis (hypokalemic)
Cellular metabolic toxins
    Alcohol
    Heroin
    Amphotericin B
Unavailability of adequate substrate or oxygen
    Ischemic compression–crush syndrome
    Intense muscular activity
    Heat stress
    Succinylcholine
Intrinsic muscle disease
    Dermatomyositis
    Progressive muscular dystrophies
    Infections (influenza and Coxsackie virus)

syndrome has been associated with other myopathic entities including muscular dystrophy[76] and central core myopathy, the majority of patients probably have a mild or subclinical myopathy that is yet to be clearly defined. Inheritance is probably autosomal dominant, although penetrance is often incomplete.[77]

The incidence of malignant hyperthermia is reported as 1 in 15,000 instances of induced anesthesia in children, about five times that in adults. These statistics do not reflect the true incidence of susceptibility, since 50 percent of patients who have had the syndrome have had prior anesthesia without the syndrome developing.[78]

The underlying defect seems to be an idiopathic increase in the sarcoplasmic concentration of calcium ion.[79] As a consequence, during anesthesia with inciting drugs, total body oxygen consumption in susceptible patients is two to three times that of normal patients, and body temperature rises to as high as 43°C at a rate up to 1°C every 5 minutes. It is most frequently associated with the administration of halogenated inhalational anesthetic drugs and the muscle relaxant succinylcholine. Physical or emotional stress can trigger the syndrome in awake subjects, as can psychotropic drugs.[80] Both recrudescence and an initial attack can occur during recovery from general anesthesia.[81–84]

Development of the syndrome can vary from insidious to fulminant. Features of the slowly developing entity include tachycardia and other arrhythmias. Arterial blood gas analysis will demonstrate metabolic acidosis and an inappropriately low oxygen tension. Hyperpnea occurs owing to rising carbon dioxide production; core temperature begins to rise, while muscle rigidity occurs late in the crisis.

The more fulminant form of the disease is usually associated with administration of succinylcholine, fol-

lowed by a halothane anesthetic. The onset of muscle rigidity occurs immediately after the relaxant, and may be global or limited to the masseter muscles. Tracheal intubation may be difficult or impossible, but sometimes is readily accomplished. Cardiac arrhythmia and a malignant hypermetabolic state with vasoconstriction and cyanosis rapidly ensue unless prompt therapy is rendered. Masseter spasm may be the sole indication of an imminent crisis, and the anesthetic must be aborted immediately if this occurs—70 percent of such individuals have been shown to be susceptible to the entity.[85–87]

Rhabdomyolysis occurs later in the course of the syndrome, producing gross elevations in serum creatine kinase and myoglobin. Electrolyte disturbances are severe, with acute hyperkalemia and hypocalcemia developing from altered muscle cellular permeability to these ions. During the post-crisis diuresis the reverse occurs, with hypokalemia and hypercalcemia ensuing. Renal failure is common, as is disseminated intravascular coagulation. The mortality is approximately 7 percent even with optimal therapy.

Management of the crisis must be prompt. The volatile anesthetic agents must be discontinued immediately, and exposed circuitry replaced. Hyperventilation with oxygen must match metabolic requirements, with a minute ventilation of at least three times normal. Sodium bicarbonate is indicated for the metabolic acidosis, while active cooling by surface and body cavity is begun. Chilled saline is the recommended intravenous fluid. Cardiovascular monitoring is imperative, and arrhythmias should be treated with procainamide if they are not abolished by metabolic correction. Volume loading and osmotic diuretics are given to induce a brisk diuresis to avoid myoglobin deposition and renal failure. Intravascular monitoring of cardiac filling and arterial pressures are desirable, and vascular access is necessary for frequent blood gas and biochemical monitoring. Glucose should be given as energy substrate. Surgical procedures must be terminated as soon as possible, but the patient should not be moved until the crisis is terminated.

Dantrolene sodium is currently the drug of choice.[88, 89] This acts directly on skeletal muscle and probably blocks transfer of the excitation from the sarcolemmal membrane to release calcium from storage sites in the sarcoplasmic reticulum. There is no effect on cardiac muscle. Responses to treatment have occurred at doses between 1 and 10 mg/kg intravenously. For practical purposes an initial dose of 3 mg/kg should be given;[90] if this is unsuccessful, the patient should then be given 10 mg/kg. Serious cardiopulmonary depression does not usually occur at that dosage, unless there is potentiation by other drugs. Verapamil, a potent calcium channel blocker, is particularly dangerous in this situation.[91]

Preoperative preparation with dantrolene is recommended for patients known or suspected to have malignant hyperthermia. For elective surgery the drug can be given orally at 4 to 8 mg/kg per day for 1 or 2 days, with the last dose given 2 hours before anesthesia. For emergency surgery the administration of 2.5 mg/kg intravenously is recommended. The elimination half-life is 12 hours.[90] It has been reported that such prophylaxis is not absolute protection from the syndrome,[92, 93] so all other precautions are indicated.

Patients known to be susceptible to malignant hyperthermia, and their relatives, need not be denied anesthesia. Drugs not associated with the syndrome include barbiturates, narcotics, diazepam, droperidol, nitrous oxide, and ester-type local anesthetics. The use of amide-type local anesthetics and ketamine is controversial, but probably safe. Skeletal muscle paralysis can be accomplished with pancuronium. Reversal of paralysis with atropine and neostigmine has not been reported to be associated with difficulties. Since calcium flux across the sarcoplasmic membrane may be regulated by the cyclic-AMP system, the use of sympathomimetics is not recommended.[89]

The muscles from patients with susceptibility to malignant hyperthermia may be structurally and biochemically normal upon biopsy. Although the frequency of musculoskeletal abnormalities such as scoliosis, strabismus, and hernia is reported as greater in patients with malignant hyperthermia, there is nothing diagnostic in their presence. A high index of suspicion must exist whenever there is a family or personal history of anesthetic or surgical disaster. Muscle enzyme elevations in the serum, while increased in 70 percent of subjects, may be normal in 30 percent of those with documented susceptibility.[94] The level of CPK may also be elevated by exercise or other myopathic conditions, and hence its value is limited. HLA typing of family members susceptible to the condition has not proved useful.[95] Since this disease may represent a generalized defect of membrane function, evaluation of more accessible membranes such as those of blood platelets has been attempted in vitro.[96] However, the results have not been sufficiently reliable to prove diagnostic.[97, 98]

It has been shown that caffeine is capable of producing contracture of skeletal muscle in vitro, by causing the release or efflux of calcium from the sarcoplasmic reticulum. It was demonstrated that muscle from patients with malignant hyperthermia undergoes a hypercontracture to caffeine, and that this can be potentiated by halothane and blocked by dantrolene. This forms the basis for the only currently reliable test for susceptibility.[99] Skeletal muscle is obtained by open biopsy and suspended between force transducers in a physiologic bath. Susceptible muscle demonstrates a contracture of 1 gram at a much lower caffeine concentration (1 to 2 mM caffeine) than does normal muscle ($\geq$ 4 mM). Halothane, when bubbled through the bath of susceptible individuals, may also elicit a large contracture. Patients demonstrating either of these phenomena are susceptible to malignant hyper-

thermia and are described as having H-type phenotypes. The combined use of caffeine and halothane to elicit a response defines the K-type phenotype and a more equivocal susceptibility to the disease.[100, 101] While the diagnostic testing is perhaps imperfect and depends considerably on laboratory interpretation and biopsy characteristics,[102] there have been few false negative results reported from any laboratory. Those who have been H-typed are conclusively susceptible; K-type responders should be assumed to have a variant of the disease but to be nevertheless susceptible in the presence of inciting drugs.

REFERENCES

1. Swainman KF, Wright FS: Pediatric Neuromuscular Diseases. St. Louis, C.V. Mosby Co., 1979.
2. Dubowitz V: Muscle Disorders in Childhood. Philadelphia, W.B. Saunders Co., 1978.
3. Ellis FR: Neuromuscular disease and anesthesia. Br J Anaesth 46:603, 1974.
4. Azar I: The response of patients with neuromuscular disorders to muscle relaxants: a review. Anesthesiology 61:173, 1984.
5. Tobey RE: Paraplegia, succinylcholine, and cardiac arrest. Anesthesiology 32:359, 1970.
6. Beach TP, Stone WA, Hamelberg W: Circulatory collapse following succinylcholine: report of a patient with diffuse motor neuron disease. Anesth Analg 50:431, 1971.
7. Stone WA, Beach TP, Hamelberg W: Succinylcholine-induced hyperkalemia in dogs with transsected sciatic nerves or spinal cords. Anesthesiology 32:515, 1970.
8. Cooperman LH: Succinylcholine-induced hyperkalemia in neuromuscular disease. JAMA 213:1867, 1970.
9. Hyperkalemia following succinylcholine administration in neurologic disorders: a review. Can Anaesth Soc J 18:199, 1971.
10. Rosenbaum KJ, Neigh JL, Strobel GE: Sensitivity to nondepolarizing muscle relaxants in amyotrophic lateral sclerosis: report of two cases. Anesthesiology 35:638, 1971.
11. Desmond J: Paraplegia: problems confronting the anesthesiologist. Can Anaesth Soc J 17:435, 1970.
12. Gode GR: Paraplegia and cardiac arrest: case reports. Can Anaesth Soc J 17:452, 1970.
13. Ciliberti BJ, Goldfine J, Rovenstine EA: Hypertension during anesthesia in patients with spinal cord injuries. Anesthesiology 15:273, 1954.
14. Drinker AS, Helrich M: Halothane anesthesia in the paraplegic patient. Anesthesiology 24:399, 1963.
15. Tanaka H, Uemura N, Toyama Y: Cardiac involvement in the Kugelberg-Welander syndrome. Am J Cardiol 38:528, 1976.
16. Edwards AE, Bras JF: The enhancement of neurologic signs under anesthesia. Br J Anaesth 42:337, 1970.
17. Lichtenfeld P: Autonomic dysfunction in Guillain-Barré syndrome. Am J Med 50:72, 1971.
18. Perel A, Reche A, Davidson JT: Anesthesia in the Guillain-Barré syndrome. Anaesthesia 32:257, 1977.
19. Summer E: Porphyria in relation to surgery and anesthesia. Ann Roy Coll Surg Engl 56:81, 1975.
20. Ward RJ: Porphyria and its relation to anesthesia. Anesthesiology 26:212, 1965.
21. Mustajoki P, Heinonen J: General anesthesia in "inductible" porphyrias. Anesthesiology 53:15, 1980.
22. Huxtable R: Cardiac pharmacology and cardiomyopathy in Friedreich's ataxia. J Can Sci Neurol 5:83, 1978.
23. McCaughey TJ: Familial dysautonomia as an anesthetic hazard. Can Anaesth Soc J 12:558, 1965.

24. Meridy HW, Creighton RE: General anaesthesia in eight patients with familial dysautonomia. Can Anaesth Soc J 18:563, 1971.

25. Bortels JM: Familial dysautonomia. JAMA 212:318, 1970.

26. Kritcheman MM, Swartz J, Papper E: Experience with general anesthesia in patients with familial dysautonomia. JAMA 170:529, 1959.

27. Inkster JS: Anaesthesia for a patient suffering from familial dysautonomia. Br J Anaesth 43:509, 1971.

28. Filler J, Smith AA, Stone S, et al.: Respiratory control in familial dysautonomia. J Pediatr 66:509, 1965.

29. Humble RM: Pheochromocytoma, neurofibromatosis, and pregnancy. Anesthesia 22:296, 1967.

30. Fisher MD: Anesthetic difficulties in neurofibromatosis. Anaesthesia 30:648, 1975.

31. Massaro D, Katz S, Mathews MJ, et al.: Von Recklinghausen's neurofibromatosis associated with cystic lung disease. Am J Med 38:233, 1965.

32. Bourke E, Fatenby PBB: Renal artery dysplasia with hypertension in neurofibromatosis. Br J Med 3:681, 1971.

33. Magbagbeola JA: Abnormal responses to muscle relaxants in a patient with von Recklinghausen's disease. Br J Anaesth 42:710, 1970.

34. Manser J: Abnormal responses in von Recklinghausen's disease. Br J Anaesth 42:183, 1970.

35. Drachman DB: Myasthenia gravis. N Engl J Med 298:136, 1978.

36. Appel SH, Almon RR, Levy N: Acetylcholine receptor antibodies in myasthenia gravis. N Engl J Med 293:760, 1975.

37. Flacke W: Treatment of myasthenia gravis. N Engl J Med 288:27, 1973.

38. Head JM: Respiratory failure after thymectomy for myasthenia gravis. Ann Surg 160:123, 1964.

39. Lake CL: Curare sensitivity in steroid-treated myasthenia gravis. Anaesth Analg 57:132, 1978.

40. Davies DW, Steward DJ: Myasthenia gravis in children and anesthetic management for thymectomy. Can Anaesth Soc J 20:253, 1973.

41. Leventhal SR, Orkin F, Hirsh R: Prediction of the need for postoperative mechanical ventilation in myasthenia gravis. Anesthesiology 53:26, 1980.

42. Grant RP, Jenkins LC: Prediction of the need for postoperative mechanical ventilation in myasthenia gravis: thymectomy compared to other surgical procedures. Can Anaesth Soc J 29:112, 1982.

43. Dalal FY, Bennett EJ, Gegg WS: Congenital myasthenia gravis and minor surgical procedures. Anaesthesia 27:61, 1972.

44. Wahlin A, Havermark KG: Enflurane anesthesia in patients with myasthenia gravis. Acta Anaesth Belg 2:215, 1974.

45. Sanyal SK, Tierney RC, Rao PS, et al.: Systolic time interval characteristics in children with Duchenne's progressive muscle dystrophy. Pediatrics 70:958, 1982.

46. Jenkins JG, Bohn D, Edmonds JF, et al.: Evaluation of pulmonary function in muscular dystrophy patients requiring spinal surgery. Crit Care Med 10:645, 1982.

47. Milne B, Rosales JK: Anesthetic considerations in patients with muscular dystrophy undergoing spinal fusion and Harrington rod insertion. Can Anaesth Soc J 29:250, 1982.

48. Cobham JG, Davis HS: Anesthesia for muscular dystrophy patients. Anesth Analg 43:22, 1964.

49. Richards WC: Anesthesia and serum creatine phosphokinase levels in Duchenne's pseudohypertrophic muscular dystrophy. Anaesth Intens Care 1:150, 1972.

50. Wislicki L: Anaesthesia and post-operative complications in progressive muscular dystrophy. Anaesthesia 17:482, 1962.

51. Kelfer HM, Singer WD, Reynolds RN: Malignant hyperthermia in a child with Duchenne muscular dystrophy. Pediatrics 71:118, 1983.

52. Seay AR, Ziter FA, Thompson JA: Cardiac arrest during induction of anesthesia in Duchenne muscular dystrophy. J Pediatr 93:88, 1978.

53. Henderson WAV: Succinylcholine-induced cardiac arrest in unsuspected Duchenne muscular dystrophy. Can Anaesth Soc J 31:444, 1984.

54. Lewandowski KB: Strabismus as a presenting sign of subclinical muscular dystrophy predisposing to rhabdomyolysis and myoglobinuria. Can Anaesth Soc J 29:372, 1982.

55. Oka S, Igarashi Y, Takagi A, et al.: Malignant hyperpyrexia and Duchenne muscular dystrophy: a case report. Can Anaesth Soc J 29:627, 1982.

56. Brownell AKW, Paasuke RT, Elash A: Malignant hyperthermia in Duchenne muscular dystrophy. Anesthesiology 58:180, 1983.

57. Jacob JG, Varkey GP: Curare sensitivity in ocular myopathy. Can Anaesth Soc J 13:449, 1966.

58. Seay AR, Ziter FA: Malignant hyperthermia in a patient with Schwartz-Jampel syndrome. J Pediatr 93:83, 1978.

59. Dundee JW: Thiopentone in dystrophia myotonica. Anesth Analg 31:257, 1952.

60. Ravin M, Newmark Z, Saviello G: Myotonia dystrophica—an anesthetic hazard. Anesth Analg 54:216, 1975.

61. Mitchell MM, Ali HH, Savarese JJ: Myotonia and neuromuscular blocking agents. Anesthesiology 49:44, 1978.

62. Meyers MB, Barash PG: Cardiac decompensation during enflurane anesthesia. A patient with myotonia atrophica. Anesth Analg 55:433, 1976.

63. Eng GD, Epstein BS, Engel WK, et al.: Malignant hyperthermia and central core disease in a child with congenital dislocating hips. Arch Neurol 35:189, 1978.

64. Denborough MA, Dennett X, Anderson R: Central core disease and malignant hyperpyrexia. Br Med J 1:272, 1973.

65. Heard SO, Kaplan RF: Neuromuscular blockade in a patient with nemaline myopathy. Anesthesiology 59:588, 1983.

66. Cox JM: Anesthesia and glycogen storage disease. Anesthesiology 29:1221, 1968.

67. Kaplan R: Pompe's disease presenting for anesthesia. Anesth Rev 7:21, 1980.

68. Melnick B, Chang JL, Larson CE, et al.: Hypokalemic familial periodic paralysis. Anesthesiology 58:263, 1983.

69. Siler JN, Discavage WJ: Anesthetic management of hypokalemic periodic paralysis. Anesthesiology 43:489, 1975.

70. Horton B: Anesthetic experiences in a family with hypokalemic periodic paralysis. Anesthesiology 47:308, 1977.

71. Egan TJ, Klein R: Hyperkalemic familial periodic paralysis. Pediatrics 24:761, 1959.

72. Robotham JL, Haddow JE: Rhabdomyolysis and myoglobinuria in childhood. Pediatr Clin North Am 23:279, 1976.

73. Ryan JF, Hagen LJ, Heyman AI: Myoglobinemia after a single dose of succinylcholine. N Engl J Med 285:824, 1971.

74. Schaer H, Steinman B, Jerusalem S, et al.: Rhabdomyolysis induced by anesthesia with intraoperative cardiac arrest. Br J Anaesth 49:495, 1977.

75. Younker D, De Vore M, Hartlage P: Malignant hyperthermia and glucose-6-phosphate dehydrogenase deficiency. Anesthesiology 60:601, 1984.

76. McKishnie JD, Muir JM, Girvan DP: Anesthetic induced rhabdomyolysis. Can Anaesth Soc J 30:295, 1983.

77. King JO, Denborough MA, Zapp PW: Inheritance of malignant hyperpyrexia. Lancet 1:365, 1972.

78. Britt BA, Kalow W: Malignant hyperthermia: a statistical review. Can Anaesth Soc J 17:293, 1970.

79. Blanck TJ, Gruener R, Suffecool S, et al.: Calcium uptake by isolated sarcoplasmic reticulum: examination of halothane inhibition, pH dependence, and calcium dependence of normal and malignant hyperthermic human muscle. Anaesth Analg 60:492, 1981.

80. Gronert GA, Thompson GL, Onofrio BM: Human malignant hyperthermia: awake episodes and correction by dantrolene. Anesth Analg (Paris) 59:377, 1980.

81. Mathieu A, Bogosian AJ, Ryan JF, et al.: Recrudescence after survival of an acute episode of malignant hyperthermia. Anesthesiology 51:454, 1979.

82. Schulte-Sasse U, Hess W, Eberlien HJ: Postoperative malig-

nant hyperthermia and dantrolene therapy. Can Anaesth Soc J 30:635, 1983.

83. Grinberg R, Edelist G, Gordon R: Postoperative malignant hyperthermia episodes in patients who received safe anesthetics. Can Anaesth Soc J 30:273, 1983.

84. Kripke BJ, Blanck TJ, Sizemore DA, et al.: Association of post-anaesthetic hyperthermia with abnormal muscle characteristics. Can Anaesth Soc J 30:290, 1983.

85. Flewellen EH, Nelson TE: Masseter spasm induced by succinylcholine in children: contracture testing for malignant hyperthermia. Can Anaesth Soc J 29:42, 1982.

86. Flewellen EH, Nelson TE: Halothane-succinylcholine induced masseter spasm: indicative of malignant hyperthermia susceptibility? Anesth Analg 63:693, 1984.

87. Badgwell JM, Heavner JE: Masseter spasm heralds malignant hyperthermia—current dilemma or merely academia gone mad? Anesthesiology 61:230, 1984.

88. Kolb ME, Horne ML, Martz R: Dantrolene in human malignant hyperthermia: a multicenter study. Anesthesiology 56:254, 1982.

89. Gronert GA: Malignant hyperthermia. Anesthesiology 53:395, 1980.

90. Flewellen EH, Nelson TE, Jones WP, et al.: Dantrolene dose response in awake man: implications for management of malignant hyperthermia. Anesthesiology 59:275, 1983.

91. Saltzman LS, Kates RA, Corke BC, et al.: Hyperkalemia and cardiovascular collapse after verapamil and dantrolene administration in swine. Anesth Analg 63:473, 1984.

92. Fitzgibbons DC: Malignant hyperthermia following preoperative oral administration of dantrolene. Anesthesiology 54:73, 1981.

93. Ruhland G, Hinkle AJ: Malignant hyperthermia after oral and intravenous pretreatment with dantrolene in a patient susceptible to malignant hyperthermia. Anesthesiology 60:159, 1984.

94. Ellis FR, Clarke IMC, Modgill M, et al.: Evaluation of creatine phosphokinase in screening patients for malignant hyperpyrexia. Br Med J 3:511, 1975.

95. Lutsky I, Witkowski J, Henschel E: HLA typing in a family prone to malignant hyperthermia. Anesthesiology 56:224, 1982.

96. Solomons C, McDermott N, Mahowald M: Screening for malignant hyperthermia with a platelet bioassay. N Engl J Med 303:642, 1980.

97. Rosenberg H, Fisher CA, Reed S, et al.: Platelet aggregation in patients susceptible to malignant hyperthermia. Anesthesiology 55:621, 1981.

98. Giger U, Kaplan R: Halothane-induced ATP depletion from patients susceptible to malignant hyperthermia and from controls. Anesthesiology 58:347, 1983.

99. Britt BA, Frodis W, Scott E, et al.: Comparison of the caffeine skinned fibre tension (CSFT) test with the caffeine-halothane contracture test in the diagnosis of malignant hyperthermia. Can Anaesth Soc J 29:550, 1982.

100. Rosenberg H, Reed S: In vitro contracture tests for susceptibility to malignant hyperthermia. Anesth Analg 62:415, 1983.

101. Nelson TE, Flewellen EH, Gloyna DF: Spectrum of susceptibility to malignant hyperthermia—diagnostic dilemma. Anesth Analg 62:545, 1983.

102. Brownell AKW, Szabo M: The in vitro caffeine contracture test: influence of the muscle histochemical profile on test results. Can Anaesth Soc J 29:218, 1982.

INDEX

Note: Page numbers in *italics* refer to illustrations; page numbers followed by (t) refer to tables.